Occupational and Environmental Neurotoxicology

Occupational and Environmental Neurotoxicology

Robert G. Feldman, M.D.

Professor of Neurology and Pharmacology
Chairman, Department of Neurology
Director of the Occupational and Environmental Neurology Program
Boston University School of Medicine
Boston, Massachusetts

Professor of Environmental Health
Boston University School of Public Health
Boston, Massachusetts

Lecturer on Occupational Health
Harvard University School of Public Health
Boston, Massachusetts

Lecturer on Neurology
Harvard University Medical School
Boston, Massachusetts

To Olga with best wishes for a happy and successful career in neurology — it has been a joy working with you —

Boston 1998

Lippincott - Raven
PUBLISHERS
Philadelphia • New York

Cover art courtesy of Charles Reynolds

The hexagonal figure on the cover represents a benzene ring; the beams suggest peripheral nerve fibers; the network of fibers indicate central nervous system synaptic connections; the center of the design is the nucleus of a neuron, while the crystalline shapes in the background represent possible chemical neurotoxicants.

Acquisitions Editor: Joyce-Rachel John
Developmental Editor: Michelle LaPlante
Manufacturing Manager: Kevin Watt
Production Manager: Robert Pancotti
Production Editor: Jonathan Geffner
Cover Designer: Karen Quigley
Indexer: Sandra King
Compositor: Compset
Printer: Maple Press

Printed in the United States of America

9 8 7 6 5 4 3 2 1

Library of Congress Cataloging-in-Publication Data

Feldman, Robert G., 1933–
    Occupational and environmental neurotoxicology / by Robert G.
Feldman.
        p. cm.
    Includes bibliographical references and index.
    ISBN 0-7817-1739-6
    1. Neurotoxicology.   2. Industrial toxicology.   3. Environmental toxicology.   I. Title.
    [DNLM: 1. Nervous System Diseases—chemically induced.   2. Nervous
System—drug effects.   3. Occupational Exposure.   4. Environmental
Exposure.   WL 140 F312o 1998]
    RC347.5.F45   1998
    616.8—dc21
    DNLM/DLC
for Library of Congress   98-13524
                                                                                      CIP

For my dear wife, Gail Poliner Feldman

Contents

Forewords

Occupational and Environmental Medicine

Millions of Americans are exposed every day to neurotoxins. Workers are exposed to organic solvents, lead, and pesticides. And despite recent substantial reductions in environmental lead contamination, there are still an estimated one million children in the United States with elevated blood lead levels at increased risk of neurologic injury.

Of the more than 70,000 chemical substances used commercially in the United States, fewer than 20% have been tested for their potential neurotoxicity, and only a handful have been evaluated thoroughly. In this context, it seems likely that there are many thousands of Americans exposed to chemicals whose potential to cause injury to the nervous system is not known. The suspicion exists, therefore, that some fraction of neurologic disease in the American population is caused by exposures to these unknown neurotoxicants.

Chronic exposure to chemicals in the environment has been shown to cause chronic neurologic disease. For example, a syndrome closely resembling Parkinson's disease develops in workers, such as miners, exposed to excessive levels of the metal manganese. A Parkinson syndrome has also been described among young adults who used the synthetic heroin substitute, MPTP. Chronic exposure to lead can cause irreversible declines in intelligence and learning as well as behavior problems. Prolonged exposure to some solvents can produce dementia. Unresolved to date is whether exposures to neurotoxins can result in Alzheimer's disease, parkinsonism or other chronic disorders of the nervous system. The available evidence suggests that toxic substances in the environment may contribute to the incidence of these diseases. The problem is complicated by the fact that latency periods lasting as long as many decades may elapse between exposure and occurrence of illness. Much research remains to be done.

This splendid volume, *Occupational and Environmental Neurotoxicology* by Robert G. Feldman, offers clinicians—generalists as well as specialists—a clear guide through the diagnostic difficulties that surround recognition of disease that is caused by chemicals in the environment. The book clearly and accurately reviews the current information on patterns of exposure and pathophysiology. It presents clear guidance that will assist in making accurate diagnoses of these disorders.

This comprehensive and well-organized book represents a great introduction to the subject of occupational and environmental neurotoxicology for the medical student or resident. It will also serve as an invaluable reference for the general medical practitioner, the practicing neurologist, and the occupational and environmental medicine physician.

Philip J. Landrigan, M.D.

Neurology

The neurologist is often faced with the difficult problem of determining whether an exposure to a neurotoxic substance is responsible for a particular array of symptoms and signs. Utilizing the tried and true formula of using the history to determine the pace of the illness and the neurological examination to determine its localization, the neurologist usually can decide whether the problem is in the brain, spinal cord, or peripheral nervous system. With the judicious use of neurodiagnostic tests, it is often possible to further characterize the problem, such as the use of electromyography and nerve conduction studies to divide peripheral neuropathies into axonal and demyelinating types. Disorders that fail to yield to this sort of analysis are ordinarily considered psychological in nature.

Not having been trained in occupational and environmental medicine, the neurologist usually does not even know the sources of potential toxins, nor how to decide whether an exposure has occurred. Even when the alleged toxin is known, most neurologists have only limited experience with the neurological manifestations of the exposure. For example, most neurologists are reasonably well-versed in the neurotoxicity of ethyl alcohol and perhaps lead, but are sorely lacking in knowledge about other heavy metals, solvents, and organophosphorus compounds. Furthermore, many such patients are involved in litigation about the alleged toxin, a fact which simultaneously prejudices and intimidates many physicians who may have to submit their records to lawyers for later scrutiny.

In his book, *Occupational and Environmental Neurotoxicology*, Robert G. Feldman has provided a useful, practical, and user-friendly source of information on the twenty most important neurotoxic substances. Dr. Feldman has used his many years of experience in evaluating patients with neurotoxic exposures to cull out of the enormous and diffuse literature the information a clinician needs to approach these often difficult problems. It is rare these days to see any medical book written by a single author as is this one. This personal *tour de force* gives the reader a completely consistent approach. Each chapter contains a brief description of the substance followed by its unique sources of exposure and the recommended exposure limits and safety regulations. The metabolism of the substance is then discussed succinctly, followed by the symptoms and signs, the physical findings, and the utility of any neurodiagnostic tests. When available, the relevant neuropathology is described, ending with recommendations for treatment and/or prevention.

For the neurologist, this approach is familiar, reflecting Dr. Feldman's neurological training as he approaches these problems. This welcome volume provides the neurologist with a concise source of clinically useful information on a largely unfamiliar group of disorders using a neurological method which is comfortable for all of us. I am sure that I will consult this book frequently.

Martin A. Samuels, M.D.

Toxicology

Neurotoxicologists and neurologists are too often separated by a great disciplinary divide, across which they see the same events but stand too far apart to communicate wisely and accurately to each other—and to a public that needs to learn from both. The toxicologist develops the knowledge of chemical hazards and the basic biology of systems, from which human health risks can sometimes be extrapolated; the neurologist proceeds from the experience of diagnosing and treating patients with symptoms and disease, from which generalizations can sometimes be inferred. The toxicologist has the resources of basic research and experimental systems, but rarely sees the person or the population affected; while the physician knows individual patients or isolated cases, but rarely the context that underlies these events. These disciplines need each other almost more than any other domain of biomedical science. No experimental system presents with the complexity of human neurocognitive function, and the variations in human intellect and personality obscures our ability to recognize subtle damage.

The division between neurotoxicology and neurology is encouraged by current medical education and training. Less and less is taught of the preventable causes of neurologic and psychiatric illness or of the techniques of ascertaining environmental and occupational etiologies of disease. Despite calls for inclusion of these topics in medical education by the prestigious Institute of Medicine, few physicians receive adequate training in occupational or environmental medicine; this leads to the undercounting of diseases as clearcut as asbestosis and missed opportunities to prevent the next case.

In this book, Robert G. Feldman creates the bridge by which the science of toxicology and the practice of medicine can be joined. This bridge enables physicians and their patients to understand the nature of occupational and environmental neurotoxicology. It takes the combined wisdom of clinical practice and the perspective of a scientist, embodied in his life work, to write this book. Now that it exists, we can appreciate how greatly it has been needed. Dr. Feldman has woven the stories of individual patients into a comprehensive review of toxicology that provides instruction in how to recognize and manage toxicant-induced injury to the nervous system. For toxicologists, he explains the complexity and challenge of relating what we know about chemicals to the real concerns of affected persons. He has created both a "how to" reference and a data source that will aid not only physicians in responding to patients' concerns, but also patients in informing their physicians.

Within this text, a more fundamental agenda is revealed. Dr. Feldman is not content with curing individual cases of occupational or environmental neurotoxicology; he is committed to improving health on a more ambitious scale, through revising the public health agenda to include arming citizens with the information needed to prevent workplace poisoning, community contamination by hazardous waste, and other exposures. He provides information on environmental and occupational standards by which we can all gauge how well our workplaces and communities are protected. Because of this commitment, his book takes its place not only among notable texts but also among the few volumes of true medical advocacy, by Alice Hamilton and Harriet Hardy. Like them, Dr. Feldman recognizes that to inform is to empower, and to empower is to change.

Ellen K. Silbergeld, Ph.D.

Preface

The vulnerability of the nervous system to the effects of chemical exposure has been a focus of clinical, epidemiological, and basic neuroscience research. The risk of neurotoxic injury by chemicals is not only of great public health concern, but it is also a serious challenge to the diagnostic and therapeutic skills of clinicians who encounter such patients.

"Is the patient's neurological problem due to chemical exposure?" The information needed to confidently answer the question is not easily found in one reference source. Reports published in the neurological literature often deal with individual cases with clinical features believed to be associated with exposure to a particular chemical. Although these reports may provide detailed descriptions of the neurological examinations, data from sampling environmental levels of the suspected chemical, and/or body burden measures in blood and urine samples taken from the subject at risk for exposure, are often lacking or inadequate to substantiate a causal relationship. Conversely, in the occupational medicine literature, reports about outbreaks of neurological illness among groups of workers may provide details concerning the exposure circumstances. However, clinical descriptions about the neurological findings associated with a particular chemical exposure are often incomplete.

Occupational and Environmental Neurotoxicology was written to fill the need for a comprehensive reference text discussing the effects of exposure to potentially neurotoxic chemicals found in occupational and environmental settings. The chemical compounds selected for discussion in this book were taken from the list of neurotoxicants for which occupational standards have been recommended by the National Institute for Occupational Safety and Health (NIOSH) and from the clinical and basic science literature that cite evidence documenting neurotoxic effects. In addition, chemicals that are required to be reported as possible causes of neurologic illness by most states in the United States are included. Since it would be impossible to cover all potential neurotoxicants in this volume, certain ones have by necessity been omitted. For example, organochlorine compounds are not covered. Organochlorines (e.g., chlordane) are no longer widely used; they have been largely replaced as pesticides by organophosphorus and carbamate compounds, which are covered in this text. Although the sodium channel mechanism of the pyrethrins and their synthetic analogs, the pyrethroids, are intriguing from a neurophysiologic standpoint, the impact of these compounds on human neurological health is relatively transient and is not disabling; therefore, they are not discussed. The neurotoxicity of ethanol is not considered separately in this text, but its biochemical interactions with other neurotoxicants and the associated risks of simultaneous exposures are discussed in the various chapters. Otherwise, the chemicals listed in the table of contents include the most widely used and potentially important neurotoxic compounds found in occupational and environmental settings.

The practical clinical neurological concepts and current scientific evidence relating to the neurotoxicants reviewed in this book should be of great interest to professionals in the fields of neurology, occupational and environmental medicine, and neuroscience research, and to those involved in toxic tort proceedings who are concerned with chemical exposure-related illnesses. The clinician who examines patients exposed to hazardous chemicals may be called upon by lawyers to advise them as to whether there is sufficient clinical and scientific evidence to warrant litigation, or they may be asked to serve as expert witnesses. In such cases, the practitioner will need to turn to his or her previous clinical experience and scientific background, and to refer to the large body of relevant literature for support of a diagnosis. This book contains well-described clinical examples and up-to-date scientific data that explain many of the manifestations that result from exposure to specific neurotoxicants and will allow the clinician, in any capacity, to make a differential diagnosis with confidence.

Occupational and Environmental Neurotoxicology draws upon my many years of experience in differentiating the manifestations of neurotoxic disease from those associated with nonneurotoxic conditions.

I served as the Director of the Occupational Health Program at Boston University Medical Center and I am an investigator in the Boston Environmental Hazards Center at the Boston Veterans Administration Medical Center. While a member of the Board of Scientific Advisors of NIOSH, I participated in the development of applied research programs designed to assess individuals and populations at risk for neurotoxic exposures and to determine how to clinically measure low-level effects of exposure to neurotoxicants. Wherever possible, I have used my own patients' stories and exposure data. Many of these patients were followed in the Occupational and Environmental Neurology Program at Boston University Medical Center from the time of their acute injury for years afterward, providing information about long-term outcomes. My background in pharmacology is reflected in the discussions on the effects of exposure to chemicals. These discussions take into consideration the principles of absorption; pharmacokinetics; and tissue biochemistry, including possible transformations of the exposure substance to more toxic metabolites; and identification of those metabolites and excretion products that can be used to document exposure. The range of clinical manifestations of toxic effects among groups of exposed subjects is examined with consideration to dose–response relationships, individual susceptibilities, and thresholds of toxicity.

Early detection of occupational or environmental illness prevents further exposure and alerts others at risk to the danger. Unfortunately, by the time a chemically exposed and symptomatic person comes to medical attention, proof that a specific neurotoxicant or its metabolite has caused the adverse health effects is usually unavailable. Thus, whenever possible, it is important to monitor levels of exposure in order to avoid hazardous situations and to document exposure levels close to the time of onset of any symptoms in those cases where unsuspected or accidental exposures have occurred. Biological samples should be taken from the patients while they are still at risk or immediately after they have vacated the source of exposure. Few neurologists have the opportunity to evaluate their patients for neurotoxic illness in the settings where exposure was ongoing and where confirmatory evidence of specific neurotoxicant exposure could be collected. I have studied exposed workers on-site (in a lead mine, at lead and arsenic smelters, in lead reclamation plants, in a brass-lead alloy foundry, in houses being deleaded, in mixed solvent and spray painting shops, around degreasing operations, and at toxic waste sites). I bring to this book my first-hand experience in evaluating patients with their neurotoxic illness in the occupational and environmental settings where they were exposed to neurotoxicants.

This book was written with a unified style, avoiding redundancy and maintaining a consistent quality from chapter to chapter. The organization of *Occupational and Environmental Neurotoxicology* begins with chapters that review the symptomatic presentations of neurotoxic effects and the overall topic of occupational and environmental exposures and it presents approaches necessary in assessment of patients and others at risk. Each of the remaining chapters follows a definite format. Sections within each chapter provide information about selected chemical substances and their neurotoxic features. The *Introduction* describes the physical nature and chemical structure of the substance and indicates its importance as a neurotoxicant. *Sources of Exposure* reveals the probable locations where one might encounter or become exposed to the chemical. The next section, *Exposure Limits and Safety Regulations,* cites the official standards and exposure limits that have been set forth by various governmental agencies concerned with occupational and environmental health. Under the heading *Metabolism,* the chemical is discussed in terms of how it enters the body, how it is distributed within the body tissues, and how it reacts within the tissues and/or is transformed to other possibly more or less toxic metabolites. The excretion of the various changed or unchanged forms of the absorbed chemical(s) are also discussed. In addition to the *Symptomatic Diagnosis* section, wherein the manifestations that result from neurotoxicant exposures are described, sections on *Neurophysiological Diagnosis, Neuropsychological Diagnosis,* and *Neuroimaging* discuss confirmatory tests that document the effects of exposure on the peripheral and central nervous systems. In the *Neuropathological Diagnosis* section, the reader is provided with evidence of human tissue damage wherever possible; otherwise, results of exposures in experimental animals are shown. The pharmacological basis for impaired function and cellular damage or cell death are also discussed under this section. *Therapeutic and Preventive Measures* provides specific instructions concerning acute and long-term therapeutic interventions that are appropriate to poisonings by the particular neurotoxicant. Occupational and environmental health safety and hazard prevention strategies for exposed and at-risk individuals or populations are also discussed. Selected case descriptions and additional details of various exposure scenarios and their possible acute and long-term neurotoxic effects are included in the *Clinical Experiences* section of each chapter.

Occupational and Environmental Neurotoxicology should serve as a helpful tool for the clinician. I have tried to make the text user-friendly for all practitioners. In its preparation, I sought peer review by consulting with colleagues in the fields of neurology, environmental health, and pharmacology. Abundant references include classical descriptions and reports of current molecular biological and pharmacological research. Where a concept is controversial, multiple references are cited to offer differing points of view. I hope that this book will be useful in providing comprehensive information on occupational neurological syndromes that should be of direct value to many practitioners.

Robert G. Feldman, M.D.

Acknowledgments

Occupational and Environmental Neurotoxicology could not have been completed without the extraordinarily dedicated efforts of my Research Assistant, Ms. Marcia Ratner. Her ability to organize large volumes of references and her critical proofreading have assured accuracy in documentation of the material used, and her skills in graphic design have been crucial to the preparation of the manuscript.

I received valuable advice, encouragement, and constructive criticism regarding content accuracy and relevance of the various chapters from Edward Baker, Patricia Buffler, Roberta White, Phillipe Grandjean, James Albers, Louis Chang, Alan Ducatman, Patricia Williams, Howard Frumkin, Paula Lina, and Robert Budinsky. In addition to these friends and colleagues, there are others to whom I express my appreciation for their sharing of occupational and environmental toxicology interests and projects over the years, including Drs. David Wegman, Barry Johnson, Robert McCunney, David Ozonoff, Barry Levy, Howard Hu, David Christiani, Juhani Juntunen, Ann Fidler, Patricia Travers, Rose Goldman, Susan Proctors, Cheryl Barbanel, Ching-Ming (Joseph) Chern, Kazuhito Yamadori, and Jonathan Rutchik; Jan Schlictmann, Esq., Michael Baram, Esq., and Bruce Berger, Esq. The contribution of the residents, graduate students, and research assistants who have worked with me in the evaluating patients and doing literature searches is recognized, especially the efforts of Drs. Ike Eriator, Manisha Thakore, Michael Moritoglu, and Salmon Malik.

My appreciation is also expressed to the scientists and clinicians who provided photographic materials from their work to help me illustrate certain points in the various chapters; the courtesy of these individuals is noted in the legends of the illustrations they provided.

The administrative support provided by Boston University School of Medicine and especially the staff of the Department of Neurology was very important throughout the preparation of this book, especially that given by Robert V. Sartini, Sara Johnson, Kristan Boluch, and Josephina Maguigad.

I also derived personal support and encouragement throughout this endeavor from my long-time friend, Norman Paul, and especially from my wife, Gail; son, John; and daughter, Elise.

Robert G. Feldman, M.D.

Occupational and Environmental Neurotoxicology

CHAPTER 1

Exposure to Hazardous Chemicals

Both clinicians and the general public have become increasingly aware that neurological syndromes may result from exposures to certain chemicals and that risks of exposure to chemical hazards are ubiquitous. Occupationally and environmentally related neurotoxic illness may go undetected until the patient's symptoms and signs interfere with performance of job tasks or result in frank disability. An individual is *exposed* when a recognized or suspected contaminant found in the air, drinking water, soil, food, or surface water has been ingested, inhaled, and/or absorbed through the skin. An individual is *at-risk* when a contaminant is present but evidence of actual intake is lacking (potential exposure). That the nervous system is particularly vulnerable to the effects of exposure to chemicals is acknowledged as an important public health issue (Landrigan et al., 1994).

OCCUPATIONAL AND ENVIRONMENTAL HEALTH

Although few of the more than 70,000 chemicals in commercial use have been tested for neurotoxicity by standardized research protocols, neurotoxic effects in animals and humans have been associated with exposures to many of them. Surveys of individuals or groups of workers have reported various incidence rates of occupational and environmental illnesses. The full extent to which neurological diseases occur secondary to exposure to toxic chemicals is unknown. Approximately 40% of new cases of occupational illness reported in 1990 were due to chemical exposures and other nonmechanical causes (Bureau of Labor Statistics, 1991). Neurological and/or behavioral effects served as criteria for the recommended safe exposure limits (threshold limit values [TLVs]) for 167 of the 588 chemicals developed by the American Conference of Governmental Industrial Hygienists (ACGIH) (Anger and Johnson, 1985). A review of clinical case reports involving about 220 different chemicals showed that 149 had caused documented neurotoxicity in humans (Grandjean et al., 1991). Overall, these are probably low estimates of the number of available chemicals capable of causing neurotoxic illnesses, since most responses identified were readily apparent and were observed after high dose exposures. Milder and less obvious neurotoxic effects might have occurred at lower levels of exposure but were undetected and thus unreported. In addition to underreporting, inaccuracy of a clinical diagnosis can also result in an underestimation of persons at risk and/or those who have neurological injury.

A worker who experiences adverse effects at a low concentration of chemical exposure often leaves that job; a heartier person with less susceptibility to the effects of exposure stays on, reporting no ill effects. Such *well-worker effects* affect the outcomes of health hazard evaluations and suggest that the workplace is safe. Nonoccupational sources of exposure to neurotoxicants, such as those associated with hobbies and crafts materials or household products, must also be considered in estimating the total extent of chemically related illness. Systematic studies of low-level exposure situations using sophisticated tests sensitive to subtle neurotoxic effects will almost certainly identify additional neurotoxicants and their effects.

Even though both employers and employees increasingly heed the warnings of labels, material safety data sheets, and various federal and state agencies, many exposed and at-risk workers may still be unaware of chemical hazards at their workplace. Clinicians in the fields of neurology, occupational and environmental health, and primary care must also be prepared to recognize the risks of exposure to chemicals and their potential for causing injury to the nervous system, as well as to other organ systems. Every patient's complaints should be evaluated in the context of his or her overall occupational and environmental experiences.

In an environmental setting it is more difficult to detect a specific causative neurotoxic chemical and to determine the source of exposure than it is in an occupational one, despite an outbreak of symptoms among individuals. Exposure can be suspected in communities where chemical industries and/or chemical waste disposal sites are located,

1

or where ongoing potentially hazardous processes are located near water supply sources, even in the absence of specifically reported exposure data. A health effects study in a community or other nonoccupational setting is often prompted by the realization that there has been a release of chemicals into the environment. Relevant indicators of risk or adverse health effects may be detected by routine monitoring, health statistics, popular rumors about adverse health and exposure, or routine visits to primary care physicians, who may note a trend, such as an unusual number of cases of leukemia in a neighborhood (Lagakos et al., 1986).

Short-term, very low-level exposures are less likely to produce any health effects; acute high-level and high-intensity exposures may induce a variety of immediate and remote effects; and chronic exposures of any intensity result in a wide range of outcomes. In the latter situation, adverse health effects will depend on the general levels of contamination within an exposed community's atmosphere and/or water sources, the circumstances and exposure levels experienced, and individual susceptibilities. Evidence of toxic levels of particular chemicals (and/or their metabolites) in the tissues of an exposed individual is often lacking by the time clinical effects are noted and the contaminated environmental source investigated. Examination of selected sensitive health indices can help to determine whether the expected background rates of illnesses have increased or decreased; all clinically affected persons and those suspected of being exposed but who appear to be unaffected require careful clinical evaluation using standard measures of neurological functioning (Buffler et al., 1985).

RECOGNITION AND REGULATION OF NEUROTOXICANTS

Neurotoxicants are chemicals capable of altering the integrity of nerve cell membranes, affecting neuronal excitability, transmitter systems, and synaptic activity in the peripheral and central nervous systems; disturbing axoplasmic transport; affecting neurological functions indirectly by toxic actions on Schwann cells and peripheral myelin; damaging central myelin, oligodendroglia cells, and other supporting elements including astrocytes and microglia; and disturbing extracellular fluid volume and flow by damaging capillary endothelium (Spencer and Schaumberg, 1984). Accidental exposures and intentional poisonings in humans and experimental animals have resulted in many reports on the deleterious effects of chemicals on neurological functioning. In some instances the neurotoxic effects observed have become useful models for studying pathophysiological and biochemical mechanisms of normal neural function and disease processes. For example, acrylamide has been used in the study of peripheral nerves; organotin selectively affects neurons in the hippocampus and serves as a model for studying memory and epilepsy; aluminum has been used to create experimental epileptogenesis in animals; and 1-methyl-4 pheynl-1,2,3,6-tetrahy-

dropyridine has provided a model for Parkinson's disease and for studying the possible causes of neurodegenerative diseases. Thus, "experiments" resulting from occupational and environmental chemical exposures have stimulated research on possible relationships between neurotoxic exposures and the ecoetiology and pathophysiology of diseases heretofore considered "degenerative" (e.g., Parkinson's disease, Alzheimer's disease, and amyotrophic lateral sclerosis). Neurotoxic effects of chemical exposures are of scientific as well as economic importance (Cote and Vandenburgh, 1994).

Recognition of potential neurotoxic health hazards associated with exposure to certain chemicals depends on the clinician's knowledge of substances in and around work areas. In addition to reviews of the toxicological, clinical, and epidemiological literature describing previously reported clinical effects of exposures to known neurotoxic chemicals, reference to established handbooks and/or government-recommended occupational and environmental standards is necessary in establishing a causal basis for the findings in suspected or previously unrecognized cases of neurotoxic syndromes. Current "reference levels" for many toxic agents have been based on data obtained from past environmental monitoring. Lists of chemical substances, descriptions of exposure circumstances, and frequently reported clinical neurotoxic effects have been compiled (Sax, 1979; Clayton and Clayton, 1994; NIOSH, 1994; Meister, 1996). The most readily available reference data are the regulatory or advisory guidelines provided by national or international health and environmental agencies. In addition, information about toxic exposures and their neurotoxic and other organ toxicities can be accessed from electronic data systems (Table 1-1). The principal governmental agencies responsible for most occupational and environmental health issues (including hazard detection, regulation, and prevention through investigation, research, legislation, and enforcement) are listed below.

1. *The American Conference of Governmental Industrial Hygienists (ACGIH)* is an independent group of health specialists from governmental and nongovernmental, academic and nonacademic organizations, as well as representatives of the National Institute of Occupational Safety and Health (NIOSH) and industry who consult annually to develop consensus safety standards and exposure limits. These recommendations are revised periodically as new evidence about toxicities of individual chemicals becomes known. ACGIH and NIOSH are the two major authoritative reference sources for recommended informational, but not legally enforceable, exposure levels for chemicals in the workplace. However, these recommendations serve as a basis for the federal *permissible exposure limits* (PELs), which then are enforced by the Occupational Safety and Health Administration (OSHA) (Federal Register, 1974). The generally accepted term for ACGIH exposure concentrations is

TABLE 1-1. *Accessing toxicology information on the Internet*

Host	Address	Available information
U.S. National Library of Medicine (NLM)	http://www.nlm.nih.gov	NLM's Medline, via Grateful Med or PubMed. Access the Toxicology Data Network, which contains TOXLINE, Hazardous Substance Data Bank (HSBD), Integrated Risk Information Systems (IRIS), Registry of Toxic Effects of Chemical Substances (RTECS), and Toxic Chemical Release Inventory (TRT). NLM also has many other medically related features.
The Agency for Toxic Substances and Disease Registry (ATSDR) scientific and administrative database (HAZDAT)	http://atsdr1.atsdr.cdc.gov:8080/atsdrhome.htmlftp://ncsa.uiuc.edu	Includes data about the releases and health effects of substances from more than 1,500 Superfund hazardous waste sites released or during accidental spills. Toxicological profiles for over 160 chemicals have been prepared by ATSDR and are available through the Internet with full text search and retrieval (through FTP site).
The Extension Toxicology Network (EXTOXNET)	http://ace.orst.edu/info/extoxnet/ghindex.html	A joint effort between several universities (maintained at Oregon State University), this site contains an extensive collection of data concerning pesticide information and toxicity.
Medical, Clinical, and Occupational Toxicology Resource Home Page	http://www.pitt.edu/~martint/welcome.html	Hosted by the University of Pittsburgh School of Medicine, this site provides an exhaustive compendium of toxicologically relevant material. Includes websites and addresses of American and international toxicology professional groups, poison control centers, and related organizations. The links section is one of the most complete listings of medical, clinical, and occupational toxicology websites available.
Medscape	http://www.medscape.com	A commercial Web service for clinicians, free access to the National Library of Medicine medical databases: Medline, Aidsline, and especially Toxline. It also provides access to the Web's largest collection of freely available, full-text, clinical articles.
Environmental Protection Agency (EPA)	http://www.epa.gov	A public Web service designed to provide information on the latest EPA programs, its offices, and news. Information is presented in a mostly nontechnical, informal format designed for ease of use and understanding by the average person. It provides access to the latest information on environmental concerns.
Occupational Safety and Health Administration (OSHA)	http://www.osha.gov	A public information source describing OSHA, its mission, current standards for occupational health and safety, and offices. The site provides detailed information on government regulations concerning hazardous chemicals, as well as information on individual substances.
National Institute of Occupational Safety and Health (NIOSH)	http://www.cdc.gov/niosh/homepage.html	A division of the Centers for Disease Control. The site provides information on all aspects of NIOSH, including the Databases Homepage, which allows free access to the National Agriculture Safety Database, the Pocket Guide to Chemical Hazards, the Registry of Toxic Effects of Chemical Substances, and International Chemical Safety cards, as well as various other valuable resources.

threshold limit value (TLV). *Threshold limit value–time-weighted average* (TLV-TWA) is the airborne concentration of a given substance and condition to which most workers may be exposed for 8 hours (day after day) or for 40 hours a week (week after week) without adverse effects. *Threshold limit value-ceiling* (TLV-C) means that any exposure should not exceed the designated allowable concentration, even for an instant. *Threshold limit value–short-term exposure limit* (TLV-STEL) means that exposure to this concentration of a substance should be no longer than 15 minutes in duration, provided that a given episode of exposure does not exceed the TLV-TWA for the substance, that no more than four such short-term exposures occur during a day, and that each exposure episode is separated from the other by at least 60 minutes.

2. *The National Institute for Occupational Safety and Health (NIOSH)* is associated with the Centers for Disease Control of the United States Public Health Service; it conducts clinical, laboratory, and epidemiological studies of employees allegedly exposed to potentially hazardous substances. These studies may include workplace inspections, measurement of air, water, and biological samples of possible intoxicants, and determination of the incidence of occupational illness among employees. NIOSH develops criteria, recommends standards for chemicals that lack PELs, and reviews those with existing PELs. NIOSH defines a *recommended exposure limit* (REL) for various chemical substances. These RELs are occupational exposure limits considered to be protective of worker health over a lifetime. RELs are expressed as a TWA exposure for up to 10 hours a day during a 40-hour work week, as a STEL that should not exceed a specified sampling period such as 15 minutes, or as a ceiling limit that should not be exceeded unless specified over a given period, in some cases even instantaneously (NIOSH, 1992).

3. *The Occupational Safety and Health Administration (OSHA)* is part of the Department of Labor; it has the legislative authority to set standards, inspect work sites to observe conditions, and enforce compliance with these standards by both employers and employees. OSHA establishes legally enforceable PELs for specific chemicals used in U.S. industry (Federal Register, 1974).

4. *The Agency for Toxic Substances and Disease Registry (ATSDR)* maintains a registry of exposures to chemicals and the possibly associated illnesses at hazardous waste sites and chemical spill locations; it also supports activities that protect the public from toxic chemical exposure. The ATSDR conducts research about the health effects of hazardous materials and publishes comprehensive reports on various environmentally hazardous substances (in *Toxicological Profiles* and *Case Studies in Environmental Medicine*), and maintains electronic databases through the National Library of Medicine. In addition, it provides a 24-hour emergency response capability (Federal Register, 1989; Mitchell, 1994) to assist the clinician in detecting adverse health effects associated with exposure to toxic chemicals.

5. *The United States Environmental Protection Agency (EPA)* regulates hazardous industrial wastes from the point of generation through disposal and protects citizens who are thought to be at risk of exposure. The EPA identifies hazardous waste, tracks its presence in the environment, and establishes standards for managing waste disposal facilities. It issues permits for the production, storage, handling, transport, and disposal of hazardous waste (including solid, liquid, and semiliquid waste) and gaseous materials generated from industrial, commercial, mining, agricultural, and community sources considered by the EPA to be capable of causing injury to humans or to the environment. Environmental criteria can be obtained from the U.S. EPA regional office or by referring to related EPA reports, such as *Air Quality Criteria for Lead* (EPA, 1986; OTA, 1989).

DOCUMENTING EXPOSURE

Exposure refers to the quantity or concentration of a substance present in the environment that is assumed to be absorbed by an individual who is in the area. Exposure involves both the intensity and the duration of a chemical encountered, and it should be distinguished from dose, which is the amount of chemical actually absorbed by an individual; (the body-burden) dose is determined not only by the exposure circumstances and the availability of the toxicant, but also by the roles played by the personal hygiene (e.g., protective clothing and washing), behavior (e.g., intentional inhaling for euphoric effects), and biological characteristics (e.g., genetically determined protective enzymes) of the exposed person (Checkoway, 1989; Johnson, 1992). Exposure may be recent or it may have occurred in the past. In fact, an acute exposure may be considered the illness-producing event but in actuality may be only another recent episode in a chronic series of exposure episodes. An individual may report neurological symptoms experienced as a result of a specific acute exposure episode (e.g., chemical spill accident), but he or she may have had chronic exposure (e.g., exposure over many years in the workplace or through environmental sources such as drinking and bathing contaminated water). Sometimes the source of toxic exposure cannot be determined.

Obtaining information about current chemical exposures often requires careful and comprehensive industrial hygiene (IH) investigations by trained IH personnel utilizing appropriate and sensitive monitoring equipment. On-site evaluation of current exposure data at the workplace should include descriptions of the work tasks, the processes, the working conditions, and the nature of raw materials used as well as any intermediate products and other sources of exposure and potential hazards. Ambient air samples, taken for analysis of content and concentration of relevant chemicals used within the at-risk subjects' work area and found in an individual's breathing space, are of value in estimating the actual amount inhaled during the job or throughout one or several work shifts. Job activities should also be reviewed with plant personnel to learn where the worker was located while working and on break, exactly how the job assignments are expected to be safely carried out, and how hazards are dealt with (if they exist) (World Health Organization, 1986; Cohen, 1992).

Personal sampling (i.e., direct measurement of the concentration of toxicants near the individual's breathing zone) provides the most information about possible exposure to inhalant neurotoxicants. Quantifiable personal measurements can include personal air sampling monitoring (i.e., following an individual in the potential exposure area over time) and/or the use of biological markers (e.g., biochemical, histological, or physiological indicators of neurotoxicant exposure or effect). However, if it is not possible to obtain direct personal sampling exposure measures, it may be necessary to use more indirect means to estimate exposures. These surrogate measures may include *area sampling* at designated high-risk work sites or in a possibly polluted residence. Calculations of drinking water exposure are based on estimated intake levels, distance measurements of a residence from the sources of possible hazardous waste or industrial pollution, and length of residence or duration of employment in the at-risk areas. Environmental exposure to hazardous substances or contaminated water, soil, or air is also determined through either area or personal sampling (Johnson, 1992; ATSDR, 1992a,b). Concentrations of a chemical in the air, measured by environmental monitoring methods, often do not correlate closely with actual amounts absorbed by an exposed person because certain physical and biological factors are not accounted for (e.g., variation in the concentration of chemicals at different locations and points in time, solubility and particle size characteristics, use of personal protection devices, workload demand effects on respiratory volume, individual nutritional status and body composition); all these affect the uptake of chemical in the body (Aito et al., 1988).

In some cases measurement of biological markers has distinct advantages over environmental monitoring. Biological markers are indicators of total uptake, reflecting intake from multiple routes and fluctuating exposures over time (Wilcosky and Griffith, 1990; see Chapter 3). However, biological monitoring is of little value for assessing exposure to substances that are poorly absorbed or that exhibit toxic effects at the sites of first contact, such as skin or mucous membranes (Ashford et al., 1990; Lauwerys, 1991). Therefore, environmental and biological monitoring should be viewed as complementary methods. Confirmation of exposure to a specific chemical agent and documentation of its effect in a clinical setting gains greater probability when the suspected toxic substance and the alleged exposed subject(s) are found in the same location; when measurements detecting the chemical in atmospheric samples (e.g., ambient air, soil, water, foods, etc.) as well as levels of the chemical or its metabolites (biological markers) are found in the tissues of the patient; when clinical manifestations are reasonable and are compatible with the duration of employment and the temporal sequence of

documented exposure and the emergence of symptoms (i.e., the exposure preceded the onset of clinical effects); and finally, when all other nontoxic explanations for neurological manifestations have been satisfactorily raised and eliminated.

Sometimes current and past time-related exposure levels and the presenting clinical symptoms cannot be linked because the contamination circumstances have changed by the time environmental measurements can be made and the exposure data obtainable may be inadequate to ascertain the previous exposure level. An estimate of exposure will require mathematical modeling methods. Quantification of cumulative exposures is required for determining a probable dose–response relationship in cases of neurotoxic illness arising after prolonged exposures from both occupational and environmental sources. Mathematical modeling using "historical" exposure records may be the only way to estimate a patient's cumulative exposure dose. This cumulative dose represents a time-integrated measure that is the summation of concentrations over time. For example, for a particular job during a specific period, the exposure can be quantified by multiplying the actual working time at that job (vacations and leaves not included), the rate of intake of that agent (e.g., inhalation rate for airborne contaminants), and the level of the agent during that period. Then, by adding up each exposure at each job, the cumulative exposure to that specific agent for this patient can be estimated (Checkoway et al., 1989). Past monitoring data may not be available, limiting exposure status to measures of the current level of an identifiable chemical in the environment and then making assumptions to estimate this person's past exposure.

Semiquantitative estimates of cumulative exposure can be obtained by indirect means. For example, a hydrogeologic model was used in a study of solvent-contaminated drinking water to simulate movement of the solvent leak plume and water flow within the distribution system so that an estimation of past exposure to contaminated well water could be made, using the average amount of drinking water consumed per day to represent the rate of intake (Wrensch et al., 1990). A similar and much easier method using an *exposure factor* to average out the dose over the exposure interval is also suggested for cases of more intermittent exposures (ATSDR, 1992b). In addition to studies of hazardous waste sites, these quantitative measures have been applied in occupational epidemiology studies to approximate the total exposed dose and can readily be applied to the clinical evaluation of exposed individuals to estimate exposure dose.

REFERENCES

Agency for Toxic Substances and Disease Registry (ATSDR). Determining contaminants of concern. In: *Public Health Assessment Guidance Manual.* Atlanta, GA: ATSDR, 1992a.
Agency for Toxic Substances and Disease Registry (ATSDR). Appendix D: estimation of exposure dose. In: *Public Health Assessment Guidance Manual.* Atlanta, GA: ATSDR, 1992b.

Aitio A, Jarvisalo J, Riihimaki V, Hernberg S. Biologic monitoring. In: Zene C, ed. *Occupational medicine,* 2nd ed. Chicago: Year-Book Medical Publishers, 1988:178–197.

Anger WK, Johnson BL. Chemicals affecting behavior. In: O'Donoghue JL, ed. *Neurotoxicity of industrial and commercial chemicals,* vol. 1, Boca Raton, FL: CRC Press, 1985:51–148.

Ashford NA, Spadafor CJ, Hattis DB, Caldart CC. *Monitoring the worker for exposure and disease: overview and definitions.* Baltimore: The Johns Hopkins University Press, 1990.

Buffler PA, Crane M, Key MM. Possibilities of detecting health effects by studies of populations exposed to chemicals from waste disposal sites. *Environ Health Perspect* 1985;62:423–456.

Bureau of Labor Statistics. Results of Bureau of Labor Statistics Survey on U.S. Occupational Injuries, Illnesses in 1990. Washington, DC: U.S. Department of Labor, 1991.

Checkoway H, Pearce N, Crawford-Brown DJ. Characterizing the workplace environment. In: Checkoway H, Pearce N, Crawford-Brown DJ, eds. *Research methods in occupational epidemiology.* New York: Oxford University Press, 1989:18–45.

Clayton GD, Clayton FE (eds). *Patty's industrial hygiene and toxicology,* 4th ed. New York: John Wiley & Sons, 1994:5046.

Cohen BS. Industrial hygiene measurement and control. In Rom W, ed. *Environmental and occupational medicine,* 2nd ed. Boston: Little, Brown, 1992:1389–1404.

Cote IL, Vandenburg JJ. Overview of health effects and risk assessment issues associated with air pollution. In: Isaacson RL, Jensen KF, eds. *The vulnerable brain and environmental risks, vol. 3: Toxins in air and water.* New York: Plenum Press, 1994:231–245.

Environmental Protection Agency (EPA). *Air quality criteria for lead.* EPA Report no. EPA-600/8-83-028aF-DF. Research Triangle Park, NC: Environmental Criteria and Assessment Office, USEPA, 1986.

Federal Register, Agency for Toxic Substances and Disease Registry. *Statement of organization, functions and delegations of authority.* 1989;54:33617.

Federal Register. Occupational Safety and Health Administration. *Occupational safety and health standards.* 1974;39:23502.

Grandjean P, Sandoe SH, Kimbrough RD. Non-specificity of clinical signs and symptoms caused by environmental chemicals. *Hum Exp Toxicol* 1991;10:167–173.

Johnson BL. A precision exposure assessment. *J Environ Health* 1992; 55:6–9.

World Health Organization (WHO). *Early detection of occupational diseases.* Geneva: WHO, 1986:243–251.

Lagakos SW, Wessen BJ, Zelen M. An analysis of contaminated well water and health effects in Woburn, Massachusetts. *J Am Stat Assoc* 1986;81:583–596.

Landrigan PJ, Graham DG, Thomas RD. Environmental neurotoxic illness: research for prevention. *Environ Health Perspect* 1994;102 [suppl. 2]:117–120.

Lauwerys R. Occupational toxicology. In: Klaassen C, Admur M, Doull J, eds. *Cassarett and Doull's toxicology.* New York: Macmillan, 1991: 947–969.

Meister RT (ed). *Farm chemical handbook.* Willoughby, OH: Meister, 1996.

Mitchell FL. The Agency for Toxic Substances and Disease Registry. In: McCunney RJ (ed). *A practical approach to occupational and environmental medicine,* 2nd ed. Boston: Little, Brown, 1994:651–660.

NIOSH. *Recommendations for occupational safety and health: compendium of policy documents and statements.* DHHS publications no. 92-100. Cincinnati, OH: U.S. Department of Health and Human Services Publications Dissemination, DSDTT, 1992.

NIOSH. *Pocket guide to chemical hazards.* U.S. Department of Health and Human Services (NIOSH), publication no. 94-116. Cincinnati, OH: U.S. Government Printing Office, 1994.

Office of Technology Assessment (OTA). *Coming clean: superfund problems can be solved.* OTA-ITE-433. Washington, DC: U.S. Government Printing Office, 1989.

Sax NI. *Dangerous properties of industrial materials,* 5th ed. New York: Van Nostrand Reinhold, 1979.

Spencer PS, Schaumburg HH. An expanded classification of neurotoxic responses based on cellular targets of chemical agents. *Acta Neurol Scand* 1984;70[Suppl 100]:9–19.

Wilcosky TC, Griffith JD. Applications of biological markers. In Hulka BS, Wilcosky TC, Griffith JD (eds). *Biological markers in epidemiology.* New York: Oxford University Press, 1990:16–27.

Wrensch M, Swan S, Murphy P, et al. Hydrogeologic assessment of exposure to solvent-contaminated drinking water: pregnancy outcomes in relation to exposure. *Arch Environ Health* 1990;45:210–216.

CHAPTER 2

Recognizing the Chemically Exposed Person

Symptoms associated with the effects of chemicals may occur immediately after exposure, may emerge gradually with repeated or continued exposure, or may not become apparent until some time after a latency period during which neurotoxic damage has progressed to a level sufficient to cause clinically evident effects. The patient's presenting complaints will usually trigger a search for neurotoxic effects.

Early recognition of neurotoxic effects in one person (i.e., *sentinel case*) should call attention to the possibility that other exposed persons may be in the area who have not yet exhibited symptoms. A worker is often unaware of any relationship between his or her symptoms and job tasks or possible exposure to hazardous chemicals. Many accidents in the workplace are attributed to human error when they may in fact be due to impaired alertness, judgment, or sensorimotor abilities caused by chemical exposures that were overlooked by observers. Often poor attention, mood changes, memory problems, delirium, or even the appearance of drunkenness with ataxia and incoordination may be ignored by the affected person. The problem may be pointed out by coworkers or family members.

An exposed subject may experience general nonspecific malaise or feelings of unwellness (including complaints of nausea, dizziness, and headache) and accept them as "part of the job." If these symptoms are disturbing enough, the person may vacate the exposure area to get relief from the discomfort or to seek medical attention. More rapidly progressing symptoms may preclude an escape, and the hazardous condition may reach a more dramatic and serious state, leading to stupor, seizures, and coma. Some neurotoxicants may be life threatening, and others may cause reversible illness— the symptoms appear soon after the exposure and subside after leaving the exposure. In some cases recovery may be soon after the removal from exposure, and other cases may take months to years to reach amelioration or full recovery.

SYMPTOMATIC PRESENTATIONS

Prompt appearance of neurological symptoms and signs after an acute exposure to neurotoxicants is more obvious than the gradual emergence of neurological symptoms with chronic exposure or the presentation of symptoms following a latent period. In many cases, several follow-up evaluations are necessary to detect emerging symptoms, document the persistence and/or progression of postexposure symptoms, assess the resolution of symptoms, or identify residual neurological impairments or disabilities. Idiopathic (nontoxic) neurological disease usually follows a progressive course with continued development of symptoms in the absence of any identified exposure to neurotoxicants.

Nonspecific systemic effects of neurotoxicants include vegetative symptoms such as nausea, dizziness, and headache. Behavioral symptoms such as poor attention, memory troubles, and delirium are obvious when they interfere with daily tasks. Acute and sometimes reversible central nervous system (CNS) symptoms precede the onset of the signs of peripheral neuropathy. Neurological dysfunction (motor weakness, sensory loss, or altered mental status) results from damage to specialized areas of the brain, spinal cord, and peripheral nerves. Similar neurological signs and symptoms arise from the same principal neuroanatomical structures and thus resemble those associated with primary neurological diseases. Unless a clinician is alert to the possibility that the symptoms occurred following exposure to neurotoxicants, the illness may be attributed to a common neurological disorder, and an occupational or environmental illness may be undiagnosed (Table 2-1). For example, exposure to carbon disulfide, carbon monoxide, and manganese, which affect basal ganglia function, can result in a clinical picture suggestive of Parkinson's disease. Individuals exposed to certain solvents and metals have developed peripheral neuropathy not unlike that seen in patients with a history of alcoholism or diabetes. Neurotoxic symptoms of chemical exposure may be direct or indirect, reversible or irreversible, depending on the chemical structure of the specific neurotoxicant involved, the nature and duration of exposure, the amount (body burden) of the chemical(s) absorbed, and its selective effects on the peripheral nervous system and CNS. The diagnosis of a neurotoxic syndrome following

TABLE 2-1. *Chemical exposures and associated neurotoxic disorders*

Neurotoxin	Source of exposure	Clinical diagnosis
Metals		
Arsenic	Pesticides Pigments Antifouling paint Electroplating industry Seafood Smelters Semiconductors	*Acute:* encephalopathy *Chronic:* peripheral neuropathy
Lead	Solder Lead shot Illicit whiskey Insecticides Auto body shop Storage battery manufacturing Foundries, smelters Lead-based paint Lead pipes	*Acute:* encephalopathy *Chronic:* encephalopathy and peripheral neuropathy
Manganese	Iron, steel industry Welding operations Metal-finishing operations Fertilizers Manufacturers of fireworks, matches Manufacturers of dry cell batteries	*Acute:* encephalopathy *Chronic:* parkinsonism
Mercury	Scientific instruments Electrical equipment Amalgams Electroplating industry Photography Felt making	*Acute:* headache, nausea, onset of tremor *Chronic:* ataxia, peripheral neuropathy encephalopathy
Tin	Canning industry Solder Electronic components Polyvinyl plastics Fungicides	*Acute:* memory defects, seizures, disorientation *Chronic:* encephalomyelopathy
Solvents		
Carbon disulfide	Manufacturers of viscose rayon Preservatives Textiles Rubber cement Varnishes Electroplating industry	*Acute:* encephalopathy *Chronic:* peripheral neuropathy, parkinsonism
n-hexane, methyl butyl ketone	Paints Lacquers Varnishes Metal-cleaning compounds Quick-drying inks Paint removers Glues, adhesives	*Acute:* narcosis *Chronic:* peripheral neuropathy
Perchloroethylene	Paint removers Degreasers Extraction agents Dry cleaning industry Textile industry	*Acute:* narcosis *Chronic:* peripheral neuropathy, encephalopathy
Toluene	Rubber solvents Cleaning agents Glues Manufacturers of benzene Gasoline, aviation fuel Paints, paint thinners Lacquers	*Acute:* narcosis *Chronic:* ataxia, encephalopathy

TABLE 2-1. *Continued*

Neurotoxin	Source of exposure	Clinical diagnosis
Trichloroethylene	Degreasers Painting industry Varnishes Spot removers Process of decaffeination Dry cleaning industry Rubber solvents	*Acute:* narcosis *Chronic:* encephalopathy, cranial neuropathy
Insecticides Organophosphates	Agricultural industry: manufacturing and application	*Acute:* cholinergic poisoning *Chronic:* ataxia, paralysis, peripheral neuropathy
Carbamates	Agricultural industry: manufacturing and application Flea powders	*Acute:* cholinergic poisoning. *Chronic:* tremor, peripheral neuropathy

chemical exposure must be differentiated from a neurological disease of nonneurotoxic etiology, not associated with chemical exposure. The diagnostician needs an understanding of the pathogenesis of the neurological symptoms and signs and a knowledge of the pharmacology of the substances that are capable of affecting certain nervous tissues.

Clinical manifestations reflect damage or alteration in normal function in affected target cellular elements, such as neurons, glial cells, myelin sheaths, or blood vessels. Metabolic impairments and often cell death result when natural protective mechanisms fail to detoxify a potentially hazardous substance and to eliminate it, either unchanged before it causes damage or after tissue biochemistry has changed it to an excretable nontoxic metabolite. Symptoms appear when detoxification of the absorbed chemicals has been inadequate or has failed completely; the body burden of an absorbed neurotoxicant or its metabolites then reaches a critical threshold level above which intracellular oxidative processes and energy production of particular cellular targets may become impaired. Alteration in protein or lipid content of cell membranes, ionic imbalances, defective neurotransmitter activity, or damage to capillary endothelium are some of the mechanisms that lead to neurologic dysfunction. Disturbances in the rate of axoplasmic transport and accumulation of neurofilaments are associated with the swelling of axons and dying back of the nerve cells. Reversible functional alterations may be responsible for clinical manifestations and the subclinical effects that can be detected by electroencephalography, evoked potentials, or peripheral nerve conduction velocity testing. Irreversible damage to neural systems may interfere with function so much that an exposed person's ability to perform ordinary daily activities and job tasks cannot be carried out as before. Suspicion that neurotoxic illness may explain a patient's presenting complaints should lead to a clinical diagnosis within the context of occupational and environ-

mental exposures. The diagnostic process integrates the clinician's observations and the results of tests on physiological, anatomical, and behavioral functions, along with his or her acumen and judgment accumulated from experience with similar cases; information contained in the literature and computer data banks is also used. (Fig. 2-1)

Headache

Despite its vagueness and nonspecificity as a symptom, the differential diagnosis of headache must include the effects of exposure to noxious substances. Headache is frequently associated with acute exposure to metal fumes and solvent vapors. In some instances, the mechanism for pain is brain swelling (from tin or lead); in others, transient hypoxia or vasodilation (from zinc, tellurium, manganese, and nickel) may account for the pain.

Two men worked in an electroplating plant using solutions of nickel chloride, nickel sulfate, and hypophosphate; they both developed severe frontal headache following an accident at work. The process involved mixing a solution and heating it to the correct operating temperature. As the temperature reached 150°F, spontaneous decomposition occurred. The gaseous contamination of the environment was detected as an unpleasant odor escaping into a poorly ventilated workplace. The solution and contaminants were secured, and the men were excused from work and sent home. Itching of the exposed skin on the arms and face soon occurred. Several hours later, they both developed severe headache, nausea, and vomiting and required medical attention. It was learned that the usual mixture of 70 gallons of water, 5 gallons of nickel chloride/sulfate, and 14.5 gallons of hypophosphate had instead been 14.5 gallons of hydrogen peroxide. The men were observed in our clinic. Severe headache was reported, and visual field testing showed increased blind

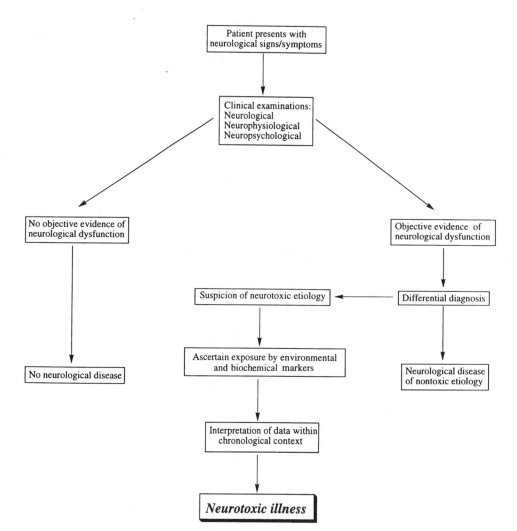

FIG. 2-1. Algorithm. Diagnosis of neurotoxic illness.

spots consistent with the appearance of papilledema. The acute and intense exposure to nickel resulted in the characteristic itch, the subsequent cerebral edema, and the accompanying severe headache.

Computed tomogram in both men revealed small ventricles, consistent with cerebral edema (pseudotumor). The cerebrospinal fluid pressures were 200 mm in one man and 170 mm in the other. Nickel concentrations in 24-hour urine were 27.3 and 45 mg/L in case 1 and 8 mg/liter in case 2. Both men were treated with penicillamine (250 mg four times a day) to reduce the body burden of nickel. Within 4 to 5 days after instituting chelation, improvement in the headaches began, with complete recovery by the end of the month. The output of nickel in case 1 prior to chelation was 1.4 mg/day; during the first week of chelation, it was 4.2 mg/day. Prior to chelation, the output of case 2 was 0.4 mg/day, and his average output for 4 days of chelation was 4.0 mg/day.

Memory and Behavioral Disturbances

In the occupational setting, many accidents attributed to human error may in fact be due to impaired alertness, judgment, or sensorimotor abilities—the result of undetected chemical exposures. Subtle changes in mental functioning due to intoxication often go unrecognized unless looked for using sophisticated neuropsychological test batteries. Lead poisoning was associated with signs of toxic encephalopathy and peripheral neuropathy until more stringent controls in the workplace, coupled with government regulations and stricter environmental standards, led to a decline in cases of industrial lead poisoning. Subtle changes in neurologic dysfunction, such as disturbances of affect, psychomotor function, and nerve conduction, have been reported among workers whose blood concentrations of lead seem relatively low. Overt manifestations of lead-related neurotoxicity, including ataxia, confusion, convulsions, weakness, and paresthesias of the extremities are less often seen. Intoxication with other metals such as manganese is manifested earliest by neuropsychological disturbances, including euphoria, apathy, hallucinations, flight of ideas, compulsivity, agitation, and verbosity. Inorganic mercury poisoning has been known to produce irritability, poor concentration, memory deficiencies, anxiety, and depression.

Effects of solvent exposure on the CNS may manifest as a mental disorder, an impairment in psychologic functioning, or nerve damage. The acute, narcotic effects of solvent exposure have been known for a long time, since many solvents were at one time used as anesthetic agents. Symptoms resulting from acute exposure to solvents include feelings of intoxication, difficulty concentrating, and dizziness. Headache, nausea, and vomiting are also known to occur following exposure. Chronic neurotoxic effects from solvent exposure are characterized by fatigue, irritability, affect lability, depression, and short-term memory disturbances, as well as impairments in psychomotor speed, attention, and complex verbal reasoning.

Exposure to high concentrations of toluene and trichloroethylene (TCE) can cause narcosis and anesthesia. Chronic exposure to TCE has been reported to cause losses in coordination, impairment of tactile senses, an intolerance to alcohol, tremor, and anxiety. Chronic exposure to toluene has been reported to cause fatigue, confusion, weakness, nervousness, and paresthesia of the skin. The features of solvent encephalopathy are illustrated by the case of a 42-year-old optician who had worked for 5 years developing new procedures and techniques in the production of optical surfaces. He heated TCE and toluene in an ultrasonic cleaner to clean the optical surfaces. He frequently left the tops off the solvent containers and often leaned over the ultrasonic cleaner and breathed in the solvent vapors. Sometimes he did not leave this room, where he worked alone, for 2 to 3 days at a time.

At the end of 5 years, he began to notice memory problems and concentration difficulties. In addition, he felt he had a decreased attention span, problems with recall, tremors in both hands, numbness and tingling in all extremities, and emotional lability. While driving home from work, he found it necessary to pull over to the side of the road to sleep and would be unable to recall the length of time he had been there. He was evaluated clinically and with a neuropsychological test battery for his memory and concentration difficulties. This examination revealed decreased attention span and poor short- and long-term memory. His sensory examination showed diminished vibration in the toes and over the lower extremities below the knees. He consistently interpreted pinprick as being dull except over his face. In addition, he had diminished proprioception in the feet and diminished graphesthesia in his palms. While he was symptomatic, his electroencephalogram showed excessive amounts of bilateral theta (slow waves) activity. Nerve conduction velocity studies demonstrated

slowed motor conduction velocities suggestive of peripheral neuropathy; articularly, sensory conduction velocities were slowed and amplitudes were reduced, indicative of axonal (solvent) neuropathy. Neuropsychological testing revealed significant depression, variable psychomotor speed, slightly impaired verbal fluency, and memory deficits. These findings were suggestive of bilateral frontotemporal dysfunction with lesions involving the amygdala and hippocampus. His clinical and laboratory tests demonstrated behavioral as well as the peripheral nervous system findings which resulted from exposure to an organic neurotoxicant solvent.

Numbness, Tingling, and Weakness of Extremities

Complaints of numbness and tingling or weakness are early signs of peripheral neuropathy, often prompting individuals to seek a neurologist's evaluation. The myelin sheath and/or axon are the targets of neurotoxins. Peripheral nervous system symptoms occur after exposure to certain metals (lead, arsenic, and thallium) and solvents (methyl butyl ketone and n-hexane). TCE has a predilection for cranial nerves, especially the distribution of the trigeminal nerve, producing loss of sensation over the face.

Segmental demyelination affects the myelin sheath with relative sparing of the axon. The process results in slowed nerve conduction velocities and later may lead to muscle denervation and atrophy, in part as a result of disuse. Recovery is rapid once remyelination begins and is usually complete in mild to moderate neuropathies. Axonal degeneration results from a metabolic imbalance of the entire neuron. Degeneration of the distal portion of the nerve fiber is evident; degeneration of the myelin sheath may occur secondarily. Unlike segmental demyelination, nerve conduction rates are usually normal, and distal muscles show stages of denervation. Recovery is slow and incomplete. The development of clinical features of peripheral neuropathy is insidious, occurring after several months of exposure with increased absorption and accumulation of lead. Numbness and tingling of the fingers and toes are the initial symptoms, followed by motor weakness. Detection at an early stage of neuropathy allows for a significant degree of recovery from lead neuropathy, if exposure is ended and excess lead is removed from the body tissues by chelation. Weakness, sensory changes, and paresthesia persist if the combined myelin–axonal degeneration has already occurred.

Although the symptoms and signs of peripheral nerve disease are consistent with either axonal or demyelinating processes, or a combination of the two, the cause of the neuropathy cannot be determined solely on clinical grounds. However, the selective toxicities of various chemicals for axonal or Schwann cell targets may point to a particular neurotoxicant exposure. For example, arsenical neuropathy initially presents as loss of sensation in the feet and hands. Dysesthesias are common. Position and vibration sensation are usually impaired, and there is reduced perception to painful stimuli. Motor impairment is gradual in its onset, involving the small muscles of the feet and hands. The site of toxicity is intracellular, causing axonal change, and fragmentation of myelin occurs after axonal degeneration takes place. Sensory fibers are affected before motor fibers, and distal fibers are attacked before proximal portions. Once axonal damage and secondary myelin degeneration have occurred, there is little chance of regeneration and clinical recovery.

REFERENCES

Feldman RG, Travers PH. Environmental and occupational neurology. In: Feldman RG (ed). *Neurology: a physician's guide.* New York: Thieme Stratton, 1984:191–213.

Feldman RG. Effects of toxins and physical agents on the nervous system. In: Bradley WG, et al., eds. *Neurology in clinical practice,* vol 2. Stoneham, MA: Buttersworth-Heinemann, 1991:1185–1209.

CHAPTER 3

Approach to Diagnosis

To make a diagnosis of neurotoxic disease, a critical and consistent strategy is needed to assess a patient's daily functioning, to document physical findings on clinical examinations, and to account for all possible confounding variables within occupational and environment circumstances. This process of evaluation begins with a careful occupational, environmental, and medical history and is followed by careful physical and neurological examinations. The use of selected diagnostic tests (neurophysiological, neuropsychological, neuroimaging, and biochemical) for confirmation and substantiation of clinical findings is also important (Feldman and Travers, 1984; Feldman et al., 1994). The same techniques used in the everyday practice of medicine are employed in diagnosing neurotoxic illnesses.

OCCUPATIONAL, ENVIRONMENTAL, AND MEDICAL QUESTIONNAIRE

A well-designed questionnaire provides a standard outline for the interview and for subjects to use in reporting symptoms, exposures, and perception of the problem (see Appendix, page 466). It serves as a useful chronicle of the emergence of medical complaints in relation to the suspected exposure. Questions are asked about all chemical substances that could be present in the patient's environment, especially those known to cause certain symptoms. Because many people are unaware of common exposures or are not familiar with the names of the chemicals with which they work, it is helpful to list the names of specific chemicals (trade names or jargon references are often more familiar) on the questionnaire. To assess all possible sources of potential risk of exposure to an individual(s), inquiries must be made about conditions in the workplace, the home, and the general environment. It is important to review past exposure histories and information about current production activity at work that might affect exposure levels of suspected neurotoxicants. The patient should be asked about use of personal protection equipment (e.g., masks, gloves, special work clothes) and current and past jobs. Subjects should also be asked about hobby and home repair materials and products.

The patient's self-reporting questionnaire should be followed up with a face-to-face probing interview and record review, first of all to establish that the patient actually supplied the information and that it was not provided by someone else such as the employer, a relative, or an attorney. In addition, a personal interview can bring out additional contributing events or conditions. Direct questions are often necessary to detect concurrent personal use of the many legal medications and illegal chemicals that can cause neurotoxic effects. In addition to prescribed medications, some natural components in foods or food additives have been associated with specific neurotoxic syndromes. Psychoactive effects can result from the use of alcohol, cocaine, toluene (in glue sniffers), and amphetamines, among others (Sterman and Schaumburg, 1980; Juntunen, 1982; Goetz, 1985; Abou-Donia, 1992).

The questionnaire and interview should be used to collect information about current and past medical complaints; to review past and present places of residence(s); to summarize family medical and social history; and to record data on educational and occupational backgrounds. Information should be listed chronologically and considered in relation to all possible past and recent exposures to the suspected source or to other possible sources of neurointoxicants, occupational and nonoccupational, such as passive intake of polluted water through domestic water usage (showering and bathing, swimming, and consumption of water through cooking and drinking).

Since questionnaires involve self-reporting and therefore may be biased, it is best to have external referents for checking the validity of the subject's responses. For verification of occupational exposure at previous job sites, it may be necessary to review past employers' records about the employee, including work histories and production records, as well as safety compliance documents. In-house environmental monitoring programs for specific chemical exposures may be in place to detect actual or possible exposures in the workplace. Material Safety Data Sheets, operating manuals, industrial processes records, and any information provided from various sources to the employer and through the employer to the employees concerning possible chemical hazards and relevant safety precautions should be reviewed.

A *time-exposure-symptoms (T-E-S) line* (see Chapter 16, Fig. 16-10) can be constructed from the responses to the interview and questionnaire. This chronology should begin with prenatal information, if available (to include congenital issues), and then proceed through birth and the developmental, childhood, and young adult years to identify possible injuries and illnesses, as well as abuses of drugs or prior exposures to chemicals up to the present. Exposure data (including environmental sample measurements and tissue sample concentration levels of all chemicals relevant to suspected exposure periods) should also be placed along the T-E-S line. In the absence of any other reasonable explanation, a presumptive diagnosis of neurotoxic disease can be made by the coincidence of the exposure episodes and the appearance of illnesses along the T-E-S line. A firm clinical diagnosis with a causal conclusion is made as in any other patient–doctor encounter. Substantiation of the relationship of clinical manifestations to exposure to particular chemicals can be made by reference to previously reported cases found in the scientific literature and various databases. If no such previous reports exist, then exposure data verification and the recorded events along the T-E-S line are the rationale for reaching a clinical conclusion and causative diagnosis (see Chapter 16, Fig. 16-10).

NEUROLOGICAL EXAMINATION

An algorithm (see Chapter 2, Fig. 2-1) for systematically sorting out neurological symptoms and signs leading to a diagnosis of neurotoxic or nonneurotoxic disease begins with the physician suspecting neurotoxicant involvement. Clinical examination assesses the extent of impairment or disability and obtains findings with which to infer an anatomical site of dysfunction for the complaints. Blood pressure, pulse rate, and respiratory rate are taken, chest sounds are listened to, and the skin and mucous membranes of conjunctiva and/or oral pharynx are examined. Appropriate laboratory analyses including blood, urine, x-ray, brain imaging, and electrophysiological [electrocardiogram (EKG) and electroencephalogram (EEG)] tests are performed if needed to exclude possible nonneurotoxic explanations. Such explanations may include thyroid disease, diabetes, anemia, liver or kidney disease, collagen vascular disorders, cardiac or cerebrovascular disease, or any condition that may produce similar symptoms. Preexisting diseases such as diabetes, renal, or hepatic disorders and chronic pulmonary insufficiency may contribute to the clinical effects of exposure (Feldman and Pransky, 1988; Baker et al., 1990).

Specific symptoms and signs such as motor weakness, sensory loss, or altered mental status arise from disturbances in the functions of specialized cells of the brain, spinal cord, and peripheral nerves. Deviations from ex-

pected performance levels found on examination of an individual are considered *abnormalities*. Similar neurological signs and symptoms are expressions of common damaged neural structures, regardless of the specific etiology of the given malady. Thus neurological symptoms due to neurotoxic exposures may resemble those found in primary neurological illness.

Mental Status

To ensure good communication, the neurological examination should begin with an assessment of the patient's ability to comprehend, to follow directions, to solve problems, to perform coordinated motor functions, and to perceive and identify sensations of various modalities. The patient's mental status is evaluated by screening tests of speech and language and by tests of attention, memory, and cognitive performance. Formal neuropsychological tests are usually required and are performed as part of the series of diagnostic tests (see Neuropsychological Diagnosis section below).

Motor Control, Strength, and Posture

Motor function examination provides information on the functioning of the cerebral cortex and its connections through the subcortical, brainstem, cerebellar, and spinal cord pathways to the effector muscles, which produce intended actions. Abnormality in the motor cortex will result in weakness of the contralateral limbs, whereas basal ganglia dysfunction may alter muscle tone and speed of response, causing bradykinesia. Midbrain and brainstem structures control coordination of cranial nerve functions such as conjugate eye movement, articulation of speech, and swallowing. Impaired cerebellar functioning may result in ataxia and unsteadiness of gait appearing as unsteadiness of the trunk or simply as tremor of the outstretched extremities and head. Tremors may occur as a result of cerebellar and vestibular dysfunction, appearing during action, or as a result of basal ganglia dysfunction, appearing during rest and disappearing during action. Loss of muscle tone and total paralysis suggest disease in the lower motor neurons. In such instances, muscle atrophy occurs as well. Spinal cord function is best measured through combined sensory and motor examinations. The loss of sensation to pain and temperature suggest anterior spinal cord dysfunction, whereas position and light touch represent anatomical structures in the posterior columns or dorsal portion of the spinal cord. Weakness in the arm and leg indicate disturbance in the spinal pathways on the same side if a lesion exists below the foramen magnum. Observations of gait, posture, muscle tone, fine motor control, and coordination are recorded. Motor and sensory functions of peripheral and cranial nerves are tested. Spinal cord reflexes and various special reflexes of upper motor neuron and basal ganglia systems are evaluated.

Sensations and Reflex Pathways

Loss of pain and temperature occurs on the side of the body opposite to the affected spinal cord and central spinothalamic pathways that convey these sensations. The peripheral nerve is a bundle of fibers consisting of motor axons arising in the anterior horn cells of the lower motor neurons in the spinal cord ventral horn and transcending long distances from the spinal cord to the individual muscles these fibers innervate. The motor fibers connect with the muscle cells at the neuromuscular junction. The nerve trunk carries sensory fibers back into the spinal cord. These afferent fibers bring information from the sensory receptors in the skin, muscles, and joints to the spinal cord. There, after passing over synapses in the dorsal root ganglion, pain and temperature sensation is conducted by long fibers ascending in the ventral spinal thalamic tracts. Light touch, position, and vibration sensations are carried in the dorsal columns of the spinal cord. A complete lesion in a peripheral nerve denervates the muscle in a similar fashion as would occur with lower motor neuron disease, but the latter would also be accompanied by sensory loss in the distribution of the affected peripheral nerve.

Reflex testing is used to determine the intactness and functional continuity of afferent and efferent nerve pathways. Reflex activity involves the central nervous system (CNS) as well as the peripheral nervous system. CNS reflexes are manifested by behavioral responses such as a startled head-turning response to a sound in the ear or stimulation of vestibular reflexes by changes in body posture in relation to gravity or induction of nystagmus by installation of cold water in the external ear. A light placed on the eye results in a constriction of the pupil after the light stimulus has traversed the cornea and lens to the retina; the impulse then travels by way of the optic nerve, optic chiasm, and lateral geniculate ganglion and connects with the parasympathetic nuclei. From there the efferent pathways from the midbrain travel via the fibers of the pupillary constrictor muscles and cause contractions in response to the light stimulation, completing this reflex loop.

Tendon reflexes are elicited by tapping, thus stretching the tendons at the biceps, triceps, gastrocnemius, and quadriceps muscles. Both symmetry and intensity of reflexes are important in determining neurological impairment and spinal root levels affected. Asymmetrical reflexes must be explained. Bilateral reduction in reflexes in the lower extremities compared with the upper extremities suggests the possibility of peripheral nerve disease. Increased reflexes in the extremities suggests a release of upper motor neuron control and therefore the possibility of a CNS lesion. The concomitant signs of abnormal postures of response, such as the upgoing toe when the bottom of the foot is stroked, similarly indicate a release of upper motor neuron control. Such a response, known as the Babinski sign, may be unilateral when there is a contralateral cerebral lesion, or ipsilateral with a corticospinal pathway lesion.

Significance of Findings

The neurological examination following exposure to neurotoxic substances may be consistent with the expected findings for a specific location of damage in the central, peripheral, or autonomic nervous systems. Encephalopathy due to neurotoxicants does not exhibit focal signs. However, asymmetrical lesions and brain edema similar to that seen in head injury or cerebrovascular accidents are sometimes seen in lead, tin, and mercury intoxication. In addition, the symptoms of dementia associated with multi-infarct disease, vitamin B_{12} deficiency, and Alzheimer's disease must be considered in the differential diagnosis of toxic encephalopathies (White, 1987). Although movement disorders observed on neurological examination such as bradykinesia, chorea, or resting tremor may appear to be similar to those seen in traumatic brain injury, hypoxia, Parkinson's disease, or Huntington's disease, similar movement disorders can result from intoxication (e.g., due to carbon monoxide, carbon disulfide, or manganese exposures).

Exposure to toxic agents can result in impaired peripheral nervous system functions. Peripheral neuropathy generally presents with gradual onset of symptoms such as intermittent tingling and numbness (paresthesias) and may progress to the inability to perceive sensation and/or to spontaneous development of increased sensations, often of an unpleasant nature (dysasthesias). Muscle weakness and eventual muscle atrophy result from damage to the motor neurons and nerve fibers.

Based on the structural components of the nerve primarily involved, toxic polyneuropathies may be subdivided into axonopathies, myelinopathies, and neuronopathies. The most common pattern seen in metabolic or toxic neuropathies is distal axonopathy with segmental demyelination occurring as a secondary effect. Objectively, insensitivity to pinpoint and touch suggests peripheral neuropathy. Two-point discrimination, position, vibration, and temperature sensation may also be impaired. Depending on the severity of the neuropathy, electrophysiological measurements may be necessary to confirm the diagnosis and characterize the type of pathology present.

Physical findings may not be present in some patients who have been exposed to inhalant neurotoxicants and/or their vehicle solvents. In such patients, acute symptoms subside but never quite go away completely; recurrent complaints appear later involving the autonomic nervous system (e.g., vasomotor instability, sleep disturbances, gastrointestinal complaints, dizziness, vague symptoms of weakness and fatigue, irritability, and headache). These symptoms and often disabling behavioral changes recur for months to years after the cessation of the original exposure. Severe emotional responses such as phobias and anxiety attacks occur along with some of these symptoms when the subject comes in low-level contact with the same or similar chemical odors that were associated with the original illness. The visceral response may occur even before the subject is aware of the presence of a noxious substance. Usually no clinically abnormal neurological signs are found on physical examination, and these patients are often thought to be neurotic or at least suffering the effects of a posttraumatic stress disorder (PTSD) originally triggered by the first exposure. Neuropsychological tests may reveal some abnormal responses in addition to the disturbances in mood. Because symptoms seem to recur when the patient is challenged by a variety of chemicals, these patients have been described as suffering from sensitivity to multiple chemicals, or *multiple chemical sensitivity syndrome* (Schottenfeld and Cullen, 1985; Cullen et al., 1987; Weiss, 1998). Another controversial syndrome (consisting of a variety of nonspecific neurological, musculoskeletal, and autonomic nervous system complaints) for which chemical exposure has been suggested as a causal condition are the symptoms reported in Persian Gulf War veterans. Despite serious epidemiological and methodological flaws in early studies (Landrigan, 1997), a neurotoxic basis has been postulated (Haley et al., 1997; Haley and Kurt, 1997). Reported or perceived exposure to chemical warfare could represent a unique set of factors that could be responsible for an environmental illness. These include effects of hazardous exposures, ingestion of anti-nerve gas prophylactic medications (i.e., pyridostigmine), and possible connections between health status and subsequent psychological stress. In the latter case the development of PTSD, along with deteriorating health in returning Persian Gulf War veterans could be operational in influencing descriptions and recollections of experiences; however, this does not exclude the possibility of actual hazardous exposures (Wolfe et al., 1998). In such large survey studies with so many uncertain variables, it is difficult to reach conclusions. The exact mechanisms for these maladies have not yet been established.

NEUROPHYSIOLOGICAL DIAGNOSIS

Clinical neurophysiological tests document the functions of the brain, the cranial nerves, and the peripheral nerves by recording the bioelectrical responses of these tissues using highly sophisticated and sensitive electronic equipment. Conventional techniques are employed using standard clinical measures; interpretation is based on laboratory and/or population study control values. Proper application of electrodes, control for artifacts, and use of the amplifiers and recording equipment are essential in obtaining reliable and meaningful data in exposure subjects and all clinical patients. The neurophysiological data gathered from patients under various recording circumstances can serve as biological markers of effect (see Biochemical Diagnosis and Use of Biologic Markers sections).

A recognizable deficit in perception may be difficult to detect in a given person; when such individual deficits are analyzed in tested groups, an apparently abnormal threshold measure may be statistically insignificant and considered normal, or, conversely, significant group differences may appear. Values for electrophysiological parameters that

fall within 1 to 2 standard deviations (SD) from the laboratory or control group mean are accepted as "normal." Values above 2 SD from the mean are considered "abnormal" in clinical settings; a more limited range of acceptable values is used from time to time for tests with greater degrees of variability in response, such as the direct response (R1) of the electrically induced blink reflex test (Kimura, 1989; Feldman et al., 1988; 1994). Dysfunction may exist among many, but not all, of the nerve fibers in a peripheral nerve, without slowing the overall conduction velocity enough to place the calculated value outside 2 SDs. In such instances, the frequency distribution of each electrophysiological parameter studied can be evaluated to determine the actual SD from the mean instead of expressing these data in their measured units. Computerized transformation of variable nonlinear data provides a way to assess relative degrees of impairment, rather than the actual speed (conduction velocity) in meters per second. For instance, results that fall between 2.5 to 2.9 mean related value (MRV; clinically equivalent to "mild") can be referred to as grade I; those between 3 and 3.4 MRV as grade II; and those between 3.5 and 3.9 MRV (clinically equivalent to "severe") as grade III, with an absent response considered to be grade IV (Jabre and Sato, 1990). The test results then indicate changes from baseline and yet are still within the "normal" range of 2 SD for each test parameter; changes in the MRV over time, however, would reveal relative impairments, incomplete damage, progression of dysfunction, or evidence of recovery following an injury to the nerve fibers. Subclinical neurotoxic effects can be detected, and peripheral neurotoxic effects can be monitored serially using the MRV method (Feldman et al., 1994).

Subclinical toxic neuropathy may be detected by the results of electrical testing of a group of exposed persons, although no one patient among them exhibits overt clinical neurotoxic effects. In this situation, analysis of the results obtained from the group requires different statistical approaches, such as those for central tendencies (means, modes, and medians). The statistical power of field studies of individuals suspected to have toxic neuropathy may uncover a significant degree of neurotoxic effect below values usually accepted as clinically normal in individuals seen in office practice (Arezzo and Schaumburg, 1989). Subgrouping and unit analysis have been used to define relationships between exposure and neurophysiological impairments as measured by electrophysiological techniques (Seppalainen and Anti-Poika, 1983; Feldman et al., 1979).

Electroencephalography

Bioelectric potentials arising from neurons of the cerebral cortex and modulated by thalamic nuclei and the reticular activating system are transmitted by complex synaptic networks throughout the cerebral hemispheres. These generated magnetic fields can be recorded from scalp electrodes on the surface of the skull. Sensitive electronic equipment amplifies and displays patterns of mixed frequencies, amplitudes, and their topographical distributions over the cranium. The resulting EEG provides real-time monitoring of electrophysiological activity of the brain during the duration of the sampling. A routine EEG usually takes 20 to 40 minutes with the patient lying in a resting position on a bed or lounge chair. Continuous recording with ambulatory equipment during the performance of tasks as well as during controlled behavioral studies can also be performed and provides an opportunity to observe acute EEG changes under given circumstances. The EEG has predictable patterns under normal waking, drowsing, and sleeping states. Mixtures of fast (beta and alpha) and slow (theta and delta) frequencies appear in the frontal, temporal, and occipital areas. When the symmetry, amplitude, frequencies, and patterns of the EEG are different from the normal configurations, impairment in brain function, referred to as encephalopathy, is diagnosed. A paroxysmal quality in the wave forms, associated with sharp, spiked discharges, indicates epileptic activity; diffuse slowing of the background (alpha) rhythm with disappearance of normal resting frequencies suggests metabolic or toxic encephalopathy; a marked asymmetry of amplitude and/or frequencies suggests a lateralized pathology; a concentration of sharp, slow, and/or paroxysmal waves in a particular area may indicate an underlying focal structural lesion, such as a tumor, cerebrovascular infarct, stroke, or old trauma. Early in the course of progressive dementia in Alzheimer's disease, the EEG is normal. As in other neurodegenerative diseases, greater amounts of slowing and disorganization appear as progression of the disease occurs.

Increased amounts of slow wave activity occur during exposure to neurotoxicants that have CNS effects. Performance on neuropsychological testing can be observed during EEG monitoring. The EEG tracing returns to a normal pattern after the patient's removal from exposure to CNS neurotoxicants, although behavioral manifestations may persist clinically, or be detectable on further formal neuropsychological testing. Abnormalities in the EEG are indicators of the physiological state of the brain only at the time of recording, and the patterns are not specific to any particular causal substance. As with all laboratory tests, the significance of the EEG report depends on correlation with other clinical information and examinations. In the differential diagnosis of neurotoxic syndromes and nonneurotoxic, neurological disease, the EEG is most helpful when an abnormality is seen during or in proximity in time to exposure, since the EEG becomes normal in reversible encephalopathy when the patient is away from the suspected neurotoxic environment. The persistence of an EEG disturbance long after exposure ceases suggests that the cause is not neurotoxic, unless severe encephalopathy had existed.

Evoked Potential Testing

Electrical cortical potentials (i.e., responses) are produced by the stimulation of specific afferent pathways and are recorded from the surface of the brain through the skull and the scalp utilizing electrodes and highly sensitive amplifying electronic equipment. *Sensory evoked potentials* (SEPs), recorded after stimulation of peripheral sensory nerve fibers in the extremities and/or direct recording over the dorsal columns of the spinal cord, are commonly used to assess the integrity and function of sensory pathways. The SEPs consist of the visually evoked potentials, the brainstem auditory evoked potentials, and the somatosensory evoked potentials.

Visual evoked potentials (VEPs) examine the pathway and integrity of the optic system, from the optic nerve and the chiasm, over the optic tract in projection to the geniculate nuclei, and to the calcarine cortex, all of which are involved in transmitting the VEP after a stimulus has been applied at the retina. Because the optic pathways decussate at the chiasm, the bioelectric response posterior to the chiasm contains transmitted impulses from both eyes when one eye is not covered during stimulation. Therefore, care must be taken in eliciting a VEP. Two types of VEPs are clinically elicited: (a) flash VEPs (FVEPs), a crude test that recognizes the presence of light perception and is useful in testing uncooperative subjects and children to see if the light signal is getting into the brain; and (b) pattern shift visual evoked potentials (PSVEPs), elicited by presenting a checkerboard pattern that flickers on and off at a rate of 2 Hz. Each eye is tested separately. In both forms, the latency between stimulus and response is approximately 100 ms, recordable over the occipital region and termed the P100 peak. Both forms have been used to study the effects of exposure to neurotoxins (Rebert, 1983; Otto and Hudnell, 1993) in man and animals.

Brainstem auditory evoked potentials (BAEPs) are recordable following presentation of a clicking sound used as a stimulus in one ear, while the other ear is masked with white noise. Recording electrodes are placed over the earlobes and the vertex of the head. Activation of the auditory (eighth cranial) nerve occurs over about 10 ms, generating a complex wave form visible by oscilloscope, which relates to specific sites along the auditory pathway (Chiappa, 1992). Wave I activates the acoustic nerve; waves II and III reflect the activation of structures in the pontomedullary region; the sources of waves IV and V are less clearly defined but appear to be related to functions of the upper pons and low midbrain. The absolute latencies of each wave are recorded, but interpeak latencies of waves I to III, III to V, and I to V are more consistent and reproducible and therefore are utilized in clinical testing. BAEPs have been useful in studies of neurodegenerative diseases of the brainstem and of demyelinating processes such as multiple sclerosis. They are also helpful in detecting insults caused by ototoxic substances (Otto and Fox, 1993).

Somatosensory evoked potentials (SSEPs) are recorded from scalp electrodes placed over the sensory cortex after activation of the peripheral sensory or mixed nerve. The stimulus is conveyed centrally in peripheral nerve fibers to dorsal columns in the spinal cord, producing a propagated potential that is then projected to the contralateral cortex. The absolute latencies can be influenced by limb length and the presence of peripheral neuropathy, and therefore technique is important in obtaining reliable measures. SSEPs are usually tested in both upper and lower extremities; interpeak latencies are more consistent and can help to localize pathology along the path of the peripheral nerve through the spinal cord, brainstem, and thalamus to the cortex. Since many neurotoxicants affect peripheral nerves, it is commonly the distalmost sites of sensory conduction that are slowed and affect the cortically evoked SSEPs in patients exposed to neurotoxicants. Therefore, it is uncertain whether SSEPs offer any advantage over standard nerve conduction velocities, except for studies of conduction through the spinal cord posterior columns and when proximal nerve blocks or asymmetrical problems are being considered in the differential diagnosis (Arrezzo et al., 1985).

Nerve Conduction Studies

The conduction characteristics of a nerve fiber are determined by the nerve cell body and axon, its axoplasm, and its myelin sheath. Transcutaneous electrical stimulation of a particular nerve results in contraction of the muscle to which the nerve conducts impulses. The twitch of the muscle recordable by electrodes is either attached to the skin over the muscle or inserted (sterile needle electrode), into the muscle belly. Muscle action responses (potentials) are transmitted from the electrodes to an amplifier system and displayed on an oscilloscope screen, or printed out on a permanent recording device. Generally accepted and conventional clinical electrophysiological procedures should be used to measure and report electromyographic and nerve conduction data (Liveson and Ma, 1992). Differences in techniques and instrumentation, as well as variables among study population often account for inconsistencies in the nerve conduction and other neurophysiological parameter data collected and its interpretation.

Appropriately applied tests of nerve conduction and muscle activity can help to localize sites of impaired function, whether in the individual nerve, nerve root, plexus, or motor neurons. In addition, degrees of impairment correspond to the proportion of abnormally conducting myelinated nerve fibers, whether the amplitude or speed is more affected and whether sensory or motor fibers are more involved; subsequently, on serial studies, patterns of recovery or persistence of abnormality tell about prognosis after neurotoxic peripheral nerve damage. These tests can also provide information about the pathophysiological bases for neurological findings, such as axonal, demyelinating, myopathy, or neurogenic atrophy.

A peripheral nerve is composed of axons of many neuron groups in bundles consisting of thousands of individual nerve fibers of various sizes. The thicker the myelin sheath, the larger the fiber diameter. The amount of myelin surrounding each nerve axon determines the speed of conduction of that axon: the less myelin, the slower the conduction time; the more myelin, the faster the conduction time. The fastest firing nerve fibers deliver impulses earlier than do the slower fibers, which conduct the later arriving impulses. A recordable complex nerve action potential involves all the conducted nerve action potentials of the various fiber sizes in that nerve (Yokoyama et al., 1990). The proportion of larger fibers, and therefore faster firing fibers, determine the faster speeds of an evoked and conducted compound nerve impulse, traveling between the point of stimulation and the recording site of the response.

The delay in milliseconds between the applied stimulus and an observed motor or sensory response is called the *latency*. If the number of larger fibers is reduced because of demyelination, as occurs in lead neuropathy, the latency between the stimulus and the recorded response will be prolonged. A prolonged latency reflects the later appearing responses of the remaining smaller and more slowly conducting fibers' ability to conduct the impulses. If some axons are damaged, nerve impulses will be conducted only by the axons that remain undamaged, with the resultant bioelectric potential recording showing an overall reduction in the *amplitude* (expressed in microvolts) of an evoked nerve action potential, or evidence of absence of any evoked nerve action potential. *Conduction velocity* expressed in meters/second, is the travel speed of an evoked nerve action potential between a proximal (S1) and a distal (S2) site of stimulation and a common reference site (R), at which recording electrodes are placed to detect bioelectric potentials or muscle contraction responses. The conduction velocity value is calculated by subtracting the latency measured from S2 to R from the latency determined between S1 to R, and then dividing this difference (in milliseconds) into the distance (in millimeters) measured between the two sites (S1 to S2) of stimulation. The quotient is the conduction velocity expressed in meters/second.

Three additional physiological parameters offer information about the central connections of peripheral nerve fibers: the *F-wave*, the *H-reflex*, and the *blink reflex*. The *F-wave* is a long-latency muscle action potential obtained following supramaximal stimulation of motor axons. It is generally accepted that the F-wave is elicited by antidromic stimulation of the anterior horn cell at the axonal hillock. The F-wave is therefore always preceded by an M-wave. F-waves are routinely performed in the same procedure as the motor nerve conduction study, using a slower sweep speed and a higher gain and stimulating the distal stimulation site. Ten impulses are delivered. The shortest latency potential is identified and selected as the F-wave for latency measurement. A prolonged or absent F-wave is considered abnormal.

The *H-reflex* is the electrical equivalent of a monosynaptic stretch reflex. It is obtained by selectively stimulating the Ia fibers, which recruit the anterior horn cell or cells and generate a late response in the muscle, usually obtained before the direct motor response or M-wave. The H-reflex can be obtained by stimulating the posterior tibial nerve at the popliteal fossa. The response is recorded from the muscle, between the two heads of the gastrocnemius muscles. Minimal and maximal amplitude responses are obtained and the latency is measured from stimulus artifact to take-off of the potential deflections. H-reflexes can also be obtained in the forearm muscles, most notably, the flexor carpi radialis muscle.

The electrically or percussion-induced *blink reflex* tests the circuitry carried by the afferent fibers of the fifth cranial nerve and its synapse, directly with the ipsilateral efferent seventh cranial nerve fibers and indirectly with both contralateral and ipsilateral seventh cranial nerve nuclei after a central (late) response. The blink reflex is elicited by stimulation of the supraorbital branch of the fifth nerve as it enters through the supraorbital foramen. On the ipsilateral side, both direct and indirect responses are seen. The direct response (R1) has a latency of about 10.5 ms and is mono- or biphasic in configuration. The indirect response (R2 ipsilateral) has a variable latency of about 30.5 ms and is polyphasic. On the contralateral side, only an indirect, long-latency (R2 contralateral) polyphasic response is seen with a latency of about 30.5 ms.

Vibrotactile sensory threshold testing evaluates a patient's ability to perceive a vibrating stimulus. It can be performed clinically by using a tuning fork (128 Hz) placed over a toe or finger pad, the joints of the foot, or ankle, tibia, finger, or wrist. This clinical examination depends on the subjective ability of the patient to indicate to the examiner that he or she has felt the vibration and/or can detect when it diminishes and disappears. Quantitative standardized methods, sometimes referred to as quantitative sensory testing, use electronic equipment to assess the function of the large fibers of a peripheral nerve that carry the sensation of position and vibration (Arezzo et al., 1983; Gerr and Letz, 1988; Berger et al., 1992), by delivering various amplitudes of vibration through two probe posts applied to the skin over a finger pad or an extremity joint, while the frequency of vibration remains constant at 100 Hz. By forced choice method the subject is required to report when he or she perceives or does not perceive one or both poles vibrating. After a series of repeated ascending and descending tests of threshold (method of limits), an average is calculated from the values of the thresholds detected for the final four trials of each test series. Testing in an exposed individual soon after an exposure followed by subsequent serial testing after removal from exposure provides evidence of possible impairment and then recovery of vibrotactile sensation perception.

Other means of testing peripheral nerve conduction include measuring the *distribution of conduction velocities* (Yokoyama et al., 1990), which quantifies the conduction properties of the fiber population of a nerve utilizing mathematical modeling of the electric signal derived from a single nerve fiber. In addition, a *near nerve recording* technique (Buchtal and Rosenfalck, 1966) was developed as a sensitive way for detecting abnormalities of slower conducting fibers.

Electromyography (EMG) can be used to assess motor unit function, that is, the integrity of the motor neuron, its axon, and the muscle cell it supplies. The time at which an EMG examination is performed in relationship to a toxic exposure is very important in the interpretation of the results of this test. Denervation of motor units is necessary before the muscle cells begin to develop abnormal spontaneously discharging potentials; an EMG will detect a reduced number of motor units as evidence of denervation of the motor units. As toxic neuropathy develops and neuromuscular clinical signs emerge, greater EMG changes are recordable. A pattern of muscle action potentials recorded from a muscle in conjunction with a full volitional contraction will reveal the relative dropout of units when there has been denervation and therefore loss of connection between the motor neuron, its axon, and the muscle fiber it supplies. Denervated muscle fibers exhibit spontaneous bioelectric discharges, called *fibrillations,* which can be recorded from a needle electrode inserted into the muscle when it is at rest. *Polyphasic potentials* are recorded from a previously denervated muscle that has become reinnervated; fibrillations may or may not be present depending on whether or not active denervation is occurring and how much regeneration has taken place.

Fibrillations and Positive Waves

When a muscle fiber is denervated, the acetylcholine receptors spread all across the muscle fiber to attract new innervation to the denervated muscle fiber from adjacent nerves. The muscle fiber thus becomes more sensitive to the free acetylcholine and is depolarized and repolarized spontaneously as these neurotransmitter molecules reach it. Each single depolarization is electrically detected as a single muscle fiber action potential recorded as a fibrillation or a positive wave. These discharge in a highly rhythmic manner and usually start and stop abruptly. As the muscle is reinnervated, both fibrillations and positive waves decrease in numbers and eventually disappear when the reinnervation is successfully completed.

Motor Unit Action Potentials

Following denervation, reinnervation is usually accomplished by collateral sprouting with the denervated muscle cells (fiber) seeking new nerve sprouts from adjacent nerves. This reinnervation alters the motor unit in two ways: on the one hand, the motor unit now contains more muscle fibers; on the other hand, the newly acquired muscle fibers are asynchronous with those of the host unit and indeed among themselves. The newly formed end plates may not be stable in the beginning, and many of them never reach maturity. Their respective muscle fibers either die or attract innervation from another source. This process of acquiring new muscle fibers and forming new end plates begins in the first 2 months after nerve injury and results in a prolongation of the motor unit potential duration and an increase in the number of phases of the discharge potential. The duration is prolonged simply because there are more fibers to depolarize; the increase in the number of phases is due to the lack of synchronization between the host fibers and the newly acquired fibers.

NEUROPSYCHOLOGICAL DIAGNOSIS

The neurobehavioral effects of exposure to neurotoxicants can be classified according to the clinical manifestations, the temporal profile of the symptoms, and the nature of recovery or residual deficits (Baker and White, 1985) (Table 3-1). For example, a brief exposure to volatile and aromatic substances, such as glues or varnish, in poor ven-

TABLE 3-1. *Classification of toxic encephalopathies*

I. Acute organic mental disorders
  A. Acute intoxication
    1. Duration: minutes to hours
    2. Residua: none
    3. Symptoms: CNS depression, psychomotor or attentional deficits
  B. Acute toxic encephalopathy
    1. Symptoms: confusion, coma, seizures
    2. Pathophysiology: cerebral edema, CNS capillary damage, hypoxia
    3. Residua: possible permanent cognitive deficit
II. Chronic organic mental disorders
  A. Organic affective syndrome
    1. Symptoms: mood disturbance (depression, irritability, fatigue, anxiety)
    2. Duration: days to weeks
    3. Residua: none
  B. Mild chronic toxic encephalopathies
    1. Symptoms: fatigue, mood disturbance, cognitive complaints
    2. Course: insidious onset; duration: weeks
    3. Cognitive deficits: may include attentional impairment, motor slowing or incoordination, visuospatial deficits, short-term memory loss
    4. Residua: improvement may occur in absence of exposure, but permanent mild cognitive deficits can be seen
  C. Severe chronic toxic encephalopathy
    1. Symptoms: cognitive and affective change sufficient to interfere with daily living
    2. Cognitive deficits: same as in mild chronic toxic encephalopathy but more severe
    3. Neurological deficits: abnormalities seen on some neurophysiological (EMG, EEG) or neuroimaging (CT, MRI) measures
    4. Course: insidious onset, irreversible
    5. Residua: permanent cognitive dysfunction

CNS, central nervous system; CT, computed tomography; EMG, electromyography; MRI, magnetic resonance imaging; EEG, electroencephalography.
Modified from White et al., 1991, with permission.

tilation circumstances, or ingestion of common ethyl alcohol (ethanol), produces (i) an *acute organic mental disorder;* in this group the symptoms of (a) *acute intoxication* are mild, transient, and reversible. When the acute intoxication is associated with permanent residual cognitive impairment, the condition is termed (b) *acute toxic encephalopathy;* this may be overwhelming and may result in coma or even death. However, subacute toxicity (duration of days to weeks) is sometimes incorrectly attributed to primary psychiatric illness, because the features are mostly disturbances of mood and affect. More prolonged behavioral symptoms of depression, irritability, fatigue, and anxiety are referred to as (ii) *chronic organic mental disorders,* which include (a) *organic affective syndrome,* (b) *mild chronic toxic encephalopathies,* and (c) *severe chronic toxic encephalopathies.* However, when the onset of mood disturbances and cognitive impairments is insidious, it is often very difficult to confirm the deficits without using formal neuropsychological tests. Consideration of other findings on neurological examination along with the results of formal neuropsychological testing allows the clinician to reconcile discrepancies and to corroborate the test results, especially in the patients with mild chronic toxic encephalopathies. In severe chronic toxic encephalopathy the cognitive and affective disturbances interfere with independent daily living and performing meaningful employment is impossible, usually permanently.

Formal Neuropsychological Testing

Toxic encephalopathy in adults is usually characterized by impairments in one or more of the following behavioral functional areas: attention, executive function, fluency (verbal or visual), motor abilities, visuospatial skills, learning and short-term memory, and mood and adjustment. Formal neuropsychological testing can define the character of a deficit; test results can then be related to other information gathered from clinical and social evaluations. A qualified neuropsychologist, experienced in testing patients with occupational and environmental neurotoxicant exposures, will recognize the importance of designing a test battery that will control for demographic and cultural variables, premorbid cognitive status, changes in mood state and perceptual experiences, energy levels, and personality and motivational influences. In referring a suspected neurotoxicant-exposed subject for tests, the following questions may be asked of the neuropsychologist: (a) do the deficits in testing results explain problems exhibited by the patient in daily life? (b) do the findings suggest the existence of other disorders (neurological, psychiatric, motivational, developmental, medical)? and (c) are the test results consistent with those described in the literature or previously observed in other cases of neurotoxicant exposures?

The test battery must be sensitive and specific enough to detect the effects of neurotoxicants to which the patient is suspected of having been exposed. In clinical situations, it is generally desirable to select neuropsychological tests that will assess as many functions as possible and provide a profile of the abilities and deficits of a particular person. Certain neurotoxicants affect neurons of the hippocampus, basal ganglia, cerebellum, frontal lobes, or occipital cortex; others affect white matter. Each anatomical site of adverse effect contributes to a clinical picture, and the performance patterns of results and deficits obtained are defined by neuropsychological testing. Neuropsychological test raw data are scored by a qualified diplomate neuropsychologist, using standardized and validated methods for each test instrument. From the analysis of these scores, impairments in specific behavioral domains are identified (White et al., 1992).

The purpose of using formal neuropsychological test batteries in the differential diagnosis of toxic encephalopathies is to characterize the patient's premorbid cognitive status and identify any coexisting psychiatric, medical, and neurological disorders; and to differentiate the specific effects of exposure to various neurotoxicants in the presence of multiple exposures, substance abuse, or prescription drug use. These tests can also obtain evidence of hypochondriasis, malingering, and the presence or absence of psychiatric disorders, especially somatoform disorders. In patients with suspected toxic exposure, underlying long-standing learning disability may become apparent on testing of cognitive and academic skills. Usually no previous test results are available to use as a basis of comparison, so serial testing (from after exposure to a sufficient length of time for recovery) is necessary in many instances. An underestimation of neurotoxicant-induced behavioral changes in patients with superior premorbid intelligence and an overestimation of such changes in patients with below average premorbid intelligence commonly occurs. The cultural background and language skills of patients for whom English is not their native language may require interpreters and appropriate translation. It is also important to recognize an exposed individual who may have had other neurological impairments such as a prior head injury, alcohol abuse, or other primary neurological disease. These are usually assessed by the clinical neurological examination and neuroimaging studies.

Batteries of neuropsychological tests designed to diagnose solvent-induced encephalopathy (Baker and White, 1985) are administered in the standardized manner for each person suspected of exposure (Table 3-2). The neurobehavioral effects of exposure to neurotoxicants in adults is usually characterized by impairments in one or more of the following functional areas: *intelligence, attention, executive function, fluency (verbal or visual), motor abilities, visuospatial skills, learning and short-term memory, and mood and adjustment* (White et al., 1992). Individual differences are most likely to occur between individuals in intensity of exposure, duration of exposure, and exposures to multiple neurotoxicants. Developmental variables (e.g., age at exposure, cognitive maturity at exposure) and individual subject variables (e.g., differences in fragile cognitive skills, preexisting cognitive deficits or neuropsychiatric disorder, educational history, socioeconomic status) are important contributors to the subject's clinical picture following exposure.

Intelligence

Patients with a moderate to severe chronic toxic encephalopathy (Table 3-1) may show a mild decline in Verbal IQ due to decrements in performance on reasoning tasks, diminished digit spans, and/or concreteness in vocabulary definitions, while Performance IQ may be more significantly affected due to impaired performance on any of the tasks (but especially Block Design, Digit Symbol, and Picture Arrangement). Effects on a highly verbally mediated test such as the Peabody Picture Vocabulary Test would be unusual unless the exposure produced a stroke or an anoxia.

Attention and Executive Function

Deficits in simple attention, cognitive tracking, and cognitive flexibility are commonly seen in patients with exposures to various neurotoxicants. In patients with a mild acute reversible encephalopathy or mild chronic residual encephalopathy, these findings may represent the primary or only manifestations of the encephalopathy.

Cognitive tracking is often a significant problem for toxicant-exposed patients. The Trails A or B test is frequently sensitive to the tracking problems observed in these patients, although Digit Span (backwards), Mental Control, Recurrent Series Writing (MN) and the Wechsler Adult Intelligence Scale–Revised (WAIS-R) Arithmetic subtest and the Paced Auditory Serial Addition Task are also sensitive. The Stroop test has been of variable utility in exposure subjects, in part because there is great variability in patients' abilities to carry out the task demands; some patients who experience problems with other executive tasks perform well on the Stroop. Cognitive flexibility is also often affected in toxic encephalopathy. Although some patients show effects on both tracking and flexibility, others show a dissociation between these two types of dysfunction, exhibiting one but not the other. It has been impossible to predict which type of deficit will be seen: it does not appear to be related to type of exposure or even severity. Difficulties in cognitive flexibility may be seen on the Wisconsin Card Sorting Test, Categories Test, Trails B, and WAIS-R subtests requiring abstract reasoning.

Simple attention in some cases can be impaired on Continuous Performance Test, although Digit Spans or Visual Spans are also helpful.

Motor Skills

Motor skills may be minimally affected, and deficits may not be detectable in some patients with identifiable

Table 3-2. *Functional domains in toxic encephalopathies: selected neuropsychological tests*

Domain	Description	Implications
Intelligence		
Wechsler IQ tests (WAIS-R, WCIS, WPPSI)	IQ measures	Overall level of cognitive function compared with population norms
Peabody Picture Vocabulary Test	Single word comprehension	Measure of verbal intelligence in adults; can be sensitive to exposure in children
Stanford-Binet	IQ measure	Similar to Wechsler tests
Wide Range Achievement Test	Academic skills in arithmetic, spelling, reading	Estimate of premorbid ability patterns in adults; can be sensitive to exposure in children
Attention, executive functioning		
Digit Span (WAIS-R)	Digits forward and backward	Measures simple attention and cognitive tracking
Arithmetic (Wechsler tests)	Oral calculations	Assesses attention, tracking, and calculation
Trail Making Test	Connect-a-dot task requiring sequencing and alternating sequences	Measures attention, sequencing, visual scanning, and speed of processing
Continuous Performance Test	Acknowledgment of occurrence of critical stimuli in a series of orally or visually presented stimuli	Assesses attention
Paced Auditory Serial Addition	Serial calculation test	Sensitive measure of attention and tracking speed
Wisconsin Card Sorting Test	Requires subject to infer decision-making rules	Tests ability to think flexibly
Verbal, language		
Information (Wechsler tests)	Information usually learned in school	Estimate of native abilities in adults
Vocabulary (Wechsler tests)	Verbal vocabulary definitions	Estimate of verbal intelligence; sensitive to concreteness associated with brain damage (including toxic encephalopathy)
Comprehension (Wechsler tests)	Proverb definitions, social judgment, problem solving	Sensitive to reasoning skills; can be impaired after exposure to neurotoxicants
Similarities (Wechsler tests)	Inference of similarities between nominative words	Sensitive to reasoning skills; can be impaired after exposure to neurotoxicants
Controlled Oral Word Association	Word list generation within alphabetical or semantic categories	Assesses flexibility, planning, arousal, processing speed, ability to generate strategies; somewhat sensitive to exposure
Boston Naming Test	Naming of objects depicted in line drawings	Sensitive to aphasia; also sensitive to native verbal processing deficits or those acquired through childhood exposure
Reading Comprehension (Boston Diagnostic Aphasia Exam)	Direct, screening test of simple reading comprehension	Sensitive to moderate to severe dyslexia, usually insensitive to exposure in adults
Writing Sample	Patient writes to dictation or describes a picture	Assesses graphomotor skills, spelling
Visuospatial, visuomotor		
Picture completion (Wechsler tests)	Identification of missing details in line drawings	Measures perceptual analysis
Santa Ana Formboard Test	Knobs in a formboard are turned 180 degrees with each hand individually and both hands together	Measures motor speed and coordination
Finger Tapping	Speed of tapping with each index finger	Sensitive to manual lateralized motor speed
Memory		
Logical Memories: Immediate and Delayed Recall (IR, DR) (Wechsler Memory Scales)	Recall of paragraph information read orally on an immediate and 20-min delayed recall	Sensitive to new learning and retention of newly learned information

Table 3-2. *Continued*

Domain	Description	Implications
Verbal Paired Associate Learning: DR (Wechsler Memory Scales)	Two paired words are presented in a list of pairs; subject must recall second word; test is presented on immediate and delayed recall	Measures abstract verbal list IR, learning, retention
Figural Memory (Wechsler Memory Scales)	Multiple choice recognition of using recognition (not recall) performance measures	Assesses visual recognition memory
Digit Symbol (Wechsler Tests)	Coding task requiring matching symbols to digits	Complex task assessing motor speed, visual scanning, working memory, incidental learning
Picture Arrangement (Wechsler Tests)	Sequencing of cartoon frames to represent meaningful stories	Measures visual sequencing, ability to infer relationships from visuospatial/social stimuli
Block Design (Wechsler Tests)	Assembly of 3-D blocks to replicate 2-D representation of designs	Assesses abstract visual construction ability and planning
Object Assembly (Wechsler Tests)	Assembly of puzzles	Measure of concrete visual construction skills, Gestalt recognition
Boston Visuospatial Quantitative Battery	Drawings of common objects spontaneously and to copy	Measures construction abilities, motor functioning
Hooper Visual Organization Test	Identification of correct outline of drawings of cut-up objects	Sensitive to Gestalt integration processing
Rey-Osterreith Complex Figure (copy condition)	Drawing of a complicated abstract visual design	Sensitive to deficits in visuospatial planning and construction
Visual Paired Associate Learning, IR, DR (Wechsler Memory Scales)	Six visual designs are paired with six colors; recognition memory is tested immediately after the six are presented on learning trials and delayed recall	Test of abstract visual learning using recognition (not recall) performance measures
Visual Reproductions, IR, DR (Wechsler Memory Scales)	Visual designs are drawn immediately after presentation and on delayed recall	Measures visual learning and retention
Delayed Recognition Span Test	Based on delayed nonmatching to sample paradigm, discs are moved about on a board to assess recognition memory for words, color, spatial locations	Assesses new learning
Peterson Task	Words or consonants are presented and must be recalled after a period of distraction	Measures sensitivity to interference in new learning
California Verbal Learning Test	Subject is presented with a list of 16 words (which can be semantically related) over multiple learning trials and with an interference list	Provides multiple measures of new learning, recall, recognition memory, use of strategies, and sensitivity to interference
Rey-Osterreith (IR, DR)	Complex design is drawn from IR immediately after it has been copied and at a 20-min delayed recall	Assesses memory for information that is difficult to encode verbally
Personality, mood		
Profile of Mood states	65 single-word descriptors of affective symptoms are endorsed by degree of severity on six scales	Sensitive to clinical mood disturbance and to affective changes secondary to toxicant exposure
Minnesota Multiphasic Personality Inventory (R)	True-false responses provided on personality inventory summarized on multiple clinical dimensions	Provides description of current personality function; some scales sensitive to exposure; screening for inconsistency and malingering

WAIS-R, Wechsler Adult Intelligence Scale–Revised; WISC, Wechsler Intelligence Scale for Children; WPPSI, Wechsler Preschool and Primary Scale of Intelligence.

toxic encephalopathy. Some patients show slowed performance only on relatively complex tasks such as Formboard tests or Digit Symbol but not on simpler tasks such as Finger Tapping, whereas others have such impaired motor function that it is obvious on all tasks with a manual motor component, including Trails and constructional tasks. This is especially true of patients who develop postural and tone abnormalities (e.g., parkinsonian) secondary to exposure to organic solvents, carbon disulfide, or carbaryl and of patients with cerebellar dysfunction secondary to exposure to mercury or toluene. The Finger Tapping test is sometimes genuinely impaired in toxin-exposed patients.

Language/Verbal Skills

Adult patients with toxic encephalopathy involving central myelin often show problems in verbal fluency or word retrieval. This may manifest in reduced scores on word list generation test, such as the FAS, verbal fluency task. Problems with retrieval on naming tasks require increased latencies to respond, but primary dysnomia or paraphasic errors attributable to toxic exposure are seen in cases in which exposure has led to a cerebral infarction. Hesitancies may be noted in free speech, and patients with exposure affecting the basal ganglia or cerebellum may be dysarthric and/or hypophonic. Motor aspects of writing may be affected, although linguistic aspects of writing and reading remain intact. Exposure to neurotoxicants may affect language capabilities in children, depending on the age of exposure, to at least age 10 or later. Verbally mediated reasoning tests such as WAIS-R Similarities and Comprehension are also frequently sensitive to neurotoxic effects. Although it is our impression that Similarities is a more reliable measure of such reasoning deficits and although some patients show deficits on both tasks, there is interindividual variability in sensitivity of the tasks, with some patients showing effects on only one of them.

Visuospatial Abilities

Visuospatial abilities deficits are seen following exposure to most types of neurotoxicant, including heavy metals, pesticides, organic solvents, and gases such as carbon monoxide, probably due to the vulnerability of subcortical and cerebellar structures to the effects of neurotoxicants. The WAIS-R visuospatial subtests, especially Block Designs and Object Assembly, are sensitive to toxic exposure, producing a mild to moderate encephalopathy. The Rey-Osterreith construction, Hooper Visual Organization Test, Degraded Stimuli, and Embedded Figures tasks are also useful at times. When evaluating individual patients, it becomes clear that primary problems in visuospatial analysis and organization occur in some of these patients as well as toxicant-induced changes in visual acuity, neurophthalmo-

logical function, manual motor dexterity, tactile sensitivity, cognitive flexibility, and psychomotor speed, which may all contribute to impaired scores observed on many traditional neuropsychological visuospatial tasks.

Memory

Memory (short-term) can be affected at several levels, including efficient encoding of new information, ability to inhibit interference during learning, retrieval of encoded information, and retention of encoded information. Many patients with toxic exposures show difficulty in learning new information due to problems in attending to tasks and perhaps to apathy or diminished motivation. Such patients show ineffective or retarded learning curves. Often there is exquisite sensitivity to interference, which can be well documented with the Peterson task paradigm (in which information is retrieved from memory following a distracter task). Because retrieval can be uneven, recognition memory paradigms should be used to assess ability to retain new information adequately. Even using recognition memory tasks, some patients with toxic exposures show significant forgetting of newly learned information over time, suggesting that the exposure has affected the limbic system. Other patients show uneven encoding and retrieval consistent with white matter or basal ganglia dysfunction. Because of the divergent patterns of memory impairment possible following toxic exposure, we use a rather extensive memory battery in assessing these patients. This may be particularly necessary if there is concurrent alcohol abuse and occupational or environmental exposure to neurotoxicants.

A neuropsychological diagnosis can be made only after important confounders have been considered. Test results are interpreted on the basis of previously defined normative scores, which take into consideration key variables such as age, gender, and education. Common patterns of premorbid function in adults include consistent levels of performance across all kinds of intellectual tasks, ranging from superior to subnormal, long-standing superiority of verbal over nonverbal abilities, long-standing superiority of nonverbal over verbal skills, and developmentally based problems with attention and executive function. Identification of specific types of behavioral impairments of the patient's test results may suggest to the neuropsychologist, through his or her knowledge of brain–behavior relationships, probable cerebral structures that are most likely affected; also, toxic encephalopathy may be differentiated in this fashion from other neuropsychiatric disorders (White et al., 1992). The ultimate neuropsychological diagnosis, therefore, will depend on the patient's exposure circumstances and neurological findings interpreted within the context of the examiner's previous clinical experience in evaluating similar cases and his or her knowledge of similar cases in the literature. Interpretations of these findings are used by the neurologist in formulating an overall clinical diagnosis.

BIOCHEMICAL DIAGNOSIS AND THE USE OF BIOLOGICAL MARKERS

To corroborate a diagnosis of neurotoxic illness, a chemical and/or its metabolite should be found in tissues of an exposed person (Aitio et al., 1988). A biological marker is an indicator of alteration in cellular structure, biochemical process, and/or system function as measured in a biological sample. In clinical neurotoxicology such markers can represent the severity of various effects and possibly also stages of progression of clinical disease following exposure. Three types of biological markers are useful in making a diagnosis of neurotoxic illness: biological markers of exposure, biological markers of effect, and biomarkers of susceptibility (National Research Council, 1992; Chern et al., 1995). Regulatory standards are yet to be set for many biochemical markers and other biological markers of effect, such as neurophysiological or neuropsychological test results.

Biologic markers of exposure are measures of (a) internal dose (ID), (b) the biologically effective dose (BED), or (c) the product of an interaction between a substance and some target molecules or other nervous system receptor. For example, electrophilic compounds, such as ethylene oxide, can covalently bind with nucleophilic centers (e.g., amino groups) in molecules to form adducts. An adduct is the product formed by the covalent binding of an electrophilic alkylating agent (e.g., EtO) with a nucleophilic center (e.g., amino group) in the molecule (e.g., DNA) (Landrigan et al., 1984; Walker et al., 1990). This occurs with hemoglobin, DNA, RNA, and the cytoskeletal proteins of neurons. These adducts can be used as biological markers of exposure by reason of the persistent binding between the chemical moiety absorbed and biological tissue. Basic pharmacokinetic principles such as absorption, distribution, excretion, and metabolism (as well as individual variations in gender and age and—in physiological functions involving blood flow—membrane permeability, respiratory rate, and nervous system accessibility) can all affect the measures of ID and/or BED.

Biological markers of effect are measurable biochemical or physiological alterations within the nervous system that can be associated with an established or potential health impairment or disease. They include markers of early biological effects, markers of altered structure and function changes more closely related to the development of disease, and markers of clinical disease; they can be any qualitative or quantitative change from a baseline or expected level of appearance or performance that indicates impairment or damage resulting from a given chemical exposure (NRC, 1992). In the clinical setting, the results of neurophysiological studies, neuropsychological tests, and neuro-

imaging studies serve as important biological markers of effects of chemical exposure on the nervous system.

Biomarkers of susceptibility are indicators of increased (or decreased) risk; they can affect the measurement and interpretation of other biomarkers along the continuum from exposure to disease.

A biological marker of susceptibility reflects an individual's level of sensitivity and the nature and severity of the developing symptoms resulting from exposure to a particular chemical(s). It is an indicator of the relative characteristics of a person who has been exposed. Some individuals have a lower threshold to exposure effects than do others; a preexisting disease state or concurrent condition may affect the metabolism of certain neurotoxicants, thus increasing the internal dose or the biologically effective dose. Biological markers of susceptibility include genetically determined mechanisms of absorption, tissue biochemistry, and excretion; immunoreaction; low organ reserve capacity; or other identifiable factors that can influence the effect of the neurotoxic substances (NRC, 1992).

The clinical relevance of biological marker data should be interpreted cautiously. Also, it is important to recognize that different chemicals may have similar detoxification pathways resulting in the common detectable metabolic products. For example, exposure to either trichloroethylene or perchloroethylene can result in urinary excretion of the same metabolites (e.g., trichloroethanol and trichloroacetic acid). Thus, in using biological monitoring, it is necessary to understand the biochemical processes involved and to recognize that certain biological markers may result from exposure to several different but structurally related chemicals. Relevant reference values have been established for many chemicals considered to be neurotoxic. Biological exposure indices for substances found in the workplace have been recommended and periodically updated by the American Conference of Governmental Industrial Hygienists (Lauwerys, 1991; ACGIH, 1995).

Interpretation of Biological Marker Data

The *sensitivity* and *specificity* of each biological marker must be considered to be used reliably in a clinical setting as an indication of neurotoxicant exposure. Sensitivity is the ability of a marker to identify correctly those subjects who, because of exposure to a suspected neurotoxicant, possess symptoms and/or signs of concern detectable by measuring this particular biological marker. It is determined by calculating the proportion of the exposed or diseased persons who demonstrate the marker of exposure or effect. Specificity is the ability to identify correctly and separate out those who have not been exposed because they do not possess detectable symptoms and/or signs of disease or effects of exposure to neurotoxicants. Specificity of a marker is determined by calculating the proportion of the unexposed or nondiseased persons who do not demonstrate the marker of exposure or effect (Hennekens and Buring, 1987; NRC, 1992).

The predictive value of a marker to define an exposure and an effect accurately is determined not only by factors that determine the validity of the test itself (i.e., sensitivity and specificity), but also by the characteristics of the population to which the test is applied, in particular the prevalence of the exposure status or the symptoms and signs of disease. Because exposure to neurotoxic substances can result in a range of biological side effects, there is a need to define clearly the critical effect(s) being considered as a previously observed outcome of exposure to the suspected neurotoxicant. The positive predictive value of a biological marker derives from its presence or amount of the marker among those persons who actually have been exposed and/or who have illness (Wilcosky and Griffith, 1990; Schulte, 1991). The higher the prevalence of the exposure or disease, the more likely it is that a positive test (i.e., indicated by the marker) is predictive of exposure or disease. Thus, the validation study of markers indicative of exposure or effect requires information on specificity, sensitivity, and prior knowledge of the disease rate or exposure rate (Needleman, 1987).

Finally, for a biological marker to be useful in the clinical setting, certain practical issues regarding collection of the appropriate sample should be considered: (a) availability of a marker from an appropriate specimen; (b) appropriate timing of sample collection; and (c) the correct device for sample collection.

NEUROIMAGING

Neuroimaging techniques provide objective data concerning brain structures. These highly sophisticated, computerized radiological methodologies demonstrate the outlines of the cerebral hemispheres and ventricular systems and also differentiate between cerebral cortex and white matter structures. The sensitivity of neuroimaging techniques in the detection of neurotoxic effects is limited. Nonetheless, there have been reports of clinical correlations between images obtained with magnetic resonance imaging (MRI), single-photon emission computed tomography (SPECT), and positron emission tomography (PET) in the presence of exposure to various neurotoxicants.

For example, MRI findings in two patients with exposure to carbon monoxide showed high signal intensity areas in the globus pallidus (Horowitz et al., 1987). Following severe carbon monoxide encephalopathy with unconsciousness, three patients had abnormalities on T_2-weighted, but not T_1-weighted MRI or computed tomography (CT); a fourth patient showed hyperintensity in the globus pallidus bilaterally (Murata et al., 1993). The severity of cerebral white matter involvement seen on MRI following chronic toluene exposure correlated with changes in neuropsychological performance (Filley et al., 1990). MRI changes were noted in subcortical and temporal areas, but not in cortical

gray matter, following exposure to 2,6-dimethyl-4-heptenone (White et al., 1993). Associations have been made between MRI changes and exposure to organolead in gasoline (Prockop and Karampelas, 1981) and to inorganic mercury (White et al., 1993). In a welder with manganese exposure, there were hyperintense signals in the basal ganglia on T_1-weighted MRI, whereas normal T_2 signals were seen. There was complete resolution 6 months after an exposure ended. A SPECT scan performed at the time of the first MRI also showed decreased uptake in the cortex, with local decreases in basal ganglia (Nelson et al., 1993).

Some authors have suggested that SPECT scans may have value in assessing neurotoxic effects in humans (Callendar et al., 1993), but Triebig and Lang (1993), in reporting results of cerebral blood flow, SPECT, CT, and MRI tests in patients with toxic encephalopathies following exposure to solvents, noted that their results were not significant and were possibly inconclusive. It was thought that the chronic low-dose exposure produces physiological disruption measured by neuropsychological testing, without showing measurable degrees of brain structure effect, as defined by CT.

A PET scan utilizing [18]S-2-deoxyglucose in a 31-year-old man exposed to tetrabromoethane, a halogenated aliphatic hydrocarbon, showed a significant decrease in uptake in multiple areas of the brain; no abnormalities were seen on CT or EEG studies. However, neurobehavioral assessments did reveal deficits in learning ability, memory, and psychomotor speed, which seemed to be related to the deficits seen on PET scan.

FORMULATING A DIAGNOSIS

The diagnosis of environmental neurotoxic illness rests on the ability of a clinician to recognize that certain environmental agents can cause adverse biological responses in nervous tissues at critical levels of exposure and absorption. A high index of suspicion is needed to detect individual cases or outbreaks of neurotoxic illness in communities, especially in the absence of a dramatic accident or obvious hazardous waste spill (Buffler et al., 1985).

Deviations from expected performance levels, considered normal in standard references or as baselines in comparable control groups, are defined as abnormalities. In this way, the clinician determines whether or not clinical impairments exist in central and/or peripheral nervous system function. Conventional and standardized clinical neuropsychological test batteries, neurophysiological measures of cranial and peripheral nerve function, and neuroimaging techniques are then used to obtain objective evidence and thus confirmation of any neurological abnormalities.

Analyses of environmental exposure sample concentrations of neurotoxicants and biological markers of neurotoxicant effects are necessary to ascertain the risk of ongoing exposure in relation to the emergence of symptoms in an individual patient or in a group of exposed persons.

Confirmation of a neurotoxic origin of the clinical findings depends on the presence of biological markers such as specific chemical levels in tissues, blood, urine, feces, hair, and nails, as well as measures of neurotoxicants in air, water, and soil, which serve as necessary exposure data proving the presence of suspected neurotoxicants. In some instances, metabolites or other biological markers (such as abnormalities in sperm count and motility, enzyme levels, or histopathological evidence of pathology on peripheral nerve biopsy tissue, muscle biopsy, or autopsy specimens) are necessary to support the historical information regarding the patient's exposure.

An overall clinical diagnosis of neurotoxic disease is arrived at by considering the relative importance of each parameter of function that falls within the limits, or exceeds the expected limits, of testing and observations for unaffected or "normal" subjects. Along with supporting historical information and biological and exposure marker data, the clinical findings are placed into the context of the other parameters obtained on various standardized neuropsychological testing and quantified neurophysiological measures to formulate a diagnosis.

In the clinical practice of medicine, it is unlikely that each patient will be compared with a matched control subject. It is the frequency and severity of reported symptoms and observed physical findings that lend support to the impression of clinical impairment. The "normal" is an ideal set of clinical findings derived from the experiences of many previous examinations of nonaffected persons, which serve as a reasonable database for comparison. The accumulated clinical data may not meet specific conventional criteria of an epidemiological design; however, each parameter has value in reaching a diagnosis. Thus, the results of studying exposure effects on individuals or small groups of individuals are valuable in recognizing neurotoxicity in the causation of neurological disorders, as long as each of the observations and measurements is made with care and accuracy.

Strategies and protocols have been developed for collecting relevant information and evidence to establish a diagnosis of occupational and environmental disease. A constellation of neurological effects ranging from subclinical or barely perceptible sensory deficits to gross behavioral abnormalities may characterize an exposed population. Appropriate and sensitive procedures must be applied for detecting and characterizing disturbances in neurological and behavioral functions, as well as documenting the nature and extent of any hazardous conditions. Such multiple parameter screening procedures parallel the process of human assessment that incorporates various findings of clinical neurological examinations, electrophysiological measurements of peripheral and central nervous system functions, and observations and test scores of standardized neuropsychological studies; such assessment leads to a clinical diagnosis. This approach is similar to that used by the United States Environmental Protection Agency: a multitiered laboratory approach is used for testing neurotoxicity in animals, and a variety of measurements are integrated into a health or safety indices.

Boston University Environmental Neurology Assessment

In an effort to standardize a procedure for clinical assessment of neurotoxic disease in individuals as well as in groups, we have developed the Boston University Environmental Neurology Assessment (BUENA) (Table 3-3). The BUENA is an approach to the diagnosis of neurotoxic disease that has been used in evaluating workers suspected of having been exposed to various neurotoxicants; it has been used during health hazard evaluations of members of communities in which hazardous pollutants were found in drinking water sources (Feldman et al., 1988, 1994). This protocol lists specific essential questions to be answered, extending the algorithm (see Chapter 2, Fig. 2-1) to a more detailed documentation of observations and eliminating as many confounding variables as possible to make diagnostic conclusions. The BUENA raises questions to be answered about a patient or group of patients with suspected neurotoxic illness and prompts the examiner to consider the following: Do the reported symptoms suggest impairment of the nervous system? Are these complaints substantiated by clinical neurological examination, by neurophysiological tests, and/or by neuropsychological tests? Are the findings due to a primary neurological disease or other nontoxic and idiopathic medical condition, or are they associated with exposure to occupational or environmental hazards? Is there evidence of environmental (air, water, soil), or workplace contamination by neurotoxicants? Do blood, urine, feces, hair, or fingernail analyses confirm absorption by body tissues of these same neurotoxicants? Are the clinical findings and the laboratory data reliable and significant enough to establish a causal relationship between documented effects and the affected person's ascertained exposure to specific neurotoxicants? What confounding variables might influence the outcomes of any diagnostic tests studies and affect conclusions on diagnosis and prognosis?

Although the data collected by the BUENA do not meet conventional criteria of an epidemiological design, they are nevertheless useful from scientific, clinical, and legal points of view. Furthermore, as strongly supported by Rothman et al. (1992), reanalysis and metaanalysis of observed associations between suspected risk factors and medical conditions provide valid and useful evidence. If it were practical to design a more conventional epidemiological study, then all the parameters, including concurrent control subjects and exposure data measures for much larger groups of subjects, would be needed for proper statistical analysis. Thus, without an elaborate epidemiological design to which traditional statistical analyses can be applied, the results of studying small groups or well-studied exposed people can be valuable in supporting the concept that environmental factors play a role in causing

TABLE 3-3. *Boston University Environmental Neurology Assessment (BUENA)*

I. **Are the data sufficient to identify any or all complaints as being caused by a neurotoxin?**
   A. *List complaints* and relate them on a time line identifying all possible chemical exposures, episodes, and their sources (work, home, hobby).
      1. Identify symptoms and functional changes expressed, experienced, or observed by others; list examples of mood, anxiety, sleep disturbances, and effect on quality of life.
      2. Cite time of onset, duration, and intensity of all complaints. Characterize symptoms as to worsening or remitting in relation to exposure and away from exposure sources (e.g., work week, weekend, time of shift, on vacation).
      3. Evaluate subject's family/genetic health, special sensitivities, and possible congenital factors.
   B. *List all substances* and how they are used (at workplace, home, hobbies).
      1. Obtain chemical names (not trade label names), material safety data sheets, and other identifying data concerning each chemical substance.
      2. Review workplace information available (e.g., OSHA-mandated material safety data sheets and employer training program materials; employer's medical records and exposure records, which, if kept by employer, must be made available under OSHA rules. Review, if available, the following: employer's TSCA 8c and 8e reports to EPA, employer's community right to know reports to local officials re: hazardous materials made, used, or sorted on site.)
   C. *Obtain environmental and industrial hygiene air or drinking water samplings measures* to prove the presence of suspected or other chemicals in the alleged sources. *Current levels* are important, and levels taken in relationship to occurrence of complaints is essential.
   D. *Obtain urine and/or blood samples from the suspected exposed and/or affected* individuals and from known unexposed control patients of similar age and occupation, especially at time of complaints, to *establish body burden of chemical.*
   E. For suspect chemicals, *develop information on dose–response relationships, animal studies, toxicological and epidemiological studies.*
II. **Are the complaints substantiated by clinical neurological physical examination; standardized neuropsychological and neurophysiological tests; and appropriate blood and urine analyses?** Also, are the complaints corroborated by epidemiological, toxicological, animal studies; by NIOSH or OSHA or EPA studies of the workforce or community; by employer studies and reports to EPA or OSHA (e.g., TSCA 8c and 8e reports)?
III. **Are the findings due to a primary neurological disease or other medical condition?**
IV. **Are the findings on examination explained by any other causal factors** in past medical history or previous and/or current unrelated exposures to substances from sources other than the one under consideration, or are they due to a primary neurological disease or other medical condition?
   A. Time line of past jobs, residences.
   B. Time line of past medical history.
V. **Analyze individual cases for confirmatory studies;** group data for cluster analysis and/or population statistical study.
VI. **Identify and critically review previously published and/or reported case reports, case control studies, population studies, and animal studies concerning the alleged neurotoxins and relate documentation to case data.**
VII. **Estimate the damage consequences for the subject:** disease, anxiety, loss of consort, functional impairments, need for special education or counseling or medical surveillance, need for medical therapeutic measures, job disability, loss of earnings, etc.
VIII. **Reevaluate after reasonable absence from all neurotoxic exposure** to assess course of progression, recovery, or persistent impairment and/or disability.

OSHA, Occupational Safety and Health Administration; TSCA, Toxic Substances Control Act; EPA, Environmental Protection Agency; NIOSH, National Institute of Occupational Safety and Health.
From Feldman, 1993, with permission.

neurological disorders. By using a consistent protocol and conventional test instruments, the neurophysiological and neuropsychological performance in many patients, and in groups of patients exposed to the same neurotoxicant, can be compared for possible generalizations. This approach formalizes techniques as they are used in the everyday practice of medicine, in which the goal is to assess impairments of an individual within the environment. In this context, differing from the traditional epidemiological study, the clinician takes the position that even a small probability of serious illness must not be dismissed and deserves a thorough assessment.

A clinical diagnosis in a patient is arrived at by an intellectual process that integrates all available information in a systematic manner. This process should be the same whether used in the day-to-day practice of clinical medicine or in the special circumstances of evaluating self-referred individuals who may have neurotoxic disease and who are involved in litigation. Sets of physiological, anatomical, and behavioral concepts and principles accumulated from experience and derived from a database of previously published reports and conventionally accepted clinical norms known to the examiner serve as a frame of reference for evaluating these abnormalities and formulating a diagnosis and possible causal explanation for the reported unwellness.

REFERENCES

Abou-Donia MM. Nutrition and neurotoxicology. In: Abou-Donia MB, eds. *Neurotoxicology.* Boca Raton, FL: CRC Press, 1992:319–335.

Aitio A, Jarvisalo J, Riihimaki V, Hernberg S. Biologic monitoring. In: Zene C, ed. *Occupational medicine,* 2nd ed. Chicago: Year-Book Medical Publishers, 1988:178–197.

American Conference of Government Industrial Hygienists (ACGIH). *Documentation of the threshold limit values and biological exposure indices,* 5th ed. Cincinnati, OH: ACGIH, 1988.

American Conference of Governmental Industrial Hygienists (ACGIH). *Threshold limit values (TLVs) for chemical substances and physical agents and Biological Exposure Indices (BEIs).* Cincinnati, OH: ACGIH, 1995.

Arezzo JCV, Schaumburg HH. Screening for neurotoxic disease in humans. *Trans Am Coll. Toxicol* 1989;8:147–155.

Arezzo JC, Schaumburg HH, Petersen CA. Rapid screening for peripheral neuropathy: a field study with the Optacon. *Neurology* 1983;33:626–629.

Arezzo JC, Simson R, Brennan NE. Evoked potentials in the assessment of neurotoxicity in humans. *Neurobehav Toxicol Teratol* 1985;7: 299–304.

Baker EL, Feldman RG, French J. Environmentally related disorders of the nervous system. *Med Clin North Am* 1990;74:325–345.

Baker EL, White RF. *Chronic effects of organic solvents on the central nervous system and diagnostic criteria.* World Health Organization (Copenhagen) and Nordic Council of Ministers (Oslo). Washington, DC: U.S. Department of Health and Human Services, Public Health Service, 1985.

Berger AR, Schaumburg HH, Schroeder C, Apfel S, Reynolds R. Dose response, coasting, and differential fiber vulnerability in human toxic neuropathy; a prospective study of pyridoxine neurotoxicity. *Neurology* 1992;42:1367–1370.

Buchthal F, Rosenfalck A. Evoked action potentials and conduction velocity in human sensory nerves. *Brain Res* 1966;3:1–122.

Buffler PA, Crane M, Key MM. Possibilities of detecting health effects by studies of populations exposed to chemicals from waste disposal sites. *Environ Health Perspect* 1985;62:423–456.

Callender TJ, Morrow L, Subrainanian K, et al. Three-dimensional brain metabolic imaging in patients with toxic encephalopathy. *Environ Res* 1993;60:295–319.

Chiappa K. Evoked potentials. In: Chiappa K, ed. *Clinical medicine,* 2nd ed. New York: Raven Press, 1992.

Chern C-M, Proctor SP, Feldman RG. Exposure assessment in clinical neurotoxicology: environmental monitoring and biologic markers. In: Chang L, Slokker W Jr, eds. *Neurotoxicology: approaches and methods.* San Diego: Academic Press, 1995:695–709.

Cullen MR. The worker with multiple chemical sensitivities: an overview. In: Cullen M, ed. *Workers with multiple chemical sensitivities.* Philadelphia: Hanley and Belfus, 1987:655–662.

Feldman RG, Pransky GS. Neurologic considerations in worker fitness evaluation. In: *Comprehensive approaches to worker fitness and risk evaluations, occupational medicine: state of the art review,* vol 3. Philadelphia: Hanley and Belfus, 1988:299–308.

Feldman RG, Travers PH. Environmental and occupational neurology. In: Feldman RG, ed. *Neurology: the physician's guide.* New York: Thieme-Stratton, 1984:191–212.

Feldman RG, White RF, Eriator II, et al. Neurotoxic effects of trichloroethylene in drinking water: approach to diagnosis. In: Isaacson RL, Jensen KF, eds. *The vulnerable brain and environmental risks,* vol 3, *Toxins in air and water.* New York: Plenum Press, 1994:3–23.

Feldman RG, Niles CA, Kelly-Hayes M, et al. Peripheral neuropathy in arsenic smelter workers. *Neurology* 1979;29:939–944.

Feldman RG, Chirico-Post JA, Proctor SP. Blink reflex latency after exposure to trichloroethylene in well water. *Arch Environ Health* 1988; 43:143–148.

Filley CM, Heaton RK, Rosenberg NL. White matter dementia in chronic toluene abuse. *Neurology* 1990;40:532–534.

Gerr F, Hershman D, Letz R. Vibrotactile threshold measurement for detecting neuropathy: reliability and determination of age- and height-standard normative values. *Arch Environ Health* 1990;45:148–154.

Goetz CG. Dietary toxins and miscellaneous drugs: neurotoxins in clinical practice. In: Weintraub M, ed. *Neurologic illness: diagnosis and treatment.* New York: Spectrum, 1985:313–339.

Haley RW, Kurt TL. Self-reported exposure to neurotoxic chemical combinations in the Gulf War: a cross sectional epidemiological study. *JAMA* 1997;277:231–237.

Haley RW, Kurt TL, Hom J. Is there a Gulf War Syndrome? Searching for syndromes by factor analysis of symptoms. *JAMA* 1997;277:215–222.

Hennekens CH, Buring JE. Screening. In: Mayrent SL, ed. *Epidemiology in medicine.* Boston: Little, Brown, 1987:327–345.

Horowitz AL, Kaplan R, Sarpel G. Carbon monoxide toxicity: MR imaging in the brain. *Radiology* 1987;162:787–788.

Jabre JF, Sato L. The expression of electrophysiologic data as mean related values (MRVs). *Muscle Nerve* 1990;13:861–862.

Juntunen J. Alcoholism in occupational neurology: diagnostic difficulties with special reference to the neurological syndromes caused by exposure to organic solvents. *Acta Neurol Scand* 1982;66(Suppl 92): 89–108.

Kimura J. The blink reflex. In: Kimura J, ed. *Electrodiagnosis in disease of nerve and muscle—principles and practice.* Philadelphia: FA Davis, 1989:323–351.

Landrigan PJ. Illness in Gulf War veterans: causes and consequences. *JAMA* 1997;277:259–261.

Lauwerys R. Occupational toxicology. In: Klaassen C, Admur M, Doull J, eds. *Casarett and Doull's toxicology.* New York: Macmillan, 1991: 947–969.

Liveson J, Ma D. *Laboratory reference for clinical neurophysiology.* Philadelphia: FA Davis, 1992.

Murata S, Asaba H, Hiraishi K, et al. Magnetic resonance imaging findings in carbon monoxide intoxications. *Neurology* 1993;3:128–131.

National Research Council (NRC). *Environmental neurotoxicology.* Washington, DC: National Academy Press, 1992.

Needleman HL. Introduction: biomarkers in neurodevelopmental toxicology. *Environ Health Perspect* 1987;74:149–151.

Nelson K, Golnick J, Kom T, et al. Manganese encephalopathy: utility of early magnetic resonance imaging. *Br J Ind Med* 1993;50:510–513.

Otto DA, Fox DA. Auditory and visual dysfunction following lead exposure. *Neurotoxicology* 1993;14:191–208.

Otto DA, Hudnell HK. The use of visual and chemosensory evoked potentials in environmental and occupational health. *Environ Res* 1993; 62:159–171.

Prockop LD, Karampelas D. Encephalopathy secondary to abusive gasoline inhalation. *J Fla Med Assoc* 1981;68:823–824.

Rebert CS. Multisensory evoked potentials in experimental and applied neurotoxicology. *Neurobehav Toxicol Teratol* 1983;5:659–671.

Rothman K, Weiss N, Robbins J, Neutra R, Stellman S. Amicus Curiae. William Daubert v. Merrill Dow Pharmaceuticals Inc., U.S. Supreme Court No. 92-102. December 2, 1992.

Schottenfeld RS, Cullen M. Occupation-induced post traumatic stress disorders. *Am J Psychiatr* 1985;142:198–202.

Schulte P. Contribution of biological markers to occupational health. *Am J Ind Med* 1991;20:435–446.

Seppalainen AM, Anti-Poika M. Time course of electrophysiological findings for patients with solvent poisoning. *Scand J Work Environ Health* 1983;9:15–241.

Sterman AB, Schaumburg HH. Neurotoxicity of selected drugs. In: Spencer PS, Schaumburg HH, eds. *Experimental and clinical neurotoxicology.* Baltimore: Williams & Wilkins, 1980:593–612.

Triebig G, Lang C. Brain imaging techniques applied to chronically solvent-exposed workers: current results and clinical evaluation. *Environ Res* 1993;61:239–250.

Weiss B. Behavioral properties of chemical sensitivity syndromes. *Neurotoxicology* 1998; 19:259–268.

White RF. Differential diagnosis of probable Alzheimer's disease and solvent encephalopathy in older workers. *Clin Neuropsych* 1987;1: 153–160.

White RF, Feldman RG, Proctor SP. Neurobehavioral effects of toxic exposures. In: White RF, ed. *Clinical syndromes in adult neuropsychology: The practitioner's handbook.* New York: Elsevier, 1992:1–51.

White RF, Feldman RG, Moss MB, et al. Magnetic resonance imaging (MRI), neurobehavioral testing, and toxic encephalopathy: two cases. *Environ Res* 1993;61:117–123.

Wilcosky TC, Griffith JD. Applications of biological markers. In: Hulka BS, Wilcosky TC, Griffith JD, eds. *Biological markers in epidemiology.* New York: Oxford University Press, 1990:16–27.

Wolfe J, Proctor SP, Davis DJ, et al. Health symptoms reported by Persian Gulf War veterans two years after return. *Am J Ind Med* 1998;33: 104–113.

Yokoyama K, Feldman RG, Sax DS, et al. Relation of distribution of conduction velocities to nerve biopsy findings in *n*-hexane poisoning. *Muscle Nerve* 1990;13:314–320.

CHAPTER 4

Lead

Lead (plumbum; Pb) is a bluish gray metal found in the earth. Deposits of lead ore commonly consist of lead sulfide (plumbus sulfide; galena; PbS), lead sulfate (anglesite; $PbSO_4$), and lead carbonate (cerussite; $PbCO_3$). Lead chlorophosphate [pyromorphite; $PbCl_2 \cdot 3Pb_3(PO_4)$] also occurs in nature. Lead ores are found as conglomerates with the ores of other metals including silver, zinc, copper, and iron (Beliles, 1994). Lead occurs in oxidation states of 2^+ and 4^+ and reacts with carbon, oxygen, nitrogen, sulfur, and the halides to form a variety of inorganic and organic compounds. Inorganic compounds include lead oxide (Pb_3O_4); lead chloride ($PbCl_2$); lead chlorate [$Pb(ClO_3)_2$]; and lead acetate [$Pb(CH_3COO)_2$], also known as sugar of lead. Stable organic lead compounds such as tetramethyl and tetraethyl lead are formed from tetravalent lead (Pb^{4+}) (Sax, 1979) (Table 4-1).

The mining and use of lead over the past centuries have resulted in increases in lead concentrations in surface soils; lead is ubiquitous (Murozumi et al., 1969; ATSDR, 1997). Analysis of the concentration of naturally occurring stable isotopes of lead (e.g., Pb 204, 206, 207, and 208) in meteorites and in samples taken at various levels of the ice sheets of the frozen polar regions in Greenland provides a record of lead accumulation from the atmosphere over the years: less than 0.0005 μg/kg ice at geological levels corresponding to 800 B.C. to more than 0.2 μg/kg of ice at geological levels corresponding to the year 1965 A.D., 400 times the levels found in the ice sheet corresponding to 800 B.C. (Murozumi et al., 1969; Doe, 1970).

In keeping with efforts to reduce further lead accumulation and to minimize the health hazards of lead exposure, the manufacture and use of lead-containing products have been limited. Steps taken have included the establishment of exposure standards limiting the production and usage of lead-containing products, the monitoring and reduction of lead content in drinking water, and reductions in the use of fuels containing organic lead as an octane-raising additive (Brody et al., 1994; EPA, 1996a,b). A regulation prohibiting the sale or use of leaded gasoline in the United States was instituted in 1995 (EPA, 1991, 1996b). The percentage of food contain-

ers manufactured in the United States that contain lead solder seams declined from 47% in 1980 to 0.9% in 1990. In 1995 the Food and Drug Administration issued a ruling prohibiting the use of lead solder in the manufacture of cans used for the packaging of food but allowed the sale of existing stocks of lead-soldered cans for an additional year (FDA, 1995). Other factors contributing to a decrease in environmental lead and therefore background blood lead levels include the Consumer Products Safety Commission's ban on lead-based paint and lead-soldered plumbing for residential use. Lead oxide is no longer added to house paints, toys, and ceramic tableware, and water conveyance pipes are carefully examined for lead content; those containing lead are replaced or avoided. In addition, the number of occupied dwellings built before 1940 that contained lead-based paint decreased from 24.2 million (30.3% of dwellings) in 1980 to 20.8 million (22.2% of dwellings in 1989) (CDC, 1994a). Requirements now exist for the training and education of workers involved in lead paint–related work, such as its removal from old houses and other cleanup projects (Feldman, 1978). These abatement efforts resulted in a decrease in the average blood lead concentrations in many areas of the world, especially in the United States and in several European countries. The blood lead levels of persons younger than 75 years showed a 78% reduction since they were first recorded during the second National Health and Nutrition Examination Survey (NHANES II) and the subsequent time they were recorded during the NHANES III, phase I (1976 to 1980). The prevalence of BLLs greater than 10 μg/100 mL among children aged 1 to 5 years old also decreased substantially, from 88.2% during NHANES II to 8.9% during NHANES III, phase I. Although surveillance programs conducted by state health departments mandated by the Lead-Based Paint Poisoning Prevention Act of 1971 have decreased the risks of lead poisoning significantly, cases of elevated blood lead levels among adults as well as children continue to be documented (HUD, 1990; Hu et al., 1990; Sokas et al., 1995, 1997). Although many cases of lead poisoning (plumbism) occur among adults following work-related exposures, children are the most vulnerable to the effects of lead expo-

TABLE 4-1. *Physical characteristics of some common lead compounds*

Compound	Form	Color
Metallic lead	Malleable metal	Bluish gray
Lead acetate	Crystals	White
Lead azide	Needles	Colorless
Lead chloride	Crystals	White
Lead chlorate	Monoclinic crystals	Yellow
Lead chromate	Crystals	Yellow
Lead fluoride	Solid	Colorless
Lead iodate	Solid	White
Lead nitrate	Crystals	White
Lead oxide	Powder	Bright red
Lead sulfate	Rhombic crystals	White
Lead sulfide	Metallic crystals	Silvery
Tetraethyl lead	Oily liquid	Colorless
Tetramethyl lead	Liquid	Colorless

Data from Sax, 1979.

sure. Permanent neurological impairments are associated with incidents of *in utero* and/or childhood exposures (Mushak, 1992; Olden, 1993; White et al., 1993; Aschengrau et al., 1994; McDonald and Potter, 1996).

Exposures to neurotoxic levels of lead whether among children or adults are costly to both the individual and the general public. Intake of inorganic lead from various sources (occupational exposures, food containing inorganic lead, and the release of inorganic lead from consumer products including toys) can produce acute and chronic neurological and systemic effects (Bucy and Buchanan, 1935; Byers and Lord, 1943; Hess, 1961; Seppäläinen et al., 1975; Feldman et al., 1973; Feldman, 1982). The nervous system is especially vulnerable to the effects of lead. Thus, an awareness of the potential sources of exposure, the established and recommended exposure limits, and the early signs and symptoms of lead poisoning are very important to the health maintenance of individuals and groups of people who are at risk.

SOURCES OF EXPOSURE

Inorganic Lead

Mining and processing of lead has taken place throughout recorded history. An estimated 300 million metric tons of lead have been taken from the earth over the past 5,000 years (Mushak, 1992). Lead for commercial use is extracted from lead ore and recovered from secondary sources such as scrap metal recycling (e.g., reclamation from used automobile batteries). Lead mines in the United States produced 384,000 metric tons of lead in 1995. An additional 972,000 million metric tons of lead available for consumption in the United States in 1995 was acquired by the recycling of lead-containing materials such as old batteries. Lead recovered from scrap lead acid batteries accounted for 89%

(867,000 metric tons) of the lead produced from secondary sources in 1995 (USGS, 1995).

Hernberg (1975) defined categories of high- and moderate-risk operations for occupational settings according to the likelihood of being exposed to lead. *High-risk* operations include activities in which metallic lead or lead-coated materials are burned and lead fumes are generated in high concentration such as smelting, welding, and cutting of lead and lead painted constructions, spray painting, mixing of lead salt stabilizers used in the production of plastics, mixing of crystal glass mass, sanding or scraping of lead paint, burning of lead in enamel workshops, and repairing of automobile radiators. Workers at *moderate risk* include lead miners, solderers, plumbers, cable makers, wire platers, type founders, stereo typesetters, automobile factory workers, automobile repair mechanics, autobody mechanics, ship repair workers, lead founders, lead glass blowers and lead crystal glass producers, stained glass workers, and pottery glazers. Instructors and other persons who work at indoor pistol firing ranges are also at risk of exposure to inorganic lead (Anania et al., 1974; Landrigan et al., 1975; Anderson et al., 1977; Ozonoff, 1994).

Occupational exposure to inorganic lead occurs among miners and smelter workers (Buchthal and Behse, 1979). The processes used in the primary smelting (i.e., refining of lead ore) and secondary smelting (i.e., reclamation from alloys to a purer metal) are hazardous operations that can result in significant exposure to workers and others who may be passively exposed to lead distributed as particulate matter in the atmosphere and water and redeposited in the surrounding soil (Federal Institute for Minerals Research and German Institute for Economic Research, 1972; Weitzman et al., 1993; Sexton et al., 1993). Monthly lead emissions from a smelter in Shoshone County, Idaho, averaged 8.3 metric tons from 1955 through 1964 and 11.7 metric tons from 1965 through September of 1973 but increased to 35.3 metric tons from October, 1973 through September, 1974, following a fire in the main filtration facility (Landrigan et al., 1976). Twenty-four-hour high-volume sampling of ambient air lead levels revealed the highest air lead levels immediately adjacent to the smelter, and the levels increased three- to fourfold from 1971 through 1974, corresponding to increases in smelter emissions (Fig. 4-1). As a result of distribution by prevailing winds, surface soil samples and local vegetation obtained from locations throughout the valley in June of 1974 showed lead content highest near the smelter and trailing off with increasing distance away from the stack. Peak values were 9,000 mg/kg for soil and 3,478 mg/kg for vegetation. Since samples of the public drinking water in the area all revealed acceptable lead concentrations (below 0.05 mg/L), the particulate airborne lead concentrations were considered the only significant source of lead exposure to the population studied.

Foundry workers, construction and demolition workers, and metal salvage yard personnel are exposed to lead oxides when they use oxyacetylene torches to cut metal

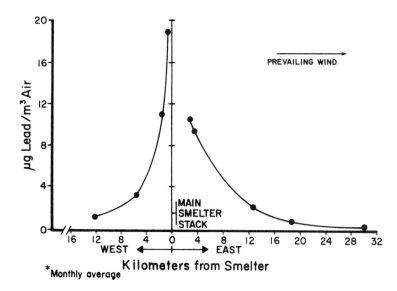

FIG. 4-1. Relationship between ambient air lead levels and distance from the main smelter stack of a lead smelter. Airborne lead particulates accumulated more toward the west, where thermal inversions are frequent because of the geography of the intermountain valley of the South Fork of the Coeur d'Alene River, and decreased more quickly with the prevailing winds blowing in the easterly direction. (From Landrigan et al., 1976, with permission.)

painted with "red lead primer" as well as other paints containing inorganic lead as pigments (Rieke, 1969; Feldman et al., 1977; Feldman, 1978; Grandjean and Kon, 1981; Baker et al., 1984; Marino et al., 1989; Nosal and Wilhelm, 1990). Malleable inorganic lead is used as a dent filler in the autobody manufacturing and repair industries (Lilis et al., 1982). Risk of toxic exposure exists among automobile radiator workers who are exposed to organic lead fumes during repairs (Goldman et al., 1987). Workers in the battery manufacturing and reclamation industries are exposed to inorganic lead (Hess, 1961; Kumar et al., 1987; Kentner et al., 1994). Small amounts of lead are used in the manufacture of chemicals and glass and ceramic products and as paint pigments (USGS, 1995).

Increased blood lead levels have been detected in the children and spouses of lead-exposed workers (Baker et al., 1977; Otto et al., 1985; Gittleman et al., 1994; Chiaradia et al., 1997). Twelve of 16 children of lead-exposed workers had blood lead levels greater than 10 μg/100 mL, and 3 had blood lead levels greater than 40 μg/100 mL (Gittleman et al., 1994). Indirect and passive maternal exposures through contact with contaminated work clothing brought into the home have also been associated with prenatal exposure to lead and low birth weights (Min et al., 1996). Together, these findings emphatically attest to the need for proper hygienic habits in lead-exposed workers.

Inorganic lead halides and oxides are released into the environment with combustion of organic lead compounds, such as tetramethyl and tetraethyl lead. Decomposition rate of methyl lead to inorganic lead is very low (about 4%), whereas nearly 99% of ethyl lead in the environment is decomposed to inorganic lead (Carson et al., 1987). Grass samples taken near a heavily trafficked highway before the use of organic lead additives in gasoline was restricted showed a mean lead content of 250 mg/kg at the roadside and 100 mg/kg in grass samples taken at a distance of 24 m from the roadside (NAS, 1972). Sediments in the beds of

lakes, rivers, and streams contain more lead than is found suspended in these bodies of water. Only colloidal lead is taken up with the water absorbed by plants. Street dust from residential and commercial areas in 77 Midwestern cities in the United States contained concentrations of lead ranging from 1,600 to 2,400 mg/kg (NAS, 1972). Determination of lead concentrations in dust samples from residences in the United Kingdom revealed a geometric mean of greater than 500 μg/g. The concentration of organic lead in the dust in these households was also found to correlate with blood lead levels in the children living there (Thornton et al., 1990).

Epidemiological studies to determine sources of lead exposure among children are often difficult to perform, and data analysis must take into account many variables in addition to the blood lead levels alone, such as estimates of intake from various sources (air, soil, dust, food, and paint), as well as socioeconomic factors (Baghurst et al., 1992). Despite the attention paid to the dangers of lead in the environment, including the workplace and the home, lead paint is still present in many older homes and the ground soil around them; both sources continue to pose ongoing health hazards, especially for children (Feldman et al., 1973; Feldman, 1978; Feldman and White, 1992; Binder, 1992; Aschengrau et al., 1994). The risk of lead poisoning is far greater among children living in single-parent households, in which financial constraints can result in the family living in older and often rundown housing with peeling lead paint and lead-soldered pipes (Bailey et al., 1994).

Daily dietary intake of lead varies from one country to another and with individual eating habits, age, occupation, and personal hygiene habits (GESAMP, 1985; Coulston et al., 1972a,b,e). Significant exposures occur in many so-called underdeveloped countries (Grandjean, 1993; Romieu et al., 1994; Saxena et al., 1994; Polizopoulou et al., 1994), as well as in the United States, where approximately 1.7 million children aged 1 to 5 years old were reported in 1991 to have BLLs greater than 10 μg/100 mL (CDC, 1994a). Dietary intake in infants is influenced by whether or not the child is breast-fed (Moore et al., 1982). Consumption of lead-contaminated illicitly distilled whiskey and wine continues to be a source of nonoccupational intake; these are affected by the containers in which the beverages are distilled and/or aged (Whitfield et al., 1972). Daily intake of lead, as documented by blood and hair levels, is greater among persons who use tobacco (Wolfsperger et al., 1994; Sokas et al., 1997).

Intake of inorganic lead from various sources including occupational exposures, hobbies and crafts, food containing lead, and the release of lead from consumer products including toys and ceramic glazed products leads to acute and chronic biological effects. Concern for the health and welfare of children exposed to inorganic lead-contaminated housing and soil as well as adults working in inorganic lead-related industries has led to careful monitoring of those individuals known to be at risk for exposure and to improved hygienic conditions; an occasional case of inorganic lead intoxication occurs through unsuspected sources (Table 4-2).

Organic Lead

Previous studies performed when the sale of gasoline containing organic lead compounds was legal revealed annual emissions of 7,000 tons of organic lead compounds into the atmosphere (Grandjean and Nielsen, 1979). The mean values at various sites for vapor-phase organic lead concentrations in the air near highways and in tunnels were 1 to 78 ng/m³ and 20 to 120 ng/m³, respectively. American values were generally higher than European values. Or-

ganic lead vapor concentrations in the center of six U.S. cities ranged from 100 to 800 ng/m³ (mean: 230 ng/m³). A mean of 100 ng/m³ was reported for the center of Los Angeles; levels reported for European cities are typically similar. However, the level reported for Toronto, Ontario was only 14 ng/m³ (Nielsen, 1984). Although the use of organic lead compounds as gasoline additives is now prohibited in the United States (EPA, 1996a) and thus these compounds are no longer as significant a threat to the health of the general public in this country as previously, the clinician must be familiar with the clinical manifestations of organic lead poisoning. Furthermore, in those regions of the world where leaded gasolines are still used, consumers continue to be exposed while using automobiles, power lawnmowers, motor boats, chain saws, and motors used for pumping water and generating electricity.

Atmospheric fallout and discharges from industrial and municipal facilities contribute organic leads to the aquatic environment. The average concentration of lead in the surface and ground water in the United States ranges from 5 to 30 ppm (EPA, 1986). Accidental spills of organic lead compounds also contribute to increased concentrations of lead in water. For example, surface water lead concentrations in the Adriatic Sea were 5 to 6 ppb (background lead values were 0.02 to 0.2 ppb) in 1976, 2 years after the sinking of a cargo ship carrying lead antiknock compounds. Lead concentrations of 1 to 15 ppb were found at 90 m deep, and concentrations in the sediment on the sea floor reached 2.5 to 16.8 ppm. Tetraalkyl lead may be taken up by aquatic organisms, or they may simply volatize (Chau and Wong, 1984). Tetramethyl lead accumulates in marine life. Biddlinger and Gloss (1984) indicated from their review on trophic transfer of metals and organics in aquatic ecosystems that there is no evidence of biomagnification of lead concentration in finfish. However, shellfish may pose a hazard since oysters exposed to water with lead concentrations as little as 2 ppb may accumulate more than 2 ppm of lead in their tissues, the limit set by the Canadian Food and Drug Directorate. Biomethylation does not appear to be a prominent means of mobilizing inorganic lead from marine sediments (Carson et al., 1987).

Organic lead compounds are more readily taken up by plants than is inorganic lead and can become part of the food chain. The water solubilities of tetraethyl lead and tetramethyl lead are 100 and 15 ppm, respectively (Beijer and Jernelöv, 1984). When added to soil, mixtures of tetraethyl lead and tetramethyl lead are quickly converted to the more highly water-soluble trialkyl lead and dialkyl lead species. Lead (as tetraethyl lead or tetramethyl lead) added to potting soil can be detected in vegetative parts and grains of spring wheat: 2.0 ppm dry weight in the grain when 1 ppm was added and 19.5 ppm when 10 ppm was added. At 10 ppm, grain yield was only 22% of the controls; when 100 ppm lead was added as tetraalkyl lead, the yield was further depressed and no grain was produced; 350 ppm lead was found in the wheat straw. Adding 100 ppm as $Pb(NO_3)_2$, on the other hand, gave little uptake by

TABLE 4-2. *Unusual sources of exposure to inorganic lead*

Source of inorganic lead	Reference
Lead shot retained in the appendix following unwitting ingestion of contaminated beef	Hillman, 1967
Ambient air at a pistol firing range	Anderson et al., 1977
Ingestion of hair spray containing lead	Raasch et al., 1983
Gunshot wounds	Dillman et al., 1979
Lead leaching from crystal cocktail glasses	Dickinson et al., 1972
Lead leaching from ceramic glaze	Harris and Elsea, 1967
Consumption of lead-contaminated home-made cider	Walls, 1969
Herbal medicines	Chan et al., 1977
Precious metal assayer	Samuel and Baxter, 1986
Art conservator	Fischbein et al., 1982
Consumption of illicit whiskey	Whitfield et al., 1972
Consumption of flour contaminated with lead	Panariti and Berxholi, 1998

the plants: 3.8 ppm dry weight in the straw, 2.2 ppm in the glumes (chaff), and 0.57 ppm in the grain, compared with values of 1.3, 1.2, and 0.03 in straw, chaff, and grain, respectively, of the controls (Diehl et al., 1983).

Significant lead poisoning was encountered early in the days when manufacturing and blending antiknock fluids containing organic lead compounds with gasoline was considered a "safe" industry (Hamilton et al., 1925). The National Institute of Occupational Safety and Health (NIOSH) estimated that approximately 875,000 workers (including gasoline service station attendants and workers who use leaded gasoline in chain saws, lawnmowers, and power tools) had been exposed to organic lead compounds while on the job in 1982 (Grandjean, 1984). Cleaning storage tanks containing residual leaded gasoline is extremely hazardous and has resulted in severe human exposure to organic lead (Cassell and Dodds, 1946; Beattie et al., 1972). Ambient air in such tanks can contain as much as 65 mg/m^3 of organic lead. Prolonged exposure to only 1.5 mg/m^3 caused seven deaths among workers cleaning aviation fuel tanks. Auto mechanics, drivers, and World War II soldiers involved in can filling and stacking have also suffered organic lead poisoning. Accidental poisonings have also been reported in several persons exposed to an organic lead production waste during its transport and attempted reprocessing (Grandjean, 1984).

Alkyl leads are rapidly dealkylated in the environment. Alkyl lead compounds in the atmosphere may be degraded by photolysis and reactions with hydroxyl radicals ($\cdot$OH), ozone, NO_2, SO_2, and O_2. The reaction with $\cdot$OH predominates over photolysis and the reaction with ozone. Degradation proceeds by way of trialkyl lead and dialkyl lead species to elemental lead (Chau and Wong, 1984). However, thermal decomposition in the presence of oxygen will yield oxidized lead compounds instead of elemental lead. Thus the result is increased environmental levels of inorganic lead.

EXPOSURE LIMITS AND SAFETY REGULATIONS

Inorganic Lead

The *Occupational Safety and Health Administration* (OSHA) has established a permissible exposure level (PEL) of 0.05 mg/m^3 for inorganic lead compounds, including elemental lead, lead oxides, and lead salts (OSHA, 1995) (Table 4-3). NIOSH's recommended exposure limit (REL) for inorganic lead is 0.1 mg/m^3. The NIOSH immediately dangerous to life or health (IDLH) exposure limit for inorganic lead is 100 mg/m^3 (NIOSH, 1997). The *American Conference of Governmental Industrial Hygienists* (ACGIH) has recommended a threshold limit value (TLV) of 0.05 mg/m^3 for inorganic lead (ACGIH, 1995).

The *Department of Housing and Urban Development* (HUD) has recommended a hazard level guideline for inorganic lead in bare soil of 2,000 μg/g (2,000 ppm); in high-contact play areas the soil lead concentration should not ex-

TABLE 4-3. *Established and recommended occupational and environmental exposure limits for lead compounds in air and water*

	Air (mg/m^3)[a]	Water (mg/L)[a]
Odor threshold*	—	—
OSHA		
PEL (8-hr TWA)		
Inorganic lead	0.05	—
Organic lead	0.075[b]	—
NIOSH		
REL (10-hr TWA)		
Inorganic lead	0.1	—
Organic lead	0.075[b]	—
IDLH		
Inorganic lead	100	—
Organic lead	40[b]	—
ACGIH		
TLV (8-hr TWA)		
Inorganic lead	0.05	
Tetraethyl lead	0.1[b]	
Tetramethyl lead	0.15[b]	—
EPA		
MCL		
Inorganic lead	—	TT
MCLG		
Inorganic lead	—	0.0

OSHA, Occupational Safety and Health Administration; PEL, permissible exposure limit; TWA, time-weighted average; NIOSH, National Institute of Occupational Safety and Health; REL, recommended exposure limit; IDLH, immediately dangerous to life or health; ACGIH, American Conference of Governmental Industrial Hygienists; TLV, Threshold Limit Value; EPA, Environmental Protection Agency; MCL, maximum contamination level; MCLG, maximum contamination level goal; TT, use of water treatment technique required by EPA.

[a]Unit conversion: *tetraethyl lead,* 1 ppm = 13.45 mg/m^3; *tetramethyl lead,* 1 ppm = 11.11 mg/m^3; 1 ppm = 1 mg/L.

[b]SKIN designation, indicating potential for dermal absorption.

Data from *Amoore and Hautala, 1983; OSHA, 1995; ACGIH, 1995; EPA, 1996; NIOSH, 1997.

ceed 400 μg/g (400 ppm) (HUD, 1995). The *Environmental Protection Agency* (EPA) and HUD have both recommended the following guidelines for triggering the removal of indoor dust because of increased lead concentrations: 100 μg/ft^2 for dust on uncarpeted floors; 500 μg/ft^2 for dust on interior window sills; and 800 μg/ft^2 for dust in window troughs (EPA, 1995; HUD, 1995). Additional information on the established and recommended guidelines for the prevention of lead poisoning is accessible via the Internet at the website of the National Lead Information Center at **http://www.nsc.org/ehc/lead.htm.**

Organic Lead

The OSHA PEL for tetramethyl and tetraethyl lead is 0.075 mg/m^3 (OSHA, 1995) (Table 4-3). The NIOSH REL for both tetramethyl and tetraethyl lead is also 0.075 mg/m³. The NIOSH IDLH concentration for both tetramethyl and tetraethyl lead is 40 mg/m³ (NIOSH, 1997). The ACGIH has recommended TLVs of 0.1 mg/m³ for tetraethyl lead and 0.15 mg/m³ for tetramethyl lead (ACGIH, 1995). All three organizations have assigned a "SKIN" designation to these two organic lead compounds, indicating that dermal absorption contributes significantly to an exposed individual's body burden and the risk of toxic effects (OSHA, 1995; NIOSH, 1997; ACGIH, 1995).

METABOLISM

Tissue Absorption

Inorganic Lead

The size of the inorganic lead particles, the chemical medium within which they are contained, and the structure of the particular inorganic lead compound all influence absorption kinetics. For example, lead acetate is more readily absorbed via the lungs than is lead chromate in an alkyd resin paint matrix (Eaton et al., 1984). Smaller particles (less than 1 μm in diameter) are deposited in the lower respiratory tract, where they are then absorbed across the pulmonary alveoli (Morrow et al., 1980; Hodgkins et al., 1991). Larger particles are deposited in the upper respiratory tract, taken up by macrophages, and subsequently brought back up the oral cavity by cilia and swallowed (Kehoe, 1987). Pulmonary absorption of the portion of inorganic lead deposited in the lower respiratory tract is nearly complete (Altshuler et al., 1964; Booker et al., 1969; Ogata et al., 1973; Morgan and Holmes, 1978), and the lead concentration in blood begins to rise immediately following inhalation of inorganic lead (Tola et al., 1973). Total daily absorption of inorganic lead in five male volunteers exposed to ambient air concentration of 0.002 mg/m³ was 14 μg (Rabinowitz et al., 1977). The clearance half-life for inorganic lead in the lungs is approximately 8 hr (Jacobi, 1964; Hursh et al., 1969; Booker et al., 1969).

Approximately 10% to 20% of an ingested dose of inorganic lead is absorbed from the gastrointestinal (GI) tract of adults (Chamberlain et al., 1978). GI absorption of lead is significantly greater in children than in adults (Hursh and Suomela, 1968). Approximately 50% of an ingested dose of inorganic lead is absorbed via the GI tract in children; adults absorb less than 20% via this route (Chamberlain et al., 1978; Hammond, 1982). This point is of major clinical importance since the primary source of intake for children is via the mouth due to pica (Hammond, 1982). GI absorption in adults is increased at least fivefold during fasting conditions (Chamberlain et al., 1978; Heard and Chamberlain, 1982). GI absorption of inorganic lead is also greater in those individuals whose diet is deficient in iron, phosphate, calcium, and/or vitamin D (Kello and Kostial, 1973; Quartermen et al., 1975; Heard and Chamber, 1982). GI absorption of inorganic lead was decreased in human volunteers when calcium and phosphate was added to their diet (Heard and Chamberlain, 1982).

Dermal absorption of inorganic lead can contribute significantly to the individual's total body burden, especially during occupational exposure situations in which high concentrations of inorganic lead dust are encountered (Moore et al., 1980; EPA, 1986; Stauber et al., 1994). Contact dermatitis has been reported following exposure to hair dyes containing lead acetate (Edwards and Edwards, 1982).

Organic Lead

Tetraalkyl lead compounds are lipophilic and thus are readily absorbed by the lungs following inhalation exposures and are soon circulating in the bloodstream. Intentional inhalation of gasoline vapors containing tetraalkyl lead for the acute euphoric effects has been associated with an increased body burden of lead (Law and Nelson, 1968; Valpey et al., 1978; Marsh, 1985). The acute psychotropic effect, however, is probably more the effect of the volatile organic solvents (e.g., toluene, n-hexane, and methyl n-butyl ketone) than the absorbed lead content. Heard et al. (1979) exposed human volunteers to radiolabeled tetraalkyl lead and found that at least 30% of the inhaled dose was absorbed via the lungs. Total retention is increased with increasing pulmonary ventilation rate (Wells et al., 1975).

Ingestion of organic lead compounds also contributes to the total body burden of lead (Schepers, 1964; Bolanowska et al., 1967). Studies in rabbits suggest that the GI absorption of tetraethyl lead is slower than is its absorption via the dermal route (Kehoe, 1927, 1987). Tetraethyl lead is more rapidly absorbed via the GI tract of rhesus monkeys than is tetramethyl lead (Heywood et al., 1979).

Dermal absorption of the more lipid-soluble organic lead compounds has been reported in humans and following experimental exposures of rodents (Hamilton et al., 1925; Laug and Kunze, 1948; Hayakawa, 1972; Gething, 1975). Dermal absorption of organic lead compounds is significantly greater than that of inorganic lead compounds (Kehoe et al., 1933; Laug and Kunze, 1948).

Tissue Distribution

Inorganic Lead

Blood lead levels remain elevated after cessation of exposure, reflecting the increased body burden and indicating the potential for accumulation of lead after multiple or chronic exposures (Sokas et al., 1997). Balance and postmortem studies indicate that an average person retains approximately 10 μg of lead a day and passively accumulates a total body burden of approximately 219 mg from the environment after 60 years of life (Thompson, 1971; Barry, 1975). The total body burden of inorganic lead reflects the accumulated amounts absorbed from all sources. Nonoccupationally exposed males carry higher body burdens (mean: 164.8 mg) than do females (mean 103.6 mg) (Barry, 1975; Brody et al., 1994); and both levels were considerably less, however, than those found in seven occupationally exposed males whose mean total body burden of inorganic lead was 566.4 mg (Barry, 1975).

Lead is found in three tissue compartments: blood, soft tissues, and bone (Rabinowitz et al., 1976). Approximately 90% of the absorbed inorganic lead in blood is bound to erythrocytes (Booker et al., 1969; Everson and Patterson, 1980). Soft tissue (muscle and parenchymal organs) concentrations of inorganic lead range from less than 0.1 ppm in muscle tissue to over 2 ppm in the wall of the aorta. The half-life for lead in the blood and soft tissues has been determined experimentally to be approximately 40 days in human volunteers exposed to inorganic lead (Rabinowitz et al., 1976). Inorganic lead accumulates in bone with normal aging. Most of the body burden of inorganic lead is found in bone and accounts for up to 90% of the total body burden in adults. Children have a lower capacity to retain lead in bone than do adults; only about 70% of the body burden of inorganic lead is found in the bone of children, and a higher percentage of an absorbed dose of lead is retained in the soft tissue of children (Barry, 1975, 1981). There are two physiological storage compartments for inorganic lead in bone; one is mobilizable and the other is not. In the first compartment the lead is mobilizable at approximately the same rate as in the soft tissue and thus is readily exchanged with the blood compartment. In the second (dense bone), the lead is essentially inert, with small amounts released daily and a half-life of approximately 25 years (Rabinowitz et al., 1976, 1977; Pounds and Rosen, 1986). The gradual release of lead from bone serves as a continuous source of exposure. Increased mobilization of lead from dense bone can occur during pregnancy, at which time it readily crosses the placenta, exposing the fetus. The infant is also exposed through the mother's milk (Gulson et al., 1997). Mobilization of bone lead also occurs in association with osteoporosis (Berlin et al., 1995) (see Clinical Experiences section).

Inorganic lead readily crosses the blood–brain barrier (BBB) and has been found in the brain tissue of persons with and without histories of occupational exposure to lead (Whitfield et al., 1972; Barry, 1975; Goyer, 1990; Ng et al., 1994; Selvín-Testa et al., 1994). For example, the total brain lead concentrations were 0.58 and 1.02 μg/g in two adults who died of encephalopathy following consumption of lead-contaminated home-brewed alcohol (moonshine) (Whitfield et al., 1972). Regional concentrations vary: the mean concentrations of inorganic lead in the basal ganglia and cerebral cortex of 10 occupationally exposed male adults were 0.29 and 0.65 μg/g, respectively. The lead concentration in the cerebral cortex after exposure was 1.02 μg/g. In comparison, the mean concentrations of inorganic lead in the basal ganglia and cerebral cortex of the unexposed human brain are 0.09 and 0.1 μg/g, respectively. These increased brain tissue lead levels were not age related (Barry, 1975).

Studies on regional distributions of inorganic lead within the human brain have also shown increased concentrations in the hippocampus (Nielsen et al., 1978; Grandjean, 1978) as well as the frontal and temporal cortices (Niklowitz, 1975). Experimental studies in animals exposed to inorganic lead also indicated that a greater accumulation of inorganic lead occurs in the hippocampus (Fjerdingstad et al., 1974; Danscher et al., 1976). Autoradiography revealed the highest lead concentrations in the hypothalamus of the mouse after injection with radioactive lead (Lever and Scheffel, 1998). Selvín-Testa et al. (1994) showed that chronic exposure of rats to inorganic lead induces astrogliosis in the hippocampus and cerebellum. Taken together, these findings suggest that lead is concentrated in several specific brain regions and that region-specific neuropathological findings may reflect variances in the distribution of inorganic lead within the brain as well as the variable vulnerability of specific brain regions, which may have a great deal to do with the neurotoxic effects expressed as developmental neurobehavioral abnormalities (Holtzman et al., 1984; Petit et al., 1983; Scott and Lew, 1986) (see Neuropathological Diagnosis section).

Organic Lead

Organic lead compounds are found in the lipid fraction of the blood and are rapidly distributed throughout the body, with highest concentrations found in well-perfused lipid-rich tissues such as the brain. Although these compounds contribute only a minor proportion of the total lead exposure of most humans, their lipophilic properties facilitate their entry into various body tissues, including the central nervous system (CNS), where they have significant toxic potential (Beattie et al., 1972; Grandjean and Nielsen, 1979; Bondy, 1988). Highest concentrations of the tetraethyl lead metabolite triethyl lead were found, in decreasing order, in the liver, blood, kidney, brain, and muscle tissues of rats that had been injected with tetraethyl lead (10.3 mg/kg body weight). The concentration of triethyl lead in the blood of these same animals declined rapidly beginning on day 3 post exposure, whereas the concentration of triethyl lead in their brains gradually increased from day 1 through day 8 post exposure, after which the concentration of triethyl lead in the brain began to decrease. The concentration of triethyl lead in blood and brains of these animals was at equilibrium on day 16 post exposure (Bolanowska, 1968).

Relatively higher concentrations of lead are found in the human brain following exposure to tetraethyl lead than are typically seen following exposures to inorganic lead compounds, reflecting the affinity of organic lead compounds for the lipid-rich tissue of the human CNS. Nielsen et al. (1978) documented higher organic lead concentrations in the brains of urban dwellers than in rural populations, suggesting greater exposure to environmental sources of lead in urban locales. Postmortem determination of tissue contents of triethyl lead in three persons who died following exposure to tetraethyl lead showed highest concentrations in the liver, kidney, and brain, respectively (Cassells and

Dodds, 1946; Bolanowska et al., 1967). Both volatile and nonvolatile forms of lead are found in the brain and other human tissues on postmortem examination of persons who have died following exposure to organic lead compounds (Norris and Gettler, 1925). The ratio of volatile to nonvolatile lead compounds in postmortem tissue samples reflects the metabolism of the particular organic lead to inorganic lead and the duration of time since cessation of exposure (Norris and Gettler, 1925; Bolanowska, 1968).

Tissue Biochemistry

Inorganic Lead

Inorganic lead reacts with sulfhydryl, carboxyl, phosphate, and amino groups *in vivo*. The sulfhydryl-containing enzymes of the heme biosynthetic pathway are especially susceptible to the effects of inorganic lead (Goering, 1993) and are the targets of lead's critical effect on the hematopoetic system. Inorganic lead impairs heme synthesis and shortens the life span of erythrocytes. Lead inhibits the activity of pyrimidine 5'-nucleotidase. Paglia et al. (1975) have suggested that impairment of pyrimidine 5'-nucleoti-

dase activity may be responsible for the basophilic stippling and premature erythrocyte hemolysis seen with lead poisoning. Inorganic lead has also been shown to inhibit the activity of δ-aminolevulinic acid dehydrogenase (ALA-D) and coproporphyrinogen oxidase (Hernberg and Nikkanen, 1970; Millar et al., 1970; Nordman and Hernberg, 1975; Goering, 1993) (Fig. 4-2). Lead appears to inhibit the activity of ALA-D by preventing the normal binding of zinc ions with the sulfhydryl groups of this heme biosynthetic enzyme (Goering, 1993). The activity of ferrochelatase is also depressed by inorganic lead (Lamola et al., 1975a,b), leading to interference with the incorporation of iron into the porphyrin ring and resulting in depression of heme formation. Zinc is subsequently incorporated into the site, displacing iron and resulting in formation of zinc protoporphyrin (ZPP) (Fig. 4-2). Inhibition of the aforementioned enzymes by lead results in elevated blood and urine levels of the associated heme precursors ALA, coproporphyrin III, and ZPP (Hernberg et al., 1970; Tutunji and Al-Mahasneh, 1994).

Inhibition of heme synthesis also interferes with the activity of other heme-containing enzymes such as cytochrome P-450 and mitochondrial cytochrome oxidase,

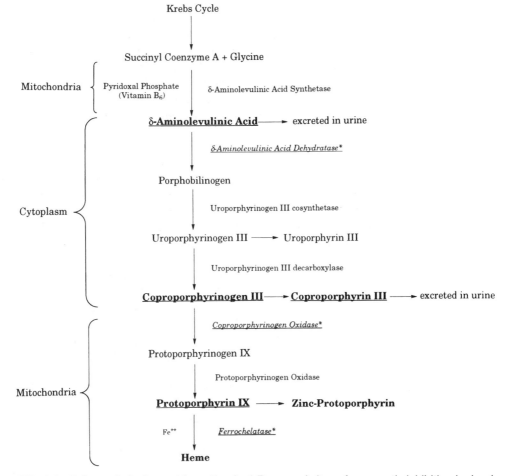

FIG. 4-2. Schematic for heme biosynthesis. *,Proposed sites of enzymatic inhibition by lead.

thereby interfering with biotransformation of other neurotoxicants and cellular respiration, respectively (Goering, 1993; Jover et al., 1996). Furthermore, inorganic lead interrupts neuronal biochemistry and alters the release of neurotransmitters from presynaptic nerve endings. For example, Minnema and colleagues have shown that inorganic lead increases the spontaneous release of dopamine, acetylcholine, and γ-aminobutyric acid (GABA) in the CNS of the rat (Minnema and Michaelson, 1986; Minnema et al., 1986, 1988).

The acute and chronic neurological effects of inorganic lead have been attributed in part to its apparent displacement of calcium ions (Silbergeld et al., 1974; Sandhir and Gill, 1993; Hegg and Miletic, 1996), and its transport into the cell through calcium channels (Simons and Pocock, 1987). The calcium-dependent regulatory enzyme protein kinase C is activated by inorganic lead (Markovac and Goldstein, 1988). *In vivo* exposure to lead increases the activity of calmodulin by 45% (Sandhir and Gill, 1993). Lead interferes with calcium ion currents by acting on voltage-gated calcium channels (Hegg and Miletic, 1996). Inorganic lead has an inhibitory effect on Ca^{2+} adenosine triphosphatase (ATPase) activity, resulting in an increase in intracellular calcium (Sandhir and Gill, 1993). Elevated levels of intracellular calcium normally trigger exocytosis. However, there is also evidence that cell death can be induced by excessive levels of intracellular calcium (Halliwell, 1989). The alterations in intracellular calcium concentrations induced by inorganic lead have also been shown to interfere with mechanisms involved in memory, learning, and neurodevelopment. This may occur as a result of lead's ability to compete with calcium for binding sites. Inorganic lead has been shown to compete with calcium for binding sites on N-methyl-D-aspartate (NMDA) receptors (Marchioro et al., 1996). The role of the glutaminergic system and in particular the NMDA receptor in the long-term potentiation model of learning and the demonstrated effects of lead on the NMDA receptor suggest that mimicking of calcium by inorganic lead may contribute to the cognitive impairments associated with exposure to inorganic lead (Marchioro et al., 1996) (see Neurophysiological, Neuropsychological, and Neuropathological Diagnosis sections).

Increased blood levels of ALA resulting from inhibition of ALA-D have also been implicated as a mechanism of inorganic lead neurotoxicity. ALA crosses the BBB into the brain, where it disrupts GABAergic neurotransmission (Müller and Snyder, 1977; Silbergeld and Lamon, 1982; Solliway et al., 1995). Autooxidation of ALA can produce free radicals, which can subsequently react with membrane lipids and cellular macromolecules (Monteiro et al., 1991).

Concurrent exposure to other neurotoxicants can influence the metabolism and neurotoxicity of lead compounds. The neurotoxic effects of lead are enhanced by current intake of ethanol. Current exposure to ethanol and lead acetate resulted in relatively increased levels of lead in the blood, liver, and brain tissue of rats. In addition, current exposure to lead acetate and ethanol inhibited the activity of alcohol and aldehyde dehydrogenase. Moreover, brain tissue levels of norepinephrine were significantly increased and levels of dopamine and 5-hydroxytryptamine were decreased by concurrent exposures to lead and ethanol (Flora and Tandon, 1987).

Organic Lead

Recent studies on the human metabolism of organic lead compounds have been remarkably sparse. However, earlier studies showed that tetramethyl lead is less toxic than tetraethyl lead (Gething, 1975); the latter is believed to be a toxic metabolite in persons poisoned by tetraalkyl leads (Cremer, 1959; Cremer and Calloway, 1961). The differences in the toxicities of tetramethyl lead and tetraethyl lead appear to be related to the rate at which each is demethylated to diethyl lead *in vivo;* tetramethyl lead is dealkylated more rapidly than is tetraethyl lead in rats (Cremer and Calloway, 1961; Hayakawa, 1972). Metabolism of tetraalkyl leads to trialkyl leads occurs mainly in the liver. Posner et al. (1978) showed that liver microsomal proteins can convert tetraethyl lead to triethyl lead. Further degradation, to dialkyl lead compounds, also occurs in the liver, and the predominant metabolite excreted after human exposure to tetraethyl lead is diethyl lead. However, the dialkyl lead compounds do not appear to be of toxicological significance (Posner et al., 1978; Turlakiewicz and Chmielnicka, 1985). Turlakiewicz and Chmielnicka (1985) reported findings suggesting that the dealkylation of organic lead compounds is inducible. However, the metabolism of organic lead compounds may also result in the formation of free radicals that can induce lipid peroxidation. The existence of this proposed mechanism of toxicity was demonstrated experimentally in rats injected with triethyl lead; the rats exhaled ethane and ethylene (markers of lipid peroxidation) soon afterward (Ramstoeck et al., 1980).

Triethyl lead intoxication results in decreased responses in behavioral tests of pain in animals. Hong et al. (1983) found that five daily doses of 2.5 mg/kg triethyl lead caused a large decrease in metenkephalin in the septum of rats. Since opioid peptides are known to mediate pain perception effects, these data suggest a mechanism for the analgesic and behavioral findings seen following exposure to organic lead.

Trisubstituted organic lead compounds are more effective than inorganic lead in inhibiting a dopamine-sensitive adenylate cyclase in the brain (Wilson, 1982). The trialkyl lead compounds interfered directly with the dopamine receptor linked to adenylate cyclase (D_1 receptor). Wilson (1982) also reported that both basal and dopamine-stimulated adenylate cyclase activities were affected, although the latter was about three to five times more sensitive than the former. It is not certain whether the responsible mechanism is a membrane effect or a specific reaction on D_1 dopamine receptors, but this biochemical effect might be involved in the parkinsonian symptoms seen in some lead-exposed patients (see Clinical Experiences section).

Excretion

Inorganic Lead

The size of the airborne particle of inorganic lead determines whether it will be absorbed via the lungs or swallowed; a smaller percent of the total dose is excreted in the feces following exposure to smaller particles as fewer smaller particles are deposited in the upper respiratory tract, cleared by ciliary action, and subsequently swallowed (Booker et al., 1969). The appearance of inorganic lead in the feces following exposure by inhalation reflects the intake of larger particles, which collected in the upper respiratory tract and oral pharynx and were swallowed. Approximately 90% of an ingested dose of inorganic lead is not absorbed and is excreted unchanged in feces (Kehoe et al., 1943; Booker et al., 1969). Following cessation of exposure, fecal excretion of inorganic lead quickly returns to basal levels, whereas urinary excretion remains elevated until the excess body burden has been eliminated from the blood and soft tissues and the mobilizable fraction in bone (Kehoe et al., 1943; Rabinowitz et al., 1976).

Urinary excretion accounts for approximately 75% of an absorbed dose of inorganic lead; 15% is excreted in the bile, and less than 10% is found collectively in the hair, nails, sweat, saliva, and breast milk (Murthy and Rhea, 1971; Moore et al., 1982). Approximately 4% of an absorbed dose of inorganic lead is excreted in the urine within the first 24 hours after exposure, after which average daily urinary output drops to approximately 1% of the absorbed dose. The urinary excretion half-life is approximately 45 days (Hursh and Suomela, 1968; Hursh et al., 1969; Booker et al., 1969; Campbell et al., 1984). Urinary excretion rates increase during chronic exposures to inorganic lead (Kehoe et al., 1943) (see Preventive and Therapeutic Measures section).

Organic Lead

The metabolism and excretion of organic lead compounds is influenced by the length of the alkyl chains. For example, human exposure to tetraethyl lead at 0.15 mg/m^3 produced urine levels of more than 0.1 ppb, whereas 0.3 mg/m^3 was required for tetramethyl lead to produce urine lead levels greater than 0.1 ppb (Linch et al., 1970; Linch, 1975). Most of an absorbed dose of tetraethyl lead is excreted in the urine of humans as diethyl lead (Yamamura et al., 1981; Turlakiewicz and Chmielnicka, 1985). Yamamura et al. (1981) showed that diethyl lead accounted for about 50% total lead excreted in the urine of a tetramethyl-lead-poisoned patient 21 and 23 days after the exposure incident. About 2% was triethyl lead, and the rest was ele-

mental Pb^{2+}. By day 28, however, diethyl lead content was accounted for only 10% of the total urinary lead.

CLINICAL MANIFESTATIONS

Symptomatic Diagnosis

Inorganic Lead

The rate of accumulation of lead with exposure determines the clinical picture. Recognition of the early symptoms of lead exposure can minimize toxic effects, reduce neurological damage, and thus prevent permanent impairments among susceptible individuals exposed to levels that may have been considered safe (Damm et al., 1993). The nervous system, along with the hematopoetic, gastrointestinal, renal, cardiovascular, endocrine, and reproductive systems, is the target of the toxic effects of inorganic lead (Thould, 1961; Seppäläinen and Hernberg, 1972; Lilis et al., 1978; Feldman, 1982, 1996; Yokoyama et al., 1997). Porphyrias must be included in the differential diagnosis of inorganic lead poisoning, as these conditions can produce many of the GI and neurological clinical signs and symptoms, and biochemical markers of lead toxicity (Dyer et al., 1993).

Acute Exposure

Acute neurological effects of occupational inhalation exposure to lead oxide or lead sulfide vapors occurs where molten lead is found (i.e., during reclamation, smelting, and alloy production processes, as well as during the cutting of lead-painted steel materials). Exposed workers experience nonspecific subjective symptoms of inorganic lead poisoning including abdominal colic, constipation, anorexia, vomiting, headaches, lightheadedness, dizziness, forgetfulness, anxiety, depression, irritability, excessive sweating, and muscle and joint pain (Thould, 1961; Hanninen et al., 1979; Feldman, 1982). The acute symptoms subside following cessation of exposure and the reduction of blood lead levels. Repeated acute exposures or chronic exposures lead to more persistent neurological manifestations including peripheral neuropathy, muscle wasting, and overt neuropsychological impairment. An example is a 34-year-old man worked on a steel structure demolition crew and often cut lead-painted metal pipes with an acetylene torch. He began to complain of constipation and abdominal cramps, and he later developed frequent headaches, lightheadedness, and dizziness (Feldman, 1982). Because these early symptoms were nonspecific, their occurrence was not attributed to his work exposure to inorganic lead fumes and he continued to work. His symptoms progressed and included attention and memory problems; he found that he would easily forget the names of people he had recently met and that he could no longer concentrate well enough to play cribbage, which was formerly his favorite game. A diagnosis of lead neuropathy and encephalopathy was not made until he developed marked extremity weakness, which affected his ability to hold his heavy tools. A blood lead level of 80 μg/100 mL was discovered at that time.

Encephalopathy following acute exposure and the intake of inorganic lead is the most serious consequence of plumbism in children. Although lead encephalopathy is seen more frequently in children with oral intake of inorganic lead in paint chips and soil by pica, it also occurs among adults who have been exposed to inorganic lead from various occupational and nonoccupational sources including the ingestion of lead-contaminated moonshine whiskey (Byers and Lord, 1943; Hess, 1961; Thould, 1961; Whitfield et al., 1972; Needleman et al., 1979; Feldman, 1982; Kumar et al., 1987; Guijarro et al., 1989; Panariti and Berxholi, 1998) (see Table 4-2). Seizures and coma are seen in both children and adults with inorganic lead encephalopathy, and death occurs in the most severe cases (Hess, 1961; Thould, 1961; Perlstein and Attala, 1966; Jacobziner, 1966; Whitfield et al., 1972; Feldman, 1982; Panariti and Berxholi, 1998). The encephalopathy of inorganic lead can be associated with a constellation of symptoms similar to those of a cerebellar mass lesion—increased intracranial pressure with brain edema (Feldman, 1982; Perelman et al., 1993). Neuroimaging studies are useful in the differential diagnosis of suspected cases of lead encephalopathy and intracranial mass lesions (Whitfield et al., 1972; Perelman et al., 1993) (see Fig. 4-5 on page 54). However, reports of findings on neuroimaging studies that mimic mass lesions indicate that the clinician must interpret neuroimaging studies with caution; these should always be considered along with the patient's exposure history and the laboratory test results (Goldings and Stewart, 1982; Pappas et al., 1986; Perelman et al., 1993) (see Neuroimaging section).

Whitfield et al. (1972) summarized the clinical picture of acute lead encephalopathy in the adult after reviewing 27 cases. Urine lead levels were elevated in all patients. Twenty-one (77%) of the patients were anemic, and 70% had marked basophilic stippling of erythrocytes. A gingival lead line was noted in 7 of 15 (47%) of those patients specifically examined for this marker of lead exposure. Cerebrospinal fluid protein content was elevated in 17 of 27 (63%). In nearly all these patients the source of lead was determined to be illicit moonshine whiskey contaminated with inorganic lead that had leached from the batteries used to fabricate the makeshift still. The neurological symptoms varied in severity. Ten patients (40%) were either comatose or semicomatose on admission to the hospital. Eighteen (66%) patients had recurrent seizures that were refractory to barbiturates, diphenylhydantoin, and intravenously administered diazepam but that did respond to chelation with calcium disodium ethylenediamine tetraacetic acid (Ca-EDTA). Lateralized neurological signs were noted in 8 of 27 (35%) patients and included focal motor seizures (5 of 8), hemiparesis (2 of 8), and Babinski sign (1 of 8). Other presenting symptoms seen included confusion (2 of 27),

dizzy spells (2 of 27), lethargy (2 of 27), headache (2 of 27), disorientation, and bilateral blindness (1 of 27).

Chronic Exposure

Perlstein and Attala (1966) reported recurrent seizures in 20% (85 of 425) of children who had been chronically exposed to inorganic lead; 85% of these children had generalized grand mal seizures. Although seizures are a common symptom in lead-poisoned children, the differential diagnosis should nevertheless include other possible etiologies such as cerebral tumor, trauma, subdural hematoma, and meningitis. *In utero* and/or early childhood exposure to lead has also been associated with persistent cognitive deficits (Byers and Lord, 1943; Perlstein and Attala, 1966; Needleman et al., 1990). A childhood episode of severe acute inorganic lead encephalopathy is associated with significant brain damage and persistent cognitive deficits of chronic encephalopathy (Perlstein and Attala, 1966; Feldman and White, 1992).

The symptoms of lead-induced peripheral neuropathy develop insidiously during chronic exposure and reflect the accumulation of lead in the body of an exposed individual. The amount of lead intake generally correlates with the gradual progression in severity of the neuropathy from the subclinical stages to clinically overt signs and symptoms. Recognition of the early and usually subtle sensorimotor symptoms of inorganic lead neuropathy can signal the need for removal of the individual from further exposure and can thus prevent the development of more severe and possibly irreversible nervous system damage. Peripheral neuropathy is typically seen in adults with chronic exposure to inorganic lead and blood lead levels above 70 μg/100 mL (Buchthal and Behse, 1979). Of 25 workers with maximum blood lead levels between 50 and 69 μg/100 mL, 11 reported difficulty walking in the dark; this symptom was reported by only 2 of 20 workers with maximum blood lead levels less than 49 μg/100 mL and only 1 unexposed control subject (Hanninen et al., 1979). Chronic exposure to lead appears to affect the median and ulnar nerves preferentially, and thus patients with inorganic lead neuropathy often present with muscle weakness of the upper extremities and slowing of nerve conduction velocities in the median and/or ulnar nerves (Imbus et al., 1978; Seppäläinen et al., 1975; Feldman, 1982; Bordo et al., 1982). Exposure to lead has also been associated with lower motor neuron damage, but a definite causal relationship to idiopathic motor neuron diseases such as amyotrophic lateral sclerosis has not been established (Simpson et al., 1964; Chancellor et al., 1993; Ng et al., 1994; Ahlskog et al., 1995). Clinical as well as neurophysiological and neuropathological evidence indicates that inorganic lead exposure produces a polyneuropathy affecting upper and lower extremities of exposed individuals (Feldman et al., 1973; Buchthal and Behse, 1979; Hanninen et al., 1979; Feldman, 1982). The isolated mononeuropathies common among laborers are due to secondary compression injuries to the nerves most accessible to trauma. The pathophysiology of lead neuropathy increases susceptibility to damage by repetitive trauma and compression.

Organic Lead

Organic lead poisoning is now relatively uncommon and is primarily seen among workers in the petroleum industry who are involved in the manufacture of organic lead compounds such as tetraethyl lead and in the blending and handling of leaded gasolines (Machle, 1935; Cassells and Dodds, 1946; Boyd et al., 1957; Sanders, 1964a,b; Beattie et al., 1972). Stringent industry safety measures have significantly reduced the number of cases of occupational exposure to toxic levels of organic lead (Machle, 1935; Sanders, 1964a,b; Beattie et al., 1972). However, nonoccupational exposures to toxic levels have continued to occur among those who sniff leaded gasoline for its euphoric effects (Young et al., 1977; Valpey et al., 1978; Hansen and Sharp, 1978; Robinson, 1978; Coulihan et al., 1983; Brown, 1983). The trialkyl metabolites, trimethyl lead and triethyl lead, of the antiknock agents tetramethyl lead and tetraethyl lead are potent neurotoxicants. The clinical syndrome caused by organic lead exposure in humans is different from inorganic lead poisoning because of its prominent CNS presentations rather than peripheral neuropathy and milder CNS effects (Cassells and Dodds, 1946; Sanders, 1964a,b; Seshia et al., 1978; Le Quesne, 1982). The clinical picture typically includes marked irritability, insomnia, disturbing dreams, hallucinations, anorexia, nausea, vomiting, tremulousness, and ataxia. Constipation, abdominal colic, pallor, peripheral neuropathy, and myalgia typical of inorganic lead poisoning are not as common following exposure to organic lead (Machle, 1935; Cassells and Dodds, 1946; Boyd et al., 1957; Young et al., 1977; Valpey et al., 1978; Hansen and Sharp, 1978; Robinson, 1978; Brown, 1983) (Table 4-4).

Acute Exposure

The general pattern following acute exposure to toxic doses of organic lead consists of lowered threshold to external stimuli with increased responsiveness and emotional disturbances (agitation in humans and increased aggressiveness in rats) proceeding to tremors, convulsions, and death (Bolanowska et al., 1967). Other common symptoms include nausea, vomiting, diarrhea, confusion, memory disturbances, dysarthria, auditory and visual hallucinations, troublesome dreams, insomnia, and anorexia (Cassells and Dodds, 1946; Boyd et al., 1957; Beattie et al., 1972; Goldings and Stewart, 1982). Severe tremulousness with choreiform movements and associated gait disturbances is frequently seen in the more severe cases of acute organic lead poisoning. Patients presenting with severe behavioral disturbances, hallucinations, tremulousness, and/or ataxia should be chelated to hasten their recovery (see Preventive and Therapeutic Measures section). The severity of the behavioral disturbances, tremu-

lousness, and ataxia all closely reflect the patient's current blood lead levels (Machle, 1935; Boyd et al., 1957). Symptoms of mild acute organic lead poisoning have been reported at blood lead levels as low as 51 μg/100 mL and typically resolve without therapeutic interventions (e.g., chelation) within a period of several days to a few weeks (Machle, 1935; Boyd et al., 1957; Beattie et al., 1972). Cassells and Dodds (1946) described a young man who developed insomnia and diarrhea 2 weeks after he began cleaning sludge from the inside of gasoline storage tanks that had previously contained leaded gasoline. One week later he began to show signs of confusion and irritability, and his speech pattern was wordy and rambling. He was admitted to the hospital 13 days after the onset of his symptoms, at which time he was violent, suicidal, disoriented as to time and place; he required constant nursing supervision. Deep tendon reflexes were diminished, cranial nerves normal, and plantar response flexor. The patient also had incontinence of bowel and bladder. Laboratory studies at that time showed a urine lead level of 44 μg/100mL and no stippling of red blood cells. His condition deteriorated during the first 2 weeks that he was in the hospital, during which time he developed hallucinations and muscle twitching. The patient began to show signs of recovery during his third week in the hospital; his mental status gradually improved, the muscle twitching ceased, his sleep pattern returned to normal, and he regained control of his bladder and bowel. His urinary lead had decreased to 8.6 μg/100 mL. He showed amnesia for his illness and could only remember that during it he had had bad dreams. On discharge from the hospital he had slight stiffness in both knees, but he was otherwise considered clinically recovered.

Chronic Exposure

Chronic exposure to organic lead compounds is frequently seen among persons who sniff gasoline for its euphoric effects, but the recognition of lead intoxication due to gasoline sniffing is difficult because exposures to the other ingredients (e.g., n-hexane, toluene, petroleum byproducts) in gasoline also produce neurological symptoms. Chronic exposure to organic lead compounds is associated with the insidious onset of a constellation of symptoms similar to those seen following severe acute organic lead exposures but also including symptoms more frequently associated with exposure to inorganic lead. These include abdominal pains, nausea, vomiting, anorexia, hallucinations, attention and short-term memory deficits, nystagmus, tremulousness, ataxia, incoordination, chorea, hyperactive deep tendon reflexes, seizures, and electroencephalographic abnormalities (Law and Nelson, 1968; Young et al., 1977; Valpey et al., 1978; Brown et al., 1983). Responses to tests of sensation are typically normal (Law and Nelson, 1968; Valpey et al., 1978). Basophilic stippling of red blood cells has been reported following chronic exposure to organic lead and may reflect the metabolism of organic lead

TABLE 4-4. *Clinical manifestations of organic lead poisoning[a]*

Age (yr)/sex	Exposure source	Biochemical diagnosis	Symptoms/signs	Other findings	Reference
21/M	Gasoline sniffing	Blood Pb: 269 μg/100 mL; occasional basophilic stippling	Agitation, poor attention and short-term memory; oriented to time, person, and place; tremulousness, ataxia; brisk reflexes; good muscle strength; clinical improvement following chelation	Abnormal EEG	Brown, 1983
16/M[b]	Gasoline sniffing	Blood Pb: 146 μg/100 mL; some basophilic stippling	Hallucinations; tremulousness, ataxia; clinical improvement following chelation	Abnormal EEG	Boeckx et al., 1977
14/F[b]	Gasoline sniffing	Blood Pb: 142 μg/100 mL; basophilic stippling	Frightened; no hallucinations; oriented to time, person, and place; tremulousness, ataxia; chorea; deep tendon reflexes were 2+; good muscle strength; clinical improvement following chelation	Abnormal EEG	Young et al., 1977
41/F[b]	Gasoline sniffing	Blood Pb: 110 μg/100 mL	Agitation; confusion; hallucinations; disturbing dreams; nausea, vomiting; anorexia; short-term memory impairment; oriented to time, person, and place; tremulousness, mild ataxia; hyperactive deep tendon reflexes; normal sensory response; clinical improvement following chelation	Abnormal EEG	Law and Nelson, 1968
14/M[b]	Gasoline sniffing	Blood Pb: 100 μg/100 mL; no basophilic stippling	Hallucinations; oriented to time and place; tremulousness; ataxia; negative Rhomberg's sign; clinical improvement following chelation	Abnormal EEG	Boeckx et al., 1977
46/m[b]	Cleaning gasoline storage tanks	Blood Pb: 92 μg/100 mL	Agitation; confusion; insomnia; disturbing dreams; nausea; vomiting; abdominal pain; headache; dizziness; tremor in fingers	Normal EEG	Beattie et al., 1972

TABLE 4-4. *Continued*

Age (yr)/sex	Exposure source	Biochemical diagnosis	Symptoms/signs	Other findings	Reference
31/M	Cleaning gasoline storage tanks	Blood Pb: 89 µg/100 mL; no basophilic stippling	Agitation; confusion; hallucinations; insomnia; nausea; vomiting; tremor in hands; dizziness; clinical improvement following chelation	Normal EEG	Boyd et al., 1957
47/M[b]	Cleaning gasoline storage tanks	Blood Pb: 80 µg/100 mL	Agitation; insomnia; nausea; vomiting; abdominal pain; tremor in fingers; subsided spontaneously after 2 weeks	Abnormal EEG showing focal sharp activity in right anterior temporal region indicative of a cortical abnormality in that region	Beattie et al., 1972
39/M[b]	Cleaning gasoline storage tanks	Blood Pb: 66 µg/100 mL	Agitation; abdominal pain; clinical improvement following chelation		Beattie et al., 1972
53/M[b]	Cleaning gasoline storage tanks	Blood Pb: 64 µg/100 mL	Vomiting; mild aching in both shoulders		Beattie et al., 1972
28/M	Cleaning gasoline storage tanks	Blood Pb: 63 µg/100 mL; no basophilic stippling	Insomnia; nightmares, diarrhea; vomiting; anorexia; metallic taste; headache, giddiness	Normal EEG	Boyd et al., 1957
25/M	Cleaning gasoline storage tanks	Blood Pb: 56 µg/100 mL; no basophilic stippling	Irritability; impairment of concentration; insomnia; hallucinations; nightmares, abdominal pain; nausea; vomiting; anorexia	Normal EEG	Boyd et al., 1957
41/M	Cleaning gasoline storage tanks	Blood Pb: 51 µg/100 mL; no basophilic stippling	Dryness of throat; vomiting; anorexia, insomnia; tremor in hands; mood swings; clinical improvement following chelation	Normal EEG	Boyd et al., 1957

EEG, electroencephalogram.
[a]Clinical findings and blood lead levels in eight cases of organic lead poisoning.
[b]See text for a more complete description of this case.

compounds to inorganic lead (Young et al., 1977; Brown, 1983). Chelation therapy reduces the symptoms of exposure and hastens recovery (Law and Nelson, 1968; Boeckx et al., 1977; Young et al., 1977; Brown, 1983).

Neurophysiological Diagnosis

Inorganic Lead

In those persons chronically exposed to lower concentrations of inorganic lead the neuropathy and encephalopathy may remain subclinical for years or may become overt following a brief period of higher level exposure. In cases of chronic exposure to higher concentrations of inorganic lead, the differential diagnosis of muscle weakness in the extremities can usually be made purely on the results of clinical and laboratory findings (Simpson et al., 1964). Neurophysiological testing can be used to detect and document subclinical electrical changes and the early neuropathy before the exposed individual develops overt symptoms, thereby preventing acute and/or persistent neurological illness among populations exposed to inorganic lead; such testing is useful as a biological marker of effect from an epidemiological standpoint for determining low-level effects of exposure to inorganic lead (Catton et al., 1970; Feldman, 1973; Seppäläinen et al., 1975; Seppäläinen and Hernberg, 1980; Bordo et al., 1982).

Electroencephalography (EEG) can document the effects of inorganic lead encephalopathy. The EEG in patients with acute inorganic lead poisoning typically shows diffuse slowing and paroxysmal abnormalities (Smith et al., 1963; Simpson et al., 1964; Feldman, 1982; Seppäläinen, 1984). The EEG of a 39-year-old man who was occupationally exposed to inorganic lead revealed symmetrical slowing of the dominant rhythm (7.5 to 8 Hz) and occasional bursts of theta activity in both temporal leads, but there was no evidence of focal or paroxysmal activity (Simpson et al., 1964). A follow-up EEG performed 3 years later revealed the return of the alpha rhythm. In another patient, a 34-year-old man who developed memory and concentration problems following chronic exposure to inorganic lead, the EEG showed bilateral theta activity and a poorly organized and relatively slow (8 to 9 Hz) alpha rhythm (Feldman, 1982). The findings in this patient exemplify the clinical importance of performing complete neurophysiological and neuropsychological evaluations in suspected cases of lead poisoning.

EEG in children reveals the seizure activity associated with current and remote exposures to inorganic lead. Follow-up EEG studies were made in 10 children aged 6 to 11 years who had experienced acute inorganic lead encephalopathy as infants (age range: 9 to 40 months; mean age: 24 months). Five of these children had experienced recurrent seizures following the exposure, and in three children the seizures were still occurring. EEG revealed focal and/or paroxysmal abnormalities in 7 of 10 children. By contrast, the EEG studies were normal in children with elevated blood lead levels but who did not develop overt symptoms of encephalopathy. These findings demonstrated the clinical utility of using EEG studies for documenting pathology and predicting the prognosis of symptomatic children exposed to inorganic lead. Burchfield et al. (1980) evaluated the EEG findings in asymptomatic children with high ($n = 22$) and low ($n = 19$) dentin lead levels. When compared with the low dentin group, the EEGs of the high dentin lead group showed a significant decrease in alpha activity in the parietal and occipital lobes and had a consistently higher percentage of delta activity in the central, parietal, and occipital lobes. In addition, using the findings on these EEG studies, these researchers were able to identify correctly individuals by their exposure groups. Group distinctions were improved to highly significant levels ($p = 0.0002$) when using the EEG findings in combination with the results of neuropsychological testing.

Evoked potentials (EP) can be used to document some of the central nervous system effects of inorganic lead (Seppäläinen, 1978; Otto et al., 1981; Hirata and Kosaka, 1993; Otto and Fox, 1993). *Brainstem auditory evoked potentials* (BAEPs) have been used to document the effects of

inorganic lead poisoning in children and adults (Otto et al., 1985; Robinson et al., 1985; Holdstein et al., 1986). Otto et al. (1981) measured the BAEPs and sensory-evoked slow-wave potentials in 49 children with blood levels of 6 to 59 µg/100 mL (mean: 28 µg/100 mL) and found a correlation between the amplitude of the slow waves and blood lead levels. No correlation was found between the sensory evoked slow-wave potentials and blood lead levels at 5-year follow-up when these children had blood lead levels of 6 to 30 µg/100 mL (mean: 14 µg/100 mL), indicating that the effect found at initial testing was reversed by the reduction in body burden of lead (Otto et al., 1985). However, the BAEPs in these same children at the 5-year follow-up revealed a significant positive linear relationship between the initial blood lead levels and the latencies of waves III and V. These findings indicate that childhood exposure to inorganic lead can disrupt functioning in auditory pathways rostral to the cochlear nucleus and that this effect persists even after blood lead levels have been reduced. Such hearing impairment must contribute to whatever learning disabilities an affected lead-exposed child must deal with as the result of permanent encephalopathy (Feldman and White, 1992).

Somatosensory evoked potentials (SSEP) amplitudes were significantly correlated with blood lead levels in lead-exposed workers (Seppäläinen, 1978). The amplitude of the N18 peak was highest among those workers whose blood lead levels were between 50 and 70 µg/100 mL. Hirata and Kosaka (1993) found a significant positive correlation between blood lead levels and interpeak latency between components N13 and N20 of short-latency SSEPs. These authors also found a significant positive relationship between the N145 component of visual evoked potentials and lead exposure duration. Araki et al. (1987) did not find a prolongation of the N13–N20 or N20–N23 latencies of short-latency SSEPs when comparing the results from lead-exposed workers (mean blood lead concentration of 42 µg/100 mL) with those of unexposed controls. However, these authors did find a significant prolongation of the N1, P2, N2, and N9 SSEP component latencies. In addition, the latencies between N9 and N13 (somatosensory tract from brachial plexus to medulla) were also significantly ($p < 0.01$) prolonged by exposure to inorganic lead. A correlation between alterations in biological exposure indices (urinary coproporphyrins and blood lead levels) and the prolongation of N9 latencies was also revealed by this study; increased blood lead levels and decreased ALA-D activity were correlated with prolongation of N9 latencies. These findings indicate that short-latency SSEPs can be used to document changes in peripheral nervous system functioning in adults occupationally exposed to low levels of inorganic lead.

Nerve conduction studies (NCS) can be used to detect subclinical neuropathy and to document the severity of clinical neuropathy in cases of occupational and nonoccupational exposure to inorganic lead (Fullerton and Harrison, 1970; Catton et al., 1970; Seppäläinen and Hernberg,

1972; Seppäläinen et al., 1975; Feldman et al., 1977; Seppäläinen and Hernberg, 1980; Bordo et al., 1982; Schwartz et al., 1988; Wong et al., 1991). Feldman et al. (1977) demonstrated subclinical effects of lead exposure in demolition workers. Those workers involved in cutting lead-painted steel with acetylene torches showed significantly slower mean motor conduction velocities than did nonburners and unexposed controls, although nonburners also showed slowed nerve conduction velocity (NCV) relative to unexposed controls. These changes were correlated with blood lead levels and free erythrocyte protoporphyrin (FEP) (Fig. 4-3; see Clinical Experiences section).

NCS were performed on 26 workers (18 men and 8 women) who had been exposed to inorganic lead at a storage battery manufacturing factory for durations of 13 months to 17 years (mean: 4.6 years) (Seppäläinen et al., 1975). Motor nerve conduction velocity (MNCV) studies were made in the median, ulnar, deep peroneal, and posterior tibial nerves. Sensory nerve conduction velocity (SNCV) studies were made in the median and ulnar nerves. The conduction velocity of the slower motor fibers (CVSF) in the ulnar nerve was also determined. Neurophysiological testing results from the exposed workers were compared with those from a group of 26 age- and sex-matched controls. During the 4-year period prior to the study the workers' blood lead levels ranged from 20 to 70 μg/100 mL, and their urine ALA levels were consistently below 20 mg/L during this same period. Mean blood lead and urine ALA levels measured on the day of testing were 40.2 μg/100 mL and 7.4 mg/L, respectively. These are relatively low levels of lead body burden among occupationally exposed populations. Motor conduction velocities were reduced in the median and ulnar nerves of the exposed workers. The most significant reductions were seen in CVSF studies in the ulnar nerves. These findings confirmed an early report (Seppäläinen and Hernberg, 1972) indicating that CVSF is a particularly sensitive test for detection of the effects of lead exposure on peripheral nerve functioning.

NCS also indicate that a dose–response relationship exists between exposure to inorganic lead and the development of peripheral neuropathy (Seppäläinen et al., 1975, 1979; Seppäläinen and Hernberg, 1980). Seppäläinen and Hernberg (1980) noted a dose–response relationship while performing a prospective study in previously unexposed workers entering an industry in which the potential for lead exposure exists. The study group consisted of 24 workers who had initial NCS performed within 6 weeks after they began working with inorganic lead. The mean blood lead level in these workers at that time was 15.7 μg/100 mL (control group mean blood lead level: 10.5 μg/100 mL), and the mean blood ZPP level in the workers was 40.5 μg/100 mL (control mean blood ZPP level: 41.7 μg/100 mL). The blood lead and ZPP levels of the exposed workers increased to 30.2 μg/100 mL and 74.4 μg/100 mL, respectively, during the first year of exposure, but both levels

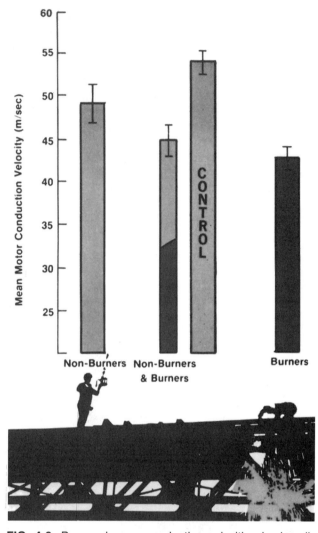

FIG. 4-3. Peroneal nerve conduction velocities in demolition workers (nonburners, burners, and control) showing relation of job task to motor nerve conduction velocity as indicator of lead neuropathy. (From Feldman et al., 1977, with permission.)

remained stable during the second year of exposure. Reexaminations were performed after 1 and then 2 years of exposure to inorganic lead. At that time the motor and sensory nerve conduction velocities in the median and ulnar nerves of the lead-exposed workers showed a tendency toward a decrease, but this difference was not significant when compared with the controls. However, when the exposed workers were divided into high- and low-exposure groups based on blood lead levels (high: more than 30 μg/100 mL; low: less than 30 μg/100 mL), a significant decrease in motor nerve conduction velocity and motor distal latency was seen in the median nerves of the high-exposure group.

Similar dose–response relationships between blood levels of lead and conduction velocity in peripheral nerves were observed in children. Several important relationships between lead level and biological effects were noted in a study of children exposed to particulate lead emissions from a smelting plant. These included a significant negative relationship between blood lead level and hematocrit; increased FEP levels and anemia; and a statistically significant dose–effect relation between conduction velocity and blood lead level (Landrigan et al., 1976) (Fig. 4-4).

Nerve conduction studies documented subclinical peripheral nervous system effects of low-level exposure to inorganic lead from paint chip pica among 24 children aged 19 months to 10 years (Feldman et al., 1973). Eighteen of the 24 subjects had blood lead levels greater than 40 µg/g (40 µg/100 mL) of whole blood (see Biochemical Diagnosis section). The mean peroneal motor nerve con-

duction velocity in the exposed children was significantly ($p < 0.001$) decreased (mean: 42.33 m/sec; laboratory normal mean 52.78 m/sec). These findings demonstrated subclinical effects of chronic low-level exposure to inorganic lead in children and indicate that such studies are useful in determining safe levels and thus in preventing the development of irreversible CNS effects.

NCS revealed a relationship between the incidence of peripheral neuropathy and maximum exposure dose within the 2-year period prior to the study in 62 lead smelter workers (Bordo et al., 1982). The workers ranged in age from 17 to 51 years old and were exposed to lead for durations of 2 to 10 years. Individual mean blood lead levels for

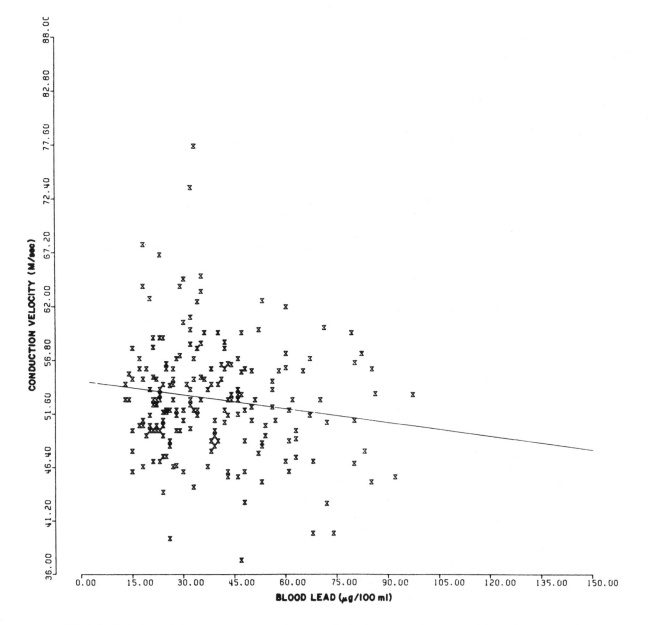

FIG. 4-4. Relationship between nerve conduction velocity in peroneal nerve and blood lead levels in children living near a lead smelter. (From Landrigan et al., 1976, with permission.)

all subjects were less than 50 μg/100 mL over the previous 2 years before the studies; renovations in the facility resulting in a reduction of exposure levels and the institution of a program of regular biological monitoring also began 2 years prior to the study. The workers' exposure to inorganic lead was considered to be significantly higher before these changes were made. To study the relationship between maximum blood lead levels and the development of peripheral neuropathy, the workers were divided into three groups based on maximum blood lead levels reported during the past 2 years (group 1: blood lead less than 50 μg/100 mL; group 2: blood lead 50 to 69 μg/100 mL; group 3: blood lead more than 70 μg/100 mL). The smelter workers were also divided into two groups based on their durations of exposure to lead (group 1: 2 to 5 years; group 2: 5 to 10 years) to investigate the relationship between duration of exposure to inorganic lead and the development of peripheral neuropathy. Twenty-seven hospital maintenance workers without occupational exposure to lead served as control subjects. The NCS were made in the median, peroneal, and sural nerves of these workers. The NCS documented subclinical sensorimotor polyneuropathy in these smelter workers. Maximum blood lead levels within the 2-year period prior to the study were correlated with severity of the neuropathy, but the severity of the neuropathy did not increase with increasing duration of exposure. Details of the results of this study led to the conclusions that in these workers (a) neurophysiological abnormalities associated with exposure to inorganic lead were detected even when maximum blood lead levels had not exceeded 50 μg/100 mL and were more marked at higher blood lead levels, indicating a dose–response effect of inorganic lead; (b) the onset of the neuropathy was rapid and was related to exceeding a threshold exposure level of approximately 50 μg/100 mL; neither the onset of the neuropathy nor the severity of the neuropathy appeared to be related to exposure duration; and (c) the neuropathy was more pronounced in the upper extremities, a finding similar to that of Seppäläinen et al. (1979). No relationship was found between duration of exposure to inorganic lead and the incidence of peripheral neuropathy in these workers.

The distribution of nerve conduction velocities (DCV) has been used to determine the effect of lead on specific fiber populations in the median nerve of workers exposed to inorganic lead (Araki et al., 1986). The subjects included 20 men who had been employed at a gun metal foundry for a mean duration of 10 years and whose current blood lead levels ranged from 22 to 59 μg/100 mL (mean: 39 μg/100 mL); the mean age of these workers was 48 years (age range: 34 to 59 years). None of the subjects had clinical signs or symptoms indicative of lead poisoning. The workers were divided into high (blood lead levels > 40 μg/100 mL) and low (blood lead levels < 40 μg/100 mL) exposure groups and were compared with 20 unexposed controls. The conduction velocities in the slower conducting fibers of the median nerves of the exposed workers were inversely related to the workers' current blood lead levels.

Exposure to zinc appeared to have a protective effect; an increase in conduction velocities in the faster fibers of the median nerves of the lead-exposed workers were correlated with current blood zinc levels, which ranged from 73 to 111 μg/100 mL (mean: 88 μg/100 mL).

Electromyography (EMG) can be used to document denervation of muscle fibers in patients with inorganic lead exposure–induced neuropathy (Simpson et al., 1964; Seppäläinen et al., 1975; Buchthal and Behse, 1979). Simpson et al. (1964) found EMG abnormalities in a 39-year-old man who developed marked weakness and muscle atrophy in both hands following chronic exposure to inorganic lead while cutting lead-painted metal with an acetylene torch. The EMG studies in this patient were made in the first dorsal interosseous muscles bilaterally and in the right extensor digitorum longus. In each muscle there was marked insertion activity and mild spontaneous fibrillations, but no fasciculation potentials were noted. Occasional long-duration polyphasic units were recorded in the right extensor digitorum longus. The number of units recruited was reduced in all three muscles tested. Supramaximal electrical stimulation of the right ulnar nerve was used to assess the response of the first dorsal interosseous muscle of the right hand. The latency of response was within normal limits, and when the muscle was stimulated 50 times per second with supramaximal current, the evoked potential of the muscle did not show a decrement, suggesting lower motor neuron involvement rather than peripheral neuropathy. At the time the initial EMG studies were made, this patient's blood lead level was only 28 μg/100 mL, and his urine lead excretion rate was only 87 μg/24 hr (normal less than 120 μg/24 hr). Nevertheless, because of his exposure history, the patient was therapeutically chelated. A follow-up EMG study performed 1 year later showed discrete motor units in the first dorsal interosseous muscle bilaterally under voluntary control. These were normal in size and contour, and there was no spontaneous activity (i.e., fibrillations). At 3 years after cessation of exposure, follow-up studies showed further clinical improvement in both hands, but no further improvement was noted on the EMG studies performed at that time.

EMG abnormalities were seen in nine of 11 storage battery factory workers (blood lead levels less than 70 μg/100 mL) whose NCV studies in the ulnar and median nerves showed evidence of subclinical neuropathy (Seppäläinen et al., 1975). Evidence of denervation (fibrillations) was present in five of these nine workers. Other abnormalities consistent with a loss of motor units noted on EMG included absence of a full interference pattern at maximal contraction and abnormally prolonged durations of motor units. The EMG studies in 7 of 20 workers exposed to inorganic lead showed an increased incidence of polyphasic potentials in the anterior tibial muscle without fibrillation potentials or positive sharp waves, suggesting regeneration and no further active neuropathy and muscle denervation (Buchthal and Behse, 1979). These studies demonstrate that lead poisoning can clinically and electrophysiologically mimic idiopathic motor neuron disease; it exemplifies the importance of taking a complete exposure history when making the differential diagnosis and performing serial EMGs and also doing careful follow-up examinations (see Clinical Experiences section).

Posturography studies, analysis of postural sway using a microprocessor-based force platform system, indicate that neurological effects of childhood lead exposure persist (Bhattacharya et al., 1995). Results of postural sway analysis in 63 6-year-old children with mean blood lead levels of 20.7 μg/100 mL revealed a significant relationship between increased postural sway and postnatal blood lead levels (Bhattacharya et al., 1990). Posturography in a 15-year-old boy who had been exposed to lead at the age of 2 years and 2 months (blood lead: 56 μg/100 mL; FEP: 430 μg/100 mL) revealed increased postural sway compared with unexposed controls (Bhattacharya and Linz, 1991). These findings suggest that assessment of postural stability may be a sensitive measure of the subclinical neurological effects of childhood lead poisoning (Bhattacharya et al., 1995).

Postural stability was assessed in 60 battery manufacturing workers who had been exposed to lead for a mean duration of 7 years (range: 3 months to 30.5 years) (Chia et al., 1996). Sixty unexposed subjects were also tested and served as controls. Mean blood lead concentration for the lead-exposed workers at the time of testing was 36 μg/100 mL (range: 6.4 to 64.5 μg/100 mL), and while mean blood lead concentration for the controls was 6.3 μg/100 mL (range: 3.1 to 10.9 μg/100 mL). Cumulative exposure indices, based on previous blood lead levels, were established for the lead-exposed workers. The results of this study revealed a significant positive correlation between blood lead levels during the past 2 years and impairment of postural stability in the lead-exposed workers. However, no correlation was found between current blood lead levels or total cumulative blood lead and postural stability, suggesting that the effects of lead exposure on postural stability are not immediately manifested and may be reversible in adults. Linz et al. (1992) reported impairment of postural stability in a 37-year-old construction worker who had been exposed to inorganic lead (blood lead: 109 μg/100 mL). Follow-up testing of postural stability after a 5-day course of chelation with Ca-EDTA revealed improved postural stability. Taken together, these findings suggest that lead affects pathways involved in postural stability (i.e., peripheral nerves, posterior columns of spinal cord, and vestibular mechanisms) in adults as well as children and that the effects in children are persistent whereas the effects in adults may be reversible.

Yokoyama et al. (1997) used computerized static posturography to assess spinocerebellar effects of current and past exposure to lead in 49 chemical factory workers exposed to lead stearate. Current blood lead levels in these subjects ranged from 7 to 36 μg/100 mL (mean: 18 μg/100 mL). Maximum past blood lead levels ranged from 11 to 113 μg/100 mL (mean: 47.7 μg/100 mL). The workers were compared with 23 unexposed male control subjects. The exposed workers showed significantly greater postural sway frequency both with eyes open and closed when compared with the controls. Multiple regression analysis of the data indicated that with eyes open postural sway in the anterior–posterior direction at frequencies of 0.5 to 2 Hz was significantly related to current blood lead levels, whereas with eyes closed postural sway in the medio-lateral direction was significantly related to lead exposure in the past. These findings indicate that subclinical changes in vestibulo-cerebellar functioning occur at a mean blood lead level of 18 μg/100 mL, and that persistent changes in anterior cerebellar lobe functioning occur at mean blood lead levels of 47.7 μg/100 mL.

Organic Lead

Electroencephalography (EEG) can be used to document the acute encephalopathy associated with exposure to organic lead. Saito (1973) performed EEG studies in rats exposed to either leaded (tetraethyl lead) or unleaded gasoline by intraperitoneal injection. The estimated dosage of organic lead in the rats exposed to the leaded gasoline was 16 mg/kg. Baseline EEG recordings were made 1 day before dosing. The EEG recordings in the rats exposed to tetraethyl lead revealed an increase in alpha activity on day 7 post exposure; the EEGs made on day 10 post exposure revealed an increase in slow activity (theta and delta). These findings suggest that tetraethyl lead has a biphasic effect on the CNS of rats.

The EEG of a 14-year-old girl who sniffed leaded gasoline for the euphoric effects showed slowing of the dominant (alpha) rhythm (Young et al., 1977). The EEG of a 15-year-old boy who developed tremulousness and hallucinations following several years of sniffing leaded gasoline (blood lead level on admission: 165 μg/100 mL) showed marked slowing that was more pronounced in the left hemisphere (Goldings and Stewart, 1982). The patient was chelated with Ca-EDTA and British antilewisite (BAL), following which his blood lead level was reduced to 36 μg/100 mL. A repeat EEG was performed after completion of chelation therapy and revealed return of the alpha activity. In a similar case, diffuse abnormalities of moderate severity were seen on the initial EEG of a 21-year-old man with a 9-year history of sniffing gasoline. The severity indicated by these findings were also notably reduced at a follow-up EEG performed subsequent to chelation therapy (Brown, 1983). The improvement of the EEG pattern after chelation therapy demonstrates the usefulness of the EEG for differentiating the persistent encephalopathy seen among solvent abusers from the more reversible effects of acute encephalopathies associated with lead poisoning.

Nerve Conduction Studies (NCS) in persons exposed to organic lead reveal abnormalities in peripheral nervous system functioning. Mitchell et al. (1996) performed NCS in 31 of 58 organic lead manufacturing workers who had been exposed to organic lead for a mean duration of 14.7 years. The mean lifetime blood level among these workers was 26.1 μg/100 mL. Eleven (35.5%) workers had mixed sensorimotor polyneuropathy. It is possible that the neuropathy in these subjects was not entirely attributable to organic lead exposure but rather to a combination of inorganic lead effects and an organic solvent neuropathy (e.g., *n*-hexane or methyl *n*-butyl ketone) from a component of the gasoline mixture (see Clinical Experiences section).

Neuropsychological Diagnosis

Inorganic Lead

Exposure to high concentrations of inorganic lead is associated with acute encephalopathy in adults and children (Byers and Lord, 1943; Hess, 1961; Simpson et al., 1964; Kumar et al., 1987; Feldman and White, 1992; White et al., 1993, 1996; Bleecker et al., 1997). Performance on neuropsychological tests of attention, visuospatial functioning, and memory (particularly visual memory) is frequently impaired. Residual cognitive deficits and behavioral disturbances have been reported in survivors of childhood lead poisoning (Bellinger et al., 1994). Language function is typically spared in adults but is often impaired in those individuals who were exposed to inorganic lead as children (Byers and Lord, 1943; Simpson et al., 1964; Needleman et al., 1979; White et al., 1993). Foundry workers exposed to inorganic lead also showed neuropsychological test deficits in memory (Paired Associate Learning) and in visuomotor tasks (Santa Ana Dexterity Test) deficits (Baker et al., 1984, 1985).

Although many investigators have found lower intelligence quotient (IQ) scores among children exposed to inorganic lead, many of these findings have not reached statistical significance, prompting other investigators to argue that a strict dose–response relationship cannot be established (Harvey et al., 1984; Fergusson et al., 1988). Nevertheless, metaanalysis of the data from 24 major studies suggests that children's IQ scores are inversely related to lead body burden (Needleman and Gatsonis, 1990). Furthermore, from a practical standpoint, a 4- to 6-point reduction in IQ scores results in a shift in the mean IQ curve such that the proportion of children with severe deficits (IQ less than 80) is increased, whereas the percentage of children with IQ scores in the superior range (IQ more than 125) is reduced (Needleman et al., 1979; CDC, 1991).

The effects of ongoing lead exposure in children were reported by Winneke et al. (1985). These authors measured umbilical cord blood lead levels (range: 4 to 31 μg/100 mL), maternal blood lead levels (range 4 to 30 μg/100 mL), and current blood lead levels (range 3.9 to 22.8 μg/100 mL) in 114 6- and 7-year-old children born into families living near a lead-zinc smelter. Each child was

given a battery of neuropsychological tests including the Wechsler Intelligence Scale for Children, the Bender visual performance test, and tests of simple, choice, and serial reaction time. Serial reaction times were correlated with the children's current blood lead levels. Performance IQ was also mildly impaired. Current blood lead levels were better correlated with performance than were maternal or umbilical cord blood lead levels.

Bellinger et al. (1987) studied the relationship between early cognitive development and pre- and postnatal exposure to inorganic lead in a group of 249 children. The children were assigned to exposure groups based on umbilical cord blood lead levels: low (less than 3 μg/100 mL), medium (6 to 7 μg/100 mL), and high (more than 10 to 25 μg/100 mL). Cognitive development was assessed semiannually, from birth to 2 years of age, using the Bailey Scale of Infant Mental Development (BSIMD). Cognitive performance was most impaired among the infants in the high exposure group. Bellinger et al. (1990) reported recovery of function by age 5. Dietrich et al. (1990) also found a statistically significant relationship between pre- or postnatal inorganic lead exposure and decreased scores on subtests of the BSIMD. The mean prenatal blood lead levels in these children were 8.0 μg/100 mL, but 25% of the infants had at least one postnatal serial blood lead level of 25 μg/100 mL or higher. No statistically significant effects of exposure to inorganic lead were found at follow-up testing when these children were 2 years of age, again suggesting recovery of function. However, these findings suggesting recovery function should be interpreted with caution as the neuropsychological tests used by these authors may not be sensitive enough to reflect accurately the more subtle and persistent cognitive deficits associated with childhood exposure to low levels of inorganic lead.

Byers and Lord (1943) reported persistent neuropsychological impairments in persons who were exposed to inorganic lead as children. The overall pattern of dysfunction is very similar to that seen in adults, but language functioning was also impaired. The neuropsychological testing of these children revealed impaired performance on tests of memory (e.g., Digit Spans), visuospatial abilities (e.g., Block Designs), concept formation (e.g., Picture Completion) in 19 of 20 cases. White et al. (1993) reported the results of the comprehensive neuropsychological assessment of 18 adults (7 male and 11 female) who had been exposed to lead as children 50 years earlier. All the exposed subjects were under the age of 4 years at the time of exposure; the mean age of the exposed subjects at the time of neuropsychological testing was 54.4 years (SD: 2.7 years). Eighteen age- and sex-matched subjects with no history of lead exposure served as controls. The blood lead levels of the exposed subjects were not reported, but a review of their medical charts showed that all the exposed subjects exhibited lead lines on the radiograph of at least one long bone and that each child had presented with symptoms consistent with overt lead poisoning, indicating that blood lead levels in all cases had exceeded 60 μg/100 mL. All participants were required to complete a questionnaire on past medical, occupational, and recreational histories as well as their use of alcohol and tobacco. The neuropsychological test battery used included four subtests from the Wechsler Adult Intelligence Scale–Revised (WAIS-R); the Wechsler Memory Scale (WMS); Trails A and B (attention and visuomotor functioning); FAS word list generation test (verbal fluency); Raven progressive matrices (nonverbal reasoning); finger tapping (motor speed); and the Profile of Mood States (POMS). Results of neuropsychological testing revealed significant deficits on the Picture Completion subtest of the WAIS-R and the Logical Memories subtest of the WMS. In addition, the lead-exposed subjects showed impaired performance on Raven progressive matrices and Trails B. No performance deficits were noted on the less complex tests of attention and memory such as Digit Spans. These findings are consistent with persistent impairment of functioning in the cognitive domains of attention and executive functioning, concept formation, and short-term memory. Furthermore, these reveal deficits in performance on complex cognitive tasks that may impede the exposed individual's ability to learn new information. Although such subtle cognitive deficits may not be apparent during most activities of daily living, they can interfere with the exposed individual's academic and occupational achievements and advancement. Subtle cognitive deficits such as those reported in this study are particularly significant among those individuals whose premorbid IQ is below average.

Neuropsychological testing can also be used to detect and document the subclinical and clinical CNS effects of inorganic lead poisoning in adults. A 31-year-old woman who had personally undertaken the job of deleading her recently purchased home developed symptoms indicative of inorganic lead encephalopathy after approximately 9 months of exposure (Feldman, 1982). Her blood lead level was 146 μg/100 mL whole blood. Neuropsychological testing revealed poor attention and impaired memory for new material, especially visual information. Specific tests revealing impairments of CNS function included Digit Span, Digit Symbol, and Block Design. A similar pattern of performance was seen in a 19-year-old man who had worked as a professional deleader for approximately 10 months (Feldman, 1982). His blood levels ranged from 70 to 100 μg/100 mL whole blood. A short while prior to testing he became forgetful and noted feeling "spacy," as if things did not register properly in his mind. Neuropsychological testing revealed impaired attention, short-term memory, and visuomotor functioning. The most severe deficits were noted on tests of visuospatial ability and visual memory. Specific tests revealing impaired functioning included Digit Span, Digit Symbol, Block Design, and Picture Arrangement. Tests of vocabulary were within expectation.

The neuropsychological impairments associated with chronic exposure to lead are often persistent. The neuropsychological assessment of a 39-year-old man who de-veloped encephalopathy and muscle weakness in his upper extremities, both of which were related to his occupational exposure to lead while burning lead-painted metals, revealed impaired performance on tests of memory and abstract reasoning (Simpson et al., 1964). His performance on tests of language function was within expectation. An EEG performed at that time revealed diffuse slowing. The patient began to show clinical improvement following chelation therapy, and there was marked improvement in muscle power 6 months later. At follow-up examination 3 years later, the EEG pattern had returned to normal, and the patient showed further improvement in muscle strength. However, there was little if any improvement in the patient's mental status (see Clinical Experiences section).

Baker et al. (1984, 1985) performed neuropsychological assessments in 99 asymptomatic foundry workers with blood lead levels that ranged from 15 to 80 μg/100 mL and ZPP levels that ranged from 16 to 203 μg/100 mL. Domains assessed included verbal ability, memory, psychomotor functioning, and mood. Performance on tests of psychomotor and memory functions revealed impaired performance among those workers with blood lead levels greater than 50 μg/100 mL. These deficits were not ameliorated by a reduction in lead levels. By contrast, a comparison of responses on the POMS before and after the reductions in lead exposure levels revealed considerably fewer reports of tension, anger, depression, fatigue, and confusion among those workers whose blood lead levels had initially been greater than 50 μg/100 mL. No comparable improvement in POMS scores was seen among those workers whose initial blood lead levels were less than 50 μg/100 mL.

Organic Lead

The severity of the encephalopathy associated with organic lead poisoning has been related to the patient's body burden of lead as reflected by measurement of blood inorganic lead levels (Law and Nelson, 1968; Beattie et al., 1972; Boeckx et al., 1977; Valpey et al., 1978). The CNS effects of exposure to organic lead are those of toxic psychosis, with alterations in consciousness, orientation, and motivation, as well as disturbances in thinking. Organic lead encephalopathy has been associated with acute attention and short-term memory deficits (Boyd et al., 1957; Sanders, 1964a,b; Law and Nelson, 1968; Brown, 1983).

Boyd et al. (1957) reported concentration and memory impairments in a 25-year-old man who had been occupationally exposed to leaded gasoline for only 6 weeks. The patient's symptoms were ameliorated by removal from exposure and chelation therapy. Law and Nelson (1968) reported on the cognitive functioning of a 41-year-old woman who presented with symptoms of organic lead poisoning (blood lead level: 110 μg/100 mL) and an 8-month history of sniffing leaded gasoline for its euphoric effects. Assessment of this patient revealed her to be well oriented with intact remote memory, but her attention span and short-term memory functioning were severely impaired. The patient could not subtract serial 7s from 100 and was unable to perform several other simple arithmetic problems, indicating attention deficits. In addition, her performance on delayed recall tests of short-term memory functioning indicated that she also had severe deficits in this cognitive domain. Her attention and memory functioning as well as her other symptoms of lead poisoning were improved by chelation therapy. In a similar case, formal neuropsychological testing in a 21-year-old man revealed a decrease in his full-scale IQ from a score of 84 at age 13 years to less than 70 when tested after a 9-year history of sniffing leaded gasoline and with a current blood lead level of 269 µg/100 mL (Brown, 1983). An EEG at that time showed severe diffuse abnormalities. Follow-up bedside assessments of this patient's cognitive functioning, performed after one course of chelation therapy (blood lead levels: 165 µg/100 mL), revealed a moderate improvement in short-term memory functioning. Follow-up EEG performed at that time was also improved but still showed a mild background abnormality.

Few studies specifically evaluating the persistence and/or the severity of the cognitive effects of chronic low-level exposure to organic lead in humans have been reported. Mitchell et al. (1996) evaluated neuropsychological functioning in 39 of 58 organic lead manufacturing workers with a mean age of 44.5 years and a mean exposure duration of 14.7 years. The mean lifetime blood lead level among these workers was 26.1 µg/100 mL. Eighteen (46.2%) of the workers had neuropsychological performance deficits. The most common cognitive domains affected were attention, memory, and psychomotor speed. These 18 workers all subsequently underwent additional testing to rule out the existence of metabolic, infectious, or structural etiologies of their performance deficits. No alternative explanation for the neuropsychological deficits seen in any of these workers was found (see Clinical Experiences section).

Biochemical Diagnosis

The use of biological markers for diagnosing increased body burden of lead, whether clinical manifestations are obvious or not, requires careful attention to the time of sampling in relation to the suspected time of exposure (Table 4-5).

Blood lead levels are the preferred method for determination of lead poisoning following recent exposure to inorganic and/or organic lead compounds. However, variations in whole-blood lead, plasma lead, and serum lead are dependent upon methodological and procedural factors. For example, hemolysis contributes significantly to plasma and serum levels (Smith et al., 1998). The mean background blood lead level among nonoccupationally exposed adults in the United States is less than 5 µg/100 mL whole blood (5 µg/100 g whole blood) (Seppäläinen and Hernberg, 1980; Bordo et al., 1982; Brody et al., 1994; Sokas et al.,

TABLE 4-5. *Biological exposure indices for lead*

Determinant	Urine (µg/g creatinine)	Blood (µg/100 mL)[a]	
	Lead	Lead[b]	ZPP
Start of shift	150	30	100
During shift	150	30	100
End of work shift	150	30	100

ZPP, zinc protoporphyrin.
[a]Blood lead unit conversion: 1 µg/100 mL = 0.04826 µmol/L.
[b]See text.
Data from ACGIH, 1995.

1997). The Centers for Disease Control has specifically recommended determination of blood lead levels for the documentation of low-level (less than 25 µg/100 mL) exposures in children (CDC, 1991) (see Table 4-5). A persistent increase in blood lead levels is seen among workers with prior exposures to lead, indicating accumulation and recirculation of lead from storage compartments in soft tissue and bone (Rabinowitz et al., 1976, 1977; Sokas et al., 1997). Blood lead levels reflect concentrations of mobilizable lead in soft tissues and thus are best for documenting more recent exposures.

However, only about 2% of the total body burden of lead is found in the blood, and the exposed individual's total body burden cannot be determined from blood lead levels alone. A relationship between acute blood lead levels and changes in neurological function cannot always be established. The debate concerning maximum acceptable body burden, particularly in children, continues (Feldman et al., 1973; Seppäläinen et al., 1975; Bordo et al., 1982; Needleman, 1993). In 1965 chronic exposure to an ambient air lead particulate concentration of up to 0.15 mg/m³ and a blood lead level of 60 µg/100 mL was considered safe (Kehoe, 1969). The OSHA now requires biannual biological monitoring of all workers at risk for occupational exposure to lead; if a worker's blood lead level exceeds 40 µg/100 mL, the monitoring frequency must be increased from every 6 months to every 2 months until two consecutive measurements are below 40 µg/100 mL (OSHA, 1995). The ACGIH has recommended that blood lead levels of occupationally exposed adults not be allowed to exceed 30 µg/100 mL. To protect the fetus from the risk of developmental effects of lead, the blood lead levels of pregnant women should not exceed 10 µg/100 mL regardless of whether they are occupationally or environmentally exposed to lead (CDC, 1991; ACGIH, 1995). In addition, seasonal effects on blood lead levels among poor pregnant women may result in important intrauterine risks and sometimes underestimates of exposure hazard if sampling does not consider them (Schell et al., 1997).

The prevalence of increased lead absorption, as indicated by blood lead levels and hematological evidence among children (1 to 9 years old) living near a lead smelter was compared with matched children in two control areas (Landrigan et al., 1976). Blood lead levels greater than 40 μg/100 mL were found in 385 (41.9%) of the 919 children examined. Blood lead levels increased with proximity to the smelter stack. Ninety-eight percent (170 of 172) of the children living within 1.6 km of the smelter had blood lead levels greater than 40 μg/100 mL, the highest being 164 μg/100 mL (Fig. 4-4). A strong correlation was found between blood lead levels and estimated exposure to lead in the air, soil, and dust. Blood lead levels were also found to increase with the duration of residence near the smelter. Furthermore, a correlation between FEP and blood lead levels was found, indicating an effect of lead on the biochemistry of erythrocyte formation. A significant negative relationship also existed between blood lead levels and hematocrit values.

Urine lead analysis is a noninvasive method of monitoring for inorganic and organic lead exposure. The ratio of urine lead level to blood lead level (BLL) is higher following exposure to organic lead compounds than it is with exposure to inorganic lead compounds. This distinction can be used to determine whether exposure has been to an inorganic or an organic lead compound (Sanders, 1964a,b). Regardless of the source (i.e., inorganic or organic lead) urine lead levels should not exceed 150 μg/g creatinine in adults exposed to either inorganic and organic lead (ACGIH, 1988) (Table 4-5). Urine lead levels fluctuate with changes in renal functioning and diet and therefore are not as direct a reflection of current exposure as is the BLL. Because urine lead levels are a less accurate estimate of body burden, urine lead is not recommended as a biological exposure index (BEI) for monitoring women of child-bearing age, as this method will not adequately protect the fetus from exposure to toxic levels of lead. Chelation with Ca-EDTA mobilizes the body burden of lead from stores in soft tissues and bone, and determination of urine lead output during the first day of chelation can confirm a diagnosis of lead poisoning if the ratio of micrograms of lead excreted in the urine to the milligrams of Ca-EDTA administered exceeds 0.6 (Chisolm and Harrison, 1956; Markowitz and Rosen, 1991).

Enzymes and products of heme synthesis are useful biological markers of increased body burden of inorganic and organic lead. Lead inhibits the activity of several essential enzymes of the heme biosynthetic pathway including ALA-D, coproporphyrinogen oxidase, and ferrochelatase (see Fig. 4-2, page 37) (Hernberg and Nikkanen, 1970; Millar et al., 1970; Nordman and Hernberg, 1975; Goering, 1993). Lead exposure is associated with decreased blood levels of ALA-D, coproporphyrinogen oxidase, and ferrochelatase and thus these parameters can be used to confirm an exposure (Hernberg et al., 1970; Tutunji and Al-Mahasneh, 1994). Furthermore, the inhibiting effects of lead on these enzymes causes a backup of heme precursors, which can also be used as biological markers of exposure. Exposure to lead results in elevated blood and urine levels of the heme

precursors ALA and coproporphyrin III (Tutunji and Al-Mahasneh, 1994). Increased blood levels of ZPP reflect inhibition of ferrochelatase activity (Lamola et al., 1975a; 1975b; ACGIH, 1988). Red blood cells containing ZPP are extremely fluorescent and thus their presence in the blood can be used to document exposures to lead. Blood ZPP levels reflect chronic lead exposure more closely than do blood lead levels (Chisolm et al., 1975; Fischbein et al., 1980; Valciukas et al., 1981). Background blood ZPP levels in nonoccupationally exposed persons range from 20 to 50 μg/100 mL (Piomelli, 1973; Seppäläinen and Hernberg, 1980; Suga et al., 1981; Valciukas et al., 1981; Franco et al., 1984). The ACGIH-recommended BEI for blood ZPP is 100 μg/100 mL (ACGIH, 1988).

The relationship between blood ZPP and FEP levels is linear and thus blood FEP levels can also be used to document lead exposures (Watson et al., 1958; Joselow and Flores, 1977; Lamola et al., 1975a, Karacic et al., 1980). However, the clinician should be aware that blood FEP levels are also elevated in patients with erythropoietic protoporphyria and iron-deficient anemia (Lamola et al., 1975b). Elevation of FEP alone, especially in females, is not conclusive evidence of lead exposure (Lamola and Yamane, 1974; Lamola et al., 1975a; 1975b; ACGIH, 1988). In addition, FEP levels also do not accurately reflect low-level exposures to lead and thus are not recommended for risk assessment in children; blood levels are the preferred method for monitoring children (CDC, 1991). Thus, an accurate diagnosis of lead exposure, particularly in children, depends on recognition of the clinical effects of lead exposure, determination of an exposure source, and measurement of blood ZPP and lead levels.

Basophilic stippling is another hematologic effect of lead poisoning that is seen on a blood smear and that can be used as a biological marker of lead poisoning. Exposure to lead is associated with shortened erythrocyte life span and an increase in the number of reticulocytes with basophilic stippling (i.e., coarse or fine granules composed of RNA and resulting from aggregation of ribosomes) (Paglia et al., 1975). Although these parameters are not sensitive to low-level exposures, they can be used as adjunct biological markers of inorganic and organic lead exposure (Young et al., 1977; Brown, 1983).

Lead levels in dentin, hair, nails, and bone can also be used as adjunctive biological markers of increased body burden of lead reflecting lead accumulated from past and recent exposures. The less mobilizable lead contents in the dentin of teeth and in hair and nails persist long after exposure has ended (Barry, 1975; Wolfsperger et al., 1994; Gerhardsson et al., 1995; Powell et al., 1995; Hac and Krechniak, 1996). The lead content in the dentin of deciduous as well as permanent teeth can be used to document remote exposures to lead in both children and adults (Altshuler et al., 1964; Needleman and Shapiro, 1974; Frank et al., 1988; Bercovitz and Laufer, 1991; Damm et al., 1993; Gulson, 1996). Increased dentin lead levels have been reported in children living in deteriorated housing as well as those living near other sources of lead exposure (Needleman and Shapiro, 1974; Damm et al., 1993; Bellinger et al., 1994; Gulson, 1996). Increased dentin lead levels have been associated with acute and persistent cognitive deficits, particularly in the domains of attention and executive functioning (Damm et al., 1993; Bellinger et al., 1994). The content of lead in the nails of children exposed to lead is significantly higher than that found in adults, possibly due to age-related differences in the retention of lead in dense bone (Barry, 1975).

Lead is incorporated into the keratin molecules in the hair. Analysis of hair for lead content requires that the sample be thoroughly cleaned to remove external contamination by the apposition of environmental background lead particles (Barry, 1975). The presence of lead along the hair shaft corresponds to the appropriate time of exposure. Evidence of recent exposures are proximal, and that of remote exposures are found in the more distal parts of the shaft. Hair lead levels are distributed relatively evenly if exposure has been continuous, whereas episodic exposures result in sectional differences in hair lead contents (Baloh, 1974; Watt et al., 1995). The mean concentration of lead in hair of nonexposed persons ranges from less than 1 to 5 μg/g (5 ppm) (Watt et al., 1995; Schuhmacher et al., 1996). Mean hair lead concentrations in 502 residents of Tarragona Province, Spain decreased from 8.8 to 4.1 ppm over a 5-year period following a reduction in the use of leaded gasolines (Schuhmacher et al., 1996). A maximum hair lead concentration of 16 ppm was found in a patient presenting with subacute lead poisoning (Watt et al., 1995). Hair lead concentrations are elevated in smokers (Wolfsperger et al., 1994).

Skeletal radiological studies can also be used to confirm a diagnosis of inorganic lead poisoning. Dense metaphyseal bands in long bones, particularly around the knee joint, are indicative of an elevated body burden of inorganic lead. Multiple metaphyseal bands reflect the patient's history of remote as well as current inorganic lead exposures (Woolf et al., 1990). Hu et al. (1994) used a cadmium 109 K radiographic fluorescence instrument to make *in vivo* measurements of bone lead concentration. These investigators determined that the concentration of lead in bone is associated with a decrease in hematocrit and hemoglobin levels in patients with low blood lead levels, indicating that this technique can be used to document low-level exposures to lead.

Cerebrospinal fluid pressure and protein content may be abnormal in cases of inorganic lead encephalopathy. The spinal fluid pressure may be elevated, and protein may be increased (Hess, 1961; Feldman, 1982). The cerebrospinal fluid protein content was 318 mg/100 mL in a 9-month-old infant who died of lead encephalopathy (Pappas et al., 1986). In a 40-year-old man who developed encephalopathy following exposure to the inorganic lead from old batteries, the lumbar puncture revealed an opening pressure of 225 and a closing pressure of 180 mm of water and a protein content of 107 mg/100 mL (Hess, 1961). Repeat lumbar puncture 10 days later revealed a normal opening pressure,

but spinal fluid protein content had increased to 148 mg/100 mL. Fourteen days later the pressure was again normal and the protein content had fallen to 20 mg/100 mL.

Neuroimaging

Magnetic resonance imaging (MRI) and computed tomography (CT) can be used to differentiate inorganic and organic lead poisoning from meningitis, from mass lesions such as a cerebellar tumor, and from other etiologies of encephalopathy (Goldings and Stewart, 1982; Pappas et al., 1986; Perelman et al., 1993) (see Fig. 4-5, page 54). The findings on neuroimaging studies must always be interpreted with caution. The results of the neuroimaging studies are not diagnostic of lead effects and should never be considered in context with the biochemical documentation of the patient's body burden of lead, current clinical manifestations, and clinical response to specific therapeutic interventions such as chelation therapy.

Inorganic Lead

The morphological changes associated with the edema of acute inorganic lead encephalopathy are revealed by CT scan and MRI (Pappas et al., 1986; Perelman et al., 1993). The CT scan of a 9-month-old boy who presented with irritability and decreasing responsiveness revealed dilation of the temporal horns of the lateral ventricles, compression of the fourth ventricle, and low attenuation of the white matter tracts of the cerebellum, reflecting the morphological changes associated with the brain edema induced by exposure to inorganic lead (Pappas et al., 1986).

Although CT scan reveals the morphological changes associated with the edema induced by inorganic lead poisoning, the image produced by MRI may be more diagnostically accurate. MRI allows multidimensional images that are of particular advantage in the diagnosis of posterior fossa pathology (Iwata et al., 1986). For example, the conventional and the enhanced CT scans in a 36-month-old girl who developed tremors and ataxia following a 2-month history of paint chip pica revealed what appeared to be a posterior fossa mass (Harrington et al., 1986). However, a suboccipital craniotomy in this patient revealed edematous but otherwise normal cerebellar tissue. Similarly, the CT scan of a 47-year-old man who developed encephalopathy following exposure to inorganic lead revealed left to right ventricle shift and what appeared to be a mass lesion in the left temporal area (Powers et al., 1977). However, at craniotomy no mass could be found. The diagnosis of inorganic lead encephalopathy in this adult was not confirmed until postmortem studies revealed an elevated brain lead content (right cerebrum: 322 μg/100 g wet weight; left cerebrum 181 μg/100 g wet weight; normal less than 80 g/100 g wet weight). Perelman et al. (1993) used MRI to confirm the differential diagnosis of lead encephalopathy in a 2 1/2-year-old boy who presented with a 1-month history of behavioral disturbances, vomiting, and abdominal colic; his blood lead level was 95 μg/100 mL. The CT scan of this patient revealed displacement of the fourth ventricle and what appeared to be a cerebellar mass lesion that was isodense to the cerebellar white matter. An MRI was performed to confirm the diagnosis and revealed an enlarged edematous cerebellum and protrusion of the cerebellar tonsils into the foramen magnum but no evidence of a cerebellar tumor. The child responded clinically to combined chelation with BAL and Ca-EDTA. Follow-up MRI performed 1 month later was normal (Fig. 4-5).

Organic Lead

The CT scan of a 15-year-old boy who developed tremulousness and hallucinations and whose EEG showed slowing of the dominant rhythm following recreational exposure (sniffing gasoline) to organic lead (blood lead level: 165 μg/100 mL) revealed no gross morphological abnormalities (Goldings and Stewart, 1982).

Neuropathological Diagnosis

Inorganic Lead

Central Nervous System

Cerebral edema is the principal gross neuropathological finding in the CNS of persons dying of inorganic lead en-

cephalopathy (Whitfield et al., 1972). The edema is associated with arterial hypertension and purpuric hemorrhagic extravations. The brain is swollen and soft, with flattened gyri and narrow sulci (Powers et al., 1977) (Fig. 4-6). The gray matter appears thicker and more translucent than normal (Blackman, 1937; Whitfield et al., 1972; Powers et al., 1977; Wong et al., 1991). The leptomeninges are congested (Popoff et al., 1963). The cerebellum may be preferentially affected by acute swelling (Bucy and Buchanan, 1935; Biemond and Van Creveld, 1939; Popoff et al., 1963; Tonge et al., 1977; Pappas et al., 1986).

Microscopic examination of the brain reveals vascular changes in the gray and white matter, which include capillary narrowing as well as dilation and capillary thrombi; necrotic vessels are also present. The toxic effects of lead on the endothelial cells of brain capillaries also increase the permeability of the BBB (Goldstein, 1984). The normal cellular architecture is disrupted by the edema; nerve fibers are stretched and torn by the infiltrating exudate. There is typically a ring of glial proliferation seen around areas of focal necrosis (Blackman, 1937; Nordberg, 1975; Wong et al., 1991). There are often focal and diffuse changes in the white matter including fragmentation of myelin sheaths and reactive astrocytosis (Popoff et al., 1963). Glial cells containing lipid globules and yellowish brown granules are seen around the arterioles in the white matter. Diffuse neuronal loss is seen throughout the gray matter, including neurons of Ammon's horn of the hippocampus. The basal

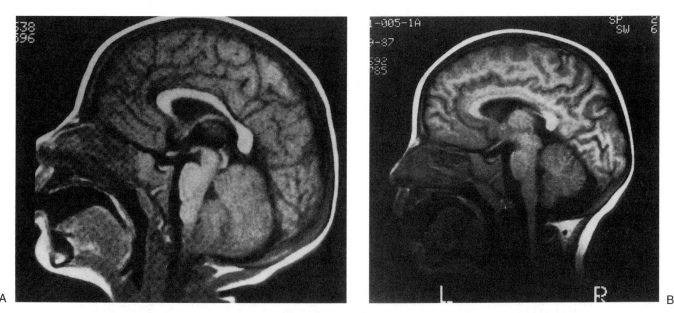

FIG. 4-5. The MRI of a 2½-year-old boy whose initial CT scan showed evidence of a cerebellar mass. The MRI of this patient ruled out a cerebellar mass and confirmed the differential diagnosis of edema related to lead poisoning. **A:** T_1-weighted image showing an enlarged cerebellum and disappearance of the fissurae cerebelli. The cerebellar tonsils are in a low position at the levels of the foramen magnum, and the fourth ventricle is compressed. **B:** Follow-up MRI (T_1-weighted image) performed 1 month after chelation therapy and removal from further exposure shows a normal-sized cerebellum with the return of the fissurae cerebelli. (From Perelman et al., 1993, with permission.)

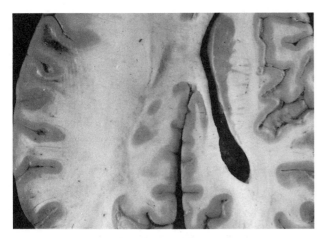

FIG. 4-6. Horizontal section of the brain of a 47-year-old man who died following consumption of illicit whiskey that was contaminated with inorganic lead. Left posterior frontal and parietal lobes are enlarged, wet, and soft; the ventricle is collapsed and the gyri are flattened. (From Powers et al., 1977, with permission.)

ganglia, pons, and medulla show focal areas of necrosis. Marked loss of Purkinje cells is seen in the cerebellum. The remaining Purkinje cells of the cerebellum are vacuolated, and the Purkinje cell layer is spongy (Blackman, 1937; Popoff et al., 1963). Focal necrosis of the cerebral cortex is also seen. Large astrocytes with vesicular nuclei and hyaline cytoplasm are seen in the gray and white matter of the cerebral cortex. Various stages of neuronal degeneration and patchy demyelination and proliferation of glia are also noted. Vascular congestion is occasionally seen, and perivascular monocytic and polymorphonuclear leukocytic infiltrations are seen around the smaller capillaries (Blackman, 1937).

Experimental studies of the developmental effects of inorganic lead exposure on the CNS in rats revealed neuropathological changes including edema and focal perivascular hemorrhages in the gray matter of the cerebellum. Gitter cells, together with degeneration and loss of Purkinje cells, were observed. Regional atrophy, cavitation, and degeneration of the white matter were also noted (Clasen et al., 1974; Hirano and Kochen, 1976). Chronic postnatal exposure of rats to inorganic lead at concentrations below those that produce overt intoxication induces astrogliosis in cells of the hippocampus and cerebellum (Selvín-Testa et al., 1994). The cells in the hippocampus undergo extensive postnatal development, and studies on the developmental effects of lead in rats indicate that the dentate gyrus of the hippocampus is particularly sensitive to the effects of inorganic lead (Petit et al., 1983), possibly because lead displaces zinc, which is normally found in high concentrations in the hippocampus (Fjerdingstad et al., 1974; Campbell et al., 1982). Lead-containing intranuclear inclusion bodies are seen in astrocytes, a finding suggesting that proliferation of astrocytes may be a neuroprotective response (Goyer et al., 1971; Holtzman et al.,

1984). Scott and Lew (1986) have suggested that neuronal and nonneuronal cells undergoing mitosis are particularly vulnerable to the effects of lead. This hypothesis may account for the differential susceptibility of the developing and mature CNS to the effects of inorganic lead.

Peripheral Nervous System

The neuropathological effects of inorganic lead on the peripheral nervous system include primary segmental demyelination and secondary axonal degeneration (Dyck et al., 1977; Low and Dyck et al., 1977; Ohnishi et al., 1977; Buchthal and Behse, 1979; Wong et al., 1991). Postmortem examination of a 2-month girl who died following acute lead poisoning revealed segmental demyelination of the median nerve (Wong et al., 1991). Buchthal and Behse (1979) performed sural nerve biopsies in eight lead smelter workers in whom neurophysiological evidence of neuropathy had previously been documented. One of the eight workers, a 58-year-old man who was exposed to lead for 13 years, had clinically overt signs and symptoms of peripheral neuropathy while the other seven workers were asymptomatic. Microscopic examination of the teased fibers from the man with overt neuropathy did not show evidence of active segmental demyelination, although areas of segmental remyelination were noted (Fig. 4-7). The findings in this man are consistent with his history of two previous severe acute exposures during which he experienced nausea, vomiting, constipation, abdominal colic, and the onset of polyneuropathy. The first incident occurred after he had been working with lead for only 1 year, at which time laboratory tests revealed a uring lead level of 185 μg/L and basophilic stippling of red blood cells. The second incident occurred approximately 1 year before the current investigation, at which time laboratory tests again revealed basophilic stippling of red blood cells and a urine lead level of 200 μg/L. Light microscopic studies of the teased fibers from the seven asymptomatic workers revealed morphological evidence of paranodal demyelination and reduced diameters of the myelin sheaths at the internodes, although the width of the internodes was normal. A slight increased incidence of remyelination was also noted. Electron microscopic studies of the myelinated nerve fibers from this same group showed increased numbers of bands of Büngner, indicating remyelination. Among the unmyelinated fibers there was an increased incidence of fibers currently undergoing degeneration; these fibers were characterized by a loss of organelles.

Ultrastructural studies of inorganic lead-induced peripheral neuropathy reveal necrotic endothelium, basement membrane reduplication, reactive pericytes, and mural thickening of vessels (Myers et al., 1980). Dyck et al. (1977) noted that elevated endoneurial pressure and edema occur at approximately the same time as does the onset of segmental demyelination in rats exposed to inorganic lead. Myers et al. (1980) identified intranuclear inclusion bodies reflecting the deposition of

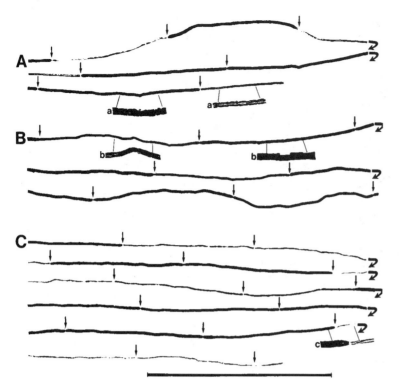

FIG. 4-7. Sural nerve biopsy from a 58-year-old lead-smelter worker who developed overt polyneuropathy after exposure to inorganic lead (current BLL: 50 μg/100 mL) (see text). **A–C:** Sections of the same teased nerve fiber revealing normal and smaller diameters of the myelin sheath and reflecting areas of prior segmental demyelination and remyelination. Inset figures (*a, b,* and *c*) are higher magnifications of fibers showing areas of normal and smaller diameter myelin sheaths. The magnification is indicated by the scale at the bottom of the figure; it is 1 mm for **A, B,** and **C;** and 0.3 mm for *a, b,* and *c.* The perpendicular arrows indicate nodes of Ranvier. (From Buchthal and Behse, 1979, with permission.)

lead in Schwann cells and suggesting that lead may also have a direct toxic effect on Schwann cells; lead-induced intranuclear inclusion bodies have also been found in renal tubular cells (Goyer and Wilson, 1975).

The increase in the permeability of the blood–nerve interface may be an adaptive response to demyelination and associated changes in the osmolity of the endoneurial microenvironment (Weerasuriya et al., 1990). Studies show that the accumulation of lead in the endoneurium and onset of edema precede changes in the permeability of the blood–nerve interface (Windebank et al., 1980; Weerasuriya et al., 1990). Sobue and Pleasure (1985) have shown that inorganic lead inhibits the proliferation of Schwann cells, indicating that a direct toxic effect may be responsible for the morphological changes associated with exposure to inorganic lead.

Animal studies have also revealed segmental demyelination and axonal degeneration following exposure to inorganic lead (Lampert and Schochet, 1968; Fullerton, 1966; Dyck et al., 1977; Ohnishi et al., 1977). The degree of axonal involvement is related to the severity of the lead neuropathy. *In vitro* studies indicate that Schwann cells are more sensitive to the effects of inorganic lead than are neurons (Scott and Lew, 1986). Ohnishi and Dyck (1981) have shown that lead reduces Schwann cell mitosis by 50%. These findings suggest that the peripheral axonopathy reported by some investigators may be secondary to a concomitant decrease in the availability of neuronotropic factors. Dyck et al. (1977) reported that Schwann cells in rats are randomly affected by inorganic lead, indicating that segmental demyelination is a primary event and is not sec-ondary to axonal degeneration. The myelin sheaths begin to disintegrate at the nodes of Ranvier in rats; electron micrographs reveal separation of the myelin lamellae. The basement lamina remains intact. Repeated demyelination and remyelination leads to the formation of onion bulbs around the affected axons (Lampert and Schochet, 1968).

Ohnishi et al. (1977) performed morphometric analyses of the neuropathy in rats exposed to a diet containing 4% lead carbonate for 3 and 6 months. Microscopic examinations of teased sural and peroneal nerve fibers from these animals revealed segmental demyelination that occurred with about the same frequency in proximal and distal segments of the axons. After 3 months, approximately one-third of the teased myelinated fibers showed segmental demyelination; after 6 months of exposure, approximately four-fifths of the myelinated fibers showed such changes, indicating that the severity of the neuropathy in cases of inorganic lead poisoning is related at least in part to the duration of exposure. Similar results were reported by Lampert and Schochet (1968).

A considerable body of evidence indicates that lead is substituted for calcium *in vivo* (Silbergeld et al., 1974; Sandhir and Gill, 1994; Albano et al., 1994; Hegg and Miletic, 1996). Inorganic lead is apparently transported into the cell through calcium channels (Simons and Pocock, 1987). Holtzman et al. (1984) have suggested that inorganic lead may impair mitochondrial function by competing with calcium. The calcium-dependent regulatory enzyme, protein kinase C, is activated by inorganic lead (Markovac and Goldstein, 1988). *In vivo* exposure to lead increases the activity of calmodulin by 45% (Sandhir and

Gill, 1994). Lead apparently interferes with calcium currents by acting on voltage-gated calcium channels (Hegg and Miletic, 1996). Inorganic lead has an inhibitory effect on Ca^{2+} ATPase activity, resulting in an increase in intracellular calcium (Sandhir and Gill, 1994; Albano et al., 1994).

Calcium has been identified as a second messenger in neuronal transmission; elevated levels of intracellular calcium normally trigger exocytosis. Altered calcium homeostasis interferes with cellular processes such as the release of neurotransmitters. There is also evidence that cell death can be induced by excessive levels of intracellular calcium (Halliwell, 1989). Inorganic lead has also been shown to interfere with mechanisms involved in memory, learning, and neurodevelopment. Inorganic lead has been shown to compete with calcium for binding sites on NMDA receptors (Marchioro et al., 1996). The role of the glutaminergic system, in particular on the NMDA receptor in the long-term potentiation model of learning, and the demonstrated effects of lead on the NMDA receptor suggest that mimicking of calcium effect by inorganic lead may contribute to the cognitive impairments associated with exposure to inorganic lead (Marchioro et al., 1996).

Organic Lead

Most information available about the neuropathological changes associated with severe acute organic lead poisoning derives from experimental studies and not human postmortem reports. For example, experimental exposure to tetraalkyl lead by inhalation in rats and dogs resulted in brain lead levels at time of death of 10 μg/g. Morphological changes observed in these animals included various degenerative changes affecting neurons in the spinal cord, medulla oblongata, pons, cerebellar cortex, midbrain, thalamus, basal ganglia, and neocortex (Davis et al., 1963; Schepers, 1964). Lesions are seen in the hippocampus, amygdaloid nucleus, caudate, and thalamus, and changes in various brainstem nuclei including the red nucleus have been noted following exposure of rats to triethyl lead and trimethyl lead (Seawright et al., 1980). Exposure to trialkyl lead is associated with mitochondrial swelling. Another neuropathological finding noted in trialkyl lead is the accumulation of multilaminar bodies in the parykaryon (Seawright et al., 1984).

Ultrastructural studies of the brains of rabbits exposed to organic lead compounds revealed that initial changes occur in the nuclei of neurons, which showed irregular nuclear membranes, condensation, and increased osmiophilia of the chromatin. Hypertrophy of the Golgi complex, marked swelling and loss of cristae of mitochondria, dilation of the endoplasmic reticulum, degeneration of the rough endoplasmic reticulum, and dispersion of the polyribosomes followed the nuclear changes. Proliferation of neurofibrils in the cytoplasm was noted in many of the affected neurons. Astrocytes in the affected region were frequently swollen (Niklowitz, 1974, 1975; Manthos et al., 1980).

Chang et al. (1984) and Walsh et al. (1986) compared the neurotoxic effects of triethyl lead and trimethyl lead in rats. Triethyl lead induced mitochondrial changes in the dorsal root ganglion neurons; these neuropathological changes were associated with sensory disturbances. Accumulations of lysosomes and disintegration of Nissl substance were also noted. By contrast, trimethyl lead exposure was associated with extensive chromolytic and degenerative changes in large brainstem neurons and anterior horn cells. Neuronal swelling and necrosis were observed in the hippocampus after both triethyl and trimethyl lead exposure.

The neuropathological effects of alkyl lead on the developing brain have been studied experimentally following both pre- and postnatal exposures. The neonatal brain shows more morphological changes than the adult brain following exposure to organic lead. Brain growth is depressed by neonatal exposure to triethyl lead, and it appears that the oligodendrocyte viability, and hence myelin formation, is particularly sensitive to these effects of triethyl lead (Konat and Clausen, 1974; Konat et al., 1976).

PREVENTIVE AND THERAPEUTIC MEASURES

Workers at risk of exposure to lead (inorganic or organic) should undergo regular biological monitoring according to the guidelines mandated by OSHA. Signs must be posted in all areas where the potential for exposure to lead concentrations above the current PEL exists. Respirators must be provided and used by those workers at risk of exposure to higher concentrations (more than 0.5 mg/m³) (OSHA, 1995). Gloves and protective garments should be worn by workers at risk of exposure to organic lead compounds. The work area should be maintained as free of lead accumulations as possible. Vacuuming is the preferred cleaning method; compressed air should not be used to displace accumulations of lead (OSHA, 1995; HUD, 1995). To minimize ingestion of lead compounds, workers should always wash their hands before eating and should not eat or drink in the work area. To prevent contamination of the employee's home and exposure of family members to lead, workers exposed to lead compounds should shower and change into clean clothing before leaving work; work clothing should be laundered at the work site (Baker et al., 1977; Rice et al., 1978; Ghiaradia et al., 1997).

Workers involved in the deleading and/or restoration of older buildings should wear dust masks and gloves at all times. Whenever possible, the lead-painted surface should simply be covered. Persons involved in the removal of lead-based paint should follow the HUD guidelines. Suggested methods of lead paint removal include heat guns, as well as sanders and blasters that are equipped with a high-efficiency particulate air vacuum system, and/or wet scraping. Open flame burning and traditional power sanding and abrasive blasting techniques all release lead particulate into the atmosphere and are prohibited by HUD. Dry scraping is permitted when necessary but is not recommended for similar reasons (HUD, 1995). Following removal, the paint chips, particles, and dust must be properly disposed of. Additional current and accurate information on the prevention of lead poisoning is accessible via the Internet at the website of the National Lead Information Center at ***http://www.nsc.org/ehc/lead.htm.***

If biological monitoring reveals an elevated body burden of lead in an asymptomatic worker, he or she should immediately be removed from further exposure to lead. When overt symptoms of peripheral neuropathy are seen, the worker should be chelated. However, prophylactic chelation of occupationally exposed individuals is not recommended (Baker et al., 1980; OSHA, 1995).

Early recognition of exposure to inorganic lead is essential to the prevention of permanent neurological sequelae in children. Whereas parents, physicians, politicians, and attorneys are impressed by the catastrophic symptoms of childhood lead poisoning such as recurrent seizures, coma, and respiratory arrest, the early and less severe symptoms frequently go unrecognized or ignored (Greengard, 1966). Thus the pediatrician and primary care physician as well as other professionals involved in the welfare of children, need to be aware of the subtle early clinical manifestations of inorganic lead poisoning as well as the most current biochemical, neurophysiological, and neuropsychological methods available for detection and documentation of subclinical effects (see Biochemical, Neurophysiological, and Neuropsychological Diagnosis sections).

Physicians should always inquire about a child's history of pica and other mouthing behaviors. If the history is positive, the physician should inform the parents of the risks of lead poisoning associated with pica. Children with a history of pica should be watched closely and discouraged from eating soil that may be contaminated with paint chips. Individuals responsible for the welfare of children should also be aware of the early symptoms of poisoning including irritability, abdominal colic, constipation, anorexia, vomiting, and/or pallor. When reasonable suspicion of lead poisoning exists, the child should be referred to a physician and appropriate laboratory analysis performed to determine the child's body burden of lead.

Biochemical testing for lead should also be made if the child has a positive history of pica and any early symptoms of lead poisoning (Jacobziner, 1966). Because iron deficiency can enhance absorption of lead, children with blood lead levels greater than 20 µg/100 mL should also be tested for iron deficiency. The Ca-EDTA provocative chelation test can be used to confirm lead poisoning. An iron deficiency can alter the outcome of the provocative chelation test and therefore should not be done on iron-deficient patients (Markowitz et al., 1990). Before provocative chelation is begun, the patient must empty his or her bladder. Following evacuation of the bladder the patient can be administered 500 mg/m^2 of Ca-EDTA in 5% dextrose infused over 1 hr. Alternatively, the same dose of Ca-EDTA can be administered intramuscularly in solution with 0.5% procaine. The urine excreted over the next 8 hr must be collected in a lead-free apparatus (CDC, 1991). The total urinary excretion of lead is divided by the amount of Ca-EDTA given. An 8-hr Ca-EDTA provocative chelation test is considered positive if the lead excretion ratio is greater than 0.6 (Markowitz and Rosen, 1991).

The mortality rate among lead-poisoned children presenting with seizures is high (Pappas et al., 1986). Brain edema should be managed urgently by restriction of water intake and administration of mannitol or corticosteroids (Perelman et al., 1993). The use of anticonvulsants in the management of seizures associated with inorganic lead poisoning is generally not satisfactory, but diazepam may be administered empirically (Hess, 1961; Jacobziner, 1966; Powers et al., 1977; Kumar et al., 1987; Perelman et al., 1993). Although the use of NMDA receptor blockers such as felbamate seems warranted in light of the ability of inorganic lead to alter glutaminergic activity, there is evidence that this type of antiepileptic drug may exacerbate the acute porphyria associated with lead poisoning (Hahn et al., 1997). In addition, studies indicate that NMDA receptor blockers may exacerbate epileptic activity in children (Stafstrom et al., 1997). Children with blood lead levels greater than 70 µg/100 mL represent an acute medical emergency and should be chelated immediately (CDC, 1991). Chelation therapy should be administered to reduce the patient's body burden of lead and to hasten alleviation of the brain edema. Combined administration of BAL and Ca-EDTA is recommended for the treatment of acute lead encephalopathy in children and adults. The course is started with BAL at 3 to 5 mg/kg deep i.m.; subsequently, beginning 4 hr later, BAL and Ca-EDTA are administered simultaneously but in separate deep i.m. sites every 4 hr for the next 5 days at doses of 3 to 5 mg/kg and 25 mg/kg, respectively. Chelation with Ca-EDTA alone can be used in patients presenting with lead neuropathy. Intramuscular or intravenous administration of Ca-EDTA in divided doses of 50 to 75 mg/kg every 12 hours for a 3- to 5-day course with a 2- to 3-week rest between courses until the patient's blood lead levels are within normal range is recommended.

Chelation of children with blood lead levels less than 45 µg/100 mL can be accomplished orally with meso-2,3-dimercaptosuccinic acid (DMSA; succimer) and penicillamine (CDC, 1991). Although multiple courses of chelation will temporarily reduce the individual's body burden of lead, the long-term case management of lead poisoning requires a permanent reduction in exposure and correction of the toxic hazards (Chisolm, 1990; CDC, 1991).

Long-term management of children who survive the acute encephalopathy associated with inorganic lead poisoning must be tailored to the specific case. When impaired cognitive functioning and/or behavioral problems results in poor performance in school, specific interventions ranging from tutoring in milder cases to special education programs for more severely affected children may be necessary (Byers and Lord, 1943; Feldman and White, 1992; White et al., 1993).

CLINICAL EXPERIENCES

Group Studies

Inorganic Lead

Neurobehavioral Manifestations among Lead Foundry Workers

A longitudinal epidemiological study performed by Baker et al. (1984; 1985) evaluated the effects of inorganic lead on the neuropsychological and neurophysiological functioning of foundry workers before and after a marked reduction in employee lead exposure. The initial evaluations were performed immediately before the institution of an OSHA-mandated reduction in lead exposure levels. Ninety-nine asymptomatic workers and 61 unexposed controls were tested at that time. Blood lead levels in the exposed workers at the initial evaluations ranged from 15 to 80 µg/100 mL, and ZPP levels ranged from 16 to 203 µg/100 mL. Lead melters were exposed to the highest concentrations of inorganic lead and had mean blood lead levels of 66.4 µg/100 mL (range: 43 to 80 µg/100 mL) and mean ZPP levels of 118.9 µg/100 mL (range: 22 to 138 µg/100 mL).

SNCVs were slowed and amplitudes reduced in the sural nerves of these workers. In addition, this finding was correlated with current and cumulative exposure indices of these inorganic lead–exposed workers. MNCV studies in the peroneal and ulnar nerves of these workers were within normal ranges. Neuropsychological assessments of these workers documented acute and persistent deficits (see Neuropsychological Diagnosis section).

Subacute Effects of Lead-Oxide Fumes in Demolition Workers

Burners on a demolition job had average exposures of as high as 15.0 mg/m³, 100 times the proposed standard and 10 times the level for which the usual respirators are considered adequate. The average personal breathing zone air concentration for 32 burner workers was 4.36 mg/m³, whereas the mean was 0.23 mg/m³ for 12 measurements of nonburner workers employed in the vicinity of the burning. These nonburners included laborers and supervisory personnel. The blood lead levels of the burners ranged from 44 to 100 µg/100 mL (mean: 79.5 µg/100 mL). The nonburners had a mean blood lead level of 48.8 µg/100 mL (range: 24 to 75 µg/100 mL). The nonburners offered no complaints, whereas the burners experienced nausea, abdominal discomfort, mood change and irritability, sleeplessness, fatigue, headache, and numbness and tingling of the extremities. Only four of the burners had no

complaints. None of the workers had diabetes, although four burners and one nonburner had a significant intake of alcohol. The burners had an average hematocrit of 41.4%, and the nonburners had an average of 44.0% (normal: 45% to 52%). The mean FEP of the burners was 1134 µg/100 mL red blood cells; for the nonburners, it was 714 µg/100 mL. The normal value is 46.9 ± 14.9 µg/100 mL. Thus, although there was not a significant difference between the hematocrit levels of the burners and nonburners, both groups had FEP values considerably different from normal. FEP was positively correlated with blood lead levels ($r = 0.73$; $p < 0.001$). Peroneal MNCV of the 13 burners had a mean of 43.2 m/sec, and was significantly different ($p < 0.02$) from the mean (49.0 m/sec) of six nonburners. Each group, as well as the combined worker groups, differed from the control mean (54.09 ± 5.96 m/sec) for men of the same age. All the nonburners had been on the job for 4 to 10 months, but the burners had as little as 1 month of exposure before symptoms and other signs of increased body burden of lead appeared. When a worker had abnormalities in two of three variables (blood lead level, FEP, or MNCV) and also complained of some symptoms, he or she was considered intoxicated and was referred for chelation therapy. Such chelation not only confirmed the diagnosis but also effectively treated the individual. Experienced burners always burn with their back to the wind, and thoughtful foremen will try to have the yard work done upwind from the burning and not down the airstream, to lessen possible hazards. These studies exemplify the need to practice such safety measures and provide evidence of MNVC slowing, and thus subclinical neuropathy, in individuals with subacute low-level exposure to lead (Feldman et al., 1977).

Organic Lead

Peripheral Neuropathy after Chronic Exposure to Organic Lead

A group study of the effects of chronic low-level exposure to organic lead compounds was conducted by Mitchell et al. (1996). A total of 58 organic lead manufacturing workers with a mean age of 44.5 years and a mean exposure duration of 14.7 years participated in the study. The mean lifetime blood lead level among these workers was determined from historical data and was found to be 26.1 µg/100 mL. Clinical, neuropsychological, and neurophysiological assessments were performed. The most frequently reported symptoms included memory loss, insomnia, irritability, joint pain, paresthesia, nightmares, and fatigue; the GI symptoms associated with exposure to inorganic lead were rarely reported. Neuropsychological testing was performed in 39 workers and revealed deficits in 18 (46.2%). Nerve conduction studies were performed in all workers reporting symptoms of peripheral nervous system dysfunction or showing clinical evidence of abnormal peripheral nervous system functioning.

Nerve conduction studies documented sensorimotor poly-neuropathy in 11 of the 31 workers tested.

As noted elsewhere in this chapter, the occurrence of peripheral neuropathy following exposure to organic lead in gasoline cannot exclude the possibility of neurotoxic effects of other ingredients. However, in these subjects such confounders in gasoline were not present and the neuropathy was considered a lead effect, whether directly from organic lead or its inorganic metabolites.

Individual Studies

Inorganic Lead

Acute Encephalopathy Associated with Unexplained Mobilization of Stored Lead

Acute encephalopathy characterized by irritability, insomnia, confusion, and ataxia was seen in a 72-year-old man who had retired from a lead foundry 7 years prior to the onset of his symptoms (Guijarro et al., 1989). Blood lead levels of this patient were elevated (90 μg/100 mL), and basophilic stippling of erythrocytes was noted on the blood smear. An EEG performed on admission revealed diffuse slow waves. Clinical as well as electrophysiological improvement in the patient's status was seen following chelation therapy. Acute inorganic lead encephalopathy in this adult patient was indicated by the presence of biological markers of lead exposure, and the diagnosis was supported by his favorable response to chelation therapy. No new exogenous source of inorganic lead was found, suggesting that the increased blood lead level was probably due to the release of mobilizable lead from endogenous storage compartments in bone.

Urban Lead Miners; Deleading Old Houses

Public health initiatives to remove lead paint from old housing to protect children from exposure often results in occupational hazards to the workers involved in the abatement process. Instructions to the workers often include recommendations to use dry scraping as the fastest and most economical method, and to employ sanding, sandblasting, and wire brushing only for exterior applications since these methods create dangerous levels of dust particles in interior environments. Burning with an open flame is very hazardous because it creates dangerous lead fumes. Liquid stripper has no advantage over dry scraping. An urban lead miner (deleader) must be protected from lead intake by proper use of adequate exhaust ventilation in work areas; use of protective clothing that is not worn home; use of respirators with appropriate filters (changed at appropriate intervals); and proper and frequent washing before eating. Careful handling and disposal of waste materials, which are also a source of potential exposure, are necessary. Periodic medical surveillance including blood lead and ZPP levels should be performed to determine the need to remove the worker from exposure until the levels recede (Feldman, 1978).

Case 1. A 35-year-old man was admitted to the hospital because of a generalized convulsion. He had been working for 6 months as a deleader removing lead paint from interior walls with sanding machines, burning equipment, and chemical solvents. He admitted that he did not wash his hands before eating and that he only sporadically wore a mask or gloves. For a period of 3 months, he had complained of frequent headaches, indigestion, and stomach discomfort. He had experienced an unintentional weight loss of 3.6 to 4.5 kg. Physical examination after recovery from the convulsion was normal. The hematocrit was 20%, and the hemoglobin 9.1 g/100 mL; moderate basophilic stippling was present on red-cell smear. Because of the man's occupation, the blood lead level was measured and found to be 600 μg/100 g of whole blood. Therapy was instituted using 3 g of Ca-EDTA and 1.3 g of BAL for 5 days. The blood level came down to 76 μg/100 g on the seventh day (Feldman, 1978).

Case 2. A 24-year-old man, who had been using a propane torch and an electric sander to remove lead-based paint from the woodwork of old houses for the past three months, complained of severe abdominal pain of one week's duration. Based on his complaints, an appendectomy was performed before the diagnosis of lead poisoning was made. The patient still had symptoms after surgery, at which time the physical examination was unremarkable except for a thin, bluish line seen at the gingival margin of several front lower teeth. The hemoglobin was 11 g/100 mL and the hematocrit 33%. Basophilic stippling was noted on a red-cell smear. The patient's blood lead level was 264 μg/100 mL. A 24-hour urine sample contained 11,931 μg of lead per liter. Aminolevulinic acid content of the urine was 78 mg per 24 hours (normal: less than 7 mg per 24 hours). Chelation therapy using Ca-EDTA was instituted, after which the patient showed marked clinical improvement (Feldman, 1978).

Abdominal Cramps, Sickle Cell Disease, and Lead Poisoning

Nerve conduction studies documented overt peripheral neuropathy in a 10-year-old boy who had been exposed to inorganic lead and who presented with headaches, lethargy, abdominal colic, and a high steppage gait (Imbus et al., 1978). The patient's medical history included a diagnosis of sickle cell anemia. The patient had been experiencing abdominal cramps for nearly 5 years prior to his developing the steppage gait; however, the abdominal cramps, as well as his headaches and lethargy, had all previously been attributed to the sickle cell anemia. A history of pica was obtained from the patient's parents and subsequent laboratory tests revealed a blood lead level of 130 μg/100 mL and elevated urine coproporphyrins. Radiographs of the distal metaphysis of the femurs, tibia, fibula, radius, and ulna showed dense bands consistent with heavy metal exposure. MNCV studies revealed marked slowing in the ulnar (32 m/sec; normal range: 52.36 to 68.84 m/sec) and median (24 m/sec; normal range: 50.29 to 64.29 m/sec) nerves. Muscle action potentials could not be elicited by supramaximal shocks in the peroneal nerves.

Extrapyramidal Syndrome, Dementia, and Lower Motor Neuron Disease

A 57-year-old man had worked for 20 years coating wire. His recent work involved running wire off a spool through an acid flux bath into a tub of molten lead (Feldman et al., 1977). He then pulled the wire out of the tub with bare hands to attach it to a spindle for rewinding. The tubs containing molten lead were heated, and fumes and smoke were given off into an open room where he worked without benefit of a mask. Not infrequently, he ate his lunch and drank his beverage with one hand while he guided the wire throughout the coating procedure with the other. He complained of chronic "stomach trouble," and for 3 years had noted a metallic taste, difficulty swallowing, nausea, and increasing abdominal cramps.

Over a period of 2 to 3 years, his family observed that he had become withdrawn and forgetful and appeared easily confused by ordinary tasks. A definite movement disorder gradually developed; his left arm did not swing with walking, his gait became hesitant and stiff, writing became difficult and erratic, and his speech was hesitant. Physical examination disclosed rigidity of all extremities, more left than right, and increased reflexes, without Babinski signs. At rest, he held his hands in a flexed dystonic posture but had no tremor. Sensation was intact. His family physician found a blood lead level of 160 μg/100 mL of blood and a hematocrit value of 45%. He did not have diabetes, malnutrition, or alcoholism. The left deltoid and biceps muscles showed atrophy, and surface fasciculations were evident. EMG studies in the gastrocnemius, quadriceps, first dorsal interosseus, and abductor pollicis brevis muscles showed denervation potentials, fibrillations, and reduced numbers of motor potentials. Atrophy of the interosseus muscles was noted in both hands, although ulnar MNCV was normal. MNCV studies were done in the right median (55 m/sec), right ulnar (60 m/sec), right peroneal (44 m/sec), and left peroneal (42 m/sec) nerves.

Following Ca-EDTA infusion (25 mg/kg for 3 days), the urine lead level was 640 μg/L, and at a second 24-hour collection it was 1,560 μg/L; a third 24-hour urine specimen contained 1,080 μg/L. Two years later, he was asymptomatic and was once again able to serve as treasurer of his church. Conduction velocity in the right peroneal nerve was 50 m/sec, and muscle tone and strength returned to normal. Denervation was no longer evident by EMG (Feldman et al., 1977).

Lead Glass Hobby: Subacute Lead Toxicity and Long-Term Follow-up (25 Years)

A 36-year-old woman had a hobby of making lead-solder and glass ornaments in her kitchen (Feldman et al., 1977). She developed the history described below after 2

years of careless and uninformed use of the craft materials. Lead strips are used to outline pieces of colorful glass and to hold them in place. The patient was unaware of the dangers of handling lead and soldering seams in the absence of proper precautions and safety measures; inadequate handwashing and poor room ventilation led to her exposure by vapor inhalation and ingestion along with food. Symptoms of nausea, abdominal cramps, malaise, headache, irritability, paresthesia of the hands and feet, and weakness in the hands brought her to her physician. A blood lead test of 58 μg/100 mL of whole blood, an FEP test of 106 μg/100 mL of red blood cells (normal: 20 to 50 μg/100 mL), slowed peroneal-nerve conduction velocity (41 m/sec), and a history of exposure to lead were all factors justifying a trial of chelation. Ca-EDTA was given in two divided doses totaling 2.0 g. A baseline 24-hour urine contained 20 μg/L; postchelation urine contained 2,100 μg/L in 24 hours.

The patient stopped her work for a month and returned to work after she had improved her precautionary measures by using disposable gloves and a face mask and installing a better ventilation system in her working area. The nausea and cramping disappeared over several weeks, and after 6 to 8 weeks the paresthesia subsided. Strength was returning to her hands at that time. Periodic evaluations continued to document recovery, including return of normal NCV. For the next 15 years, the patient was successfully employed as a personnel executive. She apparently did not exhibit any neurobehavioral symptoms that interfered with her work. Formal neuropsychological testing was not performed at follow-up.

Approximately 22 years after her lead intoxication, the patient began to complain of muscle cramping, fatigue with exertion, and weakness in her lower extremities. Neurological examination using MNCVs showed bilateral median motor nerve slowing in the carpal tunnels, mild slowing on the left and moderate on the right ulnar nerves, and slowing of the common peroneal nerve on the right. Symptoms of paresthesia and pain were reported in her hands, the right more than the left. She often sat with her thin legs crossed and typed at a keyboard for long hours. It was concluded that this patient had developed multiple nerve entrapment sites and that her underlying recovered lead neuropathy had increased the susceptibility of the nerves to compression. Symptoms similar to those seen in postpolio syndrome (cramps, weakness, and fatigue) in this patient as she became deconditioned with age could be explained in part by the denervation and reinnervation of the muscles associated with the earlier lead neuropathy.

She had also had fractures of the small bones of her foot, which resulted from minor force incurred while stepping off a curb. She was followed up, and bone mineral density tests showed decreased measurements in the left hip and spine, which was consistent with osteopenia in this 58-year-old woman who had had a hysterectomy at age 29 and who did not take hormone replacements or calcium supplements. The relatively severe and premature osteoporosis seen in this patient may have resulted in considerable mobilization of lead stored in dense bone. Although a single blood lead level taken at follow-up was not elevated, the contribution of prolonged exposure to lead (released from bone over time) to this patient's complaints of cramps, weakness, and fatigue cannot be ruled out.

Organic Lead

Gasoline Sniffing Leading to Organic Lead Encephalopathy

Young et al. (1977) reported the case of a 14-year-old girl with a 2-year history of sniffing leaded gasoline. On admission, the patient exhibited rapid, jerky, and purposeless movements in all four extremities and was severely ataxic. The patient was unable to perform a finger to nose test or rapid alternating movements on command. Her muscle strength was normal. Cognitively she was oriented, cooperative, and denied having hallucinations. Her blood lead level was 142 μg/100 mL. The patient was chelated with Ca-EDTA and BAL for 5 days and then with penicillamine for an additional 15 days. Following chelation therapy the patient's blood lead levels dropped to 60 μg/100 mL, and she showed marked clinical improvement. After discharge, her parents enrolled her in a local boarding school with hopes of improving her wayward behavior. The patient was readmitted 3 months later, at which time she was severely ataxic and stated that she had returned to sniffing gasoline because she did not like the boarding school. Her blood lead level at that time was 110 μg/100 mL. She underwent a second course of chelation therapy, after which her blood lead level dropped to 10 μg/100 mL. At the time of discharge her neurological symptoms had disappeared. The patient resumed sniffing gasoline shortly after discharge and was readmitted 3 months later with severe ataxia and a blood level of 62 μg/100 mL. She received a third course of chelation therapy after which her neurological symptoms again improved. The patient was subsequently transferred to a different boarding school; she stated that she was much happier there. She did not return to sniffing gasoline and has been free of cerebellar symptoms since.

REFERENCES

Agency for Toxic Substances and Disease Registry (ATSDR). *Toxicological profile for lead.* Washington: U.S. Department of Health and Human Services, Public Health Services, 1997.

Agency for Toxic Substances and Disease Registry (ATSDR). 1997.

Ahlskog JE, Waring SC, Kurland LT, et al. Guamanian neurodegenerative disease: investigation of the calcium metabolism/heavy metal hypothesis. *Neurology* 1995;45:1340–1344.

Albano E, Bellomo G, Benedetti A, et al. Alterations in hepatocyte Ca^{2+} homeostasis by triethylated lead (Et_3Pb^+): are they correlated with cytotoxicity? *Chem Biol Interact* 1994;90:59–72.

Altshuler B, Nelson N, Kuschner M. Estimation of lung tissue dose from the inhalation of radon and daughters. *Health Phys* 1964;10:1137–1161.

American Conference of Governmental Industrial Hygienists (ACGIH). *Documentation of the Threshold Limit Values and Biological Exposure Indices,* 5th ed. Cincinnati, OH: ACGIH, 1988.

American Conference of Governmental Industrial Hygienists (ACGIH). *Threshold limit values (TLVs) for chemical substances and physical agents and biological exposure indices (BEIs).* Cincinnati, OH: ACGIH, 1995–1996.

Anania TL, Lucas JB, Seta JH. *Lead exposure at an indoor firing range.* Cincinnati, OH: National Institute for Occupational Safety and Health, Technical Publication, 1974.

Anderson KE, Fischbein A, Kestenbaum D, et al. Plumbism from airborne lead in a firing range: an unusual exposure to a toxic heavy metal. *Am J Med* 1977;63:306–312.

Araki S, Yokoyama K, Murata K, Aono H. Determination of distribution of conduction velocities in workers exposed to lead, zinc, and copper. *Brit J Ind Med* 1986;43:321–326.

Araki S, Murata K, Aono H. Central and peripheral nervous system dysfunction in workers exposed to lead, zinc, and copper: a follow-up study of visual and somatosensory evoked potentials. *Int Arch Occup Environ Health* 1987;59:177–187.

Aschengrau A, Beiser A, Bellinger D, et al. The impact of soil lead abatement on urban children's blood lead levels: phase II from the Boston Lead-in-Soil Demonstration Project. *Environ Res* 1994;67:125–148.

Baghurst PA, Tong S-L, McMichael AJ, et al. Determinants of blood lead concentrations to age 5 years in a birth cohort of children living in the lead smelting city of Port Pirie and surrounding areas. *Arch Environ Health* 1992;47:203–210.

Bailey AJ, Sargent JD, Goodman DC, et al. Poisoned landscapes: the epidemiology of environmental lead exposure in Massachusetts children 1990–1991. *Soc Sci Med* 1994;39:757–766.

Baker EL, Folland DS, Taylor TA, et al. Lead poisoning in children of lead workers: home contamination with industrial dust. *N Engl J Med* 1977;296:260–261.

Baker EL, Goyer RA, Fowler BA, et al. Occupational lead exposure, nephropathy, and renal cancer. *Am J Ind Med* 1980;1:139–148.

Baker EL, Feldman RG, White RF, et al. Occupational lead neurotoxicity: a behavioral and electrophysiological evaluation. Study design and year one results. *Br J Ind Med* 1984;41:352–361.

Baker EL, White RF, Pothier LJ, et al. Occupational lead neurotoxicity: improvement in behavioral effects after reduction of exposure. *Br J Ind Med* 1985;42:507–516.

Baloh RW. Laboratory diagnosis of increased lead absorption. *Arch Environ Hlth* 1974;28:198–208.

Barry PSI. A comparison of concentrations of lead in human tissues. *Br J Ind Med* 1975;32:119–139.

Barry PSI. Concentrations of lead in the tissues of children. *Br J Ind Med* 1981;38:61–71.

Beattie AD, Moore MR, Goldberg A. Tetraethyl-lead poisoning. *Lancet* 1972;1:12–15.

Beijer K, Jernelöv A. Microbial methylation of lead. In: Grandjean P, Grandjean EC, eds. *Biological effects of organolead compounds.* Boca Raton, FL: CRC Press, 1984:13–20.

Beliles RP. The metals. In: Clayton GD, Clayton FE, eds. *Patty's industrial hygiene and toxicology,* 4th ed., vol II. New York: Wiley Interscience, 1994:2065–2087.

Bellinger D, Leviton A, Waternaux C, et al. Longitudinal analyses of prenatal and postnatal lead exposure and early cognitive development. *N Engl J Med* 1987;316:1037–1050.

Bellinger D, Leviton A, Sloman J. Antecedents and correlates of improved cognitive performance in children exposed in utero to low levels of lead. *Environ Health Perspect* 1990;89:5–11.

Bellinger D, Hu H, Titlebaum L, Needleman HL. Attentional correlates of dentin and bone levels in adolescents. *Arch Environ Health* 1994;49:98–105.

Bercovitz K, Laufer D. Age and gender influence on lead accumulation in root dentine of human permanent teeth. *Arch Oral Biol* 1991;36:671–673.

Berlin K, Gerhardsson L, Börjesson J, et al. Lead intoxication caused by skeletal disease. *Scand J Work Environ Health* 1995;21:296–300.

Bhattacharya A, Linz DH. Postural sway analysis of a teenager with childhood lead intoxication—a case study. *Clin Pediatr* 1991;30: 543–548.

Bhattacharya A, Shukla R, Bornschein R, et al. Lead effects on postural balance of children. *Environ Health Perspect* 1990;89:35–42.

Bhattacharya A, Shukla R, Dietrich K, et al. Effect of early lead exposure on children's postural balance. *Dev Med Child Neurol* 1995;37: 861–878.

Biddinger GR, Gloss SP. Importance of trophic transfer in the bioaccumulation of chemical contaminants in aquatic ecosystems. *Residue Rev* 1984;91:103–145.

Biemond A, Van Creveld S. On the cerebellar form of saturnism encephalopathy. *Acta Paediatr Scand* 1939;27:51–62.

Binder S. Hazards of low level lead exposure recognized. *Am J Public Health* 1992;82:1043–1044.

Blackman SS. The lesions of lead encephalopathy in children. *Bull Johns Hopkins Hosp* 1937;31:1–61.

Bleecker ML, Lindrigen KN, Ford DP. Differential contribution of current and cumulative indices of lead dose to neuropsychological performance by age. *Neurology* 1997;48:639–645.

Boeckx RL, Postl B, Coodin FJ. Gasoline sniffing and tetraethyl lead poisoning in children. *Pediatrics* 1977;60:140–145.

Bolanowska W. Distribution and excretion of triethyllead in rats. *Br J Ind Med* 1968;25:203–208.

Bolanowska W, Piotrowski J, Garczynski H. Triethyllead in the biological material in cases of acute tetraethyllead poisoning. *Arch Toxikol* 1967;22:278–282.

Bondy SC. The neurotoxicity of organic and inorganic lead. In: Bondy SC, Prasad KN, eds. *Metal Toxicity.* Boca Raton, FL: CRC Press, 1988:1–18.

Booker DV, Chamberlain AC, Newton D, Stott AN. Uptake of radioactive lead following inhalation and injection. *Br J Radiol* 1969;42:457–466.

Bordo B, Massetto N, Musicco M, et al. Electrophysiologic changes in workers with "low" blood lead levels. *Am J Ind Med* 1982;3:23–32.

Boyd PR, Walker G, Henderson IN. The treatment of tetraethyl lead poisoning. *Lancet* 1957;1:181–185.

Brody DJ, Pirkle JL, Kramer RA, et al. Blood levels in the U.S. population from phase 1 of the Third National Health and Nutrition Examination Surveys. *JAMA* 1994;272:284–291.

Brown A. Petrol sniffing lead encephalopathy. *NZ Med J* 1983;96:421–422.

Buchthal F, Behse F. Electrophysiology and nerve biopsy in men exposed to lead. *Br J Ind Med* 1979;36:135–147.

Bucy PC, Buchanan DN. The simulation of intracranial tumor by lead encephalopathy in children. *JAMA* 1935;27:244–250.

Burchfield JL, Duffy FH, Bartels PH, Needleman HL. The combined discrimination power of quantitative electroencephalography and neuropsychological measures in evaluating central nervous system effects of lead at low levels. In: Needleman HL, ed. *Low level lead exposure: the clinical implications of current research.* New York: Raven Press, 1980:75–89.

Byers RK, Lord EE. Late effects of lead poisoning on mental development. *Am J Dis Child* 1943;66:471–494.

Campbell BC, Meredith PA, Moore MR, Watson WS. Kinetics of lead following intravenous administration in man. *Toxicol Lett* 1984;21:231–235.

Campbell JB, Woolley DE, Vijayan VK, Overman SR. Morphometric effects of postnatal lead exposure on hippocampal development of the 15-day-old rat. *Dev Brain Res* 1982;3:595–612.

Carson BL, Stockton RA, Wilkinson RR. Organomercury, -lead, and -tin compounds in the environment and the potential for human exposure: In: Tilson HA, Sparber SB, eds. *Neurotoxicants and neurobiological function: effects of organoheavy metals.* New York: John Wiley & Sons, 1987:1–79.

Cassells DAK, Dodds EC. Tetra-ethyl lead poisoning. *BMJ* 1946;2:681–685.

Catton MJ, Harrison MJG, Fullerton PM, Kazantzis G. Subclinical neuropathy in lead workers. *BMJ* 1970;2:80–82.

CDC. *Preventing lead poisoning in young children: a statement by the Centers for Disease Control—October, 1991.* Atlanta, GA: Centers for Disease Control, 1991.

CDC. *Blood lead levels—United States, 1988–1991. MMWR* 1994a;43:545–548.

Chamberlain A, Heard C, Little MJ, et al. Investigations into lead from motor vehicles. Harwell, United Kingdom: United Kingdom Atomic Energy Authority. Report no. AERE-9198. The dispersion of lead from motor vehicle exhausts. *Philos Trans R Soc Lond A* 1978;290:557–589.

Chan H, Billmeier GJ Jr, Evans WE, Chan H. Lead poisoning from ingestion of Chinese herbal medicine. *Clin Toxicol* 1977;10:273–281.

Chancellor AM, Slattery JM, Fraser H, Warlow CP: Risk factors for motor neuron disease: a case-control study based on patients from the Scottish Motor Disease Register. *J Neurol Neurosurg Psychiatry* 1993;56:1200–1206.

Chang LW, Tilson HA, Walsh TJ. Neuropathological changes induced by triethyl and trimethyllead compounds. *Toxicologist* 1984;4:164.

Chau YK, Wong PTS. Organic lead in the aquatic environment. In: Grandjean P, Grandjean EC, eds. *Biological effects of organolead compounds.* Boca Raton FL: CRC Press, 1984:21–31.

Chia SE, Chia HP, Ong CN, Jeyaratman J. Cumulative concentrations of blood lead and postural stability. *Occup Environ Med* 1996;53:264–268.

Chiaradia M, Gulson BL, MacDonald K. Contamination of houses by workers occupationally exposed in a lead-zinc-copper mine and impact on blood lead concentrations in the families. *Occup Environ Med* 1997;54:117–124.

Chisolm JJ Jr. Evaluation of the potential role of chelation therapy in treatment of low to moderate lead exposures. *Environ Health Perspect* 1990;89:67–74.

Chisolm JJ, Harrison HE. The exposure of children to lead. *Pediatrics* 1956;18:943–957.

Chisolm JJ Jr, Barrett MB, Harrison HV. Indicators of internal dose of lead in relation to derangement in heme synthesis. *Johns Hopkins Med J* 1975;137:6–12.

Clasen RA, Hartmann JF, Starr AJ, et al. Electromicroscopic and chemical studies of vascular changes and edema of lead encephalopathy. *Am J Pathol* 1974;74:215–224.

Coulihan JL, Hirsh W, Brillman J, et al. Gasoline sniffing and lead toxicity in Navajo adolescents. *Pediatrics* 1983;71:113–117.

Coulston F, Goldberg L, Griffin TB, Russell JC. The effects of continuous exposure to airborne lead. I. Exposure of rats and monkeys to particulate lead at a level of 21.5 µg/m³. Final Report to the U.S. Environmental Protection Agency. Washington: EPA, 1972a.

Coulston F, Goldberg L, Griffin TB, Russell JC. The effects of continuous exposure to airborne lead. II. Exposure of man to particulate lead at a level of 10.9 µg/m³. Final Report to the U.S. Environmental Protection Agency. Washington: EPA, 1972b.

Coulston F, Goldberg L, Griffin TB, Russell JC. The effects of continuous exposure to airborne lead. IV. Exposure of man to particulate lead at a level of 3.2 µg/m³. Final Report to the U.S. Environmental Protection Agency. Washington: EPA, 1972c.

Cremer JE. Biochemical studies on the toxicity of tetraethyllead and other organo-lead compounds. *Br J Ind Med* 1959;16:191–199.

Cremer JE, Callaway S. Further studies on the toxicity of some tetra and trialkyl lead compounds. *J Ind Med* 1961;18:277–282.

Damm D, Grandjean P, Lyngbye T, et al. Early lead exposure and neonatal jaundice: relation to neurobehavioral performance at 15 years of age. *Neurotoxicol Teratol* 1993;15:173–181.

Danscher G, Fjerdingstad EJ, Fjerdingstad E, Fredens K. Heavy metal content in subdivisions of the rat hippocampus (zinc, lead and copper). *Brain Res* 1976;112:442–446.

Davis RY, Morton AW, Lawson EE, et al. Inhalation of tetramethyl lead and tetraethyl lead. *Arch Environ Hlth* 1963;6:473–479.

Dickinson L, Reichert EL, Ho RC, et al. Lead poisoning in a family due to cocktail glasses. *Am J Med* 1972;52:391–394.

Diehl KH, Rosopulo A, Kreuzer W, Judel GK. Behavior of tetraalkylleads in the soil and their uptake by plants. *Z Pflanzenernaehr Bodenkd* 1983;146:551–559.

Dietrich KN, Succop PA, Bornschein RL, et al. Lead exposure and neurobehavioral development in later infancy. *Environ Health Perspect* 1990;89:13–19.

Dillman RO, Crumb CK, Lidsky MJ. Lead poisoning from gunshot wound. Report of a case and review of the literature. *Am J Med* 1979;66:509–514.

Doe BR. *Lead isotopes, minerals, rocks, and inorganic materials.* Monograph Series of Theoretical and Experimental Studies No. 3. New York: Springer-Verlag, 1970.

Dyck PJ, O'Brien PC, Ohnishi A. Lead neuropathy; 2. Random distribution of segmental demyelination among "old internodes" of myelinated fibers. *J Neuropathol Exp Neurol* 1977;36:570–575.

Dyer J, Garrick DP, Inglis A, Pye IF. Plumboporphyria (ALAD deficiency) in a lead worker: a scenario for potential diagnostic confusion. *Br J Ind Med* 1993;50:1119–1121.

Eaton DL, Kalman D, Garvey D, et al. Biological availability of lead in paint aerosol. 2. Absorption, distribution, and excretion of intratracheally instilled lead paint particles in the rat. *Toxicol Lett* 1984;22: 307–313.

Edwards EK Jr, Edwards EK. Allergic contact dermatitis to lead acetate in a hair dye. *Cutis* 1982;30:629–630.

Environmental Protection Agency (EPA). *Air quality criteria for lead.* Research Triangle Park, NC: US Environmental Protection Agency,

Office of Research and Development, Office of Health and Environmental Assessment, Environmental Criteria and Assessment Office. EPA 600/8-83-028F, 1986.

Environmental Protection Agency (EPA). *Quarterly summary of lead phasedown reporting data.* Washington, DC: United States Environmental Protection Agency, Office of Mobile Sources, Office of Air and Radiation, 1991.

Environmental Protection Agency (EPA). Guidance on identification of lead-based paint hazards. *Federal Register* 1995;60:47248–47257.

Environmental Protection Agency (EPA). Drinking water regulations and health advisories. EPA 822-R-96-001. Washington: Office of Water, 1996a.

Environmental Protection Agency (EPA). Code of Federal Regulations; 40 Ch. 1 (7-1-96 edit). Washington: Office of the Federal Register, National Archives and Records Administration, 1996b:480–481.

Everson J, Patterson CC. "Ultra-clean" isotope dilution/mass spectrometric analysis for lead in human blood plasma indicate that most reported values are artificially high. *Clin Chem* 1980;26:1603–1607.

Federal Institute for Minerals Research and German Institute for Economic Research. Supply and Demand for Lead, pp 1–47 (translated into English by Lead Development Association, 34 Berkeley Square, London W16AJ, April, 1972): cited by Tsuchiya K. Lead. In: Friberg L, Nordberg GF, Touk VB, eds. *Handbook of the toxicology of metals,* vol 2. Amsterdam: Elsevier Science Publishers, 1986:288–353.

Feldman RG. Urban lead mining: lead intoxication among deleaders. *N Engl J Med* 1978;298:1143–1145.

Feldman RG. Neurological picture of lead poisoning. *Acta Neurol Scand* 1982;66[Suppl 92]:185–199.

Feldman RG. Clinical manifestation of neurotoxic exposure to metals. In: Samuels MA, Feske S, eds. *Office practice of neurology.* New York: Churchill Livingston, 1996:1065–1069.

Feldman RG, Haddow J, Chisolm J. Chronic lead intoxication in urban children. In: Desmedt J, Korger S, eds. *New developments in electromyography and clinical neurophysiology.* Basel, Switzerland: Karger, 1973:313–317.

Feldman RG, Hayes MK, Younes R, Aldrich FD. Lead neuropathy in adults and children. *Arch Neurol* 1977;34:481–488.

Feldman RG, White RF. Lead neurotoxicity and disorders of learning and attention. *J Child Neurol* 1992;7:354–359.

Fergusson DM, Fergusson JE, Horwood LJ, Kinzett NG. A longitudinal study of dentine lead levels, intelligence, school performance and behavior. *Child Psychol Psychiatr* 1988;29:793–809.

Fischbein A, Thornton JC, Lilis R, et al. Zinc protoporphyrin, blood lead and clinical symptoms in two occupational groups with low-level exposure to lead. *Am J Ind Med* 1980;1:391–399.

Fischbein A, Wallace J, Anderson KE, et al. Lead poisoning in an art conservator. *JAMA* 1982;247:2007–2009.

Fjerdingstad E, Danscher G, Fjerdingstad EJ. Zinc content in hippocampus and whole brain of normal rats. *Brain Res* 1974;79:338–342.

Flora SJ, Tandon SK. Effect of combined exposure to lead and ethanol on some biochemical indices in the rat. *Biochem Pharmacol* 1987;36:537–541.

Food and Drug Administration (FDA), Department of Health and Human Services. Lead-soldered food cans. *Federal Register* 1995 Jun 27:60: 33106–33109.

Franco GG, Tempini G, Forte R. Reference values of erythrocyte zinc-protoporphyrin in monitoring occupational exposure to lead. *Quad Sclavo-Diagn* 1984;20:28–38.

Frank RM, Sargentini-Maier ML, Leroy MJ, Turlot JC. Age-related lead increase in human permanent teeth demonstrated by energy dispersive x-ray fluorescence. *J Trace Elem Electrol Health Dis* 1988;2:175–179.

Fullerton PM. Chronic peripheral neuropathy produced by lead poisoning in guinea-pigs. *J Neuropathol Exp Neurol* 1966;25:214–236.

Fullerton PM, Harrison MJG. Subclinical lead neuropathy in man. *Bull Am Assoc Electromyogr Electrodiagn* 1970;17:25.

Gerhardsson L, Englyst V, Lundstrom NG, et al. Lead in tissues of deceased lead smelter workers. *J Trace Elem Med Biol* 1995;9:136–143.

GESAMP. Reports and Studies #22, IMO/FAO/UNESCO/WMO/WHO/IAEA/UN/UNEP Joint Group of Experts on the scientific aspects of marine pollution. Geneva: World Health Organization, 1985.

Gething J. Tetramethyl lead absorption: a report of human exposure to a high level of tetramethyl lead. *Br J Ind Med* 1975;32:329–333.

Gittleman JL, Engelgau MM, Shaw J, et al. Lead poisoning among battery reclamation workers in Alabama. *J Occup Med* 1994;36:526–532.

Goering PL. Lead-protein interactions as a basis for lead toxicity. *Neurotoxicology* 1993;14:45–60.

Goldings AS, Stewart M. Organic lead encephalopathy: behavioral change and movement disorder following gasoline inhalation. *J Clin Psychiatry* 1982;437:70–72.

Goldman RH, Baker EL, Hannan M, Kamerow DB. Lead poisoning in automobile radiator mechanics. *N Engl J Med* 1987;317:214–218.

Goyer RA. Lead toxicity: a problem in environmental pathology. *Am J Pathol* 1971;64:167–182.

Goyer RA. Transplacental transport of lead. *Environ Health Perspect* 1990;89:101–105.

Goyer RA, Wilson MH. Lead-induced inclusion bodies—results of ethylene diamine tetraacetic acid treatment. *Lab Invest* 1975;32:149–156.

Grandjean P. Regional distribution of lead in human brains. *Toxicol Lett* 1978;2:65–69.

Grandjean P. Organolead exposures and intoxications. In: Grandjean P, Grandjean EC, eds. *Biological effects of organolead compounds.* Boca Raton, FL: CRC Press, 1984:227–241.

Grandjean P. International perspectives of lead exposure and lead toxicity. *Neurotoxicology* 1993;14:9–14.

Grandjean P, Nielsen T. Organolead compounds: environmental health aspects. *Residue Rev* 1979;72:97–148.

Grandjean P, Kon SH. Lead exposure of welders and bystanders in a ship repair yard. *Am J Ind Med* 1981;2:65–70.

Grengard J. Lead poisoning in childhood: signs, symptoms, current therapy, clinical expressions. *Clin Pediatr* 1966;5:269–276.

Guijarro C, García Díaz JD, Herrero O, Aranda JL. Acute encephalopathy in adult as delayed presentation of occupational lead intoxication. *J Neurol Neurosurg Psychiatry* 1989;52:127–128.

Gulson BL. Tooth analyses of sources and intensity of lead exposure in children. *Environ Health Perspect* 1996;104:306–312.

Gulson BL, Jameson CW, Mahaffey KR, et al. Pregnancy increases mobilization of lead from maternal skeleton. *J Lab Clin Med* 1997;130: 51–62.

Hac E, Krechniak J. Lead levels in bone and hair of rats treated with lead acetate. *Biol Trace Elem Res* 1996;52:293–301.

Hahn M, Gildemeister OS, Krauss GL, et al. Effects of new anticonvulsant medications on porphyrin synthesis in cultured liver cells: potential implications for patients with acute porphyria. *Neurology* 1997;49:97–106.

Halliwell B. Oxidants and the central nervous system: some fundamental questions. Is oxidant damage relevant to Parkinson's disease, Alzheimer's disease, traumatic injury and stroke? *Acta Neurol Scand* 1989; 126:23–33.

Hamilton A, Reznikoff P, Burnham GM. Tetra-ethyl lead. *JAMA* 1925;84:1481–1486.

Hammond PB. Metabolism of lead. In: Chisolm JJ, O'Hara DM, eds. *Lead absorption in children: management, clinical and environmental aspects.* Baltimore, MD: Urban and Schwarzenberg, 1982:11–20.

Hänninen H, Mantere P, Hernberg S, et al. Subjective symptoms in low-level exposure to lead. *Neurotoxicology* 1979;1:333–347.

Hansen KS, Sharp FR. Gasoline sniffing, lead poisoning, and myoclonus. *JAMA* 1978;240:1375–1376.

Harrington JF, Mapstone TB, Selman WR, et al. Lead encephalopathy presenting as a posterior fossa mass. Case report. *J Neurosurg* 1986;65: 713–715.

Harris RW, Elsea WR. Ceramic glaze as a source of lead poisoning. *JAMA* 1967;202:544–546.

Harvey PG, Hamlin MW, Kumar R, Delves HT. Blood lead, behavior and intelligence test performance in preschool children. *Sci Total Environ* 1984;240:45–60.

Hayakawa K. Microdetermination and dynamic aspects of in vivo alkyl-lead compounds. Part II. Studies on the dynamic aspects of alkyllead compounds in vivo. *Jpn J Hyg* 1972;26:526–535.

Heard MJ, Chamberlain AC. Effect of minerals and food on uptake of lead from the gastrointestinal tract of humans. *Hum Toxicol* 1982;1: 441–445.

Heard MJ, Wells AC, Newton D, et al. Human uptake and metabolism of tetra ethyl and tetramethyl lead vapour labelled with 203Pb. In: *International Conference on Management and Control of Heavy Metals in the Environment, London, England, September.* Edinburgh, United Kingdom: CEPO Consultants, LTD., 1979:103–108.

Hegg CC, Miletic V. Acute exposure to inorganic lead modifies high-threshold voltage-gated calcium currents in rat PC12 cells. *Brain Res* 1996;738:333–336.

Hernberg S. Toxic metals and their compounds: lead. In: Zenz C, ed. *Occupational medicine: principles and practical applications.* Chicago: Yearbook Medical Publishers, 1975:715–769.

Hernberg S, Nikkanen J. Enzyme inhibition by lead under normal urban conditions. *Lancet* 1970;1:63–64.

Hernberg S, Nikkanen J, Mellin G, Lilius H. δ-Aminolevulinic acid dehydrase as a measure of lead exposure. *Arch Environ Health* 1970;21:140–145.

Hess JW. Lead encephalopathy simulating subdural hematoma in an adult. *N Engl J Med* 1961;264:382–384.

Heywood RR, James RQ, Pulsford AH, et al. Chronic administration of alkyl lead solution to the rhesus monkey. *Toxicol Lett* 1979;4:119–125.

Hillman FE. A rare case of chronic lead poisoning: polyneuropathy traced to lead shot in the appendix. *Ind Med Surg* 1967;36:488–492.

Hirano A, Kochen JA. Further observations on the effects of lead implantation in rat brains. *Acta Neuropathol* 1976;34:87–93.

Hirata M, Kosaka H. Effects of lead on neurophysiological parameters. *Environ Res* 1993;63:60–69.

Hodgkins DG, Rogins TG, Hinkamp DL, et al. The effect of airborne lead particle size on worker blood-lead levels: an empirical study of battery workers. *J Occup Med* 1991;33:1265–1273.

Holdstein Y, Pratt H, Goldsher M, et al. Auditory brain stem evoked potentials in asymptomatic lead-exposed subjects. *J Laryngol Otol* 1986;100:1031–1036.

Holtzman D, DeVries C, Nguyen H, et al. Maturation of resistance to lead encephalopathy: cellular and subcellular mechanisms. *Neurotoxicology* 1984;5:97–124.

Hong JS, Tilson HA, Hudson P, Ali SF, Wilson WE, Hunter V. Correlation of neurochemical and behavioral effects of triethyllead chloride in rats. *Toxicol Appl Pharmacol* 1983;69:471–479.

Housing and Urban Development, U.S. Department of (HUD). Comprehensive and workable plan for the abatement of lead-based paint in privately owned housing: report to Congress. Washington: HUD, 1990.

Housing and Urban Development, U.S. Department of (HUD). Guidelines for the evaluation and control of lead-based paint hazards in housing. Selected chapters, 11: Interim controls; 12: Abatement; 13: Encapsulation; 14: Cleaning. Washington: HUD, 1995.

Hu H, Milder FL, Burger DE. X-ray fluorescence measurements of lead burden in subjects with low-level community lead exposure. *Arch Environ Health* 1990;43:335–341.

Hu H, Watanabe H, Payton M, et al. The relationship between bone lead and hemoglobin. *JAMA* 1994;272:1512–1517.

Hursh JB, Schraub A, Sattler EL, Hofmann HP. Fate of ^{212}Pb inhaled by human subjects. *Health Phys* 1969;16:257–267.

Hursh JB, Suomela J. Absorption of 212Pb from the gastrointestinal tract of man. *Acta Radiol [Ther](Stockh)* 1968;7:108–120.

Imbus CE, Warner J, Smith E, et al. Peripheral neuropathy in lead-intoxicated sickle cell patients. *Muscle Nerve* 1978;1:168–171.

Iwata K, Nakagawa H, Hoshino D, Matsuo T. Magnetic resonance imaging in the diagnosis of the posterior fossa and the spinal column. *Acta Radiol Suppl* 1986;369:747–749.

Jacobziner H. Lead poisoning in childhood: epidemiology, manifestations, and prevention. *Clin Pediatr* 1966;5:277–286.

Joselow MM, Flores J. Comparison of zinc protoporphyrin and free erythrocyte protoporphyrin in whole blood. *Health Lab Sci* 1977;14:126–128.

Jover R, Lindberg RL, Meyer UA. Role of heme in cytochrome P450 transcription and function in mice treated with lead acetate. *Mol Pharmacol* 1996;50:474–481.

Karacic V, Prpic-Majic D, Telisman S. The relationship between zinc protoporphyrin (ZPP) and "free" erythrocyte protoporphyrin (FEP) in lead-exposed individuals. *Int Arch Occup Environ Health* 1980;47:165–177.

Kehoe RA. On the toxicity of tetraethyl lead and inorganic lead salts. *J Lab Clin Med* 1927;7:554–560.

Kehoe RA. Experimental studies on the inhalation of lead by human subjects. *Pure Appl Chem* 1969;3:129–144.

Kehoe RA. Studies of lead administration and elimination in adult volunteers under natural and experimentally induced conditions over extended periods of time. *Food Chem Toxicol* 1987;25:425–493.

Kehoe RA, Thamann F, Cholak J. On the normal absorption and excretion of lead. *J Ind Hyg* 1933;15:257.

Kehoe RA, Cholak J, Hubbard DM, et al. Experimental studies on lead absorption and excretion and their relation to the diagnosis and treatment of lead poisoning. *J Ind Hyg Toxicol* 1943;25:71–78.

Kello D, Kostial K. The effect of milk diet on lead metabolism in rats. *Environ Res* 1973;6:355–360.

Kentner M, Fischer T, Richter G. Changes in external and internal lead load in different working areas of a starter battery production plant in the period 1982–1991. *Int Arch Occup Environ Health* 1994;66:23–31.

Konat G, Clausen J. The effect of long-term administration of triethyl lead on the developing rat brain. *Environ Physiol Biochem* 1974;4:236–242.

Konat G, Offner H, Clausen J. Triethyllead-restrained myelin deposition and protein synthesis in the developing rat forebrain. *Exp Neurol* 1976;52:58–65.

Kumar S, Jain S, Aggarwal CS, Ahuja GK. Encephalopathy due to inorganic lead in an adult. *Jpn J Med* 1987;26:253–254.

Lamola AA, Joselow M, Yamane T. Zinc protoporphyrin (ZPP): a simple sensitive fluorometric screening test for lead poisoning. *Clin Chem* 1975a;21:93–97.

Lamola AA, Piomelli S, Poh-Fitzpatrick MG, et al. Erythrocyte protoporphyria and lead intoxication: the molecular basis for difference in cutaneous photosensitivity. II. Different binding of erythrocyte protoporphyrin to hemoglobin. *J Clin Invest* 1975b;56:1528–1535.

Lamola AA, Yamane T. Zinc protoporphyrin in erythrocytes of patients with lead intoxication and iron deficiency anemia. *Science* 1974;186:936–938.

Lampert PW, Schochet SS. Demyelination and remyelination in lead neuropathy. Electron microscopic studies. *J Neuropathol Exp Neurol* 1968;27:527–545.

Landrigan PJ, Baker EL, Feldman RG, et al. Increased lead absorption with anemia and slowed nerve conduction in children near a lead smelter. *J Pediatr* 1976;89:904–910.

Landrigan PJ, McKinney AS, Hopkins LC, et al. Chronic lead absorption. Result of poor ventilation in an indoor pistol range. *JAMA* 1975;234:394–397.

Laug EP, Kunze FM. The penetration of lead through the skin. *J Ind Hyg Toxicol* 1948;30:256–259.

Law WR, Nelson ER. Gasoline-sniffing by an adult. Report of a case with the unusual complication of lead encephalopathy. *JAMA* 1968;204:144–146.

Le Quesne P. Metal-induced disease of the nervous system. *Br J Hosp Med* 1982;28:501–505.

Lever SZ, Scheffel U. Regional distribution of ^{203}PbCl$_2$ in the mouse after intravenous injection. *Neurotoxicol* 1998;19:197–208.

Lilis R, Eisinger J, Blumberg W, et al. Hemoglobin, serum iron, and zinc protoporphyrin in lead-exposed workers. *Environ Health Perspect* 1978;25:97–102.

Lilis R, Valciukas JA, Kon S, et al. Assessment of lead health hazards in body shop of an automobile assembly plant. *Am J Ind Med* 1982;3:33–51.

Linch AL. Biological monitoring for industrial exposure to tetraethyl lead. *Am Ind Hyg Assoc J* 1975;36:214–219.

Linch AL, Wiest EG, Carter MD. Evaluation of tetraalkyl lead exposure by personnel monitor surveys. *Am Ind Hyg Assoc J* 1970;31:170–179.

Linz DH, Barret ET, Pflauamer JE, Keith RE. Neuropsychological and postural sway improvement after Ca^{++}EDTA chelation for mild lead intoxication. *J Occup Med* 1992;34:638–641.

Low PA, Dyck PJ. Increased endoneurial fluid pressure in experimental lead neuropathy. *Nature* 1977;269:427–428.

Machle WF. Tetra-ethyl lead intoxication and poisoning by related compounds of lead. *JAMA* 1935;105:578–585.

Manthos A, Kerameous-Faroglou C, Kovatsis A. Electron microscopic study of the effects of triethyllead administration on the brain and retina of the rabbit. *Annu Fac Med Aristotelian Univ Thessaloniki (Greece)* 1980;13:853–903.

Marchioro M, Swanson KL, Aracava Y, Albuquerque EX. Glycine and calcium-dependent effects of lead on N-methyl-D-aspartate receptor function in rat hippocampal neurons. *J Pharmacol Exp Ther* 1996;279:143–153.

Marino PE, Franzblau A, Lilis R, Landrigan PJ. Acute lead poisoning in construction workers: the failure of current protective standards. *Arch Environ Health* 1989;44:140–145.

Markovac J, Goldstein GW. Lead activates protein kinase C in immature rat brain microvessels. *Toxicol Appl Pharmacol* 1988;96:14–23.

Markowitz ME, Rosen JF. Need for the lead mobilization test in children with lead poisoning. *J Pediatr* 1991;119:305–310.

Markowitz ME, Rosen JF, Bijur PE. Effects of iron deficiency on lead excretion in children with moderate lead intoxication. *J Pediatr* 1990;116:360–364.

Marsh DO. The neurotoxicity of mercury and lead. In: O'Donoghue JL, ed. *Neurotoxicity of industrial and commercial chemicals*. Boca Raton, FL: CRC Press, 1985;159–169.

McDonald J, Potter N. Lead's legacy? Early and late mortality of 454 lead-poisoned children. *Arch Environ Health* 1996;51:116–121.

Millar JA, Cummings RLC, Battistini V, et al. Lead and δ-aminolaevulinic acid dehydratase levels in mentally retarded children and in lead-poisoning suckling rats. *Lancet* 1970;2:695–698.

Min Y-I, Correa-Villasenor A, Stewart PA. Parental occupational lead exposure and low birth weight. *Am J Ind Med* 1996;30:569–578.

Minnema DJ, Michaelson IA. Differential effects of inorganic lead and delta-aminolevulinic acid in vitro on synaptosomal gamma-aminobutyric acid release. *Toxicol Appl Pharmacol* 1986;86:437–447.

Minnema DJ, Greenland RD, Michaelson IA. Effects of in vitro inorganic lead on dopamine release from superfused rat striatal synaptosomes. *Toxicol Appl Pharmacol* 1986;84:400–411.

Minnema DJ, Michaelson IA, Cooper GP. Calcium efflux and neurotransmitter released from rat hippocampal synaptosomes exposed to lead. *Toxicol Appl Pharmacol* 1988;92:351–357.

Mitchell CS, Shear MS, Bolla KI, Schwartz BS. Clinical evaluation of 58 organolead manufacturing workers. *J Occup Environ Med* 1996;38:372–378.

Monteiro HP, Bechara EJH, Abdualla DSP. Free radical involvement in neurological porphyrias and lead poisoning. *Mol Cell Biochem* 1991;103:73–83.

Moore MR, Goldberg A, Pocock SJ, et al. Some studies of maternal and infant lead exposure in Glasgow. *Scot Med J* 1982;27:113–122.

Moore MR, Meredith PA, Goldberg A. Lead and heme biosynthesis: In Singhal RL, Thomas JA, eds. *Lead toxicity.* Baltimore, MD: Urban and Schwarzenberg, 1980:79–117.

Morgan A, Holmes A. The fate of lead in petrol-engine exhaust particulates inhaled by the rat. *Environ Res* 1978;15:44–56.

Morrow PE, Beiter H, Amato F, et al. Pulmonary retention of lead: an experimental study in man. *Environ Res* 1980;21:373–384.

Muldoon SB, Cauley JA, Kuller LH, et al. Effects of blood lead levels on cognitive function of older women. *Neuroepidemiology* 1996;15:62–72.

Müller WE, Snyder SH. Delta aminolevulinic acid: influence on synaptic GABA receptor binding may explain CNS symptoms of porphyria. *Ann Neurol* 1977;2:340–342.

Murozumi M, Chow TJ, Patterson C. Chemical concentration of pollutant aerosols, terrestrial dusts, and sea salts in Greenland and Antarctic snow strata. *Geochim Cosmochim Acta* 1969;33:1247–1294.

Murthy GK, Rhea US. Cadmium, copper, iron, lead, manganese, and zinc in evaporated milk, infant products, and human milk. *J Dairy Sci* 1971;54:1001–1005.

Mushak P. Defining lead as the premiere environmental health issue for children in America: criteria and their quantitative application. *Environ Res* 1992;59:281–309.

Myers RR, Powell HC, Shapiro HM, Costello ML, Lampert PW. Changes in endoneurial fluid pressure, permeability, and peripheral nerve ultrastructure in experimental lead neuropathy. *Ann Neurol* 1980;8:392–401.

National Academy of Sciences (NAS). *Lead: Biologic effects of atmospheric pollutants.* Washington: National Academy of Sciences, 1972:1–32.

National Institute for Occupational Safety and Health (NIOSH). *Pocket guide to chemical hazards.* Washington: U.S. Department of Health and Human Services, CDC, 1997.

Needleman HL, Shapiro IM. Dentine lead levels in asymptomatic Philadelphia school children: subclinical exposure in high and low risk groups. *Environ Health Perspect* 1974;7:27–31.

Needleman HL. The current status of childhood low-level lead toxicity. *Neurotoxicology* 1993;14:161–166.

Needleman HL, Gatsonis CA. Low-level lead exposure and the IQ of children. A meta-analysis of modern studies. *JAMA* 1990;263:673–678.

Needleman HL, Gunnoe C, Leviton A, et al. Deficits in psychological and classroom performance of children with elevated dentine lead levels. *N Engl J Med* 1979;300:689–695.

Needleman HL, Schell A, Bellinger D, et al. The long-term effects of low doses of lead in childhood. An 11-year follow-up report. *N Engl J Med* 1990;322:83–88.

Ng Y-W, Snitch P, Pamphlett R. Spinal cord uptake of lead injected into muscle. *Neurotoxicology* 1994;15:315–320.

Nielsen T. Atmospheric occurrence of organolead compounds. In: Grandjean P, Grandjean EC, eds. *Biological effects of organolead compounds.* Boca Raton, FL: CRC Press, 1984:43–62.

Nielsen T, Jensen KA, Grandjean P. Organic lead in normal human brains. *Nature* 1978;274:602–603.

Niklowitz WJ. Ultrastructure effects of acute tetraethyllead poisoning on nerve cells in the rabbit brain. *Environ Res* 1974;8:17–36.

Niklowitz WJ. Neurofibrillary changes after acute experimental lead poisoning. *Neurology* 1975;25:927–934.

Nordberg G. *Effects and dose-response relationships of toxic metals.* Amsterdam: Elsevier, 1975:1–111.

Nordman CH, Hernberg S. Blood lead levels and erythrocyte delta-amino-levulinic acid dehydratase activity of selected population groups in Helsinki. *Scand J Work Environ Health* 1975;1:219–232.

Norris C, Gettler AO. Poisoning by tetra-ethyl lead: post mortem findings. *JAMA* 1925;85:818–820.

Nosal RM, Wilhelm WJ. Lead toxicity in the shipbreaking industry: the Ontario experience. *Can J Public Health* 1990;81:259–262.

Occupational Safety and Health Administration (OSHA). Code of Federal Regulations, 29, 1910.1000/.1047. Washington: Office of the Federal Register, National Archives and Records Administration, 1995:411–431.

Occupational Safety and Health Administration (OSHA). 1995.

Ogata M, Tanaka A, Yokomura E, et al. Intake of lead particles through lung alveoli by lead fume inhalation. *Acta Med Okayama* 1973;27:211–219.

Oh SJ: Lead neuropathy. *Arch Phys Med Rehabil* 1975;56:312–317.

Ohnishi A, Dyck PJ. Retardation of Schwann cell division and axonal regrowth following nerve crush in experimental lead neuropathy. *Ann Neurol* 1981;10:469–477.

Ohnishi A, Schilling K, Brimijoin WS, et al. Lead neuropathy. 1) Morphometry, nerve conduction, and choline acetyltransferase transport: new finding of endoneurial edema associated with segmental demyelination. *J Neuropathol Exp Neurol* 1977;37:499–517.

Olden K. Environmental risks to the health of American children. *Prev Med* 1993;22:576–578.

Otto DA, Benignus VA, Muller KE, Barton CN. Effects of age and body lead burden on CNS function in young children. I. Slow cortical potentials. *Electroencephalogr Clin Neurophysiol* 1981;52:229–239.

Otto DA, Fox DA. Auditory and visual dysfunction following lead exposure. *Neurotoxicology* 1993;14:191–208.

Otto D, Robinson G, Baumann S, et al. 5-Year follow-up study of children with low-to-moderate lead absorption: electrophysiological evaluation. *Environ Res* 1985;38:168–186.

Ozonoff D. Lead on the range. *Lancet* 1994;343:6–7.

Paglia DE, Valentine WN, Dahlgren JG. Effects of low-level lead exposure on pyrimidine 5'-nucleotidase and other erythrocyte enzymes. Possible role of pyrimidine 5'-nucleotidase in the pathogenesis of lead-induced anemia. *J Clin Invest* 1975;56:1164–1169.

Panariti E, Berxholi K. Lead toxicity in humans from contaminated flour in Albania. *Vet Hum Toxicol* 1998;40:91–92.

Pappas CL, Quisling RG, Ballinger WE, Love LC: Lead encephalopathy: symptoms of cerebellar mass lesion and obstructive hydrocephalus. *Surg Neurol* 1986;26:391–394.

Perelman S, Hertz-Pannier L, Hassan M, Bourrillon A. Case report. Lead encephalopathy mimicking a cerebellar tumor. *Acta Pediatr* 1993;82:423–425.

Perlstein MA, Attala R. Neurological sequelae of plumbism in children. *Clin Pediatr* 1966;5:292–298.

Petit TL, Alfano DP, LeBoutillier JC. Early lead exposure and the hippocampus: a review and recent advances. *Neurotoxicology* 1983;4:79–94.

Piomelli S. A micromethod for free erythrocyte porphyrins: the FEP test. *J Lab Clin Med* 1973;81:932–940.

Polizopoulou Z, Roubies N, Karatzias H, Papasteriades AP. Incidence of subclinical lead (Pb) exposure in cattle of an industrial area of Greece. *J Trace Elem Electrol Health Dis* 1994;8:49–52.

Popoff N, Weinberg S, Feigin I. Pathologic observations in lead encephalopathy: with special reference to the vascular changes. *Neurology* 1963;13:101–112.

Posner HS, Damastra T, Nriagu JO. Human health effects of lead. In: Nriagu JO, ed. *The biogeochemistry of lead in the environment, Part B.* Amsterdam: Elsevier, 1978:173–223.

Pounds JG, Rosen JF. Cellular metabolism of lead: a kinetic analysis in cultured osteoclastic bone cells. *Toxicol Appl Pharmacol* 1986;83:531–545.

Powell JJ, Greenfield SM, Thompson RP, et al. Assessment of toxic metal exposure following the Camelford water pollution incident: evidence of acute mobilization of lead into drinking water. *Analyst* 1995;120:793–798.

Powers JM, Rawe SE, Earlywine GR. Lead encephalopathy simulating cerebral neoplasm in an adult. *J Neurosurg* 1977;46:816–819.

Quarterman J, Morrison JN. The effects of dietary calcium and phosphates on the retention and excretion of lead in rats. *Brit J Nutr* 1975;34:351–362.

Raasch FO, Rosenberg JH, Abraham JL. Lead poisoning from hair spray ingestion. *Am J Forensic Med Pathol* 1983;4:159–164.

Rabinowitz MB, Wetherill GW, Kopple JD. Kinetic analysis of lead metabolism from respiration by normal man. *J Lab Clin Med* 1976;90:238–248.

Rabinowitz MB, Wetherill GW, Kopple JD. Magnitude of lead intake from respiration by normal man. *J Lab Clin Med* 1977;90:238–248.

Ramstoeck ER, Hoekstra WG, Ganther HE. Trialkyl lead metabolism and lipid peroxidation in vivo in vitamin E- and selenium-deficient rats, as measured by ethane production. *Toxicol Appl Pharmacol* 1980;54:251–257.

Rice C, Fischbein A, Lilis R, et al. Lead contamination in the homes of employees of secondary lead smelters. *Environ Res* 1978;15:375–380.

Rieke FE. Lead intoxication in shipbuilding and shipscrapping 1941 to 1968. *Arch Environ Health* 1969;19:521–539.

Robinson GS, Baumann S, Kleinbaum D, et al. *Effects of low to moderate lead exposure on brainstem auditory evoked potentials in children: environmental health document 3.* Copenhagen: World Health Organization Regional Office for Europe, 1985:177–182.

Robinson RO. Tetraethyl lead poisoning from gasoline sniffing. *JAMA* 1978;240:1373–1374.

Romieu I, Palazuelos E, Avila MH, et al. Sources of lead exposure in Mexico City. *Environ Health Perspect* 1994;102:384–389.

Saito K. Electroencephalography studies on petrol intoxication: comparison between nonleaded and leaded white petrol. *Br J Ind Med* 1973;30:352–358.

Samuel AM, Baxter PJ. An unusual source of lead exposure in a precious metal assay worker. *Br J Ind Med* 1986;43:420–421.

Sanders LW. Tetraethyllead intoxication. *Arch Environ Health* 1964a;8:82–88.

Sanders LW. Tetraethyllead intoxication. *Arch Environ Health* 1964b;8:270–277.

Sandhir R, Gill KD. Alterations in calcium homeostasis on lead exposure in rat synaptosomes. *Mol Cell Biochem* 1994;131:25–33.

Sax NI. *Dangerous properties of industrial chemicals,* 5th ed. New York: Van Nostrand Reinhold, 1979.

Saxena DK, Singh C, Murthy RC, et al. Blood and placental lead levels in an Indian city: a preliminary report. *Arch Environ Health* 1994;49:106–110.

Schell LM, Stark AO, Gomez MI, Grattan WA. Blood lead level by year and season among poor pregnant women. *Arch Environ Health* 1997;52:286–291.

Schepers GWH. Tetraethyl and tetramethyl lead. *Arch Environ Health* 1964;8:277–295.

Schuhmacher M, Belles M, Rico A, et al. Impact of reduction of lead in gasoline on blood and hair lead levels in the population of Tarragona Province, Spain 1990–1995. *Sci Total Environ* 1996;184:203–209.

Schwartz J, Landrigan PJ, Feldman RG, et al. Threshold effect in lead-induced peripheral neuropathy. *J Pediatr* 1988;112:12–17.

Scott B, Lew J. Lead neurotoxicity: neuronal and non-neuronal cell survival in fetal and adult DRG cell cultures. *Neurotoxicology* 1986;7:57–68.

Seawright AA, Brown AW, Aldridge WN, et al. Neuropathological changes caused by trialkyllead compounds in the rat. *Dev Toxicol Environ Sci* 1980;8:71–74.

Seawright AA, Brown AW, Ng JC, Hrdlicka J. Experimental pathology of short-chain alkyllead compounds. In: Grandjean P, Grandjean EC, eds. *Biological effects of organolead compounds.* Boca Raton, FL: CRC Press, 1984:178–206.

Selvín-Testa A, Loidl CF, López-Costa JJ, et al. Chronic lead exposure induces astrogliosis in hippocampus and cerebellum. *Neurotoxicology* 1994;15:389–402.

Seppäläinen AM. Diagnostic utility of neuroelectric measures in environmental and occupational medicine. In: Otto D, ed. *Multidisciplinary perspectives in event-related brain potential research.* Proceedings of the Fourth International Congress on Event-Related Slow Potentials of the Brain. Washington, DC: US Environmental Protection Agency EPA-600/9-77-043, 1978:448–452.

Seppäläinen AM. Electrophysiological evaluation of central and peripheral neural effects of lead exposure. *Neurotoxicology* 1984;5:43–52.

Seppäläinen AM, Hernberg S. Sensitive technique for detecting subclinical lead neuropathy. *Br J Ind Med* 1972;29:443–449.

Seppäläinen AM, Herberg S. Subclinical lead neuropathy. *Am J Ind Med* 1980;1:413–420.

Seppäläinen AM, Herberg S, Kock B. Relationship between blood lead levels and nerve conduction velocities. *Neurotoxicology* 1979;1:313–332.

Seppäläinen AM, Tola S, Herberg S, Kock B. Subclinical neuropathy at "safe" levels of lead exposure. *Arch Environ Health* 1975;30:180–183.

Seshia SS, Rjani KR, Boeckx RL, Chow PN. The neurological manifestations of chronic inhalation of leaded gasoline. *Dev Med Child Neurol* 1978;20:323–334.

Sexton K, Olden K, Johnson BL. Environmental justice: the central role of research in establishing a credible scientific foundation for informed decision making. *Toxicol Ind Health* 1993;9:685–727.

Silbergeld EK, Fales JT, Goldberg AM. Lead: evidence for a prejunctional effect on neuromuscular function. *Nature* 1974;247:49–50.

Silbergeld EK, Lamon JM. Effects of altered porphyrin synthesis on brain neurochemistry. *Neurobehav Toxicol Teratol* 1982;4:635–642.

Simons TJ, Pocock G. Lead enters bovine adrenal medullary cells through calcium channels. *J Neurochem* 1987;48:383–389.

Simpson JA, Seaton DA, Adams JF. Response to treatment with chelating agents of anaemia, chronic encephalopathy, and myelopathy due to lead poisoning. *J Neurol Neurosurg Psychiatry* 1964;27:536–541.

Smith HD, Baehner RL, Carney T, Majors WJ. The sequelae of pica with and without lead poisoning. *Am J Dis Child* 1963;105:609–616.

Smith DR, Ilustre RP, Osterloh JD. Methodological considerations for the accurate determination of lead in human plasma and serum. *Am J Ind Med* 1998;33:430–438.

Sobue G, Pleasure D. Experimental lead neuropathy: inorganic lead inhibits proliferation but not differentiation on Schwann cells. *Ann Neurol* 1985;17:462–468.

Sokas RK, Simmens S, Sophar K, et al. Lead levels in Maryland construction workers. *Am J Ind Med* 1997;31:188–194.

Sokas RK, Weller SC, Stolley PD. Predictors of lead stores in male veterans. *J Environ Pathol Toxicol Oncol* 1995;14:53–59.

Solliway BM, Schaffer A, Pratt H, et al. Visual evoked potentials N75 and P100 latencies correlate with urinary delta-aminolevulinic acid, suggesting gamma-aminobutyric acid involvement in their generation. *J Neurol Sci* 1995;134:89–94.

Stafstrom CE, Tandon P, Hori A, et al. Acute effects of MK801 or kainic acid–induced seizures in neonatal rats. *Epilepsy Res* 1997;26:335–344.

Stauber JL, Florence TM, Gulson BL, et al. Percutaneous absorption of inorganic lead compounds. *Sci Total Environ* 1994;145:55–70.

Suga RS, Fischinger AJ, Knoch FW. Establishment of normal values for zinc protoporphyrin (ZPP) using hematofluorometer: correlation with normal blood lead values. *Am Ind Hyg Assoc J* 1981;42:637–642.

Thompson JA. Balance between intake and output of lead in normal individuals. *Br J Ind Med* 1971;28:189–194.

Thornton I, Davies DJA, Watt JM, Quinn MJ. Lead exposure in young children from dust and soil in the United Kingdom. *Environ Health Perspect* 1990;89:55–60.

Thould AK. Lead encephalopathy. *Proc R Soc Med* 1961;54:228–229.

Tola S, Hernberg S, Asp S, Nikkanen J. Parameters indicative of absorption and biological effect in new lead exposure: a prospective study. *Br J Ind Med* 1973;30:134–141.

Tonge JI, Burry AF, Soral JR. Cerebellar calcification: a possible marker of lead poisoning. *Pathology* 1977;38:289–300.

Turlakiewicz Z, Chmielnicka J. Diethyllead as a specific indicator of occupational exposure in tetraethyllead. *Br J Ind Med* 1985;42:682–685.

Tutunji MF, Al-Mahasneh QM. Disappearance of heme metabolites following chelation therapy with meso 2,3-dimercaptosuccinc acid (DMSA). *Clin Toxicol* 1994;32:267–276.

United States Geological Survey (USGS). Mineral industry surveys: lead. Annual Review. Reston, VA: U.S. Department of the Interior, U.S. Geological Survey. 1995:1–22.

Valciukas JA, Lilis R, Petrocci M. An integrated index of biological effects of lead. *Am J Ind Med* 1981;2:261–272.

Valpey R, Sumi SM, Copass M, Goble GJ. Acute and chronic progressive encephalopathy due to gasoline sniffing. *Neurology* 1978;28:507–510.

Walls AD. Home-made cider: source of lead-poisoning. *BMJ* 1969;1:98.

Walsh TJ, McLamb RL, Bondy SC, et al. Triethyl and trimethyl lead: effects on behavior, central nervous system morphology and concentrations of lead in blood and brain of rat. *Neurotoxicology* 1986;7:21–34.

Watson RJ, Decker E, Lichtman HC. Hematologic studies of children with lead poisoning. *Pediatrics* 1958;21:40.

Watt F, Landberg J, Powell JJ, et al. Analysis of copper and lead in hair using the nuclear microscope; results from normal subjects, and patients with Wilson's disease and lead poisoning. *Analyst* 1995;120: 789–791.

Weerasuriya A, Curran GL, Poduslo JF. Physiological changes in the sciatic nerve endoneurium of lead-intoxicated rats: a model of endoneurial homeostasis. *Brain Res* 1990;517:1–6.

Weitzman M, Aschengrau A, Bellinger D, et al. Lead-contaminated soil abatement and urban children's blood lead levels. *JAMA* 1993;269: 1647–1654.

Wells AC, Venn JB, Heard MJ. Deposition in the lung and uptake to blood of motor exhaust labelled with [203]Pb. *Inhaled Particles* 1975;4:175–189.

White RF, Diamond R, Proctor S, et al. Residual cognitive deficits 50 years after lead poisoning during childhood. *Br J Ind Med* 1993;50: 613–622.

White RF, Feldman RG, Proctor SP. Behavioral syndromes in neurotoxicology. In: Fogel BS, Schiffer RB, Rao SM, eds. *Neuropsychiatry.* Philadelphia: Williams & Wilkins, 1996:959–971.

Whitfield CL, Ch'ien LT, Whitehead JD. Lead encephalopathy in adults. *Am J Med* 1972;52:289–298.

Wilson WE. Dopamine sensitive adenylate cyclase inactivation by organolead. *Neurotoxicology* 1982;3:100–107.

Windebank AJ, McCall JT, Hunder HG, Dyck PJ. The endoneurial content of lead related to the onset and severity of segmental demyelination. *J Neuropathol Exp Neurol* 1980;39:692.

Winneke G, Beginn U, Ewert T, et al. Comparing the effects of perinatal and later childhood lead exposure on neuropsychological outcome. *Environ Res* 1985;38:155–167.

Wolfsperger M, Hauser G, Gossler W, Schlagenhaufen C. Heavy metals in human hair samples from Austria and Italy: influence of sex and smoking habits. *Sci Total Environ* 1994;156:235–242.

Wong VCN, Ng THK, Yeung CY. Electrophysiologic study in acute lead poisoning. *Pediatr Neurol* 1991;7:133–136.

Woolf DA, Riach IC, Derweesh A, Vyas H. Lead lines in young infants with acute lead encephalopathy: a reliable diagnostic test. *J Trop Pediatr* 1990;36:90–93.

Yamamura Y, Arai F, Yamauchi H. Urinary excretion pattern of triethyllead, diethyllead and inorganic lead in the tetraethyllead poisoning. *Ind Health* 1981;19:125–131.

Yokoyama K, Araki S, Murata K, et al. Subclinical vestibulo-cerebellar, anterior cerebellar lobe and spinocerebellar effects in lead workers in relation to current and past exposure. *Neurotoxicology* 1997;18:371–380.

Young RSK, Grzyb SE, Crismon L. Recurrent cerebellar dysfunction as related to chronic gasoline sniffing in an adolescent girl. *Clin Pediatr* 1977;16:706–708.

CHAPTER 5

Arsenic

Arsenic (arsenicals, As) is obtained from arsenopyrite and other arsenic-containing ores. It is found in the atmosphere, in soil, in plants, and in water, eventually appearing in the food chain of humans and other animals (Gorby, 1988). It exists in several valence states (-3, $+3$, and $+5$), permitting reactions with other metals, hydrogen, oxygen, and carbon, resulting in the formation of inorganic trivalent arsenic compounds (e.g., arsenic trioxide, arsenic trichloride, and sodium arsenide), pentavalent inorganic arsenic compounds (e.g., arsenic pentoxide, arsenic acid, and calcium arsenate), and organic arsenical compounds such as sodium arsanilate (Atoxyl), arsanilic acid, methylarsonic acid, dimethylarsinic acid (cacodylic acid), arsenobetaine, and arsenocholine (NAS, 1977; Lawrence et al., 1986). Arsine gas (AsH_3, arsenic hydride, arseniuretted hydrogen) is a colorless compound with a mild, garlic-like odor (Sax, 1979). Arsenic found in body tissues reflects its intake and absorption from external sources. There is evidence that trace levels of arsenic are essential to normal biological functioning and that arsenic may play a role in methionine metabolism (Uthus, 1994). Adverse effects on the nervous system as well as other organ systems occur when exposure exceeds that which is biologically necessary and tolerable; the clinical manifestations associated with arsenic poisoning include neuropathy, neuropsychological disturbances, and death.

SOURCES OF EXPOSURE

Arsenic trioxide is generated in nonferrous (e.g., copper) metal production (Fitzgerald, 1983; ATSDR, 1993). Arsenic and arsenic trioxide are no longer produced in the United States. Nevertheless, large amounts of arsenic trioxide continue to be imported annually. Total import of arsenic into the United States has ranged from 36 million pounds in 1985 to 69 million pounds in 1989 (ATSDR, 1993). The majority (74%) is used in the formulation of wood preservatives, another 20% is used in the production of agricultural chemicals such as pesticides and herbicides, and the remaining 6% is used in the production of

glass and nonferrous alloys and in the electronics industry (ATSDR, 1993).

Arsenic has been used therapeutically since the days of Hippocrates (460 to 377 B.C.) in the traditional remedies of various cultures throughout the world (Mitchell-Heggs et al., 1990; Malachowski, 1990). Because it is odorless, tasteless, and quite toxic, arsenic has been used both as a homicidal and a suicidal agent. Its more practical current uses are in products such as pesticides (e.g., lead arsenate, calcium arsenate, and sodium arsenite), herbicides (e.g., monosodium arsenate and dimethylarsinic acid), wood preservatives (e.g., zinc and chromium-copper-arsenate), and glass and enamel production. Other applications include paper dyes; leather manufacture; defoliants; food additives for cattle, poultry, and swine; drugs; and nerve gases. Gallium arsenide is an artificial crystal used in the manufacture of integrated circuits (Webb et al., 1984); arsine gas is used to make computer microchips (Lowe et al., 1992).

Arsenic exposure occurs in approximately 1.5 million workers, half of whom are directly involved in commercial processes such as mining, refining, chemical and pharmaceutical production, and the application of arsenic-containing pesticides mean yearly intake of arsenic in 43 copper-smelter workers was estimated to be 25 mg (Lagerkvist and Zetterlund, 1994). Inhalation is the main route of entry for airborne arsenic particulate associated with occupational exposure. In a Swedish copper smelter, the average air concentration of arsenic was determined to be between 0.06 and 2 $\mu g/m^3$ (Lundgren, 1954). The average arsenic concentration in the air in a Japanese copper refinery was 0.006 to 0.011 $\mu g/m^3$ under normal ventilation conditions, and 0.08 to 0.19 $\mu g/m^3$ under nonventilated conditions (Kodama et al., 1976).

Arsenic concentrations in atmospheric dust are usually insignificant, except where large quantities of particulate arsenic (e.g., arsenic trioxide) are released from certain situations. Arsenic-treated wood and arsenic-containing fossil fuels are well-known sources of airborne arsenic pollution when burned as a fuel at electric power stations or burned inadvertently at family barbecues (Bencko and Symon, 1977; NIOSH, 1983; Peters et al., 1984; Gratt and Levin, 1994; Geschke et al., 1996). In the United States, background levels of arsenic in soil are generally less than 20 ppm. Arsenic was found in soil polluted by a copper smelter in the Mill Creek area of Montana at concentrations averaging over 400 ppm (Binder, 1988). Arsenic concentrations as high as 21,000 ppb have been reported in soil contaminated by arsenic-containing pesticide (Feinglass, 1973). Arsenic concentration in well water is usually below 10 ppb, although higher levels can result from the release of arsenic from bedrock (Grantham and Jones, 1977). Arsenic concentrations of up to 4,781 ppm were found in well water in Ester Dome, Alaska (Kreiss et al., 1983). Groundwater contamination occurs from the run-off (migration) of arsenic from waste disposal sites. Drinking water often contains arsenic as arsenate. Arsenite may be found in water under anaerobic conditions. Organic arsenicals, such as methylarsonic acid and dimethylarsinic acid, are rarely found in water supplies. However, when found, they either are formed from inorganic arsenic through microbial activity or are introduced through the application of arsenic-containing herbicides which then find their way into the water supply (Ridley et al., 1977; ATSDR, 1993).

The general population ingests arsenic in food and water. Meat, fish, and poultry account for 80% of the dietary arsenic intake in an average American adult. Seafood and algae also contain high concentrations of organic arsenic in the form of arsenobetaine and arsenocholine, the so-called fish arsenic. Fish arsenic is commonly found in shellfish, cod fish, and haddock and is relatively nontoxic to humans (Sabbioni et al., 1991). Fish arsenic is rapidly excreted after ingestion without detection of residual toxic metabolites; and unlike inorganic arsenic, fish arsenic does not accumulate in hair (Vahter et al., 1983; Brown et al., 1990). Wine made from grapes sprayed with arsenic-containing pesticides may have appreciable levels of arsenic. Smokers may also inhale small amounts of arsenic due to pesticide residue on tobacco leaves. Accidental and intentional ingestion of arsenic continues to be reported in the medical and forensic literature (NIOSH, 1975; EPA, 1977; Milham and Strong, 1974; Feldman, 1982; Polissar et al., 1990; Civantos et al., 1995; Geschke et al., 1996).

EXPOSURE LIMITS AND SAFETY REGULATIONS

The *Occupational Safety and Health Administration* (OSHA) requires medical surveillance and maintenance of exposure records by all employers in situations where arsenic is used. This may be done by examining only the workers who complain of symptoms; otherwise, workers considered at risk undergo periodic examinations and tests of biological exposure indices (BEIs) (Weeks et al., 1991). The OSHA has established an 8-hour time-weighted average (TWA) permissible exposure limit (PEL) of 0.01 mg/m^3 for inorganic arsenic. The OSHA PEL for organic arsenic is 0.5 mg/m^3. The PEL for arsine gas is 0.2 mg/m^3

TABLE 5-1. *Established and recommended occupational and environmental exposure limits for arsenic in air and water*

	Air (mg/m^3)[a]	Water (mg/L)[a]
Odor threshold		
Arsine*	1.6	0.000035
OSHA		
PEL (8-hr TWA)		
Inorganic	0.010	—
Organic	0.5	—
Arsine	0.2	—
PEL ceiling (15-min TWA)		
Inorganic	—	—
Organic	—	—
Arsine	—	—
NIOSH		
REL (10-hr TWA)		
Inorganic	Carcinogen	—
Organic	—	—
Arsine	Carcinogen	—
STEL (15-min TWA)		
Inorganic	0.002	—
Organic	—	—
Arsine	0.002	—
IDLH		
Inorganic	5	—
Organic	—	—
Arsine	10	—
ACGIH		
TLV (8-hr TWA)		
Inorganic	0.01	—
Organic	0.01	—
Arsine	0.16	—
STEL (15-min TWA)		
Inorganic	—	—
Organic	—	—
Arsine	—	—
USEPA		
MCL	—	0.05
Inorganic		
Organic		
Arsine		
MCLG	—	—
Inorganic		
Organic		
Arsine		

[a]Unit Conversion: 1 mg/L= 1 ppm.
OSHA, Occupational Safety and Health Administration; PEL, permissible exposure limit; TWA, time-weighted average; NIOSH, National Institute for Occupational Safety and Health; REL, recommended exposure limit; STEL, short-term exposure limit; IDLH, immediately dangerous to life or health; ACGIH, American Conference of Governmental Industrial Hygienists; TLV, threshold limit value; USEPA, United States Environmental Protection Agency; MCL, maximum contamination level; MCLG, maximum contamination level goal.
Data from *Amoore and Hautala, 1983; OSHA, 1995; ACGIH, 1995; EPA, 1996; NIOSH, 1997.

(OSHA, 1995). The *National Institute for Occupational Safety and Health's* (NIOSH) recommended short-term exposure limit (STEL) for inorganic arsenic is a 15-minute TWA of 0.002 mg/m^3. The NIOSH considers inorganic arsenic to be a carcinogen and recommends respirators anytime exposure exceeds their recommended STEL. The NIOSH STEL for arsine gas is 0.002 mg/m^3 (NIOSH, 1997). The *American Conference of Governmental Industrial Hygienists* (ACGIH) recommends an 8-hour-TWA threshold limit value (TLV) for inorganic arsenic of 0.01 mg/m^3. The ACGIH TLV for arsine gas is 0.16 mg/m^3 (ACGIH, 1995) (Table 5-1).

Because of the many accidental poisonings in children (Fuortes, 1988), the *United States Environmental Protection Agency* (USEPA) proposed cancellation of all registered uses of inorganic arsenic for nonwood preservative purposes, except for the use of calcium arsenate as a turf herbicide, lead arsenate as a grapefruit growth regulator, sodium arsenite as a grape fungicide, and arsenic acid as a crop desiccant. Arsenic is listed by the USEPA as a hazardous air pollutant, and therefore its emission from copper smelters, glass manufacturing plants, and other arsenic-using facilities has been limited since 1986; however, although many states have established acceptable ambient air thresholds, there is currently no national ambient air standard for arsenic (ATSDR, 1993). The Food and Drug Administration (FDA) has set "no tolerance levels" (NTLs) for arsenic in food except as by-products in animals treated with veterinary drugs. Levels of permissible arsenic in foods range from 0.5 ppm in eggs and uncooked edible tissues of chicken and turkey to 2 ppm in certain uncooked edible products of pigs (ATSDR, 1993). The USEPA maximum contamination level (MCL) for inorganic arsenic in drinking water is 0.05 mg/L (USEPA, 1996) (see Table 5-1).

METABOLISM

Tissue Absorption

Pulmonary absorption of arsenic occurs following exposure to arsine gas and arsenic particulate (e.g., As$_2$O$_3$ (Jones, 1907; Lagerkvist et al., 1986). The amount of arsenic absorbed by inhalation of dust depends on the size of the airborne particles containing arsenic. Small particles are readily absorbed across the pulmonary alveoli. Airborne dust in copper–arsenic smelters contains particulate arsenic of approximately 5 μm in size that can be deposited in the airways and lungs (Brune et al., 1980; Leffler et al., 1984). Some larger-size particles remain in the upper respiratory passages of the lungs and do not reach the more vascular and absorptive alveolar surfaces as do the smaller particles. Other large particles are transferred by mucociliary clearance from the lungs by way of the oral pharynx and swallowing to the gastrointestinal (GI) tract from which they are subsequently absorbed.

GI absorption of arsenic is determined by the solubility of the particular arsenical compound. For example, highly soluble compounds such as monomethylarsonic acid and sodium arsenite and arsenic trioxide are almost completely absorbed from the GI tract following ingestion, while less soluble arsenic compounds such as arsenic triselinide are not as well absorbed (Mappes, 1977; Mahieu et al., 1981; Buchet et al., 1981).

Dermal absorption of arsenic compounds also occurs. For example, sodium arsenate is absorbed through the skin at a rate as high as 33 μg/cm^2/hr (Dutkiewicz, 1977).

Tissue Distribution

After uptake into the bloodstream, arsenic binds to the globin portion of hemoglobin, leukocyte membranes, or plasma proteins (Schoolmeester and White, 1980). Blood levels of inorganic arsenic decline rapidly and are detectable for only 2 to 4 hours after exposure. However, the methylated metabolites of inorganic arsenic (e.g., monomethylarsonic acid and dimethylarsinic acid) are detectable in the blood for more than 24 hours after ingestion (Hindmarsh and McCurdy, 1986; Moyer, 1993). As arsenic clears from the blood, it is distributed to the liver, spleen, kidney, lungs, and GI tissues, with less accumulation in muscle and nervous tissue. The specific pattern of distribution of arsenic depends on (a) tissue blood perfusion and (b) the affinity of the particular tissue for the arsenic compound and its metabolites (Mann et al., 1996). Arsenic in the trivalent (arsenite) form binds to sulfhydryl groups, while pentavalent arsenic (arsenate) is substituted for phosphates *in vivo* (Klaassen, 1990). For example, arsenite binds with sulfhydryl groups (—SH) in keratin-rich tissues such as skin, hair, and nails, while arsenate accumulates in bone and teeth by replacing phosphate (Levinsky et al., 1970; Schoolmeester and White, 1980; Fesmire et al., 1988). Median concentrations of arsenic measured in the brains of otherwise healthy people who died in accidents were reported as 0.013 mg/kg dry weight (range: 0.001 to 0.036 mg/kg) (Liebscher and Smith, 1968). Clearance of arsenic from the brain is slow. Higher concentrations of arsenic are found in the white matter than in the gray matter of the brain. Arsenic is also found in the myelin of the peripheral nerves. This distribution reflects arsenic's accumulation in neural tissues high in lipids, phospholipids, and/or phosphatides (Larsen et al., 1977).

Inorganic arsenic readily crosses the placenta and subsequently affects the fetus (Lugo et al., 1969; Ferm, 1977; Hood et al., 1988). In contrast, studies suggest that organic arsenic compounds such as arsphenamine do not as easily cross the placenta and are considerably less toxic to the fetus (Eastman, 1931; Kantor and Levin, 1948; Ferm, 1977; Willhite and Ferm, 1984; Hood et al., 1988). Methylation of inorganic arsenic is presumed to decrease its toxic effect on the fetus as well as on the mother (Hood et al., 1988). Nevertheless, *in utero* exposure to inorganic and organic arsenicals has been associated with teratogenic effects and neonatal death in humans and laboratory animals (Lugo et al., 1969; Willhite and Ferm, 1984). At high levels of maternal exposure to inorganic arsenic, detoxification mechanisms may become saturated and neonatal death may result (Hood et al., 1988). High concentrations of arsenic were found in the brain of a newborn infant who died after having been exposed *in utero* to inorganic arsenic ingested by the mother (Lugo et al., 1969).

Tissue Biochemistry

Reduction of the less toxic arsenate (As^{5+}) to the more toxic arsenite (As^{3+}) by the actions of glutathione is essential to the detoxification process; arsenic must be in the trivalent state to be methylated (Vahter and Envall, 1983; Buchet and Lauwerys, 1987; Delnomdedieu et al., 1994). This reaction is followed by biomethylation (Buchet and Lauwerys, 1985; Goyer, 1986). *S*-Adenosylmethionine is the methyl donor for biotransformation of inorganic arsenic to mono- and dimethylarsenic acid compounds (Buchet and Lauwerys, 1985). Dimethylarsenic is the major metabolite of arsenic in humans (40% to 60%) (Tam et al., 1979; Vahter, 1986; Buchet et al., 1981; Mann et al., 1996). The efficiency of the methylation process decreases as arsenic intake increases and as glutathione stores are depleted (Buchet and Lauwerys, 1987; Mann et al., 1996). Therefore, as the capacity for methylation is exceeded by the body burden of arsenic, increased retention occurs in soft tissue. Tolerance to slowly accumulated inorganic arsenic occurs over time by induction of the methylation process (Chhuttani and Chopra, 1979). Subjects with poor nutritional status have a lower capacity to methylate and to detoxify inorganic arsenic (DeWolff and Edelbroek, 1994). Impairment of inorganic arsenic methylation has been reported in patients with hepatic insufficiency (Buchet et al., 1984). Genetic polymorphisms have been identified at the S-transferase gene loci that can increase an individual's susceptibility to the toxic effects of arsenic (Strange et al., 1998). In contrast to inorganic arsenic, the organic arsenic compounds do not undergo extensive metabolism (Buchet et al., 1981).

The biochemical mechanism of toxicity is dependent on the valence state of arsenic. For example, arsenate has been shown to uncouple mitochondrial respiration, while arsenite has been shown to bind to sulfhydryl groups of biological ligands such as lipoic acid (Klaassen, 1990) (see Neuropathological Diagnosis section).

Excretion

Arsenic is excreted mainly by the kidneys, with very little appearing in feces and even less found in the skin, hair, nails, and sweat (Buchet and Lauwerys, 1987; Ishinishi et al., 1986). Urinary excretion of inorganic arsenic is maximal approximately 10 hours after ingestion of inorganic arsenic whether as arsenate or arsenite, returning to normal after 20 to 30 hours; urinary monomethylarsenic and dimethylarsenic acid levels peak at 40 to 60 hours after ingestion, returning to baseline in 6 to 20 days (Moyer, 1993). The biological half-life of inorganic arsenic is about 10 hours, with 50% to 80% excreted in 3 days (Goyer,

1986). Elimination of arsenic from most tissues is complete within 2 to 4 weeks. The arsenic that remains in the body after 4 weeks is bound to sulfhydryl groups (—SH) in keratin-rich skin, hair, and nails (Levinsky et al., 1970; Fesmire et al., 1988). The measurement of urinary levels of methylated arsenic acid is helpful in determining whether excessive arsenic intake comes from food or from occupational and environmental exposure (Johnson and Farmer, 1991; Moyer, 1993).

The organic arsenic forms found in fish and crustaceans, arsenobetaine and arsenocholine, are not biotransformed *in vivo* and are rapidly excreted, unchanged, in the urine (Goyer, 1986). Organic arsenic is excreted completely within 1 to 2 days after ingestion. Following a single oral ingestion of seafood, 50% of the fish arsenic (arsenobetaine) is eliminated within 20 hours in humans (Johnson and Farmer, 1991), with total clearance in 48 hours (ATSDR, 1993).

CLINICAL MANIFESTATIONS AND DIAGNOSIS

Symptomatic Diagnosis

The clinical manifestations associated with exposure to arsenic-containing compounds depends on the route of intake, dose, and duration of exposure, as well as on the physiochemical state of the arsenic (i.e., inorganic, organic, gas, liquid, or particulate) (Heyman et al., 1956). For example, organic arsenic compounds such as arsenobetaine are considerably less toxic than are inorganic arsenic compounds such as arsine gas and arsenic trioxide (Sabbioni et al., 1991).

Acute Exposure

Arsine gas is the most toxic form of the arsenic compounds with an instantly lethal dose of 250 ppm (800 mg/m^3) (NIOSH, 1979). The effects of acute exposure to high concentrations of arsine gas are mostly hemolytic, although peripheral neuropathy with associated clinical symptoms of paresthesias and muscle weakness has been reported (Jones, 1907; Dudley, 1919; DePalma, 1969; Fowler and Weissberg, 1974). Following acute exposure to arsine gas, there is generally a 2- to 24-hour delay before the occurrence of the acute clinical manifestations of intoxication, which include dizziness, headache, nausea, vomiting, and shortness of breath. In more severe cases, these symptoms are accompanied by a hemolytic reaction with intravascular hemolysis and jaundice; the skin often has a bronze tint (Jones, 1907; Dudley, 1919; DePalma, 1969; Fowler and Weissberg, 1974; Goyer, 1986). Hemoglobinuria, proteinuria, and hemolytic anemia are common; the urine is often dark red in color 4 to 6 hours after inhalation of arsine gas (Jones, 1907; Dudley, 1919; DePalma, 1969; Fowler and Weissberg, 1974). Death due to renal failure induced by accumulation of products of hemolysis follows the most severe exposures to arsine gas (Jones, 1907). In those patients who survive the acute effects of exposure to arsine gas, horizontal stratifications of the fingernails (leukonychia, Mee's lines) appear within 2 to 3 weeks and signs of peripheral neuropathy appear within 4 weeks (DePalma, 1969; Levinsky et al., 1970).

Acute ingestion of arsenic is often followed by a similar constellation of nonspecific symptoms that include nausea, vomiting, abdominal pain, watery and/or bloody stool, fever, acute renal failure, seizures, coma, cardiac arrhythmias, rhabdomyolysis, and sometimes death (St. Petery et al., 1970; O'Shaughnessy and Kraft, 1976; Sanz et al., 1989; Ghariani et al., 1991; Civantos et al., 1995). Fluid and electrolyte imbalance, autonomic nervous system involvement with hypotension, cardiac arrhythmias, respiratory failure, and death due to cardiac arrest occur in severe cases of arsenic ingestion (Fincher and Koerker, 1987; Campbell and Alvarez, 1989; Civantos et al., 1995). However, the hemolytic reaction that is associated with inhalation of arsine gas is not seen following ingestion of arsenic compounds. Mee's line and hyperkeratosis appear 4 to 6 weeks after ingestion of inorganic arsenic salts (Jenkins, 1966). Acute exposure of sufficient intensity is typically followed by tingling, burning, and often painful paresthesias, indicative of peripheral neuropathy within 7 to 14 days and progressing to a maximum sensory and motor affliction within 4 to 5 weeks (Jenkins, 1966; Tay and Seah, 1975; O'Shaughnessy and Kraft, 1976; LeQuesne and McLeod, 1977; Murphy et al., 1981; Fesmire et al., 1988; Geschke et al., 1996) (Table 5-2). Paresthesias initially appear in the lower extremities and eventually involve the upper extremities as well (Jenkins, 1966; Chhuttani and Chopra, 1979; Oh, 1991). Objective evidence of sensory deficits are detectable with tests of pinprick and touch and show a "glove and stocking" distribution. Position and vibra-

tion sense are reduced in the feet and may be the earliest detectable clinical evidence of peripheral neuropathy (Conomy and Barnes, 1976). Patients rarely lack objective sensory symptoms (Dudley, 1919; Heyman et al., 1956; St. Petery et al., 1970; Jenkins, 1966). Tendon reflexes are diminished or disappear early, especially in the ankles (Jenkins, 1966; St. Petery et al., 1970; Chhuttani and Chopra, 1979). Muscle weakness occurs, especially in the lower extremities (St. Petery et al., 1970; O'Shaughnessy and Kraft, 1976). Cranial nerve impairment has also been reported following acute exposure to inorganic arsenic salts (Geschke et al., 1996).

Early clinical and electrodiagnostic features are indistinguishable from those of Guillain–Barré syndrome, typically presenting with symmetrical muscular weakness of the most distal muscles and sometimes extending more proximally but rarely involving the shoulder or pelvic girdle (St. Petery et al., 1970; Donofrio et al., 1987; Gherardi et al., 1990). Bilateral footdrop is a common clinical manifestation (St. Petery et al., 1970; O'Shaughnessy and Kraft, 1976). Although sensory symptoms predominate during the clinical course, weakness and atrophic muscles may persist in severe cases of arsenic neuropathy. Slow and incomplete recovery occurs over several years, during which the patients often require leg braces and sensory input adaptations for walking (O'Shaughnessy and Kraft, 1976). Abnormalities of various neurophysiological parameters persist in some cases for 6 to 8 years or more after acute arsenic exposure (Schenk and Stolk, 1967; Tay and Seah, 1975; O'Shaughnessy and Kraft, 1976; LeQuesne and McLeod, 1977; Fincher and Koerker, 1987; Morton and Caron, 1989; Windebank, 1993).

O'Shaughnessy and Kraft (1976) described the sequence of affection and recovery over a period of 3 years after an acute intentional ingestion of an unknown quantity of sodium arsenate in addition to 30 mg of flurazepam in the suicide attempt of a 19-year-old woman. On admission to the hospital 12 hours after ingestion the patient was stuporous and unable to answer questions. She had already vomited and had "rice water" stools. Her blood pressure was 80/52. She was given oxygen, intravenous fluids, and British antilewisite (BAL), 5 mg/kg intramuscularly. The BAL was administered for 14 days, during which time the patient had been in coma and had developed renal failure, left bundle branch block, and a plural effusion. Her electroencephalogram showed a diffusely slow record, consistent with encephalopathy. Her renal function returned to normal by the eleventh day, but bone marrow showed suppression of red cell precursors. The latter recovered by the fourteenth day, when it was noted that her persistent problem was muscle weakness in all limbs, more distal than proximal and most prominent in the legs. Reduced muscle strength continued for the following 42 weeks, before improvement was seen in

TABLE 5-2. *Clinical manifestations of acute arsenic poisoning and the time of their appearance after an exposure*

Immediate to hours	Hours to days	Weeks to months
Metallic taste	Proteinuria	Alopecia
Extreme thirst	Hematuria	Renal failure
Cough, dyspnea	Hemolysis	Hyperkeratosis
Pulmonary edema	Jaundice	Stomatitis
Nausea	Delirium	Sensory/motor
Vomiting	Hallucinations	neuropathy
Diarrhea		Encephalopathy
Abdominal pain		
Hematemesis		
Confusion		
Seizures		
Headache		

the first in proximal upper and lower extremities. Muscle strength in the more distal muscles of the arms was then considered fair (initially poor), whereas the strength in the lower extremities had improved from trace–poor to poor–fair. Muscle strength was normal in the proximal and distal muscles of the upper extremities and in the proximal muscles of the lower extremities at follow-up 146 weeks postexposure. Persistent distal weakness caused the patient to walk with a bilateral footdrop slap and necessitated the use of lower leg braces. Nerve conduction studies documented the progression of the peripheral neuropathy in this patient (see Neurophysiological Diagnosis section).

Acute intravenous administration of organic arsenical remedies for syphilis and other diseases were used in the 1930s and 1940s before the introduction of more specific therapies such as penicillin. As a result, many cases of hemorrhagic necrosis of the central nervous system (CNS) were reported as "hemorrhagic encephalopathies," "cerebral purpura," "toxic myelitis," "pericapillary encephalorrhagia," and, most commonly, "arsenical encephalopathy." Call and Gunn (1949) described a case of arsenical encephalopathy in a 34-year-old man who died after receiving two intravenous injections of arsphenamine, 1 week apart, for treatment of his syphilis. No adverse effects were experienced after the first injection; however, 48 hours after the second treatment, the patient complained of symptoms of the "flu," followed by the development of disorientation, lethargy, incoordination, and somnolence over the next 12 hours. By then he had right-sided pyramidal signs, bilateral Babinski signs, and papilledema. He became comatose by 72 hours and died 1 week after the last arsphenamine treatment (see Neuropathological Diagnosis section).

Chronic Exposure

Chronic exposure to inorganic arsenic compounds, whether by inhalation or ingestion, causes nonspecific symptoms including: cardiovascular abnormalities; acrocyanosis; gangrene of the lower extremities ("black foot disease"); mucosal irritation; dermal changes of hyperpigmentation and epithelial hyperplasia with hyperkeratosis; anemia; and disturbances of hepatic function (Dewar and Lenihan, 1956; Glazener et al., 1968; Tseng, 1977; Lagerkvist et al., 1986). Inflammation and ulceration of the nasal septum and conjunctivitis result from prolonged and/or intense exposure to airborne arsenic (Lagerkvist et al., 1986). In addition, exposure to arsenic is also strongly associated with an increased risk of cancer of skin, lung, and of the hepatic, lymphatic, and hematopoietic systems (Tseng, 1977; Järup et al., 1989; ATSDR, 1993). Mee's lines are usually not seen in cases of chronic arsenic exposure, unless severe acute episodes have also occurred. The onset of peripheral neuropathy associated with chronic exposure to arsenic occurs insidiously and may go unnoticed for as long as 2 years (Goldstein et al., 1984; Feldman et al., 1979; Windebank, 1993).

Cranial nerve involvement has been reported following inhalation of arsine gas as well as following chronic ingestion and inhalation of inorganic arsenic salts (Dudley, 1919; Zaloga et al., 1985; Geschke et al., 1996). Reports of cranial neuropathies following chronic arsenic exposure have involved the auditory nerves with perceptive hearing loss (Yamashita et al., 1972; Hotta, 1989; Bencko and Symon, 1977) and impairment of the optic nerve (Hotta, 1989; Schenk and Stolk, 1967), oculomotor nerve (Chhuttani et al., 1967), facial nerve (Friedman and Olson, 1941; Zaloga et al., 1985) and vestibular nerve (Diamant, 1958). Olfactory abnormalities such as hyposmia and anosmia have also been described (Hotta, 1989). Exposed persons may experience a metallic or garlic-like taste (Garb and Hine, 1977). Involvement of the phrenic nerve has also been reported (Bansal et al., 1991).

Encephalopathy following both acute and chronic exposures to arsenic presents as headache, emotional distress, and cognitive impairments that often include attention deficit and impairment of short-term memory function (Heyman, 1956; Freeman and Couch, 1978; Danan et al., 1984; Beckett et al., 1986; Morton and Caron, 1989; Klaassen, 1990). Twenty percent of arsenic exposure cases present with acute behavioral disturbances (Schoolmeester and White, 1980). Seizures and coma have also been reported (Kantor and Levin, 1948; Talwalkar et al., 1976; Haller et al., 1986; Ortel et al., 1987; Fincher and Koerker, 1987). Chronic encephalopathy is more common after exposure to organic arsenic (Kantor and Levin, 1948; Call and Gunn, 1949; Windebank, 1993); however, with use of sensitive neuropsychological test batteries, subtle cognitive disturbances as well as disturbances of personality and affect have also been documented after exposure to inorganic arsenic (Yamashita et al., 1972; Bolla-Wilson and Bleecker, 1987; Morton and Caron, 1989; White and Proctor, 1995). Encephalopathy after chronic exposure to inorganic arsenic may include visual and auditory hallucinations, paranoid delusions, confusion, irritability, drowsiness, and delirium (Schenk and Stolk, 1967; Bolla-Wilson and Bleeker, 1987; Hotta, 1989; Morton and Caron, 1989). Arsenic encephalopathy usually improves after removal from exposure; however, in some cases, persistent abnormalities including psychosis have been reported (Schenk and Stolk, 1967; Freeman and Couch, 1978; Fincher and Koerker, 1987; Morton and Caron, 1989).

Neurophysiological Diagnosis

Electroencephalography (EEG) of patients exposed to arsenic is typically normal, but slowing of the alpha rhythm occurs in those patients presenting with acute encephalopathy (Talwalkar et al., 1976; Danan et al., 1984; Beckett et al., 1986; Ortel et al., 1987; Fincher and Koerker, 1987; Fesmire et al., 1988). However, the contribution of metabolic disturbances (e.g., acute renal failure with associated uremic encephalopathy) must be considered when interpreting the EEG of patients exposed to arsenic (Lugo et al., 1969; O'Shaughnessy and Kraft, 1976). For example, the EEG of a 19-year-old woman who developed acute renal failure after she ingested an unknown quantity of arsenic showed diffuse slowing of the background rhythm (O'Shaughnessy and Kraft, 1976). The EEG of a 50-year-old man who developed encephalopathy after exposure to arsenic (urine arsenic 41 μg/L; normal 0 to 20 μg/L) revealed slowing of the alpha rhythm; other laboratory tests including blood urea nitrogen (BUN) were normal. His mental status improved following chelation therapy with BAL, but the results of a follow-up EEG were not reported in this case (Bolla-Wilson and Bleecker, 1987). Bilateral slowing in EEG rhythms was observed in a 25-year-old man and a 45-year-old woman, both of whom were being treated with organic arsenicals for bronchial asthma. Follow-up at 2 weeks after cessation of treatment showed marked improvement in the clinical conditions and in the background EEG rhythms of both patients (Talwalkar et al., 1976). In a more severe case of arsenic encephalopathy involving a 20-year-old man who became comatose after he ingested 1 g of sodium arsenite, the initial EEG also showed diffuse slowing (theta). However, at follow-up 3 months after exposure the EEG showed complete absence of alpha activity with a background rhythm of only 1.5 to 5 Hz (delta). One year later, the patient was semiconscious and the dominant rhythm had increased (5 to 7 Hz). No epileptiform activity was noted. A computed tomography scan of this patient's brain documented diffuse cortical atrophy (Fincher and Koerker, 1987). In contrast, the EEG of a 41-year-old man who attempted suicide by ingesting 8 to 9 g of powdered arsenic was normal; this patient did not develop arsenic encephalopathy (Goebel et al., 1990). Similarly, a 30-year-old woman ingested arsenic trioxide and developed peripheral neuropathy and abnormalities on neuropsychological tests but showed no abnormalities on EEG (Danan et al., 1984).

Visual evoked potentials (VEPs) and *brainstem auditory evoked potentials* (BAEPs) have also been used to document the CNS effects of arsenic. The VEPs of a 20-year-old man who was comatose after he ingested 1 g of sodium arsenite were absent at testing 4, 12, and 24 months after exposure. However, the BAEPs in this patient at 1 year after exposure were normal, and he responded to noise and verbal stimulation (Fincher and Koerker, 1987). The BAEPs of a 41-year-old man who attempted suicide by ingesting 8 to 9 g of powdered arsenic but did not develop arsenic encephalopathy were within normal limits (Goebel et al., 1990).

Nerve conduction studies and electromyography (EMG) have been used to document peripheral neuropathy following acute and chronic exposures to arsenic (O'Shaughnessy and Kraft, 1976; LeQuesne and McLeod, 1977; Feldman et al., 1979; Fincher and Koerker, 1987; Lagerkvist and Zetterlund, 1994; Greenberg, 1996). Electrophysiological evidence, typical of axonal degeneration, has been found in cases of arsenic-exposure-induced peripheral neuropathy. These include low- to absent-amplitude recordings of the sensory potentials, prolonged sensory latencies, reduced conduction velocities, and absent F-waves (O'Shaughnessy and Kraft, 1976; Oh, 1991). Serial tests of arsenic-exposed individuals have demonstrated progressively slower motor conduction velocities, reaching a maximum impairment approximately 90 days after exposure (O'Shaughnessy and Kraft, 1976; Murphy et al., 1981).

Nerve conduction studies documented the progression of the peripheral neuropathy in a 19-year-old woman who attempted suicide by ingesting an unknown quantity of sodium arsenate in addition to 30 mg of flurazepam (see above). Progression of the neuropathy was followed over a 3-year period (O'Shaughnessy and Kraft, 1976). Initial nerve conduction studies at 2 weeks after exposure showed a right median nerve conduction velocity (NCV) of 42 m/sec, a right ulnar NCV of 43 m/sec, and a right peroneal NCV of 29 m/sec. Neurological examination at that time showed good muscle strength in the upper extremities and fair–good strength in the lower extremities. In addition, touch and pressure sensation were reduced and the patient was experiencing painful paresthesias. NCV studies showed worsening at follow-up 13 weeks after exposure, with a median NCV of 28 m/sec and an ulnar NCV of 39 m/sec; nerve conduction velocities could not be obtained following stimulation of the peroneal nerve at that time. EMG studies performed at that time in the anterior tibialis and extensor digitorum brevis muscles showed fibrillations and many positive waves. In addition, no voluntary motor unit action potentials could be elicited. Neurological examination at that time revealed reduced strength in the distal upper and lower extremities. Gradual recovery in the upper extremities was noted by 42 weeks (median NCV = 42 m/sec; ulnar NCV = 52 m/sec). However, stimulation of the peroneal nerve still failed to evoke a response. The EMG study of the first dorsal interosseous muscle also documented regeneration of peripheral nerve fibers in the upper extremities and showed 50% recruitment with no positive waves or fibrillations. However, positive waves and fibrillations were still seen in the anterior tibialis and extensor digitorum brevis muscles. In addition, recruitment in the anterior tibialis had improved to only 10% of normal, and no voluntary motor potentials could be elicited in the extensor digitorum brevis. Neurological examination showed normal muscle strength in the proximal upper extremities, but strength was still reduced distally in the upper and lower extremities. Nerve conduction velocities in the median and ulnar nerves was normal at follow-up 146 weeks after exposure. No evoked potential could be obtained after surface stimulation of the peroneal nerve and recording over the area of the extensor digitorum brevis, but a low-amplitude (6 mV) long latency (5.5 msec) response was obtained with a needle recording in the anterior tibialis muscle. Neurological examination showed normal muscle strength in the arms, but strength was still reduced distally in the legs. This study demonstrates regeneration of peripheral nerve components following an intense acute exposure to arsenic and shows how the length of the nerve fiber correlates with the electrophysiological and clinical prognosis.

In a similar case, a 41-year-old vintner attempted suicide by ingesting 8 to 9 g of arsenic (Goebel et al., 1990). Within a few hours, he developed vomiting and diarrhea, and he was treated at a local hospital for shock and aneuria with hemodialysis. Upon admission to the hospital the patient's urinary level of arsenic was 7.5 mg/L as baseline; following BAL, 100 mg b.i.d., urinary excretion increased to 9.2 mg/L after 2 days, and it decreased to 0.2 mg/L after 14 days. Ten days after ingestion, the patient noticed numbness in his feet; this spread proximally, involving his upper extremities within several days. Tendon reflexes were absent in the legs and diminished in the arms. Sensation to touch and pinprick were reduced below the knees and were impaired to the level of the elbows. Vibration sense was absent in ankles and fingers, and it diminished in knees and wrists. Diffuse hyperkeratotic areas over the soles and transverse white stria of the fingernails (Mees' lines) were present.

Eight weeks after the initial ingestion of arsenic, NCV studies were performed (Table 5-3). The EMG studies performed in this patient at that time revealed a few fibrillations in the distal leg muscles, but motor unit potential abnormalities were not noted. Serial follow-up nerve conduction and electromyographic studies taken over a 4-year exposure-free period documented regeneration without signs of further degeneration and recovery with the return of sensory conduction in the median, ulnar, and sural nerves. Motor nerve conduction velocity studies also showed recovery.

Nerve conduction studies in a group of arsenic-exposed smelter workers showed prolonged conduction velocities in motor and sensory fibers (Table 5-4) (Feldman et al., 1979). Average values for conduction velocities and amplitudes were computed for all workers. Except for differences in peroneal motor conduction velocity, the average conduction velocities of the arsenic-exposed workers showed no consistent patterns. Nevertheless, with the exception of the sural nerve amplitude, the lowest values were always found in the arsenic-exposed group. In addition, evoked sensory potentials were not elicited and conduction velocities were slower than the lower limit of the normal range (40 m/sec) in 12 workers (Table 5-4). Statistical analyses are often needed to demonstrate subclinical neuropathy in arsenic-exposed populations (Lagerkvist

TABLE 5-3. *Serial nerve conduction studies after acute arsenic ingestion in humans*

		Time after exposure		
	Normal	8 weeks	2 years	4 years
Sensory conduction				
Median nerve				
Velocity (m/sec)	45–72	No response	58.0	63.0
Amplitude (mV)	>5.0	No response	4.0	4.0
Ulnar nerve				
Velocity (m/sec)	42–58	No response	57.0	56.0
Amplitude (mV)	>7.0	No response	5.0	12.0
Sural nerve				
Velocity (m/sec)	40–58	No response	40.0	NA
Amplitude (mV)	>4.0	No response	2.5	NA
Motor conduction				
Median nerve				
Distal latency (m/sec)	2.4–4.0	2.7	3.1	3.0
Velocity (m/sec)	48–64	49.0	50.0	59.0
Amplitude proximal (mV)	>7.0	10.0	16.5	17.0
Amplitude distal (mV)	>7.0	12.0	16.5	17.0
Ulnar nerve				
Distal latency (m/sec)	1.8–3.2	2.1	2.8	2.4
Velocity (m/sec)	46–75	50.0	55.0	61.0
Amplitude proximal (mV)	>7.0	12.0	15.5	16.5
Amplitude distal (mV)	>7.0	13.0	16.0	17.0
Peroneal nerve				
Distal latency (m/sec)	2.4–4.8	4.2	4.0	4.2
Velocity (m/sec)	42–58	36.0	40.0	41.0
Amplitude proximal (mV)	>3.0	2.5	4.0	4.0
Amplitude distal (mV)	>3.0	3.2	4.0	3.9

NA, not available.
Modified from Goebel et al., 1990, with permission.

TABLE 5-4. *Average conduction velocities (m/sec) and amplitudes (µV) by intensity of exposure in arsenic workers*

Exposure	n	Ulnar motor wrist–elbow (m/sec)	Ulnar motor elbow–axilla (m/sec)	Ulnar sensory (m/sec)	µV	Peroneal motor (m/sec)	µV	Sural sensory (m/sec)	µV
Arsenic high	37	55.6	63.5	50.4	6.4	44.9	4.7	41.4	10.7
Arsenic low	33	54.4	63.3	50.6	8.2	44.8	4.3	41.3	12.7
Control	28	56.1	61.5	52.2	8.4	47.1	6.9	43.5	11.4
Other	13	53.9	62.2	49.4	10.3	47.4	5.4	41.6	10.9
Total	111								

Modified from Feldman et al., 1979, with permission.

and Zetterlund, 1994; Feldman and Jabre, 1997). The mean conduction velocity may be reduced in an arsenic-exposed population differing significantly from the mean conduction velocity in a nonexposed control group, yet it may still fall within the normal range (2 SD). In other words, an individual patient's nerve conduction velocity can be recorded as normal in spite of subclinical effects of exposure. Simple analysis confirmed statistically significant differences between the exposed groups and the control groups, although there were only weak correlation coefficients of association. Discriminant analysis of the relationship between tissue concentration of arsenic, ulnar sensory action potential amplitude, and slower peroneal motor nerve conduction velocity showed that the arsenic workers could be separated from the nonarsenic workers (69.1% correct classification) and that the nonarsenic group could be separated from the arsenic group (67.5% correct classification).

Other reports have described clinical and subclinical neuropathy in arsenic-exposed copper-smelter workers (Singer et al., 1982; Blom et al., 1985; Lagerkvist and Zetterlund, 1994). Lagerkvist and Zetterlund (1994) evaluated 43 workers exposed to arsenic trioxide for a period of 13 to 45 years. It was determined that the peripheral nerves are affected more by long-term exposure than by short-term fluctuations in arsenic levels. Furthermore, the normal decrease in NCV that occurs with aging may be enhanced by previous exposure to arsenic.

Neuropsychological Diagnosis

Acute and chronic exposure to arsenic has been associated with impairment of cognitive functioning. Attention and short-term memory function are frequently impaired in arsenic-exposed persons (Danan et al., 1984; Peters et al., 1986; Bolla-Wilson and Bleecker, 1987; Morton and Caron, 1989). Decreased memory, drowsiness, confusion, delirium, and even symptoms suggestive of schizophrenia have been described following exposure to inorganic arsenic (Bolla-Wilson and Bleecker, 1987). Lassitude, fatigability, and anxiety have been noted on examination of affect and personality in patients chronically exposed to arsenic (McCutchen and Utterback, 1966). Neuropsychological testing has also revealed nonspecific effects on visuospatial abilities in arsenic-exposed patients. The Block Designs and Object As-

sembly subtests of the Wechsler Adult Intelligence Test–Revised (WAIS-R) are sensitive to mild and moderate arsenic encephalopathy (White and Proctor, 1995). Language and general intellectual function are typically spared in adults exposed to arsenic (Bolla-Wilson and Bleecker, 1987).

Neuropsychological assessment of a 30-year-old female dental surgeon who intentionally ingested arsenic trioxide in a suicide attempt showed impaired attention and short-term memory function. At follow-up evaluation 11 months after exposure, her performance on neuropsychological testing was considered recovered and normal (Danan et al., 1984).

Neuropsychological assessment of a woman who had inhaled arsenic as sawdust and vapors from the burning of chromate–copper–arsenate-treated wood (elevated arsenic levels in hair and nails) showed consistent disturbances in short-term memory on the Wechsler Memory Scale (Peters et al., 1986) (see Clinical Experiences section). The neuropsychological assessment of a 50-year-old chemical engineer who was occupationally exposed to inorganic arsenic revealed impairments of functioning on tests of attention and psychomotor speed (e.g., simple reaction time and Digit Symbol test) and on tests of verbal memory (e.g., Logical Memories, Consonant Trigrams, and Rey Auditory Verbal Learning Test). Visual memory and language function were spared. Although this patient's performance on tests of verbal memory remained below expectation, improved functioning in other neuropsychological domains was seen at follow-up 4 and 8 months after exposure (Bolla-Wilson and Bleecker, 1987). Neuropsychological assessment of a worker who was exposed to arsenic fumes from hot pressurized lumber for 14 months revealed impaired cognitive functioning, especially on tests of attention and short-term memory. A follow-up 5 months after cessation of exposure revealed significant improvement in all areas of cognitive functioning (Morton and Caron, 1989).

Biochemical Diagnosis

Monitoring of the urinary concentrations of the inorganic metabolites of arsenic is the recommended biological exposure index (BEI) for workers exposed to arsenic. The urinary concentrations measured at the end of the work week should not exceed 50 mg/g creatinine (ACGIH, 1995) (Table 5-5). Urine concentrations of arsenic serve as

TABLE 5-5. *Biological exposure indices for arsenic (ACGIH, 1995)*

	Urine	Blood	Alveolar air
Determinant:	Inorganic arsenic	Arsenic	Arsenic
Start of shift:	Not established	Not established	Not established
During shift:	Not established	Not established	Not established
End of shift at end of workweek:	50 µg/g creatinine	Not established	Not established

Data from ACGIH, 1995.

a better indicator of exposure than do blood concentrations, especially 24 hours or more after the end of exposure. In the case of arsenic poisoning, a blood sample reflects the intake only if taken within the first 2 to 4 hours after exposure, since arsenic clears from the blood rapidly (Moyer, 1993). Even if blood levels are not elevated, other tissues may contain arsenic. Roses et al. (1991) reported of a massive epidemic of acute arsenic (sodium arsenite) poisoning in 718 persons in Argentina. Urine samples were obtained from 307. Symptoms of exposure increased with urine arsenic concentrations; and an increased incidence of diarrhea, vomiting, and systemic symptoms was seen among those persons with urine arsenic concentrations greater than 75 µg/dL.

An elevated cerebrospinal fluid (CSF) protein level of 99.3 mg/dL (normal 20 to 45 mg/dL) was reported in a 41-year-old vintner who had ingested 8 to 9 g of arsenic. This abnormality of the CSF may reflect the severe neurotoxic effects of arsenic in this patient but other explanations must be considered in such cases as well (Goebel et al., 1990).

The use of hair arsenic analysis is a convenient way to estimate cumulative exposures; however, extraneous contamination on the hair shaft by adherence of environmental pollutants and/or hair treatments may exaggerate actual exposure levels and thus may not as accurately reflect the internal arsenic dose as does determination of urine arsenic levels. For this reason, hair analysis alone is not a reliable means of making a biochemical diagnosis of increased arsenic intake (Feldman and Baker, 1979). Arsenic does accumulate in hair and nails over time; therefore, the proximal portion of the hair may contain increased levels of arsenic in cases of recent exposure, while the more distal segment reflects a more remote exposure. Increased arsenic levels in the whole shaft suggests ongoing chronic exposure.

Analysis of blood, urine, hair, and fingernails for arsenic was performed on copper smelter workers who were chronically exposed to arsenic trioxide. The workers were divided into three groups according to personal sampling of atmospheric arsenic levels: those at risk for high exposure, those at risk for low exposure, and a control group. Blood levels were not a useful indicator of exposure, but a definite relationship was demonstrated between the incidence of elevated arsenic levels in the urine and the intensity of exposure (Table 5-6). The average urine sample concentration for 37 workers at high-arsenic sites was 98 ppb, with 22 men registering levels higher than 50 ppb. Only one of the workers from a low-arsenic exposure site had a urine level higher than 50 ppb. The sites of employment in the plant with greater opportunity for exposure had more effect on the quantity of arsenic excreted in the urine than did the duration of employment. The high-exposure group, employed for an average of 14.5 years, had an average urine arsenic concentration of 378.1 ppb; the low-exposure group, employed for an average of 16.4 years, had an average of 74.1 ppb. Not surprisingly, the average arsenic concentrations in fingernails and hair were higher in the high-exposure group than in the low-exposure group, and both had higher levels than the control subjects (Table 5-7). In addition, a correlation was found between the levels of arsenic in urine, nails, and hair of these workers and the occurrence of clinical, subclinical, or no peripheral neuropathy (Fig. 5-1).

Neuroimaging

Magnetic resonance imaging (MRI) and computed tomography (CT) can be used to document the CNS effects of arsenic exposure and to detect changes arising from secondary brain swelling and/or vascular events associated with the encephalopathy. The CT scan is typically normal following acute arsenic exposure with associated encephalopathy (Danan et al., 1984). However, in those cases of higher levels of arsenic exposure with severe acute en-

TABLE 5-6. *Distribution of urine arsenic levels in workers by intensity of exposure*

Exposure	Workers (n)	Urine arsenic levels (ppb)						
		Nondetectable	<10	10–19	20–29	30–49	50–99	>100
Arsenic high	37	1	2	2	3	7	11	11
Arsenic low	33	14	6	3	7	2	0	1
Control group	41	33	2	4	1	0	1	0
Total	111	48	10	9	11	9	12	12

Modified from Feldman et al., 1979, with permission.

TABLE 5-7. *Average arsenic quantity (ppm) in nails and hair reflects intensity of workplace exposure levels*

Exposure	Nails	Hair
High exposure	72.8	182.6
Low exposure	21.1	8.9
Control	1.2	0.6

Modified from Feldman et al., 1979, with permission.

cephalopathy the CT scan may reveal areas of edema and necrosis due to vascular occlusions and hemorrhages (Call and Gunn, 1949; Jenkins, 1966). For example, the CT scan 1 month after exposure in a 20-year-old man who ingested 1 g of sodium arsenite revealed moderate ventricular enlargement. A follow-up CT scan of this patient made 6 months after exposure revealed marked cortical atrophy (Fincher and Koerker, 1987) (see Neuropathological Diagnosis section).

Neuropathological Diagnosis

The effects of inorganic and organic arsenic compounds on the brain are similar (Jenkins, 1966). Severe arsenical encephalopathy appears to be related to the development of vascular occlusions with subsequent tissue hypoxia, demyelination, gliosis, and necrosis. Perivascular hemorrhages or "ring hemorrhages" are common and often coalesce to form larger areas of hemorrhage. Gross pathological examination of the brain reveals petechial hemorrhages and lesions of the white matter in the centrum semiovale, corpus callosum, internal capsule, thalamus, and pons. Microscopically small blood vessels including arterioles and capillaries are occluded by thrombi. Marked areas of necrosis are evident in the white matter of nearly all brain regions, while the gray matter is typically less affected. Microscopic examination of the white matter often reveals vacuolation associated with demyelination (Call and Gunn, 1949).

Nerve biopsies of patients with arsenic poisoning show prominent pathological changes including degenerated fibers and a marked reduction in the number of myelinated fibers. Silver staining demonstrates absent or diminished axons and fragmented axons (Chhuttani et al., 1967). Axons of all sizes are affected initially, followed by secondary demyelination, although segmental demyelination is rarely seen. Occcasional appearances of onion bulbs are thought to represent a Schwann cell response to axonal degeneration (Windebank, 1993). Sensory fibers are affected before motor fibers, and distal fibers are affected before proximal fibers (Jenkins, 1966). The dying back of long axons eventually involves spinal cord pathways and anterior horn cells (Ohta, 1970; Goebel et al., 1990).

A very carefully done serial neurophysiological study (Goebel et al., 1990) of polyneuropathy following acute arsenic intoxication utilizing nerve conduction studies (see Table 5-3) as well as two sequential sural nerve and gas-

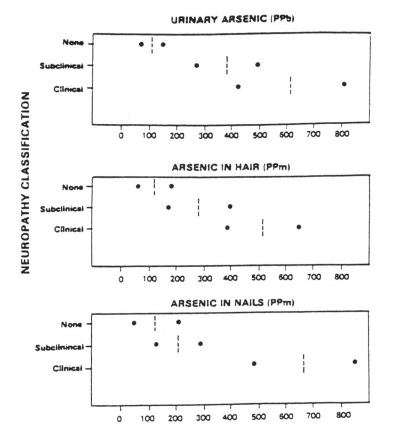

FIG. 5-1. Mean concentrations of arsenic in urine, hair, and nails by neuropathy classification. (Modified from Feldman et al., 1979, with permission.)

trocnemius muscle biopsies provided evidence of symmetrical involvement with acute wallerian degeneration of myelinated fibers and subsequent incomplete recovery following chelation (BAL) therapy in a 41-year-old man. A nerve biopsy done early in the course of recovery was compared with one done 4 years later. The initial biopsy revealed that numerous nerve fibers among the population of large myelinated nerve axons had undergone acute degeneration (Fig. 5-2A). This was further demonstrated in single teased fibers (Fig. 5-2B). A few scattered macrophages were present. There was no demyelination or remyelination, onion bulb formation, regeneration, metachromatic granules, or amyloid. Electron microscopy studies confirmed light microscopic features. Schwann cell processes containing debris of myelinated axons indicated the loss of

nerve fibers and the presence of macrophages (Fig. 5-3A). Remnants of once myelinated fibers were occasionally seen (Fig. 5-3B). In addition, a few myelinated axons contained intraaxonal lamellar and amorphous inclusions as well as smooth membrane cisternae. Swelling of unmyelinated axons was also observed, and sometimes only the remnants of Schwann cells around a large empty space indicated the former presence of a nerve fiber (Fig. 5-3C). Many single small, unmyelinated axons were superficially located between the basal lamina and the tiers of Schwann cell processes, suggesting regeneration (Fig. 5-3D). Fibroblasts, Schwann cells, and endothelial cells contained membrane-bound bodies that appeared partly electron-lucent and partly electron-dense. The electron-dense part was generally confined to a peripheral segment and, on higher magnification, could be seen to

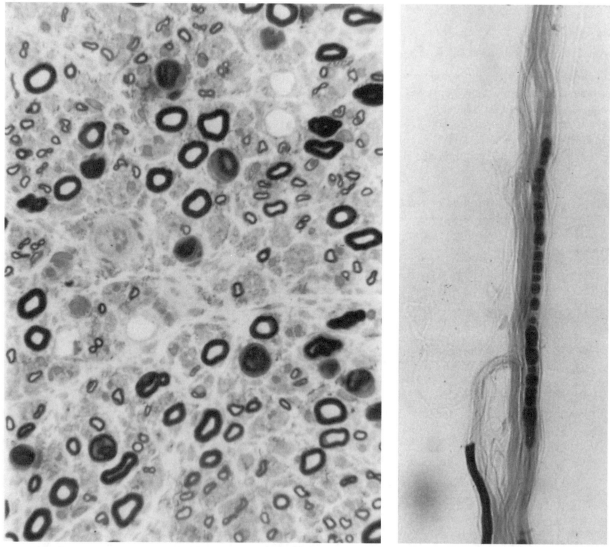

A

B

FIG. 5-2. Light microscopies of sural nerve biopsies from a 41-year-old vintner who developed polyneuropathy after acute arsenic intoxication. **A:** First sural nerve biopsy showing the numerous nerve fibers among the population of large myelinated nerve axons that had undergone acute degeneration (original magnification, ×430). **B:** Teased sural nerve fiber from first biopsy further demonstrating acute degeneration (original magnification, ×450). (Modified from Goebel et al., 1990, with permission.)

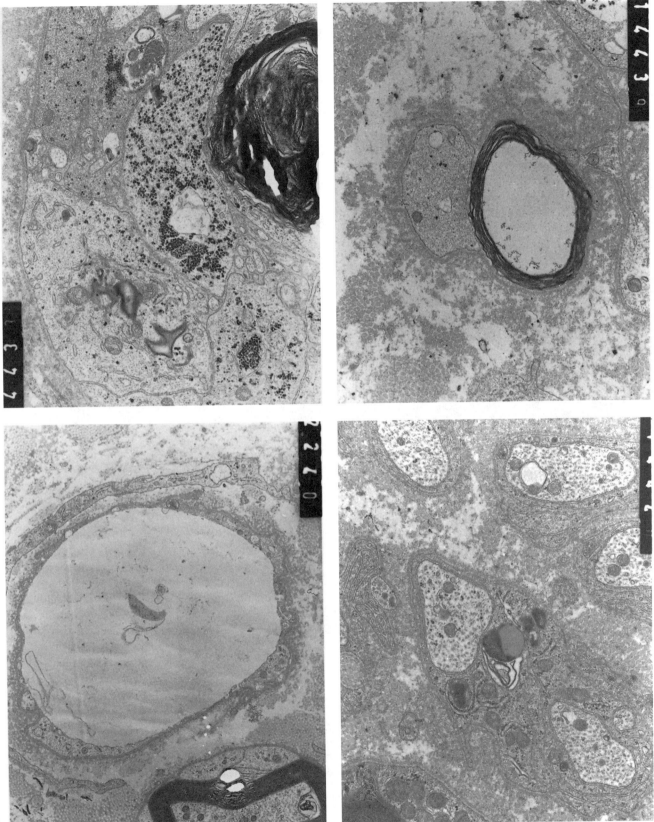

FIG. 5-3. Electron microscopy of first sural nerve biopsy 8 weeks after acute arsenic intoxication: **A:** Schwann cell processes containing debris of myelinated axons indicating the loss of nerve fibers and the presence of macrophages (original magnification, ×22,000). **B:** Remnants of once myelinated fibers (original magnification, ×25,872). **C:** Swelling of unmyelinated axons and the remnants of Schwann cells around a large empty space indicating the former presence of a nerve fiber (original magnification, ×8,624). **D:** Many single small, unmyelinated axons superficially located between the basal lamina and the tiers of Schwann cell processes suggesting regeneration (original magnification, ×39,600). (Modified from Goebel et al., 1990, with permission.)

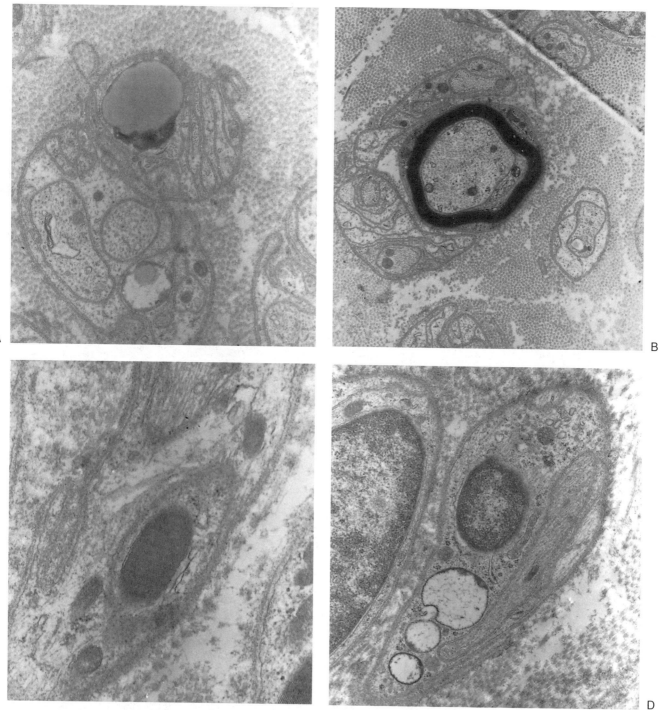

FIG. 5-4. Electron microscopy of second sural nerve biopsy 2 years after acute arsenic intoxication. **A:** Loss of primary unmyelinated axons (original magnification, ×20,559). **B:** Schwann cell processes containing unmyelinated axons arranged around a myelinated axon (original magnification, ×14,200). **C:** Inclusions in Schwann cells of unmyelinated axons consisting of membrane-bound closely packed filaments or tubules (original magnification, ×68,040). **D:** Presence of vacuolar inclusions that were membrane-bound with some electron-dense material attached to the inner margin of the vacuoles (original magnification, ×19,602). (Modified from Goebel et al., 1990, with permission.)

consist of a granular matrix and a few membranes. In the basement membranes of the perineurium, various-sized electron-dense spheroids were visible; frequently these were surrounded by a minute halo, indicating the possible deposition of calcium. Laser microprobe mass analysis (LAMMA) of the initial nerve biopsy documented the presence of arsenic; arsenic was not found on LAMMA of the second biopsy specimen.

The second biopsy showed persistence of a loss of large and small myelinated axons without signs of acute wallerian degeneration, primary axonal damage, or acute demyelination. However, occasional regeneration was seen. A teased fiber occasionally contained a thinner, myelinated segment. Electron microscopic study of the second biopsy indicated loss of primary unmyelinated axons because Schwann cell processes appeared arranged in plates surrounded by a common basal lamina (Fig. 5-4A). In addition, Schwann cell processes containing unmyelinated axons were arranged around a myelinated axon (Fig. 5-4B). There were many membrane-bound inclusions, often of a lamellar type in Schwann cells of myelinated and unmyelinated axons either outside of the myelin sheath or between the myelin sheath and axon. Inclusions in Schwann cells of unmyelinated axons consisted of membrane-bound closely packed filaments or tubules (Fig. 5-4C). Other inclusions appeared vacuolar and were membrane-bound with some electron-dense material attached to the inner margins of the vacuoles (Fig. 5-4D). The lack of an arsenic peak on LAMMA on the second biopsy of the sural nerve indicates that acute arsenic deposition in peripheral myelinated nerve fibers is reversible.

Interference with cellular metabolism by arsenic compounds results in distal axonal degeneration (dying back neuropathy). The mechanism by which arsenic interferes with cellular processes, and thus the arsenical compounds' ability to induce peripheral neuropathy, is determined by the valence state of the arsenic ion. Trivalent arsenic is significantly more toxic than pentavalent arsenic. Nevertheless, arsenate can disrupt cellular processes by substituting for phosphate in vivo (Klaassen, 1990). However, and perhaps of greater toxic importance, is that pentavalent arsenic is metabolized to the trivalent form in vivo (Vahter and Envall, 1983; Buchet and Lauwerys, 1987; Delnomdedieu et al., 1994). Cellular respiration mechanisms mediated by nicotinamide adenine dinucleotide (NAD)-linked substrates are sensitive to the effects of trivalent arsenic (Peters and Sanadi, 1961). Arsenite has an affinity for sulfhydryl groups and has been shown to inhibit the activity of sulfhydryl-containing enzymes such as pyruvate dehydrogenase, succinic dehydrogenase, and alpha glutarate oxidase (Bansal et al., 1991; Gherardi et al., 1990; Donofrio et al., 1987). Mechanisms involved in the toxicity of arsenic compounds include: (a) inhibition of sulfhydryl-containing enzymes in the body, especially by trivalent arsenite, which causes renal tubular damage; (b) arsenite binding to dihydrolipoic acid, a cofactor for pyruvate dehydrogenase leading to an

interruption of glucose metabolism; and (c) arsenolysis, in which pentavalent arsenic ions competitively substitute for phosphate in biochemical reactions, disrupting oxidative phosphorylation by replacing the stable phosphoryl with less stable arsenyl compounds (Schoolmeester and White, 1980; ATSDR, 1993). The latter mechanism leads to (a) rapid hydrolysis of high-energy bonds in compounds such as adenosine triphosphate (ATP) and (b) the loss of energy needed for critical steps in cellular metabolism (Moyer, 1993). The organelles of peripheral neurons and their axons are sensitive to the inhibition of energy supply and are affected early in the course of arsenic intoxication (Ohta, 1970). Secondary demyelination occurs after axonal degeneration takes place. The sensory fibers are affected before the motor fibers, and the distal portions are affected before the proximal fibers (Jenkins, 1966).

The clinical manifestations of arsenic encephalopathy and peripheral neuropathy are similar to those of thallium toxicity and riboflavin deficiency (Cavanagh, 1985; Windebank, 1986). Interference with pyruvate decarboxylation has been implicated as a common mechanism of toxicity. A similarity has also been noted between the effects of arsenic and those seen in thiamine deficiency, which have been attributed to the ability of arsenic to prevent the transformation of thiamine into acetyl-CoA and succinyl-CoA, thus blocking the tricarboxylic acid (Krebs) cycle (Sexton and Gowdey, 1963; Politis et al., 1980).

The underlying mechanism of arsine gas toxicity differs from that of the other arsenic compounds. It is a potent hemolytic agent, it rapidly fixes to red cells, and it produces irreversible cell membrane damage. In addition, red blood cell destruction by arsine produces indirect renal damage. At high levels, arsine produces direct cytotoxicity to multiple organ systems associated with sudden death. Once arsine is inhaled, it breaks down and then it releases inorganic arsenic into the bloodstream (NIOSH, 1979). Thus, prolonged nonfatal exposure to arsine produces many of the same symptoms of chronic inorganic arsenical exposure including peripheral neuropathy (Jones, 1907; Dudley, 1919; DePalma, 1969; Fowler et al., 1974; Wilkerson et al., 1975; Garb and Hine, 1977).

PREVENTIVE AND THERAPEUTIC MEASURES

Signs should be posted in all areas where the potential for exposure to inorganic arsenic exists (OSHA, 1995). Compressed air should not be used to clean floors and other surfaces contaminated with arsenic compounds. Respirators should be provided to employees who are potentially exposed to high concentrations of inorganic arsenic (e.g., arsenic trioxide) and arsine gas (OSHA, 1995). Biological monitoring, especially measuring urine arsenic levels, contributes to early detection of neurological effects.

Suspected cases of acute arsenic poisoning must be treated quickly, even before ascertaining a biochemical diagnosis. Multisystem symptomatology appears within 30 minutes of acute arsenic ingestion. The need to respond to the medical emergency (treating hypovolemia from hemolysis and vascular extravasation, dehydration, electrolyte imbalance, and cardiac irregularity) often displaces the importance of waiting for the results of a contemporary blood sample for possible toxic causative agents. Patients with suspected acute arsenic poisoning require rapid stabilization of their fluids and electrolytes in an intensive care setting (ATSDR, 1993). Monitoring for cardiac arrhythmia as well as renal failure is important (Civantos et al., 1995). Following acute ingestion, residual arsenic should be removed from the stomach of the patient after he or she is stabilized. This should be accomplished by gastric lavage and the use of a cathartic to prevent further intestinal absorption (Schoolmeester and White, 1980). Administration of activated charcoal and the combination of tincture of ferric chloride (300 mL) and sodium carbonate (30 mg) in 120 mL of water are possible effective antidotes (Schoolmeester and White, 1980). Hemodialysis may be necessary in those cases where there is associated renal failure (ATSDR, 1993).

Parenteral administration of chelating agents serves to inactivate toxic arsenicals. Chelation given before neuropathy develops brings about the best results (Murphy et al., 1981). Dimercaprol (2,3-dimercaptopropanol) or British antilewisite (BAL) is a recommended chelating agent for arsenic. The earlier dimercaprol is administered, the greater the chance of preventing serious irreversibility effects of arsenic intoxication (Heyman et al., 1956). An initial intramuscular dose of 3 to 5 mg/kg body weight can be given, followed by repeat doses every 4 hours for 2 days, every 6 hours on the third day, and then twice daily for 10 days or until symptoms have subsided. Other chelating agents used orally in children with heavy metal poisoning are dimercaptosuccinic acid (DMSA) and D-penicillamine (ATSDR, 1993). These oral chelating agents can be used in patients who do not have GI symptoms such as vomiting and diarrhea (Kersjes et al., 1987). D-Penicillamine is less effective in arsenic poisoning because of its monothio structure as compared to the dithio-containing chelators such as BAL and DMSA. Because of the serious effects of arsine gas poisoning, exchange transfusion may be needed to replace the hemolyzed red cells (ATSDR, 1993). In such cases, BAL is not considered helpful (Goyer, 1986).

Aggressive initial therapy including resuscitation, chelation with BAL, and hemodialysis resulted in survival of a 30-year-old man who had ingested a massive dose of arsenic in an apparent suicide attempt (see Clinical Experiences section). A time line documented a rapid fall in serum and urine arsenic levels during the treatment with hemodialysis and BAL. The serum levels and urinary output in this patient appeared to be influenced by BAL therapy (Fesmire et al., 1988). Within the first 24 hours after ingestion, serum arsenic levels fell rapidly. The urinary arsenic level was also elevated (22,000 µg/L) during the first 24 hours after exposure and fell gradually over the next week to 7,000 µg/L and was 600 µg/L at 16 days after in-

gestion. It is difficult to determine from the data presented in this case the contribution made by dialysis therapy to the excretion of arsenic. Furthermore, the urinary levels are not reported in relation to creatinine excretion; therefore, comparison of the three specimens is not possible. Nevertheless, the data reported in this case study do suggest the existence of a correlation between the excretion of large amounts of arsenic and the prompt administration of multiple therapeutic interventions as soon as possible following ingestion of inorganic arsenic.

The most important aspect of the treatment of patients with arsenic poisoning is the identification of the toxic source and the subsequent removal of the person at risk. Repeated hospital admissions (eight) were reported in a victim of recurrent arsenic poisoning over several years; the source of exposure had not been determined and eliminated. It is unwise to discharge without following up patients contaminated by arsenic of obscure source. Health department or other officials should be called upon to inspect the suspected toxic environment (Hutton and Christians, 1983; ATSDR, 1993).

The sooner chelation therapy is administered in relation to the exposure episode, the better the exposed individual's prognosis for recovery from arsenic neuropathy or encephalopathy (Chhuttani et al., 1967; Murphy et al., 1981; Fesmire et al., 1988). Complete recovery may occur in mild cases; patients with more severe poisoning, however, will retain motor disability or cognitive impairment for years with slow recovery, if any. Even then, residual findings may persist (Chhuttani et al., 1967; Yamashita et al., 1972; O'Shaughnessy and Kraft, 1976; Fincher and Koerker, 1987; Windebank, 1993). Once the nervous system is damaged, functional recovery may not follow chelation therapy (Heyman et al., 1956; Jenkins, 1966; Yamashita et al., 1972). Some patients will require vocational rehabilitation while others may require appropriate prostheses or long-term supervision and care (Heyman et al., 1956; O'Shaughnessy and Kraft, 1976; Fincher and Koerker, 1987).

CLINICAL EXPERIENCES

Group Studies

High- and Low-Risk Work Sites in a Copper Smelter: Clinical and Subclinical Neuropathy

A double-blind controlled study design was used to examine individuals currently exposed to arsenic trioxide in a copper-smelting factory (Feldman et al., 1979). Evidence of clinical and subclinical injury was sought in 70 workers from the copper-smelting site, 41 "nonarsenic" workers, 28 workers from an aluminum factory, and 13 volunteers who were residents of the town in which the smelting plant was located but who had no direct exposure risk. A 5-year average of periodic urinary sample tests that showed more or less than 200 ppb determined whether the worker was at high or low risk for arsenic exposure.

The subjects were given neurological and neurophysiological examinations by several neurologists who were unaware of the particular arsenic exposure risk of any given individual. Administrators of the neurological examinations were not the same ones who performed the neurophysiological examinations. Samples of blood, urine, hair, and fingernails obtained from each subject were analyzed for arsenic and other heavy metals by standard laboratory analytical chemistry methods. The results of these tests were disclosed to the investigators only after all of the clinical and electrophysiological studies had been completed on each subject.

The clinical examination considered (a) weakness or gait disorder, (b) numbness, (c) painful or burning paresthesias, (d) reduced perception of sensation to pinprick, (e) reduction or absence of vibratory perception, and (f) reduction or absence of tendon reflexes. Based on these six criteria, categories of clinical neuropathy were defined as follows: sensory, motor, or mixed sensory and motor. Clinical neuropathies were identified in 40 of the 111 subjects. In 16 of these, there were other possible explanations for the condition, such as frostbite in one, diabetes in three, and severe alcoholism in the remaining 12. The workers from the high-level arsenic site (10 subjects) and those from the low-level arsenic site (eight subjects) had greater incidence of sensory neuropathy than the control group (four subjects). Among all arsenic workers, there were three cases of motor neuropathy; there were no cases among the nonarsenic workers. There were five cases of mixed sensory and motor neuropathy in arsenic workers and none in the nonarsenic workers.

In 12 men exposed to arsenic, the NCVs were slower than the lower limit of the normal range (40 m/sec). For all nerves tested with the exception of the sural nerve amplitude, the lowest values were always found in the arsenic-exposed group (see Table 5-4). The average values of electrical measurements (conduction velocities and amplitudes) were computed for all participants grouped by classifications of "clinical neuropathy," "subclinical neuropathy," and "no neuropathy." Clinical neuropathy was based on physical examination only. Subclinical neuropathy exhibited either one or more reduced velocities and two or more nerves with reduced amplitudes. All subjects with no neuropathy were classified as normal. Although simple analysis confirmed statistically significant differences between exposed groups and the control groups, there were only weak correlation coefficients of association.

A statistically significant relationship was found between arsenic load and clinical or subclinical evidence of neuropathy in workers exposed in the copper-smelting plant. This relationship was dose-dependent. A limited multivariate analysis was performed to determine the relationship between neurological response and arsenic levels of urine, hair, and nails as well as demographic variables including place of employment, age, smoking history,

urine creatinine and specific gravity, and carboxyhemoglobin as a percentage of hemoglobin. Lower sensory amplitude and slower peroneal velocity were associated with higher arsenic levels in urine, hair, and nails ($p < 0.01$). Lower peroneal amplitudes distally and proximally were also associated with higher arsenic levels in urine, hair, and nails. Discriminant analysis showed that the arsenic workers could be separated from the nonarsenic workers (69.1% correct classification) and that the nonarsenic group could be separated from the arsenic group (67.5% correct classification). Canonical analysis was performed to evaluate the individual values of the arsenic levels in blood, hair, nails, and urine, as one group of variables, with the neurological measurements constituting the other group. With this method, lines of regression of the two macrovariables (arsenic levels and macroneurological variables) showed that the control group and the low-arsenic-site group fell within the expected range for normal populations with minimal or no exposure to arsenic. The group with nonarsenic causes coincided with the group of high-arsenic-site workers—that is, if the common denominator was neuropathy, clinical or subclinical. This epidemiological and clinical study demonstrates a dose response relationship between neurological outcome and the level of arsenic encountered at various work sites within a copper smelter.

Past Exposure to Arsenic: Long-Term Follow-Up

Lagerkvist and Zetterlund (1994) found clinical and subclinical neuropathy in arsenic exposed copper-smelter workers. A group of 43 workers who had been exposed to arsenic trioxide for 13 to 45 years were evaluated. The results were compared with those obtained from a group of 46 referents; both the study patients and the referents had been tested 5 years earlier by Blom, Lagerkvist, and Linderholm. The mean urinary level of inorganic arsenic and its metabolites (monomethylarsonic acid and dimethylarsinic acid) and blood levels for arsenic and lead were measured for all subjects. The daily absorption of arsenic was calculated at about 100 μg, with a mean estimated absorption of 25 mg/year. The exposed workers reported more symptoms and had more general medical complaints than the referents. Nine workers and six referents retired. Four of the workers and no referents developed diabetes. Of the referents, one was hospitalized for dementia, one died of liver cancer, and two died of myocardial infarction. Of the exposed workers, one died of myocardial infarction, one refused to be retested, and another who had reduced conduction time in the past was dropped from the study because it appeared that his neuropathy was hereditary. It was concluded that adverse effects of arsenic on peripheral nerves result from long-term exposure rather than from short-term elevations in exposure levels.

Evaluation of a Community Consuming Arsenic-Contaminated Well Water

High levels of arsenic (arsenate) were found in well water in Ester Dome, Alaska (Kreiss et al., 1983). A total of 147 persons who ingested well water with arsenic concentrations above or below the maximum level of 15 μg/L participated in an epidemiological study. Of these, 132 persons had a home well, although five denied ever drinking well water, having brought in a portion of their drinking water from other sources. Well-water arsenic concentrations ranged from 1 to 4,781 μg/L, with a mean of 347.3 and a median of 41 μg/L. Arsenic concentrations in water hauled or available from pipe sources ranged from 0 to 32 μg/L, with a mean of 4.8 and a median of 1.4 μg/L. To account for the variability in amounts and sources of water consumed, an index of arsenic ingestion was calculated by adding the arsenic present in the usual quantity of well water consumed to that present in the usual quantity of other types of water consumed. The index of arsenic ingestion ranged from 0.0 to 4,521.0 μg/day. Urine arsenic concentrations in the group ranged from 6 to 4,964 μg/L, with a median of 50.9 μg/L.

Of the 147 persons receiving neurological examinations, six showed symptoms and physical findings compatible with mild sensory neuropathy. Of these, two had conditions associated with neuropathy other than exposure to neurotoxicants, such as diabetes and Raynaud's disease. Of the four remaining persons, one had a calculated daily arsenic ingestion of 3,437 μg and the other three were in the lowest arsenic exposure group. Of the six persons found to have sensory neuropathy, only the diabetic and one in the control group met rigorous criteria of neuropathy—that is, impairment of two sensory modalities and reduced deep tendon reflexes. The remaining persons had either subjective complaints such as hyperpathia of the soles of the feet or single abnormalities on neurological examination such as decreased pinprick sensations on the feet or hands. The proportion of persons having abnormal nerve conduction velocity did not differ significantly among the different arsenic exposure groups.

The effects of ingesting arsenic in well water on peripheral nerve function appears to be less than those seen in workers exposed to arsenic in a copper-smelting factory, as in the studies described above. The special statistical methods applied to the copper-smelter workers were not used for the people exposed to arsenic in drinking water in the Alaskan study. Therefore, it cannot be stated whether the long-term effects of exposure to arsenic in well water are as intense or as hazardous as those from arsenic inhaled in the smelting factory. In the copper-smelter workers exposed to arsenic, the neurological hazard was clearly defined, and severity of peripheral neuropathy was correlated with dosage as estimated by the arsenic content in urine, hair, and fingernails.

Burning Arsenic-Treated Wood: Effects of Arsenic Exposure on a Family

Eight members of a rural Wisconsin family were exposed to arsenic by burning wood treated with chromium–copper–arsenate (Peters et al., 1984). These people inhaled the arsenic in the smoke released from the burning of scraps of this treated wood in their poorly ventilated wood-burning space heater. A mother, father, and their six children (ages: 1 to 30 years) experienced sensory hyperesthesias, muscle cramps, recurrent pruritic conjunctivitis, bronchitis, and pneumonitis. The children exhibited a measles-like rash. All the family members complained of malaise, poor concentration, and decreased sensation in the hands and feet. The symptoms were worst in the winter months, lightening somewhat in the summer. During the third year of illness, headaches and blackouts occurred in the parents, the two youngest children had recurrent generalized seizures, the mother had a premature birth, and everyone including the children developed alopecia. In June of 1982 air samples from their house were tested for carbon monoxide and formaldehyde with negative results. Well water was also examined for possible toxicants, but none were found.

The father received an initial examination for thallium intoxication, the results of which were negative. Urine samples were analyzed for thallium, arsenic, mercury, copper, and lead. These tests revealed no evidence of increased metal output. Hair samples taken from the parents, however, revealed 12 to 87 ppm of arsenic, and levels of arsenic in the fingernails of the entire family ranged from 105 to 5,066 ppm. The living area of the house was subsequently found to contain ashes and dust particles with concentrations of over 1,000 ppm of pentavalent arsenate.

Individual Case Studies

Sawdust and Arsenic: Cognitive Change and Neuropathy

As a winter pastime, a 62-year-old male physician made outdoor wooden furniture and a deck, in sections, in the basement of his house. He planned to assemble them outside in the spring. He apparently did not know that the wood had been treated with arsenate as a preservative. Gradually, over 2 to 3 months' time, he experienced difficulty walking in the dark and a prickly sensation in his feet. These paresthesias in his feet soon also developed in his hands. Two months later, an examination showed impaired vibration sensation over the toes, poor performance in tandem gait, and a Romberg sign. Stocking and glove impairments of all sensory modalities with decreased knee and absent ankle tendon reflexes manifested themselves. The physician's patients and colleagues began finding him forgetful and irritable. A diagnosis of sensorimotor polyneuropathy was confirmed by NCVs, which showed normal distal sensory latencies with markedly decreased to absent amplitude recordings of sensory action potentials. Motor NCV studies showed normal distal latencies and velocities, but the amplitude of the compound motor action potentials (CMAPs) was reduced mildly over the hands and significantly over the feet.

When his dog died mysteriously, the physician learned that the wood he had been using had been treated with chromated copper arsenate. Tests for diabetes, malignancy, and nutritional deficiency and a history for exposure to other neurotoxicants, including alcohol, were all negative. Samples taken at the time of his neurological examination showed the patient's urine arsenic output was 58 μg per 24 hours (lab normal range: 0 to 100 μg per 24 hours) and his scalp hair contained 67 μg per 100 g (lab normal range: 0 to 65 μg per 100 g). Analysis of the arsenic content of the wood shavings and dust found in the basement workshop yielded results of 2,500 ppm and 460 ppm, respectively. Measurement of the arsenic in the dust taken from a ceiling beam and the furnace filter yielded results of 180 ppm and 75 ppm, respectively.

Despite a thorough environmental cleanup of the physician's house, a follow-up neurological examination 1 year later revealed persistence of sensorimotor polyneuropathy. A second NCV study demonstrated persistence of axonal sensorimotor neuropathy, worse in the distal legs. Neuropsychological testing at that time revealed difficulties in sustained attention and memory, as well as complex visuospatial organization and judgment.

A course of chelation therapy with penicillamine was given, though it was approximately 1 year after the end of exposure and late in the course of illness (2 years and 8 months after the onset of his symptoms). The total urinary arsenic level did not increase with chelation, and the patient's clinical conditions failed to improve. Neuropsychological evaluation a year later, showed impaired performance on tests of attention, memory, complex reasoning, and visual sequencing. Follow-up communication from the patient almost 10 years after his exposure to arsenic-treated wood revealed the persistence of peripheral sensation loss, paresthesias, and some, but not complete, cognitive improvement (R. G. Feldman, personal observation).

Long-Term Effects After Cutting Arsenic-Treated Wood

Peters et al. (1986) described a 42-year-old female construction worker who experienced nosebleeds, itching skin, heaviness of the chest, epigastric distress, and memory problems 3 days after she began power-sawing wood treated with chromium–copper–arsenic. Despite these symptoms she continued to work with the arsenic-treated wood for an additional 3 weeks. Her symptoms gradually subsided over the following months as she continued to work on tasks other than cutting arsenic-treated wood. One year later, she returned to the power-sawing of arsenic-treated wood and immediately experienced lightheadedness and near blackouts, painful aching of the legs, a

metallic taste in the mouth, nosebleeds, and burning in the stomach. She stopped working after 3 days. The acute symptoms disappeared and she was not examined until 1 month later. No overt physical or neurological abnormalities were observed, and nerve conduction and electromyography studies showed negative findings.

This patient's urine arsenic level was normal, but the levels in her hair (130 μg/g; normal: <0.65 μg/g) and nails (1,352 μg/g; normal: 0.9 to 1.8 μg/g) were significantly increased. A neuropsychological test 5 months after cessation of exposure revealed impairment of short-term verbal memory. The neuropathic changes became increasingly more evident as the neurological effects of an increased body burden of arsenic developed, even after the acute exogenous exposure had ended. Repeat NCV study 10 months after exposure showed decreased sensory action potentials, compatible with her clinical complaints of tingling in her fingers. Arsenic levels were still elevated in the hair (10.4 μg/g) and nails (23.3 μg/g) of this patient at a follow-up 1 year after cessation of exposure.

Recovery After Removal from Exposure to Arsenic

A 27-year-old male worker (Morton and Caron, 1989) at a wood treatment plant gradually developed, over 1 year's time, exertional dyspnea, chest tightness, headaches, irritability, poor concentration, and forgetfulness. His occupational history indicated that he had been exposed to ammoniated copper arsenate fumes in his workplace for 18 months. A 24-hour urinary inorganic arsenic level was 115 μg/L (normal: <20 μg/L). After a second measurement 1 month later of 61 μg/L, he was relocated to a new job without further exposure to arsenic fumes.

The only abnormal finding on physical examination was a distinct purplish flush over the patient's malar eminences and shoulders. Neurological examination showed a slight decrease of pain sensation over radial aspects of the forearms extending distally to the dorsum of his index finger but was otherwise negative. Mental status examination revealed difficulty with calculation and with repeating numbers backward. He was also noted to show signs of depression, which worsened to include a suicidal tendency about 2 months after the exposure ended. Neuropsychological testing conducted 1 month after exposure showed moderate impairment of concentration, new learning, and short-term memory, plus considerable mental confusion and anxiety. A follow-up neuropsychological evaluation 4 months later showed significant improvement in both cognitive and psychiatric functions. He returned to "light duty" work in a location with little or no further exposure to arsenic.

Ingestion of Arsenic Trioxide: Myopathy and Death

A 23-year-old man was admitted to the emergency department 1 hour after ingesting 20 g of arsenic trioxide. His blood arsenic level measured at 3 and 8 hours after ingestion was 0.98 mg/L and 1.85 mg/L, respectively. He was initially alert and asymptomatic. Intramuscular BAL (3 mg/kg every 4 hours) was given, and syrup of ipecac (30 mL twice) was administered to induce vomiting. Arterial hypotension (BP: 90/50 mmHg) developed 8 hours after admission but responded to dopamine infusion and plasma expanders. Nine hours later his serum creatine kinase level was 1,223 u./L (normal: 17 to 148 u./L), and creatinine was 300 μmol/L (normal: 53 to 133μmol/L). Over the next 24 hours, the patient's liver enzymes increased markedly with alanine aminotransferase at 519 u./L, aspartate aminotransferase at 550 u./L, and a total bilirubin level of 77 μmol/L (normal: <17 μmol/L). He subsequently went into renal failure. The rhabdomyolysis progressive worsened over the next several days (serum creatine kinase 31,350 u./L) and he died of ventricular fibrillation 80 hours after ingestion of the arsenic (Sanz et al., 1989).

Muscle biopsy revealed perifascicular hypercontracted fibers, myofibrillar disruption, mitochondrial abnormalities, and abundant cytoplasmic vacuoles containing lipids. Autopsy disclosed brain edema, intraalveolar lung hemorrhage, intracellular cholestasis and hepatic fatty degeneration, ulceration of gastric mucosa, and vacuolar degeneration of the renal tubules. The heart showed tissue destruction with loss of striation and inflammatory infiltrates. Tissue destruction was also observed in the pectoral muscles, with striation loss and centralization of the nucleus (Fernandez-Sola et al., 1991).

This case illustrates that acute arsenic poisoning damages skeletal muscle as well as myocardium. Skeletal muscle cramping may occur after arsenic intoxication (Schoolmeester and White, 1980), but rhabdomyolysis is an uncommon observation. Side effects of dimercaprol therapy do not include myoglobinuria.

Lifesaving Measures After Acute Ingestion of Arsenical Rodenticide

A 30-year-old man was found unresponsive by his family; he could be aroused only by vigorous stimulation (Fesmire et al., 1988). When more alert he admitted ingesting "Blue Ball Rat Killer" and ethanol. The rodenticide, which contained 1.5% arsenous oxide (2,150 mg metallic arsenic per 6 ounces), was washed down with ethanol. In addition, he admitted to using intranasal cocaine. Emergency medical technicians were summoned and arrived promptly. They administered 2 mg naloxone and 50 mL of a 50% dextrose solution. The patient became more responsive en route to the hospital emergency room, where upon arrival he was described as lethargic but at times combative.

On examination in the hospital emergency department (ED) the patient was oriented to persons and time. His pupils were equal and reacted to light. Tendon reflexes were 2+ and symmetrical. Sensory exam was normal. Electrocardiogram (ECG) showed sinus tachycardia. A blood test for toxic substances detected arsenic (44.4 μg/dL; lab normal 2.9 μg/dL), and 24-hour urine arsenic level was 21,900 μg/L (lab normal: <50 μg/L). In addition, cocaine was present in the initial screen. Emergency therapeutic measures were instituted, including: intravenous naloxone infusion (2 mg/hr); gastric lavage with tap water until clear, followed by instillation of 60 g activated charcoal and 30 g magnesium sulfate. Twenty-five minutes after his arrival in the ED the patient received 300 mg (4 mg/kg) BAL intramuscularly (IM). Approximately 1.5 hours later the patient developed abdominal tenderness and bloody nasogastric aspirate and heme-positive stools.

Hemodialysis was begun 4 hours after admission, although there was no evidence of renal failure at that time; dialysis was administered in two courses of 6 and 4 hours, respectively, 18 hours apart. Chelation with BAL was continued through dialysis at a dose of 250 mg IM every 4 hours for the first 12 hours, with subsequent doses at every 6 hours. During the first week of treatment the patient was quite ill with disseminated intravascular coagulation and gastrointestinal bleeding. On the fourth day the patient developed complications of BAL therapy that included blespharospasm, tachycardia, hypertension, and diaphoresis. The BAL dose interval was increased from 6 to 12 hours at this time, and the patient's complications resolved. On the fifth day, BAL was discontinued and the patient was started on D-penicillamine (250 mg every 6 hours).

Throughout this intensive use of chelating agents (BAL and D-penicillamine) the patient received supportive fluid and electrolyte replacement. The patient became hypertensive during the second week of treatment and was administered parenteral hydralazine. Renal tubular acidosis was treated with sodium bicarbonate by infusion. Intestinal ileus developed on day 9, at which time D-penicillamine was discontinued; by day 11 the gastrointestinal ileus had resolved and D-penicillamine was reinstated for additional 3 days to complete the initial 14 days of chelation therapy.

The patient entered into a deep coma on day 10 and remained comatose until day 16, following which recovery of sensorium continued. By day 18, the patient was alert but unable to move his extremities. He appeared indifferent to his condition of severe sensory and motor impairment. He continued to receive chelation therapy (three 5-day courses of D-penicillamine) for the next 4 weeks. Diagnostic studies during the same time period revealed normal EEG and CT scan, but nerve conduction studies on day 19 showed a moderate reduction in velocity. Hyperkeratosis and Mee's lines became evident and hypertension persisted. The peripheral neuropathy, cognitive impairments, and affective indifference persisted for more than 6 months. Formal neuropsychological tests were not reported for this case.

This description of the detailed therapeutic measures taken acutely after ingestion of a large amount of inorganic arsenic demonstrates the success of aggressive intervention, probably preventing immediate death in this patient. However, this case also demonstrates that the central and peripheral nervous system as well as renal effects of arsenic can persist for more than 6 months and may possibly remain as permanent residua of acute poisoning.

REFERENCES

Agency for Toxic Substances and Disease Registry (ATSDR). *Toxicological profile for arsenic.* Atlanta: US Department of Health and Human Services, Public Health Service, 1993.

American Conference of Governmental Industrial Hygienists (ACGIH). *Threshold limit values (TLVs) from chemical substances and physical agents and biological exposure indices (BEIs).* Cincinnati, 1995.

Bansal SK, Haldar N, Dhand UK, Chopra JS. Phrenic neuropathy in arsenic poisoning. *Chest* 1991;133:878–880.

Beckett WS, Moore JL, Keoch JP, Bleecker ML. Acute encephalopathy due to occupational exposure to arsenic. *Br J Ind Med* 1986;43:66–67.

Bencko V, Symon K. Test of environmental exposure to arsenic and hearing changes in exposed children. *Environ Health Perspect* 1977;19:95–101.

Binder S. The case for the NEDEL (the no epidemiologically detectable exposure level) [News]. *AJPH* 1988;78:589–590.

Blom S, Lagerkvist B, Linderholm H. Arsenic exposure to smelter workers. Clinical and neurophysiological studies. *Scand J Work Environ Health* 1985;11:265–269.

Bolla-Wilson K, Bleecker ML. Neuropsychological impairment following inorganic arsenic exposure. *J Occup Med* 1987;29:500–503.

Brown RM, Newton D, Pickford CJ, et al. Human metabolism of arsenobetaine ingested with fish. *Hum Exp Toxicol* 1990;9:41–46.

Brune D, Nordberg G, Wester PO. Distribution of 23 elements in the kidney, liver and lungs of workers from a smeltery and refinery in North Sweden exposed to a number of elements and of a control group. *Sci Tot Environ* 1980;16:13–35.

Buchet JP, Lauwerys R. Study of inorganic arsenic methylation by rat liver *in vitro;* relevance for the interpretation of observations in man. *Arch Toxicol* 1985;57:125–129.

Buchet JP, Lauwerys R. Study of factors influencing the *in vivo* methylation of inorganic arsenic in rats. *Toxicol Appl Pharmacol* 1987;91:65–74.

Buchet JP, Lauwerys R, Roels H. Comparison of the urinary excretion of arsenic metabolites after a single oral dose of sodium arsenite, monomethyl arsonate or dimethyl arsinate in man. *Int Arch Occup Environ Health* 1981;48:71–79.

Buchet JP, Geubel A, Pauwels S, Mahieu P, Lauwerys R. The influence of liver disease on the methylation of arsenite in humans. *Arch Toxicol* 1984;55:151–154.

Call RA, Gunn FD. Arsenical encephalopathy. Report of a case. *Arch Pathol* 1949;48:119–128.

Campbell JP, Alvarez JA. Acute arsenic intoxication. *Am Fam Physician* 1989;40:93–97.

Cavanagh JB. Peripheral nervous system toxicity: a morphological approach. In: Blum T, Manzo L, eds. *Neurotoxicity.* New York: Marcel Dekker, 1985:1–44.

Chhuttani P, Chopra J. Arsenic poisoning. In: Vinken PJ, Bruyn GW, eds. *Handbook of clinical neurology, vol 36: Intoxication of the nervous system, part I.* Amsterdam: North-Holland, 1979:199–216.

Chhuttani PN, Chawla LS, Sharma TD. Arsenical neuropathy. *Neurology* 1967;17:269–274.

Civantos DP, Lopez Rodriguez A, Aguado-Borruey JM, Narvaez JA. Fulminant malignant arrhythmia and multiorgan failure in acute arsenic poisoning [Letter]. *Chest* 1995;108:1774–1775.

Conomy JJ, Barnes KL. Quantitative assessment of cutaneous sensory function in subjects with neurologic disease. *J Neurol Sci* 1976;30:221–235.

Danan M, Dally S, Conso F. Arsenic-induced encephalopathy. *Neurology* 1984;34:1524.

Delnomdedieu M, Basti MM, Otvos JD, Thomas DJ. Reduction and binding of arsenate and dimethylarsinate by glutathione: a magnetic resonance study. *Chemico-Biol Interact* 1994;90:139–155.

DePalma AE. Arsine intoxication in a chemical plant: report of three cases. *J Occup Med* 1969;11(11):582–587.

Dewar WA, Lenihan JMA. A case of chronic arsenical poisoning: examination of tissue samples by activation analysis. *Scott Med J* 1956;1:236–238.

DeWolff FA, Edelbroek PM. Neurotoxicity of arsenic and its compounds. In: *Handbook of clinical neurology: intoxications of the nervous system,* part I, vol 20(64). Amsterdam: Elsevier, 1994:283–291.

Diamant H. The toxic action of some compounds on the inner ear and its vestibular connections. *Arch Otolaryngol* 1958;67:546–552.

Donofrio PD, Wilbourn AJ, Albers LW, Rogers L, Salanga V, Greenberg HS. Acute arsenic intoxication presenting as Guillain–Barré-like syndrome. *Muscle Nerve* 1987;10:114–120.

Dudley SF. Toxemic anemia from arseniuretted hydrogen gas in submarines. *J Ind Hyg* 1919;1:215–232.

Dutkiewicz T. Experimental studies on arsenic absorption routes in rats. *Environ Health Perspect* 1977;19:173–177.

Eastman NJ. The arsenic content of the human placenta following arsphenamine therapy. *Am J Obstet Gynecol* 1931;21:60–64.

EPA. Selected noncarcinogenic effects of industrial exposure to inorganic arsenic. EPA 560/6-77-018, 1977.

Feinglass EJ. Arsenic intoxication from well water in the United States. *N Engl J Med* 1973;288:828–829.

Feldman RG. Central and peripheral nervous system in effects of metals: a survey. In: Juntunen J, ed. *Occupational neurology. Acta Neurol Scand* 1982;66[Suppl 92]:143–166.

Feldman RG, Baker EL. Therapy of arsenical encephalopathy [Letter]. *Neurology* 1979;29:753.

Feldman RG, Jabre JF. Analysis of electrophysiological studies in arsenic exposure. In: Abernathy CO, ed. *Arsenic: exposure and health effects.* London: Thomson Science Publishers, 1997:145–157.

Feldman RG, Niles CA, Sax DS, Dixon WJ, Thompson DJ, Landau E. Peripheral neuropathy in arsenic smelter workers. *Neurology* 1979;29:939–944.

Ferm VH. Arsenic as a teratogenic agent. *Environ Health Persp* 1977;19:215–217.

Fernandez-Sola J, Nogue S, Grau JM, Casademont J, Munne P. Acute arsenical myopathy: morphological description. *Clin Toxicol* 1991;29:131–136.

Fesmire FM, Schauben JL, Roberge RJ. Survival following massive arsenic ingestion. *Am J Emerg Med* 1988;6:602–606.

Fincher RME, Koerker RM. Long-term survival in acute arsenic encephalopathy: follow-up using newer measures of electrophysiological parameters. *Am J Med* 1987;82:549–552.

Fitzgerald L. Arsenic sources, production and application in the 1980's. In: Lederer WH, Fensterheim RJ, eds. *Arsenic: industrial, biomedical, environmental perspectives.* New York: Van Nostrand Reinhold, 1983:3–9.

Fowler BA, Weissberg JB. Arsine poisoning. *N Engl J Med* 1974;291:1171–1174.

Freeman JW, Couch JR. Prolonged encephalopathy in arsenic poisoning. *Neurology* 1978;28:853–855.

Friedman A, Olsen C. Bilateral paralysis of the facial and masticatory nerves following arsenic poisoning. *Bull LA Neurol Soc* 1941;6:85–86.

Fuortes L. Arsenic poisoning. *Iowa Med* 1988;78:571–574.

Garb LG, Hine CH. Arsenical neuropathy residual effects following acute industrial exposure. *J Occup Med* 1977;19:567–568.

Geschke AM, Lynch V, Rouch GJ, Golec R. Arsenic poisoning after a barbeque [Letter]. *Med J Aust* 1996;165:296.

Ghariani M, Adrien ML, Raucoules M, Bayle J, Jacomet Y, Grimaud D. Acute arsenic poisoning. *Ann Fr Anesth Reanim* 1991;10:304–307.

Gherardi RK, Chariot P, Vanderstigel M, Malapert D, Verroust J, Astier A, Brun-Buisson C, Schaeffer A. Organic arsenic-induced Guillain–Barré like syndrome due to melarsoprol: a clinical, electrophysiological, and pathological study. *Muscle Nerve* 1990;13:637–645.

Glazener FS, Ellis JG, Johnson PK. Electrocardiographic findings with arsenic poisoning. *Calif Med* 1968;109:158–162.

Goebel HH, Schmidt PF, Bohl J, Tettenborn B, Kramer G, Gutmann L. Polyneuropathy due to acute arsenic intoxication: biopsy studies. *J Neuropathol Exp Neurol* 1990;49:137–149.

Goldstein NP, McCall JT, Dyck PJ. Metal neuropathy. In: Dyck PJ, Thomas PK, Lambert EH, Bunge R, eds. *Peripheral neuropathy.* Philadelphia: WB Saunders, 1984:1227–1240.

Gorby MS. Arsenic poisoning. *West J Med* 1988;149:308–315.

Goyer R. Toxic effects of metals. In: Klaassen C, Admur M, Doull J, eds. *Casarett and Doull's toxicology: the basic science of poisons.* New York: Macmillan, 1986:582–635.

Grantham DA, Jones JF. Arsenic contamination of water wells in Nova Scotia. *J Am Water Works Assoc* 1977;69:653–657.

Gratt LB, Levin L. Exposure assessment for arsenic concentrations from electric power stations. In: Chappell WR, Abernathy CO, Cothern CR, eds. *Arsenic exposure and health*. Northwood, O.K.: Science and Technology Letters, 1994:71–82.

Greenberg SA. Acute demyelinating polyneuropathy with arsenic ingestion. *Muscle Nerve* 1996;19:1611–1613.

Haller L, Adams H, Merouze F, Dago A. Clinical and pathological aspects of human trypanosomiasis (*T.b. gambiense*) with particular reference to reactive arsenical encephalopathy. *Am J Trop Med Hyg* 1986;35:94–99.

Heyman A, Pfeiffer JB, Taylor HM. Peripheral neuropathy caused by arsenical intoxication: a study of 41 cases with observations on the effects of BAL (2,3-dimercapto-propanol). *N Engl J Med* 1956;254:401–409.

Hindmarsh JT, McCurdy RF. Clinical and environmental aspects of arsenic toxicity. *CRC Crit Rev Clin Lab Sci* 1986;23:315–347.

Hood RD, Vedel GC, Zaworotko MJ, Tatum FM. Uptake, distribution, and metabolism of trivalent arsenic in the pregnant mouse. *J Toxicol Environ Health* 1988;25:423–434.

Hotta N. Clinical aspects of chronic arsenic poisoning due to environmental and occupational pollution in and around a small refining spot. *Jpn J Const Med* 1989;53:49–69.

Hutton JT, Christians BL. Sources, symptoms, and signs of arsenic poisoning. *J Fam Pract* 1983;3:423–426.

Ishinishi N, Tsuchiya K, Vahter M, Fowler B. Arsenic. In: Friberg L, Nordberg GH, Vouk V, eds. *Handbook on the toxicology of metals*, 2nd edition. Amsterdam: Elsevier, 1986:43–83.

Järup L, Pershagen G, Wall S. Cumulative arsenic exposure and lung cancer in smelter workers: a dose-response study. *Am J Ind Med* 1989;15:31–41.

Jenkins RB. Inorganic arsenic and the nervous system. *Brain* 1966;89:479–498.

Johnson LR, Farmer JG. Use of human metabolic studies and urinary arsenic speciation in assessing arsenic exposure. *Bull Environ Contam Toxicol* 1991;46:53–61.

Jones NW. Arseniureted hydrogen poisoning: with report of five cases. *JAMA* 1907;48:1099–1105.

Kantor HI, Levin PM. Arsenical encephalopathy in pregnancy with recovery. *Am J Obstet Gynecol* 1948;56:370–374.

Kersjes MP, Maurer JR, Trestrail JH, McCoy DJ. An analysis of arsenic exposure referred to the Blodgett Regional Poison Center. *Vet Hum Toxicol* 1987;29:75–78.

Klaassen C. Heavy metals and heavy metal antagonists. In: Goodman Gilman A, Rall TW, Nies AS, Taylor P, eds. *Goodman and Gilman's: The pharmacological basis of therapeutics*. Elmsford, NY: Pergamon Press, Section 18, 1990:1602–1605.

Kodama Y, Ishinshi N, Kunitake E, Imanusu T, Nobutomo K. Arsenic. In: Nordberg GF, ed. *Effects and dose-response relationships of toxic metals*. Amsterdam: Elsevier, 1976:464–470.

Kreiss K, Zack MW, Feldman RG, Landrigan PJ, Boyd MH, Cox DH. Neurologic evaluation of a population exposed to arsenic in Alaskan well water. *Arch Environ Health* 1983;38:116–121.

Lagerkvist BJ, Zetterlund B. Assessment of exposure to arsenic among smelter workers: a five year follow-up. *Am J Ind Med* 1994;25: 477–488.

Lagerkvist BJ, Linderholm H, Nordberg GF. Vasopastic tendency and Raynaud's phenomenon in smelter workers exposed to arsenic. *Environ Res* 1986;39:465–474.

Larsen NA, Pallenberg H, Damsgaard E, Heydorn K. Topographical distribution of arsenic, manganese, and selenium in the normal human brain. *J Neurol Sci* 1977;32:437–451.

Lawrence JF, Michalik P, Tam G, Conacher HBS. Identification of arsinobetaine and arsenocholine in Canadian fish and shellfish by high performance liquid chromatography with atomic absorption detection and confirmation by fast atom bombardment mass spectrometry. *J Agric Food Chem* 1986;34:315–319.

Leffler P, Gerhardsson L, Brune D, Nordberg G. Lung retention of antimony and arsenic in hamsters after intratracheal instillation of industrial dust. *Scand Work Environ Health* 1984;10:245–251.

LeQuesne PM, McLeod JG. Peripheral neuropathy following a single exposure to arsenic. *J Neurol Sci* 1977;32:437–451.

Levinsky WJ, Smalley RV, Hillyer PN, Shindler RL. Arsine hemolysis. *Arch Environ Health* 1970;20:436–440.

Liebscher K, Smith H. Essential and nonessential trace elements. A method of determining whether an element is essential or nonessential in human tissue. *Arch Environ Health* 1968;17:881–890.

Lowe J, Kreiger GR, Radis SR, Sullivan JB Jr. Assessing community risk from the sudden release of a toxic gas. In: Sullivan JB, Krieger GR,

eds. *Hazardous Materials Toxicology, Clinical Principles of Environmental Health*. Baltimore: Williams & Wilkins, 1992:451–462.

Lugo G, Cassady G, Palmisano P. Acute maternal arsenic intoxication with neonatal death. *Am J Dis Child* 1969;117:328–330.

Lundgren KD. Lesions of respiratory tract in smelting workers. *Nord Hyg Tidskr* 1954;3:66–81.

Mahieu P, Buchet JP, Roels HA, et al. The metabolism of arsenic in humans intoxicated by AS_2O_3: its significance for the duration of BAL therapy. *Clin Toxicol* 1981;18:1067–1075.

Malachowski M. An update on arsenic. *Clin Lab Med* 1990;10:457–472.

Mann S, Droz P-O, Vahter M. A physiologically based pharmacokinetic model for arsenic exposure. II. Validation and application in humans. *Toxicol Appl Pharmacol* 1996;140:471–486.

Mappes R. Experiments on excretion of arsenic in urine. *Int Arch Occup Environ Health* 1977;40:267–272.

McCutchen JJ, Utterback RJ. Chronic arsenic poisoning resembling muscular dystrophy. *South Med J* 1966;59:1139–1145.

Milham S, Strong T. Human arsenic exposure in relation to a copper smelter. *Environ Res* 1974;7:176–182.

Mitchell-Heggs CAW, Conway M, Cassar J. Herbal medicine as a cause of combined lead and arsenic poisoning. *Hum Exp Toxicol* 1990;9:195–196.

Morton WE, Caron GA. Encephalopathy: an uncommon manifestation of workplace arsenic poisoning? *Am J Ind Med* 1989;15:1–5.

Moyer TP. Testing for arsenic. *Mayo Clin Proc* 1993;68:1210–1211.

Murphy MJ, Lyon LW, Taylor JW. Subacute arsenic neuropathy; clinical and neurophysiological observations. *J Neurol Neurosurg Psychiatry* 1981;44:896–900.

NAS. *Medical and biologic effects of environmental arsenic*. Washington, DC: National Research Council, National Academy of Sciences (NAS), 1977.

National Institute for Occupational Safety and Health (NIOSH). *Occupational exposure to inorganic arsenic: new criteria*. Washington, DC: US Department of Health Education and Welfare, 1975.

National Institute for Occupational Safety and Health (NIOSH). *Arsine (arsenic hydroxide) poisoning in the workplace*. Current Intelligence Bulletin 32. Cincinnati: US Department of Health and Human Services, Centers for Disease Control, 1979.

National Institute for Occupational Safety and Health (NIOSH). *Industrial hygiene surveys of occupational exposure to wood preservative chemicals*. Cincinnati: US Department of Health and Human Services, Centers for Disease Control, 1983.

National Institute for Occupational Safety and Health (NIOSH). *Pocket guide to chemical hazards*. US Department of Health and Human Services, Centers for Disease Control and Prevention. Cincinnati: NIOSH Publications, 1997.

Occupational Safety and Health Administration (OSHA). Code of Federal Regulations 29: Part 1910.1000. Washington, DC: Office of the Federal Register National Archives and Records Administration, 1995.

Oh SJ. Electrophysiological profile in arsenic. *Neuropathy* 1991;54:1103–1105.

Ohta M. Ultrastructure of sural nerve in a case of arsenical neuropathy. *Acta Neuropathol* 1970;16:233–242.

Ortel TL, Bedrosian CL, Simel DL. Arsenic poisoning and seizures. *N Carolina Med J* 1987;48:627–630.

O'Shaughnessy E, Kraft GH. Arsenic poisoning: long-term follow-up of a nonfatal case. *Arch Phys Med Rehab* 1976;57:403–406.

Peters HA, Croft WA, Woolson EA, Darcey BA, Olson MA. Seasonal arsenic exposure from burning chromium-copper-arsenate-treated wood. *JAMA* 1984;251:2393–2396.

Peters HA, Croft WA, Woolson EA, Darcey B, Olson M. Hematologic, dermal, and neuropsychological disease from burning and power sawing chromium-copper-arsenic (CCA) treated wood. *Acta Pharmacol Toxicol* 1986;59[Suppl 7]:39–43.

Peters JM, Sanadi DR. Effects of arsenite and cadmium ions on xanthine oxidase. *Arch Biochem Biophys* 1961;93:312–313.

Polissar L, Lowry-Coble K, Kalman DA, et al. Pathways of human exposure to arsenic in a community surrounding a copper smelter. *Environ Res* 1990;53:29–47.

Politis MJ, Schaumburg HH, Spencer PS. Neurotoxicity of selected chemicals. In: Spencer PS, Schaumburg HH, eds. *Experimental and clinical neurotoxicology*. Baltimore: Williams & Wilkins, 1980:613.

Ridley WP, Dizikes L, Cheh A, Wood JM. Recent studies on biomethylation and demethylation of toxic elements. *Environ Health Perspect* 1977;19:43–46.

Roses OE, Garcia-Fernandez JC, Villaamil EC, et al. Mass poisoning by sodium arsenite. *Clin Toxicol* 1991;29:209–213.

Sabbioni E, Fischbach M, Pozzi G, Pietra R, Gallorini M, Piette JL. Cellular retention, toxicity and carcinogenic potential of seafood arsenic. I. Lack of cytotoxicity and transforming activity of arsenobetaine in the BALB/3T3 cell line. *Carcinogen* 1991;12:1287–1291.

Sanz P, Corbella J, Nogue S, Munne P, Rodriguez-Pazos M. Rhabdomyolysis in fatal arsenic trioxide poisoning. *JAMA* 1989;262:3271.

Sax NI. Dangerous properties of industrial chemicals, 5th ed. New York: Van Nostrand Reinhold, 1979.

Schenk V, Stolk P. Psychosis following arsenic (possibly thallium) poisoning: a clinical–pathological report. *Psychiatr Neurol Neurochir* 1967;70:31–37.

Schoolmeester WL, White DR. Arsenic poisoning. *South Med J* 1980;73:198–208.

Sexton GB, Gowdey CW. Relation between thiamine and arsenical toxicity. *Arch Dermatol Syph* 1963;56:634–647.

Singer R, Valciukas JA, Lilis R. Nerve conduction velocity assessment of copper smelter workers. In: *Health hazards among copper smelter workers. Report to the National Institute of Environmental Health Sciences.* New York: Environmental Sciences Laboratory, Mount Sinai School of Medicine of the City University of New York, 1982:126–142.

Strange RC, Lear JT, Fryer AA. Polymorphism in glutathione S-transferase loci as a risk factor for common cancers. *Arch Toxicol Suppl* 1998;20:419–428.

St Petery J, Gross C, Victoria BE. Ventricular fibrillation caused by arsenic poisoning. *Am J Dis Child* 1970;120:367–371.

Talwalkar PG, Narula DV, Bhat RR. Arsenic encephalopathy (a report of two cases). *J Assoc Phys Ind* 1976;24:869–871.

Tam GK, Charbonneau SM, Bryce F, et al. Metabolism of inorganic arsenic (^{74}As) in humans following oral ingestion. *Toxicol Appl Pharmacol* 1979;50:319–322.

Tay C-H, Seah C-S. Arsenic poisoning from anti-asthmatic herbal preparations. *Med J Aust* 1975;2:424–428.

Tseng W-P. Effects and dose-response relationship of skin cancer and blackfoot disease with arsenic. *Environ Health Perspect* 1977;19:109–119.

United States Environmental Protection Agency (USEPA). Drinking water regulations and health advisories. EPA, 822-R-96-001, Office of Water, 4304, Washington, DC, February 1996.

Uthus EO. Arsenic essentiality and factors affecting its importance. In: Chappell WR, Abernathy CO, Cothern CR, eds. *Arsenic exposure and health.* Northwood: Science and Technology Letters, 1994:199–208.

Vahter M. Environmental and occupational exposure to inorganic arsenic. *Acta Pharmacol Toxicol* 1986;59:31–34.

Vahter M, Envall J. In vivo reduction of arsenate in mice and rabbits. *Environ Res* 1983;32:14–24.

Vahter M, Marafante E, Dencker L. Metabolism and excretion of arsenobetaine in mice, rats, and rabbits. *Sci Tot Environ* 1983;30:197–211.

Webb DR, Wilson SE, Carter DE. In vitro solubility and in vivo toxicity of gallium arsenide. *Toxicol Appl Pharmacol* 1984;76:96–104.

Weeks JL, Levy BS, Wagner GR. Strategies for prevention. In: Weeks JL, Levy BS, Wagner GR, eds. *Preventing occupational disease and injury.* Washington, DC: American Public Health Association, 1991:3–10.

White RF, Proctor SP. Clinico-neuropsychological assessment methods in behavioral toxicology. In: Chang LW, Slikker W, eds. *Neurotoxicology: approaches and methods.* New York: Academic Press, 1995:711–726.

Wilkerson SP, McHugh P, Horsely S, Tubbs H, Lewis M. Arsine toxicity aboard the Asia freighter. *Br Med J* 1975;3:559–563.

Willhite CC, Ferm VH. Prenatal and developmental toxicology of arsenicals. *Adv Exp Med Biol* 1984;177:205–228.

Windebank AJ. Specific inhibition of myelination by lead in vitro: comparison with arsenic, thallium, and mercury. *Exp Neurol* 1986;94(1):203.

Windebank AJ. Metal Neuropathy. In: Dyck PJ, Thomas PK, eds. *Peripheral neuropathy,* vol 2, 3rd ed. Philadelphia: WB Saunders, 1993:1549–1570.

Winship KA. Toxicity of inorganic arsenic salts. *Adverse Drug React Acute Poison Rev* 1984;3:129–160.

Yamashita N, Doi M, Nishio M, Hojo H, Tanaka M. Current state of Kyoto children poisoned by arsenic tinted Morinage dry milk. *Jpn J Hyg* 1972;27:364–399.

Zaloga GP, Deal J, Spurling T, Richter J, Chernow B. Case report: unusual manifestations of arsenic intoxication. *Am J Med Sci* 1985;289:210–214.

CHAPTER 6

Mercury

Mercury (Hg) is extracted from ore [cinnabar (HgS)] by a roasting process. Elemental mercury (Hg^0), a liquid at room temperature, is also called quicksilver or liquid silver because of its appearance. Mercury exists in a total of three oxidation states, and thus it also forms univalent (mercurous) and bivalent (mercuric) compounds. Mercuric chloride ($HgCl_2$) is readily dissolved, ionized, and absorbed, and it is more toxic than the relatively insoluble mercurous chloride (Hg_2Cl_2). Organic mercury compounds including short- and long-chain alkyl as well as aryl mercurial compounds are also formed. The phenyl mercury compounds are much less toxic than the alkyl mercury compounds (Sax, 1979). Methylmercury is relatively stable in contrast to other organic mercury compounds (Fig. 6-1). The toxic effects of exposure to inorganic mercury have been known for many centuries (Kark, 1994), while the importance of organic mercury intoxication of the nervous system has only more recently been recognized (Marsh, 1994). Exposure to mercury has been associated with neurological and immunological effects (Kark, 1994; Marsh, 1994; Pelletier et al., 1994).

SOURCES OF EXPOSURE

Elemental mercury is used in barometers, thermometers, and gauges. Inorganic mercury has been used in cosmetics, dyes, mirrors, jewelry, and medications (Kark, 1994). Mercuric salts are used in gold, silver, and bronze plating processes. Mercury is found in electronic equipment, such as batteries, switches, rectifiers, and mercury vapor lamps. Inorganic mercury is used in photography, antiseptics, tanning processes, embalming, the manufacturing of felt, and as a preservative of wood. Exposure to elemental mercury vapor occurs in the choralkali industry during the manufacture of chlorine (Langolf et al., 1978; Lamm and Pratt, 1985). Natural gas from certain sites has been reported to contain elemental mercury, and thus significant exposures to elemental mercury can occur among workers involved in the inspection and maintenance of equipment at these sites (Boogaard et al., 1996). Metallic mercury is used in dental amalgam. Mercury in dental amalgam has been questioned as a potential source of low-level chronic exposure to mercury and, therefore, as a workplace health hazard among members of the dental profession (Iyer et al., 1976; de Freitas, 1981; Bloch and Shapiro, 1982). Approximately 70,000 workers are exposed to mercury in the United States annually (ATSDR, 1994). The proportion of adults exposed to industrial levels of elemental mercury vapor who develop symptoms of intoxication is estimated to be approximately 10% to 20% (Kark, 1994).

Nonoccupational exposures to organic mercury occur during the use of fungicides, bactericides, and disinfectants (Key et al., 1977). Topical application of ammoniated mercury ointment has been associated with peripheral neuropathy (Kern et al., 1991). Occupational (e.g., painters) as well as nonoccupational (e.g., residents) exposures to mercury occur during the use of latex paints that contain phenyl mercuric acetate as a preservative. For example, the ambient air mercury concentrations were significantly higher in homes which had recently been painted with latex paints containing phenyl mercuric acetate. In addition, the urine mercury concentrations of residents living in homes that had recently been painted with latex paints, as well as persons who had recently applied latex paints, were significantly higher than that of unexposed controls (Agocs et al., 1990). Elemental, inorganic, and organic mercury are excreted in breast milk, and thus the breast-fed children of women who are currently or have recently been exposed to mercury may also be exposed to toxic amounts of mercury (Amin-Zaki et al., 1974; Yoshida et al., 1992; Sundberg and Oskarsson, 1992; Grandjean et al., 1995). Mercury vapor is released from dental amalgams during brushing and chewing as the surfaces of teeth grind together and apply pressure to the filling material (Gay et al., 1979; Vimy and Lorscheider, 1990; Aposhian et al., 1992; Skare and Enqvist, 1994; ATSDR, 1994; Barregård et al., 1995; Trepka et al., 1997). This represents a very small contribution to the total body burden of mercury and is similar to that estimated to be taken in with food and drink (Brune and Evje, 1985; Berglund, 1990). The average daily dose of elemental mercury inhaled from the re-

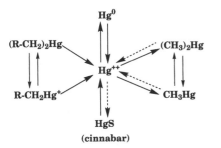

FIG. 6-1. Simplified scheme of transformation pathways of mercury, accounting for the various molecular forms found in nature (R denotes an aryl, a long-chain alkyl, or an alkoxy–alkyl radical).

lease of vapor from the dental amalgams in people with re-construction work has been estimated to be about 1% (1.7 μg) of the amount obtained from exposure to the National Institute for Occupational Safety and Health recommended exposure limit (NIOSH) REL of 50 μg/m³ (0.05 mg/m³). The World Health Organization (WHO) has concluded that mercury from dental amalgam is a significant contributor to the overall body burden of mercury in the general population (WHO, 1991). In individuals who had no other known source of mercury exposure, their baseline blood and urine mercury levels were reduced after the removal of their amalgam fillings (Barregård et al., 1995) (see section on Exposure Limits and Safety Regulations). Despite assurance of the safety of mercury containing amalgam fillings (Brune and Evje, 1985; Berglund, 1990; Barregård et al., 1998), serious questions still are raised about an association between mercury and a variety of neurological, immunological, and endocrinological syndromes that occur among persons with dental amalgams containing mercury (Clausen, 1993; Pleva, 1994; Siblerud and Kienholz, 1994; Fuortes et al., 1995).

Mercury compounds are released into water from rocks and sediment, and they are also released into the general environment as a result of contamination by industrial processing and waste disposal (Kurttio et al., 1998). Average mercury concentration in unpolluted marine waters is less than 2 ng/L (Fowler, 1990), and mercury levels in unpolluted fresh water are generally less than 5 ng/L (Gilmore and Henry, 1991). Methylation of mercury by microorganisms in sediment, soil, and water leads to organic mercurials in domestic water sources, which enter the human food chain through plants and fish (ATSDR, 1989). From time to time, public health advisories have been issued about mercury-contaminated fish. Such a warning was given in Michigan when the methylmercury content in fish exceeded the levels of concern in three out of four of the inland lakes tested (NRC, 1991).

Ambient air concentrations of mercury vary according to the conditions of the site sampled. For example, the average annual air concentration of mercury in the United States has been reported to be 10 to 20 ng/m³, with higher concentrations in industrialized areas (EPA, 1980). Ambi-

ent air levels as high as 10 to 15 mg/m³ have been reported near industrial sites such as mercury mines and refineries (ATSDR, 1994).

EXPOSURE LIMITS AND SAFETY REGULATIONS

People and experimental animals vary in their ability to tolerate different levels of exposure to mercury. Individual

TABLE 6-1. *Established and recommended occupational and environmental exposure limits for mercury in air and water*

	Air (mg/m³)[a]	Water (mg/L)[a]
Odor threshold*	—	—
OSHA		
PEL (8-hr TWA)		
Inorganic mercury	—	—
Organic mercury	0.01	
PEL ceiling		
Inorganic mercury	0.1	
Organic mercury	0.04	
NIOSH		
REL (10-hr TWA)		
Inorganic mercury	0.05	—
Organic mercury	5	
STEL		
Inorganic mercury	0.1	
Organic mercury	0.03	
IDLH		
Inorganic mercury	10.0	
Organic mercury	2.0	
ACGIH		
TLV (8-hr TWA)		
Inorganic mercury	0.025	—
Alkyl compounds	0.01	
Aryl compounds	0.1	
STEL ceiling		
Alkyl compounds	0.03	
USEPA		
MCL		
Inorganic mercury	—	0.002
MCLG		
Inorganic mercury	—	0.002

[a]*Unit Conversion:* 1 ppm = 8.43 mg/m³; 1 ppm = 1 mg/L.
OSHA, Occupational Safety and Health Administration; PEL, permissible exposure limit; TWA, time-weighted average; NIOSH, National Institute for Occupational Safety and Health; REL, recommended exposure limit; STEL, short-term exposure limit; IDLH, immediately dangerous to life and health; ACGIH TLV, American Conference of Governmental Industrial Hygienists threshold limit value; USEPA-MCL, United States Environmental Protection Agency; MCL, maximum contamination level; MCLG, maximum contamination level goal.
Data from *Amoore and Houtala, 1983; ACGIH, 1995; OSHA, 1995; EPA, 1996; NIOSH, 1997.

response to a given mercury exposure dose is affected by the circumstances of exposure, personal hygiene, diet, and concomitant exposures to other chemicals, including alcohol. The exposed individual's biological susceptibility is linked to the efficacy of various intrinsic protective detoxifying mechanisms. Safe levels of mercury exposure have been derived from careful analysis of prior exposure outcomes in individual case reports, epidemiological studies of occupational and accidental exposures, and controlled animal experiments.

The *Occupational Safety and Health Administration* (OSHA) has established an 8-hour time-weighted average (TWA) permissible exposure limit (PEL) for organic mercury compounds of 0.01 mg/m³, with a 15-minute TWA ceiling of 0.04 mg/m³. The OSHA TWA–PEL for inorganic mercury vapor is 0.05 mg/m³, with a TWA ceiling of 0.1 mg/m³ (OSHA, 1995). The NIOSH has set its 10-hour TWA REL for organic mercury compounds at 0.01 mg/m³, with 15-minute short-term exposure limit (STEL) of 0.03 mg/m³. The NIOSH has set its REL for inorganic mercury vapor at 0.05 mg/m³ with an STEL of 0.1 mg/m³ (NIOSH, 1997). The *American Conference of Governmental Industrial Hygienists* (ACGIH) has set an 8-hour TWA threshold limit value (TLV) of 0.01 mg/m³ for alkyl mercury compounds and a TLV of 0.1 mg/m³ for aryl mercury compounds. The ACGIH TLV for inorganic mercury compounds is 0.025 mg/m³ (ACGIH, 1995). The NIOSH recommended immediately dangerous to life or health (IDLH) level for elemental or inorganic mercury is 10 mg/m³, and for organic (alkyl) mercury compounds it is 2 mg/m³. Because of the potential for dermal absorption, skin exposure should be prevented through the use of protective clothing and goggles (NIOSH, 1994) (Table 6-1).

The *Environmental Protection Agency's* (EPA) maximum contamination level (MCL) for drinking water is 0.002 mg/L. The EPA maximum contamination level goal (MCLG) for drinking water is 0.002 mg/L (EPA, 1996). The *Food and Drug Administration's* (FDA) permissible level for bottled water is 0.002 mg/L (FDA, 1989). The maximum contamination level in seafood products is 1.0 mg/kg (1.0 ppm) (ATSDR, 1994) (see Table 6-1).

METABOLISM

Tissue Absorption

Mercury exposure in humans is pervasive, and individuals exposed to mercury accumulate this metal (Chang, 1977; Lorscheider and Vimy, 1990). Differences in the solubility of the particular mercury compound influence its absorption. Elemental mercury vapor is highly lipophilic, resulting in prompt absorption across the alveolar membranes into the systemic circulation (Teisinger and Fiserova-Bergerova, 1965; Cherian et al., 1978; Barregård et al., 1992). Less soluble inorganic compounds such as mercuric chloride must first be oxidized to more soluble compounds before being absorbed. Short-chain alkyl mercury compounds are also lipid-soluble and are easily absorbed

across the alveolar membrane following inhalation. The vapors of the aryl mercury compound, phenyl mercuric acetate, are very easily absorbed across the pulmonary alveoli, with up to 80% of an inhaled dose retained. Ethanol reduces the absorption of mercury vapor (Neilsen Kudsk, 1965, 1969a, 1969b).

Liquid elemental mercury is poorly absorbed from the gastrointestinal tract and is excreted unchanged in feces (Wright et al., 1981; Campbell et al., 1992). The inorganic mercury salts are also not well absorbed after ingestion (Clarkson, 1971; Rahola et al., 1973). For example, only 20% of an oral dose of mercuric chloride is absorbed, while large amounts remain bound to the gastrointestinal mucosa (Nielsen, 1992). In contrast, organic mercury compounds are almost completely (90%) absorbed after ingestion because of their increased lipid solubility (Angle and McIntire, 1974; Shapiro et al., 1982).

Cutaneous absorption of metallic mercury, inorganic mercury, and organic mercury compounds occurs (Swaiman and Flagler, 1971; Gotelli et al., 1985; Hursh et al., 1989; Kern et al., 1991). Total dermal absorption is determined by the amount of skin exposed and the duration of exposure as well as the particular mercury compound's ability to penetrate the skin. For example, studies in five volunteers subjected to acute (27 to 43 minutes) dermal exposure to radioactive elemental mercury vapor (^{203}Hg) demonstrated that transdermal uptake contributes about 2.6% to an individual's total exposure dose (Hursh et al., 1989). Chronic dermal exposure by topical application of ammoniated mercury ointment has been associated with a significant increase in body burden (blood mercury: 128 μg/L; normal <15 μg/L) and the development of peripheral neuropathy (Warkany and Hubbard, 1953; Kern et al., 1991). Infants who wore diapers treated with a phenylmercury fungicide had higher concentrations of mercury in their urine than did unexposed infants (Gotelli et al., 1985).

Retention of all mercury compounds is affected by interactions with other chemicals. For example, ethanol reduces retention of elemental mercury vapor in humans and has been shown to inhibit the uptake of mercury by red blood cells *in vitro* and *in vivo* (Neilsen Kudsk, 1965; Magos et al., 1973; Hursh et al., 1980).

Tissue Distribution

Inorganic Mercury

Distribution of mercury in the parenchymal organs, muscles, and adipose tissue is similar after exposures to elemental mercury and inorganic mercury salts; however, accumulation within the central nervous system (CNS) is greater following exposure to elemental mercury vapor than to inorganic mercury (Berlin et al., 1966; Chang and Hartman, 1972a; Kosta et al., 1975). Elemental mercury is highly lipophilic and thus can readily cross the blood–brain barrier (BBB). High concentrations of mercury were found in the brains of mice exposed to elemental mercury vapor (Berlin et al., 1966). Although the majority of an absorbed dose of elemental mercury is oxidized to Hg^{2+} in the red blood cells by the hydrogen peroxide catalase system before it can cross the BBB, a small amount is able to enter the CNS unchanged. Elemental mercury which has crossed the BBB is subsequently oxidized by the hydrogen peroxide catalase system within the CNS to Hg^{2+}. The divalent cation formed in this reaction rapidly binds to thiol-containing ligands, resulting in its fixation within the CNS (Aschner and Aschner, 1990) (Fig. 6-2). Thus, the total amount of mercury retained in the CNS of a person who has been exposed to elemental mercury vapor is dependent in part on the rate at which the individual's endogenous hydrogen peroxide catalase system can convert it to the divalent form (Magos, 1980; Aschner and Aschner, 1990). In contrast, inorganic mercury salts, whether in the Hg^+ or Hg^{2+} oxidation state, are protein-bound in plasma and do not as readily cross the BBB. Nevertheless, accumulation of mercury within the CNS has been demonstrated following exposure to inorganic mercury compounds (Chang and Hartman, 1972a; Kosta et al., 1975). Postmortem determinations of mercury contents in the brains of miners exposed to inorganic mercury ($n = 6$) and unexposed controls ($n = 5$) revealed average wet tissue concentrations of 0.70 ppm (range: 0.18 to 1.50 ppm) and 0.0042 ppm (range: 0.001 to 0.007 ppm), respectively (Kosta et al., 1975).

Organic Mercury

Approximately 90% of the methylmercury in human blood is found in the red blood cells (Kershaw et al., 1980). Methylmercury is lipid-soluble and crosses the BBB by passive diffusion. In addition, methylmercury binds to thiol-containing ligands and subsequently crosses the BBB by active transport (Thomas and Smith, 1982; Aschner and Aschner, 1990) (see Tissue Biochemistry section). Despite these two methods of transport, the mercury content in the brain tissue following exposure to methylmercury is less than that found in the liver and kidneys (Campbell et al., 1992) (Fig. 6-3). Release of methylmercury from small diffusible thiol-containing ligands and its subsequent irreversible binding to larger nondiffusible ligands within the CNS contributes to its accumulation in the brain. In addition, some of the methylmercury that has crossed to the BBB is converted by demethylation to the inorganic form (Aschner and Aschner, 1990). Brain tissue concentrations of inorganic mercury are significantly higher following chronic exposure to methylmercury than following an acute exposure, suggesting that demethylation of methylmercury results in the accumulation of inorganic mercury within the CNS (Friberg and Mottet, 1989). Inorganic mercury in the CNS has a biological half-life measured in several years, in

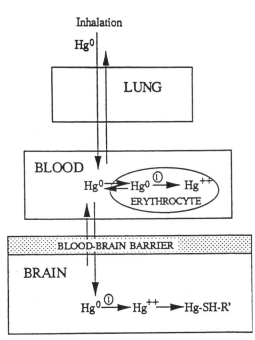

FIG. 6-2. Transport of elemental mercury vapor (Hg^0). Diffusion occurs across alveolar membrane into the systemic circulation where it is oxidized to Hg^{2+} by erythrocytes. Minute amounts of Hg^0 cross the blood–brain barrier into the central nervous system, where it is then oxidized to Hg^{2+} and fixates to —SH-containing ligands. (From Aschner and Aschner, 1990, with permission.)

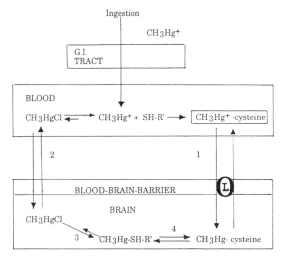

FIG. 6-3. Transport model for methylmercury. Methylmercury chloride traverses the gastrointestinal membrane by virtue of its lipid solubility, accounting for continuous absorption of methylmercury chloride from the stomach into the systemic circulation where a rapid exchange of CH_3Hg^+ to —SH-containing ligands takes place. Methylmercury cysteine conjugates are transported on the Na^+-independent system L (1). An infinitesimal amount may also be transported in the form of methylmercury chloride (2). Rapid exchange of methylmercury between chloride and —SH groups (3 and 4) may account for the concentrative mechanism of this organometal within the cells. The approximate relative rate constants of these reactions are indicated by the length of the arrows (not to scale). (From Aschner and Aschner, 1990, with permission.)

contrast to days or weeks for methylmercury (Aschner and Aschner, 1990). The persistence of mercury in the brain following cessation of exposure to methylmercury was demonstrated in survivors of the Minamata Bay outbreak by postmortem studies (Takeuchi et al., 1989; Eto et al., 1992). Methylmercury also readily crosses the placenta. The tissue distribution of phenylmercury immediately following cessation of exposure resembles that of methylmercury.

Phenylmercury crosses the BBB and placenta but accumulates to a lesser degree than does methylmercury. Phenylmercury is metabolized more rapidly than is methylmercury, and thus 1 week after cessation of exposure to phenylmercury the distribution of mercury more closely resembles that which is seen following exposure to inorganic mercury (Daniel et al., 1972; Nordberg, 1976).

Mercury has been detected in portmortem brain and spinal tissue from control subjects without an identifiable source of exposure (Khare et al., 1990). Higher levels of mercury are found in gray matter (neurons) than in white matter (myelin) (Cassano et al., 1969; Ganser and Kirschner, 1985). With the exception of the calcarine cortex, which is especially vulnerable to methylmercury, other neural structures are affected by both inorganic and methylmercury (Chang, 1977). Mercury has been detected within the cytoplasm of Schwann cells 12 to 24 hours after an initial administration of either methylmercuric chloride or inorganic mercuric chloride by injection, ingestion, or inhalation (Chang and Hartman, 1972a). A glycoprotein species (molecular weight: 21 kDa) extracted from the myelin fractions of peripheral nerves of humans, rodents, and rabbits exhibited a high affinity for methylmercury *in vitro* (Ozaki et al., 1993). However, *in vivo* studies have demonstrated that all mercurials and particularly mercuric chloride have a relatively low affinity for the peripheral nerve myelin of mice (Ganser and Kirschner, 1985). Mercury is primarily found in the nuclei and cytoplasm of motor neurons and in glial cells (Kasarkis et al., 1993; Takeuchi, 1972).

Distribution of all mercury compounds is affected by interactions with other chemicals. For example, after 15 days of exposure to mercuric chloride, in addition to administered ascorbic acid, more mercury was found in tissues that were saturated by ascorbic acid than was detected in those which were not saturated by ascorbic acid (Blackstone et al., 1974). Selenium affects the distribution of mercury in the brain as well as in other tissues (Kosta et al., 1975; Cavanagh, 1988; Møller-Madsen and Danscher, 1991; Bjorkman et al., 1995). Mercury content in the thalamus, hypothalamus, and brainstem nuclei was higher in rats treated with selenium and methyl mercuric chloride than in those not treated with selenium (Møller-Madsen and Danscher, 1991). The content of mercury in dorsal root ganglion cells of rats was increased by coadministration of selenium, elemental mercury, or methylmercury (Schionning et al., 1997). When studied using the electron microscope, the mercury was found to be localized in lysosomes. Postmortem measurement of selenium and mercury levels were made in several organs and tissues in three groups of people: (a) five miners known to have high exposure to inorganic mercury, (b) two people living in the mining town but who had not worked in the mines, and (c) two persons who lived far from the mercury mines and who were also never known to be exposed to mercury (Kosta et al., 1975). In the tissues samples from groups 1 and 2, those tissues with the highest concentrations of mercury (i.e., thyroid, pituitary, kidney, and brain) also had higher concentrations of selenium, and the molar ratio of mercury to selenium was 1 : 1. When tissue mercury content of an organ was less than 2 μg/g, selenium bore no relationship to the mercury content, and the selenium content was substantially less than in organs where mercury was high. These findings suggest that selenium may have a protective effect in persons exposed to methylmercury (Skerfving, 1978; Møller-Madsen and Danscher, 1991; Goyer, 1997).

Tissue Biochemistry

The mercuric salts (oxides, sulfides, and halides) are not highly lipid-soluble and thus do not easily cross the BBB (Gutknecht, 1981). In contrast, elemental mercury and organic mercury compounds, which are highly lipid-soluble, can readily pass through the BBB by passive diffusion (Lackowicz and Anderson, 1980) (see Figs. 6-2 and 6-3).

Metabolism of an organic mercury compound to the inorganic form determines its neurotoxicity. For example, although phenylmercury readily crosses the BBB by passive diffusion, it is also rapidly metabolized in the liver to benzene and inorganic mercury (Hg^{2+}) (Daniel et al., 1972). This rapid metabolism results in less accumulation of phenylmercury within the CNS after chronic exposures and thus lower neurotoxicity (Gage and Swan, 1961). Likewise, methoxyethylmercury is rapidly metabolized to ethylene and Hg^{2+} resulting in the relatively low neurotoxicity of this organic mercurial (Daniel et al., 1971). In contrast, the metabolism of the highly neurotoxic compound methylmercury to Hg^{2+} and methane is relatively slow, and thus more of this organic mercurial remains available to enter the CNS where it can produce its neurotoxic effects (Gage and Swan, 1961; Yasutake et al., 1989).

The active transport of methylmercury across the BBB is directly linked with the transport of thiol-containing amino acids across this same structure. Complexes of methylmercury bound to cysteine and glutathione (GSH) were identified in the blood, and methylmercury–glutathione complexes have been found in the brain, liver and bile following exposure (Rabinstein and Fairhurst, 1975; Naganuma and Imura, 1979; Kajiwara et al., 1996). A study by Kerper et al. (1992) suggests that γ-glutamyltranspeptidase hydrolyzes the methylmercury–glutathione complex in plasma to a methylmercury–cysteine complex. The methylmercury–cysteine complex has been demonstrated to penetrate the BBB more rapidly than other methylmercury–amino acid compounds (Thomas and Smith, 1982; Hirayama, 1980;

1985). Once mercury has crossed the BBB, it is able to cause neurotoxic effects.

Interactions with other chemicals alters the toxicity of mercury. For example, acute ethanol ingestion inhibits the uptake of elemental mercury by red blood cells, thereby reducing absorption and neurotoxicity (Neilsen Kudsk, 1965, 1969a, 1969b). Cobalt chloride, in divided doses given to rats before an injection of mercurous chloride, protected half the animals against renal lesions and all of them against death (Gabbiani et al., 1967). Vitamin E has been shown to reduce the effects of methylmercury; reduction of oxidative damage produced by methylmercury may be the mechanism responsible for a protective effect (Ganther, 1980; Nath et al., 1996). Selenium has been shown to reduce the functional toxicity of methylmercury in rats (Møller-Madsen and Danscher, 1991) (see Neuropathological Diagnosis section).

Excretion

Liquid elemental mercury passes through the gastrointestinal tract and is found unchanged in the feces (Campbell et al., 1992). Approximately 10% of an absorbed dose of elemental mercury vapor is expired unchanged (Rothstein and Hayes, 1964; Hursh et al., 1976; Cherian et al., 1978), and less than 1% of the body burden is excreted in the urine as elemental mercury (Stopford et al., 1978). The majority of an absorbed dose of elemental mercury vapor is metabolized to inorganic mercury, after which excretion occurs mainly in the urine and to a lesser extent in the feces. In addition, mercury cysteine and large neutral methionine complexes are found in the urine after exposures to elemental and inorganic mercury (Henderson et al., 1974). The biological half-life for the elimination of metallic and inorganic mercury from urine and blood is approximately 1 month, suggesting that accumulation of mercury occurs during chronic exposures (Rahola et al., 1973; Hursh et al., 1976; Kershaw et al., 1980; Suzuki et al., 1992; Bluhm et al., 1992).

Organic mercury compounds are metabolized to inorganic mercury and to the corresponding alkyl and aryl derivatives (Daniel et al., 1971, 1972). The majority of an absorbed dose of methylmercury is excreted in the bile and feces as a methylmercury glutathione complex (Norseth and Clarkson, 1970). The portion of an absorbed dose of methylmercury that is metabolized to inorganic mercury is conjugated with cysteine and glutathione and subsequently excreted in the urine (Yasutake et al., 1989). Methylmercury is also demethylated by intestinal flora, following which the inorganic mercury is excreted in feces (Nakamura et al., 1977; Rowland et al., 1980). However, a portion undergoes biliary–hepatic recirculation, resulting in the relatively long biological half-life of methylmercury (Dutczak et al., 1991). The biological half-life for elimination of methylmercury from the blood in humans is approximately 2 months, indicating that elimination of methylmercury is slower than it is for inorganic mercury

(Rahola et al., 1973; Hursh et al., 1976; Kershaw et al., 1980). Methylmercury is also excreted in breast milk (Amin-Zaki et al., 1974; Grandjean et al., 1995). Inorganic mercury derived from metabolism of phenylmercury and methoxyethylmercury salts is excreted primarily in the urine (Daniel et al., 1972; Gotelli et al., 1985). However, these compounds, which are much more readily metabolized to inorganic mercury than is methylmercury, have correspondingly shorter elimination half-lives (Gage and Swan, 1961; Daniel et al., 1971, 1972; Nielsen, 1992).

CLINICAL MANIFESTATIONS AND DIAGNOSIS

Symptomatic Diagnosis

Inorganic Mercury

Acute inhalation of elemental mercury vapor is irritating to the nasal pharynx and upper respiratory tract and causes acute pneumonitis, bronchitis, and bronchiolitis and without an accurate history of exposure may be mistaken for a viral infection (Jaeger et al., 1979; Bluhm et al., 1992). Inflammation of the oral mucosa may also follow acute exposures to high concentrations of elemental mercury vapor (Bluhm et al., 1992; Garnier et al., 1981; Snodgrass et al., 1981; Haddad and Sternberg 1963; Tennant et al., 1961). Impairment of pulmonary function as indicated by decreased vital capacity occurs in some exposed persons (Lilis et al., 1985; McFarland and Reigel, 1978). These respiratory symptoms, along with headache, fever, chills, chest pain, general malaise, nausea, and vomiting, are referred to as "metal fume fever syndrome" and characterize the "initial phase" of acute mercury vapor poisoning; a similar constellation of symptoms is seen after exposure to other vaporized metals. Patients who are asymptomatic during the first 4 hours following an acute exposure to mercury vapor may then develop symptoms abruptly. Neurological effects including delirium, tremor, and coma develop within 24 hours. The respiratory effects may worsen to include acute interstitial pulmonary fibrosis with resultant hypoxemia (Jaeger et al., 1979). In severe cases, rapidly progressing pulmonary edema and renal shutdown may cause the death of the exposed individual within a few days (Jaeger et al., 1979; Rowens et al., 1991; Kanluen and Gottlieb, 1991). If the initial phase is not fatal, it is followed by an "intermediate phase" during which a constellation of respiratory, gastrointestinal, urological, and CNS symptoms are frequently reported. The intermediate phase is followed by a "late phase" which is characterized by the resolution of the respiratory, gastrointestinal, and urological symptoms, while the CNS disturbances persist (Bluhm et al., 1992).

The less dramatic acute symptoms of elemental mercury exposure such as irritability and agitated responses to environmental perturbations, lethargy, confusion, mood swings with emotional lability, depression, social withdrawal, and tremor are often difficult to assign to mercury without a good history of exposure. Neuromuscular symptoms include myoclonus and fasciculations (Bluhm et al., 1992). For example, a severe acute exposure to elemental mercury vapors caused muscle weakness, fasciculations, and electromyographic evidence of motor neuron deficits, with recovery after removal from the exposure in a 54-year-old man (Adams et al., 1983). An axonal neuropathy characterized by distal muscle weakness, diffuse muscle wasting, and bilateral footdrop was described in a 14-year-old boy after he was subacutely exposed to high concentrations of elemental mercury that had been vaporized by a vacuum cleaner (Zelman et al., 1991).

Chronic inhalation of elemental mercury may be expected to cause adverse health effects if exposure exceeds the minimal risk level (MRL) of 0.3 µg/m³ (ATSDR, 1994). Complaints are at first subtle and are usually considered to be of no specific importance. They include fatigue, general weakness, loss of appetite, diarrhea, insomnia, mood changes, and tremor and have been called "micromercurialism" (Friberg and Nordberg, 1972). The tremor of mercurialism begins in the fingers and hands, and then it affects the eyelids, face, and eventually the head, neck, and torso. While usually bilateral, one side may have a more prominent tremor than the other; usually the dominant hand is more affected. The tremor is fine and rapid, and it worsens with activity and emotional excitement, resembling an essential tremor that is seen in patients with hyperthyroidism. The tremor frequency is faster and differs from the characteristic resting pill-rolling seen in Parkinson's disease. Continued exposures to mercury vapor results in worsening tremor, gingivitis, a withdrawing of social interactions, greater memory loss, and emotional lability. Prolonged exposure to elemental mercury has also resulted in disturbances of the eyes including tremor of the eyelids and discoloration of the cornea and lens as seen on slit lamp examination (Grant, 1993). In young children exposed to elemental mercury, photophobia is a common manifestation (Walsh and Hoyt, 1969). Neurobehavioral abnormalities emerge after prolonged exposure and include: cognitive impairments, especially in the areas of attention and concentration; disturbances of short-term memory; visual spatial ab-

normalities; and deficits in reasoning and problem-solving. Language function and long-term memory appears to be unaffected (Vroom and Greer, 1972; Anger, 1990; White et al., 1993) (Table 6-2).

A study of 71 workers in a factory in São Paulo, Brazil, where fluorescent lamps were manufactured found 61 (86%) to be either subchronically or chronically exposed to elemental mercury which was used in the manufacturing process (estimated shop use: 83 kg/month) (Zavariz and Glina, 1992). Most (28 workers) of the workers had been exposed for 3 years, while there were 12 who had been exposed for 6 years, three for 9 years, five for 12 years, four for 15 years, and one each for 21, 24, and more than 24 years. Poor ventilation and careless spilling of mercury on the floor of the hot workroom resulted in contamination of the work environment. And yet, the employer's sampling report indicated an ambient air mercury concentration of 0.00 mg/m³. The maintenance workers (22 workers) were the largest group affected, followed by the production assistants (17 workers) and machine operators (13 workers). One person's job was to recover spilled mercury. These people were most likely to have had contact with the elemental mercury. Other exposed workers included maintenance electricians (two), machine lubricators (two), and five persons who were involved in materials inspection, packaging, and clerical work. Nonspecific complaints included gastrointestinal symptoms (46 complaints), metallic taste (42 complaints), increased salivation (35 complaints), and bleeding gums (gingivitis) (28 complaints). Neurological symptoms included headache (55 complaints), distal paresthesias (41 complaints), insomnia (38 complaints), tremulousness (35 complaints), and fatigue (31 complaints). Behavioral symptoms were also reported and included agitation (52 complaints), irritability (48 complaints), disturbances of memory (34 complaints) and attention (25 complaints), depression (25 complaints), anxiety (18 complaints), and apathy (2 complaints). Neuropsychological assessment documented the CNS effects of mercury in these workers (see Neuropsychological Diagnosis section).

TABLE 6-2. *Urine mercury levels, initial symptoms, and degree of recovery in thermometer workers following exposure to elemental mercury*

Age (years)	Sex	Symptoms	Urine mercury (µg/24 hr)	Recovery	
				Memory	Motor
45	Male	Tremor, irritable, poor concentration	347	Poor	Excellent
47	Female	Tremor, rigidity, blurred vision, diarrhea, memory loss	345	Good	Good
33	Female	Tremor, mask face, blurred vision, diarrhea, memory loss	240	Good	Excellent
63	Female	Tremor, irritable, stocking glove sensory loss, poor concentration, diarrhea	682	Poor	Good
44	Female	Tremor, blurred vision	1,101	Poor	Good

Modified from Vroom and Greer, 1972.

Most of the exposed and symptomatic workers in this fluorescent lamp factory had been employed and exposed for 3 to 6 years. Since longevity of employment dropped off quickly after this, it might be suspected that newly hired persons and their less careful work habits contributed to their risk of exposure. Alternatively, there may have been fewer long-term employees because the effects of exposure to elemental mercury vapor had rendered them unable to continue to work under these circumstances.

Prevalence of symptoms among 84 workers chronically exposed to elemental mercury vapor at a thermometer manufacturing plant was compared with that of 79 unexposed workers from the same facility. The most frequently reported symptoms among the exposed workers included headache (29%), insomnia (25%), nervousness (23%), skin rashes (20%), emotional lability (18%), and difficulty with memory or concentration (16%). Overall, the mercury exposed plant workers reported a greater mean number of symptoms (2.9 per worker) than did the control workers (1.9 per worker). Thermometer workers were more likely to complain of a metallic taste and insomnia and were also more likely to have abnormal tests of heel-to-toe coordination and abnormal gait. Specific abnormalities seen among the thermometer workers included Romberg's sign (three workers), abnormalities in ability to perform rapid alternating movements (three workers) and one each with resting and intention tremor. None of the control plant workers demonstrated such neurological findings. All of the workers demonstrating abnormal neurologic signs also had significantly higher mean exposure index values of mercury levels (Ehrenberg et al., 1991).

Subclinical peripheral neuropathy, mainly distal and axonal, was detected in 17 thermometer factory workers who had been exposed to mercury vapors for 1 to 40 years and had high urine and blood mercury levels (Zampollo et al., 1987). Peripheral neurotoxicity in other cases exposed to either elemental or inorganic mercury has been demonstrated by others as well (Singer et al., 1987; Barber, 1978; Levine et al., 1982; Zalman et al., 1991).

Acute direct contact of inorganic mercurial salts is caustic to mucous membranes, and acute ingestion causes immediate damage to the mucosa of the mouth, oral pharynx, and gastrointestinal tract, resulting in abdominal pain, nausea, vomiting, and anorexia. Impairment of awareness, confusion, and delirium are features of metabolic encephalopathy associated with renal failure due to the acute effects of inorganic mercury poisoning. Precipitation of proteins by mercuric salts results in malnutrition. In addition, elimination of mercuric ions through the kidneys initially results in diuresis, followed by severe acute tubular necrosis. Renal shutdown and death occurs within 24 hours in 50% of acute intoxications (Winek et al., 1981; Kanluen and Gottlieb, 1991; Campbell et al., 1992).

The symptoms associated with chronic exposure to inorganic mercury and elemental mercury are similar, probably because the former breaks down to the elemental form in the environment. A common constellation of presenting symptoms includes excessive salivation or dry mouth, mental changes, and a fine, fast-frequency tremor. The tremor may be quite severe and is accentuated by activity increasing in amplitude of excursion upon activation. Some patients exhibit ataxia of gait. Increased tone and myoclonus are usually superimposed upon the tremor. Proximal involvement of both small and large peripheral nerve fibers results in a clinical picture of polyneuropathy (Zampollo et al., 1987; Singer et al., 1987), similar to that seen in Guillain–Barré syndrome (Warkany and Hubbard, 1953; Ross, 1964; Fuortes et al., 1995). Progressive motor neuropathy, in which fasciculations of muscle and atrophy are prominent, occurs in some patients (Langworth et al., 1992; Kark, 1994). These changes are associated with distal axonal degeneration and denervation atrophy in muscle. Prominent muscle weakness with relatively little sensory loss is seen in some cases of chronic mercury exposure. These findings are similar to the clinical picture of amyotrophic lateral sclerosis and should be ruled out in suspected cases of the latter (Barber, 1978). Behavioral effects including memory loss, apathy, depression, and emotional swings from grandiosity to timidity are also seen (Williamson et al., 1982; Fuortes et al., 1995).

Studies among mercury industry workers documented the effects of exposure at various levels and the persistence of neurological impairments after cessation of exposure. A dose-related increase in frequency of symptoms occurred among 567 chloralkali workers who were exposed to elemental mercury vapor at concentrations exceeding 100 $\mu g/m^3$ air (Smith et al., 1970). Similarly, an increased prevalence of neurological signs and impaired neuropsychological performance was seen in chloralkali workers whose urine mercury levels were greater than 50 $\mu g/L$ (Miller et al., 1975). Neurological signs persisted for 12.25 years after cessation of exposure to mercury vapor in a study of 77 former chloralkali workers. In addition, higher specific neurological findings included decreased peripheral sensation (13% versus 2%), postural tremor (18% versus 7%), impaired coordination (10% versus 2%), Romberg's sign (6.5% versus 0%), and tandem walking (8% versus 0%) (Anderson et al., 1993; Kishi et al., 1994).

Organic Mercury

The particular chemical structure of the organic mercury compound determines its clinical effects. The short-chain alkyl mercury compounds are volatile and lipid-soluble and thus are well absorbed through inhalation, ingestion, and dermal exposure. Ethylmercury poisoning has distinct differences from methylmercury intoxication. For example, gastrointestinal and renal effects are more prominent than are neurological symptoms. Such symptoms may also occur and include disturbances of motor function and coordination more than neurobehavioral problems (Amin-Zaki et al., 1974). The toxicity of long-chain alkyl and aryl mercury compounds more closely resembles that of inorganic mercury (Gage and Swan, 1961; Daniel et al., 1972; Campbell et al., 1992).

The earliest report of methylmercury poisoning was of four men who worked in the manufacture of mercurial seed fungicides. A period of 3 to 4 months passed between the start of their exposure and the appearance of symptoms. Initially, paresthesias affected the mouth and extremities. This was followed within a month by restricted visual fields, ataxia of gait, dysarthria, and sensory deficits in the extremities (i.e., impaired vibration sense, stereognosis, and two-point discrimination: the Hunter–Russell syndrome) (Hunter and Russell, 1954; Marsh, 1994).

The effects of acute intoxication with methylmercury were reported in members of a family who ingested pork from pigs which had consumed methylmercury-contaminated feed (Pierce et al., 1972; Curley et al., 1971). In addition to the acute symptoms of somnolence, ataxia, involuntary movements, seizures, and hyperactive reflexes which were observed initially after ingestion, neurological abnormalities persisted as long as 22 years in the surviving family members. The severity of their findings appeared to be related to the original measures of mercury in tissues (Table 6-3) (see Clinical Experiences section).

Reports of two major outbreaks in Japan and Iraq provided information about the clinical and pathological effects of methylmercury poisoning. The outbreak in the Minamata Bay area of Japan affected at least 2,500 individuals who ingested fish contaminated with methylmercury (Tamashiro et al., 1985). Clinical manifestations included difficulty with concentration, short- and long-term memory loss, emotional lability, depression, decreased intellectual abilities, and, ultimately, coma. Cerebellar signs of ataxia and stumbling gait, incoordination, and difficulty performing rapid alternating movement tasks were prominent. Paresthesias of the distal extremities and sensory loss in a stocking-glove distribution,

as well as other sensory impairments involving deafness and tunnel vision, were also noted. The most prominent features were constriction of visual fields, sensory disturbances, muscle atrophy, and cognitive disturbances. The neurological impairments worsened over a 3- to 10-year period during which many of the cases had been misdiagnosed as other neurological diseases.

Prenatal exposure to methylmercury results in severe brain damage. Although pregnant women in the Minamata outbreak experienced only mild effects such as transient paresthesia, their infants suffered severe brain damage (Harada, 1966). It took several years to prove that methylmercury was the causative agent resulting in ongoing exposure of a large population including those who were intrauterine at the time (Tsuchiya, 1992; Igata, 1991).

Poisoning occurred among Iraqi adults and children who accidentally ingested food made from grain treated with methylmercury, which was intended to be used for planting and not for eating (Rustam and Hamdi, 1974). Some victims experienced no untoward symptoms during the weeks or months of intake, despite the fact that these people had apparently ingested lethal amounts of methylmercury. The reason for a long latent period is not known (Clarkson, 1992), although it is inversely related to concentrations of mercury in blood of exposed primates (Evans et al., 1977). Because weeks or months may pass before symptoms of paresthesia, ataxia, dysarthria, and deafness are observed, this can postpone recognition of the exposure circumstances, resulting in serious brain damage or death.

Neurophysiological Diagnosis

Electroencephalography (EEG) performed in chloralkali workers subjected to low-level long-term exposure to inorganic mercury showed significantly slower rhythms

TABLE 6-3. *Neurological findings following exposure to ingested methylmercury*

Acute intoxication				Neurobehavioral findings at follow-up 22 years after exposure
Patient age (years)	Sex	Symptoms	Mercury levels (ppm)	
20	Female	Confusion, ataxia, constricted visual fields, involuntary movements, dysarthria, seizures	Urine 0.06 Serum 2.78 Hair 2,436	Verbal I.Q.[a] 86, mild attention deficit, poor coordination, slow word retrieval, central vision only
13	Male	Somnolence, involuntary movements, cortical blindness, Babinski signs, hyperactive reflexes, loss of proprioception	Urine 0.21 Serum 2.91 CSF 3.33	Verbal I.Q.[a] 99, mild attention deficit, slow word retrieval, cortical blindness, dysarthria, mild ataxia, hyperactive reflexes
50	Male	Asymptomatic, low-average intelligence	Urine 0.16 Hair 186	Severe spatial deficits, poor tandem gait
48	Female	Asymptomatic, borderline intelligence	Urine 0.18 Serum 2.9	Asymptomatic, borderline intelligence

[a]Wechsler Adult Intelligence Scale.
Modified from Davis et al., 1994.

and more attenuated amplitudes than did the EEG referents (Piikivi and Tolonen, 1989). The changes were more prominent in the occipital region, were milder in the parietal areas, and did not affect the frontal areas. A tendency was noted toward increased focal EEG disturbances in the worker population studied. Because of the differences in exposures due to work shift, job tasks, and individual susceptibilities, as well as possible preexisting cerebral conditions, these EEG findings may not be specific enough to warrant a conclusion about their causal relationship to mercury in this study. However, when all other confounders are identified and excluded, EEG abnormalities in mercury-exposed persons can be attributed to the effects of encephalopathy. The EEG of an 8-year-old girl who had been exposed to methylmercury *in utero* showed diffuse and persistent slow waves with high voltage (Eto et al., 1992).

Evoked potentials (EPs) can be used to assess CNS functions of individuals exposed to mercury. *Short-latency somatosensory evoked potential* (SSEP) studies in five patients with Minamata disease revealed complete absence of the N20 wave component; the N9, N11, N13, and N14, wave components were normal. Three of these patients showed marked cortical atrophy localized to the central sulci on CT studies consistent the SSEP results (Tokuomi et al., 1982). A correlation was found between blood mercury levels (range: 7 to 45 μg/L) and I-III interpeak latencies of BAEPs on the right side among Ecuadorian children and adults environmentally exposed to methylmercury and elemental mercury derived from the gold mining process (Counter et al., 1998). These findings suggest that mercury affects central auditory and somatosensory pathways possibly by damaging cortical neurons. Grandjean et al. (1997) did not find significant differences in the BAEPs and *visual evoked potentials* (VEPs) of 7-year-old children who had been exposed to mercury *in utero*. However, neuropsychological testing of these children did reveal significant central-nervous-system effects of their *in utero* exposure (see Neuropsychological Diagnosis section).

Nerve conduction studies (NCS) provide neurophysiological confirmation of the effects of mercury exposure on the peripheral nervous system (Markowitz and Schaumburg, 1980; Levine et al., 1982; Zampollo et al., 1987; Zelman et al., 1991). Motor nerve impairment usually occurs after longer periods of exposure to mercury vapor, whereas changes in sensory function follow short-term exposures (Gilioli et al., 1976). Neurophysiological studies of workers exposed to mercury vapors intermittently, for a period of several weeks once a year at median levels below the current OSHA PEL of 0.1 mg/m³ and with current urine levels of ≤24 μg/g creatinine, did not reveal any significant difference in motor nerve conduction velocities or tremor frequency (Boogaard et al., 1996). Levine et al. (1982) found prolonged sensory and motor distal latencies in the ulnar nerves of chloralkali workers exposed to elemental mercury whose urine mercury concentrations exceeded 500 μg/L. Albers et al. (1988) performed nerve conduction studies in 386 chloralkali workers who had been exposed to elemental mercury 20 to 35 years earlier, before testing. Prolonged sensory and motor distal latencies were seen in those workers whose biological monitoring showed one or more previous urinary mercury concentrations above 600 μg/L. Diminished vibration sensation and hypoactive tendon reflexes consistent with large fiber neuropathy were also found in these same workers. Multiple linear regression analysis revealed significant correlations between declining neurological function over time and increasing exposure level as determined by urinary mercury measurements in these workers.

Singer et al. (1987) studied 16 workers exposed to inorganic mercury (e.g., mercuric oxides and phenyl mercuric acid) and demonstrated that slowing of the median motor *nerve conduction velocities* (NCVs) correlated with increased levels of mercury in blood and urine as well as with increased prevalence of neurological symptoms. In this study, the motor-nerve fibers seemed to be more affected than the sensory fibers, contrasting with the observations of Albers et al. (1988) and Levine et al. (1982), who noted that sensory nerves were affected more than motor nerves. This discrepancy may be explained by differences in susceptibility of the motor and sensory nerves to differences in levels and durations of exposure and possibly by the age of the workers. Sensory deficits are found with short-term exposure to mercury vapor, whereas motor nerve impairments occur with longer periods of exposure (Gilioli et al., 1976; Ellingsen et al., 1993).

Electromyography (EMG) studies in 247 of the 386 workers referred to above, who had been exposed to elemental mercury vapor 20 to 35 years prior to testing, revealed increased prevalence of abnormal electrical activity in the muscle (Albers et al., 1988). A brief, intense exposure to elemental mercury in a 54-year-old man who was salvaging liquid mercury from broken thermometers was followed in 3.5 months by weight loss and progressive twitching of his shoulder muscles, accompanied by a mild tingling and numb sensation of his hands and feet (Adams et al., 1983). He had general weakness and unsteadiness of handwriting. A urinary screening test for heavy metals at that time showed an increased level of mercury (98.75 μg/L every 24 hours), while levels of arsenic and thallium were within normal limits. EMG studies confirmed the presence of denervation and reinnervation consistent with severe denervation compatible with motor neuron disease, but the course of illness and the association of the neuromuscular findings and mercury exposure suggests a possible causal relationship.

Tremorography and computerized accelerometry have also been used to document the neurological effects of mercury. EMG recordings made with surface electrodes over the dorsum of each hand documented postural tremor, more severe on the right than the left, in a 48-year-old male thermometer factory worker who had been exposed to elemental mercury while separating liquid mercury from broken glass (White et al., 1993) (Fig. 6-4) (see Neuroimaging and

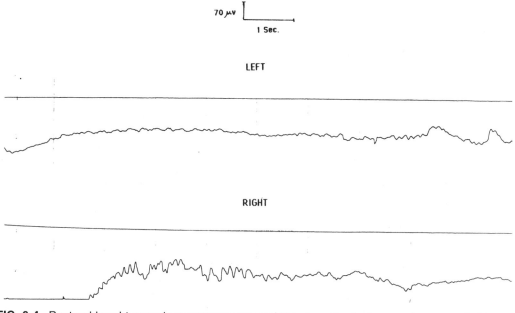

FIG. 6-4. Postural hand tremor in a mercury-exposed thermometer factory worker; recorded by surface electromyography. Note the presence of tremor, right more than left (see Clinical Experiences section for urine mercury levels).

Clinical Experiences sections). Computerized accelerometers are also useful for documenting the tremors of mercury exposure which are clinically evident, as well as those perceived only by the patient as an internal sensation of tremulousness. For example, quantitative measurements of coordination ability and performance speed, as well as the frequency and amplitude of tremor, were made on seven Danish workers acutely exposed to a spill of 0.9 kg of elemental mercury on a factory floor. Air concentrations in the contaminated room, taken 1 week after the accident, showed as much as 0.15 mg/m³ of mercury. This exceeded the Danish TLV of 0.05 mg/m³. Tremor intensity was the most sensitive parameter of acute exposure detected among the workers with mercury urine levels greater than 11 μg/L (B. Netterstrom and J. Heebøll, Danish Product Development, personal communication, 1995). This technique also has been employed to evaluate a population in the Faroe Islands exposed to mercury in their seafood, as well as to evaluate miners in the Amazon Valley who use mercury to separate gold from silt washings (PG Grandjean, personal communication, 1995).

Neuropsychological Diagnosis

Adults chronically exposed to elemental mercury demonstrate cognitive impairments, including deficits in attention and executive function, short-term memory, visuospatial ability, and motor function. Language function and long-term memory are typically spared in adults but may be impaired in persons exposed *in utero* or during childhood (Amin-Zaki et al., 1974; Anger, 1990; Eto et al., 1992; Diamond et al., 1995).

The neuropsychological effects of mercury exposure are correlated with the cumulative exposure dose. For example, digit span tests demonstrated significant impairment of attention and short-term memory that was correlated with urine mercury levels (Smith et al., 1983). Significant correlations were found between duration of exposure and impaired short-term memory function among 21 workers exposed to elemental, inorganic, and organic mercurials at a chemical manufacturing plant (Triebig and Schaller, 1982). Similarly, a correlation between length of exposure and decreased short-term memory function was found in mercury-exposed dentists (Williamson et al., 1982). In dentists with high tissue mercury levels, the Bender–Gestalt test revealed a significant impairment of visuospatial skills (Shapiro et al., 1982). A study of a thermometer manufacturing facility compared 84 mercury-exposed workers with 79 unexposed workers who served as controls. The exposed workers reported more symptoms on a questionnaire than did the controls (Ehrenberg et al., 1991). While headaches and insomnia were common, emotional lability, memory, and concentration problems were also often reported. Persistent impairments of short-term memory, coordination, and simple reaction time were seen in mercury miners more than 10 years after their removal from exposure (Kishi et al., 1993).

Neuropsychological tests in a group of 71 fluorescent lamp workers exposed to elemental mercury documented severe impairments of functioning in 55 (78%) (Zavariz and Glina, 1992). Thirteen (18.3%) were considered to show normal neuropsychological functioning on the tests. The domains most affected included attention, memory, and motor functions.

The neuropsychological assessment of 26 of 53 construction workers exposed to elemental mercury revealed acute and persistent CNS effects. Initial testing revealed impaired performance on tests of attention and executive functioning (Trails A and B; Stroop test) and motor skills (finger tapping; grooved pegboard). Severity of performance impairment was correlated with cumulative excretion of mercury. Performance on Trails A and B were improved following chelation therapy. However, performance on finger tapping and the Stroop tests remained unchanged with time away from exposure, and performance on the grooved pegboard worsened with time. These results suggest that elemental mercury affects specific cognitive domains (e.g., attention and executive functioning) and that tests of motor functioning are particularly sensitive to the persistent effects of exposure to this metal.

A case study of a 19-year-old patient with a history of chronic exposure to mercury vapors during childhood revealed persistent behavioral abnormalities indicative of developmental toxin-induced encephalopathy secondary to mercury exposure (Diamond et al., 1995). Severe cases of mental retardation following exposure to methylmercury during critical developmental periods were noted in the earlier studies of the Iraq outbreak (Amin-Zaki et al., 1974) and in the subsequent follow-up (Marsh et al., 1980). Neuropsychological development was reported to be so severely retarded in an individual exposed to methylmercury *in utero* during the Minamata outbreak that she never learned to speak (Eto et al., 1992). Unlike focal damage in adults, damage to the developing brain is diffuse and widespread, possibly resulting from interference with neuronal migration and formation of anomalous synapses (Choi et al., 1978).

Neuropsychological assessment of 7-year-old children who had been exposed *in utero* to methylmercury revealed significant performance deficits on tests of language (Boston Naming Test), attention (Continuous Performance Test), memory (California Verbal Learning test for children), and to a lesser extent in visuospatial (Bender Visual Motor Gestalt test) and motor (finger tapping) functioning. Clinical examinations and neurophysiological studies in these same children did not reveal any abnormalities that could be attributed to their *in utero* exposure to methylmercury (Grandjean et al., 1997).

Biochemical Diagnosis

Blood plasma concentration of mercury is the best measure of recent exposure to inorganic and elemental mercury.

The *American Conference of Governmental Industrial Hygienists* (ACGIH) have recommended a biological exposure index (BEI) of 15 μg/L for inorganic mercury concentration in blood at the end of the last shift of the workweek (Table 6-4) (ACGIH, 1995). Neurological symptoms of exposure to methylmercury generally appear at blood concentrations of 480 μg/L (Marsh, 1994). The plasma to red blood cell (RBC) ratio can indicate whether or not the source of mercury was inorganic or organic. A ratio of 1 : 1 indicates inorganic mercury, because it is equally distributed between the plasma and RBCs; a plasma to RBC ratio of 1 : 10 suggests organic mercury exposure. A clear correlation between the concentration of mercury in the blood and severity of symptoms was determined in the methylmercury-exposed adults in the Iraq outbreak following ingestion of contaminated bread. A threshold model was used to illustrate that more severe effects appear at higher threshold levels of methylmercury (Bakir et al., 1973). Cerebrospinal fluid mercury correlates with plasma mercury, especially in workers who have high-intensity ongoing exposure (Sälsten et al., 1994).

While blood levels are more useful than are random urine levels in assessing large exposed populations (Smith et al., 1970), serial urine measurements and the calculation of cumulative exposure indices are useful for monitoring and correlating exposure with the emergence and persistence of symptoms in individuals and/or groups of exposed persons. The ACGIH BEI for inorganic mercury in a preshift urine sample is 35 μg/g creatinine (see Table 6-4) (ACHIH, 1995). The severity of mercury intoxication cannot be accurately predicted in a given individual from the mercury concentration in a random urine sample. However, the use of multiple urine samples to determine and characterize a mercury index for each worker based on his or her previous plant urinalysis records can be used. Langworth et al. (1992) used a multiple urine sample analysis based on plant urinalysis records to characterize previous exposures in workers. The median blood mercury concentration among these workers was 11 μg/L, serum mercury concentration was 9 μg/L, and urine mercury concentration was 14.3 nmol/mmol creatinine (25.4 μg/g creatinine).

Similarly, Albers et al. (1988) used this approach, along with a medical and occupational questionnaire, a clinical examination, and neurophysiological measurements of nerve conduction velocity, to study chloralkali workers who had prior exposure to elemental mercury (20 to 35 years earlier). Multiple linear regression analysis demonstrated a consistently positive correlation between declin-

TABLE 6-4. *Biological exposure indices for mercury*

	Urine	Blood	Alveolar Air
Determinant:	Inorganic mercury	Inorganic mercury	Inorganic mercury
Start of shift:	35 μg/g creatinine	Not established	Not established
During shift:	Not established	Not established	Not established
End of shift at end of workweek:	Not established	15 μg/L	Not established

Data from ACGIH, 1995.

ing neurological performance and cumulative and peak urine mercury levels. Few subjects with high exposure had normal neurological examinations. The duration of exposure negatively correlated with all measures, indicating that most of the exposure had occurred at high levels over a short period of time. Those workers with a urinary mercury peak concentration above 850 μg/L had two- to threefold increased risk of having clinically detectable peripheral neuropathy. A patient can be used as his or her own control, with a three- to fourfold increase in 24-hour mercury concentration over baseline following chelation with D-penicillamine being indicative of an increased body burden.

Hair levels of mercury are usually 250 to 300 times the concentration found in RBCs, because mercury has an affinity for the sulfhydryl groups in the protein of hair. Hair samples should be obtained so that the longest strands can be analyzed. Total mercury in hair is the sum of the inorganic plus organic sources (Yamaguchi et al., 1975). Mercury was found in increasing concentrations in hair segments after ingestion of mercury during the epidemic methylmercury toxic occurrence in Iraq (Bakir et al., 1973; Airey, 1983). Studies of methylmercury exposure showed evidence of elevated mercury levels in 31% of blood and hair samples collected in native and northern people in 356 communities across Canada (Wheatley et al., 1979). The members of the Cree na-

tion in the communities of Northern Quebec showed an association between exposure level and neurologic abnormalities detected (Eyssen et al., 1990). Hair and urinary mercury levels were determined in residents of Papua, New Guinea. The only possible source for the elevated levels was mercury found in the fish they consumed. The hair and urine concentrations of mercury correlated significantly ($r = 0.59$) with the daily intake of mercury-containing fish (approximately 73 μg/day) (Abe et al., 1995).

Neuroimaging

Magnetic resonance imaging (MRI) has been used to assess the possible neuropathological and functional deficits thought to result from mercury intoxication (Korogi et al., 1994; White et al., 1993; Valk and van der Knapp, 1989). A report about the neurobehavioral findings in a thermometer factory worker who had significant mercury vapor exposure indicated that there were cognitive impairments which could be associated with areas of involvement of the subcortical white matter and the precentral gyri as seen on MRI. These findings included cortical atrophy, as well as diffuse and focal punctiform white matter lesions, on T2-weighted images using a 0.5-T magnet in both frontal regions (Fig. 6-5) (White et al., 1993). These changes, pre-

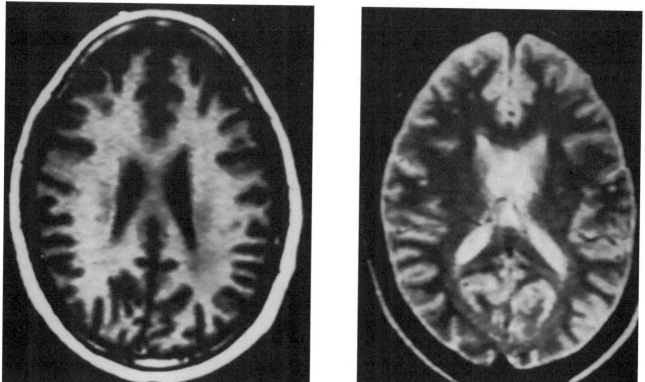

A   B

FIG. 6-5. Magnetic resonance image (0.5-T magnet) in a 48-year-old thermometer worker who had been exposed to elemental mercury for 3.5 years: **A:** T1-weighted image showing marked central and cortical atrophy. **B:** T2-weighted image demonstrating diffuse and focal punctiform white matter lesions in frontal and parietal regions (see Table 6-5).

dominantly in white matter and with no particular predilection for the cerebellum and calcarine cortex, suggest a difference in the targets of damage between elemental and methylmercury intoxication.

A magnetic resonance image was made of a patient who was exposed to methylmercury 22 years earlier by ingesting contaminated pork (hair mercury content at the time of exposure was 2,436 ppm). The magnetic resonance image revealed atrophy in the calcarine cortices, parietal cortices, and cerebellum. Similar changes in the occipital cortex were observed in the magnetic resonance image of this patient's sibling who had also consumed the contaminated pork. These changes were attributed to their earlier exposure to methylmercury (Davis et al., 1994).

MRI was performed on seven people who had been diagnosed as having Minamata disease, as a result of their having eaten methylmercury-contaminated fish between 1955 and 1958. These people have exhibited neurological manifestations of methylmercury poisoning since their exposure and have had follow-up examinations throughout the ensuing 30 years (Table 6-5). The MRI findings were essentially the same in all subjects, with varying degrees of atrophy of the cerebellar vermis, the hemispheres, and the calcarine cortex and the postcentral gyrus. The most characteristic lesion seen on MRI involved the calcarine cortex, as could be predicted by the usual anatomic pathological findings in methylmercury poisoning (Korogi et al., 1994) (Fig. 6-6). The findings of atrophy of the cerebellum and the occipital lobes in Minamata disease had been demonstrated before the use of MRI by computerized axial tomography (Matsumoto et al., 1988).

Neuropathological Diagnosis

Autopsy data from cases following toxic exposure to methylmercury by consumption of contaminated fish in Minamata Bay showed selective damage in certain anatomical areas of the brain which appear especially susceptible to damage by methylmercury (Hunter and Russell, 1954). In addition to general cerebral edema, gross examination showed atrophy of the cerebellum and the cerebral cortex (calcarine, pre- and postcentral areas). Cell loss was most severe deep in the sulci of the calcarine (visual) cortex of persons who became totally blind following exposure. Astrocytosis and glial proliferation, together with spongiform degeneration, were also observed. The remainder of the occipital cortex was spared. There was widespread granular cell loss with sparing of Purkinje cells in the cerebellum (Kurland, 1960). Neuropathologic observations of the fatal cases from the Iraq accident revealed the corticles of the cerebrum and the cerebellum to be selectively involved with focal necrosis of neurons (Rustam and Hamdi, 1974).

Postmortem studies on unborn children exposed during the poisoning in Japan and Iraq showed that high levels of brain mercury were associated with abnormal neuronal migration and deranged organization of cortical neuronal layers. In fetal brains, phagocytosis of lysed cells was followed by glial proliferation (Choi et al., 1978). Subsequent studies by Takeuchi et al. (1989) and Sakai et al. (1975) confirmed the earlier postmortem studies in Minamata victims, which demonstrated cellular loss and glial proliferation, with spongiform changes in severe cases. In particular, the tunnel vision noted clinically in patients was explained by the relative sparing of the occipital pole, with no involvement of the optic nerves or retina.

The following autopsy report describes the findings in a person who was *in utero* when her mother was exposed to methylmercury and whose autopsy was performed 29 years later when she died of related complications of chronic debilitation (Eto et al., 1992). Her mother's hair showed

TABLE 6-5. *Neurological and MRI findings in Minamata disease 30 years after exposure*

	Age (years) and sex						
	46M[a]	59M	58M	54M	52F	48F	46F
MRI (atrophy)							
Calcarine cortex	++	++	+	++	++	++	++
Postcentral gyrus	++	+	+/-	+	+	+/-	++
Cerebellar cortex	++	+	+	++	++	++	++
Cerebellar vermis	+	+	+	++	++	++	++
Brain stem	-	-	-	-	+/-	+/-	-
Neurological findings							
Constriction of visual fields	++	++	-[b]	++	++	++	+
Ataxia	+	++	+	+	+	++	+
Sensory disturbance	+	++	++	+	++	++	+

[a]See Fig. 6-6.
[b]Initially showed constriction of visual fields.
M, male; F, female; MRI, magnetic resonance imaging; -, negative; +/-, equivocal; +, mild; ++, moderate to marked.
Modified from Korogi et al., 1994.

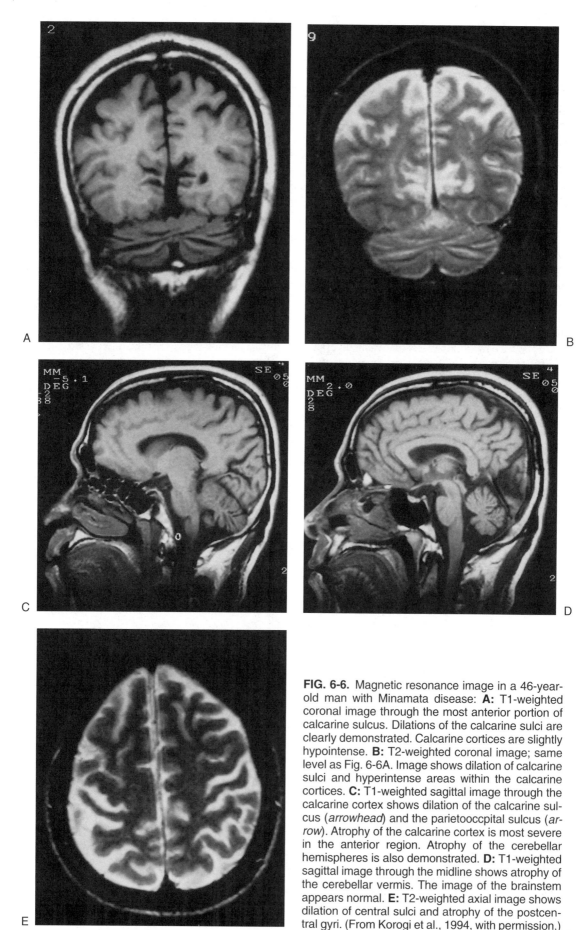

FIG. 6-6. Magnetic resonance image in a 46-year-old man with Minamata disease: **A:** T1-weighted coronal image through the most anterior portion of calcarine sulcus. Dilations of the calcarine sulci are clearly demonstrated. Calcarine cortices are slightly hypointense. **B:** T2-weighted coronal image; same level as Fig. 6-6A. Image shows dilation of calcarine sulci and hyperintense areas within the calcarine cortices. **C:** T1-weighted sagittal image through the calcarine cortex shows dilation of the calcarine sulcus (*arrowhead*) and the parietooccipital sulcus (*arrow*). Atrophy of the calcarine cortex is most severe in the anterior region. Atrophy of the cerebellar hemispheres is also demonstrated. **D:** T1-weighted sagittal image through the midline shows atrophy of the cerebellar vermis. The image of the brainstem appears normal. **E:** T2-weighted axial image shows dilation of central sulci and atrophy of the postcentral gyri. (From Korogi et al., 1994, with permission.)

101 μg/g of mercury in 1959 upon evaluation for exposure during the Minamata Bay incident. The exact transplacental dose may be estimated as elevated, but no other exposure data were available. The brain weighed 920 g and showed marked cerebral atrophy. Macroscopic examination of the brain revealed marked thinning of the corpus callosum and status marmoratus of the thalamus, neuronal loss in the calcarine, postcentral, and precentral cortices, cerebellar atrophy, and segmental demyelination of peripheral nerves. Microscopic examination revealed that the kidney, liver, and brain contained mercury granules. In the brain, the mercury granules were found in the neurons and macrophages of the cerebral cortices, the basal ganglia, ependymal cells, epithelial cells of the choroid plexus, and cerebellar and brain-stem nuclei. In addition, calcification was seen in the globus pallidus.

Electron microscopic examination showed shrunken nerve cells that had increased nuclear chromatin. Free ribosomes were scattered diffusely, with focal aggregations in the cytoplasm of neurons. Rough endoplasmic reticula (ER) were markedly decreased in number. Nissl bodies were not observed in the cytoplasm of neurons, but swollen cisternae were present in various small numbers. The Golgi apparatus was occasionally found, and its cisternae were swollen. Mitochondria were well-preserved. In the cerebellum, Purkinje cells were atrophic with high electron density. Aggregations of chromatin were present in the nuclei of the Purkinje cells, which were shrunken. The nuclear membranes were occasionally indistinct. Granule cells in the cerebellum were focally atrophic with high electron density. Parallel fibers were mixed in the molecular layer. This study, by Eto et al. (1992), showed many of the changes seen in the fetal cases examined during the Minamata investigations.

In spite of her 29-year survival, mercury was still present in the brain of Eto's patient who had been exposed to methylmercury *in utero.* While organic mercury was found in the tissues, a greater quantity of inorganic mercury was present in the specimens studied. In fact, 80% of the total mercury in the organs was in the inorganic form, suggesting that biotransformation of methylmercury to inorganic mercury occurs *in vivo* in humans (Eto et al., 1992). Such biotransformation has also been demonstrated in the brains of family members who were acutely poisoned by methylmercury following ingestion of contaminated pork (Davis et al., 1994). The pathological findings in that report showed that the cerebellum demonstrated considerable histological damage, but the damage was milder than that seen in the cerebral cortex. Damage to the basal ganglia and thalamus was also less severe than that to the cerebrum. The brain stem and spinal cord had histological changes that were mainly secondary to cortical damage. These factors support the hypothesis of Takeuchi et al. (1989), namely, that expulsion of mercury from the brain is difficult and may take longer than the biological half-life of 70 days proposed by Aberg et al. (1969) (Eto et al., 1992). Thus, the neuropathological findings in the 29-year-old patient described by Eto

et al. (1992) probably resulted from severe disruption of cytoarchitectural development during her *in utero* exposure.

Magos et al. (1985) showed that brain damage in animals correlated better with the amount of intact methylmercury or ethylmercury in the brain than with the level of inorganic mercury split off from the parent organic molecule. However, the presence of inorganic mercury following the cleavage from organic mercury may produce free radicals, leading to lipid peroxidation and cell death. The rate of cleavage would be proportional to the concentration of intact methylmercury, accounting for the observations of Magos and co-workers. In addition, reports indicate that antioxidant therapy protects against methylmercury-induced brain damage in animals (Ganther, 1980; Chang et al., 1978).

The mechanism of mercury toxicity has not been fully elucidated. However, mercury has been demonstrated to increase the permeability of the BBB (Chang and Hartman, 1972b). Oxidative injury has been proposed as a possible mechanism of mercury toxicity (Ganther, 1978; Nath et al., 1996). Oxidation–reduction reactions and the exceptional affinity of mercurials for thiol-containing ligands are important factors in its biological activity. The strong affinity of mercury for sulfhydryl groups of enzymes leads to the formation of mercaptides in compound with proteins, which inactivate sulfhydryl enzymes, thereby disrupting cellular metabolism (Carty and Malone, 1979). Methylmercury inhibits activity of the sulfhydryl enzyme choline acetyltransferase, which catalyzes the final step in acetylcholine synthesis (ATSDR, 1989). It also disrupts cellular processes including synaptic function, excitability, ion regulation, and protein synthesis. Chronic methylmercury exposure results in ultrastructural changes, with accumulation of methylmercury within mitochondria, inhibition of several mitochondrial enzymes, and depolarization of the mitochondrial membrane with inhibition of protein synthesis (Atchison and Hare, 1994). Methylmercury affects the release of Ca^{2+} from the intracellular Ca^{2+} pool, and it increases the Ca^{2+} permeability of the plasma membrane. Release of neurotransmitter from presynaptic neural terminals is affected by these changes in intracellular concentrations of Ca^{2+}. Methylmercury also blocks plasma membrane voltage-dependent Ca^{2+} and Na^+ channels, and it activates a nonspecific transmembrane cation conductance. Astroglial glutamate uptake is impaired at high concentrations of mercury, and extracellular glutamate reaches concentrations that are cytotoxic to neurons. Even low concentrations of mercury will inhibit the activity of glutamine synthetase. The CA1 pyramidal cells in the hippocampus are especially vulnerable to mercury toxicity, possibly because of their high density of *N*-methyl-D-aspartate (NMDA) receptors (Rönnbäck and Hansson, 1992).

Toxic effects on motor neurons result from either excessive mercury accumulation or inadequate mercury detoxification (Brown, 1954; Vallee and Ulmer, 1972; Adams et al., 1983; Aschner and Aschner, 1990). Mercury in spinal neurons may increase susceptibility to other neurotoxins and thereby increase vulnerability to neuronal degeneration (Kasarskis et al., 1993). Susceptibility to the biological effects of mercury may be related to the success or failure of metallothioneine (MT), a renal protein, to bind divalent metals such as mercury and thereby render them innocuous (Vallee and Ulmer, 1972). The presence of the potential mercury-detoxification moiety, MT, in motor neurons in the spinal cord suggests that metal detoxification, rather than simple accumulation, is a critical factor in the pathogenesis of amyotrophic lateral sclerosis (ALS). Impaired detoxification can result from an aberrant MT isoform within spinal motor neurons or altered MT gene expression following mercury exposure. Variations of gene control of MT or a related protein could account for differences in susceptibility to the toxic effects of mercury within different areas of the CNS (Kark, 1994). However, based on population studies, it appears unlikely that ALS results from a single environmental type of exposure (Kasarskis et al., 1993).

PREVENTIVE AND THERAPEUTIC MEASURES

Tragic outbreaks among innocent populations in several areas of the world have resulted from consumption of organic mercury–contaminated foodstuffs and improper disposal of inorganic mercury into bodies of water where methylation led to organomercurial contamination of seafood supplies. These occurrences were preventable and stress the need for proper education of those personnel responsible for the handling and disposal of mercury compounds.

Prevention is the best approach of avoiding toxicity in occupational settings. Protective clothing and goggles should be worn to prevent dermal absorption of mercury vapors (NIOSH, 1997). Work areas should be appropriately ventilated, and air sampling of the work environment should be routinely performed. A mercury vapor analyzer can be used to monitor work areas for concentrations as low as 0.001 mg/m^3. Air sampling for elemental mercury should be conducted using a solid sorbent media, low flow rate, and flameless atomic absorption (Campbell et al., 1992). In order to prevent increased volatilization, airborne dissemination, and subsequent inhalation, the vacuuming of spilled mercury should be avoided (Zelman et al., 1991; Schwartz et al., 1992; Fuortes et al., 1995). Individuals subject to increased mercury intake should be monitored and immediately removed from the source of exposure if urine mercury increases fourfold over baseline or exceeds 50 μg/L.

After an individual has been exposed to toxic levels of mercury, serial analyses of urine must be performed to ascertain that mercury excretion is satisfactory. A complete physical examination should also be performed at this time. Active treatment is necessary in any case of inorganic mercury intoxication that does not respond quickly to removal from the source of exposure (Kark, 1994). If the patient has been exposed to inorganic or elemental mercury and is symptomatic, chelation therapy with dimercaprol should begin immediately. Mercury forms a chelate complex with dimercaprol which is then elim-

inated by the kidneys (Campbell et al., 1992). Dimercaprol is administered intramuscularly in doses of 3 to 5 mg/kg every 4 to 5 hours for the first 24 hours, every 12 hours for the second 24 hours, once per day for the following 3 days, followed by a 2-day rest. The course is repeated until urine mercury level has decreased to 50 μg/L or less. Exposure to all forms of mercury, including methylmercury, may be treated with 2,3-dimercaptosuccinic acid (DMSA) or 2,3-dimercapto-propane-1-sulfonate (DMPS). DMPS, a water-soluble analog of British antilewisite (BAL), has been shown to be effective at 100 mg t.i.d. for 5 days (Torres-Alanis et al., 1995). Administration of DMSA begins with 10 mg/kg three times a day for the first 5 days, twice daily for the next 14 days, followed by 2 weeks of rest. The course of treatment is repeated until the urine levels have significantly decreased.

Bluhm et al. (1992) found DMSA to be much more effective than N-acetyl-penicillamine at increasing mercury excretion in men exposed to mercury vapor. Penicillin and D-penicillamine have also been used to treat mercury intoxication and are particularly effective in treating symptoms of acrodynia (Kark, 1994). In a thermometer factory worker who had been exposed to vapors from broken thermometers for over 3 years, two courses of oral penicillamine (250 mg every 6 hours for 10 days) were necessary to significantly reduce his elevated urine and blood levels of mercury (see Symptomatic Diagnosis section for details of the case) (Table 6-6). Hemodialysis has been used in conjunction with chelating agents to treat patients poisoned by ingestion of mercuric chloride (Kostyniak et al., 1990; Sauder et al., 1988; McLauchlan, 1991).

CLINICAL EXPERIENCES

Group Studies

Exposure to Mercury Vapor in Repairmen

Fifty-three men were acutely exposed to elemental mercury, at a chemical manufacturing plant, while they were

TABLE 6-6. *Biochemical diagnosis of mercury vapor exposure in a thermometer factory worker*[a]

Date	Urine mercury level[a]	Blood mercury level[a]
1/18/81 (Started work)	NA	NA
7/20/84 (Stopped work)	NA	NA
9/18/84	480 μg/L	0.32 μg/dL
9/25/84	690 μg/L	NA
10/1/84 (Chelation)		
10/10/84	240 μg/L	2.5 μg/dL
10/21/84 (Chelation)		
10/25/84	184 μg/L	2.0 μg/L
12/28/84	17 μg/L	4.0 μg/L
4/9/86	12 μg/L	None

[a]Before and after chelation therapy (250 mg penicillamine every 6 hours for 10 days).
NA, not available.

performing maintenance work on the metal pipes of a mercury cathode that was used as an electrolytic catalyst in the production of chlorine (Bluhm et al., 1992). Their welding equipment, oxyacetylene torches, volatized mercury which remained within the pipes being repaired. During the process, vaporization and condensation of the mercury occurred. Some of the men were working around the source of mercury vapors for 16 hours, replacing pipes and removing mercury into drains in the floor. Several men wore protective masks containing MERZORB cartridges for limited periods of time, from 30 minutes to 4 hours. Only a few of the workers wore protective suits, rubber shoes, or goggles. Twenty-six of the 53 men received detailed examinations for evidence of mercury poisoning. Seventeen were examined 19 and 36 days after the end of exposure, and nine of the workers were seen thereafter.

Several workers reported flu-like symptoms within the first few days following exposure, leading to medical evaluation. Initial symptoms in most of the men were suggestive of a viral illness, including headache, fatigue, fever, chills, and loss of appetite. Shortness of breath, nasal congestion, chest pain, and palpitations occurred in some, while others had diarrhea, abdominal cramps, tremor, and myoclonus. Irritability, depression, and forgetfulness were also common symptoms. Chest x-ray examination of those with respiratory symptoms showed evidence of edema. Patients had a clinical examination, an electrocardiogram, measurement of blood and urine mercury levels, and nerve conduction velocity studies.

Using an integrated analysis, the total mercury available for urinary excretion was modeled in each patient and was found to range from 10 to 21 mg. This represented a fraction of the total amount of exposure, which was on the order of many grams of elemental mercury. Using data from serial measurement of urinary mercury excretion, the estimate of half-life in the workers was approximately 56 days. This suggests that the cumulative urinary mercury excretion over several days reflected an ongoing mercury body burden and persistence of exposure despite removal from the source.

The follow-up of these individuals after symptomatic improvement showed that the pulmonary function as well as chest x-rays returned to normal. The clinical picture of mercury intoxication in these workers involved the initial features of metal fume fever, followed by the development of severe symptoms involving the central nervous system, respiratory system, and gastrointestinal tract. The respiratory system and gastrointestinal tract symptoms improved soon after removal from exposure, but the neurological symptoms persisted. Neuropsychological assessment of these workers documented the persistent CNS effects of elemental mercury exposure (see Neuropsychological Diagnosis section).

Unwitting Intake of Methylmercury in Contaminated Pork

Hogs inadvertently fed seed grain which had been treated with methylmercury-containing fungicide were butchered and eaten by a family over a period of 3 months (Curley et al., 1971; Pierce et al., 1972). Several children in the family became ill with neurological symptoms, which included somnolence, ataxia, constricted visual fields, involuntary movements, slurred speech, seizures, and hyperactive reflexes (see Table 6-3). An infant born to a mother who consumed the pork showed signs of CNS disorder from birth. All family members with elevated mercury levels received chelation therapy.

Twenty-two years later, surviving family members were reexamined, and neuropsychological tests and MRIs were performed. Persistent abnormalities seen upon reexamination included slow word retrieval, diminished stereognosis and graphesthesia, poor hand coordination, cortical blindness, mild ataxia, dementia, and congenital nystagmus. Evidence on MRI showed thinning of cortices of the occipital (calcerine) and parietal lobes, along with atrophy of the cerebellum (Davis et al., 1994).

Individual Case Studies

Mercury Exposure While Working in a Thermometer Factory

A 48-year-old man was exposed to vapors from elemental mercury for 3.5 years in a thermometer factory. His job required that he vacuum mercury off the floors, disassemble machines containing mercury, and operate a crusher machine that separated the mercury from broken glass for reuse. An accidental laceration with glass brought him to the emergency room, where an occupational physician became involved in his case. It was learned that he had been having various symptoms during the past 2 to 3 years which included blurred vision, ocular pain, weakness, memory loss, and occasional rage and irrational behavior. Because of his work history and an elevated urine mercury level (690 μg/L), he was chelated with penicillamine (see Table 6-6). In addition, he was removed from his job and further exposure. His follow-up urine mercury was 17 μg/L. He was evaluated again 5 months later for continuing neurological problems, at which time the findings included nystagmus, tremor, diminished reflexes, and diminished sensation to pain. His tremor was documented by electromyographic reading (see Fig. 6-4). Nerve conduction studies showed mild peripheral neuropathy. An MRI performed at this time was determined to be consistent with diffuse and focal white matter disease. The white matter lesions that appeared did not resemble those seen in multiple sclerosis (see Table 6-5).

Neuropsychological testing of this patient revealed significant deficits in attention and executive function which were marked by perseverations on all tasks including digit span, alternating sequences, and on the Wisconsin Card Sort (White et al., 1993). Visuospatial and visuomotor function tests showed problems with visuospatial analysis, coding, sequencing, and visual organization. In addition, he had difficulty with facial matching and memory tests, particularly those Wechsler Memory Scale tasks involving visuospatial materials. The patient exhibited mild problems with verbal concept formation tasks, although free speech was normal. On the Profile of Mood States (POMS) the patient reported irritability, fatigue, and confusion. His family reported that he was angry, aggressive, suicidal, and socially withdrawn. The patient also reported experiencing hallucinations and paranoia. The neuropsychological tests of this patient suggest specific problems with cognitive flexibility, cognitive tracking, visuospatial analysis, memory for visuospatial information, affect, and personality (see Neurophysiological Diagnosis and Neuroimaging sections).

Acute and Chronic Exposure to Elemental Mercury Vapors

Acute exposure to high levels of mercury primarily involves the respiratory system, resulting in dyspnea, cough, and chest pain, while long-term exposure to low levels produces tremor, neuropathy and changes in personality. The following two clinical descriptions illustrate the relationships between mercury levels and the manifestations of acute and chronic vapor exposure.

Case 1. Exposure to Mercury Vapor from Smelting Dental Amalgam. Two men and two women (ages 40 to 88) were hospitalized after experiencing nausea, diarrhea, shortness of breath, and chest pain. Upon admission to the hospital, all four patients claimed they had been exposed to freon fumes during the cleaning of an old refrigerator. Five days later, Public Health officials investigating the incident discovered mercury at the home and informed the physician, who immediately began chelation therapy with dimercaprol. Within 11 to 24 days after their exposure to mercury vapor, all four patients had died of respiratory failure despite chelation therapy.

The mercury fumes had been released into the household when one of the residents, in an attempt to recover silver, had smelted dental amalgams in a small casting furnace in the basement of their home. The fumes released during the smelting process entered into the air ducts and were circulated to the other rooms of the house, affecting the other residents.

Mercury concentrations in urine from three of the individuals ranged from 94 to 423 μg/L; serum mercury concentrations from two of the patients were 12.7 and 16.1 μg/dL. Concentration of mercury in the organs measured postmortem was greatest in the liver (as high as 2,900 μg/g), while the least was found in the brain (approximately 100 μg/g). Indoor air concentration of mercury vapor in the household was measured 11 days after the exposure and was found to be 0.885 mg/m^3 (Rowens et al., 1991; Kanluen and Gottlieb, 1991; Taueg et al., 1992).

Case 2. Children Exposed to Spilled Mercury. A young girl who was admitted to the hospital because of unsteadiness

of gait (MMWR, 1991). She was originally diagnosed as having a postinfectious viral syndrome (Guillain–Barré syndrome) and was discharged only to be readmitted 2 weeks later when she could no longer walk. At that time, an older sister was admitted with similar symptoms. It was learned that approximately 20 cm^3 of liquid mercury had been spilled in a room in which they spent a lot of time. Examination of the house using a mercury vapor analyzer detected indoor air mercury concentrations of as much as 40 μg/m^3.

A diagnosis of mercury poisoning was made to explain the findings in the girls, which included numbness in the fingers and toes, absence of tendon reflexes, elevated blood pressure, and elevated protein in cerebrospinal fluid. Chelation therapy was instituted. The presenting patient continued to have neurologic abnormalities, including visual field defects, mild upper and lower extremity weakness, and emotional lability. The older sister improved and was discharged after rehabilitation therapy. A brother living in the house was apparently unaffected. The three degrees of severity of involvement in these children suggest differences in susceptibility, as well as the doses of exposure to mercury (Diamond et al., 1995).

REFERENCES

Abe T, Ohtsuka R, Hongo T, Suzuki T, Tohyama C. High hair and urinary mercury levels of fish eaters in the nonpolluted environment of Papua New Guinea. *Arch Environ Health* 1995;50:367–373.

Aberg B, Ekman L, Falk R, Greitz U, Persson G, Snicks JO. Metabolism of methylmercury, ^{203}Hg (compounds in man): excretion and distribution. *Arch Environ Health* 1969;19:478–484.

Adams CR, Ziegler DK, Lin JT. Mercury intoxication simulating amyotrophic lateral sclerosis. *JAMA* 1983;250:642–643.

Agency for Toxic Substances and Disease Registry (ATSDR). *Toxicological profile for mercury.* Atlanta: U.S. Department of Health and Human Services, Public Health Service Agency for Toxic Substances and Disease Registry, Publication No. ATSDR/TP-89:16, 1989.

Agency for Toxic Substances and Disease Registry (ATSDR). *Toxicological profile for mercury.* Atlanta: U.S. Department of Health and Human Services, Public Health Service Agency for Toxic Substances and Disease Registry, Publication No. ATSDR/TP-93:10, 1994.

Agocs MM, Etzel RA, Parrish G, Paschal DC, et al. Mercury exposure from interior latex paint. *N Engl J Med* 1990;323:1096–1101.

Airey D. Total mercury concentrations in human hair from 13 countries in relation to fish consumption and location. *Sci Total Environ* 1983;313: 157–180.

Albers JW, Kallenbach LR, Fine LJ, et al., and the Mercury Studies Group. Neurological abnormalities associated with remote occupational elemental mercury exposure. *Ann Neurol* 1988;24:651–659.

American Conference of Governmental Industrial Hygienists (ACGIH). *Threshold limit values for chemical substances and physical agents and biological exposure indices (BEIs).* Cincinnati: American Conference of Governmental Industrial Hygienists, Technical Affairs Office, 1995.

Amin-Zaki L, Elhassani LS, Majid MA, Clarkson TW, Doherty RA, Greenwood M. Intrauterine methylmercury poisoning in Iraq. *Pediatrics* 1974;54:587–595.

Amoore JE, Hautala E. Odor as an aid to chemical safety: odor threshold compared with threshold limit values and volatilities for 214 industrial chemicals in air and water dilution. *J Appl Toxicol* 1983;3:272–290.

Anderson A, Ellingsen DG, Morland T, Kjuus H. A neurological and neurophysiological study of chloralkali workers previously exposed to mercury vapour. *Acta Neurol Scand* 1993;88:427–433.

Anger WK. Work site behavioral research results, sensitive methods, test batteries, and the transition from laboratory data to human health. *Neurotoxicology* 1990;11:629–719.

Angle CR, McIntire MS. Red cell lead, whole blood lead, and red cell enzymes. *Environ Health Perspect* 1974;7:133–137.

Aposhian HV, Bruce DC, Alter W, Dart RC, Hurlbut KM, Aposhian MM. Urinary mercury after administration of DMPS: Correlation with dental amalgam. *FASEB J* 1992;6:2472–2476.

Aschner M, Aschner JL. Mercury neurotoxicity: mechanisms of blood–brain barrier transport. *Neurosci Biobehav Rev* 1990;14:169–176.

Atchison WD, Hare MF. Mechanisms of methylmercury induced neurotoxicity. *FASEB J* 1994;8:622–629.

Bakir F, Damluji SF, Amin-Zaki L, et al. Methylmercury poisoning in Iraq. *Science* 1973;181:230–241.

Barber TE. Inorganic mercury intoxication reminiscent of amyotrophic lateral sclerosis. *J Occup Med* 1978;20(10):667–669.

Barregård L, Sallsten G, Schutz A, et al. Kinetics of mercury in blood and urine after brief occupational exposure. *Arch Environ Health* 1992;47: 176–184.

Barregård L, Sällsten G, Järvholm B. People with high mercury uptake from their own dental amalgam fillings. *Occup Environ Med* 1995;52: 124–128.

Barregård L, Ellingsen D, Alexander J, et al. Mercury exposure from dental amalgam. Risk assessment and clinical evaluation. *Tidsskrift for Den Norske Laegeforening* 1998;118:58–62.

Berglund A. Estimation by 24 hour study of the daily dose of intra-oral mercury vapor inhaled from dental amalgam. *J Dent Res* 1990;69: 1646–1651.

Berlin M, Jerskell LG, von Ubisch H. Uptake and retention of mercury in the mouse brain—a comparison of exposure to mercury vapor and intravenous injection of mercuric salt. *Arch Environ Hlth* 1966;12:33–42.

Bjorkman L, Mottet K, Nylander M, Vahter M, Lind B, Friberg L. Selenium concentrations in brain after exposure to methylmercury: relations between the inorganic mercury fraction and selenium. *Arch Toxicol* 1995;69:228–234.

Blackstone S, Hurley RJ, Hughes RE. Some inter-relationships between vitamin C (L ascorbic acid) and mercury in the guinea pig. *Food Cosmet Toxicol* 1974;12:511–516.

Bloch P, Shapiro IM. Summary of the international conference on mercury hazards in dental practice. *JADA* 1982;104:489–490.

Bluhm RE, Bobbitt RG, Welch LW, et al. Elemental mercury vapour toxicity, treatment and prognosis after acute intensive exposure in chloralkali workers. Part I. History, neuropsychological findings and chelator effects. *Hum Exp Toxicol* 1992;11:201–210.

Boogaard PJ, Houtsma A-T AJ, Journee HL, van Sittert NJ. Effects of exposure to elemental mercury on the nervous system and the kidneys of workers producing natural gas. *Arch Environ Health* 1996;51:108–115.

Brown LA. Chronic mercurialism, a case of the clinical syndrome of amyotrophic lateral sclerosis. *Arch Neurol Psychiatry* 1954;72:261–283.

Brune D, Evje DM. Man's mercury loading from a dental amalgam. *Sci Total Environ* 1985;44:51–63.

Campbell D, Gonzales M, Sullivan JB Jr. Mercury. In: Sullivan JB Jr, Krieger GR, eds. *Hazardous materials toxicology: clinical principles of environmental health.* Baltimore: Williams & Wilkins, 1992: 824–834.

Carty AJ, Malone SF. The chemistry of mercury in biological system. In: Nrigau JO, ed. *Biochemistry of mercury in the environment.* Amsterdam: Elsevier/North Holland Bio-Medical Press, 1979: 433–479.

Cassano GB, Viola PL, Ghetti B. The distribution of inhaled mercury (Hg203) vapors in the brain of rats and mice. *J Neuropathol Exp Neurol* 1969;28:308–320.

Cavanagh JB. Lesion localisation: implications for the study of functional effects and mechanisms of action. *Toxicology* 1988;49:131–136.

Chang LW. Neurotoxic effects of mercury—a review. *Environ Res* 1977; 14:329–373.

Chang LW, Hartman HA. Ultrastructural studies of the nervous system after mercury intoxication: pathological changes in the nerve fibers. *Acta Neuropathol (Berl)* 1972a;20:316–334.

Chang LW, Hartman HA. Blood–brain barrier dysfunction in experimental mercury intoxication. *Acta Neuropath (Berl)* 1972b;21:179–184.

Chang LW, Gilbert M, Sprecher J. Modification of methylmercury neurotoxicity by vitamin E. *Environ Res* 1978;17:356–366.

Cherian MG, Hursh JG, Clarkson TW, et al. Radioactive mercury distribution in biological fluids and excretion in human subjects after inhalation of mercury vapor. *Arch Environ Health* 1978;33:190–214.

Choi BH, Lapham LW, Amin-Zaki L, Saleem G. Abnormal neuronal migration, deranged cerebral cortical organizations, and diffuse white matter after cytosis astrocytosis of human fetal brain: a major effect of methylmercury poisoning *in utero. J Neuropathol Exp Neurol* 1978;37:

719–733.

Clarkson TW. Epidemiological and experimental aspects of lead and mercury contamination. *Food Cosmet Toxicol* 1971;9:229–243.

Clarkson TW. Mercury: major issues in environmental health. *Environ Health Prospect* 1992;100:31–38.

Clausen J. Mercury and multiple sclerosis. *Acta Neurol Scand* 1993;87: 461–464.

Counter SA, Buchanan LH, Laurell G, Ortega F. Blood mercury auditory neuro-sensory responses in children and adults in Nambiji gold mining area of Equador. *Neurotoxicol* 1998;19:185–196.

Curley A, Sedlak VA, Girling EF, et al. Organic mercury identified as the cause of poisoning in humans and hogs. *Science* 1971;172:65–67.

Daniel JW, Gage JC, Lefevre PA. The metabolism of methoxymethylmercury salts. *Biochem J* 1971;121:411–415.

Daniel JW, Gage JC, Lefevre PA. The metabolism of phenylmercury by the rat. *Biochem J* 1972;129:961–967.

Davis LE, Kornfeld M, Mooney SH, Fiedler KJ, Haaland KY, Orrison WW, Cernischiari E, Clarkson TW. Methylmercury poisoning: long-term clinical, radiological, toxicological, and pathological studies of an affected family. *Ann Neurol* 1994;35:680–688.

de Freitas JF. Mercury in the dental work-place: an assessment of the health hazard and safeguards. *Aust Dental J* 1981;26:156–161.

Diamond R, White RF, Gerr F, Feldman RG. A case of developmental exposure to inorganic mercury. *Child Neuropsychol* 1995;1:1–11.

Dutczak WJ, Clarkson TW, Ballatori N. Biliary–hepatic recycling of a xenobiotic gallbladder absorption of methylmercury. *Am J Physiol* 1991;260:G873–G880.

Ehrenberg RL, Vogt RL, Smith AB, et al. The effects of elemental mercury exposure at a thermometer plant. *Am J Ind Med* 1991;19:495–507.

Ellingsen DG, Morlind T, Andersen A, Kujuus H. Relation between exposure related indices and neurological and neurophysiological effects in workers previously exposed to mercury vapour. *Br J Ind Med* 1993; 50:736–744.

Environmental Protection Agency (EPA). Ambient water quality criteria for mercury. Washington, DC: US Environmental Protection Agency, Office of Water Regulations and Standards. Document no. EPA 440/5-80-058, 1980.

Environmental Protection Agency (EPA). Drinking water regulations and health advisories. In: *EPA 822-R-96-001.* Washington, DC: Office of Water, 1996.

Eto K, Oyanhei S, Itai Y, Tokunaga H, Takizawa Y, Suda I. A fetal type of Minamata disease. An autopsy case report with special reference to the nervous system. *Mol Chem Neuropathol* 1992;16:171–186.

Evans HL, Garman RH, Weiss B. Methylmercury: Exposure duration and regional distribution as determined from neurotoxicity in non-human primates. *Toxicol Appl Pharmacol* 1977;41:15–33.

Eyssen GEM, Ruedy J, Hogg S, Guernsey JR, Woods I. Validity and reproducibility of the screening examination for neurological abnormality in persons exposed to methylmercury. *J Clin Epidemiol* 1990;43:489–498.

Fagala GE, Wigg CL. Psychiatric manifestations of mercury poisoning. *J Am Acad Child Adolesc Psychiatry* 1992;31:306–311.

FDA. Quality standards for food with no identity standards: Bottled water. In: *Code of Federal Regulations. 21 CFR 103.35.* Washington, DC: Food and Drug Administration, 1989.

Foulds D, Copeland K, Franks R. Mercury poisoning and acrodynia. *Am J Dis Children* 1987;141:124–125.

Fowler BA. Critical review of selected heavy metal and chlorinated hydrocarbon concentrations in marine environment. *Mar Environ Res* 1990;29:1–64.

Friberg L, Mottet NK. Accumulation of methylmercury and inorganic mercury in brain. *Biol Trace Elem Res* 1989;21:201–206.

Friberg L, Nordberg GF. Inorganic mercury–relation between exposure and effects. In: Friberg L, Vostal J, eds. *Mercury in the environment.* Cleveland: CRC Press, 1972:113–139.

Fuortes LJ, Weismann DN, Graeff ML, Bale JF, Tannous R, Peters C. Immune thrombocytopenia and elemental mercury poisoning. *Clin Toxicol* 1995;33(5):449–455.

Gabbiani G, Baic D, Deziel C. Studies on tolerance and ionic antagonism for cadmium or mercury. *Can J Physiol Pharmacol* 1967;45:443–450.

Gage JC, Swan AAB. The toxicity of alkyl and aryl mercury salts. *Biochem Pharmacol* 1961;8:77.

Ganser AL, Kirschner DA. The interaction of mercurials with myelin: comparison of *in vitro* and *in vivo* effects. *Neurotoxicology* 1985;6: 63–78.

Ganther HE. Modification of methylmercury toxicity and metabolism by selenium and vitamin E: Possible mechanisms. *Environ Health Persp* 1978;25:71–76.

Ganther HE. Interactions of vitamin E and selenium with mercury and silver. *Ann NY Acad Sci* 1980;355:212–225.

Garnier R, Fuster JM, Conso F, Duatzenberg B, Sors C, Fournier E. Acute mercury vapor poisoning. *Toxicol Environ Res* 1981;3:77–86.

Gay DD, Cox RO, Reinhardt JW. Chewing releases mercury from fillings. *Lancet* 1979;1(8123):985–986.

Gilioli R, Bulgheroni C, Caimi L, Foa V. Correlations between subjective complaints and objective neurophysiological findings in workers of a chlor-alkali plant. In: Horvath M, ed. *Adverse effects of environmental chemicals and psychotropic drugs,* vol 2. Amsterdam: Elsevier, 1976: 157–164.

Gilmore CC, Henry EA. Mercury methylation in aquatic systems affected by acid deposition. *Environ Pollut* 1991;71(2–4):131–169.

Goldsmih RH, Soares JH Jr. Barbiturate potentiation in mercury poisoning. *Bull Environ Contam Toxicol* 1975;13:737–740.

Gotelli CA, Astolfi E, Cox C, et al. Early biochemical effects of an organic mercury fungicide on infants: "Dose makes the poison." *Science* 1985;277:638–640.

Goyer RA. Toxic and essential metal interactions. *Ann Rev Nutri* 1997; 17:37–50.

Grandjean P, Weihe P, White RF. Milestone development in infants exposed to methylmercury from human milk. *Neurotoxicology* 1995;16: 27–34.

Grandjean P, Weihe P, White RF, et al. Cognitive deficit in 7-year-old children with prenatal exposure to methylmercury. *Neurotoxicol Teratol* 1997;19:417–428.

Grant WM, Schuman JS. *Toxicology of the eye: effects on the eyes and visual system from chemicals, drugs, metals, minerals, plants, toxins and venoms; also systemic side effects from eye medications,* 4th ed. Springfield, IL: Charles C Thomas, 1993:318–323.

Gutknecht J. Inorganic mercury (Hg^{2+}) transport through lipid bilayer membranes. *J Membr Biol* 1981;61:61–66.

Haddad J, Sternberg E. Bronchitis due to acute mercury inhalation: report of two cases. *Am Rev Respir Dis* 1963;88:543–545.

Hallee TJ. Diffuse lung disease caused by inhalation of mercury vapor. *Am Rev Respir Dis* 1969;99:430–436.

Harada Y. Study group on Minamata disease. In: *Minamata disease.* Katsuma M, ed. Kumamoto, Japan: Kumamoto University, 1966:93–117.

Henderson R, Shotwell HP, Krause LA. Analyses for total, ionic and elemental mercury in urine as a basis for biological standard. *Am Ind Hyg Assoc J* 1974;38:576–580.

Hirayama K. Effects of amino acids on brain uptake of methylmercury. *Toxicol Appl Pharmacol* 1980;55:318–323.

Hunter D, Russell DS. Focal, cerebral and cerebellar atrophy in a human subject due to organic mercury compounds. *J Neurol Neurosurg Psychiatr* 1954;17:235–241.

Hursh JB, Clarkson TW, Cherian MG, Vostal JJ, Vander-Mallie R. Clearance of mercury (Hg-197, Hg-203) vapor inhaled by human subjects. *Arch Environ Health* 1976;31:302–309.

Hursh JB, Greenwood MR, Clarkson TW, Allen J, Demuth S. The effect of ethanol on the fate of mercury vapor inhaled by man. *J Pharmacol Exp Ther* 1980;214(3):520–527.

Hursh JB, Clarkson TW, Miles EF, Goldsmith LA. Percutaneous absorption of mercury vapor by man. *Arch Environ Health* 1989;44:120–127.

Igata A. Epidemiological and clinical features of Minamata disease. In: Suzuki T, Imura N, Clarkson TW, eds. *Advances in mercury toxicology.* New York: Plenum Press, 1991:439–458.

Iyer K, Goodgold J, Eberstein A, Berg P. Mercury poisoning in a dentist. *Arch Neurol* 1976;33:788–790.

Jaeger A, Tempe JD, Haegy JM, Leroy M, Porte A, Mantz JM. Accidental acute mercury vapor poisoning. *Vet Hum Toxicol* 1979;21(Suppl): 62–63.

Jaffe KM, Shurtleff DB, Robertson WO. Survival after acute mercury vapor poisoning: role of intensive supportive care. *Am J Dis Child* 1983; 137:749–751.

Kajiwara Y, Yasutake A, Adachi T, Hirayama K. Methylmercury transport across the placenta via neural amino acid carrier. *Arch Toxicol* 1996; 70:310–314.

Kanluen S, Gottlieb CA. A clinical pathological study of four adult cases of acute mercury inhalation toxicity. *Arch Pathol Lab Med* 1991;115: 56–60.

Kark RAP. Clinical and neurochemical aspects of inorganic mercury intoxication. In: de Wolff FA, ed. *Handbook of clinical neurology,* vol 20 (64): *Intoxications of the nervous system,* part 1. Amsterdam: Elsevier, 1994:367–411.

Kasarskis EJ, Ehlmann WD, Markesbery WR. Trace metals in human neurodegenerative diseases. *Prog Clin Biol Res* 1993;380:229–310.

Kern F, Roberts N, Ostlere L, Langtry J, Staughton RCD. Ammoniated mercury ointment as a cause of peripheral neuropathy. *Dermatologica* 1993;183:280–282.

Kerper LE, Ballatori N, Clarkson TW. Methylmercury transport across the blood brain barrier by an amino acid carrier. *Am J Physiol* 1992;262:R761–R765.

Kershaw TG, Clarkson TW, Dhahir PH. The relationship between blood levels and dose of methylmercury in man. *Arch Environ Health* 1980;35:28–36.

Key MM, Henschel AF, Butler J, Ligo RN, Tabershaw IR. *Occupational disease: a guide to their recognition.* US Department of Health, Education and Welfare, Centers for Disease Control, National Institute of Occupational Safety and Health, Washington, DC: US Government Printing Office, 1977:370–372.

Khare SS, Ehmann WD, Kasarskis EJ, Markesbery WR. Trace element imbalances in amyotrophic lateral sclerosis. *Neurotoxicology* 1990;11: 521–532.

Kishi R, Doi R, Fukuchi Y, et al., and the Mercury Workers Study Group. Subjective symptoms and neurobehavioral performances of ex-mercury miners at an average of eighteen years after the cessation of chronic exposure to mercury vapor. *Environ Res* 1993;62:289–302.

Kishi R, Doi R, Fukuchi Y, et al. Residual neurobehavioural effects associated with chronic exposure to mercury vapor. *Occup Environ Med* 1994;51:35–41.

Korogi Y, Takahashi M, Shinzato J, Okajima T. MR findings in seven patients with organic mercury poisoning (Minamata disease). *AJNR* 1994;15:1575–1578.

Kosta L, Byrne AR, Zelenko V. Correlation between selenium and mercury in man following exposure to inorganic mercury. *Nature* 1975; 254:238–239.

Kostyniak PJ, Greizerstein HB, Goldstein J, et al. Extracorporeal regional complexing of haemodialysis treatment of acute mercury intoxication. *Hum Toxicol* 1990;9:137–141.

Kurland LT, Faro SN, Seidler H. Minamata disease. *World Neurol* 1960; 1:370–391.

Kurttio P, Pekkanen J, Alfthan G, et al. Increased mercury exposure in inhabitants living in the vicinity of a hazardous waste incinerator: a 10-year follow-up. *Arch Environ Health* 1998;53:129–137.

Lackowicz JR, Anderson CJ. Permeability of lipid bilayers to methylmercuric chloride: quantification by fluorescence quenching of a carbazole labeled phospholipid. *Chem–Biol Interact* 1980;30: 309–323.

Lamm O, Pratt H. Subclinical effects of exposure to inorganic mercury revealed by somatosensory-evoked potentials. *Eur Neurol* 1985;24: 237–243.

Langolf GD, Chaffin DB, Henderson R, Whittle HP. Evaluation of workers exposed to elemental mercury using quantitative tests of tremor and neuromuscular functions. *Am Ind Hyg Assoc J* 1978;39:976–984.

Langworth S, Almkvist O, Söderman E, Wikström BO. Effects of occupational exposure to mercury vapor on the central nervous system. *Br J Ind Med* 1992;49:545–555.

Levine SP, Cavender GD, Langolf GD, Albers JW. Elemental mercury exposure: Peripheral neurotoxicity. *Br J Ind Med* 1982;39:136–139.

Lilis R, Miller A, Lerman Y. Acute mercury poisoning with severe chronic pulmonary manifestations. *Chest* 1985;88:306–309.

Lorscheider FL, Vimy MJ. Mercury from dental amalgam [Letter, Comment]. *Lancet* 1990;336(8730):1578–1579.

Magos L. Factors affecting the neurotoxicity of mercury and mercurials. In: Manzo L, Lery N, Lacasse Y, Roche L, eds. *Advances in neurotoxicology,* Proceedings of the International Congress on Neurotoxicology, Varese, Italy, 27–30 September, 1979. NY: Pergamon, 1980:17–25.

Magos L, Clarkson TW, Greenwood MR. The depression of pulmonary retention of mercury vapor by ethanol: identification of the site of action. *Toxicol Appl Pharmacol* 1973;26:180–183.

Magos L, Brown AW, Sparrow S, Bailey E, Snowden RT, Skipp WR. The comparative toxicology of ethyl and methylmercury. *Arch Toxicol* 1985;57:260–267.

Markowitz L, Schaumburg HH. Successful treatment of inorganic mercury neurotoxicity with *n*-acetyl-penicillamine despite an adverse reaction. *Neurology* 1980;30:1000–1001.

Marsh DO. Organic mercury: clinical and neurotoxicological aspects. In: de Wolff FA, ed. *Handbook of clinical neurology*, vol 20 (64): *Intoxications of the nervous system*, Part I. Amsterdam: Elsevier, 1994:413–429.

Marsh DO, Myers GJ, Clarkson TW, Amin-Zaki L, Al-Tikriti S, Majeed MA. Fetal methylmercury: clinical and toxicological data in 29 cases. *Ann Neurol* 1980;7:348–355.

Matthes FT, Kirschner R, Yow MD, Brennan JC. Acute poisoning associated with inhalation of mercury vapor: report of four cases. *Pediatrics* 1958;22:675–688.

Matsumoto SC, Okajima T, Inayoshi S, Ueno H. Minamata disease demonstrated by computed tomography. *Neuroradiology* 1988;30:42–46.

McFarland R, Reigel H. Chronic mercury poisoning from a single brief exposure. *J Occup Med* 1978;20:534.

McLauchlan GA. Acute mercury poisoning. *Anesthesiology* 1991;46:110–112.

Miller JM, Chaffin DB, Smith RG. Subclinical psychomotor and neuromuscular changes in workers exposed to inorganic mercury. *Am Ind Hyg Assoc J* 1975;36:725–733.

Møller-Madsen B, Danscher G. Localization of mercury in CNS of the rat. IV. The effect of selenium on orally administered organic and inorganic mercury. *Toxicol Appl Pharmacol* 1991;108:453–473.

Morbidity and Mortality Weekly Report (MMWR) 1991;40:393–395.

Naganuma A, Imura N. Methylmercury binds to a low molecular weight substance in rabbit and human erythrocytes. *Toxicol Appl Pharmacol* 1979;47:613–616.

Nakamura I, Hosokawa K, Tamra H, et al. Reduced mercury excretion with feces in germfree mice after oral administration of methylmercury chloride. *Bull Environ Contam Toxicol* 1977;17:528–533.

Nath KA, Croatt AJ, Likely S, Behrens TW, Warden D. Renal oxidant injury and oxidant response induced by mercury. *Kidney Int* 1996;50:1032–1043.

National Institute for Occupational Safety and Health (NIOSH). *Pocket guide to chemical hazards*. Washington, DC: US Department of Health and Human Services, Centers for Disease Control and Prevention, 1997.

National Research Council (NRC). *Environmental epidemiology*, vol 1: *Public health and hazardous wastes*. Washington, DC: National Academic Press, 1991:205.

Neilsen Kudsk F. The influence of ethyl alcohol on the absorption of methylmercury vapor from the lungs of man. *Acta Pharmacol Toxicol* 1965;23:263–274.

Neilsen Kudsk F. Uptake of mercury vapor in blood *in vivo* and *vitro* from Hg-containing air. *Acta Pharmacol* 1969a;27:149–160.

Neilsen Kudsk F. Factors influencing the *in vitro* uptake of mercury vapor in blood. *Acta Pharmacol* 1969b;27:161–172.

Nielsen JB. Toxicokinetics of mercuric chloride and methylmercuric chloride in mice. *J Toxicol Environ Health* 1992;37:85–122.

Nordberg GF, ed. *Effects and dose response of toxic metals*. New York: Elsevier/North Holland, 1976:24–32.

Norseth T, Clarkson TW. Studies on the biotransformation of Hg-203-labeled methylmercury chloride. *Arch Environ Health* 1970;21:717–727.

Occupational Safety and Health Administration (OSHA). *Code of Federal Regulations (29 CFR 1910.1000)*, Washington, DC: Occupational Safety and Health Administration, 1995.

Ozaki S, Ichimura T, Isobe T, Nagashima K, Sugano H, Omata S. Identification and partial characterization of a glycoprotein species with high affinity for methylmercury in peripheral nervous tissues of man and experimental animals. *Arch Toxicol* 1993;67:268–276.

Pelletier L, Castedo M, Bellon B, Druet P. Mercury and autoimmunity. In: Dean JH, Luster MI, Munson AE, Kimber I, eds. *Toxicology and immunopharmacology*. New York: Raven Press, 1994:539–552.

Pierce PE, Thompson JF, Likosky WH. Alkyl mercury poisoning in humans. Report of an outbreak. *JAMA* 1972;220:1439–1442.

Piikivi L, Tolonen U. EEG findings in chlor-alkali workers subjected to low long term exposure to mercury vapour. *Br J Ind Med* 1989;46:370–375.

Pleva J. Dental mercury: a public health hazard. *Rev Environ Health* 1994;10:1–27.

Potter S, Matrone G. Effect of selenite on the toxicity of dietary methylmercury and mercuric chloride in the rat. *J Nutr* 1974;104:638–647.

Rabinstein D, Fairhurst MT. Nuclear magnetic resonance studies of the solution chemistry of metal complexes. *J Am Chem Soc* 1975;97:2086–2092.

Rahola T, Hattula T, Korolainen A, et al. Elimination of free and protein-bound ionic mercury 203Hg^{2+} in man. *Ann Clin Res* 1973;5:214–219.

Rönnbäck L, Hansson E. Chronic encephalopathies induced by mercury or lead: aspects of underlying cellular and molecular mechanisms. *Br J Ind Med* 1992;49:233–240.

Ross AT. Mercuric polyneuropathy with albumino-cytologic dissociation and eosinophilia. *JAMA* 1964;188:830–831.

Rothstein A, Hayes AL. The turnover of mercury in rats exposed repeatedly to inhalation of vapor. *Health Phys* 1964;10:1099–1113.

Rowens B, Guerrero-Betancourt D, Gottlieb CA, Boyes RJ, Eichenhorn MS. Respiration failure following acute inhalation of mercury vapor: a clinical and histologic perspective. *Chest* 1991;99:185–199.

Rowland I, Davies M, Evans J. Tissue content of mercury in rats given methylmercury chloride orally: influence of intestinal flora. *Arch Environ Health* 1980;35:155–160.

Rustam H, Hamdi T. Methylmercury poisoning in Iraq. *Brain* 1974;97:499–510.

Sakai K, Okabe M, Eto K, Takeuchi T. Histochemical demonstration of mercury in human tissue of Minamata disease by use of autoradiographic procedure. *Acta Histochem Cytochem* 1975;8:257–264.

Sälsten G, Barregård L, Wikkelsö C, Schütz A. Mercury and proteins in cerebrospinal fluid in subjects exposed to mercury vapor. *Exp Res* 1994;65:195–206.

Sauder P, Livardjant H, Jaeger A, et al. Acute mercury chloride intoxication. Effects of hemodialysis and plasma exchange on mercury kinetics. *Clin Toxicol* 1988;26:189–197.

Sax NI. *Dangerous properties of industrial chemicals*, 5th ed. New York: Van Nostrand Reinhold Co., 1979.

Schionning JD, Eide R, Ernst E, et al. The effect of selenium on the localization of autometallographic mercury in dorsal root ganglia of rats. *Histochem J* 1997;29:183–191.

Schwartz JG, Snider TE, Montiel MM. Toxicity of a family from vacuumed mercury. *Am J Emerg Med* 1992;10:258–261.

Shapiro IM, Cornblath DR, Sumner AJ, et al. Neurophysiologic and neuropsychologic function of mercury exposed dentists. *Lancet* 1982;1(8282):1147–1150.

Siblerud R, Kienholz E. Evidence that mercury from silver dental fillings may be an etiological factor in multiple sclerosis. *Sci Total Environ* 1994;142:191–205.

Singer R, Valciukas JA, Rosenman KD. Peripheral nerve toxicity in workers exposed to inorganic mercury compounds. *Arch Environ Health* 1987;42:181–184.

Skare I, Engvist AL. Human exposure to mercury and silver released from dental amalgam restorations. *Arch Environ Health* 1994;49:384–394.

Skerfving S. Interaction between selenium and methylmercury. *Environ Health Persp* 1978;25:57–65.

Smith RG, Vorwald AJ, Patil LS, Money TF. Effects of exposure to mercury in the manufacture of chlorine. *Am Ind Hyg Assoc J* 1970;31:687–700.

Smith PJ, Langolf GD, Goldberg J. Effects of occupational exposure to elemental mercury on short term memory. *Br J Ind Med* 1983;40:413–419.

Snodgrass W, Sullivan JB, Rumack BH, Hashimoto C. Mercury poisoning from home gold ore processing: use of penicillamine and dimercaptrol. *JAMA* 1981;246:1929–1931.

Stopford W, Bundy SD, Goldwater LJ, et al. Microenvironmental exposure to mercury vapor. *Am Ind Hyg Assoc J* 1978;39:378–384.

Sundberg J, Oskarsson A. Placental and lactational transfer of mercury from rats exposed to methylmercury in their diet: speciation of mercury in the offspring. *J Trace Elem Exp Med* 1992;5:47–56.

Suzuki T, Hongo T, Yoshinaga J, et al. An acute mercuric mercury poisoning: chemical speciation of hair mercury shows a peak of inorganic mercury value. *Hum Exp Toxicol* 1992;11:53–57.

Swaiman KF, Flagler DG. Mercury poisoning with central and peripheral nervous system involvement treated with penicillamine. *Pediatrics* 1971;48:639–642.

Takeuchi T. Biological reactions and pathological changes in human beings and animals caused by organic mercury contamination. In: Hartung R, Dinman BD, eds. *Environmental mercury contamination*. Ann Arbor, MI: Ann Arbor Science, 1972:247–289.

Takeuchi T, Eto K, Tokunaga H. Mercury level and histochemical distribution in a human brain with Minamata disease following a long-term clinical course of twenty-six years. *Neurotoxicology* 1989;10:651–658.

Tamashiro H, Arakaki M, Akagi H. Mortality and survival for Minamata disease. *Int J Epidemiol* 1985;14:582–588.

Taueg C, Sanfilippo DJ, Rowens B, Szejeda J, Hesse JL. Acute and chronic poisoning from residential exposure to elemental mercury. *J Toxicol Clin Toxicol* 1992;30:63–67.

Teisinger J, Fiserova-Bergerova V. Pulmonary retention and excretion of mercury vapors in man. *Ind Med Surg* 1965;34:580.

Tennant R, Johnston H, Wells J. Acute bilateral pneumonitis associated with the inhalation of mercury vapor: a report of five cases. *Conn Med* 1961;25:106–109.

Thomas DJ, Smith CJ. Effects of coadministered low molecular weight thiol compounds on short term distribution of methylmercury in the rat. *Toxicol Appl Pharmacol* 1982;62:104–110.

Tokuomi H, Uchino M, Imamura S, et al. Minamata disease (organic mercury poisoning): neuroradiologic and electrophysiologic studies. *Neurology* 1982;32:1369–1375.

Torres-Alanis O, Garza-Ocanas L, Pineyro-Lopez A. Evaluation of urinary mercury excretion after administration of 2,3-dimercapto-1-propane sulfonic acid to occupationally exposed men. *Clin Toxicol* 1995; 33: 717–720.

Trepka MJ, Heinrich J, Krause C, et al. Factors affecting internal mercury burdens among eastern German children. *Arch Environ Health* 1997; 52(2):134–138.

Triebig G, Schaller K-H. Neurotoxic effects in mercury-exposed workers. *Neurobehav Toxicol Teratol* 1982;4:717–720.

Tsuchiya K. The discovery of the causal agent of Minamata disease. *Am J Ind Med* 1992;21:275–289.

Valk J, van der Knapp MS. Mercury intoxication. In: *Myelination and myelin disorders.* Berlin: Springer-Verlag, 1989:270–271.

Vallee BL, Ulmer DD. Biochemical effects of mercury, cadmium, and lead [Review]. *Annu Rev Biochem* 1972;41:91–128.

Vimy MJ, Lorscheider FL. Dental amalgam mercury daily dose estimated from intra-oral vapor measurements: a predictor of mercury accumulation in human tissues. *J Trace Elem Exp Med* 1990;3:111–123.

Vroom FQ, Greer M. Mercury vapor intoxication. *Brain* 1972;95:305–318.

Walsh FB, Hoyt WF. *Clinical neuro-ophthalmology,* 3rd ed. Baltimore: Williams & Wilkins, 1969.

Warkany J, Hubbard DM. Acrodynia and mercury. *J Pediatric* 1953;42: 365–386.

Wheatley B, Barbeau A, Clarkson TW, Lamphon LW. Methylmercury poisoning in Canadian Indians: the elusive diagnosis. *Can J Neurol Sci* 1979;6:417–422.

White RF, Feldman RG, Moss NB, Proctor SP. Magnetic resonance imaging (MRI), neurobehavioral testing, and toxic encephalopathy: two cases. *Environ Res* 1993;61:117–123.

Williamson AM, Teo RK, Sanderson J. Occupational mercury exposure and its consequences for behavior. *Int Arch Occup Environ Health* 1982;50:273–286.

Winek CL, Fochtman FW, Bricker JD, Wecht CH. Fatal mercuric chloride ingestion. *Clin Toxicol* 1981;18:261–266.

World Health Organization (WHO). Inorganic mercury. *Environmental health criteria,* 118. Geneva: WHO, 1991.

Wright N, Yoemen WB, Carter CE. Massive oral ingestion of elemental mercury without poisoning. *Lancet* 1981;1:206.

Yamaguchi S, Matsumoto H, Kaku S, Tateishi M, Shiramizu M. Factors affecting the amount of mercury in human scalp hair. *Am J Public Health* 1975;65:485–488.

Yasutake A, Hirayama K, Inoue M. Mechanism of urinary excretion of methylmercury in mice. *Arch Toxicol* 1989;63:479–483.

Yoshida M, Satoh H, Kojima T. Exposure to mercury via breast milk in suckling offspring of maternal guinea pigs exposed to mercury vapor parturition. *J Toxicol Environ Health* 1992;35:135–139.

Zampollo A, Baruffini A, Cirla AM, Pisati G, Zedda S. Subclinical inorganic mercury neuropathy: neurophysiological investigations in 17 occupationally exposed subjects. *Ital J Neurol Sci* 1987;8:249–254.

Zavariz C, Glina DMR. Neuropsychological clinical assessment of workers in an electric lamp factory exposed to metallic mercury. *Rev Saude Publica* 1992;26:356–365.

Zelman M, Campfield P, Moss M, Camfield C, Sweet L. Toxicity from vacuumed mercury: a household hazard. *Clin Pediatr* 1991;30:121–123.

CHAPTER 7

Thallium

Thallium (TI) is found in rock formations containing feldspar and mica, as well as in combination with lead and zinc ores (Kazantzis, 1986). It is a highly reactive heavy metal that exists in monovalent and trivalent ionic forms (Douglas et al., 1990). Elemental thallium forms compounds with acetate, oxide, carbonate, chloride, selenide, selenite, nitrate, and, most commonly, sulfate. It was originally discovered as a residue in flue dust from the burning of pyrite ore in the manufacture of sulfuric acid (Crookes, 1861), but it also occurs as a by-product of cadmium production (Aoyama et al., 1986). Thallium salt is colorless, odorless, and almost tasteless. The more water-soluble salts (thallium sulfate, thallium acetate, and thallium carbonate) have greater toxicity than the poorly soluble sulfide and iodide salts (Saddique and Peterson, 1983).

Thallium has many uses, which include: medicinal therapy for tuberculosis, syphilis, gonorrhea, and dysentery (Gettler and Weiss, 1943; Grunfeld and Henostroza, 1964; Smith and Doherty, 1964; Bank et al., 1972); use as a pesticide; use as a treatment for fungal infections; and use as a cosmetic depilatory (Heyl and Barlow, 1989). It is found in various manufacturing processes (Moeschlin, 1980) and is available throughout the world (Kazantzis, 1986; Moore et al., 1993). Factory workers chronically exposed to various salt derivatives of thallium generally develop less severe symptoms than those seen in the numerous incidents of accidental, homicidal, and suicidal intoxication (Munch, 1934; Grulee and Clark, 1951), which have led to restrictions on the sale of thallium-containing rodenticides and insecticides in the United States and other countries (USDA, 1965; Saddique and Peterson, 1983; Shabaline and Spiridonova, 1979; Moeschlin, 1980; Malbrain et al., 1997). Despite its limited availability and precautionary measures concerning its use, thallium poisonings continue to occur (Insley et al., 1986; Kravzov et al., 1993; Meggs et al., 1994) and the incidence may be underestimated due to missed or unconfirmed diagnoses (Saddique and Peterson, 1983).

The clinical differential diagnosis for otherwise unexplained neuropathies must exclude thallium as a possible cause. It is important to be familiar with the clinical and neurophysiological expression of thallium neurotoxicity, which include: axonal; axonal with secondary demyelination; multifocal conduction blocks; and primarily sensory or mixed sensorimotor impairments.

SOURCES OF EXPOSURE

Thallium is mined in the United States and in Brazil and may also be present in areas where the dust or fumes of lead, cadmium, and zinc accumulate in and around smelting plants (Kazantzis, 1986). Thallium has been detected in the environments of industries which use thallium in other processes (such as cement plants) (Dolgner et al., 1983); it has also been detected in the manufacture of tungsten filaments, jewelry, and optical glass of high refraction, in dyes and pigments, in fireworks, and in superconductor elements (Sleight, 1988). Employees may be unaware of the use of thallium rodenticides in their workplace such as slaughterhouses and food preparation plants; and incidental intake may cause illnesses, the etiology of which may be elusive unless the clinician has a high level of suspicion (Herrero et al., 1995).

The most common source of thallium poisoning is rodenticides and insecticides. Accidental ingestion by children who may mistake the thallium-treated rodenticide "wafers" for candy (Chamberlain et al., 1958; Grulee and Clark, 1951), along with the unsuspected intake of contaminated food and water by families, account for many reports of thallium poisoning (Munch et al., 1933; Munch, 1934; Moeschlin, 1980; Dolgner et al., 1983). Unwittingly "snorting" cocaine adulterated with thallium powder has resulted in severe intoxication (Insley et al., 1986). Additional sources of thallium poisoning include self-administrations in suicide attempts (David et al., 1981; Aoyama et al., 1986; Malbrain et al., 1997) and in the sinister administration to intended victims by would-be murderers (Cavanagh et al., 1974; Meggs et al., 1994).

EXPOSURE LIMITS AND SAFETY REGULATIONS

Thallium can be extremely toxic, and its use is restricted to only experienced personnel familiar with its hazards (Conley, 1957). Thallium was totally removed from use as a pesticide in the United States in 1965 (Saddigue and Peterson, 1983). However, it continues to have various industrial uses which require safety regulation. The *Occupational Safety and Health Administration* (OSHA) has established an 8-hour time-weighted average (TWA) permissible exposure level (PEL) of 0.1 mg/m³ (OSHA, 1995). The *National Institute for Occupational Safety and Healths'* (NIOSH) 10-hour TWA recommended exposure limit (REL) for thallium is 0.1 mg/m³. The NIOSH immediately dangerous to life or health (IDLH) contamination level is 15 mg/m³ (NIOSH, 1997). The *American Conference of Governmental Industrial Hygienists* (ACGIH) recommends an 8-hour TWA threshold limit value (TLV) of 0.1 mg/m³ (ACGIH, 1995) (Table 7-1). Because the risk of accumulation is so great and individual susceptibility so variable, any exposure must be monitored closely (see Biochemical Diagnosis section).

The *U.S. Environmental Protection Agency* (USEPA) has established a maximum contamination level (MCL) for thallium content in drinking water of 0.002 mg/L. The USEPA's maximum contamination level goal (MCLG) for thallium in drinking is 0.0005 mg/L (USEPA, 1996) (see Table 7-1).

TABLE 7-1. *Established and recommended occupational and environmental exposure limits for thallium in air and water*

	Air (mg/m³)[a]	Water (mg/L)[a]
Odor threshold*	—	—
OSHA		
PEL (8-hr TWA)	0.1	—
PEL ceiling (15-min TWA)	—	—
NIOSH		
REL (10-hr TWA)	0.1	—
STEL (15-min TWA)	—	—
IDLH	15	—
ACGIH		
TLV (8-hr TWA)	0.1	—
STEL (15-min TWA)	—	—
USEPA		
MCL	—	0.002
MCLG	—	0.0005

[a]*Unit conversion:* 1 mg/L = 1 ppm.
OSHA, Occupational Safety and Health Administration; PEL, permissible exposure limit; TWA, time-weighted average; NIOSH, National Institute for Occupational Safety and Health; REL, recommended exposure limit; STEL, short-term exposure limit; IDLH, immediately dangerous to life and health; ACGIH, American Conference of Governmental Industrial Hygienists; TLV, threshold limit value; USEPA, United States Environmental Protection Agency; MCL, maximum contamination level; MCLG, maximum contamination level goal.
Data from *Amoore and Hautala, 1983; OSHA, 1995; ACGIH, 1995; USEPA, 1996; NIOSH, 1997.

METABOLISM

Tissue Absorption

Thallium is well absorbed orally, dermally, and across mucous membranes and pulmonary alveoli following inhalation (Insley et al., 1986). After oral ingestion of the water-soluble salts of thallium, absorption from the gastrointestinal tract is rapid and can be detected in urine and feces within an hour (Moeschlin, 1980; de Groot and van Heijst, 1988). Dermal absorption occurs after application of ointments containing thallium (Munch, 1934; Grulee and Clark, 1951: Smith and Doherty, 1964). The rapid absorption of thallium, along with its subsequent distribution throughout the body tissues, is similar to that of potassium. Thallium readily crosses all cell membranes; but once it is inside the cell, it is less easily released than is potassium (Kazantzis, 1986).

Tissue Distribution

Thallium is almost completely absorbed from the gastrointestinal tract and equilibrates quickly in blood. Initially, thallium accumulates in the extracellular fluid, and it soon enters the intracellular space (Gefel et al., 1970; Wainwright et al., 1988). It is distributed equally between red blood cells and serum. During an initial distribution phase, which takes approximately 4 hours, thallium becomes concentrated in well-perfused tissues such as kidney, liver, heart, and muscle. Thallium readily crosses the placenta in humans and other animals (Dolgner et al., 1983).

A second distribution phase follows, lasting from 4 to 24 hours, during which thallium becomes deposited in brain, hair, and adipose tissue (Lund, 1956; de Groot and van Heijst, 1988). The proportionate tissue distribution of thallium after absorption shows considerable variation because of the site of tissue sample, the timing of the tissue analysis in relation to the phase of the absorption, the moment in the course of the half-life of already stored thallium, and the extent of recycling of thallium after excretion from salivary glands, bile, and gut reabsorption. However, it is usually constant that the kidneys are the highest and the brain is the lowest in thallium content (Cavanagh et al., 1974; Aoyama et al., 1986). Concentrations of thallium within the nervous system range from 1 to 178 μg per gram of wet tissue and differ widely depending upon the anatomical area of the nervous system being analyzed. The gray matter, rich in neurons, accumulates almost twice as much thallium as do areas devoid of neurons (Table 7-2).

Tissue Biochemistry

Thallous ions have an ionic charge and radius similar to those of potassium ions; therefore, thallium substitutes for potassium in many physiologic reactions (Gefel et al., 1970; Douglas et al., 1990; Chandler et al., 1990; Moore et al., 1993). Many toxic effects of thallium may arise from

TABLE 7-2. *Thallium concentrations within the central nervous system of a suicide victim*

Tissue	Thallium (μg/g wet tissue)
Thalamus	140.00
Caudate	107.0
Cerebellar cortex	103.3
Frontal cortex	102.0
Choroid plexus	96.9
Midbrain	86.0
First cranial nerve	68.8
Sciatic nerve	66.7
White matter	66.1
Medulla	62.0
Third cranial nerve	59.3
Sural nerve (biopsy)	53.4
Spinal cord	44.0
Trigeminal ganglion	43.9
Brachial plexus	42.7
Seventh cranial nerve	40.8
Cauda equina	40.1
Vagus nerve	38.3
Second cranial nerve	31.7
Eighth cranial nerve	28.8

Modified from Davis et al., 1981, with permission.

interference with potassium-based processes. Like potassium, thallium is primarily intracellular, and it is secreted by salivary glands, gastric epithelium, and renal tubules (Gastel, 1978). Thallous ions can enter muscle and depolarize membranes; and at high thallium concentrations, irreversible damage to muscle fibers occurs (Mullins and Moore, 1960). Thallium has a tenfold greater affinity than potassium for Na^+, K^+-adenosine triphosphatase (ATPase), and the substituting of thallium for potassium ions in this enzyme induces dephosphorylation of Na^+- and K^+-activated ATPase in brain tissue (Inturrisi, 1969). Renal clearance of thallium ions is increased by potassium ions. However, the serum thallium levels rise at the same time, indicating that potassium increases tubular excretion of thallium, but is also produces a general mobilization of tissue thallium (Gehring and Hammond, 1967). Although potassium and thallium share ion pathways through the kidney, replacement of potassium ions by thallium ions as the basis for the latter's adverse effects has not been established.

Excretion

Elimination begins about 24 hours after ingestion of a dose of thallium, although the second distribution phase during which thallium enters the nervous system is still ongoing (van Kesteren et al., 1980). As thallium is being eliminated in gastric and intestinal secretions, as well as in bile in the feces, some is being simultaneously reabsorbed through the intestines and redistributed (Rauws, 1974). Thallium is also excreted from the kidney by glomerular filtration, with some tubular reabsorption at a rate of 3.2% per day of the amount remaining in the body (Barclay et al.,

1953). Excretion of thallium in humans is a very slow process, taking weeks to months (thallium's estimated half-life is 30 days) (Kazantzis, 1986; Malbrain et al., 1997).

In animal experiments, the fecal route eliminated twice as much thallium as the renal route, and a similar excretion pattern is believed to occur in humans (Lund, 1956). In cases of thallitoxicosis in which there is decreased intestinal motility and constipation, fecal excretion is less, resulting in more reabsorption and a greater proportion of thallium eliminated by the urinary route (van der Merwe, 1972; Saddique and Peterson, 1983; Moore et al., 1993). Thallium is also excreted via saliva (Richelmi et al., 1980) and in hair (Moeschlin, 1980).

CLINICAL MANIFESTATIONS AND DIAGNOSIS

Symptomatic Diagnosis

Symptoms among workers who handle thallium ore, or are involved in its processing, and its distribution are usually immediately related to the period of exposure and disappear when it is over. However, chronic accumulation of thallium through repeated exposures may produce more serious effects. Acute gastrointestinal symptoms appear within the first few hours of ingesting thallium. Nausea, vomiting, gastric dilatation, and diarrhea containing mucus and blood are followed by anorexia and paralytic ileus. If the exposure is sufficient to cause potassium deficiency, then autonomic nervous system failure occurs along with cardiac arrhythmia and hypertension. The autonomic nervous system effects become more significant as mechanisms regulating blood pressure and cardiac rate become affected. Paresthesias and hyperesthesia of the extremities evolve over the first week and progress into obvious peripheral neuropathy by the end of the second week (Table 7-3). Multifocal motor impairments and muscle atrophy appear. Other neurological features which have been observed in human thallotoxicosis cases during the first 2 to 3 weeks after exposure include: ataxia; headache; and a variety of abnormal movements including tremor (Smith and Doherty, 1964; Stevens et al., 1974; Davis et al., 1981; Wainwright et al., 1988), choreoathetotic postures (Mathews and Anzarut, 1968), chewing movements (Cavanagh et al., 1974), myoclonus (Wainwright et al., 1988) and dystonia (Insley et al., 1986). Cranial neuropathies result in ptosis, visual disturbances, and facial muscle paralysis. Autonomic neuropathy occurs as a late effect of thallium on small unmyelinated autonomic nerve fibers (Nordentoft et al.,1998). Behavioral changes may be seen, including intellectual impairment, sleep disturbances, delusions, hallucinations, depression, decreased attentiveness, stupor, seizures, and coma (Davis et al., 1981; Bank et al., 1972; Wainwright et al., 1988; Thompson et al., 1988; Dumitru and Kalantri, 1990; Herrero et al., 1995).

Alopecia usually appears 1 to 3 weeks after exposure to thallium and occurs concurrent with other dermatological effects including erythema and dry scaliness of skin (Feld-

TABLE 7-3. *Time course of symptoms in four individuals with thallium poisoning*

Patient	Days after thallium intake				
	1	2	3	4–8	8–15
A	Numbness	Painful paresthesia; pleuritic chest pain; 2+ protein	Severe pain requiring opioids	Hypertension, tachycardia	GI bleeding, onset of hair loss
B	Numbness, constipation	Painful paresthesia; pleuritic chest pain; trace protein	Severe pain requiring opioids	Hypertension, tachycardia, T-wave changes	Onset of hair loss leading to alopecia; normalization of T-waves
C	Abdominal cramps, emesis	Abdominal cramps, diarrhea, constipation; pleuritic chest pain	Numbness		Onset of hair loss leading to alopecia; insomnia; poor concentration
D	Abdominal cramps, emesis				Constipation; mild numbness; mild pain; patient feels normal, requests discharge

Modified from Meggs et al., 1994, with permission.

man and Levisohn, 1993; Herrero et al., 1995). Excessive sweating is also common (Herrero et al., 1995). In addition, interruption in nail growth results, leading to the development of white lines (Mee's lines) across the nails (Smith and Doherty, 1964; Heyl and Barlow, 1989; Herrero et al., 1995). Recovery from acute thallitoxicosis is very slow. Permanent damage to peripheral nerves as well as severe liver and renal damage may result if the victim does not succumb to cardiac arrhythmia, renal failure, and autonomic nervous system collapse.

The effects of chronic exposure to thallium are less severe than those of acute exposure, and they follow a different time course and clinical presentation. The usual features of painful neuropathy are replaced by nonspecific symptoms such as fever, back pain, hypertension, and mental changes. Alopecia does not develop for months to years in cases of relatively low-level chronic exposure (Gefel et al., 1970; Saddique and Peterson, 1983). Early detection of chronic thallium exposure may be missed because of the nonspecific nature of the presenting gastrointestinal and neurological complaints. The differential diagnosis of thallitoxicosis includes other disorders in which peripheral neuropathy is a prominent feature, such as Guillain–Barré syndrome and diabetic neuropathy; because of erythematous scalar skin eruptions along with neuropathy, lupus erythematosus and acute intermittent porphyria are considered. The presence of dry scaly skin and neuropathy also suggests arsenic poisoning (Moore et al., 1993). Alopecia is also seen after poisoning with vincristine, chloroprene, and mercaptopurine (Moeschlin, 1980). Therefore, careful and suspicious approach to the history of evolution of symptoms in a given patient is necessary in making a correct diagnosis.

Neurophysiological Diagnosis

Electroencephalography (EEG) can be used to detect abnormalities in CNS functioning. An EEG taken during acute thallitoxicosis shows diffuse rhythms of high amplitude and low frequency. Improvement in the EEG with return to normal patterns and frequencies is seen after successful treatment (Mathews and Anzarut, 1968). With severe encephalopathy, residual EEG abnormalities may be noted (Reed et al., 1963).

Evoked potentials (EPs) can also be used to document CNS dysfunction. *Visual evoked potentials* (VEPs) were delayed (more than 110 msec) bilaterally in a thallium-exposed patient whose optic disks appeared normal but who exhibited bilateral central scotoma on the Goldmann visual field examination (Moore et al., 1993).

Nerve conduction studies (NCSs) and *electromyography* (EMG) can be used to assess peripheral nerve and muscle function and are helpful in objectively characterizing the clinical effects of thallium exposure. NCS show greater slowing of nerve-conduction velocities in the lower extremities than in the upper ones and EMG studies reveals evidence of denervation and reinervation (Wainwright et al., 1988). Serial NCS and EMG studies can be used to document axonal neuropathy, its recovery and residual permanent damage (Dumitru and Kalantri, 1990; Yokoyama et al., 1990) (Table 7-4). The electrophysiological findings usually correlate with the histological findings of thallium toxicity, which include primary axonal damage with secondary loss of myelin (Davis et al., 1981).

Electrocardiography (ECG) can be used to monitor for cardiac arrhythmia. Sinus tachycardia, lowering of amplitude or inversion of T waves as well as other S-T and T wave changes, and ventricular fibrillation are commonly seen in thallitoxicosis (Cavanagh et al., 1974; Wainwright et al., 1988).

Neuropsychological Diagnosis

Symptoms of encephalopathy following thallium exposure include hallucinations, paranoia, and impaired cognitive processing. The prognosis for recovery of mental ca-

TABLE 7-4. *Serial electromyography studies of thallium-poisoned individuals, showing varying degrees of denervation*

Muscle	Date				
	2/87	6/87	12/87	6/88	1/89
Abductor hallucis	4⁺ Fibs/PSW Reduced MU	4⁺ Fibs/PSW Absent MU	4⁺ Fibs/PSW Absent MU	4⁺ Fibs/PSW Absent MU	3⁺ Fibs/PSW Absent MU
Extensor digitorum brevis	0 Fibs/PSW Normal MU	4⁺ Fibs/PSW Absent MU	4⁺ Fibs/PSW Absent MU	3⁺ Fibs/PSW Reduced MU	1⁺ Fibs/PSW Reduced MU
Gastrocnemius	0 Fibs/PSW Normal MU	2⁺ Fibs/PSW Reduced MU	0 Fibs/PSW Normal MU	0 Fibs/PSW Normal MU	0 Fibs/PSW Normal MU
Tibialis anterior	0 Fibs/PSW Normal MU	2⁺ Fibs/PSW Reduced MU	0 Fibs/PSW Reduced MU	0 Fibs/PSW Normal MU	0 Fibs/PSW Normal MU
Vastus medialis	0 Fibs/PSW Normal MU	0 Fibs/PSW Normal MU	0 Fibs/PSW Normal MU	0 Fibs/PSW Normal MU	0 Fibs/PSW Normal MU

Fibs, fibrillations; PSWs, positive sharp waves; MU, voluntary motor unit activation. Modified from Cavanagh et al., 1974, with permission.

pacity is worse in those cases of thallium encephalopathy which have associated EEG abnormalities (Reed et al., 1963). Residual neuropsychological effects were observed 30 years after exposure in a person who survived intoxication with thallium sulfate (Barnes et al., 1984).

Persistent cognitive dysfunction associated with thallium poisoning was reported in a 20-year-old college student who had been working with thallium in the laboratory (Thompson et al., 1988). It was estimated that he had accidentally ingested approximately 3 g of thallium before he began to experience drowsiness, difficulty thinking, and paresthesia and weakness in his lower extremities. The patient's serum thallium level was 5,750 μg/L and his urine thallium concentration was 60,000 μg/L, confirming the diagnosis of thallium poisoning. Chelation therapy was promptly instituted and signs of recovery soon followed. However, agitation, confusion, and belligerent behavior emerged during his hospital stay. Detailed psychiatric evaluation of the patient, his fraternal twin brother, and his parents indicated no previous emotional instabilities, schizophrenia, or drug abuse. In fact, the patient was an outstanding student. Follow-up neuropsychological assessments were performed at 7 and 13 months after exposure. As in the first evaluation, the patient's twin brother was tested at the same time. It had always been accepted that these two boys were very similar in intelligence and talents, because their careers and school successes had been quite parallel. Tests of verbal intelligence quotient (IQ) confirmed similar premorbid intellect between the brothers. Deficits were observed in performance IQ in the patient, in part because of tremor and slowness in motor responses. Deficits were also noted in sequencing and reasoning tasks. Significant impairment was present in tests of verbal and nonverbal memory (facial recognition and delayed recall for designs). On logical memories he was severely impaired and showed no recall at all for one short story after a 1-hour delay. Tests of executive functioning also revealed impairment. There was little general improvement 6 months later (13 months after exposure). Delayed recall on the Rey–Osterreith test had moved from the 20th to the 50th percentile (the twin tested at the 90th percentile), and from less

than the 5th to the 10th to 20th percentile on the Wechsler Memory Scale (twin scored 40th to 50th percentile). His immediate recall for faces and delayed recall for designs had returned to the average level from a low of the 5th to the 10th percentile. He was faster and more accurate on picture completion and arrangement tasks than before. These findings indicated persistent cognitive deficits and that the patient's capacity to study and continue with graduate school was severely affected by his exposure to thallium.

Acute and persistent cognitive dysfunction was also reported in a 44-year-old man who developed confusion, a pustular rash on his hands and legs, alopecia, nystagmus, painful paresthesias and weakness in his upper and lower extremities, incoordination, weakness in his facial muscles, and diffuse slowing of his electroencephalogram but normal neuroimaging studies (McMillan et al., 1997). The patient's blood and urine thallium concentrations were 108 and 1,350 μg/L, respectively. Other members of the family showed less severe symptoms of thallium poisoning.

Neuropsychological assessment of this patient was first performed 3 months after cessation of exposure to thallium, at which time the tests of attention and executive functioning, verbal and visual memory (List Learning and Rey–Osterrieth), and visuospatial ability (Block Design and Object Assembly) revealed deficits. On follow-up 12 months and again 4.5 years after exposure the patient's performance had improved on tests of attention and executive functioning, verbal and visual memory, and visuospatial ability. However, verbal IQ remained significantly impaired relative to performance IQ in this patient who had not completed high school. This finding can be interpreted as being indicative of a lateralized deficit due to thallium poisoning but most likely reflects a premorbid learning disability.

Biochemical Diagnosis

The *American Conference of Governmental Industrial Hygienists* (ACGIH) has not determined a biological exposure index for thallium (ACGIH, 1995) (Table 7-5). However, analysis of a blood sample for thallium will reveal its pres-

TABLE 7-5. *Biological exposure indices for thallium*

	Urine	Blood	Alveolar Air
Determinant:	Thallium	Thallium	Thallium
Start of shift:	Not established	Not established	Not established
During shift:	Not established	Not established	Not established
End of shift:	Not established	Not established	Not established

Data from ACGIH, 1995.

ence in cases of acute and chronic exposure. The blood level of thallium can rise to between 2,000 and 3,500 µg/L in 12 to 24 hours after a dose of 1 g of thallium sulfate (Moeschlin, 1980). However, the rapid uptake of thallium by the cells of various tissues, where it can be stored before excretion by the kidneys and the intestines, makes blood an unreliable source for biochemical diagnosis. Nevertheless, blood thallium levels have been used to document exposure (Herrero et al., 1995; Malbrain et al., 1997; McMillan et al., 1997) (Fig. 7-1).

Although the presence of thallium in the urine can be documented qualitatively by a green discoloration, the most effective method for diagnosing thallium exposure is to measure urinary excretion of thallium using atomic ab-

sorption spectroscopy (Moeschlin, 1980; Brockhaus et al., 1981; Kravzov et al., 1993; Chandler et al., 1990; Malbrain et al., 1997). The normal mean urine thallium level in unexposed persons ranges from 0.3 ± 0.14 to 0.83 ± 0.54 µg/L (Dolgner et al., 1983) (Table 7-6). Urine thallium concentrations greater than 200 to 300 µg/L are considered toxic (Kazantzis, 1986; Moore et al., 1993). A *thallium-mobilization test* is helpful, especially in cases in which there is no alopecia, the baseline urine thallium level is not significantly elevated, and thallitoxicosis is strongly suspected. This is done by giving a potassium chloride load of 45 mEq orally after measuring baseline thallium levels in a 24-hour urine sample. As potassium displaces thallium from tissue

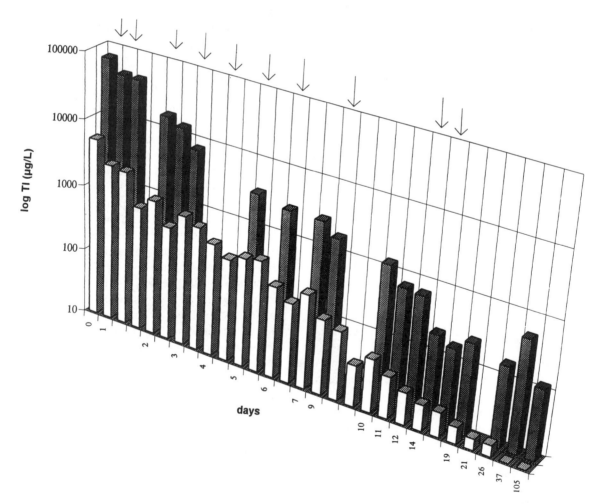

FIG. 7-1. Serum (□) and urine (□) M thallium concentrations in a 38-year-old woman following ingestion of 9 g of thallium sulfate. *Arrows* indicate day of hemodialysis. (From Malbrain et al., 1997, with permission.)

TABLE 7-6. *Urine levels (μg/L) of thallium found in persons without known exposure*

Number of individuals	Mean (± SD)	Range	Reference
149	0.3 (± 0.14)	0.02–0.7	Dolgner et al., 1983
41	0.4 (± 0.2)	0.1–1.2	Brockhaus et al., 1981
9	0.83 (± 0.54)	0.13–1.69	Weinig and Zink, 1967

Modified from Dolgner et al., 1983, with permission.

stores, the urine concentration will rise. Serial 24-hour urine collections will reflect the increased body burden if there has been accumulation of thallium (Saddique and Peterson, 1983) (see Preventive and Therapeutic Measures section).

Detection of thallium in other tissues such as saliva and hair can be used to monitor exposure. The level of salivary thallium in an intoxicated person has been reported to be as much as 15 times greater than that of the urine of the same person (Richelmi et al., 1980). Testing for thallium in and on hair can be either helpful or misleading. Contamination by external apposition of thallium particles from the environment, rather than thallium absorbed and located in the hair shaft itself, can result in overestimating the quantity of thallium in the sample. Hair samples must be thoroughly washed before drying, ashing, and dissolving, in preparation for extraction and chemical analysis (Brockhaus et al., 1981). A less analytical method of testing hair for thallium is to look for black pigmentation of the hair roots under a microscope. This pigmentation change first appears 4 days after the ingestion of thallium, and it is most noticeable in the hair of the scalp (95%) (Saddique and Peterson, 1983).

Neuroimaging

Neuroimaging studies following exposure to thallium are typically normal. McMillan et al. (1997) did not find abnormalities on the magnetic resonance imaging (MRI) or computer-assisted tomography (CT scan) studies in a 44-year-old male who developed alopecia, peripheral neuropathy, generalized slowing of his electroencephalogram, and neuropsychological deficits following exposure to thallium. His blood and urine thallium concentrations were 108 and 1,350 μg/L, respectively.

Neuropathological Diagnosis

Biochemical disturbances induced by exposure to thallium are responsible for the reversible symptoms observed in the early stages of intoxication. If the acute effects of metabolic derangements are corrected and if the amount of absorbed thallium is small enough so that its spontaneous excretion can occur before causing tissue damage, then there are few, if any, morphological changes to be seen and clinical recovery is complete.

Very few reports exist concerning the histological changes and tissue distribution of thallium early in the course of reversible thallitoxicosis (Aoyama et al., 1986). Instances of acute intoxication, which end in prompt death, show pathological changes in kidneys, liver, and lungs but relatively little nervous tissue damage (Gettler and Weiss, 1943). Most pathological studies have been done in patients several weeks after the onset of neurological symptoms or after very intense acute and fatal exposures. Engorgement of cortical blood vessels, cerebral edema, and perivascular hemorrhages, as well as various grades of chromatolysis of neurons (especially those of the pyramidal tract, third nerve nucleus, substantia nigra, and pyramidal cells of the globus pallidus) were observed at postmortem in seven people 12 to 16 days after they had ingested grain contaminated with 1% thallium sulfate (Munch et al., 1933).

Kennedy and Cavanagh (1976) (see Clinical Experiences section) had noted that chromatolysis was significantly more advanced in lumbosacral than in cervical cord. This indicates that the pathologic process started earlier in the lower limbs than in the upper limbs. Cranial nerve involvement appears to occur later, when damage to distal neurons has been underway for several days (Cavanagh, 1991). Clinical neuropathic involvement has been more significant distally than proximally. These are features which are typical of a "dying back" neuropathy. Davis et al. (1981) noted that myelin sheaths around many of the severely degenerated axons were intact or only slightly changed, suggesting a primary axonal degeneration with secondary demyelination (Figs. 7-2 and 7-3).

Different biochemical mechanisms may be operative for the various clinical manifestations of thallium toxicity. One hypothesis suggests that thallium intoxication induces riboflavin deficiency, leading to disturbances in reactions dependent upon flavoproteins and the subsequent intermediate metabolites involved in the electron transport chain and cellular energy production. Cavanagh (1991) proposed that a "metabolic lesion," resulting in decreased availability of energy to the neuron, might explain the neuropathology of thallium. This concept was based on a comparison of the neuropathy of thallium toxicity with the neuropathy of chronic thiamine deficiency and arsenic intoxication. In all three conditions, sensory nerves are affected before motor, lower limbs are affected before upper, and damage occurs to organs with high-energy requirements, such as skin and its appendages, testes, and heart. Furthermore, it is of interest that riboflavin deficiency produces a characteristic triad of peripheral neuropathy, alopecia, and cheilosis, very similar to the findings of thallotoxicosis (Saddique and Peterson, 1983; Insley et al., 1986). Schoental and Cavanagh (1977) first noted that thallium can bind with tissue riboflavin and thus lead to a deficiency in flavoproteins. Since flavoproteins are necessary in a number of metabolic reactions, including as a source of electrons in the electron transport chain, a deficiency of flavoproteins would be expected to result in impairment of cellular energy generation. Thus, flavoprotein deficiency may be the "metabolic lesion" that is causing the

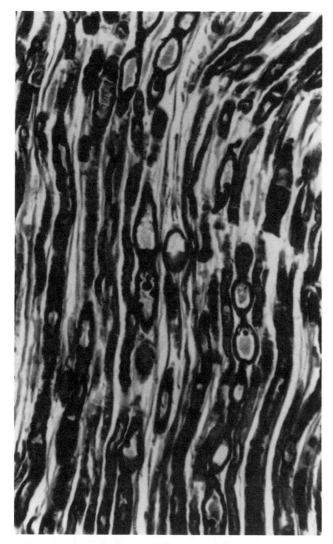

FIG. 7-2. Sural nerve biopsy following acute thallium intoxication (original magnification ×310) demonstrates axonal damage with secondary degeneration of myelin sheath after acute thallium poisoning. (Modified from Davis et al., 1981, with permission.)

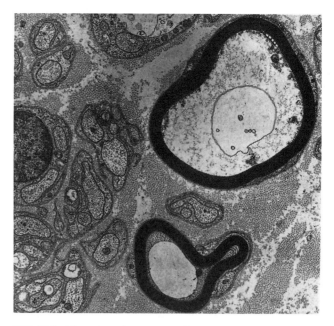

FIG. 7-3. Electron microscopy of sural nerve biopsy following acute thallium intoxication shows two small myelinated fibers (diameter <7 μm). Both fibers have a large axonal vacuole. The right axon is degenerated and the left has preserved structural elements (original magnification ×13,200 before 25% reduction). (Modified from Davis et al., 1981, with permission.)

"dying back" neuropathy and alopecia in thallotoxicosis. Another hypothesis for a possible mechanism for thallium toxicity is oxidative stress based on studies in rats given thallium (5 mg/kg) intraperitoneally for 7 days. Lipid peroxidation was significantly increased in the cerebrum, cerebellum, and in the brain stem, suggesting that uncontrolled lipid peroxidation may result in degradation of biomembranes and subcellular organelles (Hasan and Ali, 1981).

PREVENTIVE AND THERAPEUTIC MEASURES

The only prevention of thallitoxicosis is the avoidance of exposure to thallium. Among children, accidental ingestion of the candy-like thallium pesticide pellets results from the mistaken identity of the poison. Substitution of other pesticides less toxic than thallium will help reduce the risk of accidental intake. Since thallium absorption and subsequent toxicity occur even when protective gear is used (Moore et al., 1993), it is clear that occupationally exposed workers should be periodically evaluated and appropriately screened for thallium poisoning (Saddique and Peterson, 1983). Once intake has occurred and has been recognized, the first step in treating thallitoxicosis is to prevent further exposure.

If ingestion has been recent, gastric lavage should be performed (de Groot et al., 1985; Villanueva et al., 1990). Since absorption and distribution of thallium are generally complete within 24 hours, and most cases present after this window of time, treatment modalities are primarily directed toward enhancing the elimination of the metal from the body (de Groot et al., 1985). The current therapies focus on enhancing the fecal and urinary excretion of thallium (Villanueva et al., 1990; Nogué et al., 1982; Hollogginitas et al., 1980). Constipation hinders fecal elimination of thallium (van der Merwe, 1972; Moore et al., 1993). Therefore, the first step to enhance excretion is to administer laxatives (van Kesteren et al., 1980; de Groot and van Heijst, 1988). Secondly, the absorption of thallium from the gut is prevented by administration of absorptive agents, such as potassium ferric hexacyanoferrocyanate III (Prussian Blue) or activated charcoal (Kamerbeek et al., 1971; Stevens et al., 1974; Rauws and van Heijst, 1979; van Kesteren et al., 1980; Chandler et al., 1990; Villanueva et al., 1990; Kravzov et al., 1993). Both activated charcoal and Prussian Blue absorb thallium and enhance elimination via the fecal route. In Europe, Prussian Blue is the drug of choice in the treatment of thallium poisoning (Stevens et al., 1974), although other authors have suggested that activated charcoal administered in multiple doses may be superior (Lehmann and Favare, 1984).

Urinary excretion is enhanced by several methods. The oldest technique is forced diuresis with diuretics (Saddique and Peterson, 1983; de Groot et al., 1985; Villanueva et al., 1990). Potassium chloride hastens the excretion of thallium by competition with thallium in the distal renal tubule (Papp et al., 1969; Thompson, 1981; Saddique and Peterson, 1983; Insley et al., 1986). Initially there may be a transient clinical deterioration concomitant with potassium chloride therapy due to mobilization of intracellular thallium stores (Herrero et al., 1995) and impaired renal function (Bank et al., 1972), but the end result is increased thallium excretion and clinical improvement (Papp et al., 1969; Cavanagh et al., 1974). Hemodialysis is not effective for removing large amounts of thallium but may serve to hasten the reduction of the overall body burden of thallium (Pedersen et al., 1978; Van Kesteren, 1994; Malbrain et al., 1997) (Fig. 7-4).

Symptomatic, supportive, and empirical treatments including nutritional supplementation (with thiamine, riboflavin, and vitamin B$_{12}$) and physical therapy, especially in those cases where weakness and muscle atrophy associated with the peripheral neuropathy result, are suggested (Chamberlain et al., 1958; Moore et al., 1993).

CLINICAL EXPERIENCES

Group Studies

Consumption of Thallium-Contaminated Grain

A group of Mexican laborers and their families in California ingested tortillas made from a mixture of wheat flour, barley flour, and grain which had been treated with 1% thallium sulfate (Munch et al., 1933). This preparation (Thalgrain) had been intended for use in agricultural pesticide dusting. Unfortunately, the contents of a 100-pound bag were shared among the workers who used the grain as ingredients in making their food. At least 31 people were exposed. Symptoms developed within 1 to 3 days in 20 people. A total of 14 persons were hospitalized, six of whom died of thallitoxicosis within 16 days; a seventh person died 2 months later. Manifestations of involvement of the peripheral nervous system included painful extremities, with or without numbness; this was followed by muscle weakness. In the more severe cases, there were distur-

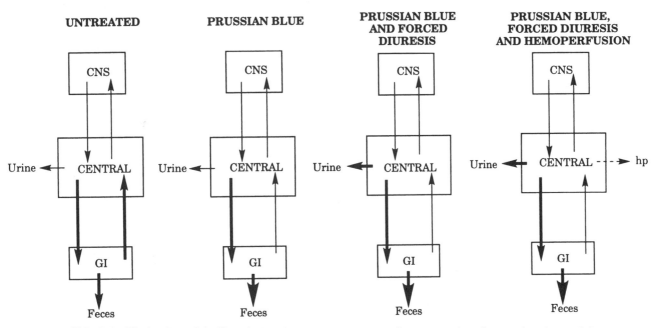

FIG. 7-4. Elimination of thallium from storage compartments in untreated and treated patients. Administration of Prussian Blue alone resulted in an elimination half-life of 3 days. Combining Prussian Blue with forced diuresis reduced elimination half-life to 2 days. When hemoperfusion was combined with Prussian Blue and forced diuresis, elimination half-life was further reduced to 1.4 days. Central nervous system (CNS); parenchymal organs, muscle, and adipose tissue (Central); gastrointestinal tract (GI). (Modified from van Kesteren et al., 1994, with permission.)

bances of sensorium, convulsions, cranial nerve palsies, and myoclonic or choreiform movements. Psychosis characterized by disorientation, marked restlessness, and confusion appeared in the less rapidly fatal cases. Tests on the unconsumed tortillas revealed that each contained approximately 1.25 to 2.0 mg of thallous sulfate. There was no way to be certain about the amount eaten by each fatal case or those who survived. Postmortem analysis of kidney, liver, heart, spleen, and intestine of the decedent confirmed the presence of thallium.

Paraoccupational Exposure to Thallium

A population living within the fall-out area around a thallium-emitting cement factory was studied by Brockhaus et al. (1981) and Dolgner et al. (1983). Twenty-four-hour urine samples were collected for determination of "unexposed" ranges of thallium in 31 people living in a nonadjacent rural area and in 10 people living in an urban area. Exposure of the "at-risk" population was determined by testing for thallium in 24-hour urine samples of 1,265 subjects and in hair samples of 1,163 subjects. Increased levels of thallium in urine (mean: 2.6 µg/g) and hair (mean: 9.5 ng/g) were seen in the population living around the cement plant, compared to the controls. Of interest, negligible amounts of thallium exposure occurred via the respiratory route. Chemical analyses of vegetables and fruits grown in the vicinity of the cement plant demonstrated contamination, probably by thallium containing dust fall-out emitted by the cement plant. Individuals who ate home-grown fruits and vegetables had higher thallium levels.

The symptoms that positively correlated with higher urinary and hair thallium levels were polyneuropathy, sleep disorders, headache, fatigue, weakness, nervousness, and muscle and joint pains. Interestingly, the classical alopecia of thallium poisoning was not correlated with high thallium levels in these subjects, indicating that this finding may be absent in chronic intake of low doses of thallium (Dolgner et al., 1983).

Homicide at a Work Site

Three men worked in the same place as a fourth man who tried to kill them with crystalline thallous acetate dissolved in water, which he poured into his coworker's tea and/or coffee (Cavanagh et al., 1974). As a result of the murderer's careful and sinister recording of the amounts of poison he administered to his victims, it is known that coworker 1 was given about 18 grains (0.93 g) in two doses; coworker 2 was given the same total amount in three doses; and coworker 3 received only 6 grains (0.31 g). Coworker 3 survived the intake of the smallest amount of thallous acetate. Autopsy studies and tissue analysis confirmed the presence of thallium and its effects in the two dead men (Table 7-7). Since the body weight of the individual must be taken into account, it is understandable that there are differences in response among the victims of thallium poisoning. These three cases illustrate that the estimated dose of thallium was lethal at a total of 0.93 g and not at 0.31 g.

Coworker 1. A 60-year-old foreman had symptoms of diarrhea and vomiting which lasted for 24 hours. A week

TABLE 7-7. *Pathological findings in victims of sinister thallium poisoning*

Age	Estimated dose ingested	Pathological findings
56	0.93 g in three doses	*Spinal cord:* scattered vacuolated fibers with myelophages in dorsal columns, indicating that an occasional nerve fiber had undergone degeneration. *Sciatic nerve:* occasional axon with granular fragmented appearance. *Sural nerve:* moderate numbers of fragmenting and granular axons, with degeneration of myelin sheath. *Vagus nerve:* moderate numbers of fragmenting and granularaxons, with degeneration of myelin sheath. *Liver:* centrilobular congestion and moderately severe fatty changes. *Kidney:* normal. *Lungs:* moderate congestion of both with edema of the right. *Heart and spleen:* normal.
60	0.93 g in two doses	*Spinal cord:* occasional fragmenting of axons in dorsal columns at cervical level, no cellular reactive changes found. *Sciatic nerve:* normal. *Lumbar dorsal root ganglion:* mild chromatolysis and one hyaline neuron. *Liver:* centrilobular necrosis with fatty change in most lobules. *Kidney:* extensive recent necrosis of cortex. *Lungs:* edema and patchy early bronchopneumonia. *Heart and spleen:* normal.
26	0.31 g in a single dose	Survived: no pathological study.

From Cavanagh et al., 1974, with permission.

later he had an episode of dizziness. He was without symptoms for 1 more week and then he developed painful paresthesias in his hands and feet. The paresthesias progressed in severity and soon were accompanied by weakness in the extremities. Over the next 6 to 10 days the weakness progressed to involve facial and bulbar musculature. Swallowing and breathing were severely affected. Perception to vibration sensation and passive movement was normal, but the feet were exquisitely painful to touch. The skin was normal and there was no hair loss. Because of a history suggesting a transient infection at the outset, the course of progressive weakness, and the presence of cerebrospinal fluid protein of 90 mg%, a diagnosis of Guillain–Barré syndrome was made. Despite positive respiratory support, the man died of cardiac arrest, approximately 3 weeks after the onset of symptoms.

The neuropathological findings in this patient showed occasional fragmented axons in the dorsal columns, but no changes in the anterior horn cells in the cervical region of the spinal cord, early chromatolytic swelling in a few anterior horn cells with microglial activity around some necrotic neurons in the lumbar region, and a suggestion of chromatolysis in neurons of the spinal root ganglia. The sciatic nerve showed no abnormalities. A diagnosis of thallium intoxication was not suspected until after the death of the second worker. At that time the cremated ashes of this patient were exhumed and analyzed. A total of 8.9 mg thallium was found in the ash and 2.5 μg/g was found in kidney tissue which had been kept in paraffin since the autopsy.

Coworker 2. A 55-year-old man who worked in the same department as coworkers 1 and 3 complained of diarrhea, vomiting, and abdominal pain lasting for approximately 1 hour. Several days later he developed burning pain in the toes of his feet and a tingling sensation in the tips of his fingers. Approximately 4 months after the death of coworker 1, this man noticed weakness of handgrip. He consulted a neurologist who noted that sensation to pinprick and to light touch over the tips of his fingers and toes was impaired; light touch caused severe hyperalgesia of the soles of both feet. There was asymmetrical weakness of the lower extremities (dorsiflexion of left foot more than right; extension of left knee). Five days later, visual impairment, nystagmus, and photophobia appeared. His condition deteriorated rapidly over the next few days, with the onset of gaze palsy, bilateral facial weakness and ptosis, and dysphagia. Global weakness of the lower extremities was present and was more pronounced distally. Intrinsic muscles of the hands were minimally weak. All tendon reflexes were absent. The patient's illness continued to progress.

An examination of his cerebrospinal fluid revealed protein of 130 mg%. Other tests included nerve conduction studies, which documented peripheral neuropathy. In particular, there was slowing of the NCVs in the lower extremities more than there was in the upper limbs. Facial nerve motor latency response was also delayed. The patient

received respiratory and electrolyte support during the next 10 days. His skin began to show scaliness and erythema, but no hair loss was noted at that time. The facial weakness, ophthalmoplegia, and the bulbar functions worsened. There were involuntary mouthing movements suggesting dyskinesia. Muscle wasting became more apparent. The patient died of cardiac arrest 19 days after the onset of his symptoms.

The diagnosis in this case also had been uncertain until the similarity to the case of coworker 1 raised serious concern about a common etiology. The neuropathy and the skin lesions were suggestive of thallium intoxication. Microscopic examination of hairs demonstrated pigmentation of the hair base. The autopsy examination looked for evidence of thallitoxicosis.

Upon postmortem examination, the brain and spinal cord were unremarkable on gross examination. Histological studies revealed swollen axons and fragmentation of myelin sheaths of the sciatic, sural, third cranial, sixth cranial, and vagus nerves. Wallerian-type axonal degeneration with secondary demyelination and proliferation of Schwann cells indicating regeneration was noted on transverse sections. Teased fiber preparations also showed wallerian-type degeneration. Dorsal spinal roots showed occasional swollen and fragmented axons; the ventral spinal roots showed no abnormality. Occasional motor neurons in the anterior gray matter of the lumbar cord were swollen due to chromatolytic response. In the dorsal columns of cervical, thoracic, and lumbar regions there were vacuolated fibers containing macrophages, indicative of degeneration. No significant abnormalities were found in the cerebellum, cerebral cortex, basal ganglia, or midbrain. The diagnosis of thallitoxicosis was confirmed by determining the concentrations of thallium in the kidney, heart, and gray matter of the brain, which were 20, 13.3, and 10 μg/g, respectively. The white matter contained 3.0 μg/g and the sciatic nerve concentration was 1.0 μg/g.

Coworker 3. A third worker, a 26-year-old clerk in the same department as the two other workers described above, received the least amount of thallium from his would-be murderer (0.31 g). He initially presented with paresthesias in both feet and chest pain. This was followed by lymphadenopathy and pharyngitis for which he was given penicillin. Vomiting, weakness, and painful paresthesias in the ankles and feet developed over the next 8 days. The paresthesia in his lower extremities was severe enough to impair his ability to walk. There was marked tenderness over the lower limbs and decreased sensation perception to light touch and pinprick over the digits of his hands and feet. His sensory symptoms began to diminish over the next 7 to 8 days.

Then suddenly, he developed malaise, tremulousness, and a tachycardia (120/minute). Two days later his hair began to come out in "fistfuls." He had no neurological findings at that time. Twelve days later, he again had a bout of diarrhea, and the numbness with sensory loss in the feet had returned. The patient was again treated supportively. Documentation of his exposure to thallium was obtained by a 24-hour urine sample taken 7 weeks after the exposure, which showed a concentration of 3.0 μg/L. Within 8 days, the patient's symptoms had remitted and hair growth had resumed. The patient made a good recovery and has remained well since.

Individual Case Studies

Tremor, Myoclonus, Facial Paresis, Hyperactive Reflexes, and Alopecia in a Child

A 3-year, 9-month-old male child from rural Iowa presented to the emergency department with a 1-week history of headache, lethargy, weakness, anorexia, lower extremity pain, and an increasingly labile affect with irritability (Mayfield et al., 1983). The neurological exam revealed an irritable child with a generalized coarse tremor, a symmetric facial paresis, bilateral ptosis, marked ataxia, hyperreflexia, and bilateral muscle weakness, more prominent in the legs. The child seemed stable for 6 days and then he had three episodes of myoclonic jerking of the extremities, suggesting severe encephalopathy. It was not until the ninth hospital day, when patchy hair loss from the head was noted, that thallium poisoning was strongly suspected. Urine thallium was 1,700 μg/L (normal: 1 to 10 μg/L). Inspection of the child's residence resulted in the discovery of a thallium sulfate rodenticide.

Although alopecia is a characteristic finding in thallitoxicosis, it usually does not appear until 1 to 3 weeks after ingestion, and therefore it should not be depended upon for making an early diagnosis. Gastrointestinal symptoms may be marked in the first few days after ingestion; but following this, neurologic symptoms (especially peripheral neuropathy) dominate the clinical picture. Facial weakness and ptosis are an early and prominent finding in the pediatric population. The tendon reflexes are preserved until late in the course of the peripheral neuropathy in thallitoxicosis. This distal symmetric anonal neuropathy in thallium poisoning is unlike the primarily demyelinative neuropathies (i.e., acute intermittent porphyria and Guillain–Barré syndrome), despite the facial paresis.

Thallium Poisoning: Successful Acute Treatment

A 38-year-old woman drank 250 mL of a suspension containing 35 g/L of thallium sulfate; her estimated total intake was 9 g of thallium (Malbrain et al., 1997). Two hours later she was brought to an emergency room (ER). Vomiting was induced en route to the hospital. In the ER, she was alert and stable (blood pressure 132/70 mmHg; pulse 74/minute; temperature 37°C). Her urine was green, indicating the presence of thallium. Gastric lavage was performed, and Prussian Blue was given via gastric tube. Lactulose was given to increase fecal excretion. In addition, plasma potassium levels were maintained in the high

normal range with supplemental potassium chloride. Hemodialysis was instituted.

The patient's serum thallium level was subsequently found to be 5,240 μg/L and her urine thallium level was 69,600 μg/L, confirming thallium intoxication. After 14 hours on hemodialysis, her serum thallium level had decreased to 2,490 μg/L. Hemodialysis was continued for 7 more days (6 hours per day), during which time her serum thallium levels continued to decrease. Hemodialysis was performed again on 9, 12, and 14 days after exposure, for a total dialysis time of 74 hours (see Fig. 7-1). Hemodialysis was discontinued when her serum level had decreased to 49 μg/dL.

The patient's clinical condition remained stable during the entire course of her treatment. However, she did have severe abdominal pain and constipation for the first 48 hours after exposure. On day 3 after exposure she complained of painful paresthesias and weakness in her legs. Neurophysiological studies on day 16 revealed evidence of sensorimotor polyneuropathy in her lower extremities. Hair loss became apparent on day 18, and she had total alopecia on day 25 after exposure.

The patient showed clinical improvement in her neuropathy 1 month after admission and treatment. At follow-up 3 weeks after discharge (7 weeks after exposure) her serum and urine thallium levels were 5.6 and 100 μg/L, respectively. At final testing 11 weeks after exposure, her serum and urine thallium levels had dropped to less than 1 and 3 μg/L, respectively. Her complaints of paresthesia and weakness were almost completely gone and her hair was regrowing.

Painful Feet and Skin Rash

The following case demonstrates that the peripheral neuropathy in thallium poisoning is characteristically very painful. These symptoms are suggestive of an early small fiber neuropathy, which later progresses to involve larger fibers.

A 45-year-old man living in Mexico presented with a 1-week history of a progressive stinging pain beginning in the plantar surfaces of both feet and progressing to mid thigh level (Dumitru and Kalantri, 1990). The patient was hospitalized complaining not only of foot pain severe enough to impede ambulation, but also of constant diffuse abdominal discomfort and constipation. By the end of the next week, mild hair loss was evident and rapidly progressed through the third week, by which time large clumps of hair were falling out. Perception of sensation to pinprick, two-point discrimination, proprioception, light touch, and vibration were intact throughout, with the exception of diminished sensation about the medial plantar aspects of both feet. Light touch evoked an exaggerated complaint of burning pain from the foot to the mid thigh (hyperesthesia). Motor examination was normal in the upper extremities. Assessment of the lower limb strength was limited by pain elicited when touching the patient. His gait was markedly impaired by pain, but no ataxia was observed. Deep tendon reflexes were present and equal in the upper and lower extremities. The profound foot pain combined with alopecia and an erythematous nontender malar rash with small pustules and perioral ulcers suggested a systemic toxic reaction.

The urinary thallium level was 1,257 μg/L (normal <10 μg/L) and the serum level was 8.5 μg/dL (normal <2 μg/dL). A sural nerve biopsy was made 4 weeks after initial presentation and revealed a moderate reduction in the large and medium-sized nerve fibers. Additionally, a number of the myelin sheaths had undergone secondary degeneration and appeared as myelin ovoids along the course of the axon. Neurophysiologic studies 10 days after initial presentation were suggestive of a progressive and profound distal axonopathy.

Dysautonomia, Encephalopathy, and Negative Blood Tests After Inhaling Thallium-Adulterated "Cocaine"

Insley et al. (1986) described a 34-year-old man who was initially hospitalized for hypertension. He also complained of persistent abdominal pain, vomiting, constipation, insomnia, and pain and weakness in both legs. Three weeks earlier, he had purchased a white powder which he thought was cocaine, and he had snorted it several times. The substance had no stimulatory or euphoric effect, but was intensely irritating to the nasal mucosa. One time after snorting the substance, the subject became unconscious and had a seizure. This was followed by a period of inappropriate behavior. He was treated and released from a local emergency department as a result of this incident. He presented to the hospital a second time complaining of abdominal pain. His blood pressure at that time was 160/100 mmHg and the pulse was 84 beats per minute. Abdominal examination was remarkable for mild tenderness. Neurologic examination revealed mild weakness of both legs with normal deep tendon reflexes and sensation. A scaly erythematous eruption was present on his trunk, arms, and legs. Over a 3-day period, alopecia developed involving the scalp, body hair, and eyebrows. A blood sample at that time was negative for thallium. Analysis of the inhaled substance by mass spectroscopy scanning electron microscopy, and x-ray diffraction revealed 99% thallium sulfate.

This case illustrates illicit drug use as a possible source of exposure to thallium and stresses the importance of a good history in the diagnosis of neurotoxicant exposures. Since the early symptoms of thallium poisoning are quite nonspecific, diagnosis may frequently be missed. In most cases of thallium poisoning, the diagnosis is not suspected until the onset of the alopecia. However, as noted previously, alopecia is usually delayed for 1 to 3 weeks after ingestion, and this often results in a delay in diagnosis and treatment. In addition, most routine "heavy metal screens" do not include thallium, and therefore the clinician who has reasonable suspicion of thallium poisoning in a patient presenting with nonspecific symptoms should request specifically for thallium levels. In this case, there was additional difficulty in confirmation of the diagnosis because the biological samples were not taken until 3 to 4 weeks after exposure and none of the biological samples demonstrated the presence of thallium. Ultimately, thallium poisoning was inferred when the substance that the patient inhaled was found to be thallium sulfate.

REFERENCES

American Conference of Governmental Industrial Hygienists (ACGIH). *Threshold limit values (TLVs) for chemical substances and physical agents and biological exposure indices (BEIs)*. Cincinnati: American Conference of Governmental Industrial Hygienists, Technical Affairs Office, 1995.

Amoore JE, Hautala E. Odor as an aid to chemical safety: odor threshold compared with threshold limit values and volatilities for 214 industrial chemicals in air and water dilution. *J Appl Toxicol* 1983; 3:272–290.

Aoyama H, Yoshida MD, Yamamura Y. Acute poisoning by intentional ingestion of thallous malonate. *Hum Toxicol* 1986;5:389–392.

Bank WJ, Pleasure DE, Suzuki K, Nigro M, Katz R. Thallium poisoning. *Arch Neurol* 1972;26:456–464.

Barclay RK, Peacock WC, Karnofsky DA. Distribution and excretion of radioactive thallium in chick embryo, rat and man. *J Pharmacol Exp Ther* 1953;107:178.

Barnes MP, Murray K, Tilley PJB. Neurological deficit more than thirty years after chronic thallium intoxication. *Lancet* 1984;1:184.

Brockhaus A, Dolgner R, Evers U, Kramer U, Soddeman H, Wiegand H. Intake and health effects of thallium among a population living in the vicinity of a cement plant emitting thallium containing dust. *Int Arch Occup Environ Health* 1981;48:375–389.

Cavanagh JB. What have we learned from Graham Frederic Young? Reflections of the mechanism of thallium neurotoxicity. *Neuropathol Apl Neurobiol* 1991;17:3–9.

Cavanagh JB, Fuller NH, Johnson HR, Rudge P. The effect of thallium salts with particular reference to the nervous system. *Q J Med* 1974; XLIII:293–319.

Chamberlain PH, Stavinoha WB, David H, Kniker WT, Panos TC. Thallium poisoning. *Pediatrics* 1958;22:1170–1182.

Chandler HA, Archbold GPR, Gibson JM, O'Callaghan P, Marks JN, Pethybridge RJ. Excretion of a toxic dose of thallium: Case report. *Clin Chem* 1990;36:1506–1509.

Conley E. Report to the council, Committee on Pesticides. *JAMA* 1957; 163:1566–1567.

Crookes W. On the existence of a new element, probably of the sulfur group. *Chem News* 1861;3:193.

Davis LE, Stadefer JC, Kornfeld M, Abercrombie DM, Butler C. Acute thallium poisoning: Toxicological and morphological studies of the nervous system. *Ann Neurol* 1981;13:38–44.

de Groot G, van Heijst ANP. Toxokinetic aspects of thallium poisoning, methods of treatment by toxin elimination. *Sci Total Environ* 1988;711: 411–418.

de Groot G, van Heijst ANP, van Kesteren RG, Maes RAA. An evaluation of the efficacy of charcoal hemoperfusion in the treatment of three cases of acute thallium poisoning. *Arch Toxicol* 1985;57:61–66.

Dolgner R, Brockhaus A, Ewers U, Weigand H, Majewski F, Soddeman H. Repeated surveillance of exposure to thallium in a population living in the vicinity of a cement plant emitting dust containing thallium. *Int Arch Occup Environ Health* 1983;52:79–94.

Douglas KT, Bunni MA, Baindur SR. Minireview: thallium in biochemistry. *Int J Biochem* 1990;22:429–438.

Dumitru D, Kalantri A. Electrophysiological investigation of thallium poisoning. *Muscle Nerve* 1990;13:433–437.

Feldman J, Levisohn DR. Acute alopecia: clue to thallium toxicity. *Pediatr Dermatol* 1993;10:29–31.

Gastel B, ed. Clinical conferences at the Johns Hopkins Hospital. *Johns Hopkins Med J* 1978;142:27–31.

Gefel A, Liron M, Hirsch W. Chronic thallium poisoning. *Israel J Med Sci* 1970;6:380–382.

Gehring P, Hammond T. The interrelationship between thallium and potassium in animals. *J Pharmacol Exp Ther* 1967;155:187–201.

Gettler AO, Weiss L. Thallium poisoning, III. Clinical toxicology of thallium. *Am J Clin Pathol* 1943;13:422–429.

Grulee C, Clark E. Thallitoxicosis in a preschool nursery. *Am J Dis Child* 1951;51:47–50.

Grunfeld OJ, Henostroza G. Thallium poisoning. *Arch Intern Med* 1964;114:132–138.

Hasan M, Ali SF. Effects of thallium, nickel, and cobalt administration on the lipid peroxidation in different regions of the rat brain. *Toxicol Appl Pharmacol* 1981;57:8–13.

Herrero T, Fernandez E, Gomez J, et al. Thallium poisoning presenting with abdominal colic, paresthesia, and irritability. *Clin Toxicol* 1995;33:261–264.

Heyl T, Barlow RJ. Thallium poisoning: a dermatological perspective. *Br J Dermatol* 1989;121:787–791.

Hollogginatas C, Ullicci P, Dricoll J, Gauerholz J, Martin H. Thallium elimination kinetics in acute thallitoxicosis. *J Anal Toxicol* 1980;4:68–74.

Insley BM, Grufferman S, Ayliffe A. Thallium poisoning in cocaine abusers. *Am J Emerg Med* 1986;4:545–548.

Inturrisi CE. Thallium activation of K+ activated phosphatases from beef brain. *Biochem Biophys Acta* 1969;173:567.

Kamerbeek HH, Rauws AG, ten Ham M, Van Heijst ANP. Dangerous redistribution of thallium by the treatment with sodium diethyldithiocarbomate. *Acta Med Scand* 1971;189:149–154.

Kazantzis G. Thallium. In: Friberg L, Nordberg EF, Vouk FV, eds. *Handbook on the toxicology of metals,* vol II: *Specific metals,* 2nd ed. Amsterdam: North-Holland/Elsevier, 1986:549–567.

Kennedy P, Cavanagh JB. Spinal changes in the neuropathy of thallium poisoning. *J Neurol Sci* 1976;29:295–301.

Kravzov J, Rios C, Altagracia M, Monroy-Moyola A, Lopez F. Relationship between physiochemical properties of Prussian Blue and its efficacy as an antidote against thallium poisoning. *J Appl Toxicol* 1993;13:213–216.

Lehman PA, Favare L. Parameters for the absorption of thallium ions by activated charcoal and Prussian Blue. *Clin Toxicol* 1984;22:331–339.

Lund A. Distribution of thallium in the organism and its elimination. *Acta Pharmacol Toxicol* 1956;12:251–259.

Malbrain MLNG, Lambrecht GLY, Zandijk E, et al. Treatment of severe thallium intoxication. *Clin Toxicol* 1997;35:97–100.

Mathews J, Anzarut A. Thallium poisoning. *Can Med Assoc J* 1968;99:72–75.

Mayfield SR, Morgan DP, Roberts RJ. Acute thallium poisoning in a 3-year-old child: a case report. *Clin Pediatr* 1983;23:461–462.

McMillan TM, Jacobson RR, Gross M. Neuropsychology of thallium poisoning. *J Neurol Neurosurg Psychiatr* 1997;63:247–250.

Meggs RJ, Hoffman RS, Shih RD, Weisman RS, Lewis RG. Thallium poisoning from maliciously contaminated food. *Clin Toxicol* 1994;32:723–730.

Moeschlin S. Thallium poisoning. *Clin Toxicol* 1980;17:133–146.

Moore D, House I, Dixon A. Thallium poisoning: diagnosis may be elusive, but alopecia is the clue. *BMJ* 1993;306(6891):1527–1529.

Mullins L, Moore RD. The movement of thallium ions in muscle. *J Gen Physiol* 1960;43:759–773.

Munch JC. Human thallotoxins. *JAMA* 1934;102(33):1929–1933.

Munch JC, Ginsberg HM, Nixon CE. The 1932 thallotoxicosis outbreak in California. *JAMA* 1933;100:1315–1319.

National Institute for Occupational Safety and Health (NIOSH): *Pocket guide to chemical hazards.* Washington, DC: US Department of Health and Human Services, CDC, 1997.

Nogué S, Mas A, Pares A, et al. Acute thallium poisoning: an evaluation of different forms of treatment. *Clin Toxicol* 1982;19:1015–1021.

Occupational Safety and Health Administration (OSHA). Code of federal regulations 29, Part 1910.1000. Washington, DC: Office of the Federal Register National Archives and Records Administration, 1995.

Papp JP, Gay PC, Dodson NV, Pollard HM. Potassium chloride in treatment of thallotoxicosis. *Ann Intern Med* 1969;71:119–123.

Pedersen RS, Olesew AW, Freund LG. Thallium intoxication treated with longterm hemodialysis, forced diuresis, and Prussian Blue. *Acta Med Scand* 1978;204:429–432.

Rauws AG. Thallium pharmacokinetics and its modification by Prussian Blue. *Arch Pharm* 1974;284:295–306.

Rauws AG, van Heijst ANP. Check Prussian Blue for antidotal efficacy in thallium poisoning. *Arch Toxicol* 1979;43:153–154.

Reed D, Crawey J, Faro S, Pieper S, Kurland L. Thallotoxicosis: acute manifestations and sequelae. *JAMA* 1963;183:516–522.

Richelmi P, Bono F, Guardia L, Ferrini B, Manzo L. Salivary levels of thallium in acute human poisoning. *Arch Toxicol* 1980;43:321–325.

Saddique A, Peterson CD. Thallium poisoning: a review. *Vet Hum Toxicol* 1983;25:16–22.

Schoental R, Cavanagh JB. Mechanisms involved in the "dying back" process—an hypothesis implicating co-factors. *Neuropathol Appl Neurobiol* 1977;3:145–157.

Shabaline LP, Spiridonova VS. Thallium as an industrial poison: review of literature. *J Hyg Epidemiol Microbiol Immunol* 1979;231:247–256.

Sleight AW. Chemistry of high temperature super-conductors. *Science* 1988;242:1519–1527.

Smith DH, Doherty RA. Thallotoxicosis: report of three cases in Massachusetts. *Pediatrics* 1964;34:480–490.

Stevens W, van Peteghem C, Heyndrick W, Barrier F. Eleven cases of thallium intoxication treated with Prussian Blue. *Int J Clin Pharmacol* 1974;10:1.

Thompson DF. Management of thallium poisoning. *Clin Toxicol* 1981;18:979–990.

Thompson C, Dent J, Saxby P. Effects of thallium poisoning on intellectual function. *Br J Psychol* 1988;153:396–399.

United States Department of Agriculture (USDA). US Department of Agriculture removes thallium sulfate from household use. National Clearinghouse Poison Control Center, 1–2: September–October, 1965.

United States Environmental Protection Agency (USEPA). Drinking water regulations and health advisories. EPA 822-R-96-001. Washington, DC: Office of Water, 1996.

van Der Merwe CF. The treatment of thallium poisoning: a report of two cases. *S Afr Med J* 1972;46:960–961.

van Kesteren RG, Rauws AG, de Groot G, van Heijst ANP. Thallium intoxication: an evaluation of therapy. *Intensive Med* 1980;17:293–297.

van Kesteren RG. Thallium. In: de Wolff FA, ed. *Handbook of Clinical Neurology,* vol 20: *Intoxications of the nervous system,* part 1. Amsterdam: Elsevier, 1994:323–329.

Villanueva E, Hernandez-Cueto C, Lachia E, Ramos R, Ramos V. Poisoning by thallium: a study of five cases. *Drug Safety* 1990;5:384–389.

Wainwright AP, Kox WJ, House IM, Henry JA, Heaton R, Seed WA. Clinical features and therapy of acute thallium poisoning. *Q J Med* 1988;69:939–944.

Weinig E, Zink P. Uber die quantitative massenspektrometrische bestimmung des normalen Thalliumgehalts im menschlichen organismus. *Arch Toxicol* 1967;22:255–274.

Yokoyama K, Araki S, Abe H. Distribution of nerve conduction velocities in acute thallium poisoning. *Muscle Nerve* 1990;13:117–120.

CHAPTER 8

Aluminum

Aluminum (Al) is a trivalent trace element that occurs as aluminum silicate, oxide, or halide. It is mined from an impure ore, bauxite, which contains aluminum oxide, water, and iron (Winship, 1992). Metallic aluminum does not occur in nature and is obtained by electrolytic processing of the aluminum oxide extracted from ore (van der Voet and De Wolff, 1994).

Aluminum is an incidental finding in adult humans who exhibit no apparent illness; it is toxic under specific circumstances and is suspected to play a role in the pathogenesis of certain neurodegenerative diseases (Greger, 1992; Sturman and Wisniewski, 1988). A possible relationship was found between the incidence rate of Alzheimer's type dementia and intake of aluminum in drinking water (Martyn et al., 1989; Wettstein et al., 1991; Crapper-McLachlan, 1989). Elevated aluminum levels have been detected in the brains of persons with amyotrophic lateral sclerosis–parkinsonism dementia complex (ALS-PDC) (Perl et al., 1982; Spencer, 1987; Kihira et al., 1993). Trembling, ataxia, and convulsions were seen following subcutaneous injection of aluminum–L-glutamate, indicating passage across the blood-brain barrier (BBB) from the peripheral circulation (Deloncle et al., 1995). Subperineural injection into rabbits induced degeneration of spinal motor neurons (Kihira et al., 1995). Experimental intracranial injection or topical application of aluminum onto the sensorimotor cortex of mice, rats, and monkeys induces epileptic seizures (Kopeloff et al., 1942, 1954; Katz, 1985). Clinical epilepsy has been associated with aluminum exposure in humans (Crapper and De Boni, 1983; Wisniewski et al., 1985; Michel et al., 1991; Wettstein et al., 1991; Simonsen et al., 1994). Brain tissue aluminum levels are elevated in patients with renal failure and encephalopathy who are receiving dialysis (Alfrey, 1986). For these reasons it is important to consider the potential neurotoxic effects of aluminum, whether exposure occurs in the workplace, in the general environment, as a result of renal dialysis, or as a finding in the brain of a patient with a pathological diagnosis of a neurodegenerative disease.

SOURCES OF EXPOSURE

Aluminum is commonly found in soil and water, especially in areas where conditions result in the release of this and other metals from the earth's mineral stores (Lukiw and McLachlan, 1995). Annual production of metallic aluminum in the United States has been greater than 4.0 million tons in the past, but a low of 3.2 million tons was reported for 1994 (Stokinger, 1981; Aluminum Association, 1996). Occupational sources of exposure include (a) dust particulates occurring during the mining of the ore; (b) dust and vapors during the smelting and recovery processes; and (c) foundry and fabrication work (Rifat et al., 1990). In addition, organoaluminum compounds are used as catalysts in polymerization processes and occur across the stages of organic synthesis, causing potential exposure and absorption through inhalation and skin contact. Trialkylaluminum compounds are sensitive to oxidation and hydrolysis in air, are very reactive when exposed to water, and are often employed as incendiary agents (Siegers and Sullivan, 1992).

Metallic aluminum is a light and sturdy material used in the construction of cooking utensils, airplanes, and automobiles (van der Voet and de Wolff, 1994). In medicinal situations, aluminum has been used as binder to regulate phosphate levels in persons with renal deficiency (Alfrey, 1989). Aluminum-containing bone cement has been used for bone reconstruction following otoneurosurgery (Hantson et al., 1995; Renard et al., 1994; Reusche et al., 1995). Aluminum compounds are used in antacid medications and in buffered analgesics (Greger et al., 1985). Aluminum acetate creams and solutions are used for relief of inflammatory conditions of the skin such as poison ivy and athlete's foot. Aluminum chlorohydrate is used in antiperspirants. In addition, aluminum salts are used in cosmetics, in the processing, preservation and packaging of foods, and in the purification of water (Crapper and De Boni, 1983).

The human diet is a major source of aluminum intake. Aluminum is commonly found in drinking water (Miller et

129

al., 1984). Farm produce, particularly root crops, contain aluminum obtained from the water taken in by the plants (Vogt et al., 1987). Aluminum is naturally present in tea (Pennington and Jones, 1989). Certain aluminum compounds (sodium aluminum phosphate and sodium aluminum silicate) are used in the baking industry as leaveners and as antiadherence additives in baking powder (van de Voet and De Wolff, 1994). In addition, using aluminum pots and pans for cooking has been shown to increase aluminum content in foods (Greger et al., 1985; Pennington and Jones, 1989; Greger, 1992). As a result of its ubiquity, the average American consumes approximately 25 mg of elemental aluminum a day, most of which is from the food additives used in grain products and processed cheeses (Pennington and Jones, 1989; Greger, 1992).

EXPOSURE LIMITS AND SAFETY REGULATIONS

The relationship between occupational exposure and systemic toxicity is unclear, but there have been efforts to establish an exposure limit of 1 mg/m³ for aluminum welding fumes intended to prevent neurobehavioral effects as well as pulmonary damage and asthma (Sjögren and Elinder, 1992). The *Occupational Safety and Health Administration* (OSHA) has established a PEL with an 8-hour time-weighted average (TWA) for total aluminum dust of 15 mg/m³, with a TWA for the respirable fraction of 5 mg/m³ (OSHA, 1995) (Table 8-1). The *National Institute for Occupational Safety and Health* (NIOSH) has recommended a 10-hour TWA exposure limit (REL) for total aluminum dust of 10 mg/m³; for the respirable fraction, it is 5 mg/m³. The NIOSH REL for aluminum pyro powders and welding fumes is 5 mg/m³. The NIOSH REL for soluble aluminum salts and organoaluminum (alkyls) is 5 mg/m³ (NIOSH, 1997). The *American Conference of Governmental and Industrial Hygienists'* (ACGIH) threshold limit value (TLV) for aluminum is an 8-hour TWA exposure to total aluminum dust of 10 mg/m³ with a TLV for the respirable fraction of 5 mg/m³. The ACGIH TLV for aluminum pyro powders and welding fumes is 5 mg/m³. For alkyl compounds and soluble salts the ACGIH TLV is 2 mg/m³ (ACGIH, 1995).

A maximum contamination level (MCL) for aluminum in water has not been established. The United States Environmental Protection Agency (USEPA) has recommended a secondary maximum contaminant level of 0.05 to 0.2 mg/L for aluminum in drinking water, below which the taste, appearance, and color should not be altered (USEPA, 1996).

METABOLISM

Tissue Absorption

Pulmonary absorption of aluminum is limited by the size of the inhaled particles (Sjögren et al., 1985; Ljunggren et

TABLE 8-1. *Established and recommended occupational and environmental exposure limits for aluminum in air and water*

	Air (mg/m³)a	Water (mg/L)a
Odor threshold*	—	—
OSHA		
PEL (8 hr TWA)		
Total Al dust	15	—
Respirable Al dust	5	—
Pyro powders	—	—
Welding fumes	—	—
Soluble salts	—	—
Alkyls	—	—
PEL ceiling (15 min, TWA)	—	—
NIOSH		
REL (10 hr TWA)		
Total Al dust	10	—
Respirable Al dust	5	—
Pyro powders	5	—
Welding fumes	5	—
Soluble salts	2	—
Alkyls	2	—
STEL (15 min TWA)	—	—
IDLH	—	—
ACGIH		
TLV (8 hr TWA)		
Total Al dust	10	—
Respirable Al dust	5	—
Pyro powders	5	—
Welding fumes	5	—
Soluble salts	2	—
Alkyls	2	—
STEL (15 min TWA)	—	—
USEPA		
MCL	—	—
MCLG	—	—
SMCL		0.05–0.2

aUnit conversion: 1 mg/L = 1 ppm.
OSHA, Occupational Safety and Health Administration; PEL, permissible exposure level; TWA, time-weighted-average; NIOSH, National Institute for Occupational Safety and Health; REL, recommended exposure limit; STEL, short-term exposure limit; IDLH, immediately dangerous to life and health level; ACGIH, American Conference of Governmental Industrial Hygienists; TLV, threshold limit value; USEPA, United States Environmental Protection Agency; MCL, maximum contamination level; MCLG, maximum contamination level goal; SMCL, secondary maximum contaminant level.
Data from *Amoore and Hautala, 1983; OSHA, 1995; ACGIH, 1995; EPA, 1996; NIOSH, 1997.

al., 1991; Greger, 1992). Only 9 μg/day (range: 3 to 15 μg/day) are taken up through the respiratory tract (Jones and Benett, 1985). Particles that are not absorbed are either entrapped by alveolar macrophages and remain indefinitely in the lungs, or are moved back up the respiratory tract by cilia to the oral pharynx where they can be swallowed (Ganrot, 1986; Alfrey, 1989). The average daily oral intake of aluminum is 25 mg (range: 1 to 100 mg/day; Greger, 1992; van der Voet, 1992). Only a small amount (0.1 to 0.5%) of the ingested aluminum load is absorbed into the blood (Recker et al., 1977; Kaehny et al., 1977b; Ganrot, 1986); a considerable amount is absorbed into the intestinal mucosa where it remains until the cells die and slough off (Ganrot, 1986). Gastrointestinal (GI) absorption is increased in persons with normal renal function during periods of high exposure (Eastwood et al., 1990). Renal failure results in greater GI uptake and retention (Cam et al., 1976; Ittel et al., 1987).

The GI absorption of aluminum is dependent partly on the acidity of the gastric secretions and their ability to dissolve aluminum compounds (Eastwood et al., 1990; Ecelbarger and Greger, 1991; Greger, 1992). At normal stomach acidity, citrate appears to be the most important modulator of aluminum absorption, involving passive paracellular pathways and mechanisms (Slanina et al., 1986; Alfrey, 1992). Enhancement of uptake and elevated plasma levels was demonstrated in rabbits following administration of an oral antacid containing aluminum hydroxide, aluminum citrate, or aluminum maltolate to (3.2-fold by the hydroxide, 2.7-fold by the citrate, and an impressive 52-fold by the aluminum maltolate) (Kruck and McLachlan, 1988). Dietary fluoride, iron, silicic acid, and calcium contents also affect the absorption and retention of aluminum in body tissues (Lote and Saunders, 1991; Lukiw and McLachlan, 1995).

Absorption of aluminum also occurs through the nasal mucosa (Roberts, 1986; Perl and Good, 1987). Aluminum acetate solution, a common astringent, is used to treat dermal inflammation. There is no evidence that aluminum can be absorbed through the skin even at high levels of exposure (Alfrey, 1989).

Tissue Distribution

Aluminum in blood is mostly (85%) bound to plasma proteins; a portion is bound to proteins with a molecular mass greater than 8,000 da; the remainder is non-protein bound and is ultrafilterable (Kaehny et al., 1977a; Kovalchik et al., 1978; Lundin et al., 1978; Trapp, 1983; Leung et al., 1985; Cochran et al., 1985; Day et al., 1991). Plasma proteins have a limited ability to bind aluminum (Kovalchik et al., 1978). The percentage of non-protein-bound ultrafilterable aluminum is increased in patients on hemodialysis who are ingesting aluminum-containing phosphate binding gels (Leung et al., 1985). Following acute aluminum loading and plasma protein saturation, aluminum begins to translocate to other tissues such as the parenchymal organs, muscle, and bone (Kovalchik et al., 1978; Crapper and De Boni, 1983).

Most aluminum in serum is bound to transferrin and albumin (Trapp, 1983; Leung et al., 1985; Martin, 1986). Aluminum complexed with transferrin or other plasma proteins can access the central nervous system (CNS) through systems normally operative for iron transport (Trapp, 1983; Goldstein and Betz, 1986; Xu et al., 1992). In addition, aluminum bound to amino acids, such as glutamate, a normal constituent of blood plasma and a neurotransmitter, crosses

from the bloodstream into the brain as an aluminum–glutamate complex (Deloncle et al., 1990). Aluminum also disrupts membrane phospholipids, allowing it to cross the BBB by passive translocation (Viestra and Haug, 1978; De Boni et al., 1980; Banks and Kastin, 1983; Ohtawa et al., 1983; Cutrufo et al., 1984; Banks and Kastin, 1985a,b; Wen and Wisniewski, 1985; Gutteridge et al., 1985; Deleers et al., 1986; Zatta et al., 1989, 1991; Kruck et al., 1991).

In humans, aluminum concentrates in bone, spleen, liver, muscle tissue, and lungs, with the highest concentrations found in the respiratory epithelium (Recker et al., 1977; Crapper and De Boni, 1983; Eastwood et al., 1990). Tissue concentrations (dry weight), measured by flameless atomic absorption, range from a mean high of 43 mg/kg for the lungs, to 1 to 4.1 mg/kg in the heart, muscle, brain (gray matter), spleen, bone, and liver (Alfrey, 1983). Retention is influenced by parathyroid hormone activity and dietary calcium (Mayor et al., 1977; Crapper and De Boni, 1983; Slanina et al., 1984; Alfrey, 1989; Ecelbarger and Greger, 1991). Tissue stores of aluminum increase in the brain and the lung with aging (McDermott et al., 1979; Alfrey, 1980).

Aluminum levels in all tissues are increased in uremic patients, whether nondialyzed or chronically dialyzed, when compared with control subjects (Alfrey, 1980; Andreoli et al., 1984). Brain aluminum is significantly higher in the gray matter of dialysis patients dying with dialysis encephalopathy than in dialysis patients dying of other causes and not diagnosed with encephalopathy, with average concentrations of 25 μg/g and 6.5 μg/g dry weight, respectively (Alfrey et al., 1976; Alfrey, 1986). The concentrations of aluminum are highest in the hippocampus (5.6 μg/g dry weight) and lowest in the corpus callosum (1.5 μg/g dry weight). The brain aluminum concentration in patients with dialysis encephalopathy is about five times greater than that in Alzheimer's disease (McDermott et al., 1978). The intracellular distribution of aluminum in experimental aluminum-induced encephalopathy and Alzheimer's disease is largely associated with chromatin of glia and large neurons, whereas aluminum is found in the cytoplasm (lysosomes) of the brain cells of patients dying of renal failure after receiving dialysis (McDermott et al., 1979; Lukiw and McLachlan, 1995).

An aluminum concentration of 2.5 μg/g (wet weight) was found in the brain of a person dying after aluminum leached from an aluminum-containing bone cement into the cerebrospinal fluid. The aluminum concentration in the brain of an unexposed control was 0.85 μg/g (Hantson et al., 1995). Electron microscopic examination of brain cells taken from the frontal cortex of a patient dying following a similar incident revealed lysosomes containing aluminum microparticles (Renard et al., 1994).

Tissue Biochemistry

Aluminum serves no known function in the human body and is not considered an essential trace element (Underwood, 1971). Aluminum exists only in the oxidation state Al^{3+} and has no oxidation–reduction chemistry under physiological conditions. Aluminum cannot be removed or manipulated by *oxidoreductive* processes, as can other biologically useful trivalent metals, such as iron (Lukiw and McLachlan, 1995). In addition, aluminum has a very small ionic radius and a strong polarizing effect on adjacent atoms (Ganrot, 1986; Martin, 1986). This makes it a strong acceptor of electrons and accounts for its preferential binding with oxygen donor groups. In biological systems, aluminum associates preferentially with phosphate and carboxylate (Lukiw and McLachlan, 1995).

The actions of aluminum within the body are dependent on its affinity to each of the ligands present, the relative availability of each ligand, and its metabolism. Because of a very high affinity for proteins, polynucleotides, and glycosaminoglycans, much of the biologically available aluminum binds to these ligands, forming macromolecular complexes. These substances are metabolically less active than the smaller, low molecular weight complexes formed by aluminum with phosphates, nucleotides, and amino acids. These later complexes metabolize slowly, which is why the toxicity may go unrecognized in short experiments (Ganrot, 1986). In some cases, aluminum forms complexes that are highly stable and are essentially permanent, such as when aluminum binds to the chromatin of cells (Ganrot, 1986; Martin, 1992; Lukiw and McLachlan, 1995).

Biochemical interactions of aluminum affect changes in a variety of ways: (a) *nuclear effects,* which increase histone–DNA binding, block adenosine diphosphate (ADP) ribosylation, alter sister chromatid exchange, decrease cell division and alter deoxynucleic acid (DNA) synthesis; (b) *cytoplasmic effects,* which decrease cellular respiration, induce changes in calmodulin, elevate cyclic adenosine monophosphate (cAMP) and cyclic guanosine monophospate (cGMP) levels, and alter iron storage by binding to transferrin; (c) *cytoskeletal effects,* such as disruption of axonal transport, altered phosphorylation of cytoskeletal proteins, and neurofibrillary degeneration; (d) *membrane effects,* which alter the physical properties of membrane lipids, enhance brain-specific lipid peroxidation, increase permeability of the BBB to neuropeptides; and (e) *synaptic and neurotransmitter effects,* which inhibit choline acetyltransferase activity and reduce acetylcholine levels. Other changes due to biochemical interactions include decreased acetylcholine binding at muscarinic receptors; reductions in the level of tyrosine hydroxylase with associated reductions in norepinephrine and dopamine; and blockage of GABA, glycine, and glutamate uptake (Crapper-McLachlan, 1989; Meiri et al., 1992). In addition, aluminum promotes the aggregation of synthetic amyloid β-protein and the deposition of amyloid on cell surfaces (Kuroda and Kawahara, 1994) and also may modulate properties of paired helical filaments in the formation of the neurofibrillary tangles and plaques in Alzheimer's disease (Shin et al., 1994) (see Neuropathological Diagnosis section).

Excretion

After ingestion, unabsorbed aluminum is excreted in feces, reaching levels of about 96% of the daily oral intake (Cam et al., 1976; Gorsky et al., 1979; Greger and Baier, 1983). In humans with normal renal function, 0.09% and 96% of the daily aluminum intake is excreted in urine and feces, respectively (Greger and Baier, 1983). Normal urinary excretion of aluminum is 0.02 to 0.05 mg a day (Ganrot, 1986). Individuals excrete the amount of aluminum absorbed that is consistent with their renal clearance (Alfrey, 1989). Renal clearance is greater when there is a larger volume of urine output (Schlatter, 1992). Excretion is decreased in patients with compromised renal functions (Alfrey, 1980; Recker et al., 1977). Urinary concentration reflects the current level as well as the duration of exposure (Sjögren et al., 1985). The half-life for urinary aluminum in welders exposed for less than 1 year is approximately 9 days, and the half-life in welders exposed for more than 10 years is at least 6 months, indicating that aluminum is stored in at least two tissue compartments and that elimination from these compartments occurs at different rates (Sjögren et al., 1988). Urinary aluminum concentrations were found to be 80 to 90 times higher in aluminum-exposed workers who were actively exposed to aluminum flake than in the nonexposed controls and no-longer-exposed aluminum workers–retirees (Ljunggren et al., 1991).

CLINICAL MANIFESTATIONS AND DIAGNOSIS

Symptomatic Diagnosis

The clinical manifestations following exposure to aluminum are influenced by the circumstances of exposure—whether occupational, environmental, or in association with renal failure. A syndrome known as *potroom palsy,* which is characterized by incoordination, poor memory, impairment of abstract reasoning, and depression has been described among aluminum smelter workers (Longstreth et al., 1985). An epidemiological investigation was conducted after potroom syndrome was reported in 25 aluminum smelting factory workers who were exposed to aluminum vapors from pots that were not properly vented for many years of operation prior to 1972, when the company began the process of installing venting hoods on the pots; installation of the pot venting hoods was completed 2 years later (Longstreth et al., 1985; Woods et al., 1989; Clapp et al., 1992; White et al., 1992, 1993; Proctor et al., 1995). The ambient air contained aluminum dust and vapors. An exposure index was calculated for each worker based on level and duration of exposure pre- and post-1972.

Self-reported CNS symptoms were found among the disability claimants and among those determined to have been highly exposed. The most common self-reported complaint was loss of balance (88%) (Table 8-2) (White et al., 1992, 1993); the deficit noted most frequently about the workers by their spouses was poor memory. Three individuals

TABLE 8-2. *Most frequently reported symptoms among 25 aluminum workers*

Symptom	Proportion of workers reporting symptom
Loss of balance	22/25
Memory loss	21/25
Joint pain	21/25
Dizziness	20/25
Numbness	20/25
Severe weakness	20/25
Poor concentration	19/25
Disturbed sleep	19/25
Parasthesias	18/25
Tremor	17/25
Headache	17/25
Anxiety	15/25
Cough	11/25

Modified from White et al., 1992, with permission.

(aged 43, 44, and 49 years old) who had worked under these conditions for 12 to 16 years reported dizziness, joint pain, severe lack of energy and strength, frequent loss of balance, and tremor. In addition, two of these three patients reported severe headaches, trouble sleeping, remembering, and concentrating; they also described "pins and needles." The critical (first) symptom to appear in each patient was incoordination. The differential diagnosis in these three most severely affected workers had included multiple sclerosis, but aluminum toxicity was deemed the most likely cause of their symptoms. Testing of motor functions in all patients revealed incoordination, intention tremor, dyssynergy of upper limb movement, and ataxic gait (potroom palsy) in 21 workers. Somatosensory function was normal in each patient. The exposure index for the period before 1972 correlated significantly with signs and symptoms of incoordination, but not for other symptoms or for the scores on the neuropsychological tests administered (White et al., 1992, 1993) (see Neuropsychological Diagnosis section).

Aluminum welders with a mean exposure duration of 17 years and median urinary concentrations of 22 μg/L reported a variety of CNS complaints, with excessive fatigue being the most common (Sjögren et al., 1996) (see Clinical Experiences section). At higher urine aluminum concentrations (mean: 250 μg/L), with a mean exposure duration of 13 years, exposed aluminum welders reported depression and difficulty with concentration (Sjögren et al., 1990, 1996).

Aluminum leached from a bone reconstruction cement (Ionocap LV) into the cerebrospinal fluid of a 54-year-old woman who underwent a right vestibular neurectomy, resulting in an encephalopathy characterized by agitation, confusion, myoclonic jerks, grand mal seizures, obtundation, and coma and culminating in death (Hantson et al., 1994, 1995).

On postoperative day 7, confusion and altered consciousness appeared. Left-sided tonic–clonic seizures developed on day 36 and soon evolved into generalized and intractable convulsions, which persisted as status epilepticus for the remainder of the patient's life until she died 80 days after the surgery. Unsuccessful therapeutic interventions included deferoxamine for 10 days from days 50 through 60, as well as administration of major antiepileptic agents. Documentation of the toxicological data from days 45 to 67 revealed the apparent aluminum body burden. Aluminum concentration in the urine increased and that in the cerebrospinal fluid (CSF) decreased after deferoxamine administration (Table 8-3). Although the postmortem microscopic examination of brain tissue in this case was unremarkable, the aluminum concentration in the brain was 2.5 μg/g (wet weight), compared with a concentration of 0.85 μg/g in the brain tissue from an unexposed cadaver (Hantson et al., 1995).

Although other instances of surgery using this aluminum-containing bone cement compound have gone without incident, and laboratory tests indicate its safety if used without access to the CSF (Reusche et al., 1995), the mechanism suggested for the encephalopathy and epileptogenesis in this case (see Clinical Experiences section) was leaching of aluminum from the unstable Ionocap LV bone cement into the CSF, allowing the aluminum subsequent access to cerebral cortical neurons. The delay of 30 to 60 days between the introduction of bone cement and clinical en-

TABLE 8-3. *Evidence of aluminum body burden following surgical bone reconstruction[a]*

Post-op day:	45	47	50[b]	53	57	58	60[b]	67
Al urine								
μg/L	92.9		51.7	78		109		206
μg/g creatinine	172.04		99.4	159.2		330.3		226.3
creatinine g/L	0.54		0.52	0.49		0.33		0.91
Al serum								
μg/100 mL	4.4	1.8	1.9	1.7	2.0	2.9	2.6	3.1
Al CSF								
μg/L	63	37		35	41			3.7

CSF, cerebrospinal fluid.
[a]Intraoperative use of an Al-containing bone cement in a case of probable toxic effect of bone cement.
[b]Ten-day course of chelation with deferoxamine started and stopped.
Modified from Hantson et al., 1995, with permission.

cephalopathy is similar to the latency seen between application of aluminum hydroxide to the cerebral cortex of experimental animals and the resulting induced epileptogenesis (Kopeloff et al., 1942, 1954; Katz, 1985).

The clinical presentation of renal failure with uremic encephalopathy begins with fatigue, drowsiness, inability to concentrate, and mild disturbances of mentation and cognition. As the severity of the syndrome progresses, the patient experiences further impairment of memory function, disorientation, and hallucinations. Eventually the patient develops dysarthria–dyspraxia of speech, myoclonus, focal and generalized seizures, coma, and ultimately death. Electroencephalograph (EEG) abnormalities generally precede clinical manifestations by several months (Glaser, 1974) (see Neurophysiological Diagnosis section). Although encephalopathy and death may occur in the most severe cases, with high blood and urine nitrogen levels, most of the symptoms resulting from uremia are reversible with the initiation of dialysis. Residual neurological deficits in well-dialyzed patients, although generally subtle, show wide variability; the adequacy of the dialysis plays an important role in the occurrence and severity of the CNS disturbances (Lazarus et al., 1996).

A syndrome known as dialysis encephalopathy (DES) has been described in uremic patients treated with intermittent hemodialysis (Alfrey et al., 1976). The signs and symptoms of DES may be exacerbated by dialysis and deferoxamine treatment (Llach and Bover, 1996). Although the cause of DES remains controversial, the syndrome has been attributed to the aluminum content of the dialysis water and to the orally ingested aluminum-containing phosphate-binding gels used to control blood phosphorous levels (Garrett et al., 1988; Alfrey, 1989; Altmann et al., 1989). Treatment of dialysate water and the avoidance of aluminum-containing phosphate binders have decreased the incidence of DES (Lazarus et al., 1996). Nevertheless, DES is still reported in uremic patients receiving dialysis with deionized water and in uremic patients who were treated with orally ingested aluminum-containing phosphate binders, but who were not receiving dialysis, indicating that retention of aluminum is increased in persons with renal insufficiency (Nathan and Pedersen, 1980; Rotundo et al., 1982; Sedman et al., 1984; Alfrey, 1989; Murray et al., 1991). Deionization of the dialysate removes other metals including mercury, lead, thallium, and tin, many of which produce a similar constellation of symptoms at toxic levels. Therefore, because of the similarities between DES and metabolic encephalopathies, as well as the possible accumulation of other potentially toxic metals in the patient with renal failure, proper diagnosis depends on the exclusion of other causes of CNS dysfunction (Fraser and Arieff, 1988).

The occurrence of dementia due to *probable* Alzheimer's disease, *possible* Alzheimer's disease, other dementias, and epilepsy in 88 county districts within England and Wales was studied in relation to the relative concentrations of aluminum found in each district's drinking water (Martyn et al., 1989). County district water records for the previous 10 years were obtained, and categorical estimates of mean water aluminum concentrations were determined. The risk of Alzheimer's disease was estimated to be 1.5 times higher in districts where the mean water aluminum concentration exceeded 0.11 mg/L than in districts where concentrations were less than 0.01 mg/L.

A dementing syndrome accompanied by parkinsonism-like motor dysfunction and muscle atrophy suggesting motor neuron disease (amyotrophic lateral sclerosis–Parkinson's disease dementia complex) has been observed in people living in an area of the southwest Pacific Ocean, where the soil and water have high levels of aluminum and manganese and extremely low levels of calcium and magnesium (Perl et al., 1982; Spencer, 1987). A causal relationship has been implied, but toxicity by aluminum or manganese has not been proven.

Neurophysiological Diagnosis

Electroencephalography documented the effects of direct aluminum toxicity in a 55-year-old man who experienced confusion and seizures with encephalopathy, resulting from CSF contact with aluminum that had apparently leached from an aluminum-containing bone cement following otoneurosurgery. His EEG was characterized by triphasic slow waves (Renard et al., 1994). Alterations in EEG are also seen in primates following topical application of aluminum hydroxide to the cerebral sensorimotor cortex (Kopeloff et al., 1954). Dose-dependent changes seen in the quantitative EEG of welders with mean urine aluminum concentrations of 76 µg/L and a mean exposure duration of 4 years included a decrease in alpha activity and an increase in theta and delta activity in the frontal area (Hänninen et al., 1994). Similar EEG abnormalities were also reported in aluminum welders by Sjögren et al. (1996). When evaluating the EEG of uremic patients with presumed DES, it is important to consider that other possible toxins associated with uremia can produce similar changes (Glaser, 1976; Fraser and Arieff, 1988). The EEG seen in patients with DES must be distinguished from that of uremic encephalopathy. The EEG of patients with DES is characterized by the presence of high-amplitude delta (slow) activity with bilateral spikes and sharp waves, intermixed with runs of more normal background activity (Hughes and Schreeder, 1980; Alfrey, 1986; Lazarus et al., 1996) (Fig. 8-1). Bilateral spike activity was found in 85% of the EEGs performed on patients presenting with clinical DES (Schreeder et al., 1983).

Visual evoked potentials (VEPs) in an aluminum foundry potroom worker exposed to aluminum for 12 years revealed delayed VEPs bilaterally, indicating disease of the optic nerve. This worker also had delayed somatosensory evoked potentials, suggesting CNS disease at the level of the medulla (Longstreth et al., 1985). Changes in both EEG and

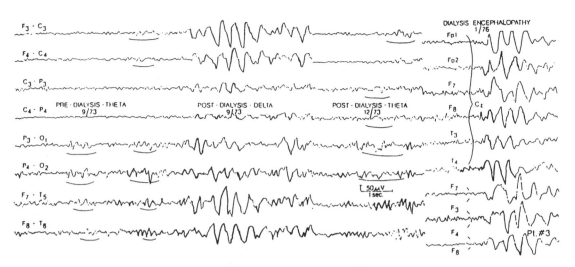

FIG. 8-1. Serial electroencephalographic studies in a patient with renal failure, demonstrating theta activity predialysis (far left), delta and theta activity postdialysis (center), and diffuse delta bursts after onset of dialysis encephalopathy (far right). (From Hughes and Schreeder, 1980, with permission.)

VEP were found in cats with aluminum encephalopathy experimentally induced by intracranial injection of aluminum (Crapper and Dalton, 1973; Crapper, 1974). Although changes in VEP have not been conclusively related to aluminum in dialysis encephalopathy, prolonged VEP latencies have been reported in uremic patients receiving hemodialysis and on peritoneal dialysis (Hughes et al., 1980).

Brainstem auditory evoked potentials (BAEPs) and event-related BAEPs (P-300) were measured in a group of 38 aluminum welders and compared with 39 unexposed controls (Sjögren et al., 1996). Latencies of P-300 did not differ significantly between the groups and were reported to be 311.4 msec in the welders and 309.4 msec in the controls. In addition, no differences were found for BAEP latencies between the exposed welders and the unexposed controls.

Nerve conduction studies in dialysis patients may reveal slowing due to neuropathy associated with chronic renal disease and azotemia (Jebsen et al., 1967) and are not necessarily attributable to aluminum toxicity.

Neuropsychological Diagnosis

The results of neuropsychological testing of individuals or groups of aluminum-exposed persons provide clinical and epidemiological information about the neurobehavioral effects of aluminum in individuals at risk of occupational exposure or increased environmental intake and in patients with renal failure.

Tremorography can be used to assess tremor in the upper and lower extremities of aluminum-exposed individuals. A cross-sectional tremorography study of 63 current ($n = 52$) and former ($n = 11$) aluminum potroom workers exposed to aluminum concentrations below the OSHA PEL did not reveal an increase in tremor frequency or amplitude when

findings were compared with those of 37 unexposed controls (Dick et al., 1997). These findings are in contrast to those of Bast-Pettersen et al. (1994), who did find a significant increase in tremor among aluminum workers when using the static steadiness test of the Halstead-Reitan battery as a measure of tremor (see Neuropsychological Diagnosis section).

Occupational Exposure

Psychomotor and intellectual abilities were assessed in 87 aluminum foundry workers (mean age: 40.7 years), who had been exposed to total ambient air dust levels of 4.6 to 11.5 mg/m³ for more than 6 years. Sixty unexposed control subjects matched for age, job seniority, and social status, as well as alcohol and drug use, were also tested. Mean urine and blood levels of the exposed workers were 45 μg/L and 137 μg/L, respectively. Total body burden of aluminum, determined in both groups by deferoxamine challenge, was found to be significantly higher in the exposed group. The possibility of toxicity resulting from an increased body burden of lead, manganese, zinc, copper, cadmium, iron, and fluoride was excluded based on blood and urine levels determined prior to and following administration of deferoxamine. Simple and complex reaction times, and performance on subscales of the Wechsler Adult Intelligence Scale (WAIS) and the Bender Visual Motor Test were assessed. All the exposed workers had impaired memory ability. In addition, the exposed group had significantly greater impairments in oculomotor coordination and prolonged complex reaction times, as well as diminished attention efficiency, mental control, and visual–motor coordination. The intelligence quotients (IQ), verbal abilities, simple reaction time, and efficiency of verbal problem solving were not significantly different between the exposed and nonexposed groups (Hosovski et al., 1990).

The neuropsychological performance of 14 aluminum smelter potroom workers and 8 aluminum foundry workers was compared with that of 16 nonexposed age matched control subjects in a cross-sectional study. The mean age for the aluminum workers and the control subjects was 63 years. Mean exposure duration for both groups of aluminum workers was 19 years. Total dust concentrations in the potroom ranged from 3.0 to 9.5 mg/m³; the average aluminum content in the total dust in the potroom was approximately 20% by weight. Mean urine aluminum concentrations for the potroom workers, the foundry workers and the controls were 12.6, 9.9, and 7.8 µg/L, respectively, although urinary concentrations of 54 and 32 µg/L determined respectively in groups of younger potroom and foundry workers from the same company may better reflect the average exposure of the older workers prior to application for retirement. Neurobehavioral functions assessed included intelligence, memory and learning, reaction time, psychomotor speed and efficiency, motor and sensory function, and neuropsychiatric symptoms. Testing of motor capacities revealed a subclinical tremor in the potroom workers, which significantly impaired performance on the Static Steadiness Test. Performance on tests of psychomotor skill and speed did not differ significantly between the groups (Bast-Pettersen et al., 1994). Tests of motor function were also used to assess the possible effects of exposure in 38 welders whose median urinary level was 59 µg/L. The performance of the welders was impaired on two of the Luria-Nebraska Motor Scales tasks (numbers 3 and 4), finger tapping speed, and the dominant hand on the pegboard test (Sjögren et al., 1996) (see Clinical Experiences section).

The question of whether or not persons with prior occupational exposure to aluminum might develop dementia of the Alzheimer's type later in life was considered in an epidemiological study of potroom workers in a large aluminum production plant (Longstreth et al., 1985; Woods et al., 1989; White et al., 1992, 1993; Proctor et al., 1995). Twenty-five workers were referred to the occupational medicine clinic for evaluation of suspected work-related illness (potroom palsy), 21 of whom had worked in the potroom, where aluminum oxide is reduced by electrolysis (White et al., 1992). High levels of aluminum particulate were emitted from the smelting pots, which had not been properly vented for many years of operation prior to 1974 when hoods were installed (Longstreth et al., 1985; Woods et al., 1989; Clapp and Coogan, 1992; White et al., 1992, 1993; Proctor et al., 1995). Neuropsychological, neurological, and electrophysiological examinations were performed on three workers who had worked in the potroom for at least 12 years. The neuropsychological test battery included the WAIS–revised (R), the Wechsler Memory Scale (WMS), and tests of problem-solving ability. The WAIS-R revealed low verbal (range: 67 to 97), performance (range: 78 to 87), and full-scale IQ scores (range: 71 to 93). WMS memory quotients ranged from 62 to 97. The performances of these three men were below expectation on tests of short-term memory and visual motor speed tasks. Severe impairment of problem-solving ability was noted in two of the three patients; the third showed mild to moderate impairment (Longstreth et al., 1985).

Neuropsychological evaluation was also performed on 20 of the 25 referred workers from the original study group and included the WAIS-R, Wide Range Achievement Test-Revised, Halstead-Reitan Neuropsychologic Battery (HRNB), and the Minnesota Multiphasic Personality Inventory (MMPI). Logical memory was assessed by immediate and 30-minute delayed recall of short stories. Immediate recall was impaired in 30% and delayed recall in 20% of the workers. Visual memory was measured by immediate and 30-minute delayed reproduction of pictorial designs and revealed impairment of immediate reproduction in 40% of the workers; 30% showed impairment on the delayed reproduction tests. On the HRNB, the workers showed impairment of speech perception (61%); memory for tactile–spatial information (53%); abstract reasoning (37%); and sustained concentration (23%). MMPI revealed depression in 17 of 19 workers tested (White et al., 1992, 1993).

Although an early investigation of workers from this same aluminum smelting plant by Woods et al. (1989) confirmed that the potroom workers were exposed to the highest levels of aluminum in the shop, an evaluation of the medical records of the disability claimants did not reveal unequivocal evidence of an occupationally related CNS health condition. However, serial follow-up assessments (Clapp and Coogan, 1992; Proctor et al., 1995) of these workers concluded that there is an increased risk for symptoms of potroom palsy and for depression-related symptoms in individuals who worked for more than 3 years in the potroom prior to 1974. However, the potroom workers did not develop evidence of Alzheimer's type dementia even though they had been exposed to high levels of aluminum in fumes and dust for many years.

Dialysis Encephalopathy

Sprague et al. (1988) administered neuropsychological tests (to assess levels of dementia, depression, and memory and language difficulties) to 16 patients with chronic renal failure to determine if a relationship exists between the appearance of neurobehavioral impairments and the use of intermittent hemodialysis. Tests used included the following: the Mini-Mental State Examination for assessment of general dementia; the Serial Digit Learning Test for assessment of memory; subtests from the Multi-Lingual Aphasia Examination, to assess language skills; and the Geriatric Depression Scale, to assess depression. Scores were adjusted for age and education. Total body aluminum concentrations in these subjects were measured by a deferoxamine infusion test (DIT). A postinfusion rise in serum aluminum of greater than 125 µg/L was considered a positive result.

Patients were divided into two groups based on the response to the DIT (positive or negative), and groups were compared by one-way analysis of variance and the Mann–Whitney U test. All patients with a positive DIT exhibited myoclonus, asterixis, and lower extremity weakness. Furthermore, patients with a positive DIT also showed significant impairment in memory testing. Neurological abnormalities were identified in all patients. Among the patients with a positive DIT, the number of neurological signs and the severity subscore were elevated. No differences were noted between those with a positive DIT and those with a negative DIT on tests of dementia, depression, or language abilities. No significant correlation was found between sex, age, presence of diabetes, mode of dialysis, years of chronic renal failure, years of dialysis, or years of aluminum ingestion, and any neurological or neurobehavioral measurement, serum aluminum level, or DIT. These changes may represent early aluminum exposure–associated neurologic dysfunction.

Biochemical Diagnosis

The ubiquitous availability of aluminum in the environment raises suspicion about earlier published data regarding "normal" or background aluminum levels in blood (Murray et al., 1991; WHO, 1994). A biological exposure index for occupational exposure to aluminum has not been established by the ACGIH (1995) (Table 8-4). Zapatero et al. (1995) found that serum aluminum levels increased with aging in healthy people, suggesting the possibility of decreased excretion or increased retention of aluminum with normal aging. Furthermore, serum levels are higher in patients with probable Alzheimer's disease than in healthy age-matched controls and in patients with other dementias (alcoholic, vascular, multiinfarct). Minor symptoms and subtle deficits in psychomotor function have been observed in persons without renal failure at mean serum aluminum levels of 59 μg/L (whole blood level of 64 μg/L) and a urinary concentration of 330 μg/L. Occasionally patients with chronic renal failure who are not receiving dialysis therapy or who had been dialyzed only with dialysate containing less than 10 μg/L develop encephalopathy.

Neurobehavioral features have been observed in hemodialysis patients whose serum aluminum concentrations

exceed 200 μg/L (De Broe and Coburn, 1990). The combination of impaired renal function and dietary exposure is sufficient to raise serum aluminum and probably contributes to the appearance of DES (Murray et al., 1991). However, serum and tissue aluminum concentrations are not always well correlated, and therefore random serum and urine aluminum levels are not sensitive enough to predict the degree of neurotoxicant effects in dialysis patients with dementia (Alfrey, 1986). Aluminum concentrations in blood and excreted in urine following provocative chelation with deferoxamine, an iron chelator that also removes aluminum, can be used to detect an increased body burden of aluminum (Milliner et al., 1984; Coburn and Norris, 1986; Abreo, 1988; Sprague et al., 1988; Salusky et al., 1991).

Exposure to aluminum welding fumes at a concentration of 7.0 mg/m³ for 8 hours increases urinary excretion from 3 μg/L (basal) to more than 100 μg/L after 1 day of exposure (Sjögren and Elinder, 1992). Urinary concentrations are also increased with chronic exposure (Sjögren et al., 1985). Based on occupational testing of postshift urine samples in welders, a serum level of 60 μg/L and a urinary concentration of 330 μg/L correspond to an ambient air level of 4.9 mg/m³ for 20 years, or 1.6 mg/m³ for 40 years and serve as good indicators of exposure to aluminum (Sjögren and Elinder, 1992).

Neuroimaging

Computed tomography (CT) and magnetic resonance imaging (MRI) can be used to demonstrate cortical atrophy and enlarged ventricles in a suspected case of Alzheimer's disease and to differentiate cases of metabolic, vascular, and other etiologies of dementia from those of neurotoxic origin (McKhann et al., 1984). The T2-weighted MRI image of a patient whose CSF was contaminated with aluminum that had leached from an aluminum-containing bone cement showed high-intensity signals in the frontobasal area, cingulum, limbic temporal cortex, and insula (Renard et al., 1994) (Fig. 8-2). MRI of a potroom worker exposed to aluminum revealed multiple hyperintensities in the white matter (White et al., 1992). CT and MRI also permit the exclusion of subdural hematomas, brain tumors, and hydrocephalus and give evidence of other diffuse myelinopathies, such as multiinfarct states.

TABLE 8-4. *Biological exposure indices for aluminum*

	Urine	Blood	Alveolar air
Determinant	Aluminum	Aluminum	Aluminum
Start of shift	Not established	Not established	Not established
During shift	Not established	Not established	Not established
End of shift at end of workweek	Not established	Not established	Not established

Data from ACGIH, 1995.

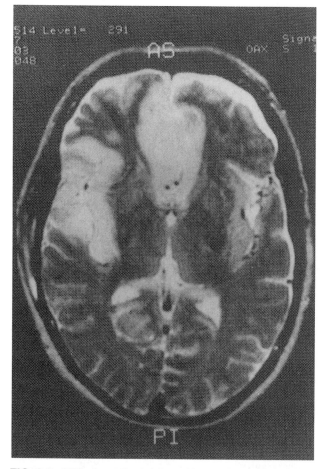

FIG. 8-2. MRI of a patient dying with encephalopathy attributed to an aluminum-containing bone cement shows high-intensity signals in the frontobasal area, cingulum, limbic temporal cortex, and insula (modified from Renard et al., 1994, with permission).

Neuropathological Diagnosis

Postmortem studies in cases of confirmed aluminum intoxication are rare. One report described a patient who died after a severe encephalopathic reaction to aluminum that leaked into his CSF after intracranial surgical use of an aluminum-containing bone cement during a vestibular neurectomy. Although aluminum concentration was elevated in the brain of this patient and brain swelling was present, microscopic examination was unremarkable, and neurofilaments appeared normal (Hantson et al., 1995) (see Symptomatic Diagnosis section).

Another case (Kobayashi et al., 1987) involved a man who had worked as an aluminum refiner for 30 years. Symptoms of dementia appeared at age 55 and progressed until he died of bronchopneumonia, 10 years after stopping his work. A postmortem examination revealed marked atrophy of the occipitotemporal lobes and senile plaques in the cerebellum. Accumulations of aluminum within the nucleus and cytoplasm of the neurofibrillary tangle-bearing

cortical neurons were demonstrated by wavelength-dispersive x-ray microanalysis. For comparison, a second patient with clinically and pathologically ascertained dementia of the Alzheimer's type, who had had no known intake of aluminum, was studied; microanalysis of brain tissue by the same method failed to disclose aluminum accumulation in the tangle-bearing neurons. Both cases exhibited clinical dementia and neurofibrillary tangles, but aluminum deposition in neurofibrillary tangles was found only in the one with known exposure.

Much of the aluminum neuropathology literature involves its possible relationship to Alzheimer's disease and dialysis encephalopathy. Aluminum has been found in the brain tissue of Alzheimer's patients, often at higher levels than in the brains of age-matched controls (Perl and Brody, 1980; Candy et al., 1986; Crapper et al., 1973) (Table 8-5). Aluminum has been detected in neurons containing neurofibrillary tangles (Perl and Brody, 1980). Furthermore, aluminum has been identified in the core of senile plaques (Candy et al., 1986). Experimental intracranial aluminum injection induces neurofibrillary degeneration in animals (Klatzo et al., 1965; Wisniewski et al., 1985; Crapper and Dalton, 1973). Formation of PHF in cases of Alzheimer's disease occurs without aluminum deposition (Kobayashi et al., 1987).

In vitro, human neuroblastoma cells treated with aluminum form complexes with ethylene diaminetetraacetic acid that accept stain by an antibody to phosphorylated t-protein (Guy et al., 1991). In Alzheimer's disease, the concentration of the phosphorylated (insoluble) form of the cytoskeletal t-protein is increased within the senile plaques and the paired helical filaments (PHFs) of the neurofibrillary tangles; the soluble form of the cytoskeletal t-protein is decreased (Garruto and Brown, 1994; Harrington et al., 1994). However, the aluminum-induced neurofibrillary degeneration produced *in vitro* and *in vivo* is dissimilar from that of Alzheimer's disease, because in the former the filaments are in "tangles," not the PHFs characteristic of Alzheimer's disease (Ganrot, 1986; Perl et al., 1982; Wisniewski et al., 1985) (Fig. 8-3). Microscopic and electron microscopic views demonstrating the neuropathological differences in the microstructure of the neurofibrillary

TABLE 8-5. *Aluminum concentrations in brain tissue of Alzheimer's disease patients and controls[a]*

Normal	Alzheimer's Disease	Reference
2.5 ± 0.3	2.7 ± 0.2	McDermott et al., 1979
0.467 ± 0.33	0.372 ± 0.2	Markesbery et al., 1981
0.23–2.7	Up to 11.5	Crapper et al., 1973
1.9 ± 0.7	0.4–10.7	Crapper et al., 1976
0.83 ± 0.12	1.37 ± 0.27	Trapp et al., 1978
1.5	Above 4	Krishnan et al., 1988

[a] μg Al/g dry weight.
Modified from Meiri et al., 1993, with permission.

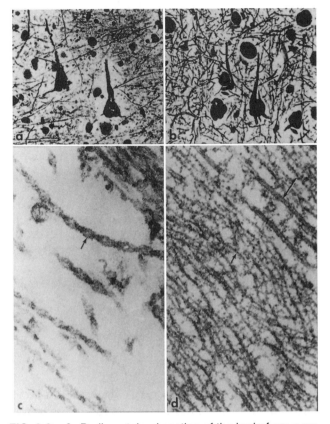

FIG. 8-3. A: Bodian-stained section of the brain from a patient with Alzheimer's disease showing neurons with neurofibrillary changes (*arrows*). **B:** Bodian stained section of a rabbit brain after intracisternal injection of aluminum chloride showing neurons with neurofibrillary changes (*arrows*). **C:** Electronmicroscopic view of paired helical neurofilaments associated with AD (*arrow*). **D:** Electronmicroscopic view of the tangles of neurofilaments induced by intracisternal injection of aluminum chloride (*upper arrow,* neurotubule; *lower arrow,* neurofilament) (see text) (modified from Wisniewski et al., 1985, with permission).

changes induced after intracisternal injection of aluminum in the rabbit brain and those associated with senile dementia of the Alzheimer's type in a human. Although neurons with neurofibrillary changes are visible on microscopic examination of tissue samples from the brains of both the rabbit after intracisternal injection of aluminum and in a patient with Alzheimer's disease, closer examination with the electronmicroscope reveals distinct differences in the ultrastructure of the neurofibrillary changes.

The truncation of τ-protein at Glu-391, a pathological finding in Alzheimer's disease, is also increased with increasing brain aluminum concentrations in renal dialysis patients (Harrington et al., 1994). Even though brain aluminum concentrations are in excess of levels that cause neurofibrillary degeneration in animals, aluminum-induced neurofibrillary degeneration is not found in cases of dialysis encephalopathy (Crapper and De Boni, 1983; Wisniewski et al., 1985; Crapper-MacLachlan, 1989; Harrington et al., 1994).

The pathogenesis of the premature occurrence of neurofibrillary tangles in otherwise neurologically normal people in the western Pacific region has been attributed to naturally occurring high levels of aluminum in their diet (Spencer, 1987). However, Kasarkis et al. (1995) did not find that aluminum concentrations were elevated in the ventral cervical spinal cords of five patients diagnosed with classic ALS when compared with five age-matched controls, in contrast to the reports from areas with indigenously high aluminum concentrations. Genetic vulnerability may be a factor in aluminum's ability to accelerate or prevent the formation of PHFs (Harrington et al., 1994).

The different solubility, stability, and hydroxylation characteristics exhibited by ligand-bound forms of aluminum are responsible for neurotoxic effects. Hydroxylated soluble polymers of aluminum, such as Al 13-28, are particularly toxic. In the range of physiological pH, the aluminate ion has a particularly high affinity for polyphosphates in biological systems, such as the cellular phosphoproteins, the internal and external face of membrane phospholipids, and the polyanionic phosphate backbone of nucleic acids (Karlik and Eichorn, 1989; Martin, 1992). Aluminum bound to acidic phospholipids, such as phosphatidylserine and phosphatidylcholine, may alter membrane properties (Wardle, 1983). Altered permeability of the BBB due to renal failure and subsequent aluminum overload may be the basis for the dialysis encephalopathy with dementia syndrome. Aluminum stimulates the peroxidation of membrane phospholipids by accelerating Fe^{2+}-dependent peroxidation (Gutteridge et al., 1985; Halliwell, 1989; Bondy et al., 1998). Aluminum also contributes to cellular oxidative stress by inhibiting the actions of superoxide dismutase, an enzyme that converts the highly reactive oxygen radical O_2^- into hydrogen peroxide and molecular oxygen (Ohtawa et al., 1983). Another target for aluminum appears to be the second-messenger cell proteins. The inhibitory effects of aluminum on the second messengers adenosine triphosphate (ATP), guanosine triphosphate (GTP), and inositol triphosphate, which are most likely due to their high phosphate content, have been demonstrated *in vitro* (Johnson and Jope, 1987, 1988; Johnson et al., 1990) and in Alzheimer's disease brains (Young et al., 1988). Aluminum also reacts with second-messenger binding proteins. For example, the GTP binding protein G_{av} is significantly inhibited by aluminum *in vitro* (Lukiw and McLachlan, 1995). The ATP-Al^{3+} may serve as an intracellular aluminum carrier, selectively shuttling this toxic element to highly specific aluminum-binding sites (Panchalingam et al., 1991). Aluminum-treated animals showed a decrease in acetylcholine receptor binding sites in the cerebral cortex, hippocampus, and corpus striatum (Julka et al., 1995). The greatest effect was observed in the hippocampus, raising the possibility that a decrease in the number of receptors in this region and the subsequent decreased transmission of nerve impulses may be responsible for neurobehavioral alterations observed following treatment with aluminum.

Plotkin and Jarvic (1986) suggest that there may be common impairments of acetylcholine (ACh) function in both Alzheimer's disease and following aluminum toxicity. For example, there is a substantial decrease in ACh following aluminum treatment rather than the expected increase in the level of ACh as a result of decreased acetylcholinesterase (AChE) activity. It is speculated that this decrease in ACh is due to either decreased recycling of choline back into the presynaptic nerve ending, or impairment of the activity of cholinacetyltransferase (ChAT). A substantial decrease (40%) in the activity of ChAT compared with controls was shown with chronic aluminum intoxication, raising the possibility that cholinotoxic effects following chronic *in vivo* administration of aluminum are a consequence of neuronal degeneration. The results indicate that the aluminum ions are not only equally potent in inducing impairment of ChAT activity and decreasing high-affinity choline uptake, but also reduce the activity of AChE, along with the level of ACh.

Although aluminum has been identified in the brains of patients with Alzheimer's disease, current opinion is that aluminum does not cause classical Alzheimer's disease, nor an effect on amyloid precursor protein expression or processing (Neill et al., 1996; Fine and Abraham, 1997).

PREVENTIVE AND THERAPEUTIC MEASURES

Because of the accumulation of aluminum and its potential for causing neurodegenerative changes, it has been suggested that the general population should limit its intake of this metal, especially older persons and those with renal disease (Zapatero et al., 1995). Proper ventilation of work areas, such as the potroom and fabricating facilities, is fundamental to the protection of workers at risk of exposure to vapors and dust containing aluminum compounds. Routine air sampling and blood and urine testing should be done to monitor levels of aluminum, with appropriate action taken at the point of recommended biological exposure indices. Those with diagnosed renal disease should be protected from exposure.

Aluminum blood levels should be monitored in persons at risk of exposure. In unexposed controls the blood level is less than 10 μg/L; concentrations over 60 μg/L in exposed persons may indicate the need for chelation therapy. Overt toxicity is often associated with blood levels of 200 μg/L. Patients with renal disease, whether on dialysis or not, should also be monitored for azotemia. EEG recordings can detect subclinical encephalopathy before any overt signs appear (Glaser, 1974; Alfrey, 1986). Use of antacids with aluminum should be restricted in persons with chronic indigestion, and the use of aluminum-based phosphate binders in chronic renal patients must be kept to a minimum. Dialysate aluminum content should not exceed 10 μg/L. Deferoxamine, 30 mg given intravenously 30 minutes before the end of dialysis, can be used to increase output of any accumulating aluminum. To enhance clearance of the deferoxamine–aluminum complex, dialysis should be performed using a high-flux membrane or with an activated charcoal filter in series with a conventional dialyzer (Lazarus et al., 1996). Repeated doses of deferoxamine given over several months reduce the body burden and in some cases reverse dialysis encephalopathy (Alfrey and Froment, 1990). Restricting intake of phosphorous and the use of calcium carbonate as a phosphate binder as an alternative to aluminum-containing phosphate binders has also been shown to decrease aluminum loading (Sedman et al., 1984). Ionomeric aluminum-containing bone cement is not recommended in those individuals with a history of renal insufficiency and when contact with the CSF can occur (Hantson et al., 1994). Removal of the cement is recommended in all symptomatic cases, and serum aluminum analysis and neurological assessment is suggested for asymptomatic patients who have had surgery involving the use of an aluminum-containing bone cement (Renard et al., 1994). Seizures should be treated with antiepileptics and correction of fluid and electrolyte levels (Lazarus et al., 1996).

CLINICAL EXPERIENCES

Group Studies

Exposure to Aluminum in Welding Fumes

The effects of aluminum on the nervous system were assessed in 38 welders (age range: 26 to 56 years) with at least 5 years of exposure to welding fumes containing aluminum (Sjögren et al., 1996). Welders were selected from companies from which information on exposure to aluminum welding fumes was available. Welders were exposed to aluminum during both metal inert gas (MIG) and tungsten inert gas (TIG) welding. The median exposure during MIG welding was 10 mg/m³. The average MIG welding time per year was 1,570 hours. Aluminum concentrations during TIG welding were 1 mg/m³. The welding time for TIG was divided by 10 to correspond to MIG welding exposure. The aluminum welders were compared with a control group consisting of 44 railway track welders (age range: 23 to 59 years) who were mainly exposed to iron and had a total of less than 25 hours of welding time exposure to aluminum, high-alloy manganese, steel, or lead. Samples of blood and urine were taken from each participant. Both welder groups were administered symptom questionnaires, and neuropsychological and neurophysiological assessments were performed. The welders exposed to aluminum reported more acute symptoms of the CNS than the control welders, with the most prominent symptom of the immediate past 6 months being fatigue.

The neuropsychological assessment included tests of short-term memory, verbal comprehension, perceptual speed, simple reaction time, finger tapping speed and endurance, psychomotor speed and coordination, eye–hand coordination, and olfactory threshold. The aluminum welders with the highest exposure (median urine aluminum concentration: 59 μg/L) were impaired on finger tapping speed in the nondominant hand. In addition, performance of the aluminum welders was impaired on tests of motor function (see Neuropsychological Diagnosis section). No significant impairment of performance was found in the other neurobehavioral domains assessed.

Neurophysiological examination included EEG, tests of diadochokinesis, and recordings of BAEPs and event-related auditory evoked potentials. EEGs were classified as normal or pathological. The proportion of pathological EEGs was 29% among the aluminum welders and only 13% among the control welders. Compared with the control welders, the welders exposed to aluminum had significantly higher amplitudes of the dominant hand on testing of rapid alternating movements (diadochokinesis). There were no differences in the latencies of BAEPs or event-related auditory evoked potentials between the welders exposed to aluminum and the control welders.

Dialysis Encephalopathy Syndrome

The medical records of 412 hemodialysis patients were reviewed. Thirty-eight (29 men and 9 women; 8.67%) fulfilled the diagnostic criteria for the dementia associated with aluminum dialysis encephalopathy syndrome (Garrett et al., 1988). These criteria included (a) a period of hemodialysis of at least 18 months or at least 150 hemodialysis sessions; (b) no other possible causes of neurological syndrome; (c) experience of two or more of the following symptoms: speech difficulty, seizures, myoclonus, or motor dyspraxia; and (d) more than five pathological fractures and/or positive aluminum staining of bone, or one of the above symptoms and three or more of the following signs/symptoms: change of mood, change in behavior, intellectual deterioration, episodic confusion related to dialysis, asterixis, serum aluminum level more than 50 μg/L, diffuse EEG abnormality, and blood transfusion on ten or more occasions over a 12-month period.

The most common neurological features included multifocal seizures ($n = 31$), disturbances of speech ($n = 30$), myoclonus ($n = 25$), gait disorder ($n = 24$), episodic confusion ($n = 22$), intellectual deterioration with poor concentration and short-term memory loss ($n = 21$), and change in personality and behavior ($n = 19$ patients). Bone pain was present in 29 patients, which accounted for many of the gait disorders. Eight of the male patients complained of impotence. The average length of time between the introduction of regular dialysis and the onset of the specific neurological syndrome was 40 months.

Nine of these patients were still alive, and seven were doing well, 35 months after successful renal transplantation; one was stable 30 months after the administration of two courses of deferoxamine for the diagnosis of aluminum encephalopathy. The other patients died after the introduction of regular dialysis 10 months after the onset of specific features of aluminum encephalopathy. These patients were very ill with renal failure and its complications, so the role played by aluminum, if any, must be considered in light of these other confounders.

Memory and Language Skills among the Elderly Exposed to Aluminum in Drinking Water

Memory and language skills were studied in 800 people between the ages of 81 and 85 who had been residents of particular districts of Zurich, Switzerland. Four hundred of these residents were from districts with low aluminum concentrations in their drinking water, and the remaining 400 were from districts with high aluminum concentrations in their drinking water. Efforts were made to ensure that each group was a valid cross section, and the possibility of the test's being skewed by a greater number of people from one or the other of the groups unwilling or unable to participate was considered unlikely. Each subject was given the mnestic and naming subtests of the Mini-Mental Status test. In addition, serum and urinary aluminum content and urinary aluminum-to-creatinine ratios were measured twice in ten clinically diagnosed Alzheimer's patients and ten controls in nursing homes in both high and low aluminum-in-water areas. A total of 12.3% of the entire test population was found to be demented, and no significant difference in incidence of dementia was found between the two groups. A consistent effect of residence in nursing homes with high or low aluminum in the drinking water could not be demonstrated (Wettstein et al., 1991).

Individual Case Studies

Aluminum Encephalopathy Following Inhalation of Aluminum Dust

A 49-year-old man who had been working in an aluminum powder factory for 13.5 years was found leaning against the wall of the workroom in a dazed and unresponsive state by his coworkers (McLaughlin et al., 1962). He remained symptomatic after that day and over the course of the next several months was reportedly forgetful and frequently had trouble finishing a conversation. However, because these symptoms did not impair his ability to perform his job, he continued to work. He began to experience brief (4-minute) attacks of clonic jerking during which he was unable to speak. Initially the attacks were infrequent and only affected his left leg, but later the left arm was involved as well and the frequency increased. Although the attacks were increasing in severity and frequency, he was not distressed by his disability and still continued to work. A clinical examination revealed mild dysarthria and weakness of the left arm and leg. EEG showed sustained high-voltage activity with a distribution that was generalized and symmetrical. However, no diagnosis was made, and the patient returned to work.

At follow-up 2 months later, the dysarthria and hemiparesis had worsened, a diagnosis of cerebral tumor was made, and the patient was admitted to the hospital. The neurological examination found the patient to be normally oriented, with no evidence of delusions or hallucinations. His speech was slurred and he was mildly dysphasic. His memory for recent events was slightly impaired. His reactions to stimulation were slow, and he had a mild left hemiparesis involving the face, arm, and leg. Tendon reflexes were increased in the left arm and leg as well. The left plantar response was equivocal. There was no objective sensory loss. The fundi were normal, and his visual fields were full. EEG showed high-voltage paroxysmal slow activity, but less than was seen at the initial examination. His blood pressure was 130/80, and there were no respiratory symptoms. Radiograph of the chest revealed slight abnormalities.

Over the course of the next 2 months, the patient had an increasing number of convulsive attacks. These were initially localized on the left side of the body but eventually developed into generalized convulsions that were followed by deep coma. The mental status of the patient continued to deteriorate, and he eventually died of bronchopneumonia.

On postmortem examination the cerebral vessels were healthy and there was no meningel thickening. The brain was edematous. The lateral ventricles were slightly dilated. No localized lesions were found. The spinal cord appeared normal on visual examination. Histological examination revealed no signs of vascular disease, syphilis, intracranial tumor, or inflammation, and nothing was seen to support a diagnosis of Pick's or Alzheimer's disease. This patient had no history of head injury or epilepsy and there was no evidence that he suffered from a deficiency disease. In addition, he had no history of alcohol or drug abuse. Sections of the brain and the lungs stained for aluminum gave positive results. Brain levels of aluminum were 17 times the normal concentration.

Based on the elevated levels of aluminum in the brain at postmortem examination, it was concluded that the progressive encephalopathy and cerebral degeneration seen in this worker were due to aluminum intoxication. Based on the elevated levels of aluminum in the lungs, the pulmonary fibrosis was attributed to aluminum as well.

Aluminum-Containing Parenteral Solutions: Seizures and Brain Aluminum Levels

A premature infant (24 weeks of gestation, 630 g) was parenterally fed solutions that contained aluminum (Bishop et al., 1989). This infant's average aluminum intake was determined to be 14 mg/day, with a total intake of aluminum from intravenous feeding of 645 mg. Convulsions occurred intermittently starting on day 10 until he died at age 3 months. At that time, samples of temporoparietal gray matter were taken and analyzed for their aluminum content and compared with those of 12 other infants who had died suddenly. Attention was paid to avoid contamination. Aluminum content of the subject's gray matter was 40.1 mg/g (wet weight), and the mean was 2.4 (1.6) mg/g wet weight of tissue for the control group. Toxicity is not proved by the finding of a high brain aluminum content, but with a history of unexplained convulsions and prolonged intravenous feeding, there is a strong probability that high aluminum intake was at least a large contributory factor.

Encephalopathy due to Aluminum-Containing Bone Cement

A 72-year-old woman was operated on for an acoustic neuroma through a translabyrinthine craniectomy. The surgical procedure was followed by the development of a retroauricular collection of CSF because of a CSF fistula. After 2 months, she developed coma and seizures, without fever or localizing signs. EEG showed bilateral anterior high-amplitude periodic triphasic slow waves. CSF protein was elevated and the aluminum concentration was 185 μg/L (normal: less than 3 to 5 μg/L); serum aluminum was 64 μg/L (normal: less than 10 μg/L). Aluminum urine excretion ranged from 150 to 200 μg/L (normal: less than 15 μg/L). The initial CT was normal, but MRI 1 month after onset of coma showed high-intensity signals in the frontobasal area, cingulum, limbic temporal cortex, and insula. Electron microscopic findings on tissue taken by stereotactic biopsy showed accumulation of lysosomes with aluminum microparticles, normal neurofilaments, and an excess of lipofuscin (Renard et al., 1994).

Attempts to remove the alleged offending aluminum-containing material were done by external lumbar CSF drainage system for 10 days (50 mL removed three times a day); deferoxamine 0.5 to 1.0 g per day for 2 months was also given. Despite this approach and the stabilization of the CSF aluminum concentration at about 20 μg/L, the patient remained in a state of chronic encephalopathy, with myoclonus, stupor, mutism, grasping, and no further clinical improvement.

REFERENCES

Abreo K. Use of deferoxamine in the treatment of aluminum overload in dialysis patients. *Semin Dial* 1988;1:55–61.

Alfrey AC. Aluminum metabolism in uremia. *Neurotoxicology* 1980;1: 43–53.

Alfrey AC. Aluminum. *Adv Clin Chem* 1983;23:69–91.

Alfrey AC. Dialysis encephalopathy. *Kidney Int* 1986;29[Suppl 18]: S53–57.

Alfrey AC. Physiology of aluminum in man. In: Gitelman HJ, ed. *Aluminum and health: a critical review.* New York: Marcel Dekker, 1989: 101–124.

Alfrey AC. Studies related to gastrointestinal absorption of aluminum. In: *Proceedings of the 2nd International Conference on Aluminum and Health, Tampa, FL*, 1992:5–6.

Alfrey AC, Froment DC. Dialysis encephalopathy. In: De Broe ME, Coburn JW, eds. *Aluminum and renal failure.* Vol 26, *Developments in nephrology.* Dordrecht: Kluwer, 1990:249–257.

Alfrey AC, LeGendre GR, Kaehny WD. The dialysis encephalopathy syndrome. Possible aluminum intoxication. *N Engl J Med* 1976;294: 184–188.

Alfrey AC, Hegg A, Craswell P. Metabolism and toxicity of aluminum in renal failure. *Am J Clin Nutr* 1980;33:1509–1516.

Altmann P, Hamon C, Blair J, Dhanesha U, Cunningham J, Marsh F. Disturbance of cerebral function by aluminum in haemodialysis patients without overt aluminum toxicity. *Lancet* 1989;2(8653):7–12.

Aluminum Association. *Wall Street Journal* 1996, May 14.

American Conference of Governmental Industrial Hygienists (ACGIH). Threshold limit values (TLVs) of chemical substances and physical agents and biological exposure indices (BEIs). Cincinnati, OH, ACGIH, 1995.

Amoore JE, Hautala E. Odor as an aid to chemical safety: odor threshold compared with threshold limit values and volatilities for 214 industrial chemicals in air and water dilution. *J Appl Toxicol* 1983;3:272–290.

Andreoli SP, Bergstein JM, Sherrard DJ. Aluminum intoxication from aluminum-containing phosphate binders in children with azotemia not undergoing dialysis. *N Engl J Med* 1984;310:1079–1084.

Banks WA, Kastin AJ. Aluminum increases permeability of the blood-brain barrier to labelled DSIP and β-endorphin—possible implications for senile and dialysis dementia. *Lancet* 1983;1:1227–1229.

Banks WA, Kastin AJ. Aluminum alters the permeability of the blood-brain barrier to some non-peptides. *Neuropharmacology* 1985a;24: 407–412.

Banks WA, Kastin AJ. The aluminum induced increase in blood-brain barrier permeability to DSIP occurs through the brain and is independent of phosphorous and acetylcholinesterase levels. *Psychopharmacology* 1985b;86:84–89.

Bast-Pettersen R, Drables PA, Goffeng LO, Thomassen Y, Torres CG. Neuropsychological deficit among elderly workers in aluminum production. *Am J Ind Med* 1994;25:649–662.

Bishop NJ, Robinson MJ, Lendon M, Hewitt CD, Day JP, O'Hara M. Increased concentration of aluminum in the brain of a parenterally fed preterm infant. *Arch Dis Child* 1989;64:1316–1317.

Bondy SC, Guo-Ross SX, Pien J. Mechanisms underlying the aluminum-induced potentiation of the pro-oxidant properties of transition metals. *Neurotoxicology* 1998;19:65–71.

Cam JM, Luck VA, East JB, de Wardener HE. The effect of aluminum hydroxide on calcium, phosphorus and aluminum metabolism in normal subjects. *Clin Sci Mol Med* 1976;51:407–414.

Candy JM, Oakley AE, Klinowski J, et al. Aluminosilicates and senile plaque formations in Alzheimer's disease. *Lancet* 1986;1:354–357.

Clapp RW, Coogan PF. *Report of a survey of Intalco workers.* Boston, MA: JSI, Center for Environmental Health Studies, May 15, 1992.

Coburn JW, Norris KC. Diagnosis of aluminum-related bone disease and the treatment of aluminum toxicity with deferoxamine. *Semin Nephrol* 1986;6:12–21.

Cochran M, Patterson D, Neoh S, Stevens B, Mazzachi R. Binding of Al by plasma of patients on maintenance hemodialysis. *Clin Chem* 1985; 31:1314–1316.

Crapper DR. Dementia: recent observations on Alzheimer's disease and experimental aluminum encephalopathy. In: Seeman P, Brown GM, eds. *Frontiers in neurology and neuroscience research.* Toronto: University of Toronto Press, 1974:97–111.

Crapper DR, Dalton AJ. Aluminum induced neurofibrillary degeneration, brain electrical activity and alterations in acquisition and retention. *Physiol Behav* 1973;10:935–945.

Crapper-McLachlan DR. Aluminum neurotoxicity: criteria for assigning a role in Alzheimer's disease. In: Lewis TE, ed. *Environmental chemistry and toxicology of aluminum.* Chelsea, MI: Lewis Publishers, 1989: 299–315.

Crapper DR, Krishnan SS, Dalton AJ. Brain aluminum distribution in Alzheimer's disease and experimental neurofibrillary degeneration. *Science* 1973;180:511–513.

Crapper DR, Krishnan S, Quittkat S. Aluminum, neurofibrillary degeneration and Alzheimer's disease. *Brain* 1976;99:67–80.

Crapper DR, De Boni U. Aluminum. In: Spencer PS, Schaumburg HH, eds. *Experimental and clinical neurotoxicology.* Baltimore: Williams & Wilkins, 1983:326–335.

Cutrufo C, Caroli S, Femmine P, et al. Experimental aluminum encephalopathy: quantitative EEG analysis and aluminum bioavailability. *J Neurol Neurosurg Psychiatry* 1984;47:204–206.

Day JP, Barker J, Evans LJA, Perks J, Seabright PJ. Aluminum absorption studied by ^{26}Al tracer. *Lancet* 1991;37:1345.

De Boni U, Seger M, Crapper-McLachlan DR. Functional consequences of chromatin bound aluminum in cultured human cells. *Neurotoxicology* 1980;1:65–81.

De Broe ME, Coburn JW, eds. *Aluminum and renal failure.* Boston: Kluwer Academic Press, 1990.

Deleers M, Servais JP, Wülfert E. Neurotoxic cations induce membrane rigidification and membrane fusion at micromolar concentrations. *Biochim Biophys Acta* 1986;855:271–276.

Deloncle R, Guillard O, Clanet F, Courtois P, Piriou A. Aluminum transfer as glutamate complex through blood-brain barrier. *Biol Trace Elem* 1990;25:39–45.

Deloncle R, Guillard O, Huguet F, Clanet F. Modification of the blood-brain-barrier through chronic intoxication by aluminum glutamate. *Biol Trace Elem Res* 1995;47:227–233.

Dick RB, Krieg EF, Sim MA, et al. Evaluation of tremor in aluminum production workers. *Neurotoxicol Teratol* 1997;19:447–453.

Eastwood JB, Levin GE, Pazianas M, Taylor AP, Denton J, Freemont AJ. Aluminum deposition in bone after contamination of drinking water supply. *Lancet* 1990;336:462–464.

Ecelbarger CA, Greger JL. Dietary citrate and kidney function affect aluminum, zinc, and iron utilization in rats. *J Nutr* 1991;121:1755–1762.

Elinder CG, Friberg L, Kjellstrom T, Nordberg G, Oberdoerster G, eds. *Biological monitoring of metals.* Geneva: World Health Organization, 1994.

Fine RE, Abraham CR. Hypothesis: β-amyloid precursor protein is a key sorting and targeting receptor for neuropeptidases. *Amyloid: Int J Exp Clin Invest* 1997;4:233–239.

Fraser CL, Arieff AI. Nervous system complications in uremia. *Ann Intern Med* 1988;109:143–153.

Ganrot PO. Metabolism and possible health effects of aluminum. *Environ Health Perspect* 1986;65:363–441.

Garrett PJ, Mulcahy D, Carmondy M, O'Dwyer WF. Aluminum encephalopathy: clinical and immunological features. *Q J Med* 1988;69: 775–783.

Garruto RM, Brown P. Tau protein, aluminum, and Alzheimer's disease. *Lancet* 1994;343:989.

Glaser GH. The EEG in certain metabolic disorders. In: Remond A, ed. *Handbook of electroencephalography and clinical neurophysiology.* Vol. 15 (Part C). North-Holland, New York: Elsevier, 1976:15C/16– 15C/25.

Goldstein GW, Betz AL. The blood brain barrier. *Sci Am* 1986;9:74–83.

Gorsky JE, Dietz AA, Spencer H, Osis D. Metabolic balance of aluminum studied in six men. *Clin Chem* 1979;25:1739–1743.

Greger JL. Dietary and other sources of aluminum intake. In: Chadwick DJ, Whelan J, eds. *Aluminum in biology and medicine.* Ciba Foundation Symposium, vol 169. Chichester: John Wiley & Sons, 1992: 26–49.

Greger JL, Baier MJ. Excretion and retention of low to moderate levels of aluminum by human subjects. *Food Chem Toxicol* 1983;21:473–477.

Greger JL, Goetz W, Sullivan D. Aluminum levels in foods cooked and stored in aluminum pans, trays, and foil. *J Food Protect* 1985;48: 772–777.

Gutteridge JMC, Quinlan GJ, Clark I, Halliwell B. Aluminum salts accelerate peroxidation of membrane lipids stimulated by iron salts. *Biochim Biophys Acta* 1985;835:441–447.

Guy SP, Jones D, Mann DMA, Itzhaki RF. Human neuroblastoma cells treated with aluminum express an epitope associated with Alzheimer's disease neurofibrillary tangles. *Neurosci Lett* 1991;121:166–168.

Halliwell B. Oxidants and the central nervous system: some fundamental questions. Is oxidant damage relevant to Parkinson's disease, Alzheimer's disease, traumatic injury or stroke? *Acta Neurol Scand* 1989;126: 23–33.

Hänninen H, Matikainen E, Kovala T, Valkonen S, Riihimäki V. Internal load of aluminum and the central nervous system function of aluminum welders. *Scand J Work Environ Health* 1994;20:279–285.

Hantson P, Mahieu P, Gersdorff M, Sindic C, Lauwerys R. Encephalopathy with seizures after use of aluminum-containing bone cement. *Lancet* 1994;344:1647.

Hantson P, Mahieu P, Gersdorff M, Sindic C, Lauwerys R. Fatal encephalopathy after otoneurosurgery procedure with an aluminum-containing biomaterial. *J Toxicol Clin Toxicol* 1995;33:645–648.

Harrington CR, Wischik CM, McArthur FK, Taylor GA, Edwardson JA, Candy JM. Alzheimer's-disease-like changes in tau protein processing: association with aluminum accumulation in brains of renal dialysis patients. *Lancet* 1994;343:993–997.

Hosovski E, Mastelica Z, Sunderic D, Radulovic D. Mental abilities of workers exposed to aluminum. *Med Lav* 1990;81:119–123.

Hughes JR, Schreeder MT. EEG in dialysis encephalopathy. *Neurology* 1980;30:1148–1154.

Hughes JR, Roxe DM, del Greco F, et al. Electrophysiological studies on uremic patients—comparison of peritoneal dialysis and hemodialysis. *Clin Electroencephalogy* 1980;11:72–82.

Ittel TH, Buddington B, Miller NL, Alfrey AC. Enhanced gastrointestinal absorption of aluminum in uremic rats. *Kidney Int* 1987;32:821–826.

Jebsen RH, Tenckhoff H, Honet JC. Natural history of uremic polyneuropathy and effects of dialysis. *N Engl J Med* 1967;277:327–333.

Jones KC, Bennett BG. Exposure commitment assessments of environmental pollutants. Report 33:4. London: London Monitoring and Assessment Research Center, Kings College, University of London, 1985.

Johnson GV, Jope RS. Aluminum alters cyclic AMP and cyclic GMP levels but not presynaptic colonergic markers in rat brain in vivo. *Brain Res* 1987;403:1–6.

Johnson GV, Jope RS. Phosphorylation of rat brain cytoskeletal protein is increased after orally administered aluminum. *Brain Res* 1988;456:95–103.

Johnson GV, Cogdill KW, Jope RS. Oral aluminum alters in vitro protein phosphorylation and kinase activities in rat brain. *Neurobiol Aging* 1990;11:209–216.

Julka D, Sandhir R, Gil KD. Altered cholinergic metabolism in rat CNS following aluminum exposure: implications on learning and performance. *J Neurochem* 1995;65:2157–2164.

Kaehny WD, Alfrey AC, Holman RE, Schorr WJ. Aluminum transfer during hemodialysis. *Kidney Int* 1977a;12:361–365.

Kaehny WD, Hegg AP, Alfrey AC. Gastrointestinal absorption of aluminum from aluminum-containing antacids. *N Engl J Med* 1977b; 296:1389–1390.

Karlik SJ, Eichhorn GL. Polynucleotide cross-linking by aluminum. *J Inorg Biochem* 1989;37:259–269.

Kasarkis E, Tandon L, Lowell MA, Ehmann WD. Aluminum, calcium, and iron in the spinal cord of patients with sporadic amyotrophic lateral sclerosis using laser microbe mass spectroscopy: a preliminary study. *J Neurol Sci* 1995;130:203–208.

Katz GV. Metals and metaloids other than mercury and lead. In: O'Donoghue JL, ed. *Neurotoxicity of industrial and commercial chemicals,* vol 1. 1985:171–191.

Kihira T, Yoshida S, Mitani K, Yasui M, Yase Y. ALS in the Kii Peninsula of Japan, with special reference to neurofibrillary tangles and aluminum. *Neuropathology* 1993;13:125–136.

Kihira T, Yoshida S, Komoto J, Wakayama I, Yase Y. Aluminum-induced model of motor neuron degeneration: subperineurial injection of aluminum in rabbits. *Neurotoxicology* 1995;16:413–424.

Klatzo I, Wisniewski HM, Streicher E. Experimental production of neurofibrillary degeneration. *J Neuropathol Exp Neurol* 1965;24:187–199.

Kobayashi S, Hirota N, Saito K, Utsayama M. Aluminum accumulation in tangle-bearing neurons of Alzheimer's disease with Balint's syndrome in a long-term aluminum refiner. *Acta Neuropathol (Berl)* 1987;74: 47–52.

Kopeloff LM, Barrera SE, Kopeloff N. Recurrent convulsive seizures in animals produced by immunologic and chemical means. *Am J Psychiatry* 1942;98:881–902.

Kopeloff LM, Chusid JG, Kopeloff N. Chronic experimental epilepsy in *Macaca mulatta. Neurology* 1954;4:218–227.

Kovalchik MT, Kaehny WD, Hegg AP, Jackson JT, Alfrey AC. Aluminum kinetics during hemodialysis. *J Lab Clin Med* 1978;92:712–720.

Krishnan SS, McLachlan DR, Krishnan B, et al. Aluminum toxicity and the brain. *Sci Tot Environ* 1988;71:59–64.

Kruck TP, McLachlan DR. Aluminum as a pathogenic factor in senile dementia of the Alzheimer's type; ion specific chelation. *Alzheimers Dis Rel Disord* 1988;2:209–228.

Kruck TPA, Lukiw WJ, McLachlan DR. Aluminum as a putative pathogenic agent in Alzheimer's disease. In: Berg JM, Karlinsky H, Lowy F, eds. *Alzheimer's disease research. Legal and ethical issues.* University of Toronto Bioethics Committee Review. Toronto: Carswell Press, 1991:120–140.

Kuroda Y, Kawahara M. Aggregation of amyloid β-protein and its neurotoxicity: enhancement by aluminum and other metals. *Tohoku J Exp Med* 1994;174:263–268.

Lazarus JM, Denker BM, Owen WF. Hemodialysis. In: Brenner BM, ed. *The kidney,* 5th ed., vol 2. Philadelphia: WB Saunders, 1996:2470–2475.

Leung FY, Hodsman AB, Muirhead N, Henderson AR. Ultrafiltration studies in vitro of serum aluminum in dialysis patients after deferoxamine chelation therapy. *Clin Chem* 1985;31:20–23.

Ljunggren KG, Lidums V, Sjögren B. Blood and urine concentration of aluminum among workers exposed to aluminum flake powders. *Br J Ind Med* 1991;48:106–109.

Llach F, Bover J. Renal osteodystrophy. In: Brenner BM, ed. *The kidney,* 5th ed., vol 2. Philadelphia: WB Saunders, 1996:2220.

Longstreth WT, Rosenstock L, Heyer NJ. Potroom palsy? Neurologic disorder in three aluminum smelter workers. *Arch Intern Med* 1985; 145:1972–1975.

Lote CJ, Saunders H. Aluminum: gastrointestinal absorption and renal excretion. *Clin Sci* 1991;81:289–295.

Lukiw WJ, McLachlan DR. Aluminum neurotoxicity. In: Chang LW, Dyer RS, eds. *Handbook of neurotoxicology.* New York: Marcel Dekker, 1995:105–142.

Lundin AP, Caruso SM, Berlyne GA. Ultrafilterable aluminum in serum of normal man. *Clin Res* 1978;26:636A.

Markesbery WR, Ehmann WD, Hossain TI, Alauddin M, Goodin DT. Instrumental neutron activation analysis of brain aluminum in Alzheimer's disease and aging. *Ann Neurol* 1981;10:511–516.

Martin RB. The chemistry of aluminum as related to biology and medicine. *Clin Chem* 1986;32:1797–1806.

Martin RB. Aluminum speciation in biology. *Ciba Found Symp* 1992; 169:5–18.

Martyn CN, Barker DJP, Osmond C, Harris EC, Edwardson JA, Lacey RF. Geographical relation between Alzheimer's disease and aluminum in drinking water. *Lancet* 1989;1:59–62.

Mayor GH, Keiser JA, Makdani D, Ku PK. Aluminum absorption and distribution: effect of parathyroid hormone. *Science* 1977;197:1187–1189.

McDermott JR, Smith AI, Ward MK, Parkinson IS, Kerr DN. Brain aluminum concentration in dialysis encephalopathy. *Lancet* 1978;1:901–904.

McDermott JR, Smith AI, Iqbal K, Wisniewski HM. Brain aluminum in aging and Alzheimer disease. *Neurology* 1979;28:809–814.

McKhann G, Drachman D, Folstein M, Katzman R, Price D, Stadlan EM. Clinical diagnosis of Alzheimer's disease: report of the NINCDS-ADRDA work group under the auspices of Department of Health and Human Services Task Force on Alzheimer's Disease. *Neurology* 1984; 34:939–944.

McLaughlin AIG, Kazantzis G, King E, Teare D, Porter RJ, Owen R. Pulmonary fibrosis and encephalopathy associated with the inhalation of aluminum dust. *Br J Ind Med* 1962;19:253–263.

Meiri H, Banin E, Roll M, Rousseau A. Toxic effect of aluminum on nerve cells and synaptic transmission. *Prog Neurobiol* 1992;40:89–121.

Michel P, Commenges D, Dartigues JF, et al. Study of the relationship between aluminum concentration in drinking water and risk of Alzheimer's disease. In: Iqbal K, McLachlan DRC, Winblad B, Wisniewski HM, eds. *Alzheimer's disease: the basic mechanisms, diagnosis and therapeutic strategies.* London: John Wiley & Sons, 1991:387–390.

Miller RG, Kopfler FC, Kelty KC, Stober JA, Ulmer NS. The occurrence of aluminum in drinking water. *J Am Water Assoc* 1984;76:84–91.

Miller JL, Hubbard CM, Litman BJ, Macdonald TL. Inhibition of transducin activation and guanosine triphosphatase by aluminum ion. *J Biol Chem* 1989;264:243–250.

Milliner DS, Nebeker HG, Ott SA, et al. Use of deferoxamine infusion test in diagnosis of aluminum-related osteodystrophy. *Ann Intern Med* 1984;101:775–780.

Murray JC, Tanner CM, Sprague SM. Aluminum neurotoxicity: a reevaluation. *Clin Neuropharmacol* 1991;14:179–185.

Nathan E, Pedersen SE. Dialysis encephalopathy in a non-dialysed uraemic boy treated with aluminum hydroxide orally. *Acta Pædiatr Scand* 1980;69:793–796.

National Institute for Occupational Safety and Health (NIOSH). *Pocket guide to chemical hazards.* Washington: US Department of Health and Human Services, CDC, 1997.

Neill D, Leake A, Hughes D, et al. Effect of aluminum on expression and processing of amyloid precursor protein. *J Neurosci Res* 1996;46:395–403.

Occupational Safety and Health Administration (OSHA). *Code of federal regulations 29: Part 1910.1000.* Washington: Office of the Federal Register National Archives and Records Administration, 1995.

Ohtawa M, Seko M, Takayama F. Effects of aluminum on lipid peroxidation in rats. *Chem Pharm Bull* 1983;31:1414–1418.

Panchalingam K, Sachedina S, Pettegrew JW, Glonek T. Al-ATP as an intracellular carrier of Al(III) ion. *Int J Biochem* 1991;23:1453–1469.

Pennington JAT, Jones JW. Dietary intake of aluminum. In: Gitelman HJ, ed. *Aluminum and health: a critical review.* New York: Marcel Dekker, 1989.

Perl DP, Brody AR. Alzheimer's disease: X-ray spectrometric evidence of aluminum accumulation in neurofibrillary tangle-bearing neurons. *Science* 1980;208:297–299.

Perl DP, Gajdusek CM, Garruto RM, Yanagihara RT, Gibbs CJ. Intraneuronal aluminum accumulation in amyotrophic lateral sclerosis and parkinsonism-dementia of Guam. *Science* 1982;217:1053–1055.

Perl DP, Good PF. Uptake of aluminum into central nervous system along nasal-olfactory pathways. *Lancet* 1987;1:1028.

Plotkin DA, Jarvic LF. Cholinergic dysfunction in Alzheimer's disease: cause or effect? *Prog Brain Res* 1986;65:91–102.

Proctor SP, Clapp RW, Coogan PF. Prevalence of depressive symptoms in a survey of aluminum workers. *New Solutions* 1995;(Summer):43–52.

Recker RR, Blotcky AJ, Leffler JA, Rack EP. Evidence for aluminum absorption from the gastrointestinal tract and bone deposition by aluminum carbonate ingestion with normal renal function. *J Lab Clin Med* 1977;90:810–815.

Renard JL, Felten D, Bequet D. Post-otoneurosurgery aluminum encephalopathy. *Lancet* 1994;344:63–64.

Reusche E, Rohwer J, Forth W, Helms J, Geyer G. Ionomeric cement and aluminum encephalopathy. *Lancet* 1995;345:1633–1634.

Rifat SL, Eastwood MR, McLachlan DR, Corey PN. Effect of exposure of miners to aluminum powder. *Lancet* 1990;336:1162–1165.

Roberts E. Alzheimer's disease may begin in the nose and may be caused by aluminosilicates. *Neurobiol Aging* 1986;7:561–567.

Rotundo A, Nevins TE, Lipton M, Lockman LA, Mauer SM, Michael AF. Progressive encephalopathy in children with chronic insufficiency in infancy. *Kidney Int* 1982;21:486–491.

Salusky IB, Foley J, Nelson P, Goodman WG. Aluminum accumulation during treatment with aluminum hydroxide and dialysis in children and young adults with chronic renal disease. *N Engl J Med* 1991;324:527–531.

Schreeder MT, Favero MS, Hughes JR, Petersen NJ, Bennett PH, Maynard JE. Dialysis encephalopathy and aluminum exposure: an epidemiological analysis. *J Chron Dis* 1983;36:581–593.

Schlatter C. Biomedical aspects of aluminum. *Med Lav* 1992;83:470–474.

Sedman AB, Wilkening GN, Warady BA, Lum GM, Alfrey AC. Encephalopathy in childhood secondary to aluminum toxicity. *J Pediatr* 1984;105:836–838.

Shin RW, Lee VM-Y, Trojanowski JQ. Aluminum modifies properties of Alzheimer's disease PHF_T proteins in vivo and vitro. *J Neurosci* 1994;14:7221–7223.

Siegers CP, Sullivan JB. Organometals and reactive metals. In: Sullivan JH, Krieger GR, eds. *Hazardous material toxicology, clinical principles of environmental health.* Baltimore: Williams & Wilkins, 1992: 929–945.

Simonsen L, Johnsen H, Lund SP, Matakainen E, Midtgård U, Wennberg A. Methodological approach to the evaluation of neurotoxicity data and the classification of neurotoxic chemicals. *Scand J Work Environ Health* 1994;20:1–12.

Sjögren B, Elinder CG. Proposal of a dose-response relationship between aluminum welding fume exposure and effect on the central nervous system. *Med Lav* 1992;83:484–488.

Sjögren B, Lidums V, Håkansson M, Hedström L. Exposure and urinary excretion of aluminum during welding. *Scand J Work Environ Health* 1985;11:39–43.

Sjögren B, Elinder CG, Lidums V, Chang G. Uptake and urinary excretion of aluminum among welders. *Int Arch Occup Environ Health* 1988; 60:77–79.

Sjögren B, Gustavsson P, Hogstedt C. Neuropsychiatric symptoms among welders exposed to neurotoxic metals. *Br J Ind Med* 1990;47:704–707.

Sjögren B, Iregren A, Frech W, et al. Effects on the nervous system among welders exposed to aluminum and manganese. *Occup Environ Med* 1996;53:32–40.

Slanina P, Falkeborn Y, Frech W, Cedergren A. Aluminum concentration in the brain and bone of rats fed citric acid, aluminum citrate or aluminum hydroxide. *Food Chem Toxicol* 1984;33:391–397.

Slanina P, Frech W, Ekström L-G, Lööf L, Slorach S, Cedergren A. Dietary citric acid enhances absorption of aluminum in antacids. *Clin Chem* 1986;32:539–541.

Spencer PS. Guam ALS/Parkinsonism-dementia: a long latency neurotoxic disorder caused by 'slow toxin(s)' in food? *Can J Neurol Sci* 1987;14:347–357.

Sprague SM, Corwin HL, Tanner CM, Wilson RS, Green BJ, Goetz CG. Relationship of aluminum to neurocognitive dysfunction in chronic dialysis patients. *Arch Intern Med* 1988;148:2169–2172.

Stokinger HE. The metals. In: Clayton GD, Clayton FE, eds. *Patty's industrial hygiene and toxicology,* 3rd ed. New York: John Wiley & Sons, 1981:1493.

Sturman JA, Wisniewski HH. Aluminum. In: Bondy SC, Prasad KN, eds. *Metal neurotoxicity.* Boca Raton, FL: CRC Press, 1988:61–68.

Trapp GA. Plasma aluminum is bound to transferrin. *Life Sci* 1983;33: 311–316.

Trapp GA, Mastri AR, Miner GD, Zimmerman RL, Neston LL. Aluminum levels in brain in Alzheimer's disease. *Biol Psychiatry* 1978;13:709–718.

Underwood EJ. *Trace elements in human and animal nutrition,* 3rd ed. New York: Academic Press, 1971.

United States Environmental Protection Agency (USEPA). *Drinking water regulations and health advisories.* EPA 822-R-96-001. Washington: Office of Water, 1996.

van der Voet GB. Intestinal absorption of aluminum. *Ciba Found Symp* 1992;139:109–122.

van der Voet GB, de Wolff FA. Neurotoxicity of aluminum. In: de Wolff FA, ed. *Handbook of clinical neurology,* vol 29, *Intoxications of the nervous system, Part I.* Amsterdam: Elsevier Science, 1994: 273–282.

Viestra R, Haug A. The effect of aluminum^{3+} on the physical properties of membranes in thermoplasma acidophilin. *Biochim Biophys Res Commun* 1978;84:134–144.

Vogt KA, Dalgren R, Ugolini F, et al. Aluminum, iron, calcium, magnesium, potassium, manganese, copper, zinc, and phosphorous in above- and below-ground biomass: II. Pools and circulation in a subalpine *Abies amabilis* stand. *Biogeochemistry* 1987;4:295–311.

Wardle EN. Aluminum intoxication. *Nephron* 1983;33:67.

Wen G, Wisniewski HM. Histochemical localization of aluminum in the rabbit CNS. *Acta Neuropathol (Berl)* 1985;68:175–184.

Wettstein A, Aeppli J, Gautschi K, Peters M. Failure to find a relationship between mnestic skills of octogenarians and aluminum in drinking water. *Int Arch Occup Environ Health* 1991;63:97–103.

White DM, Longstreth WT, Rosenstock L, Claypoole KHJ, Brodkin CA, Townes BD. Neurologic syndrome in 25 workers from an aluminum smelting plant. *Arch Intern Med* 1992;152:1443–1448.

White DM, Longstreth WT, Rosenstock L, Claypoole KHJ, Brodkin CA, Townes BD. Neurologic syndrome in 25 workers from an aluminum smelting plant: correction. *Arch Intern Med* 1993;153:2796.

Winship KA. Toxicity of aluminum: a historical review, Part I. *Adverse Drug React Toxicol Rev* 1992;11:123–141.

Wisniewski HM, Sturman JA, Shek JW, Iqbal K. Aluminum and the central nervous system. *J Environ Pathol Toxicol Oncol* 1985;6:1–8.

Woods JS, Echeverria D, Graves A, Holland J, Millberg J, White RF. *An investigation of factors influencing the neurological health of Intalco aluminum workers.* Seattle, WA: Battelle Human Research Centers, 1989.

Xu Z-C, Tang J-P, Xu Z-X, Melethil S. Kinetics of aluminum in rats IV: Blood and cerebrospinal fluid kinetics. *Toxicol Lett* 1992;63:7–12.

Young LT, Kish SJ, Li PP, Warsh JJ. Decreased brain [^{3}H]inositol 1,4,5-triphosphate binding in Alzheimer's disease. *Neurosci Lett* 1988;94: 198–202.

Zapatero MD, Garcia de Jalon A, Pascual F, Calvo ML, Escanero J, Marro A. Serum aluminum levels in Alzheimer's disease and other senile dementias. *Biol Trace Elem Res* 1995;47:235–240.

Zatta P, Perazzolo M, Bombi GG, Corain B, Nicolini M. The role of speciation in the effects of aluminum (III) on the stability of cell membranes and on the activity of selected enzymes. In: Iqbal K, Wisniewski HM, Winblad O, eds. *Alzheimer's disease and related disorders.* New York: Alan R. Liss, 1989.

Zatta P, Nicolini M, Corain B. Aluminum III toxicity and blood-brain barrier permeability. In: Nicolini M, Zatta P, Corain B, eds. *Aluminum in chemistry, biology and medicine,* vol 1. 1991;1:97–112.

CHAPTER 9

Tin

Tin (Sn) is obtained from ores such as cassiterite (SnO_2), stannite, and teallite (Stokinger, 1981). Commercial demand for this metal has increased over the years, although the quantity of tin ore mined in the United States has been relatively insignificant compared with world output. Reclamation from tin-plate scrap metal, tin cans, and other containers accounts for an estimated 25% of the tin used in the United States (Walsh and DeHaven, 1988; USGS, 1998).

Tin exists in two oxidation states (Sn^{2+} and Sn^{4+}) and forms bivalent (stannous) and quadrivalent (stannic) inorganic compounds (Stokinger, 1981; Aschner and Aschner, 1992). The most common inorganic compounds are oxides, chlorides, fluorides, and the halogenated sodium stannates and stannites (Aschner and Aschner, 1992). The relatively unstable stannous compounds are used industrially in tin plating, and the more stable stannic compounds find use in the production of glass and ceramics. Inorganic tin salts are less toxic than the organotins (Barnes and Stoner, 1959; Hiles, 1974).

The stability of tin-to-carbon bonds has provided the basis for a large and growing field of organotin chemistry. Most organotin compounds have tin in the 4+ oxidation state (Barry and Thwaites, 1983). The formation of 1 to 4 covalent bonds with carbon atoms results in mono-, di-, tri-, and tetra-organotin compounds (Magos, 1986; Aschner and Aschner, 1992). There are several hundred organotins with many applications (Piver, 1973; WHO, 1980). The toxicities of the various organotin compounds are determined by their individual chemical structure. The most widely used organotins, listed in order of their decreasing toxic potential, are: ethyl-, methyl-, propyl-, butyl-, phenyl-, hexyl-, and octyltin. The lower molecular weight compounds, trimethyltin chloride and triethyltin chloride, are primarily neurotoxic; the intermediate homologues, tripropyltin chloride, tributyltin, and triphenyltin chloride, are essentially immunotoxic; of the higher molecular weight compounds, trihexyltin is slightly immunotoxic, and trioctyltin is nontoxic (Boyer, 1989).

Organotin poisoning is an occupational hazard for chemists and others who work with these chemicals and are often unaware of their toxic potential (Foncin and Gruner, 1979; Besser et al., 1987; Colosio et al., 1991; Feldman et al., 1993). Exposure to certain organotin compounds at production sites and in research laboratories may cause adverse health effects (Besser et al., 1987; Feldman et al., 1993). When considering the neurotoxicology of organotin compounds, the effects of trimethyltin (TMT) and triethyltin (TET) are of greatest concern (Krigman and Silverman, 1984; Boyer, 1989). TMT and TET each have their own cellular targets, mechanisms of neurotoxicity, and presentation of predominant clinical features. TMT affects neurons and causes neurobehavioral changes, such as altered mood and impairment of memory, learning, and cognitive performance. TET attacks myelin, produces brain edema, and impairs motor function (Reiter and Ruppert, 1984).

SOURCES OF EXPOSURE

The content of inorganic tin in soil depends on its geological origin as well as on how much contamination has occurred due to discarding of tin-containing wastes and atmospheric fallout of tin-containing compounds derived from the biodegradation of organotin pesticides. Emissions from incineration of tin-containing wastes and the burning of fossil fuels, as well as from various industrial production processes, contribute to global and local ambient atmospheric concentrations of tin. Ambient air levels are generally low (less than 0.1 $\mu g/m^3$), except near sites of origin such as mines, smelting and industrial plants, and areas where organotin pesticides are used agriculturally (WHO, 1980; ATSDR, 1992) (Table 9-1). Bacterial biomethylation of inorganic tin compounds in estuaries increases the content of the methyltins found in water and the adjacent soil (Hallas et al., 1982). The concentration of methyltins increases with the salinity of the water. In addition, increased salinity of the water allows further methylation of TMT to tetramethyltin, increasing its solubility and volatility in the atmosphere (Guard et al., 1981).

The dioctyltin compounds, which are considered to have negligible mammalian toxicity, are used to stabilize poly-

146

TABLE 9-1. *Atmospheric tin levels*

Location	Air Sn concentration (µg/m³)	Reference
Ambient background	<0.1	ATSDR, 1992
Nonindustrial urban	0.3	WHO, 1980
Industrial	4.4	WHO, 1980
Chilean mine/foundry	14.9	Oyanguren et al., 1958

vinyl chloride (PVC) packaging materials, used for containing foods. Tributyl- and triphenyltins are widely used as biocides because of their relatively low mammalian toxicity. Tributyltin chloride in plastic-based coverings of electrical cables serves as a rodent repellant (Barry and Thwaites, 1983). Tributyltin oxide is used as a preservative for wood, paper, and cotton textiles (Barry and Thwaites, 1981; Boyer, 1989). Tributyltin oxide is also used as a mildew control agent in interior latex paints; paints containing tributyltin compounds should be used only in well-ventilated areas (Wax and Dockstader, 1995). Tributyltin benzoate is used as a germicide in hospitals (Barry and Thwaites, 1983). Paints containing tributyltin fluoride and acetate are applied to the bottoms of boats as molluscocides, fungicides, algae biocide, and antifouling agents (Barry and Thwaites, 1983; Wilkinson, 1984; Boyer, 1989). Triphenyltin acetate and hydroxide are used as pesticides, and triphenyltin chloride is used as an antifouling agent in marine paint formulations (Barry and Thwaites, 1983). The slow release of tributyl- and triphenyltin from painted surfaces, as the polymer hydrolyzes in the sea water, constitutes a serious source of alkyltin contamination of rivers, estuaries, lakes, and oceans. Elevated concentrations of tributyltin have been found in oysters, in marine mussels, in the claw muscles of crabs, and in salmon reared in sea pens treated with tributyltin oxide. Cooking reduces the tributyltin content in the salmon meat by 24% to 45% (Boyer, 1989). Varying amounts of dibutyl-, tributyl-, and triphenyltin have been found in fish and shellfish, usually in quantities considered insufficient to affect human health (Yamamoto, 1994).

Tin found in the diet of humans may result from soil intake by edible vegetation, from the residues of organotin pesticides, biocides, and fumigants on produce and, from tin released from food containers such as PVC bottles and tin-plated cans (Piver, 1973; Krigman and Silverman, 1984; Magos, 1986; Beliles, 1994). Tin has been considered to be a relatively essential dietary trace element, based on the observation that irreversible growth defects occur in rat pups fed a severely tin-deficient diet (Schwarz et al., 1970; Underwood, 1977). The average daily dietary intake of inorganic tin generally satisfies any human nutritional requirement there may be for this trace metal. Daily dietary intake varies considerably (estimated range: 1 to 38 mg) (Schroeder et al., 1964). In the United States, an average adult's daily intake of total tin compounds has been estimated at 4.003 mg: 4 mg from food, 0.003 mg from air, and undetectable amounts contributed by

drinking water (USEPA, 1987). Ingestion and dermal uptake of inorganic and organotin compounds occurs during the use of tin-containing medicinal products. Many toothpastes contain the inorganic tin salt stannous fluoride (Barry and Thwaites, 1983). Common domestic goods such as metal and glass polishes (which use tin compounds such as cassiterite as an abrasive); fingernail polish (in which tin is used as a hardener); and ceramics and textiles (where tin compounds are used in pigments) constitute additional sources of exposure to this metal (Barnes and Stoner, 1959; ATSDR, 1992). Furthermore, hobbyists as well as workers can be exposed to the vapors of tin compounds released from molten solders and other alloys (e.g., bronze and pewter).

In contrast to tributyltin and triphenyltin, TMT and TET are highly toxic to mammals. The risk of exposure to hazardous levels of TMT and TET exists for those individuals involved in the manufacture and use of these chemicals; handling of either is potentially dangerous even for the most experienced and careful workers (USEPA, 1976; Aldridge et al., 1981). TMT is an intermediate product and/or byproduct in the synthesis of other organotin compounds (USEPA, 1976; OSHA, 1978; Weast, 1981; Feldman et al., 1993; Earley et al., 1995). For example, TMT is a byproduct in the synthesis of dimethyltin dichloride, a substance used as a plastic stabilizer and surface hardener for glass (USEPA, 1976; Ross et al., 1981; Aldridge et al., 1981). TMT and TET have been used in neuroscience research laboratories to produce models of neuronal degeneration and hippocampal neurobehavioral functions, including mechanisms of memory and dementia (TMT), and in the study of cerebral edema, central myelinopathy, and neurodegeneration (TET) (Magee et al., 1957; Torack et al., 1960; Reiter and Ruppert, 1984).

EXPOSURE LIMITS AND SAFETY REGULATIONS

Environmental and occupational exposure limits set as guidelines for tin compounds are based on animal studies and clinical case reports (Table 9-2). Data from acute and chronic animal toxicity studies have shown renal, cardiac, gastric, and hematological system damage leading to death in some animals, whereas less serious or no effects were observed in others. These observations suggest that the systemic effects depend on the route, dosage, and duration of exposure, as well as on which particular tin compound is administered (ATSDR, 1992). Work site exposure measurements and reports of symptoms, as well as overt toxic effects following accidents, are important sources of experience for planning future safety programs.

The *Occupational Safety and Health Administration* (OSHA) has established an 8-hour time-weighted average (TWA) permissible exposure limit (PEL) for metallic and inorganic tin compounds (except oxides) of 2 mg/m³. The 8-hour PEL for organic tin compounds is 0.1 mg/m³ (OSHA, 1995). The *National Institute of Occupational Safety and Health's* (NIOSH) 10-hour TWA recommended exposure limit (REL) for the metallic and inorganic tin compounds

TABLE 9-2. *Established and recommended occupational and environmental exposure limits for tin compounds in air and water*

	Air (mg/m^3)	Water (mg/L)[a]
Odor threshold*	—	—
OSHA		
Inorganic		
PEL (10-hr TWA)	2.0	—
PEL ceiling (15-min TWA)	—	—
Organic		
PEL (10-hr TWA)	0.1	—
PEL ceiling (15-min TWA)	—	—
NIOSH		
Inorganic		
REL (10-hr TWA)	2.0	—
STEL (15-min TWA)	—	—
IDLH	100.0	—
Organic		
REL (10-hr TWA)	0.1	—
STEL (15-min TWA)	—	—
IDLH	25.0	—
Cyhexatin		
REL (10-hr TWA)	5.0	—
STEL (15-min TWA)		—
IDLH	80.0	—
ACGIH		
Inorganic		
TLV (8-hr TWA)	2.0	—
STEL (15-min TWA)	—	—
Organic		—
TLV (8-hr TWA)	0.1	—
STEL (15-min TWA)	—	—
USEPA		
Inorganic		
MCL	—	—
MCLG	—	—
SMCL	—	—
Organic		
MCL	—	—
MCLG	—	—
SMCL	—	—

[a]Unit conversion: 1 mg/L = 1 ppm.
OSHA, Occupational Safety and Health Administration; PEL, permissible exposure limit; TWA, time-weighted average; NIOSH, National Institute of Occupational Safety and Health; REL; recommended exposure limit; STEL, short-term exposure limit; IDLH, immediately dangerous to life or health; ACGIH, American Conference of Governmental Industrial Hygienists; TLV, threshold limit value; USEPA, U.S. Environmental Protection Agency; MCL, maximum contamination level; MCLG, maximum contamination level goal; SMCL, secondary MCL.
Data from *Amoore and Hautala, 1983; ACGIH, 1985; OSHA, 1996; USEPA, 1996; NIOSH, 1997.

is 2 mg/m^3. The NIOSH 10-hour REL for the organic tin compounds (except cyhexatin) is 0.1 mg/m^3; the 10-hour REL for cyhexatin is 5 mg/m^3. The NIOSH immediately dangerous to life and health (IDLH) concentration for the inorganic tins is 100 mg/m^3; the IDLH for the organotins (except for the cyhexatins) is 25 mg/m^3; IDLH for the cyhexatins is 80 mg/m^3 (NIOSH, 1997). The *American Conference*

of Governmental Industrial Hygienists' (ACGIH) recommended 8-hour TWA threshold limit value (TLV) for metallic and inorganic tins is 2 mg/m^3. The ACGIH 8-hour TLV for organic tins is 0.1 mg/m^3, with a 15-minute TWA short-term exposure limit (STEL) of 0.2 mg/m^3. The ACGIH 8-hour TLV for cyhexatin is 5 mg/m^3 (ACGIH, 1995).

The *United States Environmental Protection Agency* (EPA) has not established a water contamination limit for the tins (USEPA, 1996).

METABOLISM

Tissue Absorption

Inorganic Tin

Pulmonary absorption of inhaled inorganic tin appears to be negligible, as the particulate compounds become deposited in the lungs (Schroeder et al., 1964; Hiles, 1974; Magos, 1986). In general, the inorganic salts of tin are acidic, inducing repulsion and deterring further oral intake (Barnes and Stoner, 1959). Gastrointestinal (GI) absorption of inorganic tin compounds is dependent on both the valence state and the anion complement (Hiles, 1974). Most inorganic tin compounds are relatively insoluble and are poorly absorbed from the GI tract following ingestion (Barnes and Stoner, 1959; Calloway and McMullen 1966; Hiles, 1974). The uptake of inorganic tin from the small intestine appears to occur by passive diffusion (Iwai et al., 1981).

Organic Tin

In contrast to inorganic tin, the lipid-soluble organotins are readily absorbed by pulmonary, GI, and dermal routes (Magos, 1986). For example, TET and TMT are rapidly absorbed through the GI tract and the skin (Stoner et al., 1955). The extent to which GI absorption of the tetravalent organotin compounds occurs is dependent on the number and size of the alkyl and aryl groups (Magos, 1986). For example, monoethyltin and triphenyltin are poorly absorbed from the GI tract, whereas the trialkyltin compounds with short alkyl chains (e.g., TMT and TET) are readily absorbed. Tributyltin is less readily absorbed from the GI tract than TET (Iwai et al., 1982; Krigman and Silverman, 1984; Fait et al., 1994). The tissue concentrations and neurological effects of TMT are very similar after either intravenous or oral administration, indicating that TMT is nearly completely absorbed from the GI tract (Brown et al., 1979). TET given orally to rats also appears to be totally absorbed, since equivalent parenteral and oral doses produce similar effects (Barnes and Stoner, 1958).

Tissue Distribution

Inorganic Tin

Inhaled inorganic tin that is not absorbed remains in the lungs (Schroeder et al., 1964; Hiles, 1974). The majority of absorbed inorganic tin circulating in human blood is located in the red cells, with the rest found in the plasma, as it becomes distributed mainly to the bones and liver (Kehoe et al., 1940; Hiles, 1974). Inorganic tin does not readily cross the blood–brain barrier (BBB) or the placenta (Schroeder et al., 1964; Hiles, 1974).

Tissue distribution depends on the affinity of hemoglobin for the particular tin compound and on the animal species. For example, the hemoglobin affinity constant for TMT is smaller than that of TET (Rose, 1969). Human hemoglobin does not bind TET, whereas rat hemoglobin has a relatively high affinity for TET (Rose and Aldridge, 1968). A lower TMT hemoglobin binding capacity in mice and humans compared with that in rats has also been demonstrated and may explain the increased sensitivity of mice and humans to the effects of TMT (Brown et al., 1979; Aldridge et al., 1981; Brown et al., 1984).

Organic Tin

Organotin compounds are able to cross the BBB. Following intravenous administration to animals, tetraethyltin is rapidly distributed to the liver, kidney, and brain, whereas the distribution of tetrapropyltin and tetrabutyltin to these tissues occurs more slowly (Arakawa et al., 1981). Tributyltin compounds that cross the BBB are metabolized to inorganic Sn^{4+} and are retained in the central nervous system (CNS) (Iwai et al., 1981). Animal experiments show that peak brain concentrations of TMT occur within about 5 days after exposure (Cook et al., 1984c; Hasan et al., 1984). Triethyltin penetrates the BBB more readily and reaches substantially higher (4- to 25-fold) concentrations in the brain than TMT. The greater octanol–water partition coefficient of TET enhances its ability to penetrate the BBB (Cook et al., 1984c). Maximum accumulation of TET is reached in the rat brain approximately 24 hours after a single injection (Cook et al., 1984a). Twenty-four hours after a single injection of 10 mg/kg of TET, tissue concentrations were 16.0 mg/g in the liver, 3.7 mg/g in the kidneys, and 3.7 mg/g in the brain (Rose and Aldridge, 1968). Nevertheless, TMT and TET are evenly distributed across all brain regions, and the tissue concentration of tin is dose related in the rat brain (Cook et al., 1984a,b). Differences in the subcellular (synaptosome, myelin, and mitochondria) distribution as well as differences in the biophysical properties of TMT and TET may determine the severity of CNS toxicity more than total brain tin concentration (Cook et al., 1986c; Mushak et al., 1982).

Tissue Biochemistry

Inorganic Tin

Inhalation of dust containing tin results in acute bronchial irritation, and chronic inhalation of SnO_2 may produce pneumoconiosis; however, there are no specific tissue biochemical reactions unique to tin (Barnes and Stoner, 1959). Ingested inorganic tin salts combine with protein, inhibiting digestion by proteolytic enzymes; this may be a factor in the poor absorption of inorganic tin.

Organic Tin

Biotransformation (dealkylation) of the tetra- and triorganotins to di- or monoorganotin compounds occurs in the liver by the NADPH-dependent cytochrome P-450 mixed function microsomal monooxygenase system (Cremer, 1957; Bridges et al., 1967; Kimmel et al., 1980; Prough et al., 1981; Iwai et al., 1981). Tetra-substituted organotin compounds are relatively less toxic than their tri-substituted equivalents, but they are rapidly transformed to the latter more toxic compounds in the liver and brain (Cremer, 1958; Iwai et al., 1982). TMT is a stable compound and does not undergo further biotransformation by dealkylation (Cremer, 1958; Magos, 1986). The dealkylation of TET is also negligible (Iwai et al., 1982; Magos 1986). TET converts cytochrome P-450 to the inactive form (cytochrome P-420), thus reducing the enzyme's metabolic capacity (Prough et al., 1981). The dealkylation of the organotins involves free radicals, which promote lipid peroxidation, thereby altering the cell membrane fluidity and allowing Ca^{2+} to leak across (Prough et al., 1981; Halliwell, 1989). Hydroxide ions have a high affinity for the trialkyltins and form compounds that are both water and lipid soluble, allowing rapid absorption from the GI tract and passage through cellular membranes (Brown et al., 1984). Carbon-hydroxylated tin compounds are capable of altering mitochondrial function (Aldridge et al., 1977). The variable toxicity of the organotins is related in part to the lipophilicity of the particular compound; more lipophilic compounds readily cross the BBB and are also more effective membrane toxicants (Aschner and Aschner, 1992). In addition, toxicity may depend in part on the ability of the organotin compound to increase intracellular Ca^{2+} concentrations, which induces apoptosis (Viviani et al., 1995). The toxic effects of organotins do not correlate with the total amount of tin found in the brain (Mushak et al., 1982), and the different neurotoxic effects produced by TMT and TET suggest that the specific alkyl moiety of the organotin molecule contributes to the selectivity of neurotoxic effects (Magos, 1986) (see Neuropathological Diagnosis section).

The neurotoxic effect of TET includes development of severe brain edema. Exposure to TET significantly increases the water content of the brain and spinal cord. The fluid associated with this unique type of edema chemically resembles extracellular fluid but has increased levels of sodium and chloride (Katzman et al., 1963; Aleu et al., 1963; Bakay, 1965). TET does not appear to alter the BBB (Bakay, 1965). The edema fluid is apparently contained in intramyelinic vacuoles (see Neuropathological Diagnosis section) (Katzman et al., 1963).

Excretion

Inorganic Tin

Inorganic tin compounds are poorly absorbed and are excreted primarily in the feces; the small amounts of the inorganic tins that reach the general circulation are excreted through the kidneys (Hiles, 1974; Johnson and Greger, 1982).

Organic Tin

The excretion route of the organotins is determined by the absorption and metabolism of the particular compound. The less well-absorbed organotin compounds are also excreted in the feces. For example, monoethyltin given orally to rats appears only in the feces and is not detectable in urine, indicating poor absorption. Diethyltin is eliminated in the feces, and urine, and bile with the fecal fraction consisting essentially of unmetabolized diethyltin, excreted by biliary clearance, whereas the urine fraction contains metabolized monoethyltin. Following subcutaneous injection, tetraalkyltins are dealkylated to trialkyltins and excreted in the urine. Trialkyltin chloride compounds are primarily excreted in the urine, reflecting the lower susceptibility of these compounds to metabolism, as well as their greater solubility in water. Tetraalkyltin compounds that are not dealkylated are excreted in the bile (Iwai et al., 1982). Mono-, di-, and trialkyltins are principally excreted via the feces but are also found in the urine (Magos, 1986). For example, maximum urinary excretion of organotin occurred on days 4 to 10 in workers occupationally exposed to mono-, di-, and trimethyltin (Fig. 9-1) (Besser et al., 1987).

In a 36-year-old man accidentally exposed to triphenyltin acetate, a peak urinary tin excretion of 96 μg/L occurred between the fifth and the sixth day after exposure, urine concentration decreased to 30 μg/L by the eighth day, and 1 month after exposure, the value was 28 μg/L (nonexposed range: 6 to 30 μg/L) (Colosio et al., 1991). Tin disappearance from the plasma of this patient was initially concomitant with the increased urinary excretion. The plasma tin level, which was 16 μg/L on the second day, decreased rapidly up to the fourth day, with a small peak on the sixth day. The plasma level 1 month after cessation of exposure was 10 μg/L. The findings in this patient suggest that excretion of organic tin is biphasic (see Fig. 9-1).

Trimethyltin is eliminated from the brain more slowly than TET. The half-life for TMT in the adult rat brain following a dose of 6 mg/kg is 16 days, and the half-life for TET is only 8 days (Cook et al., 1984b). Tin was not detectable in the brain 12 days after cessation of chronic exposure to TET (Cremer, 1957).

CLINICAL MANIFESTATIONS AND DIAGNOSIS

Symptomatic Diagnosis

Inorganic Tin

Inorganic tin as particulate in dust or as SnO_2 in fumes causes irritation of the upper respiratory tract and mucous membranes (Barnes and Stoner, 1959; OSHA, 1978). The accumulation of inhaled and entrapped SnO_2 particles produces respiratory symptoms among exposed workers, and the chest x-rays of these workers show evidence of the radioopaque metal and often pneumoconiosis (Barnes and Stoner, 1959). Oral ingestion of inorganic tin produces acute gastric irritation and vomiting but is not responsible for neurologic effects (Magos, 1986; ACGIH, 1989).

Organic Tin

Symptoms of *organotin toxicity* are determined by the nature and complexity of the alkyl and aryl groups, as well as by activity of products formed by biotransformation. For example, the monoalkyl tins are low in toxicity and are not activated by biotransformation, whereas the tetraalkyl compounds, which as such are also relatively inactive, are biotransformed to the trialkyltins, which have been shown to produce neurological effects. Dermal and conjunctival exposure to tributyltin causes irritation and inflammation; inhalation of its vapors causes pharyngeal irritation, coughing, nausea, and vomiting. Exposure to triphenyltin, TMT, and TET results in acute symptoms of general malaise, nausea, epigastric discomfort, visual disturbances, and shortness of breath. However, much more serious manifestations of CNS impairment are seen after several days of exposure to TMT and TET, including headache, apathy, somnolence, memory loss, hallucinations, confusion, agitation, loss of consciousness, convulsions, coma, and death. Signs of cerebral cortical neuronal effect are seen after TMT exposure. TMT has been shown to produce neuropathological changes in animals, primarily affecting the limbic system with associated behavioral changes (Brown et al., 1979; Chang et al., 1982a,b; Walsh et al., 1982a,b; Messing et al., 1988; Bushnell, 1990). Abnormal motor responses and signs of the effects of increased in-

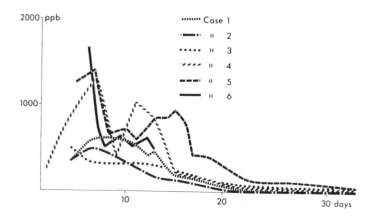

FIG. 9-1. Urinary excretion patterns of five workers exposed to TMT. Maximum excretion is reached on days 4 to 10. Note the biphasic excretion pattern. (Modified from Besser et al., 1987, with permission.)

tracranial pressure and cerebral edema are observed after exposure to TET (Fait et al., 1994).

Trimethyltin

The severity of the neurotoxic effects of TMT does not permit its study in human subjects under controlled experimental conditions; thus information has been gathered from animal experiments and accidental human exposures. *TMT syndrome* produced in rats consists of tremor, hyperactivity, aggression, self-mutilation, and spontaneous seizures (Brown et al., 1979). At higher exposure doses, TMT also induced perseverative behavior, attributable to limbic system pathology (Schwartzwelder et al., 1982). Another consistent observation in animals is impaired retention of inhibitory avoidance paradigms and long-lasting impairments in acquisition and retention of both food- and shock-motivated responses (Walsh et al., 1982a).

Seizures, memory impairment, increased aggressiveness, insomnia, and headaches are symptoms reported in humans following occupational or accidental exposure to TMT (Ross et al., 1981; Fortemps et al., 1978; Besser et al., 1987; Kreyberg et al., 1992; Feldman et al., 1993) (Table 9-3). Gaze-evoked nystagmus was described in a group of workers after a severe nonfatal exposure to TMT (Besser et al., 1987). Coma and death follow severe intoxications. The behavioral impairments resulting from severe exposure appear to be irreversible, and instances of complete recovery are unusual (Reiter and Ruppert, 1984; Besser et al., 1987; Feldman et al., 1993).

For example, a chemistry graduate student who was acutely exposed to an undetermined amount of TMT vapor during an explosion in the lab exhibited memory deficits, confusion, inappropriate affect, disorientation, depression, insomnia, reduced vigilance, and seizures (Yanofsky et al., 1991; Feldman et al., 1993). Bilateral slowing of his electro-

TABLE 9-3. *Neurological manifestations of trimethyltin intoxication*

Reference	Symptomatic diagnosis	Neurophysiological diagnosis	Biochemical diagnosis
Fortemps et al., 1978; case reports (two chemists)	Headaches, pain, memory deficits, confusion, disorientation, seizures, insomnia, anorexia, obtundation	EEG: showed low-voltage spikes and theta paroxysms	Not reported
Ross et al., 1981, 1983; epidemiologic study: compared 12 workers with high exposure and 10 with low exposure	Alternating attacks of rage and deep depression, memory problems, poor concentration, disorientation, headaches, loss of libido and motivation, sleep disturbances, fatigue, dim vision	EEG: showed abnormalities without a specific pattern. Nerve conduction studies: showed mildly reduced nerve conduction velocities	Urine tin: 20–200 ppb (levels measured 2 months after cessation of exposure)
Rey et al., 1984, and Besser et al., 1987; case reports (6 workers)	Hearing loss, seizures, amnesia, disorientation, confusion, confabulation, restlessness, aggressiveness, hyperphagia, disturbed sexual behavior, ataxia, neuropathy, blurred vision	EEG: showed prolonged bilateral theta activity localized over the temporal regions. ENG: showed bilateral gaze nystagmus and mildly saccadic pursuit eye movements. Audiometry: revealed mild hearing loss. Nerve conduction studies: revealed mild slowing of sensory nerve conduction velocity	Urine tin: 445–1580 ppb (4–8 days after exposure)
Kreyberg et al., 1992; case report: two persons with accidental ingestion of TMT-contaminated wine	Restlessness, loss of memory, agitation, episodes of unresponsiveness, nystagmus, incontinence, coma, death		Not reported
Yanofsky et al., 1991 and Feldman et al., 1993; case report: chemist with severe single exposure	Memory loss, confusion, acute delirium, disorientation, apathy, abnormal cognitive process, complex partial seizures, depression, fatigue, insomnia	EEG: bilateral and paroxysmal theta slowing predominantly over the left temporal area. SEP: normal. BAEP and VEP: normal. MRI and CT scan: normal	Urine tin (normal <18 ppb[a]): 52 ppb (17 days after exposure); 10 ppb (35 days after exposure). Serum tin (normal <3.3 ppb[a]): 13 ppb (17 days after exposure); 7.4 ppb (35 days after exposure)

EEG, electroencephalogram; ENG, electronystagmogram; TMT, trimethyltin; SEP, sensory evoked potential; BAEP, brain stem auditory evoked potential; VEP, visual evoked potential; MRI, magnetic resonance imaging; CT, computed tomography.
[a]Laboratory values for normal nonexposed subjects.

encephalogram (EEG) was consistent with toxic encephalopathy (Feldman et al., 1993). The patient exhibited more overt abnormal neurobehavior 3 days after the accident than he did immediately following the accident. This "latent period" has also been noted in animal studies (Ruppert et al., 1982; Chang, 1986; Hasan et al., 1984) and previous human exposures (Dyer et al., 1982; Walsh and DeHaven, 1988; Boyer, 1989) (see Neuropsychological Diagnosis section).

Fortemps et al. (1978), described two young chemists (aged 21 and 26 years), who were exposed to TMT while synthesizing dimethyltin chloride from metallic tin and monochloromethane at 300°C in the presence of copper. White vapors were often seen escaping from the reactor and being released into the room, but little attention had been paid to them. The men worked without masks or protective equipment, and they spent 6 to 10 hours each day in the room. After working in this situation for 2 months, one of the chemists collapsed and had the first generalized seizure of his life. He recovered from the seizure, and the initial EEG was considered normal, possibly due to postictal forced normalization. However, 3 days later, the EEG showed low voltage spikes and rare theta paroxysms. Even so, the chemist returned to work under the same exposure conditions 1 week later. A series of three generalized epileptic attacks occurred 2 months later (see Neurophysiological Diagnosis section). The second chemist was observed by witnesses to have staggered out of the chemical processing room, appearing pale and confused, with arms dangling; he suddenly fell to the ground. He became rigid and then developed a generalized tonic–clonic convulsion. He remained in a postictal sleep for 10 minutes, awoke and stood up, but was unable to recognize his coworkers, and was disoriented and combative. He continued to have amnesia for the event for at least 2 months afterwards. After these dramatic occurrences, the two chemists recalled that they had frequently disregarded an unpleasant odor and the change in taste of their cigarettes, which caused them to feel nauseous. They had also ignored recurrent episodes of memory impairment, irritability, insomnia, headache, abdominal pains, shortness of breath, and teeth pain in the absence of dental illness during the months preceding the seizures. All the symptoms disappeared after cessation of exposure to organotin compounds, and the two men were considered recovered at follow-up 1 year later.

The effects of chronic occupational exposures to TMT have been reported after large-scale accidents. Twenty-two workers were chronically exposed to low levels of TMT and dimethyltin in a poorly ventilated facility (Ross et al., 1981). For purposes of this retrospective study, the employees were assigned, according to their work task exposure histories, to *high* (n = 12) or *low* (n = 10) *probable* exposure groups. Measurement of urinary tin in each individual had not been done at the time of actual exposure. Increased frequency of neurological symptoms was noted in the high exposure group (see Table 9-3). Persistent personality changes in the high exposure group were probably due to irreversible CNS damage.

Besser et al. (1987) described industrial TMT intoxication in six workers who were exposed to a mixture of TMT, dimethyltin, and monomethyltin during the manufacture of dimethyltin from methyl chloride and inorganic tin. Spillage of di- and trimethyltin chloride caused severe irritability and rage attacks, memory loss, and disorientation in the exposed workers. The more volatile TMT vapors were inhaled while the men were cleaning the production vats and were removing the residues of product and inorganic tin. The severity of the clinical symptoms correlated with the maximum urinary excretion of organotin, with the highest urinary value (1,580 ppb) occurring in a patient who subsequently died; persistent clinical features occurred in two patients with values greater than 400 ppb. The most severely affected workers exhibited behavioral changes, loss of consciousness, seizures, and death (see Neuropathological Diagnosis section).

Triethyltin

At least 100 persons died among a group of 270 known to have ingested Stalinon, an oral bacteriocidal pharmaceutical preparation containing diethyltin iodide. It was intended as a treatment for boils and other staphylococcal skin infections. It was determined that the Stalinon unfortunately contained monoethyltin triiodione and triethyltin iodide as impurities. Triethyltin iodide was subsequently identified as the primary neurotoxic agent (Cossa et al., 1958; Alajounine et al., 1958; Barnes and Stoner, 1959; Foncin and Gruner, 1979). Only ten persons were believed to have recovered completely; the remainder had persistent neurological findings (see Clinical Experiences section).

Cossa et al. (1958) described in detail the clinical courses of 11 of the patients who had ingested the contaminated Stalinon. The symptomatology of the illness in 6 of the 11 cases for whom exposure levels were estimated are summarized in Table 9-4. Onset occurred between 2 and 25 days after taking the medication. The patients' initial symptoms included headaches, apathy, lethargy, coma, vomiting, and sometimes GI complaints (intragastric burning). Lethargy, coma, or stuporous state predominated. Nuchal rigidity and paroxysms of orbital pain suggestive of a meningitis were present. Fever was not part of the clinical picture. Mild hemiparesis, seizures, abnormal eye movements, and other motor signs were present. Vegetative and autonomic abnormalities included bradycardia and bilaterally dilated pupils. Episodes of crying and extreme anxiety were common. Papilledema was present in those patients whose headache, vomiting, and suboccipital pain also suggested brain-stem herniation. The cerebrospinal fluid (CSF) was usually normal; albumin was occasionally at the upper limit of normal.

Fatalities occurred within 2 to 11 days after onset of illness (see Neuropathological Diagnosis section). Death was sudden and rapid, and was often preceded by a period of apparent improvement. In the three surviving cases, marked clinical improvement was seen 19 to 45 days after the appearance of symptoms. The EEGs of these patients

TABLE 9-4. *Neurological manifestations of triethyltin poisoning[a]*

Case no.	Age (yr)/sex	Estimated dose of triethyltin[b] (mg)	Time to onset of symptoms	Symptoms	Prognosis
1	31/male	75/8 days	14 days after beginning treatment with Stalinon	Severe headaches; vomiting; lethargy; cardiac arrhythmia; respiratory trouble; confusion; abnormal EEG; coma and death	Died 7 days after the reported onset of symptoms
2	15/female	40/10 days	10 days after beginning treatment with Stalinon	Severe headaches; vomiting; loss of consciousness accompanied by clonic movements of the upper left extremity and urinary incontinence; abnormal EEG; apnea and death	Died 11 days after the reported onset of symptoms
3	24/female	35/4 days	4 days after beginning treatment with Stalinon	Headaches; nausea; vomiting; anorexia; papilledema, with episodes of diplopia; clonus of the left lower extremity; mild neck stiffness; abnormal EEG	Recovered; the second EEG performed 15 days after the onset of symptoms showed marked improvement; at follow-up 4 months later, the patient was doing clinically well, but the EEG was still slightly abnormal
4	26/female	45/NR	6 days after beginning treatment with Stalinon	Severe headaches; gastrointestinal problems, with abdominal bloating, fever; lethargy; agitation; mild neck stiffness; abnormal EEG	Recovered; the patient still reported experiencing headaches and nausea 2 months after the onset of symptoms; follow-up neurological examination and EEG were reported as normal
10	27/female	55/NR	2 days after cessation of treatment with Stalinon	Severe headaches; vomiting; agitation and aggression; difficulties with balance; abnormal EEG; death	Died 11 days after the reported onset of symptoms
11	22/male	55/NR	19 days after beginning treatment with Stalinon	Severe headaches; vomiting; photophobia; confusion; painful neck stiffness; lethargy; constipation; abnormal EEG; death	Died 4 days after the reported onset of symptoms

NR, duration of treatment with Stalinon not reported; EEG, electroencephalogram.

[a]Symptoms and prognosis in six persons accidentally poisoned with a triethyltin-contaminated oral pharmaceutical (Stalinon) for whom exposure levels were estimated.

[b]Estimated dose of triethyltin: based on a theoretical triethyltin concentration of 10% of the 0.015 g of diethyltindiiodide reportedly contained in each Stalinon capsule (Foncin and Gruner, 1979; Barnes and Stoner, 1958). Estimated adult oral lethal triethyltin dose is 70 mg ingested in divided doses over an 8-day period (Barnes and Stoner, 1958).

Translated from Cossa et al. (1958) by Marie H. St. Hilaire, M.D.

continued to show abnormalities for 2 to 4 months, even with apparent clinical improvement.

Neurophysiological Diagnosis

Trimethyltin

Electroencephalography documents TMT neurotoxicity, especially in patients who convulse. The EEG reflects the severity of encephalopathic change following exposure to TMT with disorganization of normal background rhythms and the emergence of bilateral theta (4- to 6-Hz) waves, often paroxysmal and developing into high-amplitude delta (2- to 3-Hz) bursts bilaterally in the temporal areas. The persistence of this epileptiform activity may continue or result in generalized clinical tonic–clonic seizures, followed by postictal slowing. Interictal EEGs show increased bilateral theta activity (4 to 6 Hz), localized over one of both temporal lobes (Fortemps et al., 1978; Besser et al., 1987). The EEG of a 26-year-old man who survived exposure to TMT showed intermittent paroxysmal epileptiform theta slowing over the left temporal area. This patient had permanent TMT-related neurological damage, with recurrent epileptic attacks (Feldman et al., 1993). His seizures were of the complex partial type and no confounding or preexisting factors for his development of epilepsy were found. The *brain stem auditory evoked response, somatosensory evoked potentials,* and *visual evoked potentials* in this patient were normal.

Although peripheral neuropathy resulting from exposure to TMT has not been substantiated in humans, paresthesias in the legs and mild slowing of *sensory nerve conduction velocity,* without sensory loss, were reported following exposure to TMT. The sural nerve conduction velocity of a 41-year-old man was 38 m/sec (normal: more than 45 m/sec); sural nerve action potential and median nerve conduction velocity were both normal (Besser et al., 1987).

Audiometry documented hearing loss of 15 to 30 dB in three of six workers exposed to TMT (Besser et al., 1987).

Triethyltin

The diffuse slow wave abnormalities on EEG following exposure to TET appears to be related to the degree of cerebral edema rather than direct neuronal effects of TET. In general, changes in the EEG tracing reflect the severity of the patient's clinical state. Changes in status can occur suddenly following exposure to TET, and the EEG findings alone should not be used to monitor or predict the clinical course (Cossa et al., 1958).

Of 11 people seen following exposure to the TET-contaminated pharmaceutical Stalinon, 9 had EEG's; six subsequently died, and three recovered (Cossa et al., 1958). In the acute stage, the patients experienced headaches, vomiting, troubles with consciousness, signs of increased intracranial pressure, cerebral hypertension, and edema. The EEG racing at that time was very poorly organized and abnormal, with bursts of high-voltage slow waves. The tracing was generally slower in the posterior regions. Asymmetrical but slow alpha (8- to 10-Hz) waves were noted in some instances; in others the alpha activity was absent. Some rapid frequencies were seen superimposed. Visual stimulation or sensory stimulation, depending on the state of the patient, provoked arousal responses. When multiple tracings were done, there were considerable variations from one day to the next. The degree of disturbed consciousness paralleled the degree of abnormalities seen on the EEG. The bioelectrical disintegration continued in certain cases until death.

In two of the patients described by Cossa et al. (1958; [cases 9 and 10 (see case 10 in Table 9-4)]), clinical abnormalities evolved with seizures, between which the states of consciousness were relatively normal. The EEG tracings during the waking intervals were only mildly abnormal, with mixed theta (4–7 Hz) and beta (12- to 15-Hz) activity, enhanced by hyperventilation (case 9). In the second patient (case 10), the tracing showed mild bursts of slowing in the posterior leads. Case 9 died 6 days after the tracing, with cerebral edema and herniation. Case 10 had very severe nuchal rigidity until she died suddenly 4 days after the EEG had shown brain-stem effects, probably due to tonsillar herniation.

There was a gradual normalization of the tracing, which was related to clinical improvement and regression of cerebral edema in those patients who survived. In one patient, the tracing remained mildly abnormal and asymmetrical despite the absence of clinical signs 4 months after intoxication. By contrast, another patient was still complaining of some symptoms 2 months later even though the EEG tracing had normalized.

Neuropsychological Diagnosis

Trimethyltin

Serial neuropsychological testing documented the clinical course of a 23-year-old man exposed to TMT (Feldman et al., 1993) (Table 9-5). Immediately after the acute intense exposure, the patient presented with a dazed affect and apparent confusion. Although he interacted with others, it was apparent that he did not grasp the severity of his condition. Three days later, his confusion and disorientation were more obvious: he did not recognize the previously familiar faces of his visitors. Neuropsychological testing revealed significant impairment in learning of new verbal and visuospatial information on the Wechsler Memory Scale–Revised (WMS-R), and performance on the visual–motor and visuospatial subtests of the Wechsler Adult Intelligence Scale–Revised (WAIS-R) was only average. A performance IQ (PIQ) of 106 was well below the PIQ of 124 earned in a school assessment 2 years prior to the accident.

Repeat (partial) neuropsychological testing done 10 days after exposure showed some recovery of cognitive function. PIQ had improved to premorbid levels. Immediate recall of verbal and visuospatial information on the WMS-R also improved, but his delayed recall was still impaired (46% on the verbal task; 23% on the visuospatial task). By the time he was discharged (18 days after exposure), his memory had not stabilized; he could not recall information presented to him. Five months after exposure, he experienced interrupted awareness on two occasions.

When seen at 19 months after exposure, neuropsychological assessment revealed very superior IQ scores (verbal IQ 126, PIQ 121). He performed at superior levels on most attention, language, and spatial tasks, but his performance was below expectation on digit symbol (a coding task). His memory quotient on the WMS-R remained below expectation at 106. Learning of narrative information was well below expectation, with forgetting on delay; multiple choice testing of recognition memory was also impaired on this task. In addition, he was also impaired in IQ for learning WMS verbal paired associates and lost 2/9 (22%) on delayed recall; learning and recall were both well below expectation for IQ on the California Verbal Learning Test (CVLT) (12/16 on Trial 5). Memory for visual designs

TABLE 9-5. *Neuropsychological test results*[a]

	Test date			
	February 1985	April 1985	October 1986	October 1988
IQ test administered	WAIS	WAIS	WAIS-R	WAIS-R
FSIQ	117		129	129
VIQ	124	124	126	118
PIQ	106		121	129
Continuous Performance Test				0 errors
Controlled Word Association Test			75th %ile	77–89th %ile
Boston Naming Test			58/60	59/60
Rey-Osterreith Complex Figure			Copy = 100th %ile	Copy = 100th %ile
			IR = 80th %ile	IR = 80th %ile
			DR = 50th %ile	DR = 50th %ile
Difficult Paired Associate Learning				
Trials 1–3				0-2-2-6
Expected scores				3-6-7-9
DR				3
Expected DR score				7
Wechsler Memory Scale				
MQ			106	120
Logical Memory				
Immediate recall	10.5	24	27	23
DR	0	13	14	20
Visual reproductions				
Immediate recall	6	13	12	12
DR	0	10	12	12
Word Triads				
Score				46/60
Expected				>54/50

WAIS, Wechsler Adult Intelligence Scale; WAIS-R, Wechsler Adult Intelligence Scale–Revised; IQ, intelligence quotient; FSIQ, full-scale IQ; VIQ, verbal IQ; PIQ, performance IQ; MQ, memory quotient; IR, immediate recall; DR, delayed recall.
Modified from Feldman et al., 1993, with permission.

was within expected limits on immediate and delayed recall. Behavioral and personality inventories revealed depression and helplessness. Neuropsychological assessment 43 months after exposure revealed an overall improvement of function on the omnibus memory test (WMS Memory Quotient 120). However, he continued to have mild memory deficits. Forgetting of verbal information was seen on WMS verbal memory tests, CVLT, and difficult paired associate learning. Performance on a memory test requiring the patient to learn new information despite interference from a distraction task (Peterson–Peterson Word Triads task) was also below expectation for IQ. He reported symptoms consistent with depressive affect on the Minnesota Multiphasic Personality Inventory. Overall, neuropsychological test findings were considered to be consistent with dysfunction localizable to the limbic system, particularly the left mesial temporal (hippocampal) area.

At follow-up 11 years after the accident, his scores on neuropsychological tests (WAIS-R) of immediate and sustained attention, processing speed, and executive functioning were all within his intellectual and educational expectations. However, his verbal fluency and his reading ability were both slightly below expectation. A very mild impairment of visuospatial ability was identified by tests of visual analysis and construction, with particular difficulties on tasks that minimized verbal facilitation; his ability to identify missing ele-

ments on the Picture Completion task was in the average range, below intellectual expectation. Testing of his short-term memory function showed impairments. His performance was diminished on tests of learning and retrieval, with greater difficulties on verbal than on visual tasks. His recognition of information was consistently better than free recall, indicating good retention of information over time. He was impaired on WMS-R verbal paired associates, and acquisition of a 16-item shopping list (CVLT) was below intellectual expectation. Performance on tests of attention and cognitive tracking ability were consistent with his intellectual ability. His mood was generally positive on tests of behavior and personality.

The neuropsychological test findings above are consistent with the descriptions by Ross et al. (1981, 1983) of verbal memory deficit and inappropriate affect and depression in organotin-exposed patients, who also had attacks of rage.

Triethyltin

Neuropsychological testing was not performed in the Stalinon (TET)-exposed people. Any residual effects in survivors that were described clinically might have reflected the combination of white matter damage and cerebral edema and herniation on formal neuropsychological measures. No formal neuropsychological test reports in humans exposed to TET have been found.

Biochemical Diagnosis

Inorganic tin is found in feces, urine, and blood. However, because the inorganic tins are poorly absorbed and relatively low in toxicity, no specific biomarkers have been established for these compounds. The ACGIH (1995) has not established biological exposure indices (BEI) for tin (Table 9-6).

Suggested and practical diagnostic biomarkers of organotin exposure include (a) blood chemistry, including alkaline phosphatase and serum transaminase; (b) urinalysis; and (c) complete blood count, including differential leukocyte counts (OSHA, 1978; ATSDR, 1992). Both TMT and TET have a low affinity for human hemoglobin, and therefore whole blood concentrations are low (Rose and Aldridge, 1968; Aldridge et al., 1981; Brown et al., 1984). Increased urinary tin levels are consistent with an increased body burden, and the severity of clinical symptoms correlates with maximal urinary excretion (Ross et al., 1981; Johnson and Greger, 1982; Besser et al., 1987). Urine organotin determinations can be performed using atomic absorption spectroscopy after toluol extraction. The average background tin concentration in 11 human urine samples was 1.0 ppb, with 18% in the methylated form (Braman and Tompkins, 1979). Maximal urine organotin levels are reached 4 to 10 days after cessation of exposure (Besser et al., 1987) (Fig. 9-1).

In the 23-year-old chemistry student referred to above, the urinary tin concentration on the 17th day after TMT exposure was 52 ppb (upper limit of normal: 18 ppb); the serum level was 13 ppb (upper limit of normal: 3.3 ppb) (Feldman et al., 1993). By the 35th day after exposure, the urinary tin concentration was down to 10 ppb, and the serum level was still elevated at 7.4 ppb. Maximum urinary levels occur at 4 to 10 days after exposure (Besser et al., 1987) (see Fig. 9-1); therefore this patient probably had a significantly higher urine tin content in the first few days after exposure than was measured in the first urine sample taken 17 days after exposure.

Neuroimaging

Magnetic resonance imaging (MRI) has been suggested as a method of documenting the cytotoxic edema induced by exposure to TET (Go and Edzes, 1975). In brain edema, there is an abnormal accumulation of water in the tissue.

Brain edema may be induced by (a) blood vessel damage with enlargement of the extracellular space (vasogenic or cold-induced); (b) a predominance of cellular swelling (cytotoxic); and (c) a movement of water into the periventricular regions (interstitial) (Rosenberg and Wolfson, 1991). The amount of water in specific brain tissues affects the relaxation times of T_1- and T_2-weighted MR images. In general, the white matter contains 12% less water than the gray matter. As a result, the relaxation times of the T2-weighted images of the white matter are relatively shorter than those of the gray matter (Edwards and Bonnin, 1991). However, following exposure to TET, the MRI of rats shows longer relaxation times on T_1- and T_2-weighted images of the white matter, possibly reflecting the intramyelinic accumulation of fluid (Gwan and Edzes, 1975).

By contrast, the brain computed tomography (CT) and MRI following exposure to TMT do not disclose any particular changes. The brain CT scan and MRI of a 23-year-old man on the third day following an acute intense exposure to TMT was normal, showing no evidence of atrophy or edema (Feldman et al., 1993). At a 4-year follow-up examination, MRI and CT scan of the brain of a 36-year-old man who had developed severe ataxia following exposure to TMT also revealed no abnormalities (Besser et al., 1987).

Neuropathological Diagnosis

TMT has been used to elucidate the cytoarchitecture of the brain and the pathogenesis of limbic seizure activity, and TET intoxication has been used as an experimental model of myelinopathies and neurodegenerative disorders and in the study of cerebral edema (Magee et al., 1957; Torack et al., 1960; Reiter and Ruppert, 1984; Walsh and DeHaven, 1988).

Trimethyltin

Histopathological studies in laboratory animals exposed to TMT have shown a preferential vulnerability of the hippocampal neurons. Early pathological changes have been noted in the pyramidal cells of areas CA1, CA3, and CA4 of the hippocampus as well as in the granule cells of the dentate gyrus (Ross et al., 1981; Ruppert et al., 1982; Valdes et al., 1983; Naalsund et al., 1985; Whittington et al., 1989; Earley et al., 1992; Allen et al., 1994). In addition, TMT induced neuronal cell necrosis in the pyriform cortex, amyg-

TABLE 9-6. *Biological exposure indices for tin*

	Urine	Blood	Alveolar air
Determinant	Tin	Tin	Tin
Start of shift	Not established	Not established	Not established
During shift	Not established	Not established	Not established
End of shift at end of workweek	Not established	Not established	Not established

Data from ACGIH, 1995.

daloid nuclei, and olfactory tuberculum (Allen et al., 1994). Damage also occurs in the entorhinal cortex, and olfactory bulbs. Loss of cholinergic neurons may be responsible for the cognitive deficits induced by TMT (Earley et al., 1995). TMT has been also shown to decrease significantly muscarinic receptor density in the hippocampus, amygdala, basal ganglia, cortex, hypothalamus, and septal area. These neuropathological alterations may contribute to the effects of TMT on memory, learning, and behavior (Earley et al., 1992; O'Connell et al., 1994; Earley et al., 1995). The damaged areas in the forebrain are those associated with learning and memory impairment in animals or dementia and amnestic syndromes in humans. Although there are many reports about the neuropathological and behavioral changes induced by TMT on animals (Fortemps et al., 1978), there have been few reports on such effects in humans (Brown et al., 1979; Ross et al., 1981; Rey et al., 1984; Boyer, 1989).

A 48-year-old woman died 6 days after she ingested an unknown quantity of wine contaminated with TMT (Kreyberg et al., 1992). Analysis of the wine showed a TMT level greater than 0.5 µg/mL. Postmortem studies showed a grossly normal-appearing brain, weighing 1,200 g with no signs of edema. Microscopic examination revealed marked neuronal swelling, with lateral displacement of the nuclei and chromatolysis in the neurons of the cerebrum, spinal cord, and spinal ganglia. Signs of recent necrosis, including pyknotic changes with increased basophilia, were seen in the neurons of the hippocampus, cerebral cortex, and basal ganglia. Several neurons in the fascia dentata of the hippocampus showed karyorrhexis. Such changes were not observed in the neurons of the brain stem or spinal cord. Purkinje cell loss was seen in the cerebellum. Neuronal necrosis and shrinkage of nuclei was present in approximately 10% of the neurons of the spinal ganglia. Electron microscopy was done on samples of hippocampus, medulla, and anterior horn cells of the spinal cord. The most prominent finding in hippocampal neurons was an accumulation of lysosomal dense bodies in the cytoplasm. The cytoplasmic zebra bodies observed by Besser et al. (1987) were not observed in the present case (Fig. 9-2). A less pronounced increase in lysosomal dense bodies was seen in the hypoglossal nuclei and the anterior horn cells. The granular endoplasmic reticulum was disorganized.

Although Kreyberg et al. (1992) attributed some of the cellular changes to hypoxia, the features described in their case are similar to neuronal changes seen in animals with experimental TMT poisoning (Bouldin et al., 1981; Brown et al., 1984; Nolan et al., 1990) and in those described in humans by Besser et al. (1987). For example, the brain described by Besser et al. (1987) in a person who died of pulmonary edema subsequent to TMT exposure revealed swollen perikarya in nerve cell bodies, loss of Nissl substance, and necrosis of temporal cortex nerve cells in some regions. Electron microscopy showed morphological alterations including zebra bodies and many vacuoles. These changes were most prominent in the temporal cortex, basal ganglia, and pontine nuclei. The cerebellar cortex showed severe loss of Purkinje cells (see Fig. 9-2).

The exact mechanisms responsible for the neurotoxic action of TMT in humans remain uncertain. Studies of the selective vulnerability of specific neuronal populations to the effects of TMT suggest that a specific gene product, stannin, is expressed by certain TMT-sensitive cells in the human brain (Krady et al., 1990; Toggas et al., 1992). Several mechanisms proposed to account for the neurotoxic effects of TMT include (a) inhibition of Ca^{2+} adenosine triphosphatase (ATPase) in a concentration-dependent manner, thereby interfering with the calcium pump and other cyclic adenosine monophosphate (cAMP) mediated processes in the brain (Yallapragada et al., 1991); (b) depression of mitochondrial respiration, which may subsequently lower the resting membrane potential of neuronal membranes and allow the release of excitatory amino acids (e.g., glutamate and aspartate) from the heavy metal-containing pathways of the hippocampus, ultimately resulting in damage to the granule and pyramidal cells innervated by these pathways (Sloviter et al., 1986; Wilson et al., 1986; Brodie et al., 1990; Aschner and Aschner, 1992); and (c) reduction in the hippocampal zinc concentration, which may lead to disinhibition and subsequent hyperexcitation of the hippocampal neuronal electrical circuitry (Chang and Dyer, 1984; Walsh and DeHaven, 1988). TMT affects uptake and levels of specific neurotransmitters and amino acids. TMT inhibits synaptosomal uptake of γ-aminobutyric acid (GABA), norepinephrine, and serotonin (Doctor et al., 1982; Costa, 1985; Earley et al., 1992). TMT produces a decrease in the concentration of GABA in the hippocampus, which may reflect alterations in convulsive thresholds (Mailman et al., 1983; Earley et al., 1992). TMT may produce memory impairment by destroying the muscarinic receptors of central cholinergic pathways (Earley et al., 1992, 1995). Increased blood levels of ammonia resulting from impaired functioning of the liver and kidneys may enhance the neurotoxic effects of TMT (Wilson et al., 1986; Walsh and DeHaven, 1988).

Triethyltin

The selective edema of the central nervous system produced by TET poisoning has peculiar characteristics that set it apart from other types of cerebral swelling. High-power microscopic examination of the human brain following TET poisoning reveals a great number of microvacuoles within the myelin lamellae (Foncin and Gruner, 1979) (Fig. 9-3).

Autopsy was performed on four patients who died following exposure to the TET-contaminated pharmaceutical Stalinon (Cossa et al., 1958). In all cases, the brain was edematous and pink. The ventricles were always small. There was hyperemia of the brain stem and herniation of cerebellar tonsils and sometimes the temporal lobes. Histologically, there were severe and diffuse lesions with acute neuronal alterations and edema in the pericellular spaces. Perineuronal edema was seen throughout the brain. There

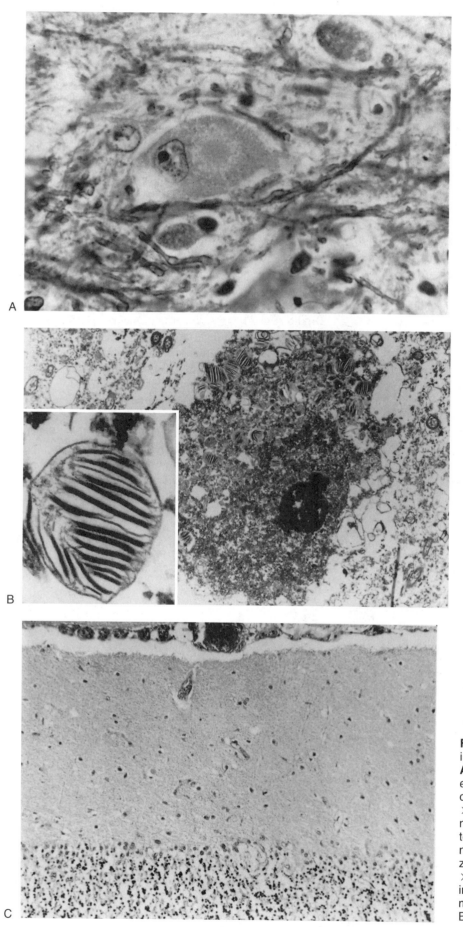

FIG. 9-2. Neuropathological changes in human following exposure to TMT. **A:** Nerve cell in the amygdala showing eccentric nucleus and cytoplasmic inclusion body (original magnification, ×650). **B:** Electron micrograph of a neuron in the amygdala, showing cytoplasmic zebra bodies (original magnification, ×7,000); inset shows single zebra body (original magnification, ×57,500). **C:** Cerebellar cortex showing loss of Purkinje's cells (original magnification, ×140). (Modified from Besser et al., 1987, with permission.)

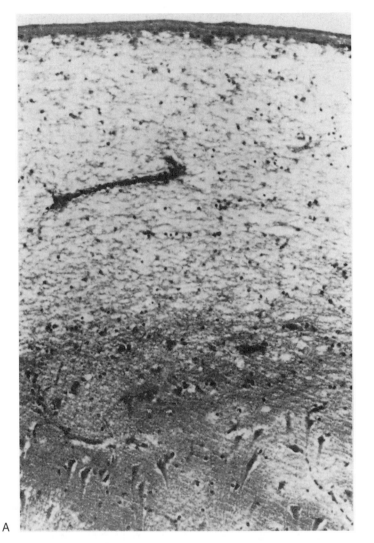

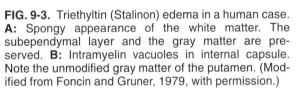

FIG. 9-3. Triethyltin (Stalinon) edema in a human case. **A:** Spongy appearance of the white matter. The subependymal layer and the gray matter are preserved. **B:** Intramyelin vacuoles in internal capsule. Note the unmodified gray matter of the putamen. (Modified from Foncin and Gruner, 1979, with permission.)

A

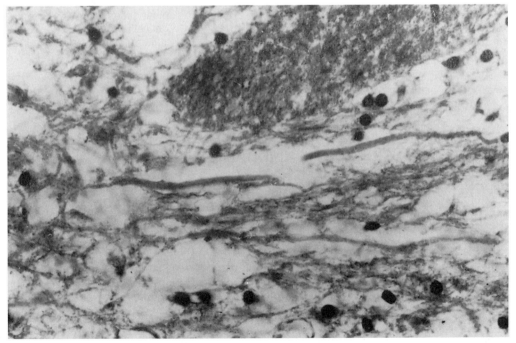

B

were also areas of interstitial edema and perivascular edema, especially in the central areas of the brain at the level of the basal ganglia, and in the floor of the fourth ventricle. The acute neurotoxic lesions were seen at the level of the cortex, the cranial nerve nuclei, and the pontine nuclei. There was atrophy and gliosis in the pyramidal layer of the cortex, and in the Purkinje cell layer of the cerebellum. The same mixture of cytotoxic and gliotic changes was seen in the area of the dentate nuclei. There was fragmentation of the neurofilaments, acute degeneration of the oligodendroglia, regressive lesions of the astrocytes, some vascular stasis in certain places reaching to extravasation, and rare petechial hemorrhage. The vessels themselves showed no alterations. There was no fatty degeneration of the vessel walls or endothelium (Table 9-7).

Bakay (1965) studied the neuropathological changes associated with TET-induced edema and their relation to the steady state and dynamic equilibrium of some of the electrolytes in albumin; he then compared these results with edema produced by thermal trauma. In rats fed TET, the first neurological signs developed 7 to 10 days after instituting the feedings. Within a few days, weakness in the hind legs progressed to complete paralysis. Interruption of TET feeding and return to normal diet was followed with complete clinical recovery within 5 days.

The pathological findings in the animals sacrificed at the time of total paralysis of the hind limbs showed enlarged and somewhat pale brains with severe cerebral edema involving the white matter of the brain and spinal cord. On coronal section, the white matter was seen to have increased moisture. There was no vascular engorgement, nor was there any evidence of petechial bleeding. The microscopic changes were localized to white matter, which was enlarged and spongy in appearance. There was a remarkable lack of glial and mesenchymal reaction in the edematous white matter. In the animals sacrificed when they showed complete clinical recovery, histological evidence of edema in the white matter was still present. Although edema was limited essentially to the white matter, vacuolar degeneration in the cytoplasm of the cells of the basal gan-

TABLE 9-7. *Neuropathological findings in humans following triethyltin poisoning[a]*

Case	Age/sex	Estimated dose of triethyltin[b] (mg)	Duration of illness from onset of symptoms until death	Neuropathological findings	
				Macroscopic examination	Microscopic examination
2	15/female	40/10 days	1 week	Edematous brain; herniation of the cerebellar tonsils	*Frontal cortex* Microvacuolization within the white matter Swelling of the oligodendroglia; swelling, vacuolization, and nuclear basophilia of the pyramidal cells No alteration of the neurofilaments Perivascular edema No meningeal abnormality *Temporal cortex* Similar alterations as the frontal cortex, but less marked Subpial edema with mild microphage activity in the arachnoid space *Optic tract and caudate nucleus* Changes in oligodendroglia and neurons Severe subependymal edema
10	27/female	55/10 days	2 weeks	The brain was congested and edematous; no sign of trauma or hematoma; hemorrhagic exudate in the ventricles	Ventricular hemorrhage; small petechial hemorrhages

[a]In two persons following ingestion of the triethyltin-contaminated pharmaceutical, Stalinon.
[b]Data from Cossa et al., 1958.

glia was noted. The lateral portions of the thalamus and the geniculate bodies showed unusually large vacuoles, which distorted the nerve cells. In addition, distinct loss of small nerve cells was seen in the striatum. These changes were attributed to increased fluid within the myelinated fibers involving the fifth and sixth cortical layers and the nuclei of the brain stem and basal ganglia along the medial portion of the internal capsule.

Bakay (1965) differentiated TET-induced cerebral edema clinically and pathologically from the cerebral edema induced by inorganic lead. The histological evidence presented by Bakay shows that the edema induced by TET exposure is essentially limited to the white matter, although neuronal swelling is seen in those portions of the gray matter that contain an abundance of myelinated fibers. Although the white matter is also severely affected in inorganic lead encephalopathy, the cortex is not spared. In addition, the vascular changes and the protein-rich exudate in the edema of inorganic lead encephalopathy are different from those caused by alkyltin and alkyl lead compounds (Popoff et al., 1963). The reason for this difference appears to be related to the fact that triethyltin intoxication produces edema that is unique in its relation to the BBB. Triethyltin produces edema in the white matter that does not stain with trypan blue, and large molecules such as albumin do not penetrate the edematous tissue from the bloodstream. Studies of the rate of uptake and radioautographic distribution of ^{131}I-labeled serum albumin showed that the BBB was essentially impermeable to ^{131}I-labeled serum albumin (Bakay, 1965). This is in striking contrast to traumatic and inflammatory edemas, which are characterized by an increased albumin content and an exchange of labeled albumin with plasma and edematous brain tissue. Bakay further showed that much smaller molecules such as glycine do not concentrate in the TET edematous white matter to any greater extent than in normal brain, in contrast to edemas produced by mechanical means; the rate of uptake and radioautographic distribution of ^{14}C-labeled glycine was identical in normal and edematous white matter. Other studies have demonstrated that the sodium and chloride content of the TET exposure-induced edema fluid is increased over that of normal extracellular fluid, reflecting a slowing in the rate of sodium exchange (Katzman et al., 1963). These results indicated that edema fluid in TET poisoning is a plasma filtrate and that it differs from the fluid of cold-induced cerebral edema and the edema produced by hypercapnic hypoxia, in both of which the fluid more closely resembles whole plasma.

The exact site at which TET binds to myelin to induce the formation of these vacuoles is unknown; however, evidence suggests that the vesicles may be derived from myelin domains engaged in the regulation of ion and fluid dynamics at the paranodal region (Lock and Aldridge, 1975; Sapirstein et al., 1993). Levels of the myelin-bound ion transport protein carbonic anhydrase are reduced by exposure to TET. Carbonic anhydrase appears to be in-

volved in the removal of accumulated fluid from within the vesicles. Rats exposed to TET and treated with a carbonic anhydrase inhibitor (acetazolamide) do not recover from TET-induced brain edema, which is usually reversible (Yanagisawa et al., 1990). Proposed mechanisms of TET-induced edema include (a) interference with cation transport by inhibition of Na^+/K^+ mediated-ATPase activity (Torack, 1965; Wassenaar and Kroon, 1973; Tosteson and Sapirstein, 1981; Watanabe, 1980); (b) altering the activity of the cAMP enzyme phosphodiesterase, potentially altering concentrations of cAMP and thus enhancing the transport of water and ions into cells (Macovschi et al., 1984); and (c) inhibiting Ca^{2+} pump activity by interacting with the Ca^{2+}-ATPase regulatory protein, calmodulin (Yallapragada et al., 1991). The biochemical effects of TET on mitochondria further contribute to its neurotoxic effects through several mechanisms, which include (a) direct binding to the mitochondrial membrane promoting oligomycinlike inhibition of mitochondrial ATPase activity (Moore and Brody, 1961; Aldridge and Street, 1964; Rose and Aldridge, 1972; Wassenaar and Kroon, 1973); and (b) promoting the exchange of halide for OH^- ions across the lipid membrane of the organelle, resulting in uncoupling of oxidative phosphorylation (Aldridge and Cremer, 1955; Aldridge, 1958; Moore and Brody, 1961; Selwyn et al., 1970; Stockdale et al., 1970; Rose and Cremer, 1970; Rose and Aldridge, 1972; Aldridge and Street, 1971; Lock, 1976; Aldridge et al., 1977). TET produces a general depletion of brain tissue concentrations of specific neurotransmitters including dopamine, norepinephrine, and serotonin (Cook, 1983). In addition, concentrations of the amino acids GABA, glutamic acid, and alanine are significantly decreased in rat brains following intraperitoneal injection of TET (Cremer, 1964). Inhibition of glucose oxidation by triethyltin has also been reported (Cremer, 1970).

PREVENTIVE AND THERAPEUTIC MEASURES

Baseline blood and urine levels should be determined for workers at risk of exposure to tin (Fait et al., 1994). The work areas where tin compounds are manufactured or used should be properly ventilated. Respirators should be used by all employees at risk of exposure to high levels of tin compounds (OSHA, 1978). Treatment of persons suspected of exposure to inorganic or organic tin compounds should be directed to minimize the acute effects and remove the possibility of continuing damage by reducing the body burden as much and as quickly as possible. The immediate irritant effects of inorganic tin salts on skin or mucous membranes are best dealt with by washing the skin and flushing the eyes with copious amounts of water to eliminate continuing contact. After oral intake, the mouth must be rinsed thoroughly to prevent damage to the mucous membranes. Ingested inorganic tins can be diluted by administration of water (Ellenhorn and Barceloux, 1988).

Although chelation using D-penicillamine or dimercaprol does not appear to increase urinary excretion of organic tin (Barnes and Stoner 1959; Ellenhorn and Barceloux, 1988), four patients administered plasmapheresis and D-penicillamine following exposure to TMT survived, suggesting that the combination of the two may be effective (Besser et al., 1987). Symptomatic treatment of epileptic seizures with therapeutic levels of carbamazepine or valproic acid should be instituted if seizures have occurred and should be continued prophylactically when reexposure to TMT is considered likely. The use of these drugs, proven in the management of limbic type seizures arising in temporal neurons, is justified since the selective hippocampal neuronal targets of TMT are likely to be damaged and to induce epileptic discharge.

Acute measures to prevent cerebral edema and subsequent tonsillar herniation must be instituted as soon as possible after TET intoxication has been diagnosed. Restriction of water intake is a relatively safe method of controlling brain edema and should be instituted immediately in suspected cases of TET intoxication and in confirmed cases if the patient has not presented signs of symptoms of exposure; blood pressure should be monitored in these patients to avoid fluid restriction–induced hypotension (Ramming et al., 1994; Zornow and Prough, 1995). If symptoms are present, osmotic diuretics such as mannitol and glycerin or steroids such as decadron, which are effective methods of managing brain edema, may be administered to lower the intracranial pressure associated with TET intoxication, although the efficacy of these therapeutic measures is unknown. Carbonic anhydrase inhibitors have been used to reduce extracellular edema, such as that in pseudotumor cerebri. However, carbonic anhydrase has been shown to be involved in the dehydration of intramyelin edema associated with TET intoxication. Thus, acetazolamide, a carbonic anhydrase inhibitor, may have adverse effects if used in the treatment of TET intoxication (Kirschner and Sapirstein, 1982; Yanagisawa et al., 1990).

CLINICAL EXPERIENCES

Trimethyltin

Group Studies

Nonfatal and Fatal Exposures to TMT while Cleaning a Synthesizing Tank

Six previously healthy industrial workers developed an acute limbic–cerebellar syndrome attributed to TMT poisoning while cleaning a tank used in the manufacture of dimethyltin. Dimethyltin is manufactured under pressure from inorganic tin and methyl chloride; TMT occurs as a byproduct. The potential of exposure is greatest when the tank is first opened and the TMT vaporizes. The cleaning process, during which these workers were exposed, involved removing "inorganic tin" from the inside of the tank with hoes and shovels. Measures taken by the workers to lessen the risks of exposure to TMT included flushing the tank with water and the use of protective clothing and masks. In addition, the workers cleaned the tank in 15-minute shifts, with each worker having a maximum of four shifts a day. Nevertheless, injury occurred, and the cases were described by Besser et al. (1987).

Case 1. A 45-year-old man was admitted to the hospital complaining of headaches and decreased hearing. He reported that for the past 4 days, he had been working outside the dimethyltin synthesizing tank, at the task of transferring the inorganic tin to a nearby container. Two days after admission, he became restless, confused, and amnesic for the events preceding his admission. He had episodes of unresponsiveness, resembling complex partial seizures. Two days later, his condition had returned to normal. EEG the following day was normal.

Case 2. A 34-year-old man noted unusual changes in his affect and occasional episodes of unresponsiveness on his third day of working inside the tank; his total time inside the tank was 2.75 hours. The next day, he began to experience tinnitus and hearing loss. Audiometry revealed hearing loss of 30 dB. He was admitted to the hospital the following day. His condition improved rapidly, and EEGs taken 4 and 9 days later were normal. In an attempt to increase urinary excretion of TMT, plasmapheresis and D-penicillamine were administered in the hospital on days 8 and 9. At follow-up 11 months later, the patient was clinically normal, but electronystagmography (ENG) revealed mild saccadic smooth pursuit eye movements. Sural nerve conduction studies were normal, with velocity of 50 m/sec and action potential amplitude of 13 μV.

Case 3. On his third day of working inside the synthesizing tank (time inside the tank: 2.75 hours), a 43-year-old man began to experience hearing loss and a pressure sensation within his ears. Audiometry performed at this time showed a hearing loss of 15 dB. Two days later he became unsteady, irritable, and aggressive and had two complex partial seizures. EEG performed 4 days later was normal. Over the course of the next 4 days, the patient became severely disoriented and amnesic. A 2-day course of plasmapheresis and D-penicillamine was administered. EEG 2 days later showed bilateral temporal slowing. The patient's clinical condition improved considerably over the next few days, although he was still mildly amnesic and experienced occasional episodes of confusion during the night. The patient subsequently became hyperphagic and remained so for the next 6 weeks. In addition, approximately 3 weeks after the onset of symptoms, the patient began experiencing paresthesias in the legs. The paresthesias continued for 5 months but were not accompanied by weakness, sensation loss, or reflex alterations. At follow-up 11 months after the incident, the patient presented as clinically normal, except for a bilateral gaze-evoked nystagmus. A single generalized nocturnal tonic–clonic seizure occurred 16 months after exposure. An EEG was taken at this time and revealed no abnormalities.

Case 4. On his second day cleaning the inside of the tank, a 41-year-old man began to experience tinnitus, hearing loss, increased thirst, and lethargy. His total time cleaning the inside of the tank was 0.75 hours. Audiometry revealed hearing loss of 30 dB. Three days after the onset of symptoms, he was disoriented, aggressive, and amnesic. The following day he became restless and wandered out of the hospital. There was no decreased consciousness, and his behavior was unresponsive to tranquilizers. Over the next 2 days, he began to experience difficulty breathing, his blood pressure was elevated, and he became somnolent. He subsequently went into respiratory arrest and was treated with dexamethasone, mechanical ventilation, plasmapheresis, and D-penicillamine. EEG performed 2 days later showed flat background activity, with rhythmic waves that were most prominent on the right. His consciousness improved over the next 8 days with an increase in appetite to the point of hyperphagia. He reported experiencing numbness in his feet and sexual dysfunction. On follow-up at 11 months, the patient still had poor impulse control as well as short- and long-term memory impairments. ENG revealed a bilateral gaze nystagmus and mildly saccadic pursuit eye movements. EEG and nerve conduction studies were normal.

Case 5. After 3 days of cleaning the tank (time inside the tank: 2.75 hours) a 34-year-old man began to develop pain in his limbs and hearing loss. The following day he was intermittently disoriented and anxious and had erythema of his chest. His condition worsened over the next 2 days, as he became more disoriented and aggressive. The next day he had several complex partial seizures and attacks of rage, during which he tried to escape out of the hospital window. Respiratory symptoms developed, leading to respiratory arrest, and he required mechanical ventilation for the next 9 days. EEG at this time showed moderate slowing of the background activity with bitemporal bursts of delta activity. Plasmapheresis and D-penicillamine were administered. Fourteen days after the onset of symptoms, he was removed from the mechanical ventilator, and all sedative drugs were discontinued. Over the course of the next several days, the patient developed severe limb and truncal ataxia, dysarthria, and gaze-evoked bilateral nystagmus. Strength, sensation, and reflexes were normal. One month after the onset of symptoms, the EEG still showed slowing of the background activity. In addition, he had periodic alternating nystagmus. At 3 months after exposure, the patient had a gaze-evoked bilateral nystagmus and was sexually aggressive, although he had no amnesia. Four years after the incident, the patient's nystagmus and dysarthria had improved, although he was still severely ataxic, wheelchair-bound, and unable to feed or dress himself.

Case 6. A 51-year-old man had worked at cleaning the tank for 3 days (time inside the tank: 2.75 hours) when he began to experience tinnitus and blurred vision. He became progressively disoriented, aggressive, and forgetful. In addition, he had erythema of the head and chest, bronchospasms, and severe peripheral cyanosis. On neuro-

logical examination, the patient was moderately ataxic, without alterations in strength, sensation, or reflexes. He later developed periods of altered consciousness and had a generalized tonic–clonic seizure. Respiratory symptoms developed, and he required mechanical ventilation. EEG at this time showed moderate slowing of background activity and intermittent and independent bitemporal paroxysmal theta activity. Three days later, the EEG showed right temporal sharp waves. The patient died 2 days later (see Neuropathological Diagnosis section).

Individual Case Studies

Long-Term Follow-up of a Chemist Exposed to TMT During an Explosion

A 23-year-old chemistry graduate student was recrystallizing an organotin compound, bis-trimethyl-stannyl acetylene, from an ether-based solvent, when it was accidentally ignited by the hot plate he was using (Yanofsky et al., 1991; Feldman et al., 1993). He was burned by the explosion and fire, and he inhaled large quantities of vapor. He was wearing safety goggles but had no respiratory protection. He quickly used the safety shower and eye wash. Help arrived, and he was taken to the hospital emergency room.

On admission examination, he was orientated to place and time. There was no lateralizing motor neurological deficit, and he was aware of the accident. He was given oxygen by mask and treated for 12% first-degree burns to the hands, upper chest, and left side of the face, 2% second-degree burns on the left side of the face and hands (distal regions), and less than 1% third-degree burns on the left earlobe and left eye. There was no acute respiratory or gastrointestinal symptomatology, and liver function tests were normal. Blood count was normal except for a slight lymphocytosis. He developed acute renal tubular acidosis, which improved with vigorous fluid and electrolyte treatment after 8 days.

During the first 72 hours after the accident, he was awake but confused and disoriented. He could not find the bathroom and appeared to have difficulty following directions. He would mumble to himself and repeat statements about the accident. He was slow to recognize his visitors. He did not recall the nurse who attended him the night before when she returned the next day. Object recall was 3/3 within 5 minutes on the fourth day after admission, but 0/3 on the fifth, 2/3 on the seventh, and 1/3 on the tenth day.

On the third day, CT of the brain was normal, with no evidence of cerebral edema. Somatosensory evoked potentials using the median and posterior tibial nerves were normal. EEG revealed 4- to 5-Hz theta waves located over the left temporal area. With drowsiness there was an increase in delta (3 to 4 Hz) activity over the left hemisphere. This asymmetry was also enhanced by hyperventilation. Definite epileptiform activity was not present at this time. At time of discharge from the hospital, 18 days after the explosion, his EEG revealed an excess of scattered slow frequencies bilaterally and theta instability over the left hemisphere, in particular.

Formal neuropsychological tests were performed while the patient was in the hospital. The WMS revealed moderate to marked impairment of recent memory function. His PIQ on the WAIS was 106. His memory waxed and waned during hospitalization, and at the time of discharge (18th day after exposure), it was not clear whether memory function was improving or not. Repeat (partial) testing a week later showed improved PIQ (124), which was more in keeping with the expected score for a science graduate student. Recent memory appeared overtly intact, and he appeared to have recovered most or all of his cognitive functions on the limited assessment completed at that time. However, while at home, he became lost in his home town, and his parents noted that he was acting strangely, appearing withdrawn and having difficulty recalling information presented to him.

Tin assay on the 17th day after accident revealed a serum TMT value of 13 ppb (upper limit for humans: less than 3.3) and 52 ppb in the urine (upper limit: 18). TMT was the only form of tin found. A repeat assay 35 days after the accident still revealed an elevated serum level (7.4 ppb) but the urine level was down to 10 ppb (analysis by GC/MS, National Medical Services, Willow Grove, PA).

When he returned to school 2 months later, he could not recall details of the research thesis he had been working on before the accident. Repeat EEG continued to show slight excess of theta activity that had a left-sided emphasis with hyperventilation.

Five months after exposure, he experienced an episode of lightheadedness followed by loss of consciousness. He was admitted an hour later when a second episode occurred. His friends described the episode thus: his eyes bulged out and he began to shake all over, nearly falling out of the chair. He was unresponsive to verbal stimuli for 2 to 3 minutes. When he appeared to recover, he did not remember the episodes. These episodes recurred at least 2 to 4 times a week. He described the "blackout" episodes as recurrent and both mild and severe. The severe episodes were characterized by a vague visual impression, with a feeling of familiarity, an unpleasant smell, and associated intense sweating and warm forearms. The spells lasted for several minutes and then disappeared as suddenly as they had appeared. Difficulties with sleeping and increased problems with concentration and recall were common problems when these spells were occurring. The mild episodes seemed to occur in a progressive fashion for about a week prior to onset of more severe spells.

Neurological examination revealed no motor or sensory deficit. EEG showed small sharp spikes suggestive of true epileptiform discharge. Repeat tests 1 week later showed the presence of intermittent paroxysmal theta slowing in the left temporal derivations suggestive of clear irritable focus in that area of the cortex. The visual evoked potential, brain stem auditory evoked response, and somatosensory evoked potential using the median and tibial nerves were all normal. Nocturnal polysomography revealed no epileptiform activity.

Neuropsychological assessment revealed superior overall cognitive functioning. His best performances were in abstract thinking (98th percentile), sequential thinking (98th percentile), and visuospatial reasoning (99th percentile). His V- and PIQ had improved, but his recall of word lists and paragraphs was inefficient, with strong primacy and recency effects and significant loss of information over time. There was also evidence of poor registration and susceptibility to retroactive interference. His memory quotient on the WMS was 106. Dysphoria was also present.

He was placed on carbamazepine (Tegretol) with the aim of achieving a blood level of 10 ppb. He claimed some improvements, with reduction in seizure frequency. During follow-up he revealed that the seizures now manifested as change in concentration with a distorted visual recall and extensive disorientation lasting only for seconds.

Neuropsychological testing at 43 months after the accident continued to show an impairment in performance on memory tasks although the memory quotient on the WMS had improved to 120. There was difficulty with acquisition and retention of new information, which was most apparent on verbal memory tasks. He continued to have residual effects in psychomotor speed and cognitive flexibility, as well as symptomatology of depression.

EEG at 43 months after the accident revealed minor left temporal theta activity with a rare sharp wave and a rare rhythmic discharge suggestive of minor epileptogenic potential. MRI of the brain was normal. There was no area of intraparenchymal abnormal signal intensity.

At follow-up 11 years after the accident he reported feeling a significant improvement, although he recognized that some of his impairments were permanent. He never finished his graduate degree. He still complained of concentration, short-term memory, language, and organizational difficulties. In addition, he stated that he fatigues easily and requires 11 to 12 hours of sleep a night. The frequency of his seizures had decreased from daily to once every several months.

Neuropsychological testing revealed persistent deficits in verbal fluency and reading ability, mild visuospatial difficulties, and impairment of short-term memory function. Tests of immediate and sustained attention, processing speed, and executive functioning were within intellectual expectation.

Although an overall improvement in his short-term memory has been noted, his spontaneous recovery in this domain seems to have reached its maximum (Table 9-5). Compensatory techniques such as mnemonic strategies may improve his performance. A comparison of his neuropsychological performance across time reveals that his visuospatial deficits had temporarily returned to superior level, but have since dropped to the high average range. Attention and tracking abilities appear to have been spared. Nevertheless, the patient continues to complain of attention and concentration difficulties. Social judgment and reasoning have returned to normal.

Triethyltin

Group Studies

The Wrong Salt of Tin Implicated in the Accidental Poisoning of 210 Persons

Two hundred and ten persons were accidentally poisoned with TET when a pharmacist inadvertently used the wrong salt of tin during preparation of the oral pharmaceutical compound known as Stalinon (Barnes and Stoner, 1959). The recommended adult treatment dose of Stalinon was 6 tablets a day, to be taken for 8 days and 3 capsules a day for children (Barnes and Stoner, 1959). The average dose of TET was estimated to be 10% of the 0.015 g of diethyltindiiodide reportedly contained in each Stalinon capsule (Foncin and Gruner, 1979; Barnes and Stoner, 1958). The median lethal dose among those exposed was 50 mg of TET (Foncin and Gruner, 1979). Most patients began to exhibit signs of intoxication within 4 days ($\approx$ 36 mg TET) (Alajouanine et al., 1958; Foncin and Gruner, 1979). The most frequently reported symptom was severe headache, associated with increased intracranial pressure (Table 9-4). Approximately 100 persons died; among the patients who survived, convalescence was slow, and many never recovered fully (Magee et al., 1957; Alajouanine et al., 1958; Cossa et al., 1958; Barnes and Stoner, 1959). One of these cases is summarized below to exemplify the clinical picture and the effects experienced by others in this group.

Individual Case Studies

Trimethyltin Encephalopathy: A Case Report

A 15-year-old girl who had been taking 4 capsules of Stalinon a day began to experience headaches after approximately 1 week of treatment (Cossa et al., 1958). She complained of these symptoms to her doctor, and treatment was stopped on the tenth day. She was hospitalized 2 days later with severe headaches, vomiting, and brief episodes of unconsciousness accompanied by clonic–tonic movements of the upper left extremity and incontinence. On general neurological examination she was considered to have normal strength, tone, reflexes, and coordination. Examination of cranial nerves also revealed no abnormalities. However, because during the interictal periods she was frequently somnolent or mute, it was difficult to get a more complete picture of her illness.

Interictal EEG showed a global disturbance of the background frequency over the entire recording. The pattern included a large proportion of slow waves with a slight right hemisphere predominance. During the first part of the tracing there was a marked predominance of slow wave activity, with bursts of sinusoidal slow waves in the frontal regions. In the other regions, polymorphic delta activity was predominant. When the patient was quiet, occasional alphalike activity was superimposed on the slow waves. The amplitude of the slow waves decreased briefly when the patient opened her eyes. When the patient was awake, the slow waves were replaced to 5 to 9 Hz activity. Three days later the patient became apneic and died (Table 9-7).

REFERENCES

Agency for Toxic Substance and Disease Registry (ATSDR). *Toxicological profile for tin.* TP-91/27. Atlanta, GA: U.S. Department of Health and Human Services, Public Health Service, 1992.

Alajouanine T, Derobert L, Thieffry S. Etude clinique d'ensemble de 210 cas d'intoxication par les sels organiques d'étain. *Rev Neurol* 1958;98: 85–96.

Aldridge WN. The biochemistry of organotin compounds, trialkyltin and oxidative phosphorylation. *Biochem J* 1958;69:367–376.

Aldridge WN, Cremer JR. The biochemistry of organo-tin compounds, diethyltin dichloride and triethyltin sulfate. *Biochem J* 1955;61:406–418.

Aldridge WN, Street BW. Oxidative phosphorylation: biochemical effects and properties of trialkyltins. *Biochem J* 1964;91:287–297.

Aldridge WN, Street BW. Oxidative phosphorylation: the relationship between the specific binding of trimethyltin and triethyltin to mitochondria and their effects on various mitochondrial functions. *Biochem J* 1971;124:221–234.

Aldridge WN, Casida JE, Fish RH, Kimmel EC, Street BW. Action on mitochondria and toxicity of metabolites of tri-*n*-butyltin derivatives. *Biochem Pharmacol* 1977;26:1997–2000.

Aldridge WN, Brown AW, Brierley JB, Verschoyle RD, Street BW. Brain damage due to trimethyltin compounds. *Lancet* 1981;2:692–693.

Aleu FP, Katzman R, Terry RD. Fine structure and electrolyte analysis of cerebral edema induced by alkyltin intoxication. *J Neuropathol Exp Neurol* 1963;22:403–413.

Allen SL, Simpson MG, Stonard MD, Jones K. Induction of trimethyltin neurotoxicity by dietary administration. *Neurotoxicology* 1994;15: 651–654.

American Conference of Governmental and Industrial Hygienists (ACGIH). *Documentation of the threshold limit values and biological exposure indices,* 5th ed. Cincinnati, OH: ACGIH, 1989.

American Conference of Governmental Industrial Hygienists (ACGIH). *Threshold limit values (TLVs) for chemical substances and physical agents and biological exposure indices (BEIs).* Cincinnati, OH: ACGIH, 1995.

Amoore JE, Hautala E. Odor as an aid to chemical safety: odor threshold compared with threshold limit values and volatilities for 214 industrial chemicals in air and water dilution. *J Appl Toxicol* 1983;3:272–290.

Arakawa Y, Wada O, Yu TH. Dealkylation and distribution of tin compounds. *Toxicol Appl Pharmacol* 1981;60:1.

Aschner M, Aschner JL. Cellular and molecular effects of trimethyltin and triethyltin: relevance to organotin neurotoxicity. *Neurosci Biochem Rev* 1992;16:427–435.

Bakay L. Morphological and chemical studies in cerebral edema: triethyl tin-induced edema. *J Neurol Sci* 1965;2:52–67.

Barnes JM, Stoner HB. Toxic property of some dialkyl and trialkyl salts. *Br J Ind Med* 1958;15:15–22.

Barnes JM, Stoner HB. The toxicology of tin compounds. *Pharmacol Rev* 1959;11:211–231.

Barry BTK, Thwaites CJ. Tin and its alloys and compounds. In: West EG, ed. *Ellis Horwood series in industrial metals.* Chichester: Ellis Horwood, 1983.

Beliles RP. The metals. In: Clayton GD, and Clayton FE, eds. *Patty's industrial hygiene and toxicology,* 4th ed., vol II, Part C. New York: John Wiley & Sons, 1994:2258–2276.

Besser R, Krämer G, Thümler R, Bohl J, Gutmann L, Hopf HC. Acute trimethyltin limbic-cerebellar syndrome. *Neurology* 1987;37:945–950.

Bouldin TW, Goines ND, Bagnell CR, Krigman MR. Pathogenesis of trimethyltin neuronal toxicity: ultrastructural and cytochemical observations. *Am J Pathol* 1981;104:237–249.

Boyer IJ. Toxicity of dibutyltin, tributyltin and other organotin compounds to humans and to experimental animals. *Toxicology* 1989;55: 253–298.

Braman RS, Tompkins MA. Separation and determination of nanogram amounts of inorganic tin and methyltin compounds in the environment. *Anal Chem* 1979;51:12–19.

Bridges JW, Davies DS, Williams RT. The fate of ethyltin and diethyltin derivatives in the rat. *Biochem J* 1967;105:1261–1267.

Brodie ME, Opacka-Juffry J, Peterson DW, Brown AW. Neurochemical changes in hippocampal and caudate dialysates associated with early trimethyltin neurotoxicity in rats. *Neurotoxicology* 1990;11:35–46.

Brown AW, Aldridge WN, Street BW, Verschoyle RD. The behavioral and neuropathological sequelae of intoxication by trimethyltin compounds in the rat. *Am J Pathol* 1979;97:59–82.

Brown AW, Verschoyle RD, Street BW, Aldridge WN, Grindley H. The neurotoxicity of trimethyltin chloride in hamsters, gerbils and marmosets. *J Appl Toxicol* 1984;4:12–21.

Bushnell PJ. Delay-dependent impairment of reversal learning in rats treated with TMT. *Behav Neurol Biol* 1990;54:75–89.

Calloway DH, McMullen JJ. Fecal excretion of iron and tin by men fed stored canned foods. *Am J Clin Nutr* 1966;18:1–6.

Chang L, Dyer R. Trimethyltin induced zinc depletion in rat hippocampus. In: Frederickson C, Howell G, eds. *Neurobiology of zinc.* New York: Alan R. Liss, 1984:275–290.

Chang LW, Tiemeyer TM, Wenger GR, McMillan DE. Neuropathology of mouse hippocampus in acute trimethyltin intoxication. *Neurobehav Toxicol Teratol* 1982a;4:149–156.

Chang LW, Tiemeyer TM, Wenger GR, McMillan DE, Reuhl KE. Neuropathology of TMT intoxication: light microscopy study. *Environ Res* 1982b;29:435–444.

Chang LW. Neuropathology of trimethyltin: a proposed pathogenic mechanism. *Fund Appl Toxicol* 1986;6:217–232.

Colosio C, Tomasini M, Cairoli S, et al. Occupational triphenyltin acetate poisoning: a case report. *Br J Ind Med* 1991;48:136–139.

Cook LL. Effects of triethyltin on brain catecholamines in the adult rat. *Toxicologist* 1983;3:135.

Cook LL, Stine KE, Reiter LW. Tin distribution in adult rat tissues after exposure to trimethyltin and triethyltin. *Toxicol Appl Pharmacol* 1984a;72:344–348.

Cook LL, Stine-Jacobs K, Reiter LW. Tin distribution in adult and neonatal rat brain following exposure to triethyltin. *Toxicol Appl Pharmacol* 1984b;72:75–81.

Cook LL, Heath SM, O'Callaghan JP. Distribution of tin in brain subcellular fractions following the administration of trimethyl tin and triethyl tin to the rat. *Toxicol Appl Pharmacol* 1984c;72:564–568.

Cossa P, Duplay J, Fischgold, et al. Encéphalopathies toxiques au Stalinon. Aspects anatomocliniques et électroencéphalographiques. *Rev Neurol* 1958;98:97–108 (translated from the French by Marie H. St. Hilaire, M.D.).

Costa LG. Inhibition of gamma-[3H] aminobutyric acid uptake by organotin compounds in vitro. *Toxicol Appl Pharmacol* 1985;79:471–479.

Cremer JE. The metabolism in vitro of tissue slices from rats given triethyltin compounds. *Biochem J* 1957;67:87–96.

Cremer JE. The biochemistry of organotin compounds. The conversion of tetraethyltin into triethyltin in mammals. *Biochem J* 1958;68:685–692.

Cremer JE. Amino acid metabolism in rat brain studied with ^{14}C-labelled glucose. *J Neurochem* 1964;11:165–185.

Cremer JE. Selective inhibition of glucose oxidation by triethyltin in rat brain. *Biochem J* 1970;119:95–102.

Doctor SV, Costa LG, Kendall DA, Murphy SD. Trimethyltin inhibits uptake of neurotransmitters into mouse synaptosomes. *Toxicology* 1982; 25:213–221.

Dyer RS, Walsh TJ, Wonderlin WF, Bercegeay M. The trimethyltin syndrome in rats. *Neurobehav Toxicol Teratol* 1982;4:127–133.

Earley B, Burke M, Leonard BE. Behavioral, biochemical and histological effects of trimethyltin (TMT) induced brain damage in the rat. *Neurochem Int* 1992;21:351–366.

Earley B, Glennon M, Leonard BE, Junien J-L. Effects of JO 1784, a selective sigma ligand, on the autoradiographic localization of M_1 and M_2 muscarinic receptor subtypes in trimethyltin treated rats. *Neurochem Int* 1995;26:559–570.

Edwards MK, Bonnin JM. White matter diseases. In: Atlas SW, ed. *Magnetic resonance imaging of the brain and spine.* New York: Raven Press, 1991:267.

Ellenhorn MJ, Barceloux DG. Metals and related compounds. In: Ellenhorn MJ, Barceloux DG, eds. *Medical toxicology: diagnosis and treatment of human poisoning.* New York: Elsevier, 1988:1062.

Fait A, Ferioli A, Barbieri F. Organotin compounds. *Toxicology* 1994;91: 77–82.

Feldman RG, White RF, Eriator II. Trimethyltin encephalopathy. *Arch Neurol* 1993;50:1320–1324.

Foncin JF, Gruner JE. Tin neurotoxicity. In: Cohen MM, Klawans HL, eds. *Handbook of clinical neurology,* vol. 36, *Intoxications of the nervous system,* Part 1. Amsterdam: North-Holland, 1979:279–290.

Fortemps E, Amand G, Bomboir A, Lauwerys R, Laterre EC. Trimethyltin poisoning: report of two cases. *Int Arch Occup Environ Health* 1978;41: 1–6.

Go KG, Edzes HT. Water in brain edema. *Arch Neurol* 1975;32:462–465.

Guard HE, Cobet AB, Coleman WM. Methylation of trimethyltin compounds by estuarine sediments. *Science* 1981;213:770–771.

Gwan K, Edzes HT. Water in brain edema. Observations by the pulsed nuclear magnetic resonance technique. *Arch Neurol* 1975;32:462–465.

Hallas LE, Means JC, Coney JJ. Methylation of tin estuarine microorganisms. *Science* 1982;215:1505–1507.

Halliwell B. Oxidants and the central nervous system: some fundamental questions. Is oxidant damage relevant to Parkinson's disease, Alzheimer's disease, traumatic injury and stroke? *Acta Neurol Scand* 1989; 126: 23–33.

Hasan Z, Zimmer L, Wooley D. Time course of the effects of trimethyltin on limbic evoked potentials and distribution of tin in blood and brain in the rat. *Neurotoxicology* 1984;27:366–379.

Hiles RA. Absorption, distribution and excretion of inorganic tin in rats. *Toxicol Appl Pharmacol* 1974;27:366–379.

Iwai H, Wada O, Arakawa Y. Determination of tri-di and monobutyltin and inorganic tin in biological materials and some aspects of their metabolism in rats. *J Anal Toxicol* 1981;5:300–306.

Iwai H, Wada O, Arakawa Y, Ono T. Intestinal uptake site, enterohepatic circulation, and excretion of tetra- and trialkyltin compounds in mammals. *J Toxicol Environ Health* 1982;9:41–49.

Johnson MA, Greger JL. Effects of dietary tin on tin and calcium metabolism of adult males. *Am J Clin Nutri* 1982;35:655–660.

Katzman R, Aleu F, Wilson C. Further observations on triethyltin edema. *Arch Neurol* 1963;9:178–187.

Kehoe RA, Cholak J, Story RV. A spectrochemical study of the normal ranges of concentration of certain trace metals in biological materials. *J Nutr* 1940;19:579–592.

Kimmel EC, Casida JE, Fish RH. Bioorganotin chemistry. Microsomal monooxygenase and mammalian metabolism of cyclohexyltin compounds including the miticide cyhexatin. *J Agric Food Chem* 1980; 28:117–122.

Kirschner DA, Sapirstein VS. Triethyl tin-induced myelin oedema: an intermediate swelling state detected by X-ray diffraction. *J Neurocytol* 1982;11:559–569.

Krady JK, Oyler GA, Balaban CD, Billingsley ML. Use of avidin-biotin subtractive hybridization to characterize mRNA common to neurons destroyed by the selective neurotoxicant trimethyltin. *Mol Brain Res* 1990;7:287–297.

Kreyberg S, Torvik A, Bjorneboe A, Wiik-Larsen W, Jacobsen D. Trimethyltin poisoning: report of a case with postmortem examination. *Clin Neuropathol* 1992;11:256–259.

Krigman MR, Silverman AP. General toxicology of tin and its organic compounds. *Neurotoxicology* 1984;5:129–140.

Lock EA. The action of triethyltin on the respiration of rat brain cortex slices. *J Neurochem* 1976;26:887–892.

Lock EA, Aldridge WN. The binding of triethyltin to rat brain myelin. *J Neurochem* 1975;25:871–876.

Macovschi O, Prigent A-F, Nemoz G, Pageaux J-F, Pacheco H. Decreased adenosine cyclic 3',5'-monophosphate phosphodiesterase activity in rat brain following triethyltin intoxication. *Biochem Pharmacol* 1984; 33:3603–3608.

Magee PN, Stoner HB, Barnes JM. The experimental production of edema in the central nervous system of the rat by triethyltin compounds. *J Pathol Bacteriol* 1957;73:107–124.

Magos L. Tin. In: Friberg L, Nordberg GF, and Vouk V, eds. *Handbook on the toxicology of metals,* vol II. Amsterdam: Elsevier, 1986:568–593.

Mailman RB, Krigman MR, Frye GD, Hanin I. Effects of postnatal trimethyltin or triethyltin treatment on CNS catecholamine, GABA and acetylcholine systems in the rat. *J Neurochem* 1983;40:1423–1429.

Messing RB, Bollweg G, Chen Q, Sparber SB. Dose-specific effects of trimethyltin poisoning on learning and hippocampal corticosterone binding. *Neurotoxicology* 1988;9:491–502.

Moore KE, Brody TM. The effect of triethyltin on oxidative phosphorylation and mitochondrial adenosine triphosphatase activation. *Biochem Pharmacol* 1961;6:125–133.

Mushak P, Krigman MR, Mailman RB. Comparative organotin toxicity in the developing rat: somatic and morphological changes and relationship to accumulation of total tin. *Neurobehav Toxicol Teratol* 1982;4:209–215.

Naalsund LV, Allen CN, Fonnum F. Changes in neurobiological parameters in the hippocampus after exposure to trimethyltin. *Neurotoxicology* 1985;6:145–158.

National Institute for Occupational Safety and Health (NIOSH). *Pocket guide to chemical hazards.* Washington: U.S. Department of Health and Human Services, CDC, 1997.

Nolan CC, Brown AW, Cavanagh JB. Regional variations in nerve cell responses to trimethyltin intoxication in Mongolian gerbils and rats: further evidence for involvement of the golgi apparatus. *Acta Neuropathol (Berl)* 1990;81:204–212.

Occupational Safety and Health Administration (OSHA). *Occupational health guideline for organic tin compounds (as tin).* Washington: U.S. Department of Labor, 1978:1–7.

Occupational Safety and Health Administration (OSHA). *Code of Federal Regulations (1910.1000).* Washington: US Department of Health and Human Services, CDC, 1995.

O'Connell A, Earley B, Leonard BE. The neuroprotective effect of tacrine on trimethyltin induced memory and muscarinic receptor dysfunction in the rat. *Neurochem Int* 1994;25:555–556.

Oyanguren H, Haddad R, Maass H. Stannosis. Benign pneumoconiosis owing to inhalation of tin dust and fume. I. Environmental and experimental studies. *Ind Med Surg* 1958;27:427–431.

Piver WT. Organotin compounds: industrial applications and biological investigation. *Environ Health Perspect* 1973;4:61–79.

Popoff N, Weinberg S, Feigin I. Pathologic observations in lead encephalopathy, with special reference to the vascular changes. *Neurology* 1963;13:101–112.

Prough RA, Stalmach MA, Wiebkin P, Bridges JW. The microsomal metabolism of the organometallic derivatives of the group-IV elements, germanium, tin and lead. *Biochem J* 1981;196:763–770.

Ramming S, Shackford SR, Zhuang J, Schmoker JD. The relationship of fluid balance and sodium administration to cerebral edema formation and intracranial pressure in porcine model of brain injury. *J Trauma* 1994;37:705–713.

Reiter LW, Ruppert PH. Behavioral toxicology of trialkyltin compounds: a review. *Neurotoxicology* 1984;5:177–186.

Rey C, Reinecke H, Besser R. Methyltin intoxication in six men: toxicologic and clinical aspects. *Vet Hum Toxicol* 1984;26:121–122.

Rose MS. Evidence for histidine in the triethyltin-binding site of rat hemoglobin. *Biochem J* 1969;111:129–137.

Rose MS, Aldridge WN. The interaction of triethyltin with components of animal tissues. *Biochem J* 1968;106:821–828.

Rose MS, Aldridge WN. Oxidative phosphorylation: the effects of anions on the inhibition of various mitochondrial functions, and the relationship between this inhibition and binding of triethyltin. *Biochem J* 1972;127:51–59.

Rosenberg GA, Wolfson LI. Disorders of brain fluids and electrolytes. In: Rosenberg RN, ed. *Comprehensive neurology.* New York: Raven Press, 1991:210.

Ross WD, Emmett EA, Steiner J, Tureen R. Neurotoxic effects of occupational exposure to organotin. *Am J Psychiatry* 1981;138:1092–1095.

Ross WD, Sholiton MC. Specificity of psychiatric manifestations in relation to neurotoxic chemicals. *Acta Psychiatr Scand* 1983;67[Suppl 303]:100–104.

Ruppert PH, Walsh TJ, Reiter LW, Dyer RS. TMT induced hyperactivity: time course and pattern. *Neurobehav Toxicol Teratol* 1982;4:135–139.

Sapirstein VS, Durrie R, Nolan CE, Marks N. Identification of membrane-bound carbonic anhydrase in white matter coated vesicles: the fate of carbonic anhydrase and other white matter coated vesicle proteins in triethyl tin-induced leukoencephalopathy. *J Neurosci Res* 1993;35:83–91.

Schroeder HA, Balassa JJ, Tipton IH. Abnormal trace metals in man: tin. *J Chroni Dis* 1964;17:483–502.

Schwarz K, Milne DB, Vinyard E. Growth effects of tin compounds in rats maintained in a trace element-controlled environment. *Biochem Biophys Res Commun* 1970;40:22–29.

Schwartzwelder HS, Helper J, Holahan W, et al. Impaired maze performance in the rat caused by TMT treatment: problem solving deficits and perseveration. *Neurobehav Toxicol Teratol* 1982;4:169–176.

Selwyn MJ, Dawson AP, Stockdale M, Gains N. Chloride-hydroxide exchange across mitochondrial, erythrocyte and artificial lipid membranes mediate by trialkyl- and triphenyltin compounds. *Eur J Biochem* 1970;14:120–126.

Sloviter RS, von Knebel Doeberitz C, Walsh TJ, Dempster DW. On the role of seizure activity in the hippocampal damage produced by trimethyltin. *Brain Res* 1986;367:169–182.

Stockdale M, Dawson AP, Selwyn MJ. Effects of trialkyltin and triphenyltin compounds on mitochondrial respiration. *Eur J Biochem* 1970;15:342–351.

Stokinger HE. Tin. In: Clayton GD, Clayton FE, eds. *Patty's industrial hygiene and toxicology,* vol 2A: *Toxicology,* 3rd ed. New York: John Wiley & Sons, 1981:1940–1968.

Stoner HB, Barney JM, Duff JI. Studies on the toxicity of triethyltin compounds. *Br J Pharmacol* '955;10:16–25.

Toggas SM, Krady JK, Billingsley ML. Molecular neurotoxicology of trimethyltin: identification of stannin, a novel protein expressed in trimethyltin-sensitive cells. *Mol Pharmacol* 1992;42:44–56.

Torack RM. The relationship between adenosinetriphosphatase activity and triethyltin toxicity in the production of cerebral edema of the rat. *Am J Pathol* 1965;46:245–261.

Torack RM, Terry RD, Zimmerman HM. The fine structure of cerebral fluid accumulation. II. Swelling produced by triethyltin poisoning and its comparison with that in the human brain. *Am J Pathol* 1960;36:273–287.

Tosteson MY, Sapirstein VS. Protein interactions with lipid bylayers. The channels of kidney plasma membrane proteolipids. *J Membr Biol* 1981;63:77–84.

Underwood EJ. *Trace elements in human and animal nutrition,* 4th ed. New York: Academic Press, 1977:449–451.

United States Environmental Protection Agency (USEPA). *The manufacture and use of selected alkyltin compounds.* Washington: EPA Office of Toxic Substances, 1976.

United States Environmental Protection Agency (USEPA). *Health effects assessment for tin and compounds. EPA/600/8-88/055.* Cincinnati OH: U.S. Environmental Protection Agency, Office of Research and Development, 1987.

United States Environmental Protection Agency (USEPA). *Drinking water regulations and health advisories.* EPA 822-R-96-001. Washington: Office of Water, 1996.

U.S. Geological Survey (USGS). *Mineral Commodity Summaries.* Washington, DC: U.S. Geological Survey, 1998:178–179.

Valdes JJ, MacTutus CF, Santos-Anderson RM, Danson R, Annua Z. Selective neurochemical and histological lesions in rat hippocampus following chronic trimethyltin exposure. *Neurobehav Toxicol Teratol* 1983;5:357–361.

Viviani B, Rossi AD, Chow SC, Nicotera P. Organotin Compounds induce calcium overload and apoptosis in PC12 cells. *Neurotoxicology* 1995;16:19–26.

Walsh TJ, DeHaven DL. Neurotoxicity of the alkyltins. In: Bondy SC, Prasad KN, eds. *Metal neurotoxicity.* Orlando, FL: CRC Press, 1988:87–107.

Walsh TJ, Gallagher M, Bostock E, Dyer RS. TMT impairs retention of a passive avoidance task. *Neurobehav Toxicol Teratol* 1982a;4:163–167.

Walsh TJ, Miller BD, Dyer RS. TMT, a selective limbic system neurotoxicant, impairs radial-arm maze performance. *Neurobehav Toxicol Teratol* 1982b;4:177–183.

Wassenaar JS, Kroon AM. Effects of triethyltin on different ATPases, 5'-nucleotidase and phosphodiesterases in grey and white matter of rabbit brain and their relation with brain edema. *Eur Neurol* 1973;10:349–370.

Watanabe I. Organotins (triethyltin). In: Spencer PS, Schaumburg HH, eds. *Experimental and clinical neurotoxicology.* Baltimore: Williams & Wilkins, 1980:545–557.

Wax PM, Dockstader L. Tributyltin use in interior paints: a continuing health hazard. *Clin Toxicol* 1995;33:239–241.

Weast RC. *CRC handbook of chemistry and physics,* 62nd ed. Boca Raton, FL: CRC Press, 1981.

Whittington DL, Woodruff ML, Baisen RH. The time course of TMT-induced fiber and terminal degeneration in hippocampus. *Neurotoxicol Teratol* 1989;11:21–33.

Wilkinson RR. Technoeconomic and environmental assessment of industrial organotin compounds. *Neurotoxicology* 1984;5:141–158.

Wilson WE, Hudson PM, Kanamatsu T, et al. Trimethyltin induced alterations in brain amino acids, amines and amine metabolites: relationship to hyperammonemia. *Neurotoxicology* 1986;7:63–74.

World Health Organization (WHO). *Tin and organotin compounds: a preliminary review. Environmental health criteria,* vol 15. Geneva: WHO, 1980.

Yallapragada PR, Vig PJS, Kodavanti PRS, Desaiah D. In vivo effects of triorganotins on calmodulin activity in the rat brain. *J Toxicol Environ Health* 1991;34:229–231.

Yamamoto I. Pollution of fish and shellfish with organotin compounds and estimation of daily intake. *Hokkaido J Med Sci* 1994;69:273–281.

Yanagisawa K, Ishigro H, Kaneko K, Miyatake T. Acetazolamide inhibits the recovery from triethyl tin intoxication: putative role of carbonic anhydrase in dehydration of central myelin. *Neurochem Res* 1990;15:483–486.

Yanofsky NN, Nierenberg D, Turco JH. Acute short-term memory loss from trimethyltin exposure. *J Emerg Med* 1991;9:137–139.

Zornow MH, Prough DS. Fluid management in patients with traumatic brain injury. [Review] *New Horizons* 1995;3:488–498.

CHAPTER 10

Manganese

Manganese (Mn) occurs in varying degrees of purity and states of oxidation. It is found combined with other chemicals such as silicon, carbon, and sulfur (NRC, 1973). Manganese-dependent enzyme activity and the catalytic properties of manganese as a transitional metal (valences -3 to $+7$) are necessary for certain biological functions, especially those concentrated in tissues rich in mitochondria. Manganese is an important essential trace element, necessary for normal development; its deficiency is associated with skeletal deformities, sterility, and neonatal death in animals (NRC, 1973; Hurley, 1981). Low blood levels of manganese have been detected in children with congenital disorders of bone development and growth (Hall et al., 1989) and with epilepsy (Papavasilou et al., 1979; Hurley, 1981; Akram et al., 1989). Maternal manganese deficiency results in depletion of catecholamines in the brain of the fetus (Mena, 1980).

The valence state of manganese is a factor in its effect on living tissues (Cotzias, 1958). Manganese neurotoxicity arises from the physiological dichotomy between the lower (Mn^{2+}) and the higher (Mn^{3+}) oxidation states. Divalent manganese acts as a powerful antioxidant, scavenging superoxide radicals; trivalent manganese produces reactive oxygen species and potentiates the autooxidation of dopamine, with the concomitant production of neurotoxic byproducts (Graham, 1978; Graham et al., 1978; Donaldson et al., 1980; Archibald and Tyree, 1987; Ali et al., 1995). Similarities in the clinical manifestations of manganese toxicity to those of Parkinson's disease (PD) have raised interest in the possibility of an environmental etiology of neurodegenerative diseases (PD in particular) that might involve transition metals such as manganese (Halliwell, 1989; Tanner and Langston, 1990; Feldman, 1992; Mergler, 1996; Blake et al., 1997; Cramner, 1998).

SOURCES OF EXPOSURE

Miners who remove manganese ore from the earth are exposed to its dust, as are the workers who handle stockpiles of the ore and the crushers who prepare the ore for smelting (Flinn et al., 1940; Huang and Quist, 1983). Man-

ganese is released during industrial processes such as metallurgical fabrication, welding, alloy manufacturing, chemical production, textile bleaching, leather tanning, and electroplating (Saric, 1986; Sjogren et al., 1996). It is an ingredient used in making potassium permanganate, manganese sulfate, and certain fungicides, germicides, and antiseptics. It is used in the production of dry-cell batteries, glass, matches, fireworks, fertilizers, animal feed, paints, and varnishes. Manganese also forms organic compounds such as manganese ethylene-bis-dithiocarbamate (maneb), an agricultural fungicide (Ferraz et al., 1988), and methyl-cyclopentadienyl manganese tricarbonyl (MMT), a yellow liquid with a faint pleasant odor used as an antiknock gasoline additive and smoke inhibitor for fuel oil (Tanaka, 1988; NIOSH, 1997; Mergler, 1996). Combustion of MMT generates manganese oxides (Ter Haar et al., 1975).

Atmospheric pollution results from the emission of particulate manganese or manganese oxide vapors from various industries and from automobiles in which MMT is used as a gasoline additive (Davis et al., 1987; Stokes, 1988; Tanaka, 1988; Loranger and Zayed, 1995; Mergler, 1996). U.S. ambient air concentrations of manganese have ranged from 5 to 60 ng/m^3 in nonpolluted rural areas to as much as 110 ng/m^3 in large urban centers where there are no foundries. Near foundries, manganese levels in thousands of nanograms per cubic meter have been reported (ATSDR, 1992).

Food is the main source of nonoccupational manganese intake, with the highest naturally occurring concentrations in wheat, rice, tea, nuts, meats, and poultry (Sittig et al., 1985). Manganese found in food sources may also be the result of residue left behind from manganese-containing insecticides (Ferraz et al., 1988). Dietary sources account for about 4 mg/day of manganese ingestion for the average adult (USEPA, 1984). Dietary habits determine an individual's daily manganese intake. For example, persons who are on a macrobiotic diet have a higher daily intake of manganese than do omnivores (Stobbaerts et al., 1995). Excess manganese may exist in drinking water as the result of local contamination due to leaching from nearby mineral formations and improper toxic waste disposal (Kawamura et al., 1941; Nordberg et al., 1985; Cawte, 1991; Zhang et al., 1995; Vieregge et al., 1996). Detrimental effects occur among the general population when exposure exceeds the quantities of manganese required for homeostasis of normal biological functions (NRC, 1973; Tanaka, 1988). Even normal dietary intake of manganese may result in manganese intoxication in individuals with decreased excretion due to chronic liver failure (Hauser et al., 1994).

EXPOSURE LIMITS AND SAFETY REGULATIONS

Although a clear dose–response relationship between exposure and the emergence of clinical manifestations may be difficult to determine, neurotoxic effects have been reported in individual cases exposed to high levels of manganese and in population studies in which people have been exposed to levels as low as 0.3 to 4.9 mg/m³ (Saric et al., 1977). The *Occupational Safety and Health Administration* (OSHA) has established a short-term permissible exposure limit (STEL) ceiling for inhalation of manganese compounds of 5 mg/m³; this is a 15-minute time-weighted average (TWA) exposure limit (OSHA, 1995) (Table 10-1). The *National Institute for Occupational Safety and Health*'s (NIOSH) 10-hour TWA recommended exposure limit (REL) for manganese is 1 mg/m³, with a 15-minute TWA STEL of 3 mg/m³ (NIOSH, 1997). The NIOSH immediately dangerous to life or health (IDLH) concentration for manganese is 500 mg/m³. The *American Conference of Governmental and Industrial Hygienists* (ACGIH) recommends an 8-hour TWA threshold limit value (TLV) for manganese of 0.2 mg/m³ (ACGIH, 1995).

OSHA has established a STEL for MMT of 5 mg/m³; this is a 15-minute TWA exposure limit (OSHA, 1995). The NIOSH REL for MMT is 0.1 mg/m³ (NIOSH, 1997). The ACGIH TLV for MMT is 0.2 mg/m³ (ACGIH, 1995). Both NIOSH and the ACGIH have assigned MMT a SKIN designation, indicating that the potential exists for considerable exposure through dermal contact (Table 10-1).

The Environmental Protection Agency (EPA) has established a secondary maximum contaminant level (SMCL) for inorganic manganese in water of 0.05 mg/L; this standard is based on the quality of taste and appearance rather than on toxicity studies (USEPA, 1996) (Table 10-1).

METABOLISM

Tissue Absorption

In workers occupationally exposed to manganese dust or vapor, intake occurs primarily through the lungs (Rodier, 1955; Aschner and Aschner, 1991; USEPA, 1984). Occupational intake of airborne manganese is highest among workers in mining, ore processing, and ferromanganese operations. The route of absorption depends on particle size. Small particles (less than 5 μm), such as manganese oxides derived from combustion of MMT, which reach the alveolar epithelium, can be absorbed through the lungs.

TABLE 10-1. *Established and recommended occupational and environmental exposure limits for manganese (Mn) in air and water*

	Air (mg/m³)	Water (mg/L)[a]
Odor threshold*		
Inorganic Mn	—	—
MMT	—	—
OSHA		
Inorganic Mn		
PEL 8-hr TWA)	—	—
PEL ceiling (15-min TWA)	5.0	—
MMT		
PEL (8-hr TWA)	—	—
PEL ceiling (15-min TWA)	5.0	—
NIOSH		
Inorganic Mn		
REL (10-hr TWA)	1.0	—
STEL (15-min TWA)	3.0	—
IDLH	500.0	—
MMT		
REL (10-hr TWA)	0.2	—
STEL (15-min TWA)	—	—
IDLH	—	—
ACGIH		
Inorganic Mn		
TLV (8-hr TWA)	0.2	—
STEL (15-min TWA)	—	—
MMT		
TLV (8-hr TWA)	0.2	
STEL (15-min TWA)	—	
USEPA		
MCL	—	—
MCLG	—	—
SMCL	—	0.05

[a]Unit conversion: 1 mg/L = 1 ppm.
MMT, methylcyclopentadienyl manganese tricarbonyl; OSHA, Occupational Safety and Health Administration; PEL, permissible exposure limit; TWA, time-weighted average; NIOSH, National Institute of Occupational Safety and Health; REL, recommended exposure limit; STEL, short-term exposure limit; IDLH, immediately dangerous to life or health; ACGIH, American Conference of Governmental Industrial Hygienists; TLV, threshold limit value; USEPA, U.S. Environmental Protection Agency; MCL, maximum contamination level; MCLG, maximum contamination level goal; SMCL, secondary MCL.
Data from *Amoore and Hautala, 1983; ACGIH, 1995; OSHA, 1995; USEPA, 1996; NIOSH, 1997.

However, most of an inhaled dose is cleared by the mucociliary lining from the lung to the oral pharynx, and then swallowed and absorbed through the gastrointestinal tract (Rodier, 1955; Mena et al., 1969; WHO, 1981; Loranger and Zayed, 1995). The solubility of the manganese compound affects its absorption (Mena et al., 1969; Brain and Valberg, 1979; Komura and Sakamoto, 1994).

Lipophilic organic manganese compounds such as MMT are more readily absorbed than are inorganic manganese compounds (Komura and Sakamoto, 1992). Divalent inorganic manganese is oxidized to trivalent manganese

(Mn^{3+}) in the alkaline condition of the duodenum; the Mn^{3+} cation is well absorbed (Cotzias, 1961). Total radioactive body-time activity studies in adults who ingested $^{54}MnCl_2$ indicate that intestinal absorption of this manganese compound is 3%; 2% of the dose is retained for 10 days; by 50 days, the total body retention of $^{54}MnCl_2$ is only 0.2% (Mena, 1980). Low-protein and iron-deficiency states increase absorption of manganese; increased calcium and phosphorus levels decrease its absorption (Mena et al., 1969; Murphy et al., 1991a). Occupational exposure to high concentrations of manganese or decreased excretion of manganese due to hepatic failure influence its distribution in the central nervous system (CNS) (Yamada et al., 1986; Prohaska, 1987; Layrargues et al., 1995). Individuals with impaired clearance of manganese resulting from liver dysfunction or portal systemic shunting show increases in blood manganese concentration and magnetic resonance imaging (MRI) findings that are indicative of increased manganese absorption (Hauser et al, 1994, 1996).

Tissue Distribution

Absorbed inorganic manganese is transported in the systemic circulation and across the blood–brain barrier (BBB) by transferrin (Aschner and Aschner, 1991). The average 70-kg man carries a total body burden of about 12 to 20 mg of manganese (Tanaka, 1988). Manganese is rapidly cleared from the plasma, with a half-life of 1.3 to 2.2 minutes (Cotzias et al., 1968). The human biological half-life for manganese in body tissues (e.g., muscle) is 2 to 8 weeks and is dependent on the preexisting body burden, with a shorter half-life seen in workers with higher tissue levels (Cotzias et al., 1968). Accumulation occurs in the brain when absorption exceeds excretion (Mena et al., 1967; Cotzias et al., 1968).

Manganese normally enters the brain across the cerebral capillaries, but at higher exposure levels entry also occurs across the choroid plexus (Murphy et al., 1991b). Manganese content in brain tissues normally averages 1 to 2 mg/g dry weight, with greater concentrations found in adults than in infants (Markesbery et al., 1984; Prohaska, 1987). The distribution of manganese in the brain is not influenced by route of intake (Newland et al., 1989). The topographical distribution of manganese in the CNS of healthy unexposed persons partly correlates with its functional association with neurotransmitters, biogenic amines, oxidative enzymes, and neuroendocrines (Donaldson, 1988). Free manganese (i.e., without a functional association) is normally distributed throughout the gray matter of the cerebral cortex and the basal ganglia, particularly in the caudate nucleus, pallidum, and putamen (Larsen et al., 1979; Mirowitz et al., 1991). The highest tissue concentrations of manganese are normally found in brain regions such as the globus pallidus and striatum, which have relatively high concentrations of neuromelanin (Maynard and Cotzias, 1955; Donaldson et al., 1981; WHO, 1981; Hintz

and Kalyaraman, 1986; Swartz et al., 1992; Olanow et al., 1996).

Manganese-induced autooxidation of dopamine initially increases the local neuromelanin content and subsequently the concentration of manganese in melanin-containing neurons in the globus pallidus (Shinotoh et al., 1995). Cell death in response to free radical damage results in a concomitant decrease in neuromelanin and a reduction in the local concentration of manganese. For example, postmortem analysis of the brain tissue in a manganese ore crusher revealed no overall increase in manganese concentration per gram of tissue (wet weight) when compared with a control. However, the distribution of manganese in the two brains was different, with the ore crusher having a greater manganese concentration in the gray matter of the cerebral cortex and a lower concentration in the basal ganglia, reflecting a marked loss of neuromelanin-rich neurons in the basal ganglia (Yamada et al., 1986). Because manganese is cleared from the brain following cessation of exposure, the duration between removal from the source of manganese exposure and the time of postmortem analysis can also influence its topographical distribution in the brain. For example, manganese concentrations were significantly ($p < 0.01$) increased in the globus pallidus of nine patients with chronic liver disease, reflecting the affinity of manganese for neuromelanin and the manganese-induced potentiation of dopamine catabolism. The subsequent accumulation of additional amounts of neuromelanin and manganese is also due to these patients' continuous exposure to manganese until death (Layrargues et al., 1995) (see Neuropathological Diagnosis section).

Manganese has also been detected in the spinal cords of patients with amyotrophic lateral sclerosis (ALS) in concentrations that differed significantly from those of controls. The significance of this in the causation of ALS is uncertain, but the possible imbalance between calcium and manganese may be associated with functional impairment and neuronal death (Kihira et al., 1990).

Experimental investigations of tissue distribution of manganese following exposure to organic manganese compounds such as MMT indicate that distribution is related to the lipophilic nature of these compounds and differs from that following exposures to inorganic manganese compounds. For example, concentrations of manganese are relatively higher in the parenchymal organs of animals exposed to MMT than in those of animals exposed to manganese chloride (Moore et al., 1974; McGinley et al., 1987; Komura and Sakamoto, 1992). In contrast to inorganic manganese compounds, organic manganese compounds readily cross the BBB by passive diffusion. Furthermore, organic manganese compounds such as MMT are metabolized to inorganic manganese compounds, which are then transported across the BBB by transferrin, indicating a potential for greater accumulation of manganese in the brain following exposure to organic manganese compounds because of these two routes of entry.

Manganese concentrations were higher in the cerebellum of mice exposed to MMT than in those of unexposed mice and mice exposed to manganese chloride, indicating that the regional distribution and accumulation of manganese in the brain is different following exposure to inorganic and organic manganese compounds (Komura and Sakamoto, 1994). The differences in distribution and accumulation of manganese seen following exposure to organic and inorganic manganese compounds may contribute to the specific neurotoxic effects produced by each (Cox et al., 1987; Fishman et al., 1987).

Tissue Biochemistry

The oxidation state of an inorganic manganese compound determines its action. For example, manganese in the 2+ oxidation state is a scavenger of free radicals and is necessary for normal brain function (Kono et al., 1976). Manganese-dependent superoxide dismutase (Mn-SOD) makes use of the variable oxidation states of manganese in mitochondrial oxygen radical metabolism (Halliwell, 1984; Ali et al., 1995). Manganese-dependent proteins play an important role in the production of certain neurotransmitters. Eighty percent of the Mn^{2+} in the brain is associated with the manganoprotein glutamine synthetase, which synthesizes glutamine. The concentration of glutamine synthetase is particularly high in glial cells, which synthesize glutamine for subsequent conversion to glutamate and γ-aminobutyric acid (GABA) in neuronal cells (Wedler and Denman, 1984). Other manganese-dependent enzymes include pyruvate carboxylase and phosphophenol pyruvate carboxykinase (Baly et al., 1985).

The acute psychosis associated with manganese poisoning may be related to an N-methyl-D-aspartate (NMDA)–glutamate receptor-mediated loss of autoreceptor presynaptic control of striatal dopamine release (Chandra et al., 1981; Cuesta de Di Zio et al., 1995) (Fig. 10-1). The acute extrapyramidal effects of manganese may involve the irreversible oxidation of dopamine to a cyclized ortho-quinone, resulting in a temporary decrease in the brain levels of dopamine (Segura-Aguilar and Lind, 1989). The chronic effects of manganese poisoning have been attributed to the generation of free radicals and cell death via apoptosis (Segura-Aguilar and Lind, 1989; Halliwell, 1989) (see Neuropathological Diagnosis section).

Absorbed organic manganese is metabolized by cytochrome P-450 enzymes in the lungs, liver, and kidneys to hydroxymethylcyclopentadienyl manganese tricarbonyl, carboxycyclopentadienyl manganese tricarbonyl, and inorganic

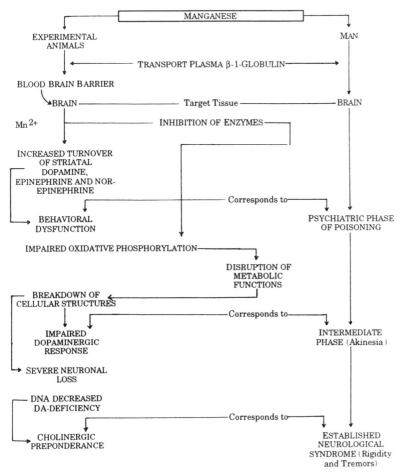

FIG. 10-1. A possible mechanism of the clinical manifestations of manganese intoxication. (Modified from Chandra, 1983, with permission.)

manganese (Moore et al., 1974; Hanzlik et al., 1980; Verschoyle et al., 1993; Komura and Sakamoto, 1994). Exposure to chemicals that inhibit or induce cytochrome P-450 activity can inhibit or enhance the metabolism of organic manganese and therefore may potentiate or attenuate toxicity (Hanzlik et al., 1980; McGinley et al., 1987; Fishman et al., 1987; Cox et al., 1987; Verschoyle et al., 1993). Animal studies indicate that exposure to organic manganese compounds such as MMT can induce seizures, which are possibly mediated by an inhibitory action of MMT on GABA-A receptor-linked chloride channels (Cox et al., 1987; Fishman et al., 1987).

Excretion

Manganese is excreted in the feces, urine, pancreatic fluid, hair, and breast milk (WHO, 1981; Saric, 1986). Excretion of inorganic manganese from the body is rapid and does not require active metabolism; inorganic manganese does not pass through the glucuronidation pathway. Most absorbed inorganic manganese rapidly appears in the bile and feces; a portion undergoes enterohepatic recirculation (Klaassen, 1974). Blood levels of manganese are increased in patients with impaired manganese clearance due to liver dysfunction (Hauser et al., 1994). Obstruction of the bile duct results in decreased fecal excretion of manganese (Papavasiliou et al., 1966; Klaassen, 1974; Marchal et al., 1993).

Only a small amount (0.1% to 1.3%) of daily intake of inorganic manganese is excreted by the kidneys into urine (Maynard and Fink, 1956). Urinary concentration of inorganic manganese is normally less than 1 mg/L (Saric, 1986), accounting for only about 0.01% of the current body burden. Urinary excretion is not increased by inorganic manganese overloading or biliary obstruction (WHO, 1981). By contrast, urinary excretion of total manganese compounds is markedly enhanced after exposure to organic manganese. For example, MMT is metabolized to hydroxymethylcyclopentadienyl manganese tricarbonyl and carboxycyclopentadienyl manganese tricarbonyl, which are both water-soluble compounds and thus are readily excreted in the urine (Hanzlik et al., 1980).

Manganese is rapidly cleared from the plasma of the blood with a half-life of 1.3 to 2.2 minutes. The clearance half-life of $^{54}MnCl_2$ is 37.5 days for the body and 54 days for the head. The human biological half-life for manganese in body tissues is dependent on the preexisting body burden, with a shorter half-life seen in workers with higher tissue levels, suggesting that excretion is increased as a protective response to excessive exposure (Cotzias et al., 1968).

CLINICAL MANIFESTATIONS AND DIAGNOSIS

Symptomatic Diagnosis

Not all people who are exposed to manganese experience clinically overt health effects and therefore many cases of manganese intoxication go unrecognized or unreported. Prevalence rates of manganese intoxication range from 4 to 25% in occupational settings at both high and low levels of exposure. A clear dose–response relationship is rarely defined (Rodier, 1955; Mena et al., 1967; Saric et al., 1977; Roels et al., 1987a; Wennberg et al., 1991). Individual susceptibility, coexisting health factors, the presence of other interacting metals, and dietary factors all contribute to toxicity at given exposure levels (Seth and Chandra, 1988; Florence and Stauber, 1989). For example, manganese encephalopathy and basal ganglia dysfunction with parkinsonian signs including rigidity, gait abnormalities, dysarthria, hypomimia, and bradykinesia have been reported in patients with chronic liver failure (Sherlock et al., 1954; Victor et al., 1965; Mena et al., 1967; Read et al., 1967; Cook et al., 1974; Huang et al., 1989; Hauser et al., 1994). In addition, patients who are naturally at risk for developing idiopathic Parkinson's disease (IPD) may be especially sensitive to the effects of manganese (Feldman, 1992; Blake et al., 1997). However, it has not been established whether or not exposure to manganese will precipitate the occurrence of progressive IPD.

Movement disorders such as IPD, Shy–Drager syndrome, Wilson's disease, nigrostriatal degeneration, olivopontine cerebellar degeneration, and supranuclear palsy must be considered in the differential diagnosis of suspected cases of manganese poisoning. In addition, exposure to other neurotoxicants known to induce extrapyramidal signs such as carbon disulfide, carbon monoxide, and dopamine antagonists like phenothiazines must be considered. Many of these conditions affect interrelated structures of the extrapyramidal system and alter dopaminergic neurotransmission, thereby producing similar clinical features that make the differential diagnosis difficult in individuals with uncertain exposure histories.

Similarities between the extrapyramidal signs of manganese intoxication and the typical features of IPD suggest a possible etiological role for manganese (Tanner and Langston, 1990; Feldman, 1992; Galvani et al., 1995; Blake et al., 1997); clear differences in the neuropathology of the two have been described, however (Barbeau, 1984; Graham, 1984; Gibb, 1988). Sufficient criteria exist for making a clinical differential diagnosis of IPD and manganese toxicity (Barbeau and Roy, 1984; Wolters et al., 1989; Feldman, 1994). For example, the extrapyramidal signs of manganese poisoning are frequently preceded or accompanied by an acute psychosis, whereas this clinical feature is not seen in patients with IPD. In addition, due to differences in underlying neuropathology, patients with IPD will respond favorably to levodopa (L-dopa) therapy, whereas responses to L-dopa in cases of manganese poisoning have been equivocal or not effective (Mena et al., 1970; Rosenstock et al., 1971; Greenhouse, 1971; Cook et al., 1974; Huang et al., 1993) (Table 10-2).

Early diagnosis of manganese intoxication is often a problem because of the nonspecific clinical features, the

TABLE 10-2. *Manganese-induced parkinsonism and Parkinson's disease: differentiating features*

	Manganese poisoning	Parkinson's disease
Age of onset	Any age	Mean age over 50 years
Onset	Subacute, acute	Usually insidious
Exposure history	History of exposure to Mn (mining, paints, batteries, fertilizers, disinfectants, or water with high Mn content)	No history of Mn exposure
Course	Acute stages are transient, increase in severity with longer duration of exposure, then stabilize; most cases do not progress after exposure is stopped	Usually progressive
Tremor	May be less likely to occur; may be postural intention.	Usually a resting tremor
Tone	Dystonia; not simple rigidity; frontal release signs (Gengenhalten); hypokinesia	Rigidity, usually cogwheel
Gait	Complex, ataxic, dystonia (cockwalk)	Bradykinetic, shuffling
Associated findings	Pyramidal signs, cognitive impairment	Pyramidal signs are rare; cognitive impairment occurs only late in course
Mn levels	May be raised or normal; may rise with chelation therapy	Usually in normal range or none detected
Therapeutic response	Poor to minimal effect of L-dopa therapy	L-dopa therapeutic; response usually good
Pathology	Lesions in pallidum, subthalamic nucleus, putamen, caudate nucleus, substantia nigra, cerebellum, pons, thalamus; Lewy bodies are rare	Pathological lesions mainly in substantia nigra, locus coeruleus, dorsal nucleus of Vagus; Lewy bodies usually present
MRI	T_1-weighted image at level of basal ganglia shows increased signal intensity in the globus pallidus; diminished width of pars compacta	Normal or diminished width of pars compacta, decreased signal intensity in the globus pallidus, reticular substantia nigra, red nucleus, and dentate nucleus
PET scan	Striatal uptake of fluorodopa normal; diminished fluorodeoxy glucose uptake	Decreased striatal uptake of fluorodopa

lack of timely environmental measures of manganese, and/or the lack of reliable biological indicators of exposure. Nevertheless, it is important for the clinician to recognize the early symptoms of manganese poisoning, especially as the late-stage features are often permanent. Whenever possible a time-based exposure history, including occupational information, documentation of environmental and/or occupational exposure levels, and biological exposure indices should be obtained to substantiate a possible relationship of symptoms to manganese exposure.

The initial manifestations of manganese poisoning are mostly behavioral and have been termed *manganese psychosis*. The clinical symptoms include mood changes, emotional lability, compulsive laughter, and hallucinations (Rodier, 1955; Mena et al., 1967). Performance on formal neuropsychological tests may also be impaired at this time. With continued exposure, the behavioral symptoms progress, and motor disturbances appear. This stage is characterized by tremor, dysarthria, gait disturbance, slowness and clumsiness of movement, and postural instability. In the later stages, the psychosis subsides, and signs of dystonia appear and are often accompanied by the onset of an awkward high-stepping dystonic gait (Rodier, 1955; Penalver, 1957; Mena et al., 1967; Barbeau et al., 1976; Chandra, 1983; Barbeau, 1984) (Fig. 10-1). The gait disturbance of manganese poisoning is in stark contrast to that of IPD, in which the patient typically presents with a shuffling gait (Table 10-2). The extrapyramidal symptoms of manganese poisoning may progress following cessation of exposure, but the progression is typically slower than that seen in IPD (Huang et al., 1993; 1998) (see Clinical Experiences section).

Case studies documenting seizure activity in humans exposed to organic manganese compounds have not been reported. Animal studies indicate that exposure to organic manganese compounds such as MMT can induce seizures (Cox et al., 1987; Fishman et al., 1987). These findings suggest that persons with preexisting seizure disorders should limit their exposure to MMT.

Neurophysiological Diagnosis

Electroencephalography (EEG) can be used to differentiate manganese encephalopathy from other neurological disorders. The EEG of patients with manganese poisoning is typically normal and therefore does not differ from that seen in cases of IPD, in which the EEG is also typically normal for the patient's age (Mena et al., 1967; Cook et al., 1974; Aminoff, 1986). Although slowing of the dominant rhythm and triphasic complexes are noted in the EEG of patients with hepatic failure, these changes are more likely due to elevated blood ammonia levels than to manganese accumulation (Aminoff, 1986; Nomiyama et al., 1991; Takeda et al., 1993).

Tremorography, the quantification of tremor in workers with a history of exposure to manganese, has been performed using a triaxial accelerometer and power spectral analysis to determine the dominant frequency and amplitude of the tremor excursions. The test requires that the individual maintain a steady resting or flexed state while holding a stylus within a ring space as the diameter is gradually decreased. There is a corresponding increase in the difficulty of the task of maintaining the stylus within the space and in the sensitivity of the meter to tremor. The manganese-exposed workers had difficulties, not encountered by unexposed controls, in this task (Roels et al., 1982, 1987a). Subclinical and clinical tremors in Danish steel workers exposed to manganese metal fumes were tested by computerized measures of coordination and tremor using the CATSYS apparatus, which also utilizes a stylus accelerometer (Gyntelberg et al., 1990; F. Gyntelberg, personal communication, 1995). No significant differences from controls were found in the asymptomatic steelworkers exposed to low levels of manganese. However, workers with subjective complaints of difficulty performing their jobs also showed evidence of poor coordination on the test.

A device consisting of a pen-based graphics tablet that emits an electronic current, which is then transformed into three-dimensional position data (MOVEMAP), was used to study residual tremor in 27 former manganese miners from Andacollo, Chile, who were previously exposed to manganese at concentrations of 62.5 to 250 mg/m^3. The miners had been retired for a minimum of 5 years, after having been employed as drillers, crushers, or utility men for an average of 20 years. The tremor acceleration parameter was higher among the manganese-exposed subjects, although tremor velocity among these subjects did not differ from that in unexposed controls (Hochberg et al., 1996).

Static posturography recordings of postural sway among manganese workers in two ore milling plants in Singapore were compared with those obtained in a nonexposed referent group using a computerized platform system (Chia et al., 1995). The workers were exposed to ore that contained 91% MnO_2, with carbon, iron, and other trace metals making up the remainder. Duration of exposure ranged from 1.1 to 15.7 years. In an earlier survey of these plants, the mean of the 8-hour TWA personal airborne manganese samples of 28 workers was 4.16 mg/m^3; 15 workers had personal exposure levels above 5 mg/m^3. However, because of a decrease in production output, the yearly mean TWA for airborne manganese concentrations had decreased over the past 10 years to less than 1 mg/m^3. The actual air exposure levels were not measured for these subjects at the time of testing. However, the current mean urine level for the exposed workers was 6.0 μg/g creatinine (range: 0.6 to 53.3 μg/g creatinine). No significant differences for the sway parameters obtained when the subject's

eyes were open were noted between the exposed workers and the unexposed referent group. However, when the eyes were closed, significant differences were observed for mean velocity of the center of pressure along the sway path and the length of the sway path. The current urine levels and thus the degree of current exposure were not significantly correlated with the findings on tests of static postural sway. However, the clinical manifestations of manganese poisoning do not necessarily correlate with current exposure levels (Cotzias et al., 1968; Chandra et al., 1974; Cook et al., 1974; Yamada et al., 1986; Tsalev et al., 1977; Roels et al., 1987b). Furthermore, 17 of the subjects who were employed for more than 5 years had probably been exposed to higher manganese concentrations in the past (see Biochemical Diagnosis section). These results suggest that past exposure to relatively low concentrations of manganese produces subclinical manifestations that probably reflect permanent damage to the basal ganglia and connections within the extrapyramidal system.

Neuropsychological Diagnosis

Formal neuropsychological testing can be used to document cognitive disorders and to detect subtle behavioral and cognitive changes due to manganese encephalopathy. Performance intelligence quotient, which is dependent on good motor functioning, is typically below expectation. Tests of psychomotor functioning such as finger tapping, the Purdue Pegboard, the Santa Ana Form Board, and Digit Symbol are sensitive to the extrapyramidal effects of manganese poisoning. Tests of reaction time reveal slowing of psychomotor speed (Iregren, 1990; Wennberg et al., 1991). Decreased attention and memory impairments are also commonly found during neuropsychological assessment of manganese-exposed persons (Grandjean, 1983; Roels et al., 1985; Hua and Huang, 1991; Lucchini et al., 1995). Language and verbal functioning are spared in manganese-exposed adults (Iregren, 1990; Hua and Huang, 1991), but children exposed to manganese may exhibit persistent language impairments (Bronstein et al., 1988; Zhang et al., 1995).

The following studies demonstrate the effects of manganese exposure on the CNS as documented by neuropsychological testing. Performance on finger tapping, simple reaction time, and digit spans was inferior in 30 foundry workers exposed to manganese levels of 0.02 to 1.4 mg/m^3 (mean: 0.25 mg/m^3) for a mean duration of 9.9 years (Iregren, 1990; Wennberg et al., 1991). Neurobehavioral assessment of 141 workers exposed to air manganese concentrations of 0.07 to 8.61 mg/m^3 (mean: 1 mg/m^3) for a mean duration of 7.1 years revealed performance deficits on tests of eye-hand coordination, reaction time, and short-term memory (Roels et al., 1985). Reaction-time impairments were noted in a group of welders exposed to 1.0 to 4.0 mg/m^3 of manganese for an average of 16 years (Siegel and Bergert, 1982). Grandjean (1983) compared 48 manganese-exposed welders with 27 unexposed control subjects and found impaired performance in the former on gestalt memory tests. Two-year exposure to air manganese levels of up to 28 mg/m³ was associated with deficits in tests of facial recognition and slowing on tests of visual constructive praxis in six workers (Huang et al., 1989).

A study by Hua and Huang (1991) compared the neuropsychological test performances of 4 workers who developed parkinsonian symptoms after a 9-year period of exposure to manganese at concentrations of more than 28 mg/m³ with those of 17 asymptomatic workers exposed to manganese at concentrations of at least 2 mg/m³ for 11.8 years, 8 patients with IPD, and 19 unexposed controls. The four workers who developed parkinsonian symptoms performed significantly worse on the Wechsler Adult Intelligence Scale–Revised (WAIS-R), facial recognition, Purdue Pegboard, and Continuous Performance tests than the unexposed controls. Although these same workers performed better on the Purdue Pegboard than did eight IPD patients, they performed worse on the facial recognition test. The 17 asymptomatic workers scored lower than the controls on the PIQ subtests of visual attention and dimensional block construction tests. These test results indicate manganese encephalopathy, with features consistent with frontal–temporal–parietal connection dysfunction. Slowness in response times and decreased fine motor control are related to basal ganglia-cortical (extrapyramidal) involvement.

Lucchini et al. (1995) reported the results of neurobehavioral testing of 58 workers from a ferromanganese alloy plant who had been exposed to manganese at concentrations of 0.027 to 2.6 mg/m³ for a mean duration of 13 years (range: 1 to 28 years). The workers were divided into three groups based on manganese exposure history, with the *high exposure* group consisting of furnace workers with previous manganese exposures of 0.12 to 2.6 mg/m³; the *medium exposure* group consisting of maintenance workers with exposures ranging from 0.072 to 0.76 mg/m³; and the *low exposure* group consisting of foremen, clerks, and laboratory technicians exposed to manganese concentrations of only 0.009 to 0.15 mg/m³. Examinations were performed during a period of 1 to 42 days absent from work. Half of the workers were tested 13 days after cessation of exposure, and the rest were evaluated over the next 29 days. Blood and urine specimens were obtained immediately before the neuropsychological test procedures. Geometric means of blood manganese for the low, medium, and high exposure groups were 6.0, 8.6, and 11.9 μg/L, respectively; mean urinary manganese levels were 1.7, 2.3, and 2.8 μg/L, respectively. Cumulative exposure indices (CEIs) were determined for each subject. Neurobehavioral effects were studied using tests of simple reaction time, complex reaction time (shapes comparison), executive function (arithmetic), perceptual speed (digit symbol), motor function (finger tapping), short-term memory (digit span), and verbal understanding (vocabulary). Impairments were most prominent in tests of motor function (finger tapping and digit symbol) and short-term memory

(digit span). The results of these tests indicate the existence of a correlation between environmental exposure levels, as represented by the individual CEI, and the development of cognitive deficits. In addition, the results of these neurobehavioral measures were correlated with the blood and urine levels of the subjects determined at the time of testing, suggesting that specimens taken a short but relevant time after exposure may better reflect actual body burden and potential manganese intoxication.

Biochemical Diagnosis

The ACGIH has not established a biological exposure index for workers exposed to manganese (ACGIH, 1995 (Table 10-3). Because it is the principal elimination route, fecal manganese content is recommended for monitoring recent exposures (WHO, 1981; ATSDR, 1992). Reported normal concentrations of manganese in individual samples of plasma or urine show a wide range of values, in part because of the low concentration of manganese in some biological specimens (e.g., blood) and in part because of the contamination of other samples (WHO, 1981). However, in population studies, a correlation emerges between urinary manganese and mean air concentration in the work place (Tanaka and Lieben, 1969; Roels et al., 1985). Urinary concentration of manganese is normally less than 1 μg/L (Saric, 1986). The rapid clearance of manganese from the blood limits its usefulness as a biomarker of toxicity (ATSDR, 1992; NIOSH, 1997). In addition, blood manganese levels are influenced by the accumulated body burden and therefore may not accurately reflect an immediate past exposure and recently acquired uptake (Cook et al., 1974; Roels et al., 1987b). Despite these limitations, blood manganese levels have been used for monitoring manganese exposure (Roels et al., 1987a; Hauser et al., 1994).

In a cross-sectional survey of 104 control subjects and 141 workers exposed to a mean manganese air level of 1 mg/m³, the average blood level of manganese in the exposed workers was more than twice the level found in the controls (Roels et al., 1987a). The survey also identified a correlation between whole blood manganese levels above 10 μg/L and the prevalence of hand tremor and impaired response to tests of hand–eye coordination, suggesting that this level may be used as a biological exposure limit. Increased blood levels of manganese, associated with MRI abnormalities and neurological dysfunctions, are seen in patients with chronic hepatic failure (Hauser et al., 1994).

Although monitoring for elevated levels of manganese in feces, blood, and urine is important for detecting current exposure, these levels do not always correlate well with the severity of manganese poisoning in a given patient. In addition, these biological markers have often returned to normal levels, whereas neurological manifestations persist after cessation of exposure (Cotzias et al., 1968; Chandra et al., 1974; Yamada et al., 1986; Tsalev et al., 1977).

TABLE 10-3. *Biological exposure indices for manganese*

Parameter	Urine	Blood	Alveolar air
Determinant	Manganese	Manganese	Manganese
Start of shift	Not established	Not established	Not established
During shift	Not established	Not established	Not established
End of shift at end of workweek	Not established	Not established	Not established

Data from ACGIH, 1995.

Mena et al. (1967) examined total body loss of radio-isotope manganese (^{54}Mn) in 14 asymptomatic working miners, 13 ex-miners with chronic manganese poisoning (CMP), and 20 unexposed controls. One of the 13 miners with CMP was studied immediately after termination of his work in the mines; the interval between termination of exposure and hospitalization for the remaining 12 varied between 2 and 25 years, with a median of 5 years. Total body turnover of ^{54}Mn was accelerated in the asymptomatic working miners, with no significant differences found between the ex-miners with CMP and the controls. These results indicate an expanded, rapidly exchanging manganese pool in actively working and exposed persons. This finding was not seen in the unexposed exminers with CMP or the controls. The results of regional counts show that the metal has a faster turnover rate in the liver than in the head or thigh.

Analyses for manganese performed on whole blood, plasma, cerebrospinal fluid, urine, hair, skin, and muscle samples confirmed that tissue concentrations of the metal were higher in active workers than in the ex-miners with CMP and that the presence of elevated tissue concentrations of manganese is not necessary for continuance of neurological manifestations of chronic manganese poisoning (Cotzias et al., 1968; Yamada et al., 1986).

Jarvisalo et al. (1983) measured manganese concentrations in the urine of five shipyard welders who had used 100 mild steel rods a day containing less than 1% manganese with a rod coating of 2% to 3% manganese for 5 to 9 years; those with the highest level of exposure had been exposed to air manganese concentrations of 0.30 and 2.30 mg/m³, and those with the lowest exposure level worked in areas with manganese levels of 0.04 to 0.014 mg/m³. Exposure was measured from urine specimens collected before and after a worker's daily shift. Although this study was unable to estimate the degree of an individual worker's exposure, the highest concentrations of manganese were seen in the urine samples taken after the workshift.

Measurement of urinary catecholamines and their metabolites is another possible means of detecting manganese exposure (Bencko and Cikrt, 1984). It can be expected that levels of catecholamines or their metabolites may also be affected by the many other factors that influence catecholamine metabolism. Nevertheless, Siqueira and Moraes (1989) reported a negative correlation between levels of urinary homovanillic acid and duration of exposure in a cross-sectional survey of 40 workers in a ferro-manganese alloy plant. Zhang et al. (1995) reported decreased plasma levels of dopamine, norepinephrine, serotonin, and acetylcholine esterase in 92 Chinese children exposed to manganese through contaminated drinking water. These children were also found to have elevated levels of manganese in hair and blood.

The measurement of manganese levels in hair can also be used to confirm exposure, but such levels vary with the degree of pigmentation of the hair shaft (Cotzias et al., 1964; WHO, 1981; Wieczorek and Oberdorster, 1989). Elevated levels of manganese were found in hair samples taken from automobile mechanics exposed to MMT and inorganic manganese (Loranger and Zayed, 1995).

Neuroimaging

Computed tomography has not been found to be extremely useful in documenting manganese poisoning. By contrast, *magnetic resonance imaging* (MRI) detected increased deposition of manganese in the basal ganglia of manganese-exposed individuals (Nelson et al., 1993) (Fig. 10-2). The T_1-weighted MR images of patients with increased blood manganese levels due to hepatic failure revealed increased signal intensity in the globus pallidus and the substantia nigra (Hauser et al., 1994; Layrargues et al., 1995). The signal intensity in the globus pallidus on T_1-weighted MR images is correlated with blood manganese levels (Hauser et al., 1996). The MRIs of nine patients receiving parenteral nutrition (mean duration: 5.3 years) for underlying illnesses such as scleroderma and Crohn's disease revealed markedly increased signal intensity on T_1-weighted images bilaterally in the globus pallidus, suggesting deposition of the intravenously administered paramagnetic trace elements, especially manganese (Mirowitz et al., 1991). Similar findings were described in children receiving prolonged parenteral nutrition (Fell et al., 1996). By contrast, the MRIs of normal individuals and of those with IPD show decreased signal intensity in the globus pallidus, substantia nigra pars reticulata, red nucleus, and dentate nucleus (Drayer et al., 1986). Serial imaging can help in tracking the time course of accumulation and documenting the extent of clearance of manganese in an individual case (Newland et al., 1989).

Newland et al. (1989) noted a marked increase in the T_1-weighted signal intensity in the basal ganglia of nonhuman

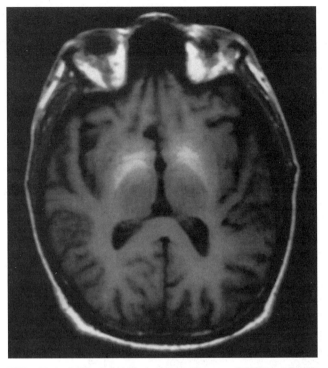

FIG. 10-2. MRI. Axial T$_1$-weighted image (TR/TE, 500/15 msec) at the level of the basal ganglia. Increased bilateral and symmetrical signal intensity in the globus pallidus reflects shortened T$_1$ relaxation due to the paramagnetic effect of Mn. (From Nelson et al., 1993, with permission.)

primates after exposure to manganese. A similar experimental MRI study by Shinotoh et al. (1995) further demonstrated that manganese is primarily distributed to brain regions high in neuromelanin content. In these studies, MRI was used to confirm the presence of manganese in the brains of rhesus monkeys following injection of manganese chloride (MnCl$_2$). The T$_1$-weighted MR images demonstrated a marked increase in signal intensity in the striatum (caudate-putamen) and to a lesser extent in the globus pallidus and substantia nigra pars reticulata. These findings were supported by the prominent neurodegenerative changes seen in the globus pallidus and substantia nigra on postmortem examination (Shinotoh et al., 1995; Olanow et al., 1996) (see Neuropathological Diagnosis section).

Single-photon emission computed tomography (SPECT) was used to document the acute reversible effects of manganese poisoning in a 52-year-old woman who presented with clinical signs of early manganese intoxication including poor balance, clumsiness, and postural instability (Lill et al., 1994). The patient's plasma manganese level was 4.8 ng/mL (lab normal: 0.40 to 0.85 ng/mL). SPECT studies of regional cerebral blood flow were documented in this patient using [99m]technetium-hexamethylpropyleneamine oxime as a tracer. Cerebral blood flow was significantly reduced in the right caudate nucleus and both thalami of this patient. At follow-up 1 year after removal from exposure, cerebral blood flow was within normal limits. Neurological examination at that

time was also normal. These findings indicate an acute impairment of basal ganglia and thalamic function associated with manganese exposure that was ameliorated following cessation of exposure. They also show that early detection and documentation of poisoning by neuroimaging studies can prevent persistent neuropathological effects.

In *positron emission tomography* (PET) studies using [18F]6-fluorodopa, the tracer is taken up by the terminals of the nigrostriatal dopaminergic system and can be used to assess the integrity of this system in manganese-exposed individuals (Brooks and Frackowiak, 1989). PET is sensitive and can provide information about the effects of manganese intoxication on the basal ganglia in humans (Fig. 10-3); it may also be helpful in differentiating manganese encephalopathy from IPD in a given patient. Using PET, Wolters et al. (1989) noted that mild "clinical parkinsonism" due to manganese exposure occurs without evidence of a profound reduction in striatal dopamine uptake, suggesting that mild neurological effects of chronic manganese poisoning result from functional disturbances in postsynaptic striatal or pallidal neurons (Donaldson and Barbeau, 1985). These findings are supported by neuropathological evidence of irreversible effects such as cell loss in the globus pallidus and explain the persistence of extrapyramidal findings in some patients after exposure has ended (Huang et al., 1993; 1998; Nelson et al., 1993).

The biochemical anatomy of the nigrostriatal dopaminergic pathway in the same animals studied by Shinotoh et al. (1995) above was investigated by PET with [11C]raclopride and [18F]6-fluorodopa; the cerebral metabolic rate of glucose was explored with [18F]fluorodeoxyglucose (Shinotoh et al., 1995). Results of the PET showed preservation of the nigrostriatal pathway. These results are quite interesting as they concur with the above report of 6FD studies in four human patients with chronic manganese intoxication (Wolters et al., 1989) and previous [11C]L-dopa PET studies in primates (Eriksson et al., 1992) (Fig. 10-3).

Collectively, the results of these studies suggest that manganese may cause parkinsonism and dystonia by damaging output pathways (e.g., globus pallidus) downstream to the dopaminergic projections, thus explaining how manganese poisoning produces the clinical features of parkinsonism and yet the lack of a therapeutic response to L-dopa (Shinotoh et al., 1995).

Neuropathological Diagnosis

Manganese damages the neuromelanin-containing cells in the basal ganglia, especially the substantia nigra; however, the cell loss in the substantia nigra is less than that which occurs in IPD and, in addition, primarily involves the pars reticulata. In IPD, specific patterns of cell loss are seen in the zona compacta of the substantia nigra; an associated reduction in the amount of dopamine in the caudate nucleus and putamen results in the clinical features. Lewy inclusion bodies, which are found in the substantia nigra

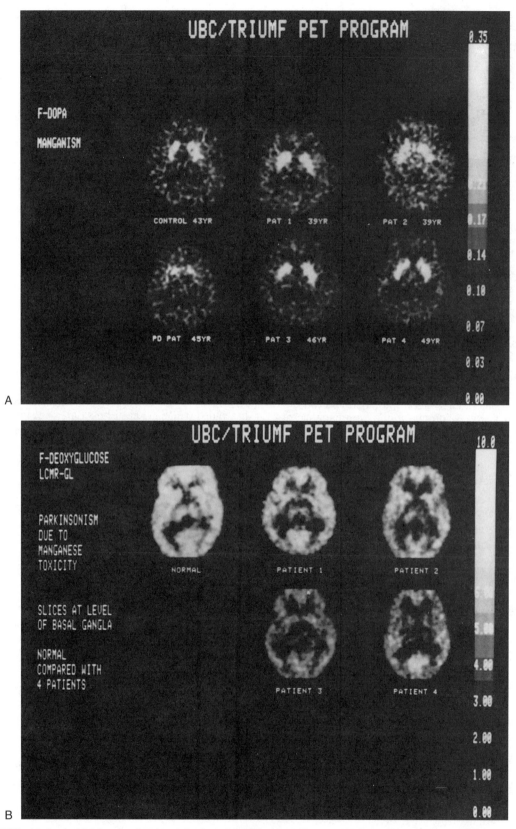

FIG. 10-3. A. Maximal striatal activity in 6-fluorodopa positron emission tomographic (PET) scans in one normal subject (control), one patient with Parkinson's disease (PD), and four patients with chronic manganism. **B.** Local cerebral metabolic rate for glucose as shown by positron emission tomography using ^{18}F-2-fluoro-2-deoxyglucose in one normal subject and four patients with chronic manganism (see text). (From Wolters et al., 1989, with permission.)

and locus ceruleus, further differentiate IPD from other conditions with similar features (Donaldson, 1988; Gibb, 1988). Unlike IPD, manganese toxicity mainly involves cell loss in the globus pallidus, substantia nigra pars reticulata, and thalamus (Graham, 1984; Barbeau, 1984) (Table 10-4).

A postmortem study of the nervous system of a 52-year-old retired manganese ore crusher previously exposed to manganese for 12 years and exhibiting extrapyramidal symptoms for 15 years showed no remarkable changes in the spinal cord or peripheral nerves (Yamada et al., 1986). Neuromelanin content in the substantia nigra zona compacta appeared normal and not depleted as would have been the case in IPD. Most of the pathological findings were in the basal ganglia. Neuronal loss was most marked in the medial segments of the globus pallidus; the lateral segments showed moderate neuronal loss. The remaining cells of the pallidum were generally shrunken. Marked decrease in myelinated fibers, moderate increase in astrocytes, and mild glial proliferation were also noted in the pallidum. In the putamen and caudate nucleus there was a moderate decrease in the number of large neurons, compared with the smaller nerve cells, which were shrunken but preserved in number. Neurons in the subthalamic nucleus and thalamus were atrophic, as they were in the mamillary bodies and nucleus gyri diagonalis in the hypothalamus. The cerebellum showed a mild decrease in granular cells. The neurons in the third and fifth layers of the cerebral cortex were atrophic.

Postmortem analysis of this patient's brain tissue for manganese content 5 years after cessation of exposure revealed no overall increase in concentration per gram of wet weight when compared with an unexposed control and a patient with IPD. Average manganese concentrations in the areas sampled were 562 ng/g wet in the brain of the manganese ore crusher; 473 to 612 ng/g wet in the control cases; and 544 ng/g wet in the brain tissue of a patient with IPD. Although no significant difference in total manganese concentration was noted, compared with that in the unexposed controls and a case with IPD, distribution of manganese in

the manganese-exposed ore crusher was greater in the gray matter of the cerebral cortex and lesser in the basal ganglia. This finding of low manganese content in the usually neuromelanin-rich basal ganglia in this patient may reflect a marked loss of neuromelanin-rich neurons in the basal ganglia and therefore a reduction in the affinity of manganese for the basal ganglia because of the reduced amount of neuromelanin present in this region (Yamada et al., 1986).

Animal studies have shown that manganese spares the nigrostriatal dopaminergic system. This was demonstrated by clinical, histological, and tissue chemistry analysis of adult rhesus monkeys that received serial intravenous injections of $MnCl_2$. Autopsies showed marked cell loss in the globus pallidus and substantia nigra pars reticulata; the zona compacta of the substantia nigra was spared. Clinical dysfunction correlated with severity of neuropathological findings (Shinotoh et al., 1995; Olanow et al., 1996). Although there was neuropathological evidence of the prominent effects of manganese in the globus pallidum of the experimental animals, which had also shown MRI signal changes soon after the $MnCl_2$ injections, tissue levels of manganese were not increased in this brain region at postmortem examination. The lack of manganese in the globus pallidus of these animals was attributed to the rapid elimination of manganese from the entire brain (Olanow et al., 1996). However, since these animals were sacrificed 5, 6, and 34 days after cessation of exposure after a minimum of 43 days of exposure to concentrations of at least 10 mg/kg and since the half-life for elimination of manganese from the head following exposure to $MnCl_2$ has been determined to be 54 days (Cotzias et al., 1968), it is also probable that the decrease in MRI signal intensity in the globus pallidus of these animals reflected a loss of neuromelanin-rich cells from this region. Consequently, the decrease in neuromelanin resulted in a concomitant decrease in the regional content of manganese detected at postmortem examination (Yamada et al., 1986).

The normal catabolism of dopamine and other catecholamines and the production of neuromelanin in the

TABLE 10-4. *Neuropathological findings in manganese encephalopathy[a]*

| Age (yr) | Location of neuronal degeneration | | | | | |
	Pallidum	Caudate nucleus	Putamen	Substantia nigra	Other lesions	Reference
33	+++	++	++	+	Pons Internal capsule Thalamus Corpus luysi Red nucleus	Ashizawa, 1927
69	+++	+++	++	NR	Thalamus	Canavan et al., 1934
46	+++	+++	+++	None	Frontal cortex Parietal cortex	Stadler, 1935
37	+++	++	++	None	Subthalamic nucleus	Parnitzke and Peiffer, 1954
43	++	NR	++	+++	Red nucleus	Bernheimer et al., 1973

[a]In five fatal cases of manganese encephalopathy. +++, marked; ++, moderate; +, slight; NR, not reported.
Modified from Barbeau et al., 1976, with permission.

brain occurs with normal aging and requires manganese in specific concentrations and oxidation states. Manganese has a high affinity for tissues high in melanin content, and the affinity of this metal for brain tissues with high concentrations of neuromelanin may account for its selective neurotoxic effect (Lydén et al., 1984). Neuromelanin, unlike cutaneous melanin, is a waste product of the nonenzymatic autooxidation of dopamine and other catecholamines (Das et al., 1978; Graham, 1984). The capacity of manganese to induce selective lesions in the neuromelanin-rich areas of the substantia nigra, globus pallidus, caudate nucleus, and putamen appears to be related to the chemical environment of these regions, in which divalent manganese is oxidized in the cytotoxic trivalent species, possibly by neuromelanin (Ambani et al., 1975; Donaldson, 1988; Swartz et al., 1992). Manganese potentiates the oxidation of critical substrates such as catecholamines, glutathione, and fatty acids, generating toxic free radicals, disrupting neuronal membrane integrity, and resulting in cell degeneration. It has been demonstrated that the accumulation of manganese in the dopamine-rich nigrostriatal pathway potentiates the autooxidation of dopamine in that system, and trivalent manganese has been shown *in vitro* to be the oxidative agent responsible for this reaction (Donaldson et al., 1981; Archibald and Tyree, 1987).

The oxidation of dopamine by trivalent manganese leads to the formation of a cyclized *ortho*-quinone and a concomitant reduction in dopamine levels. The oxidation of dopamine by trivalent manganese does not require or produce oxygen, and no reactive oxygen species are generated by this reaction (Archibald and Tyree, 1987; Segura-Aguilar and Lind, 1989). However, a one-electron reduction of the cyclized *ortho*-quinone to a semiquinone, which occurs via the actions of reduced nicotinamide adenine dinucleotide (NADH)- or NADH phosphate-dependent flavoproteins, does require oxygen and thus leads to the formation of superoxide radicals. The cyclized *ortho*-quinone formed in this reaction is normally detoxified to a hydroquinone by a two-electron reduction catalyzed by NAD(P)H:quinone oxidoreductase (DT diaphorase). Most of the hydroquinone formed in this reaction remains fully reduced; however, some is reoxidized, leading to the formation of superoxide radicals and subsequently regenerating trivalent manganese from the divalent form that was generated during the initial oxidation of dopamine. Although the two-electron reduction of the cyclized *ortho*-quinone by DT diaphorase prevents the formation of trivalent manganese, it does not open the cyclized *ortho*-quinone, and thus the irreversibility of this reaction temporarily decreases the level of dopamine, possibly producing acute neurotoxicity (Segura-Aguilar and Lind, 1989). The free radicals formed in the one-electron reduction of the cyclized *ortho*-quinone to a semiquinone contribute to the degeneration of dopaminergic cells. The death of the dopaminergic cells results in a concurrent release of neuromelanin and accompanying depigmentation of the affected region (Donaldson et al., 1980;

Graham, 1984; Donaldson and Barbeau, 1985; Segura-Aguilar and Lind, 1989). Loss of neuromelanin, which is also a scavenger of free radicals, may further potentiate the toxic effects of manganese poisoning (Barbeau, 1984; Swartz et al., 1992). The adverse effects of trivalent manganese are potentiated when other protective scavenger enzymes such as superoxide dismutase and DT diaphorase are unable to alter the oxidation potential of critical amounts of reactive oxygen species (Halliwell, 1984, 1989; Donaldson and Barbeau, 1985; Segura-Aguilar and Lind, 1989). Neurochemical changes caused by manganese, such as acute regional decreases in brain dopamine and NMDA–glutamate receptor-mediated loss of autoreceptor presynaptic control of striatal dopamine release, may precede actual structural damage to selected neural systems, producing early and often reversible symptoms of manganese intoxication (Segura-Aguilar and Lind, 1989; Cuesta de Di Zio et al., 1995).

Experimental data have shown that treatment of dopaminergic neurons (PC12 cells) with $MnCl_2$ inhibits mitochondrial complex I activity of the cellular respiratory chain, whereas glial cells (C6) are not similarly affected. These findings suggest that manganese selectively affects different cells and that the neurotoxicity of manganese may involve a direct effect on specific mitochondrial complexes of the respiratory chain as well as oxidative stress (Galvani et al., 1995). IPD has also been associated with mitochondrial respiratory dysfunction (Janetzky et al., 1994; Blake et al., 1997). These findings suggest that environmental factors such as exposure to manganese, which contribute to oxidative stress and mitochondrial respiratory dysfunction, may also contribute to the pathogenesis and accentuate the manifestations of IPD (Feldman, 1992; Blake et al., 1997).

PREVENTIVE AND THERAPEUTIC MEASURES

Information about the hazards of the manganese-containing materials and their appropriate handling must be provided by the employer along with instructions about safety precautions. Avoidance of exposure to toxic levels of manganese in the first place, or of reexposure after treatment of a recognized occurrence, is obviously the ideal approach to risk management. Lack of sufficient scientific evidence that chronic exposure to manganese does not have serious neurotoxic effects has been the basis for opposition to adding MMT to gasoline as an octane enhancer in the United States (Mergler, 1996). Preventative measures include careful handling of manganese-containing materials, proper ventilation of the work area, protective clothing and filter masks, and good personal hygiene. General health and nutritional status should be monitored. Iron deficiency and the concurrence of systemic illness can increase a worker's susceptibility to the effects of exposure to manganese. Sampling of workplace air for elevated levels of manganese and periodic analysis of stool samples should identify excess exposures to manganese. Finally, routine clinical examinations should be performed to identify possible early signs of intoxication such as neurobehavioral changes, tremor, and disturbances in muscle tone and strength. With ongoing concern, an affected worker can be removed from exposure while the symptoms are still easily reversed.

The effects of manganese exposure are dose related, and removal of an affected person from further risk of intake, regardless of the source, is the first appropriate therapeutic measure. Acute symptoms usually subside on removal from exposure, without any need for specific therapy. However, severely affected patients with extrapyramidal signs of dystonia, tremor, bradykinesia, and mental changes may exhibit permanent disability even after cessation of exposure. The body's natural ability to eliminate manganese is usually sufficient, but chelation therapy may be used to hasten excretion of any accumulated manganese (Penalver, 1957; Cook et al., 1974).

The success of chelation therapy may be limited if the treatment is given after existing neurological symptoms have become fixed (Rodier, 1955; Wynter, 1962). The efficacy of chelation depends on the method of administration, the duration of exposure before cessation and the initiation of therapy, and the chelating agent's ability to bind the metal. Intravenous administration of calcium disodium ethylenediamine tetraacetic acid (Ca-EDTA) is useful (Whitlock et al., 1966; Rosenstock et al., 1971; Sanchez et al., 1995). An increase in urinary output of manganese over baseline occurs in patients as well as in control subjects, reflecting mobilization of accumulated tissue manganese. It is therefore necessary to obtain prechelation baseline urinary output values for comparison with those obtained after chelation. The oral chelating agents dimercaptosuccinic acid and 2,3-dimercaptopropane sulfonate have seen little use in the treatment of manganese poisoning (Cook et al., 1974; Angle, 1995). Dialysis can be used in cases of severe intoxication.

The similarity between the motor signs of manganese intoxication and those of IPD prompted the use of L-dopa in cases of manganese poisoning. When dystonia is the major manifestation of manganese intoxication, high doses of L-dopa may improve fine motor control and decrease the dystonia. Rigidity and bradykinesia responded to doses of at least 3.0 g of L-dopa per day, and withdrawal of L-dopa resulted in the reappearance of a lesser degree of "parkinsonism" (Cotzias et al., 1969). This may simply have been due to the lack of further manganese exposure and recovery from the original exposure.

Rosenstock et al. (1971) observed that specific symptoms of manganese poisoning such as rigidity and tremor responded better to L-dopa than did dystonia. Six ferromanganese workers with chronic manganese-induced signs of masked facies, hypophonia, micrographia, gait disturbances, and cognitive impairment were followed after cessation of exposure. Three of the six patients showed improvement over 2 to 3 years with L-dopa therapy (Huang et al., 1993). Others, such as manganese-exposed workers who had postural abnormalities and tremor with mild rigidity or dystonia, benefited little from L-dopa even in doses as high as 5 to 9 g/day (Greenhouse, 1971; Cook et al., 1974). It is also possible that the use of L-dopa therapy for manganese intoxication may add to the neurotoxicity by increasing production of quinones and free radicals during its metabolism (Barbeau, 1984; Parenti et al., 1988).

CLINICAL EXPERIENCES

Group Studies

Manganese Miners: Acute Behavioral and Later Motor Deficits

Mena et al. (1967) summarized the neurological findings in 13 ex-miners with chronic symptoms of manganese poisoning that had persisted for less than 1 to 25 years (median: 5 years). Exposure data such as the manganese content of the ore dust or concentrations of manganese in urine samples of these workers were not reported. Each patient filled out a questionnaire and underwent a complete neurological examination.

All 13 patients reported a period of acute psychosis that included headache, auditory and visual hallucinations, compulsive behavior, impaired memory, and irritability and that lasted for at least 1 month before the onset of extrapyramidal symptoms, which included gait disturbances, dysarthria, and tremor. Persistent symptoms developed 1 to 2 years after the onset of psychosis and included tremor, clumsiness, difficulty walking, and speech disturbances. Neurological examinations revealed abnormal gait (13 of 13), increased muscle tone (nine of 13), dysarthria (eight of 13), masked facies (eight of 13), hyperactive deep tendon reflexes (seven of 13), tremor (five of 13), and cogwheel rigidity (three of 13). The tremor seen in these workers was fine, intermittent, and of small amplitude. In the individuals who were the least handicapped, speech improved to near normal within 1 year after cessation of exposure.

It was concluded from these findings that psychomotor disturbances appear as the earliest manifestation of manganese intoxication, lasting 1 to 3 months before rigidity and dystonia appear, following which the exposed individual develops motor disabilities characterized by awkward walking, dysarthria, and tremor. An expressionless face and postural rigidity suggesting parkinsonism emerge later.

Manganese Ore Crushers: Persistence of Symptoms after Cessation of Chronic Exposure

A postretirement follow-up survey and clinical neurological examination of 162 retired manganese ore miners and crushers documented the persistence of symptoms years after cessation of exposure to manganese ore dust (Sano et al., 1982). Forty-six percent had been retired for 11 to 20 years and 27% for over 20 years. Neither environmental levels nor the group's tissue levels were reported, but working conditions were known to have been poor. Twenty-eight percent of the workers had complained of subjective symptoms such as depression, irritability, fatigue, and decreased libido while they were employed; 45% had emotional and cognitive impairments for as long as 6 years after they had retired and ended exposure. Five of the retirees demonstrated definite parkinsonism 6 years after their exposure to manganese had ended, and three had tremor.

Responses to the survey and results of the neurological examinations were compared with those of 124 unexposed controls living in the same area. The following neurological findings appeared more often among the manganese-exposed group than among those not exposed: high-stepping gait, stooped posture, monotonous speech, muscle rigidity and weakness, impaired drawing, and tremor. Fifteen of the manganese-exposed group were known to have psychiatric problems. No psychiatric or parkinsonian symptoms were noted among those not exposed.

Manganese Smelting and Manganese-Alloy Manufacturing Workers: Acute and Chronic Effects Following Exposure

Case 1: A Faulty Ventilation System Resulting in High-Level Subacute Exposure

An outbreak of manganese exposure induced neurotoxicity in Taiwan's smelting and alloying industry (Wang et al., 1989). The air-cleaning device of three smelting furnaces had been malfunctioning for 8 months before it was repaired, and 8 workers who had continued to perform electrofixation (alloying or welding) without proper ventilation during this period were exposed to concentrations of manganese greater than 28.8 mg/m^3. The overall duration of manganese exposure ranged from 4 to 14 years; the interval between the onset of symptoms and their formal diagnosis ranged from 1 to 12 months. No new cases appeared in the plant after the repair of the ventilation system, when air manganese concentration was measured at 4.4 mg/m^3.

The eight workers were exposed to manganese concentrations greater than 28.8 mg/m^3 for at least 30 minutes a day, 7 days a week. Six of these workers developed motor impairments with parkinsonian features. The workers left their jobs within 5 months of diagnosis, and no further manganese exposure occurred. All patients received L-dopa for 1 to 5 years. Five years later, these same 6 workers were reevaluated (Huang et al., 1989). One of the patients had died from undetermined causes. Of the remaining five workers, three reported initial subjective improvement, but any beneficial effects were gone after 2 to 3 years of treatment. There had been no dyskinetic or wearing-off effects in response to the L-dopa. The earlier neurological symptoms in the original six workers were reviewed and compared with the presence of these symptoms at the time of the follow-up. Muscle stiffness, sleep distur-

bance, fatigue, walking backward, freezing when turning, and handwriting tended to worsen, while tremor showed improvement. All other symptoms had remained unchanged since the end of exposure.

Huang et al. (1993, 1998) attributed the apparent progression of impairments to several possible causes: (a) a slowly evolving aberrant neuronal sprouting with reorganization of neuronal networks; (b) compensatory extrapyramidal responses to unbalanced functioning among the damaged basal ganglia; (c) slow neuronal degeneration by cytotoxic free radical species generated by the neurotoxicant; and (d) continuation of gliosis within the basal ganglia. Other factors in the environment, such as high levels of carbon monoxide in the homes of the workers where unventilated wood-burning stoves are used routinely, may have contributed to the progression of extrapyramidal signs.

Case 2: Low-Level Chronic Exposure in Swedish Manganese-Alloy Workers

The effects of exposure to manganese at very low levels on 30 active and asymptomatic men working in Swedish manganese-alloy steel plants were compared with those of a reference group of 60 men unexposed to manganese (Wennberg et al., 1991). The alloy workers had at least 1 year of occupational exposure to manganese dust at concentrations of 0.03 to 1.62 mg/m^3 for 8-hour periods, depending on their job tasks and locations. Plant records of exposure levels for the 18 years preceding the study indicated consistent levels of exposure for this population.

The exposed manganese-alloy workers were compared with a group of unexposed controls. The exposed workers had more subjective complaints of reduced libido and increased lethargy. After controlling for age, sex, and education in the analysis of multiple regression, a weak dose–response relationship was identified on neuropsychological tests of reaction time, memory, and mood. Event-related auditory evoked potential (P-300) latencies were prolonged in exposed workers. A tendency toward increased latency of some of the components of the brainstem auditory evoked potential was also noted in the exposed workers.

Case 3: Incidence of Tremor among Ferromanganese Alloy Workers

Manganese ore added to iron or silicon in the presence of coke and anthracite, using a reduction process in an electric furnace, yields manganese alloy, a stronger metal. In addition to carbon monoxide and sulfur dioxide, manganese fumes linger in the environment of alloy manufacturing plants in concentrations ranging from 0.30 to 20.4 mg/m^3. Of 369 manganese-alloy workers in such conditions, 62 showed one or more neurological symptoms, including fatigue, irritability, tremor, and rigidity. Sixty-seven percent ($n = 47$) of the 62 symptomatic workers had tremor at rest and on intention (Saric et al., 1977).

Manganese Exposure in Welders and Arc Burners

The degree of exposure among welders varies according to airborne concentrations of manganese in dust in their breathing zones. In a study by Chandra et al. (1981), the urinary and plasma manganese of 20 healthy controls and 60 welders from three plants with different airborne manganese concentrations was measured and correlated with clinical features. Air manganese content was 0.44 to 0.99 mg/m^3 in plant A, 0.50 to 0.80 mg/m^3 in plant B, and 0.88 to 2.6 mg/m^3 in plant C. From plants A, B, and C respectively, five, ten, and nine welders were diagnosed as suspected cases of early manganese poisoning. The urinary content was higher in the welders with neurological symptoms than in the healthy controls; plasma manganese content was too variable to be correlated with exposure to manganese welding fumes and so could not be linked to the presence of neurological effects. The neurological effects, however, paralleled the air manganese concentrations, with the greater number of affected welders in the groups exposed to more than 0.5 mg/m^3.

Chronic Exposure to Manganese in Drinking Water

Neurobehavioral disturbances, parkinsonism, and even motor neuron disease were described among the aborigines of Groote Eylandt; manganese was found in their drinking water and body tissues (Kilburn, 1987). Elevated manganese levels were reported in the spinal cords of patients in Guam and the Kekil Peninsula in Japan, where high levels of manganese exist in the water and soil (Yase, 1972). Water manganese content of greater than 50 mg/L was associated with adverse neurological health effects in an exposed population in Greece (Kondakis et al., 1989).

Kawamura et al. (1941) reported that intake of manganese in amounts ranging from 4.2 to 13.34 mg/L caused serious subacute neurotoxicity in 16 individuals. Two of the affected persons died. On autopsy, they exhibited degeneration in the globus pallidum. The source of exposure was determined to be oral ingestion of drinking water contaminated by deteriorating buried batteries.

Contrary to the previous two reports, comparison of the fine motor functions in 41 persons (21 men and 20 women) who had continuously, for durations of 10 to 40 years, consumed well water contaminated with manganese at concentrations of 0.3 to 2.16 mg/L, with a control group of 74 subjects (41 men and 33 women) who had consumed well water with a manganese concentration of less than 0.05 mg/L for the same durations did not reveal any deficits (Vieregge et al., 1995). Mean blood manganese concentrations were 8.5 µg/L in the exposed group and 7.7 µg/L in the control group. The measures were made using an apparatus designed to document fine motor functioning in the hands by testing aiming ability, steadiness, line pursuit, and finger tapping. Although this epidemiological study did not find evidence of impairment of motor functions,

other studies have revealed impairments at similar levels of exposure to manganese through consumption of well water (Feldman, 1994).

Individual Case Studies

Acute Exposure in Two Coworkers in a Metal Plant: With Long-term Follow-up

Two men (56 and 44 years old) working side by side developed similar neurological complaints (Whitlock et al., 1966). A diagnosis of manganese intoxication in the first case raised concern about his coworker. Testing found increased manganese in the second worker as well, and both workers were removed from the poorly ventilated work area and treated with EDTA therapy. Subsequent improvement in both men, as well as correction of the ventilation problem, permitted them to return to work.

In the first case, a 56-year-old metal worker experienced progressive motor and mental impairment after 3 months of exposure. The patient appeared apathetic and confused, with decreased eye-blinking frequency. He showed the following symptoms: monotonous voice, slow and cumbersome voluntary movements, wide-based gait, impaired tandem walking, ataxia on turning, increased muscle tone, and resistance to passive stretch in all four extremities, suggesting cogwheel rigidity. Tendon reflexes were hyperactive, a right Babinski sign was present, a mild tremor was noted, as was dysmetria on finger-to-nose testing.

An extensive inquiry into the man's occupation revealed that he used an air-arc burner to cut manganese–steel castings and worked around fumes. The use of this technique prompted the testing of his urine, which revealed an elevated level of manganese (4.58 µg/L). The worker was removed from his job, and the workplace was inspected. A defective exhaust ventilation system was identified in the work area; manganese fumes had accumulated in the air. Ambient air levels of manganese were 2.3 to 4.7 mg/m^3 (electrostatic precipitator) and 0.1 to 4.5 mg/m^3 (membrane filter analysis). Concentrations in this worker's breathing zone may have been significantly higher.

Symptoms continued to progress after the worker left his job. Three months later, reevaluation showed increased weakness and hoarseness of voice and bilateral Babinski signs. Urine manganese was still elevated (1.47 µg/L). Chelation therapy was administered even though this value was lower than that of the initial spot urine sample taken during exposure on the job. After a total dose of 2 g of EDTA, a 24-hour urine collection contained 94.2 µg/L and 118 and 144.5 µg/L, respectively, on the 2 subsequent days.

Gradual improvement in strength, coordination, and mood followed the chelation over the next 3 months. A mild intention tremor persisted, but the patient was able to resume relatively normal activity. No new symptoms developed over the next 6 months of follow-up, and he returned to his job. During his absence from work, his employer had installed a new local exhaust ventilation system for removing hazardous fumes. Air samples after the installation of the system showed manganese levels of 1.8 to 2 mg/m³ (electrostatic precipitator) and 0.1 mg/m³ (membrane filter).

At a follow-up examination 4 years later the patient's symptoms, which had improved during his absence from exposure to manganese, had progressed (Tanaka and Lieben, 1969). Neurological examination at that time showed gait disturbances, tremor, and masked facies. Deep tendon reflexes were hyperactive. His speech was monotonous and hoarse.

In the second case, a 44-year-old worker complained of slowness of motor activity, night cramps, impairment of recent memory, and a change in personality. His wife described him as decidedly different, with a euphoric and carefree attitude. The patient also complained of headaches that had increased in severity over 6 months. Neurological examination revealed hypomimia, decreased eye-blink frequency, and decreased spontaneous body movements. Weakness was detected in the distal muscles, preponderantly on the right side, such that he was unable to stand on his right leg without support. His gait was slow and wide-based. Tendon reflexes were increased, as was muscle tone, with a plastic quality on stretch. Babinski signs were present bilaterally, and sensation perception was normal.

Urine manganese level was 5.48 μg/L when this patient stopped work, a month before the institution of chelation with EDTA. The prechelation baseline manganese content in a 24-hour urine collection was 4.76 μg/L, which increased to 168.6 μg/L on the first day of treatment. The patient reported improvement almost immediately. Repeat examinations recorded gradual improvement with disappearance of the plastic quality of increased muscle tone, better strength, greater animation of facial expression, and disappearance of the Babinski responses. Coordination continued to improve over the subsequent 6 months, and the patient was able to return to his previous job, where, as stated, the ventilation had been improved.

Four-year follow-up of this patient revealed that although he was still working in the same plant, he had been reassigned to a job with significantly lower levels of manganese exposure (Tanaka and Lieben, 1969). His neurological examination revealed hyperactive patellar reflex on the left. A Babinski sign was also present on the left. The patient also showed mild gait difficulties when walking backward. Tremor was no longer clinically evident and eye-blink frequency was normal. Despite residual clumsiness in his hands, the patient claimed that he was able to perform his current job without difficulty.

Chronic Manganese Poisoning in an Ore Crusher

A 37-year-old manganese ore crusher developed clumsiness of his hands and difficulty walking after 2 years of working as a manganese ore crusher (Yamada et al., 1986).

Despite these developments, he continued to work for 10 additional years, after which his deterioration forced him to stop working. A neurological examination 1 year after he retired at age 48 revealed a monotonous voice, hypomimia, emotional lability, and reduced power associated with increased muscle tone and abnormal posture in his extremities. He exhibited an awkward and dystonic "cockwalk" and an inability to walk backward. Laboratory tests at this time showed that his manganese urine level was 10.4 μg/100 mL (normal is less than 2.0 μg/100 mL); his blood manganese level was 3.4 μg/100 mL (normal is 0.4 to 2.0 μg/100 mL). Treatment with chelation (20 mg/kg EDTA) resulted in an output of 56.4 μg/100 mL of manganese in the urine. L-dopa therapy did not alleviate his symptoms. These findings, the course of the illness, and the lack of response to L-dopa were considered diagnostic of manganese intoxication, acute and chronic. The patient's disability endured, and he died of a gastric ulcer 5 years later at age 52 (see Neuropathological Diagnosis section).

Manganese-Contaminated Well Water: A Family Exposed

The following case of a young family exposed to manganese through their water supply shows how differences in individual susceptibility can determine the initial clinical presentation and prognosis. The worst affected member of this family was the child, who had been exposed during her first year of life. A similar case was reported by Bronstein et al. (1988), who described a 6½-year-old boy whose autisticlike behavior, slow speech development, and awkward gait with toe walking were attributed to exposure from his infancy through 13.5 months to water containing 0.9 mg/L of manganese. Zhang et al. (1995) also reported learning disabilities in 92 children exposed to manganese in drinking water. Blood and hair manganese levels in these children were 33.9 μg/L and 1.242 μg/g, respectively, and were significantly elevated above those of unexposed controls. Higher blood and hair manganese levels were correlated with poor school performance. In addition, the poor school performance of the exposed children was correlated with decreased plasma levels of dopamine, norepinephrine, serotonin, and acetylcholine esterase.

For the first few months after they moved into their new home, a father (32 years old), mother (25 years old), and their 1-year-old daughter used the water from their well for bathing, cooking, and drinking. Behavioral changes appeared first in the father, who began to exhibit mood changes, with irritability, memory disturbances, and loss of balance. The mother began to develop a tremor and headaches. The young daughter also had a tremor, and her hair appeared to darken. The family's clothing and dishes also seemed darker, and the water was noted to have a bad taste. When these conditions were recognized, the tap water was tested. Thorstensen Laboratory (Westford, MA) reported manganese levels ranging from 2.62 to 6.0 mg/L, which are significantly higher than the maximum contamination level (MCL) of 0.05 mg/L (USEPA, 1984). Iron content in the water was 1.7 mg/L and was also significantly higher than the EPA MCL of 0.3 mg/L. Following recognition of the elevated manganese content in their well water, the family stopped using it for anything except bathing. Plasma and urine levels of manganese taken at that time revealed that the father's plasma manganese was 56 ng/mL (lab normal: 0.04 to 0.85 ng/mL); a 24-hour urine sample contained 5.8 μg (lab normal: 0 to 0.3 μg/24 hr). The mother's 24-hour urine sample contained 0.7 μg manganese. The manganese concentration in the child's plasma was 1.5 ng/mL.

After total discontinuation of exposure to the well water, their symptoms began to disappear. By 6 to 8 weeks after cessation, the child's hair began to lighten and her tremor disappeared. The father no longer had mood changes, balance problems, or memory disturbances, and the mother's tremor was milder but persisted. Follow-up 5 years later found that the family had not used the well as a source for their water, but the mother's tremor was still slightly present, and the child's speech and general development had been delayed. The father's symptoms had disappeared completely.

Concurrent metal exposures and mineral nutrition are factors in manganese toxicity. For example, manganese levels increase with increasing blood levels of lead in young children and in occupationally exposed workers (Zielhuis et al., 1978), and coexposure to manganese and lead in iron-deficient rats causes a marked increase in lipid peroxidation in the brain (Malhotra et al., 1984). Similarly, elevated levels of iron in the water ingested by the family discussed above may have protected them somewhat against manganese.

REFERENCES

Agency for Toxic Substances and Disease Registry (ATSDR). *Toxicological profile for manganese and compounds.* TP-91/19. Atlanta, GA: ATSDR, 1992.

Akram M, Sullivan C, Mack G, Buchanan N. What is the clinical significance of reduced zinc levels in treated epileptic patients? *Med J Aust* 1989;151:113.

Ali SF, Duhart HM, Newport GD, Lipe GW, Slikker W Jr. Manganese-induced reactive oxygen species: comparison between Mn^{+2} and Mn^{+3}. *Neurodegeneration* 1995;4:329–334.

Ambani LM, Van Woert MH, Murphy S. Brain peroxidase and catalase in Parkinson disease. *Arch Neurol* 1975;32:114–118.

Aminoff MJ. Electroencephalography: general principles and clinical applications. In: Aminoff MJ, ed. *Electrodiagnosis in clinical neurology,* 2nd ed. New York: Churchill Livingston, 1986:21–75.

American Conference of Governmental Industrial Hygienists (ACGIH). Threshold limit values (TLVs) for chemical substances and physical agents and biological exposure indices (BEIs). Cincinnati, OH: ACGIH, 1995.

Amoore JE, Hautala E. Odor as an aid to chemical safety: odor threshold compared with threshold limit values and volatilities for 214 industrial chemicals in air and water dilution. *J Appl Toxicol* 1983;3:272–290.

Angle CR. Dimercaptosuccinic acid (DMSA): negligible effect on manganese in urine and blood. *Occup Environ Med* 1995;52:846.

Archibald FS, Tyree C. Manganese poisoning and the attack of trivalent manganese upon catecholamines. *Arch Biochem Biophys* 1987;256:638–650.

Aschner M, Aschner JL. Manganese neurotoxicity: cellular effects and blood-brain barrier transport. *Neurosci Biohav Rev* 1991;15:333–340.

Ashizawa R. Uber einen Sektionsfall von chronischer Manganvergiftung. *Jpn J Med Sci Trans, Int Med Pediatr Psychiatry* 1927;1:173–191.

Baly DL, Keen CL, Hurley LS. In addition, the brain contains Mn-dependent enzymes such as pyruvate carboxylase and phosphophenol pyruvate carboxykinase activity in developing rats: effect of manganese deficiency. *J Nutri* 1985;115:872–879.

Barbeau A. Manganese and extrapyramidal disorders (A critical tribute to Dr. George C. Cotzias). *Neurotoxicology* 1984;5:13–36.

Barbeau A, Inoué N, Cloutier T. Role of manganese in dystonia. *Adv Neurol* 1976;14:339–352.

Barbeau A, Roy M. Familial subsets in idiopathic Parkinson's disease. *Can J Neurol Sci* 1984;11:144–150.

Bencko V, Cikrt M. Manganese: a review of occupational and environmental toxicology. *J Hyg Epidemiol Microbiol Immunol* 1984;28:139–148.

Bernheimer H, Birkmayer W, Hornykiewicz O, Jellinger K, Seitelberger F. Brain dopamine and the syndromes of Parkinson and Huntington; clinical morphological and neurochemical correlations. *J Neurol Sci* 1973;20:415–455.

Blake CI, Spitz E, Leehy M, Hoffer BJ, Boyson SJ. Platelet mitochondrial respiratory chain function in Parkinson's disease. *Mov Disord* 1997;12:3–8.

Brain JD, Valberg PA. Deposition of aerosol in the respiratory tract. *Am Rev Respir Dis* 1979;120:1325–1373.

Bronstein AC, Kadushin FS, Riddle MW, Gilmore DA. Oral manganese ingestion and atypical organic brain syndrome and autistic behavior. *Vet Hum Toxicol* 1988;30:346.

Brooks DJ, Frackowiak RS. PET and movement disorders. *J Neurol Neurosurg Psychiatry* 1989;Suppl:68–77.

Canavan MM, Cogg S, Drinker CK. Chronic manganese poisoning: report of a case with autopsy. *Arch Neurol Psychiatry* 1934;32:501–512.

Cawte J. Environmental manganese toxicity. *Med J Aust* 1991;154:291–292.

Chandra SV. Neurological consequences of manganese imbalance. In: Dreosti IE, Smith RM, eds. *Neurobiology of the trace elements,* vol 2: *Neurotoxicology and neuropharmacology.* Clifton, NJ; Humana Press, 1983:167–196.

Chandra SV, Seth PK, Mankeshwar JK. Manganese poisoning: clinical and biochemical observations. *Environ Res* 1974;7:374–380.

Chandra SV, Shukla GS, Srivastava RS. An exploratory study of manganese exposure to welders. *Clin Toxicol* 1981;18:407–416.

Chia S-E, Gan S-L, Chua L-H, Foo S-C, Jeytaratnam J. Postural stability among manganese exposed workers. *Neurotoxicology* 1995;16:519–526.

Cook DG, Fahn S, Brait KA. Chronic manganese intoxication. *Arch Neurol* 1974;30:59–64.

Cotzias GC. Manganese in health and disease. *Physiol Rev* 1958;38:503–532.

Cotzias GC. Manganese versus magnesium: Why are they so similar in vitro and so different in vivo? *Fed Proc* 1961;20:98–103.

Cotzias GC, Papavasiliou PS, Miller ST. Manganese in melanin. *Nature* 1964;201:1228–1229.

Cotzias GC, Horiuchi K, Fuenzalida S, Mena I. Chronic manganese poisoning; clearance of tissue manganese concentrations with persistence of the neurological picture. *Neurology* 1968;18:376–382.

Cotzias GC, Papavasiliou PS, Gellene R. Modification of parkinsonism—chronic treatment with L-DOPA. *N Engl J Med* 1969;280:337–345.

Cox DN, Traiger GJ, Jacober SP, Hanzlik RP. Comparison of the toxicity of methylcyclopentadienyl manganese tricarbonyl with that of its two major metabolites. *Toxicol Lett* 1987;39:1–5.

Cramner JM. Report on the fifteenth international neurotoxicology conference. *Neurotoxicology* 1998;19:443–445.

Cuesta de Di Zio MC, Gomez G, Bonilla E, Suarez-Roca H. Autoreceptor presynaptic control of dopamine release from striatum is lost at early stages of manganese poisoning. *Life Sci* 1995;56:1857–1864.

Das KC, Abramson MB, Katzman R. Neuronal pigments: spectroscopic characterization of human brain melanin. *J Neurochem* 1978;30:601–605.

Davis DW, Hsiao K, Ingels R, Shikiya J. Origins of manganese in air particulates in California. *JAPCA* 1987;38:1152–1157.

Donaldson J, Barbeau A. Manganese neurotoxicity: possible clues to the etiology of human brain disorders. In: Gabay S, Harris J, Ho BT, eds.

Metal ions in neurology and psychiatry. New York: Alan R. Liss, 1985: 259–285.

Donaldson J, LaBella FS, Gesser D. Enhanced autoxidation of dopamine as a possible basis of manganese neurotoxicity. *Neurotoxicology* 1981; 2:53–64.

Donaldson J. Manganese and human health. In: Stokes PM, Campbell PG, Schroeder WH, et al., eds. *Manganese in the Canadian environment.* NRCC No. 26193; ISSN 0316-0114. Ottawa: NRCC Associate Committee on Scientific Criteria for Environmental Quality, 1988:93–111.

Drayer BP, Olanow W, Burger P, Johnson GA, Herfens R, Reiderer S. Parkinsonism plus syndrome: diagnosis using high field MR imaging of brain iron. *Radiology* 1986;159:493–498.

Eriksson H, Tedroff J, Thuomas KA, et al. Manganese induced brain lesion in *Macaca fascicularis* as revealed by positron emission tomography and magnetic resonance imaging. *Arch Toxicol* 1992;66:406–407.

Feldman RG. Manganese as possible ecoetiologic factor in Parkinson's disease. *Ann NY Acad Sci* 1992;648:266–267.

Feldman RG. Manganese. In: de Wolff FA, ed. *Handbook of clinical neurology: intoxications of the nervous system,* Part I, vol 20. Amsterdam: Elsevier, 1994:303–322.

Fell JM, Reynolds AP, Meadows N, et al. Manganese toxicity in children receiving long-term parenteral nutrition. *Lancet* 1996;347:1218–1221.

Ferraz HB, Bertolucci PH, Pereira JS, Lima JG, Andrade LA. Chronic exposure to the fungicide maneb may produce symptoms and signs of CNS manganese intoxication. *Neurology* 1988;38:550–553.

Fishman BE, McGinley PA, Gianutsos G. Neurotoxic effects of methylcyclopentadienyl manganese tricarbonyl (MMT) in the mouse: basis of MMT-induced seizure activity. *Toxicology* 1987;45:193–201.

Flinn RH, Neal PA, Reinhart WH, D'Allavalle JM, Fulton WB, Dooley AE. Chronic manganese poisoning in an ore crushing mill. Public Health Bulletin. No. 247. Washington: US Government Printing Office, 1940:1–77.

Florence TM, Stauber JL. Manganese catalysis of dopamine oxidation. *Sci Tot Environ* 1989;78:233–240.

Galvani P, Fumagalli P, Santagostino A. Vulnerability of mitochondrial complex I in PC 12 cells exposed to manganese. *Eur J Pharmacol* 1995; 293:377–383.

Gibb WRG. The neuropathology of parkinsonian disorders. In: Janovic J, Tolosa E, eds. *Parkinson's disease and movement disorders.* Munich: Urban and Schwartzenberg, 1988:205–223.

Graham DG. Oxidative pathways for catecholamines in the genesis of neuromelanin and cytotoxic quinones. *Mol Pharmacol* 1978;14:633–643.

Graham DG. Catecholamine toxicity: a proposal for the molecular pathogenesis of manganese neurotoxicity and Parkinson's disease. *Neurotoxicology* 1984;5:83–96.

Graham DG, Tiffany SM, Bell WR, Gutknecht WF. Autoxidation versus covalent binding of quinones as the mechanism of toxicity of dopamine, 6-hyroxydopamine, and related compounds towards C1300 neuroblastoma cells *in vitro. Mol Pharmacol* 1978;14:644–653.

Grandjean P. Behavioral toxicology of heavy metals. In: Zhinben G, Cuomo V, Racagni G, Weiss B, eds. *Applications of behavioral pharmacology in toxicology.* New York: Raven Press, 1983:331–339.

Greenhouse AH. Manganese intoxication in the United States. *Trans Am Neurol Assoc* 1971;96:248–249.

Gyntelberg F, Flarup M, Mikkelsen S, Palm T, Ryom C, Suadicani P. Computerized coordination ability testing. *Acta Neurol Scand* 1990;82: 39–42.

Hall AJ, Margetts BM, Baker DJ, et al. Low blood manganese levels in Liverpool children with Perthes' disease. *Pediatr Perinatal Epidemiol* 1989;3:131–135.

Halliwell B. Manganese ions, oxidation reactions and the superoxide radical. *Neurotoxicology* 1984;5:113–118.

Halliwell B. Oxidants and the central nervous system: some fundamental questions. Is oxidant damage relevant to Parkinson's disease, Alzheimer's disease, traumatic injury and stroke? *Acta Neurol Scand* 1989;126:23–33.

Hanzlik RP, Bhatia P, Stitt R, Traiger GJ. Biotransformation and excretion of methylcyclopentadienyl manganese tricarbonyl in the rat. *Drug Metab Dispos* 1980;8:428–433.

Hauser RA, Zesiewicz TA, Rosemurgy AS, et al. Manganese intoxication and chronic liver failure. *Ann Neurol* 1994;36:871–875.

Hauser RA, Zesiewicz TA, Martinez C, et al. Blood manganese correlates with magnetic resonance imaging changes in patients with liver disease. *Can J Neurol Sci* 1996;23:95–98.

Hintz P, Kalyaraman B. Metal ion-induced activation of molecular oxygen in pigmented polymers. *Biochem Biophys Acta* 1986;883:41–45.

Hochberg F, Miller G, Valenzuela R, et al. Late motor deficits of Chilean manganese miners: a blind control study. *Neurology* 1996;47:788–795.

Hua MS, Huang C. Chronic occupational exposure to manganese and neurobehavioral function. *J Clin Exp Neuropsychol* 1991;13:495–507.

Huang CP, Quist GC. The dissolution of manganese ore in dilute aqueous solution. *Environ Int* 1983;9:379–389.

Huang C, Chu N, Lu C, et al. Chronic manganese intoxication. *Arch Neurol* 1989;46:1104–1106.

Huang C, Lu C, Chu N, et al. Progression after chronic manganese exposure. *Neurology* 1993;43:1479–1482.

Huang C-C, Chu N-S, Lu C-S, et al. Long-term progression in chronic manganism: ten years of follow-up. *Neurology* 1998;50:698–700.

Hurley LS. Teratogenic aspects of manganese, zinc, and copper nutrition. *Physiol Rev* 1981;61:249–295.

Iregren A. Psychological test performance in foundry workers exposed to low levels of manganese. *Neurotoxicol Teratol* 1990;12:673–675.

Janetsky B, Hauch S, Youdim MBH, et al. Unaltered aconitase activity, but decreased complex I activity in substantia pars compacta of patients with Parkinson's disease. *Neurosci Lett* 1994;169:126–128.

Jarvisalo J, Olkinuora M, Tossavainen A, et al. Urinary and blood manganese as indications of manganese exposure in manual metal arc welding of mild steel. In: Brown SS, Savory J, eds. *Chemical toxicology and clinical chemistry of metals. Proceedings of the 2nd International Conference, Montreal, Canada, 19–22, July 1983.* London: Academic Press, 1983:123–126.

Kawamura R, Ikuta H, Fukuzumi S, et al., Intoxication by manganese in well water. *Kitasato Arch Exp Med* 1941;18:145–169.

Kihira T, Mukoyama M, Kazuo A, et al. Determination of manganese concentrations in the spinal cords from amyotrophic lateral sclerosis patients by inductively coupled plasma emission spectroscopy. *J Neurol Sci* 1990;98:251–258.

Kilburn CJ. Manganese, malformations and motor disorders: findings in a manganese-exposed population. *Neurotoxicology* 1987;8:421–429.

Klaassen CD. Biliary excretion of manganese in rats, rabbits and dogs. *Toxicol Appl Pharmacol* 1974;29:458–468.

Komura J, Sakamoto M. Effects of manganese forms on biogenic amines in the brain and behavioral alterations in the mouse: long-term oral administration of several manganese compounds. *Environ Res* 1992;57: 34–44.

Komura J, Sakamoto M. Chronic oral administration of methylcyclopentadienyl manganese tricarbonyl altered brain biogenic amines in the mouse: comparison with inorganic manganese. *Toxicol Lett* 1994;73: 65–73.

Kondakis XG, Makris N, Leotsinidis M, et al. Possible health effects of high manganese concentration in drinking water. *Arch Environ Health* 1989;44:175–178.

Kono Y, Takahashi M, Asada K. Oxidation of manganous pyrophosphate by superoxide radicals and illuminated spinach chloroplasts. *Arch Biochem Biophys* 1976;174:454–461.

Larsen NA, Pakkenberg H, Damsgaard E, Heydorn K. Topographical distribution of arsenic, manganese, and selenium in the normal human brain. *J Neurol Sci* 1979;42:407–416.

Layrargues GP, Shapcott D, Spahr L, Butterworth RF. Accumulation of manganese and copper in pallidum of cirrhotic patients: role in the pathogenesis of hepatic encephalopathy. *Metab Brain Dis* 1995; 10:353–356.

Lill DW, Mountz JM, Darji JT. Technetium-99m-HMPAO brain SPECT evaluation of neurotoxicity due to manganese toxicity. *J Nucl Med* 1994;35:863–866.

Loranger S, Zayed J. Environmental and occupational exposure to manganese: a multimedia assessment. *Int Arch Occup Environ Health* 1995;67:101–110.

Lucchini R, Sells L, Folli D, et al. Neurobehavioral effects of manganese in workers from a ferroalloy plant after temporary cessation of exposure. *Scand J Work Environ Health* 1995;21:143–149.

Lydén A, Larsson BS, Lindquist NG. Melanin affinity of manganese. *Acta Pharmacol Teratol* 1984;55:133–138.

Malhotra KM, Murthy RC, Srivastava RS, Chandra SV. Concurrent exposure of lead and manganese to iron-deficient rats: effect of lipid peroxidation and contents of some metals in the brain. *J Appl Toxicol* 1984;4:22–25.

Marchal G, Ni Y, Zhang X, et al. Mn-DPDP enhanced MRI in experimental bile duct obstruction. *J Comput Assist Tomogr* 1993;17:290–296.

Markesbery WR, Ehmann WD, Alauddin M, Hossain TIM. Brain trace element concentrations in aging. *Neurobiol Aging* 1984;5:19–28.

Maynard LS, Cotzias GC. Partition of manganese among organs and intracellular organelles of the rat. *J Biol Chem* 1955;214:489–495.

Maynard LS, Fink S. The influence of chelation on radiomanganese excretion in man and mouse. *J Clin Invest* 1956;35:831–836.

McGinley PA, Morris JB, Clay RJ, Gianutsos G. Disposition and toxicity of methylcyclopentadienyl manganese tricarbonyl in the rat. *Toxicol Lett* 1987;36:137–145.

Mena I. Manganese. In: Waldron H, ed. *Metals in the environment.* New York: Academic Press, 1980:119–220.

Mena I, Marin O, Fuenzalida S, Cotzias GC. Chronic manganese poisoning: clinical picture and manganese turnover. *Neurology* 1967;17:128–136.

Mena I, Horiuchi K, Burke K, Cotzias GC. Chronic manganese poisoning: Individual susceptibility and absorption of iron. *Neurology* 1969;19:1000–1006.

Mena I, Court J, Fuezalida S, et al. Modification of chronic manganese poisoning: treatment with L-dopa or 5-OH tryptophane. *N Engl J Med* 1970;282:5–10.

Mergler D. Manganese: the controversial metal. At what levels can deleterious effects occur? *Can J Neurol Sci* 1996;23:93–94.

Mirowitz SA, Westrich TJ, Hirsch JD. Hyperintense basal ganglia on T1-weighted MR images in patients receiving parenteral nutrition. *Radiology* 1991;181:117–120.

Moore W JR, Hall L, Crocker W, Adams J, Stara JF. Metabolic aspects of methylcyclopentadienyl manganese tricarbonyl in rats. *Environ Res* 1974;8:171–177.

Murphy VA, Rosenberg JM, Smith QR, Rapoport SI. Elevation of brain manganese in calcium deficient rats. *Neurotoxicology* 1991a;12:255–263.

Murphy VA, Wadhwani KC, Smith QR, Rapoport SI. Saturable transport of manganese (II) across the rat blood brain barrier. *J Neurochem* 1991b;57:948–954.

National Institute for Occupational Safety and Health (NIOSH). *Pocket guide to chemical hazards.* US Department of Health and Human Services, Centers for Disease Control and Prevention. Cincinnati, OH: NIOSH Publications, 1997.

National Research Council (NRC). *Manganese.* Publication of the Panel on Manganese Committee on Medical and Biological Effects of Environmental Pollutants. Washington: National Academy of Science, 1973.

Nelson K, Golnick J, Korn T, Angle C. Manganese encephalopathy: utility of early magnetic resonance imaging. *Br J Ind Med* 1993;50:510–513.

Newland MC, Ceckler TL, Kordower JH, Weiss B. Visualizing manganese in the primate basal ganglia with magnetic resonance imaging. *Exp Neurol* 1989;106:251–258.

Nomiyama K, Tsuji H, Ikeda K, et al. Positron emission tomography (PET) before and after treatment of hyperammonemia in a patient with decompensated liver cirrhosis. *Fuk Acta Med* 1991;82:521–527.

Nordberg GF, Goyer KA, Clarkson TW. Impact of effects of acid precipitation on toxicity and metals. *Environ Health Perspect* 1985;63:169–180.

Occupational Safety and Health Administration (OSHA). Code of Federal Regulations, 29 CFR 1910.1000. Office of the Federal Register. Washington: US Government Printing Office, 1995.

Olanow CW, Good PF, Shinotoh H, et al. Manganese intoxication in the rhesus monkey: a clinical, imaging, pathologic, and biochemical study. *Neurology* 1996;46:492–498.

Papavasiliou PS, Miller ST, Cotzias GC. Role of liver in regulating distribution and excretion of manganese. *Am J Physiol* 1966;211:211–216.

Papavasiliou PS, Kutt H, Miller ST, Rosal V, Wang YY, Aronson RB. Seizure disorders and trace metals: manganese tissue levels in treated epileptics. *Neurology* 1979;29:1466–1473.

Parenti M, Rusconi L, Cappabianca V, Parati EA, Groppetti A. Role of dopamine in manganese neurotoxicity. *Brain Res* 1988;473:236–240.

Parnitzke KH, Peiffer J. Zur klinik and pathologischen Anatomie der chronischen Braunsteinvergiftung. *Arch Psychiatr Zeitschr Neurol* 1954;192:405–429.

Penalver R. Diagnosis and treatment of manganese intoxication. *Arch Ind Health* 1957;16:64–66.

Prohaska JR. Functions of trace elements in brain metabolism. *Physiol Rev* 1987;67:858–910.

Read AE, Sherlock S, Laidlaw J, Walker JG. The neuropsychiatric syndromes associated with chronic liver disease and an extensive portal-systemic collateral circulation. *Q J Med* 1967;36:135–150.

Rodier J. Manganese poisoning in Moroccan miners. *Br J Ind Med* 1955;12:21–35.

Roels HA, Lauwerys RR, Buchet JP, et al. Comparison of renal function and psychomotor performance in workers exposed to elemental mercury. *Int Arch Occup Environ Health* 1982;50:77–93.

Roels HM, Sarhan J, Hanotiau I, et al. Preclinical toxic effects of manganese in workers from a Mn salts and oxides producing plant. *Sci Tot Environ* 1985;42:201–206.

Roels H, Lauwerys R, Buchet JP, et al. Epidemiological survey among workers exposed to manganese: effects on lung, central nervous system, and some biological indices. *Am J Ind Med* 1987a;11:307–327.

Roels H, Lauwerys R, Genet P, et al. Relationship between external and internal parameters of exposure to manganese in workers from a manganese oxide and salt producing plant. *Am J Ind Med* 1987b;11:297–305.

Rosenstock HA, Simons DG, Meyer JS. Chronic manganism. Neurologic and laboratory studies during treatment with levodopa. *JAMA* 1971;217:1354–1359.

Sanchez DJ, Gomez M, Domingo JL, Llobet JM, Corbella J. Relative efficacy of chelating agents on excretion and tissue distribution of manganese in mice. *J Appl Toxicol* 1995;15:285–288.

Sano S, Yamashita N, Kawanishi S, et al. An epidemiological survey and clinical investigations on retired workers from manganese mines and ore grinders in Kyoto prefecture. *Nippon Eiseigaku Zasshi (Jpn J Hyg)* 1982;37:566–578.

Saric M. Manganese. In: Friberg L, Nordberg GF, Vouk V, eds. *Handbook on the toxicology of metals,* 2nd ed. Amsterdam: Elsevier, 1986:354–386.

Saric M, Markicevic A, Hrustic O. Occupational exposure to manganese. *Br J Ind Med* 1977;34:114–118.

Segura-Aguilar J, Lind C. On the mechanism of the Mn^{3+}-induced neurotoxicity of dopamine: prevention of quinone-derived oxygen toxicity by DT diaphorase and superoxide dismutase. *Chem Biol Interact* 1989;72:309–324.

Seth P, Chandra SV. Neurotoxic effects of manganese. In: Bondy SC, Prasad K, eds. *Metal neurotoxicity.* Boca Raton, FL: CRC Press, 1988:19–33.

Sherlock S, Summerskill WHJ, White LP, Phear EA. Portal-systemic encephalopathy: neurological complications of liver disease. *Lancet* 1954;267:453–457.

Shinotoh H, Snow BJ, Hewitt KA, et al. MRI and PET studies of manganese intoxicated monkeys. *Neurology* 1995;45:1199–1204.

Siegel P, Bergert KD. Eine Frudiagnostische Uberwachungsmethode bei. Manganexposition. *Z Gesamte Hygiene* 1982;28:524–526.

Siqueira ME, Moraes EC. Homovanilic acid (HVA) and manganese in urine of workers exposed in a ferromanganese alloy plant. *Med Lav* 1989;80:224–228.

Sittig W, Kleindienst G, Irmisch R. Effects of food intake on CNS activity. Psychomotor performance and mood states in healthy volunteers. *Pharmacopsychiatry* 1985;18:123–126.

Sjogren B, Ingren A, Frech W, et al. Effects on the nervous system among welders exposed to aluminum and manganese. *Occup Environ Med* 1996;53:32–40.

Stadler HZ. Zur histopathology des gehirns bei manganvergiftung. *Zentrabl Gesamte Neurol Psychiatr* 1935;154:62–76.

Stobbaerts R, Robberecht H, Deelstra H. Daily dietary intake of manganese by several population groups in Belgium: preliminary reports. *J Trace Elem Med Biol* 1995;9:44–48.

Stokes PM. Summary. In: Stokes PM, Campbell PG, Schroeder WH, et al., eds. *Manganese in the Canadian environment.* NRCC No. 26193; ISSN 0316-0114. Ottawa: Associate Committee on Scientific Criteria for Environmental Quality, 1988:vii–xi.

Swartz HM, Sarna T, Zecca L. Modulation by neuromelanin of the availability and reactivity of metal ions. *Ann Neurol* 1992;32:S69–S75.

Takeda M, Tachibana H, Okuda B, Sugita M. Two cases of hepatic encephalopathy associated with a high-intensity area in the basal ganglia on T1-weighted MR images. *Jpn J Geriatr* 1993;30:709–713.

Tanaka S. Manganese and its compounds. In: Zenz C, ed. *Occupational medicine: principles and practical applications,* 2nd ed. Chicago: Yearbook Medical Publishers, 1988:583–589.

Tanaka S, Lieben J. Manganese poisoning and exposure in Pennsylvania. *Arch Environ Health* 1969;19:674–684.

Tanner CM, Langston JW. Do environmental toxins cause Parkinson's disease? A critical review. *Neurology* 1990;40:17–30.

Ter Haar GL, Griffing ME, Brandt M, Oberding DG, Kapron M. Methylcyclopentadienyl manganese tricarbonyl as an antiknock: composition and fate of manganese exhaust products. *J Am Phys Chem Assoc* 1975:25:858–860.

Tsalev DL, Langmyhr FJ, Gunderson N. Direct atomic absorption spectrometric determination of manganese in whole blood of unexposed individuals and exposed water in a Norwegian manganese alloy plant. *Bull Environ Contam Toxicol* 1977;17:660–666.

Ulrich C, Rinehart W, Brandt M, Busey W. Evaluation of the chronic inhalation toxicity of a manganese oxide aerosol. III. Pulmonary function, electromyograms, limb tremor, and tissue manganese data. *Am Ind Hyg Assoc J* 1979;40:349–353.

United States Environmental Protection Agency (U.S. EPA). *Health assessment document for manganese.* Environmental Criteria and Assessment Office. Final Report, EPA 6008-83-013F. Washington: EPA, 1984.

United States Environmental Protection Agency (U.S. EPA). *Drinking water regulations and health advisories.* EPA 822-R-96-001. Office of Water 4304, Washington: 1996.

Verschoyle RD, Wolf CR, Dinsdale D. Cytochrome P450 2B isoenzymes are responsible for the pulmonary bioactivation and toxicity of butylated hydroxytoluene, O,O,S-trimethylphosphorothioate and methylcyclopentadienyl manganese tricarbonyl. *J pharmacol Exp Thera* 1993: 266:958–963.

Victor M, Adams RD, Cole M. The acquired (non-Wilsonian) type of chronic hepatocerebral degeneration. *Medicine* 1965;44:345–396.

Vieregge P, Heinzow B, Korf G, Teichert HM, Schleifenbaum P, Mosingen H. Long-term exposure to manganese in rural well water has no neurological effects. *Can J Neurol Sci* 1995;22:286–289.

Wang JD, Huang CC, Hwang YH, Chiang JR, Lin JM, Chen JS. Manganese induced parkinsonism: an outbreak due to an unrepaired venti-lation control system in a ferromanganese smelter. *Br J Ind Med* 1989;46:856–859.

Wedler FC, Denman RB. Glutamine synthetase: the major Mn(II) enzyme in mammalian brain. *Curr Top Cell Regul* 1984;24:153–169.

Wennberg A, Iregren A, Struwe G, Cizinsky G, Hagman M, Johansson L. Manganese exposure in steel smelters; a health hazard to the nervous system. *Scand J Work Environ Health* 1991;17:255–262.

Whitlock GM, Doruso SJ, Bittenbender JB. Chronic neurological disease in two manganese steel workers. *Am Ind Hyg Assoc J* 1966;27:454–459.

Wieczorek H, Oberdorster G. Effects of chelating on organ distribution and excretion of manganese after inhalation exposure to 54MnCl$_2$ II inhalation of chelating agents. *Pol J Occup Med* 1989;2:389–396.

Wolters E, Huang CC, Clark C, et al. Positron emission tomography in manganese intoxication. *Ann Neurol* 1989;26:647–651.

World Health Organization. *Manganese, environmental health criteria,* Geneva: WHO, 1981:1–110.

Wynter JE. The prevention of manganese poisoning. *Ind Med Surg* 1962;31:308–310.

Yamada M, Ohno S, Okayasu I, Okeda R, Hatekeyama S, Watanabe H. Chronic manganese poisoning: a neuropathological study with determination of manganese distribution in the brain. *Acta Neuropathol (Berl)* 1986;70:273–278.

Yase Y. The pathogenesis of amyotrophic lateral sclerosis. *Lancet* 1972;2: 292–296.

Zhang G, Liu D, He P. Effects of manganese on learning abilities in school children. *Chin J Prevent Med* 1995;29:156–158.

Zielhuis RL, Del Castilho P, Herber RF, Wibowo AA. Levels of lead and other metals in human blood: suggestive relationships, determining factors. *Environ Health Perspect* 1978;25:103–109.

CHAPTER 11

Trichloroethylene

Trichloroethylene (TCE, TRI, trichloroethene, ethylene trichloride, acetylene trichloride) is an unsaturated chlorinated hydrocarbon (Sax, 1979; IARC, 1979; NIOSH, 1994). Trichloroethylene is derived from ethylene or acetylene. Depending upon the method, TCE and tetrachloroethylene (see Chapter 12) can be produced by the reaction of ethylene dichloride with chloride and/or hydrogen chloride and oxygen (Waters et al., 1977). The United States' TCE production capacity of 320 million pounds per year (SRI, 1987) and the several million additional pounds imported annually (CMR, 1986) together constitute the large reservoir from which this chemical is drawn for its various uses.

In its pure state [i.e., containing no less than 99.5% TCE and <0.012% decomposition-retarding stabilizers (e.g., triethylamine)], trichloroethylene is a colorless, highly volatile, nonflammable liquid (Hathway, 1980; Gennaro, 1985). Its sweet chloroform-like aroma is detectable at approximately 30 ppm (Nomiyama and Nomiyama, 1977; Amoore and Hautala, 1983). Trichloroethylene is highly fat-soluble but poorly miscible in water. Soda lime enhances its decomposition, especially when TCE is heated in the presence of air and light, to dichloroacetylene (DCA), chlorine, carbon monoxide, phosgene, and hydrochloric acid (Reichert et al., 1980). For this reason, TCE should not be heated nor allowed to come into contact with alkaline materials and should be stored in a colored bottle or other light-impervious container to prevent decomposition (Defalque, 1961; Waters et al., 1977; Greim et al., 1984).

Effects of exposure to TCE and its metabolites on various organ systems are well recognized (Anger and Johnson, 1985; Feldman, 1994; Gist and Burg, 1995). Most of the current knowledge regarding the neurotoxicity of TCE has been gained from reported cases of human exposures and animal experiments (Arlien-Søborg, 1992; ATSDR, 1993). The neurotoxic effects of TCE have been attributed to TCE itself; to trichloroethanol, a metabolite of TCE; and/or to its degradation product DCA (Defalque, 1961; Bartonicek and Brun, 1970; Henschler et al., 1970; Siegel et al., 1971; Reichert et al., 1976; Greim et al., 1984; Federal Register, 1989a, 1989b; Barret et al., 1991, 1992; ATSDR, 1993; Feldman, 1994; Leandri et al., 1995;

Szlatenyi and Wang, 1996). Regardless of which compound is the ultimate neurotoxicant, these chemicals are all derived from the parent compound and thus, whether directly or indirectly, the presence of TCE in the environment can result in neurotoxicity (Barret et al., 1991; 1992).

SOURCES OF EXPOSURE

Because of adverse effects encountered from using TCE contaminated with decomposition products, TCE is now seldom used as an anesthetic or analgesic (Humphrey and McClelland, 1944; Dillon, 1956; Crawford and Davies, 1975). However, less pure forms continue to be used in the workplace.

Trichloroethylene has many commercial uses, including degreasing of metal parts in the automotive and metal industries; as a solvent in waterless dyeing and finishing operations in the textile industry; as a refrigerant for low-temperature heat transfer (Cooper and Hickman, 1982); and, in the aerospace industry, for flushing oxygen (Kuney, 1986). Trichloroethylene is used as a degreasing and extracting solvent; as a vehicle for paint, varnish, and glue; in cleaning solutions and lubricants; and in the synthesis of other organic compounds, pharmaceuticals, polychlorinated aliphatics, flame-retardant chemicals, and insecticides (Mannsville, 1992). Some of its former uses (e.g., grain fumigant, surgical disinfectant, extractant of caffeine, and pet food additive) have been banned by the Food and Drug Administration since 1977 (IARC, 1979). Of an estimated 100,000 workers exposed to TCE, nearly 65% work in unmonitored settings (Bruckner et al., 1989). Trichloroethylene and its degradation products are released into the atmosphere during industrial processes (Waters et al., 1977) (Table 11-1).

The general population may be exposed to TCE in air, water, and food (WHO, 1985; Gist and Burg, 1995). Ambient air TCE concentrations vary depending on location and season, with lower levels often reported during the summer when higher temperatures increase degradation (ATSDR, 1993). Ambient air concentrations of TCE in U.S. cities range from 0.03 ppb in rural areas, to as high as 1.2 ppb near emission sources (Brodzinsky and Singh, 1982).

TABLE 11-1. *Degradation products of TCE under various environmental conditions*

Conditions	Products
Autoxidation	Acidic products including hydrogen chloride
Contact with strong alkali (e.g., NaOH)	Dichloroacetylene
Biodegradation	Carbon dioxide, water, chloride ions
TCE vapor in contact with hot metals or naked flame (air and water present)	Phosgene, hydrogen chloride

Modified from Waters et al., 1977, with permission.

Trichloroethylene, as well as other volatile halogenated hydrocarbons in the local atmosphere, has an affinity for foods high in fat content (e.g., oil and margarine). Access to these products is gained as a result of the inability of certain packaging materials to protect against ongoing environmental contamination (Entz et al., 1982; Entz and Diachenko, 1988). Trichloroethylene has been detected in postmortem tissue samples and in the breath of ordinary healthy persons living in nonindustrial environments (WHO, 1985; Wallace et al., 1986, 1988; ATSDR, 1993).

Intake of TCE may result from contaminated drinking and bathing water (Landrigan et al., 1987; Burg et al., 1995). Increased TCE concentration in indoor ambient air can result from the vaporization of TCE-contaminated tap water. McKone and Knezovich (1991) suggest that the use of tap water containing TCE at concentrations of 1 mg/L can result in shower, bathroom, and household air concentrations of 2.6×10^{-2} ppm, 5.1×10^{-3} ppm, and 2.3×10^{-4} ppm, respectively. Private and public water sources have been contaminated by improper toxic waste disposal (OTA, 1991; ATSDR, 1993). Well water concentrations of up to 27,300 ppb have been reported in Pennsylvania; up to 3,800 ppb in New York; and up to 1,530 ppb in New Jersey. A surface water concentration as high as 160 ppb was reported (Burmaster, 1982). Raw and finished ground water supplies in many other American cities have been found to contain TCE levels as high as 125 ppb and 53.0 ppb, respectively (Fan, 1988). Rainwater collected in Oregon was found to contain TCE at concentrations of 0.78 to 16 ppt (Ligocki et al., 1985). Intake of TCE may therefore result from occupational exposures or from a contaminated environmental source such as drinking water (Landrigan et al., 1987; ATSDR, 1993; Burg et al., 1995).

EXPOSURE LIMITS AND SAFETY REGULATIONS

The odor threshold for TCE in air is 28 ppm (Amoore and Hautala, 1983). The *Occupational Safety and Health Administration* (OSHA) has established an 8-hour time-weighted average (TWA) permissible exposure level (PEL) for TCE of 100 ppm (Table 11-2). The OSHA PEL ceiling for an 8-hour workday is a 15-minute TWA of 200 ppm, with an acceptable 5-minute maximum peak concentration

of 300 ppm within any 2-hour period of the day (OSHA, 1995). The *National Institute for Occupational Safety and Health's* (NIOSH) 10-hour TWA recommended exposure limit (REL) for TCE is 25 ppm. However, NIOSH considers TCE to be a carcinogen and recommends that exposure be limited to the lowest feasible concentration. The NIOSH immediately dangerous to life and health (IDLH) exposure level for TCE is 1,000 ppm (NIOSH, 1997). The *American Conference of Governmental Industrial Hygienists'* (ACGIH) recommended 8-hour TWA threshold limit value (TLV) for TCE, below which no narcotic effects are observed, is 50 ppm (Federal Register, 1989a; ACGIH, 1989, 1995). The ACGIH 15-minute short-term exposure-limit (STEL) is 100 ppm (ACGIH, 1995). The ACGIH and NIOSH recommended STELs for the TCE decomposition product, dichloroacetylene (DCA), are both 0.1 ppm (NIOSH, 1997; ACGIH, 1995).

The odor threshold concentration for TCE in water is 0.31 mg/L (Amoore and Hautala, 1983). The *Environmental Protection Agency* (EPA) has established a maximum contamination limit (MCL) of 0.005 mg/L for TCE in drinking water. The EPA has recommended a maximum contamination limit goal (MCLG) of 0.0 mg/L for TCE in drinking water (USEPA, 1996) (see Table 11-2). These values are based on studies of carcinogenicity rather than neurotoxicity. The be-

TABLE 11-2. *Established and recommended occupational and environmental exposure limits for trichloroethylene in air and water*

	Air (ppm)[a]	Water (mg/L)[a]
Odor threshold*	28	31
OSHA		
PEL (8-hr TWA)	100	—
PEL ceiling (15-min TWA)	200	—
PEL ceiling (5-min peak)	300	—
NIOSH		
REL (10-hr TWA)	25	—
STEL (15-min TWA)	—	—
IDLH	1,000	—
ACGIH		
TLV (8-hr TWA)	50	—
STEL (15-min TWA)	100	—
USEPA		
MCL	—	0.005
MCLG	—	0.0

[a]Unit conversion: 1 ppm = 5.46 mg/m³; 1 mg/L = 1 ppm.
OSHA, Occupational Safety and Health Administration; PEL, permissible exposure limit; TWA, time-weighted average; NIOSH, National Institute for Occupational Safety and Health; REL, recommended exposure limit; STEL, short-term exposure limit; IDLH, immediately dangerous to life and health; ACGIH, American Conference of Governmental Industrial Hygienists; TLV, threshold limit value; USEPA, United States Environmental Protection Agency; MCL, maximum contamination level; MCLG, maximum contamination level goal.
Data from *Amoore and Hautala, 1987; OSHA, 1995; ACGIH, 1995; USEPA, 1996; NIOSH, 1997.

havioral effects of low-level exposure to TCE may be experienced by an individual before any overt manifestations can be objectively measured (ATSDR, 1993; Anger and Johnson, 1985; Federal Register, 1985). Therefore, although evidence of the neurological effects of chronic low-level exposure to TCE may be lacking, subjective complaints must be considered as the earliest indicators of exposure effect.

METABOLISM

Tissue Absorption

Inhalation is the main route of entry for TCE vapors (Fernandez et al., 1977; Ellenhorn and Barceloux, 1988). The efficient absorption of TCE vapor (approximately 80%) is explained by a relatively high blood/air partition coefficient and rapid metabolism (Åstrand, 1975). Uptake following inhalation is most rapid in the vessel-rich tissues, which have the greatest blood perfusion; the poorly perfused adipose tissues require at least 6 hours to reach equilibrium (Müller et al., 1974; Fernandez et al., 1977; Sato et al., 1977; Monster et al., 1976, 1979; Perbellini et al., 1991). Total pulmonary absorption is increased by physical exercise (Monster et al., 1976). Individuals exposed to 70 ppm TCE, 4 hours daily for 5 days, showed that uptake is also influenced by variations in lean body mass. Daily uptake per kilogram lean body mass in these volunteers was 6.6 ± 0.4 mg/kg (Monster et al., 1979).

Oral intake results in extensive absorption of TCE through the gastrointestinal mucosa (Defalque, 1961). Nearly 95% of carbon-[14]-labeled TCE given orally was recovered in the expired air and urine, indicating nearly complete absorption (Prout et al., 1985). However, peak blood levels of TCE are not reached for up to 2 hours following oral intake, while peak TCE blood levels occur almost immediately after inhalation. Gastrointestinal absorption of lipophilic TCE mixed with water occurs more rapidly than when it is dissolved in corn oil (Withey et al., 1983). Although it is slower, absorption of up to 90% of TCE in solution with corn oil has been reported (Prout et al., 1985). Few experimental studies have used water rather than corn oil as a vehicle for administering TCE orally (Tucker et al., 1982; ATSDR, 1993). Oral intake data concerning neurotoxicity for humans is very limited, particularly with low doses of TCE (Isaacson et al., 1990; Feldman et al., 1994; Barton et al., 1996). Nevertheless, oral intake of TCE is toxic and can cause death (Waters et al., 1977).

A 32-year-old woman who ingested an unknown quantity of TCE (blood concentration 18 hours after the exposure was 4,500 µg/L) became comatose for 3 days and gradually recovered over the next 4 days (Perbellini et al., 1991). This case provided an opportunity to relate blood TCE concentrations to clinical symptoms and to use a physiologically based pharmacokinetic (PB-PK) model to estimate the exposure dose. A blood TCE concentration higher than 1,500 µg/L was associated with deep coma. Using blood levels and the PB-PK model these authors estimated that the patient had ingested approximately 44 mL (65 g) of TCE. The PB-PK model predicts that the concentration of TCE in the central nervous system rises rapidly during absorption and reaches peak concentrations which are approximately two times greater than that of the blood. The PB-PK model also predicts that concentrations of TCE in adipose tissue reach levels up to 100 times greater than that of the blood and that TCE levels in adipose tissue decrease slowly following cessation of exposure. The predictions of the model were supported by changes in the patient's clinical status and the long (20-hour) half-life for TCE in blood.

Dermal absorption also contributes to TCE intake and is affected by the duration of exposure and the temperature of the solvent as well as the type, surface area, and level of hydration of the skin that has been exposed. The greater the degree of hydration of the skin, either by perspiration or by immersion in water, the greater the rate of absorption (Brown et al., 1984). In addition, direct dermal contact with TCE disrupts the integrity of the stratum corneum, thereby acting to enhance its own absorption (ATSDR, 1993). In volunteers dermally exposed to pure TCE by thumb immersion, the peak concentration of TCE in expired air was only 0.5 ppm, indicating poor absorption through the skin and also indicating that dermal absorption alone would probably not result in toxicity (Stewart and Dodd, 1964; Sato and Nakajima, 1978).

Tissue Distribution

TCE is highly lipophilic, and thus its distribution throughout the body is dependent upon the lipid content as well as the extent of blood perfusion in the particular tissue (Åstrand, 1975; Wolff et al., 1982; Bergman, 1983; Anderson, 1985; Perbellini et al., 1991). High concentrations of TCE are found in the brain, kidney, lung adrenals, spleen, liver, kidneys, and adipose tissue (Cohen et al., 1958). Radioactive TCE was retained longer in body fat than in other tissues (Bergman, 1983). The total amount of accumulated organic solvent in the body is correlated with the volume of adipose tissue, which, in turn, determines the proportional biological half-life of the particular compound and its rate of elimination (Cohr, 1986). Thus, obese persons accumulate larger amounts and exhibit a longer biological half-life of the TCE body burden than do lean persons. In addition, studies indicate that at the end of exposure, TCE is redistributed: TCE concentrations in muscle and other vessel-rich tissues decrease rapidly, while its concentrations in adipose tissue continue to rise, accumulating logarithmically over several hours until reaching saturation (Fernandez et al., 1977; Savolainen, 1981; Perbellini et al., 1991). After cessation of exposure, release of TCE and its metabolites stored in adipose tissue may become a continuing source of further exposure (Cohr, 1986; Perbellini et al., 1991).

Tissue Biochemistry

Once absorbed, a portion of the TCE is retained unchanged while the majority is metabolized by the cytochrome P-450 oxidative pathway to dichloroacetyl chloride (Leibman, 1965; Allemand et al., 1978; Costa et al., 1980; Costa and Ivanetich, 1980; Bolt et al., 1982; Miller and Guengerich, 1982; Dekant and Henschler, 1983; Bruckner et al., 1989; Goeptar et al., 1995) (Fig. 11-1). The majority of the dichloroacetyl chloride formed in this reaction undergoes spontaneous intramolecular rearrangement to yield trichloroacetaldehyde (chloral). The subsequent hydrolysis of chloral yields chloral hydrate (Miller and Guengerich, 1982; Bruckner et al., 1989). The actions of alcohol dehydrogenase and chloral hydrate dehydrogenase result in the formation of trichloroethanol (TCEtOH) and trichloroacetic acid (TCAA), respectively (Cooper and Friedman, 1958; Sellers et al., 1972; Lauwerys, 1983). Trichloroethanol is subsequently conjugated with glucuronic acid before being excreted in the urine (Defalque, 1961). Two miner pathways of TCE metabolism are the dechlorination of dichloroacetyl chloride to yield dichloroacetic acid and the spontaneous intramolecular rearrangement of dichloroacetyl chloride to yield trichloroethylene epoxide. Trichloroethylene epoxide subsequently undergoes spontaneous intramolecular rearrangement to yield chloral (Hathway, 1980; Miller and Guengerich, 1982; Dekant and Henschler, 1983; Dekant et al., 1984; Green and Prout, 1985; Bruckner et al., 1989). Other products of TCE metabolism in humans include monochloroacetic acid, chloroform, glyoxylic acid, formic acid, HCl, N-(hydroxyacetyl) aminoethanol (HAAE), and carbon monoxide (Miller and Guengerich, 1982; Dekant et al., 1984; Davidson and Beliles, 1991).

The toxic effects of TCE have been attributed to the parent compound and its metabolites. Increased blood levels of unchanged TCE have been associated with sensitization of the heart to epinephrine-induced cardiac arrhythmias in rabbits, while a similar association between increased blood levels of TCEtOH and/or TCAA has not been found (White and Carlson, 1981). Disturbed physical–chemical properties of nerve membrane and/or an increase in the activity of one or more of the phosphoinositide-linked neurotransmitters have been suggested to explain the narcotic effects of TCE, an outcome used to define its neurotoxicity (Juntunen, 1986; Subramonian et al., 1989; Federal Register, 1989a; Bhakuni and Roy, 1994). The majority of the acute narcotic effects of TCE have been attributed to its metabolite TCEtOH, which has been shown to potentiate the effects of γ-aminobutyric acid (GABA), the predominant inhibitory neurotransmitter in the brain (Sellers et al., 1972; Ertle et al., 1972; Peoples and Weight, 1994). In addition, TCEtOH has also been shown to inhibit ion currents activated by excitatory amino acids involved in the excitation of neurons in the central nervous system (Peoples et al., 1990). These findings suggest that TCEtOH is responsible for the acute sedative effects associated with exposure to TCE and other chlorinated hydrocarbons such as tetrachloroethylene and 1,1,1,-trichloroethane (Sellers et al., 1972; Peoples and Weight, 1994) (see Chapters 12 and 13). The chronic effects of TCE have been attributed to

TCE epoxide, free radical damage, and the TCE breakdown product DCA and its metabolites (Reichert et al., 1976; Allemand et al., 1978; Miller and Guengerich, 1982; Gonthier and Barret, 1989; Bruckner et al., 1989; Barret et al., 1992) (see Neuropathological Diagnosis section).

Both metabolism of TCE and the acute and chronic effects of TCE are altered by concurrent exposure to other chemicals. For example, the toxicity of TCE is increased by concurrent ingestion of ethanol (Koppel et al., 1988; Sato et al., 1991). Simultaneous exposure to TCE and ethanol increases blood TCE concentrations 2.5 times and TCE in expired air increases fourfold over levels measured after exposure to TCE alone, indicating interference with metabolism and subsequent increased pulmonary excretion of the unchanged solvent (Müller et al., 1975). Both TCE and ethanol are metabolized by cytochrome P-450 enzymes and therefore, competitive inhibition can occur during simultaneous exposure to these two solvents (Müller et al., 1975; Snyder and Andrews, 1996). Ethanol and TCEtOH compete for alcohol dehydrogenase, which catalyzes the reduction of chloral hydrate to TCEtOH, as well as the oxidation of ethanol to acetaldehyde, resulting in increased blood levels of chloral hydrate and decreased excretion of TCEtOH (Bartonicek, 1963; Sellers et al., 1972; Müller et al., 1975). Furthermore, competition between chloral hydrate and acetaldehyde for aldehyde dehydrogenase is thought to be responsible for inducing the "degreaser's flush" by resulting in an accumulation of acetaldehyde (Rall, 1990). Of interest is that disulfiram, which increases blood acetaldehyde levels following ingestion of ethanol, has also been shown to inhibit the metabolism of TCE (Bartonicek and Teisinger, 1962). The metabolism of TCE is also suppressed by coexposure to other solvents such as tetrachloroethylene and toluene (Ikeda, 1974; Seiji et al., 1989). Trichloroethylene enhances the effects of barbiturates by inhibiting their metabolism (Kelly and Brown, 1974). Furthermore, the TCE metabolite, TCAA, increases the effects of anticoagulant drugs (such as warfarin) which bind to the same plasma protein sites as TCAA (Sellers and Koch-Weser, 1970). Chronic exposure to chemicals (such as phenobarbital) which induce cytochrome P-450 enzymatic activity increases the metabolism of TCE (Parkinson, 1996).

Excretion

Approximately 10% of an absorbed dose of TCE is excreted unchanged through the lungs (Fernandez et al., 1977; Monster et al., 1976, 1979; Sato and Nakajima, 1978). Measures of pulmonary excretion in volunteers following single or sequential daily exposures to TCE vapor at concentrations of 70 ppm and 140 ppm found that 7% to 17% of the total given dose was expired from the lungs unchanged, while less than 2% was expired as trichloroethanol (Monster et al., 1976, 1979). Small amounts are also expired as carbon dioxide (Dekant et al., 1984). The concentration of

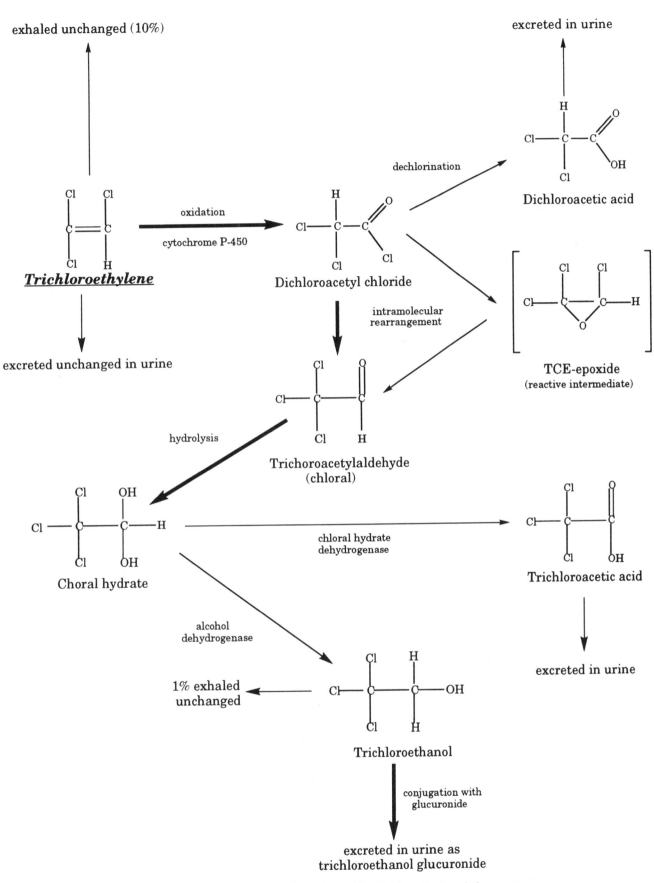

FIG. 11-1. Proposed metabolic pathways for trichloroethylene in humans.

TCE in alveolar air is related to the individual's workload during exposure, and it increases as the blood and parenchymal organs approach saturation (Monster et al., 1976). Consumption of ethanol during exposure interferes with metabolism, and it increases the concentration of TCE in alveolar air (Köppel et al., 1988). The reported long (20-hour) biological half-life of TCE in blood following accidental oral ingestion and the significant concentrations of TCE found in exhaled air as long as 18 hours after cessation of inhalation exposure in volunteers are due to the slow elimination of TCE from adipose tissue (Fernandez et al., 1977; Monster et al., 1979; Perbellini et al., 1991).

The majority (~70%) of an absorbed dose of TCE is excreted in the urine as TCEtOH glucuronide and TCAA; the urinary concentration of these metabolites is proportional to the atmospheric levels of TCE and the individual's pulmonary ventilation rate during the exposure period (Defalque, 1961; Vesterberg et al., 1976; Monster et al., 1976, 1979). Small amounts of free TCEtOH are also excreted in the urine (Vesterberg et al., 1976). Trichloroethanol appears in the urine within the first 24 hours after the start of exposure to TCE. Urinary concentrations of trichloroethanol and total trichloro compounds were both found to be proportional to the atmospheric concentration of TCE in the urine specimens from 85 male workers with daily TCE exposure levels ranging from 0.0 to 175 ppm. However, only one-third of the absorbed TCE was excreted during the workday. The concentration of TCAA in the urine of these same workers showed a linear relationship to TCE vapor concentration up to 50 ppm, after which there was a relative decrease in its excretion rate (Ikeda et al., 1972). Urinary excretion of TCAA is much slower than is elimination of trichloroethanol and trichloroethanol glucuronide (half-life of TCAA approximately 52 hours compared with 10 hours for free trichloroethanol and trichloroethanol glucuronide), and it reflects the binding of TCAA to plasma proteins (Müller

et al., 1974; Sato et al., 1977; Monster et al., 1984). There is no relationship to the amount of TCAA excreted and the degree of injury to the person (Bardodej and Vyskocil, 1956). Other possible urinary metabolites include monochloroacetic acid, chloroform, glyoxylic acid, formic acid, and HCl as well as HAAE, carbon monoxide, and other nonchloral derivatives (Fernandez et al., 1977; Monster et al., 1979; Miller and Guengerich, 1982; Dekant et al., 1984; Davidson and Beliles, 1991). Less than 10% of an absorbed dose of TCE is excreted in the feces as free TCEtOH and TCAA (Bartonicek and Teisinger, 1962).

Because TCE has a long biological half-life and the elimination of TCAA is slow, the concentration of total trichlorocompounds (TCEtOH + TCAA) in urine increases gradually during chronic exposure (Ikeda et al., 1971; Stewart et al., 1970). Exposure to TCE at 100 to 200 ppm in the workplace resulted in the appearance in urine of 30% to 50% of the absorbed amount as trichloroethanol and 10% to 30% as TCAA (Monster et al., 1979; WHO, 1985). Urinary TCE metabolite excretion was monitored in 140 workers exposed to TCE at levels below 50 ppm and in 114 nonexposed workers who served as controls. Urinary levels measured during the second half of the week revealed a linear relationship between increased exposure to TCE and the urinary concentrations of the metabolites trichloroethanol and TCAA. In addition, urinary levels of trichloroethanol were significantly higher in men than in women; TCAA levels did not differ between the sexes. The rate of TCE metabolites excreted in the urine by the end of the work shift per the amount absorbed through the lungs was determined to be 4.2%. This low rate of excretion is consistent with the long biological half-life of TCE (Inoue et al., 1989). Serial measurements of serum TCE and its metabolites were reported from a patient admitted to the hospital and followed for 7 days after he had continuously inhaled TCE vapor for its euphoric effects for 3 days. The

TABLE 11-3. *Relationship between biological exposure indices and signs and symptoms of exposure in a 35-year-old man following intentional inhalation of TCE*

| Days after exposure | Biological indices | | | Signs and symptoms of exposure |
| | Blood (µg/dL) TCEtOH | Urine (µg/dL) | | |
		TCEtOH	TCAA	
1	119	5,121	2,617	Somnolence, disorientation, agitation, ataxia, slurred speech, facial anesthesia, diplopia, cardiac arrhythmia
2	68	5,652	3,744	Somnolence, disorientation, agitation, ataxia, slurred speech, facial anesthesia, diplopia, *resolution of cardiac arrhythmia*
3	67	NR	313	Myalgia, agitation, confusion, ataxia, slurred speech, facial anesthesia, diplopia, *resolution of somnolence*
4	NR	NR	NR	Myalgia, agitation, disorientation, ataxia, slurred speech, facial anesthesia, diplopia, *resolution of diplopia*
5	55	2,842	248	Myalgia, ataxia, slurred speech, facial anesthesia, *resolution of disorientation*
6	NR	NR	NR	NR
7	NR	1,651	204	Residual trigeminal neuropathy and ataxia

TCEtOH, trichloroethanol; TCAA, trichloroacetic acid; NR, not reported.
Data from Szlatenyi and Wang, 1996.

actual amount of industrial TCE he used while "huffing" is not known. However, the prolonged elimination of metabolites which still appeared a week after no further exposure is consistent with TCE's long half-life (see Table 11-3). There were no indications of liver or renal disease in the patient; and although he had recently used cocaine, no ethanol or other volatile organic compounds were detected on careful laboratory testing (Szlatenyi and Wang, 1996).

CLINICAL MANIFESTATIONS AND DIAGNOSIS

Symptomatic Diagnosis

Acute Exposure

Subjective complaints and neurobehavioral manifestations are often the earliest indication of TCE exposure (Anger and Johnson, 1985). Experimental exposure to TCE vapor at concentrations of 50 to 250 ppm indicate that fatigue and inability to concentrate are among the earliest subjective symptoms of exposure (Ertle et al., 1972). Severe acute exposures whether by oral intake or inhalation of TCE vapors result in clinically overt as well as subjective symptoms of exposure. For example, a 29-year-old woman developed nausea, vomiting, severe headache, and loss of consciousness after she consumed approximately 15 mL of liquid TCE, which she had mistaken for cough medicine. She recovered completely in 10 days (Stephens, 1945). A similar case of acute oral intake of TCE (estimated dose: 44.0 mL) resulting in prolonged coma (3 days) and total recovery in 7 days was reported by Perbellini et al. (1991). Acute symptoms in a 26-year-old man exposed to high concentrations of TCE vapor for approximately 5 minutes while working in a confined space included dizziness, confusion, and stupor (Feldman and Lessell, 1969; Feldman et al., 1970). Acute symptoms among four workers who were exposed to TCE for 10 minutes to 2.5 hours while working inside a boiler tank of a ship included dizziness, headache, nausea, and vomiting (Buxton and Hayward, 1967). A 63-year-old laundry worker lost consciousness shortly after entering a storeroom where a bottle containing TCE had recently broken (Martinelli et al., 1984). Acute symptoms in a 20-year-old woman who was acutely exposed to high concentrations of TCE vapor included inebriation, nausea, vomiting, and loss of consciousness (Sagawa et al., 1973). Longer-duration and higher-level acute exposures to TCE vapor result in persistent neurological symptoms and death (Cohen et al., 1958; Feldman and Lessell, 1969; Lawrence and Partyka, 1981; Buxton and Hayward, 1967; Sagawa et al., 1973; Leandri et al., 1995; Szlatenyi and Wang, 1996).

Feldman and Lessell (1969) reported the persistent effects of an accidental intense exposure in a young man, which included anesthesia over the entire bilateral distribution of the fifth cranial (trigeminal) nerves. There was flattening of the nasolabial folds, reduced perception to taste, and ptosis of the left eyelid covering one-third of the iris. Corneal anesthesia was present bilaterally, visual fields were constricted, and pupillary responses were affected asymmetrically, the left pupil being smaller than the right and showing no response to near object. Recovery of facial sensation occurred in a concentric "onion-peel" pattern, with return of sensation to pain and temperature beginning at the tip of the nose and moving centripetally, suggesting that the pattern of sensation loss and recovery in the face coincides with the fiber spectra of the innervation of the face and head (Feldman et al., 1970) (Fig. 11-2). In follow-up over 18 years, further improvement was seen in visual pupillary response to a near object, although the left pupillary contraction remained sluggish (Feldman et al., 1985). Bilaterally constricted visual fields after TCE exposure were also reported by Sagawa et al. (1973) (see Neurophysiological Diagnosis section).

Similar findings have been reported by others (Lawrence and Partyka, 1981; Leandri et al., 1995; Szlatenyi and Wang, 1996). For example, Lawrence and Partyka (1981) examined a 59-year-old man who was acutely exposed to TCE while shoveling metal shavings (from an enclosed underground pit) that had recently been degreased with TCE. He worked in the pit for several hours using only a loose-fitting face mask for protection from the noxious fumes. This patient's trigeminal nerve symptoms began with numbness around the upper lip. The facial numbness spread during the course of the following 24-hour period to eventually involve his entire face, mouth, and tongue. He was admitted to the hospital 4 days later, at which time he drooled and was dysarthric. Neurological examination revealed complete anesthesia of the face and facial muscle weakness. His gag, cough, and corneal reflexes were absent. At a follow-up examination 11 years after the exposure incident the patient's speech was nasal, and he showed decreased sensation to touch, pain, and temperature over the entire distribution of the trigeminal nerve. In addition, corneal reflexes were absent bilaterally and he had a mild right ptosis.

Trigeminal neuropathy followed acute exposure to TCE vapor in a 24-year-old man (Leandri et al., 1995). With regard to the exposure dose and conditions, these authors provided only the history that the patient had been exposed to TCE and probably its breakdown products (e.g., DCA) for 15 minutes. The acute effects were not described; however, a neurological examination 1 month after the exposure revealed bilateral hypoesthesia in all three divisions of the trigeminal nerves. Thermal and tactile sensation thresholds were undetectable in divisions I and II of both trigeminal nerves. In division III, warm and cold thresholds were at least 8°C above and below skin temperature, and tactile stimulations were perceived only when above 6.10 msec. Masticatory function was slightly impaired. Subsequent examinations at 2 and 4 months after exposure showed improvement in chewing, but sensation over the face remained diminished. Neurophysiological studies in this patient suggested that the site of the lesion was in the retrogasserian root (see Neurophysiological Diagnosis section).

Acute intentional recreational euphoria-seeking inhalation of industrial quality TCE, obtained from a jewelry

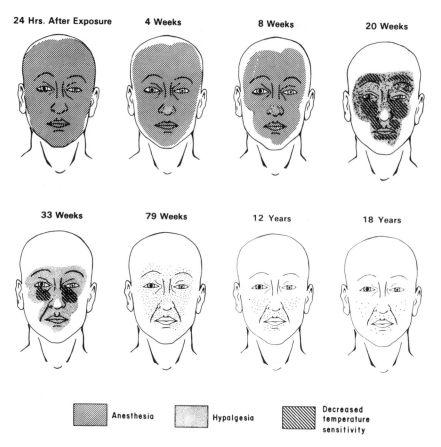

24 Hrs. After Exposure   **4 Weeks**   **8 Weeks**   **20 Weeks**

33 Weeks   **79 Weeks**   **12 Years**   **18 Years**

| Anesthesia | Hypalgesia | Decreased temperature sensitivity |

FIG. 11-2. Trigeminal distribution of facial sensation loss and recovery following acute trichloroethylene intoxication. (Modified from Feldman et al., 1985, with permission.)

manufacturing plant where it was used for degreasing, caused multiple cranial nerve palsies, cardiac dysrhythmia, and encephalopathy in a 35-year-old man (Szlatenyi and Wang, 1996). After inhaling TCE vapors continuously for 2 days, he began to develop ataxia of gait, facial anesthesia, and diplopia. Despite his symptoms he continued to inhale the solvent for another day. On the morning of the fourth day his symptoms had worsened considerably and he was admitted to the hospital. At that time he was somnolent but arousable to verbal stimuli. He was confused about his circumstances and he was oriented only to person and place. He was unsteady on his feet and his speech was slurred. He complained of diplopia, and his visual acuity without correction was 20/50 in both eyes. Evidence of limited abduction of each eye indicated sixth nerve palsies bilaterally. A mild ptosis of the left eyelid suggested a partial third nerve palsy, although the pupils were equal and reactive to light. Sensation over the face was diminished in three divisions of the trigeminal nerve bilaterally. He complained of generalized myalgia. His deep tendon reflexes were normal and the Babinski sign (upgoing toes) was present bilaterally. Urinalysis showed a trichloroethanol level of 5,121 μg/dL and a trichloroacetic acid level of 2,617 μg/dL. Serum trichloroethanol was 119 μg/mL. Toxicology screen tested positive for cocaine in the urine and serum.

An electrocardiogram performed in the emergency department showed normal sinus rhythm, but the PR segment was depressed and the ST segment was elevated. Within 12 hours, atrial fibrillation developed (rate: 150 to 170 per minute). His heart rate was controlled with metaprolol and digoxin, and after 48 hours the cardiac rhythm was again regular and normal.

Serial monitoring of serum and urine for TCE metabolites documented the correlation between clearing of TCE and its metabolites from the patient's body and resolution of his acute symptoms (Table 11-3). Diplopia was less severe and he was able to demonstrate better eye movement on the fourth day after TCE cessation of inhalation. By the fifth day, the patient was considerably better oriented. Facial numbness and ataxia were still present on the seventh day after exposure when he left the hospital against advice and was lost to follow-up.

The sensory loss over the face in this patient provides another example of the predilection of TCE's neurotoxic effects on the trigeminal nerve. As seen in other reports, the third and sixth nerves are also often affected. Of particular interest in this case is the cardiac irritability associated with TCE exposure and its possible exacerbation by the patient's use of cocaine, an adrenergic agent. Disorientation was noted, but the specifics of memory or other cognitive functioning due to TCE exposure were not documented by neuropsychological tests. The controversy of whether or not neurotoxicity is due to TCE itself or its breakdown product DCA cannot be resolved by the description of this man's use of industrial grade TCE for recreational purposes because it is not known whether the solvent had been exposed to moisture, light, and/or alkali material and, therefore, the extent to which it may or may not have decomposed. Nevertheless, it probably had not been heated the way it would have been in a degreasing tank.

Peripheral neuropathy following acute TCE exposure has generally been considered a rare occurrence (Sagawa et al., 1973; Lawrence and Partyka, 1981; Schaumburg and Berger, 1993). However, evidence of peripheral neuropathy was present on neurophysiological tests in the single case of acute toxic exposure referred to above, in whom clinical improvement was incomplete and evidence of permanent mild sensorimotor neuropathy was documented by electrodiagnostic measures years later (Feldman and Lessell, 1969; Feldman et al., 1970; Feldman et al., 1985) (see Neurophysiological Diagnosis section).

Dose effect relationships of acute exposure have been studied under controlled experimental conditions. Nomiyama and Nomiyama (1977) exposed 12 "normal" volunteers to TCE vapor at levels ranging from 0 to 201 ppm for 4 hours. At 27 ppm an odor could be detected, mucous membranes were irritated, and drowsiness occurred among members of the group. Headache was experienced by the volunteers after 2 hours of exposure to TCE at a concentration of 81 ppm. Dizziness, anorexia, and skin irritation occurred after 4 hours of exposure to 201 ppm. Stewart et al. (1970) exposed six volunteers to TCE at a level of 200 ppm for 7 hours per day for 5 days. By the fourth day, five of the six subjects experienced drowsiness and three subjects reported that it took more mental effort to carry out requested tasks. Seven volunteers who inhaled 1,000 ppm TCE for 2 hours experienced more serious visuomotor function impairment than did nonexposed control subjects (Vernon and Ferguson, 1969). In addition, two of the seven subjects exhibited performance deficits at 100 and 300 ppm, indicating increased susceptibility to the toxic effects of TCE in these individuals.

Chronic Exposure

Symptoms of chronic exposure develop insidiously whether intake occurs via pulmonary or oral routes. The National Exposure Registry (NER) has included TCE as a separate entity of the substance-specific subregistry that monitors TCE-exposed populations for the effects of long-term, low-level exposure. The TCE subregistry subset includes information on the health outcomes of 4,280 persons who have resided for at least 30 days at an address where TCE was the principal contaminant in their well water. Health outcome data collected from the TCE group revealed more self-reported adverse health conditions than were found among a comparison group (1989 National Health Interview Survey: morbidity study). Although analysis of the subregistry data do not identify a causal relationship between TCE exposure and adverse health effects among those persons interviewed, certain strong trends indicative of TCE-exposure-related effects are suggested by these population studies. A particularly noteworthy finding of this study is an increased incidence of speech and hearing disorders among children exposed to TCE (Burg et al., 1995; ATSDR, 1996). Adverse health effects related to the chronic consumption of TCE-contaminated drinking water have been reported by several authors (Ziglio et al., 1983; Logue et al., 1985; Lagakos et al., 1986; Landrigan et al., 1987; Bernad et al., 1987; Feldman et al., 1988, 1994; Barton et al., 1996). For example, subjective symptoms among residents of Woburn, Massachusetts who were exposed to TCE-contaminated well water included headache, dizziness, fatigue, irritability, insomnia, memory and concentration impairment, and paresthesias (Feldman et al., 1994) (see Clinical Experiences section).

A high incidence of nonspecific complaints including fatigue, dizziness, and inability to tolerate alcohol, in addition to pharyngitis and weight loss, in 50 workers (mean age: 43 years) exposed to undetermined concentrations of TCE for an average duration of 3.75 years was reported by Grandjean et al. (1955). Barret et al. (1987) reported symptomatic effects including dizziness (33%), headache (26%), asthenia (22%), sleep disturbances (11%), emotional irritability (10%), trigeminal nerve symptoms (18%), and sexual problems (6%), among 104 degreasers who had been occupationally exposed to TCE in a relatively high-exposure workplace with an average daily exposure time of 7 hours (mean urine TCAA concentration: 96 to 98.3 mg/g creatinine) (see Biochemical Diagnosis section). The symptomatic individuals had generally been exposed to TCE for a significantly longer time than the others in the group. Symptoms of TCE intoxication have also been reported among workers who had been exposed to relatively low levels (below the OSHA-PEL of 100 ppm) of TCE. In a study of degreasers exposed to TCE at levels of 51 to 100 ppm, the prevalence of subjective complaints and neurological findings including a heavy feeling in the head, forgetfulness, tremor and cramps in extremities, dry mouth, and nausea was found to be three times greater among the exposed workers than among a group of unexposed controls (Liu et al., 1988). The workers in this study had been divided into three exposure groups (low: 1 to 10 ppm; medium: 11 to 50 ppm; and high: 51 to 100 ppm) based on history. The prevalence of most symptoms was comparable between the groups exposed to levels of 1 to 10 ppm and 11 to 50 ppm. Although the prevalence of headache was highest (33.3%) among individuals in the low exposure group, complaints of headache decreased with increasing levels of exposure (i.e., 21.0% at 11 to 50 ppm and 12.5% at 51 to 100 ppm), possibly reflecting an anesthetic effect of TCE.

Health effects were also identified among a group of 70 female semiconductor workers, all of whom were under the age of 30 and who had been exposed to TCE for less than 2 years (Lilis et al., 1969). Of 214 determinations made of environmental air quality, 40% exceeded 10 ppm and 12% exceeded 35 ppm. Urinary TCAA concentrations were above 20 mg/L in 46% of the workers and exceeded 100 mg/L in 7.3% (see Biochemical Diagnosis section). Symptoms included dizziness (80%), headache (74%), fatigue (68%), emotional irritability (56%), anorexia (50%), sleep disturbances (46%), nausea (43%), euphoria (31%), palpitations (29%), end-of-shift sleepiness (29%), anxiety (27%), and alcohol intolerance (21%). Cardiac manifestations, such as bradycardia, premature ventricular contractions, ventricular fibrillations, and hypotension, have been reported with TCE exposure, possibly attributable to adrenergic and catecholamine sensitivity (Szlatenyi and Wang, 1996).

A possible dose–response relationship between chronic exposure to TCE and motor dyscoordination was reported using a multivariate analysis of data obtained from 99 metal degreasers (Rasmussen et al., 1993). The workers were categorized by their calculated cumulative exposures into three groups: (a) *low* mean full-time exposure (MFTE) for 0.5 years; (b) *medium* MFTE for 2.1 years, and (c) *high* MFTE for 11 years. The current mean urine TCAA level in the high MFTE group members was 7.7 mg/L. However, plant records of urine TCAA levels, which ranged from 40 to 60 mg/L, indicated that the workers in the high MFTE group had previously been exposed to much higher concentrations of TCE. Although these authors suggested a dose–response relationship between clinical neurological signs of dyscoordination, there are several methodological weaknesses in this study including the sample size, identification of which symptomatic workers were exposed to solvents other than TCE, and identification of which workers were included in the currently or recently exposed groups.

Trigeminal nerve involvement with facial hypoesthesia associated with one or more functional manifestations including dizziness, headache, motor weakness, insomnia, and sexual problems was noted among 104 chronically TCE-exposed degreasers, with an average exposure duration of 8.23 years (Barret et al., 1987). Exposure was confirmed by the presence of TCEtOH and TCAA in urine. Eighteen subjects had clinical symptoms of trigeminal neuropathy. Hypoesthesia affected the face bilaterally, and mandibular and maxillary area reflexes were absent. Among these 18 individuals, the corneal reflex was absent in five while nasopalpebral and oculopalpebral reflexes were absent in six. The subjects with trigeminal nerve symptoms were generally older and had longer durations of exposure to TCE than did the asymptomatic workers. Trigeminal sensory evoked potentials (TSEPs) documented the trigeminal neuropathy. A subject with an abnormal TSEP study was three times more likely to show clinical evidence of trigeminal neuropathy than was a subject with normal TSEP (see Neurophysiological Diagnosis section).

Chronic exposure to TCE has also been associated with peripheral neuropathy (Ohtahara et al., 1958; Takeuchi et al., 1986). Takeuchi et al. (1986) reviewed the literature and reported their own case study of a 51-year-old female degreaser with a 12-year history of exposure to TCE. Air samples of TCE at her workplace ranged from 579 to 792 ppm, with peak exposures of up to 2,099 ppm. This patient developed symptoms of peripheral neuropathy including distal paresthesias and muscle weakness in the upper and lower extremities. In addition, she experienced chronic paresthesias around her mouth, headache, fatigue, and memory impairments (Fig. 11-3). The overt signs of peripheral neuropathy seen on the neurological examination of this patient were also documented by electromyography and nerve conduction studies. Bardodej and Vyskocil (1956) also reported exposure-related effects on brachial plexus nerves as well as trigeminal nerve involvement among TCE-exposed workers (see Neurophysiological Diagnosis section).

An initial clinical diagnosis of multiple sclerosis had been made in two patients because of otherwise unexplained neurological findings that were chronic and involved asymmetrical sensory, vestibular, and behavioral changes. However, careful review of the occupational history in each instance revealed sufficient reasons to attribute the problems to chronic exposure to TCE instead of attributing them to multiple sclerosis (Noseworthy and Rice, 1988).

Neurophysiological Diagnosis

Electroencephalography (EEG) has been used to assess the acute and chronic effects of TCE intoxication. Acute ex-

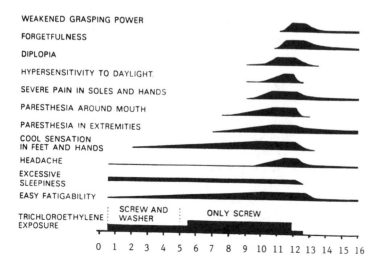

FIG. 11-3. Clinical manifestations in a 51-year-old degreaser during a 12-year exposure to trichloroethylene. The height of the blackened area indicates increased exposure intensity as her job changed from degreasing screws and washers to the degreasing-only screws, but with an increased workload. The increase in exposure appears to relate to an increase in symptoms. (Modified from Takeuchi et al., 1986, with permission.)

posure to TCE produces EEG changes consistent with the anesthetic effects of the solvent (Gevins, 1986). EEG studies in five persons chronically exposed to TCE revealed abnormalities of theta activity. In four of these five individuals, neuropsychological examination revealed memory deficits (Chalupa et al., 1960). There was a significant correlation between the degree of intoxication, EEG findings, and clinical presentations of these patients. Concurrent electrocardiographic monitoring along with EEG recording or independent recording in cases of recent TCE exposure may reveal evidence of cardiac irritability.

The EEG of a 50-year-old woman who developed drowsiness, dizziness, headache, memory disturbances, and bilateral hypoesthesia of the upper extremities after she was occupationally exposed to TCE showed a pattern of diffuse paroxysmal subcontinuous abnormalities (sharp waves) which disappeared upon sensory stimulation (Stracciari et al., 1985). Computed tomography scan at that time was normal. Follow-up neuropsychological examinations of this patient showed a gradual but significant improvement in attention and vigilance performance. However, serial EEG recordings revealed persistent severe paroxysmal abnormalities, suggesting that persistent impairment of cerebral functioning occurs after chronic exposure to TCE.

Visual evoked potentials (VEPs) were studied in human volunteers exposed to 50, 100, and 200 ppm of TCE (Stewart et al., 1974). Exposure to concentrations greater than 100 ppm continuously for 7.5 hours produced an alteration in VEP. Similar changes in second positive peak (P2) of the auditory evoked potential were observed after a 3.5-hour exposure to 50 ppm (Winneke and Kastka, 1974). Blain et al. (1992) assessed VEP in rabbits exposed to 350 and 700 ppm of TCE intermittently over 12 weeks. They reported that chronic exposure modified the VEPs in these animals and that both an increase and a decrease in wave amplitude may indicate a toxic effect. The observed modifications were related to the blood levels of trichloroethanol. N1 and P3 waves appeared most sensitive to chronic exposure. These changes in N1 amplitude can originate from the geniculocortical efferent pathways (Hetzler et al., 1981), while alterations in P3 amplitude may be the result of an inhibitory process in the visual cortex (Seppäläinen et al., 1979).

An individual experienced vertigo, tinnitus, vomiting, left facial numbness, and ataxia of gait while working with TCE in a confined space. On neurological examination 5 years later, the individual presented with tinnitus, hearing loss, horizontal nystagmus, vibratory loss in the toes, lower limb hyperreflexia, and absent abdominal reflexes. The brain-stem auditory evoked potential (BAEP) was absent on the left, and the left VEP latency was prolonged (latency: 130 msec) (Noseworthy and Rice, 1988). In a similar case of a 26-year-old man who was acutely exposed to high concentrations of TCE in a confined space, the 25-year follow-up examination showed normal VEPs (R. G. Feldman, personal observation).

Trigeminal somatosensory evoked potentials (TSEPs) were recorded in 104 TCE-exposed degreasers in a high-exposure workplace (Barret et al., 1987). Normal values used

for comparison in TSEP testing in this study were obtained from 52 healthy unexposed controls. The TSEP was obtained by electrical stimulation of the lip by using a bipolar surface electrode at a stimulation intensity of 70 to 75 V for a duration of 0.05 seconds, 500 times at 2/second. Recordings were made by a subcutaneous needle electrode placed between the vertex of the skull and the external auditory canal. A reference electrode was placed on the earlobe. The wave form obtained was analyzed for threshold of response, latencies of response, morphological changes and amplitude (Barret et al., 1982). Forty (38.4%) workers had abnormal TSEPs, with either increased latencies, modified latencies, or both. Increased response latencies were considered to be the best indication of TCE neurotoxicity, because both the duration of exposure and urine TCEtOH levels were significantly greater among workers with abnormal latencies than among those with normal latencies. In addition, when increased latencies were considered alone, the specificity of this test was estimated to be 79% versus 67% when both latencies and modified amplitude were considered as markers of pathology. Furthermore, the sensitivity of the test was lowered from 67% to 50% when modified amplitudes were considered. Barret et al. (1987) noted that among the asymptomatic workers and those with normal clinical examinations, increased latencies were seen in those who had been exposed to TCE for the longest durations, suggesting that this method can be used to detect the subclinical neurological effects of TCE exposure. Subclinical effects were also documented by this same method in 11 of 33 workers chronically exposed to TCE for a mean duration of 8.3 years (range: 3 to 22 years) (Dogui et al., 1991). The exposure was confirmed in these workers by the concentration of total trichloro compounds (TCEtOH + TCAA) in the urine which ranged from 63.7 to 86.5 mg/g creatinine (see Biochemical Diagnosis section).

A direct and possibly more accurate method of stimulating trigeminal nerve fibers and analyzing the resultant sensory evoked potentials was introduced by Leandri et al. (1985). A bipolar electrode consisting of two fine insulated steel needles with bare tips were inserted into the infraorbital foramen. The recording electrodes, fine uninsulated subcutaneous needles, were placed at the vertex of the skull and on the spinous process of the seventh cervical vertebra. Reference recordings in healthy control subjects indicate that this method of trigeminal nerve stimulation normally elicits a triphasic potential followed by two negative waves designated as W1, W2, and W3, respectively. The W1 wave form corresponds to activation of the maxillary nerve just distal to the gasserian ganglion; the W2 and W3 waves correspond to retrogasserian activation (Fig. 11-4). The TSEP obtained by this method was used to assess a case of trigeminal neuropathy which occurred in a 24-year-old man who had been exposed to high concentrations of TCE and its breakdown products for 15 minutes 1 month earlier. The TSEP showed normal latency, amplitude, and morphology of the W1 components, but the W2 and W3 wave components were absent from the recordings bilaterally (see Fig. 11-4). These findings were considered along with the results of thermal and tactile

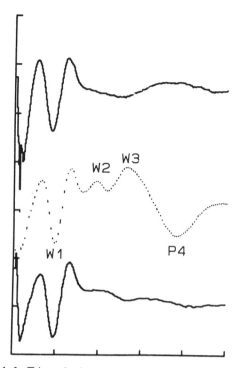

FIG. 11-4. Trigeminal somatosensory evoked potentials detected from the scalp following intraorbital stimulation in a 24-year-old man 1 month after a severe acute exposure to trichloroethylene. (From Leandri et al., 1995, with permission.)

thresholds and information obtained from trigeminal–facial nerve blink reflex studies. The normality of W1 and absent W2 and W3 components was the basis for concluding that conduction was seriously impaired at a site beyond the source of the W1 wave—that is, proximal to the gasserian ganglion. Assuming that the absence of W2 and W3 is not artifactual and that the normality of W1 reflects the intactness of cell bodies within the gasserian ganglion, the probable site of the neurotoxic action of TCE must be the retrogasserian root, if not more centrally located. These electrophysiological findings correspond with the morphological findings of demyelination and neuronal loss in trigeminal nerves (Buxton and Hayward, 1967; Cavanagh and Buxton, 1989) (see Neuropathological Diagnosis section).

Nerve conduction studies (NCS) can be used to assess damage to the trigeminal and peripheral nervous system of persons exposed to TCE. The neurophysiological clinical picture of TCE exposure will vary depending on the extent of nerve damage. NCS of the trigeminal nerve suggest that the myelin component of both large and small fibers is affected during the complete anesthesia of the face that is seen in TCE intoxication. However, when the smaller fibers of the trigeminal nerve are damaged proportionately to its larger fibers, the decrease in nerve conduction velocity of the smaller nerve fibers is greater than that of the larger fibers (Feldman et al., 1970, 1985; Feldman, 1994). A later study by Leandri et al. (1995) using TSEPs, blink reflexes, and tactile perception thresholds also showed dam-

age to medium fast conducting fibers and that small-diameter fibers were affected.

Feldman et al. (1970) documented reduced ulnar and tibial nerve conduction velocity in the distal sensory fibers and depressed reflex responses in the hand muscles of a 26-year-old man acutely exposed to TCE, as well as prolonged motor latency responses in the seventh cranial (facial) nerve. Apparently, TCE had altered the function of peripheral nerves in large and small peripheral nerve fibers. Two weeks after exposure, conduction velocity in the ulnar nerve was reduced in the distal sensory fibers and remained abnormal at 34 weeks, although clinical signs and symptoms of ulnar nerve involvement were absent. The H reflex, which normally cannot be recorded in adult hand muscles, was present in the hypothenar muscles of this individual. The conduction velocity in afferent fibers was less than that in the fastest sensory and motor fibers in the same segment. In addition, there was posttetanic potentiation of the H response but not of the F wave. Latency of the F response was the same as that of the H reflex, and the F wave was normal. Prolongation of conduction latency was recorded in the seventh cranial nerves of this individual. Serial recording of facial nerve evoked motor responses made initially at weekly and then at monthly intervals revealed prolonged latency in the orbicularis oris and orbicularis oculi early in the illness, with latency progressively decreasing over the next 18 months (Fig. 11-5).

Triebig et al. (1982) assessed motor and sensory nerve conduction velocities in the ulnar and median nerves of 24 workers who were exposed to an average of 40 ppm for a mean duration of 7 years (range: <1 to 35 years) and compared them to 24 unexposed age-matched controls without known risks of peripheral neuropathy. No significant differences between the two groups were found in this study. However, variances were large and exposure levels were quite small in this study.

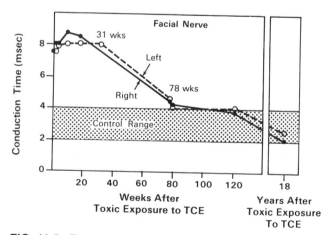

FIG. 11-5. Facial nerve motor latency responses: recovery and follow-up after a single intense accidental exposure to industrial trichloroethylene (TCE) vapors. (From Feldman et al., 1985, with permission.)

Blink reflex [trigeminal (Vth) nerve–brain-stem–facial (VIIth) nerve reflex circuit] studies which were performed 1 month after exposure, in a 24-year-old man who was acutely exposed to high concentrations of TCE for 15 minutes, showed prolonged R_1 latencies which ranged from 16.4 to 18.6 msec (normal range: 8.9 to 11.25 msec) (Leandri et al., 1995). Blink reflex studies documented the residual effects of TCE on the trigeminal nerve in a man who experienced a severe acute exposure to TCE 19 years earlier. Right and left R_1 latencies in this patient were prolonged more than three standard deviations from that of a control group at 12.7 and 14.0 msec, respectively (control mean: 10.4 ± 0.7 msec) (Feldman, 1992). The blink reflexes of 18 individuals exposed to various levels of TCE and other known neurotoxins were recorded and compared with those of 30 unexposed controls (Feldman et al., 1992). Three levels of exposure were arbitrarily defined: *extensive exposure* was used to describe cases where chronic, direct exposure to TCE occurred without proper protective equipment for more than 50% of each day's work time for 5 days per week during at least 1 year or when acute, direct exposure to TCE fumes occurred in a poorly ventilated area for more than 15 minutes; *occasional exposure* was defined as intermittent periods of working with TCE 1 to 3 days per week for less than 50% of the time during at least 1 year; those test subjects with *no exposure* differed from the *nonexposed* control subjects in that their job tasks included histories of exposure to other neurotoxins such as lead, insecticides, and organic solvents other than TCE (Fig. 11-6). The average response for each component of the blink reflex was recorded for each subject. Sub-

jects in the *extensive exposure* group demonstrated R_1 latencies of three standard deviations greater than the controls. None of the subjects from the *occasional exposure* group demonstrated increased R_1 latencies. The delayed R_1 latency in the *extensive exposure* group is consistent with the delays observed with the other pathological conditions of the trigeminal nerves (Gruener et al., 1987; Kiers and Carrol, 1990; Kimura, 1982; Hess et al., 1984).

Less striking but still statistically significant differences from unexposed controls were found in the mean R_1 blink reflex latencies in persons exposed to low levels of TCE in well water (Feldman et al., 1988) (Fig. 11-7). However, only two individuals from this population had R_1 latencies which were reduced more than three standard deviations from the mean. Thus, significant electrophysiological evidence of trigeminal nerve damage using blink reflex studies is more likely to be detected in those individuals intensely exposed to TCE in the industrial setting than in those individuals with low-level environmental exposures, such as that occurring through drinking contaminated water. In such cases, only determination of the group mean deviations may reveal evidence of subclinical effects resulting from exposure to TCE (Feldman et al., 1994).

The effects of TCE exposure on the trigeminal nerve are not always obvious because of lack of effect or technical limitations. In a study in which 31 printing workers with 16 years of low-level exposures (mean cumulative exposure of 704 ppm/year) were compared to 28 controls of similar age (Ruijten et al., 1991), no prolongation of the blink reflex was found. However, this study did show increased latency of the masseter reflex suggesting involvement of the trigeminal pathway. In addition, a slight reduction in sural nerve sensory conduction velocity, along with prolongation of the refractory period, was found in the exposed group, indicating peripheral nerve impairment.

Neuropsychological Diagnosis

Persons suspected of exposure to TCE should be evaluated with a battery of standardized and reliable neuropsychological tests, selected on their previously demonstrated

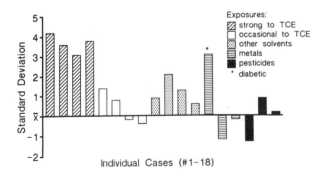

FIG. 11-6. Changes in mean blink reflex latencies according to intensity of industrial trichloroethylene (TCE) exposure. TCE-exposed subjects showed R_1 responses that were 3 × SD of the control group. Three levels of exposure: *extensive exposure,* cases where chronic, direct exposure to TCE occurred without proper protective equipment for more than 50% of each day's work time for 5 days per week during at least 1 year, or when acute, direct exposure to TCE fumes occurred in a poorly ventilated area for more than 15 minutes; *occasional exposure,* intermittent periods of working with TCE 1 to 3 days per week for less than 50% of the time during at least 1 year; *nonexposed,* subjects included those with exposure to other neurotoxicants such as lead, insecticides, and solvents other than TCE; *no exposure,* no neurotoxicant contact. (Modified from Feldman, 1994, with permission.)

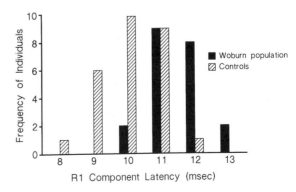

FIG. 11-7. Blink reflex: R_1 component latency means. (From Feldman et al., 1988, with permission.)

ability to assess many cognitive functions including attention, memory, reasoning, visuospatial abilities, psychomotor skills, language, and affect (Baker and White, 1985; White and Proctor, 1992). The cognitive domains most frequently affected by TCE include attention and executive functioning, short-term memory, and visuospatial ability; language and verbal skills are typically spared in adults. Children exposed to TCE may develop persistent impairment of verbal functioning which in turn appear as learning disabilities later in life (White et al., 1992; White, 1995; ATSDR, 1996).

Serial neuropsychological tests and clinical reevaluations are necessary for documenting recovery or persistence of impairments after an exposure has ended. The long-term course of recovery from acute toxic encephalopathy due to a single intense TCE exposure in a 26-year-old man was followed for over 25 years. Initial neuropsychological assessment revealed difficulty with sequential problem-solving and short-term memory deficits. Although daily functioning improved over several years, complete recovery was not seen. The patient reported persistent difficulty in maintaining attention, problems with memory and visuospatial functioning as well as depressed mood, and a sense of apathy. All of these problems interfered with his ability to perform typical activities of daily living and were documented by serial formal neuropsychological testing. At a follow-up examination 16 years after the exposure incident, his performance IQ (PIQ) was 19 points lower than his verbal IQ (VIQ) (Feldman et al., 1985). The discrepancy between the patient's PIQ and VIQ was related to significant visuospatial deficits. The deficits in visuospatial performance in this individual may be related to the prominent atrophy of the occipitoparietal areas seen on his MRI (see Neuroimaging section). Tests of short-term memory showed deficits in both immediate and delayed recall, with specific impairments seen on the Benton Visual Retention Test and on the following Wechsler Memory Scale (WMS) subtests: Logical Memories, Paired Associates, and Visual Reproductions. In addition, the Minnesota Multiphasic Personality Inventory (MMPI) indicated that the patient was also depressed, a finding that agreed with his persistent clinical symptomatology (see Clinical Experiences section).

A 62-year-old machinist chronically exposed to TCE developed profound personality changes after a brief acute exposure (Steinberg, 1981). The individual became psychotic, suffered from urine incontinence and insomnia, and was unable to ambulate or feed himself. A follow-up neuropsychological assessment 5.5 years after the incident showed specific deficits on the Digit Symbol and Object Assembly sections of the Wechsler Adult Intelligence Scale (WAIS), suggesting impairment of psychomotor functioning and visuospatial ability. Furthermore, the patient presented with a number of overt impairments in executive function, lack of insight, and low motivation, all of which were considered to be permanent residual effects of TCE intoxication.

Neuropsychological effects were noted in 50 mechanical engineers with chronic occupational exposure to TCE (Grandjean et al., 1955). Individuals were assessed with regard to attention, memory, comprehension, ideation, and affect. Results of neuropsychological testing showed a general slowing of intellectual processes ($n = 20$), diminution of fixation memory ($n = 19$), difficulty in making associations ($n = 17$), perseveration ($n = 13$), emotional instability ($n = 13$), confabulation ($n = 9$), and decreased motivation ($n = 6$). Furthermore, an increased incidence of fatigue, dizziness, and inability to tolerate alcohol were reported among this group. Neuropsychological symptoms were correlated with duration of exposure and urine levels of TCAA. No neuropsychological deficits were noted in those workers who had been dealing with TCE for only a few months.

Neuropsychological testing documented mild to moderate encephalopathy in 24 of 28 individuals who were chronically exposed to TCE-contaminated drinking and bathing water (Feldman et al., 1994). Impaired cognitive performance was seen on the following tests: WMS-R Visual Reproductions, WMS Logical Memories, Word Triads, and the Benton Visual Retention Test. Significant memory impairments were seen in 24 of 28 cases. Attention and executive function deficits were seen in 19 of 28 persons, while visuospatial deficits and manual motor function deficits were seen in 17 of 28. Language and verbal functioning among the adults was almost always within expectation. However, the neuropsychological evaluations of the children in this group indicated that developmental stage at the time of exposure is related to the type of neurobehavioral deficits seen after exposure (White et al., 1997). Children exposed before age 18 were shown to have deficits in a greater number of neuropsychological domains than individuals exposed as adults. In addition, these children showed a decrease in performance on the Boston Naming Test that was not seen in their parents. These findings suggest that exposure to TCE produces more diffuse damage to the central nervous system (CNS) in children and that children exposed to TCE are more likely to develop learning disabilities.

Biochemical Diagnosis

Measuring blood and urine levels of TCE and its metabolites (trichloroethanol and trichloroacetic acid) is a useful means of monitoring individuals chronically exposed to TCE. The recommended exposure determinant in the blood is free trichloroethanol (TCEtOH). The blood samples should be taken at the end of the work shift on the last day of the workweek, and the concentration of TCEtOH should not exceed 4 mg/L (ACGIH, 1995) (Table 11-4). The *American Conference of Governmental Industrial Hygienists* (ACGIH) does not recommend monitoring blood concentrations of unchanged TCE or trichloroacetic acid (TCAA) (ACGIH, 1995). Nevertheless, these parameters can be used to monitor exposures. Blood TCE levels decreased from 1.3 to 0.2 mg/L within 100 minutes after the end of exposure. Although blood TCE concentrations most accurately reflect the immediate past exposure, blood

TABLE 11-4. *Biological exposure indices for trichloroethylene*

	Urine		Blood	Alveolar air
Determinant:	TCAA	TCAA +TCEtOH	TCEtOH	TCE
Start of shift:	Not established	Not established	Not established	Not established
During shift:	Not established	Not established	Not established	Not established
End of shift at end of workweek:	100 mg/g creatinine	300 mg/g creatinine	4 mg/L	Not established

TCAA, trichloroacetic acid; TCEtOH, trichloroethanol; TCE, trichloroethylene.
Data from ACGIH, 1995.

concentrations of TCE in volunteers exposed to 70 ppm of TCE for 4 hours daily for 5 days were twice as high 18 hours after the fifth day than 18 hours after the first day, reflecting accumulation of the unmetabolized solvent. Furthermore, these findings indicate that TCE which has accumulated in adipose tissue can serve as a continuing internal source of exposure. The blood concentration of TCAA following the initial exposure was 5 mg/L and increased to 31 mg/L following the fifth exposure, indicating that blood TCAA concentrations more accurately reflect chronic exposures than immediate past exposures (Monster et al., 1979) (Fig. 11-8). The half-life of TCAA in blood is greater than that of trichloroethanol and TCE, because TCAA binds to plasma proteins and accumulates.

The relationship between TCE exposure dose and urinary excretion of TCAA is linear only up to 50 ppm, a finding which reflects the binding of TCAA to plasma proteins. For example, the majority of trichloroethanol derived from metabolism of a given dose of TCE is excreted during the first 24 hours after exposure, while quantities of TCAA excreted in occupationally exposed persons are higher by the end of a workweek than during the first day of contact with TCE (Müller et al., 1974; Monster et al., 1979; Inoue et al., 1989). Thus, with ongoing exposure, the concentration of TCAA excreted in urine is less reflective of the latest TCE exposure dose (Ikeda et al., 1972; Müller et al., 1974). In

volunteers exposed to TCE at a concentration of 70 ppm for 4 hours per day, the amount of TCAA excreted in urine increased over a 5-day period from an average of 10 mg per 24 hours on the first day to 82 mg per 24 hours on the fifth day, followed by a prolonged period of elimination up to 12 days (Monster et al., 1979) (Fig. 11-9). The World Health Organization (WHO) recommends that the average urinary concentration of TCAA not exceed 50 mg/L (WHO, 1981) (see Symptomatic Diagnosis and Clinical Experiences sections). The ACGIH BEI for TCAA in urine is an end-of-workweek concentration of 100 mg/g creatinine which corresponds with an average daily exposure to an 8-hour TWA ambient air TCE vapor concentration of 50 ppm. ACGIH recommends that the end-of-workweek urinary concentration of TCAA plus trichloroethanol not exceed 300 mg/g creatinine (280 mg/L) (ACGIH, 1995) (see Table 11-4).

Measuring urinary concentrations of total trichloro compounds (TCEtOH + TCAA) may be used as an alternative method of monitoring exposure (Tanaka and Ikeda, 1968; Nomiyama and Nomiyama, 1977). However, because TCEtOH reflects recent exposure and TCAA reflects cumulative exposure, this measure may provide the clinician with less information than monitoring urinary TCEtOH or TCAA alone (Monster et al., 1979).

Several studies have demonstrated the affinity of TCE for fat, based on its presence in adipose tissue even after

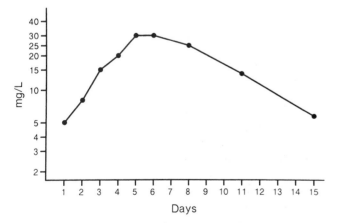

FIG. 11-8. Mean (*n* = 5) blood levels of trichloroacetic acid following exposure to 70 ppm trichloroethylene 4 hours per day for 5 days. (Modified from Monster et al., 1979, with permission.)

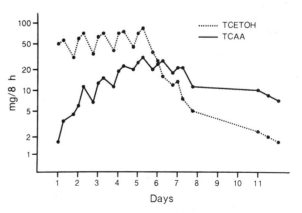

FIG. 11-9. Mean (*n* = 5) urine levels of trichloroethanol (TCETOH) and trichloroacetic (TCAA) acid per 8 hours, following exposure to 70 ppm trichloroethylene 4 hours per day for 5 days. (Modified from Monster et al., 1979, with permission.)

cessation of exposure (Savolainen et al., 1977; Bergman, 1983; Cohr, 1986). Although fat biopsy may be a way to detect stored evidence of past exposure to lipophilic organic solvents, it is an invasive procedure that is not generally considered a reliable quantitative biological indicator of body burden (Anderson, 1985).

Neuroimaging

Magnetic resonance imaging (MRI) and *computerized tomography* (CT) can be used to differentiate TCE encephalopathy from other causes of cognitive dysfunction such as Alzheimer's disease, normal pressure hydrocephalus, or multiple infarct cerebrovascular disease. The MRI at 23-year follow-up examination of a man who developed cranial and peripheral neuropathy and encephalopathy after acute intense exposure to TCE showed prominent bilateral cortical atrophy and mild vermian atrophy. The brain stem and ventricular system of this patient showed no abnormalities (R. G. Feldman, personal observation) (Fig. 11-10). The CT scan and MRI revealed no abnormalities in a technician who experienced numbness of the left side of the face for 3 weeks and permanent numbness of the dorsum of the left foot following acute exposure to TCE vapor (Noseworthy and Rice, 1988). In this case the MRI was very important because the differential diagnosis had included multiple sclerosis. Similarly, the CT scan of a 35-year-old man who developed trigeminal neuropathy after he intentionally inhaled TCE for 3 days did not reveal any abnormalities (Szlatenyi and Wang, 1996).

Neuropathological Diagnosis

The lipid-solubility of TCE allows its access to structures of the central and peripheral nervous systems, where it produces acute effects such as narcosis and irreversible effects such as demyelination and cell death. While controversy still remains concerning the specific mechanisms of TCE neurotoxicity, sufficient data in human beings and experimental animals exist to conclude that TCE produces significant morphological changes to the central and peripheral nervous systems (Barceloux, 1992; Feldman, 1994; Leandri et al., 1995). Autopsy findings in a 39-year-old man after a fatal exposure to TCE showed marked damage in the brain stem, the fifth nerve nuclei, the spinal tract, and the nerve roots. The fifth nerves had extensive demyelination and axonal degeneration. Pyknotic neurons were visible in the lateral and superior vestibular nuclei, superior olivary nuclei, and nucleus gigantocellularis. Neuronal loss was seen in the reticular formation and in the vagal, hypoglossal, and solitary nuclei. The most significant pathology was seen in the sensory trigeminal neurons, followed, in order of damage, by the facial, oculomotor, motor trigeminal, and acoustic neurons (Buxton and Hayward, 1967; Cavanagh and Buxton, 1989). Similar alterations in the myelin and axons of the trigeminal nerve have been produced experimentally by TCE and its

breakdown product, dichloroacetylene (DCA) (Barret et al., 1991; Reichert et al., 1976). Baker (1958) described damage to the Purkinje cell layer of the cerebellum, and he reported pyknotic changes with multifocal myelin swelling in the cerebral hemispheres of dogs exposed to 3,000 ppm of TCE for 60 hours. The myelin sheath of CNS neurons is a major target of TCE/DCA neurotoxicity (Barret et al., 1991, 1992; Haglid et al., 1980; Kyrklund et al., 1983, 1984), and its breakdown is apparently mediated by peroxidation of cell membrane lipids (Cojocel et al., 1989; Barret et al., 1991).

The basis of TCE-induced trigeminal neuropathy remains uncertain but is probably not entirely due to a direct neurotoxic effect of the parent compound (Gonthier and Barret, 1989; Barret et al., 1991). Vascular permeability in the trigeminal nerve nucleus has been suggested as the basis for the relative selectivity of TCE (Jacobs, 1978). Metabolic disturbances and activation of a latent viral infection have been suggested as mechanisms of toxicity (Cavanagh and Buxton, 1989). Exposure to the TCE breakdown product, DCA, is considered by several authors to be the main cause of the neurotoxic effects of TCE exposure (Siegel et al., 1971; Henschler et al., 1970; Reichert et al., 1976; Defalque, 1961). Barret et al. (1992) demonstrated that both TCE and DCA modify the lipid content of the trigeminal nerve, and they suggested that lipid peroxidation may be responsible for changes in the nerve membrane following exposure to either chemical. Studies indicate that the asymmetrical molecular conformation of TCE leads to the formation of chemically reactive metabolites and free radicals (Miller and Guengerich, 1982; Gonthier and Barret, 1989; Cojocel et al., 1989; Bruckner et al., 1989). The electrophilic metabolic intermediate TCE epoxide has been shown to irreversibly bind to cellular macromolecules and may be a potential toxic compound (Allemand et al., 1978; Bruckner et al., 1989). Electrophilic compounds have been shown to alter protein transport in neurons and to fragment DNA (Corcoran et al., 1994; Graham et al., 1995). Using electron spin resonance spectroscopy, Gonthier and Barret (1989) showed that liver and brain microsomes, which promote the enzymatic oxidation of the TCE metabolite, trichloroethanol, simultaneously produce free radicals; this may be responsible for at least some of the neurotoxic effects induced by TCE. Free radicals can induce lipid peroxidation, bind to cellular macromolecules, and fragment DNA (Cojocel et al., 1989; Halliwell, 1989; Bruckner et al., 1989; Gonthier and Barret, 1989; Bondy, 1992; Barret et al., 1992). Evidence of such effects has been obtained using nuclear magnetic resonance spectroscopy (Bhakuni and Roy, 1994).

Barret et al. (1991) demonstrated that both TCE and DCA can alter internal and external axonal diameters as well as myelin thickness in the mental branch of the trigeminal nerve, indicating that each chemical produces neurotoxic effects in the trigeminal nerve. The results of this study also showed that the myelin thickness in the largest myelinated fibers had significantly decreased in the group exposed to DCA and to a lesser extent in the TCE

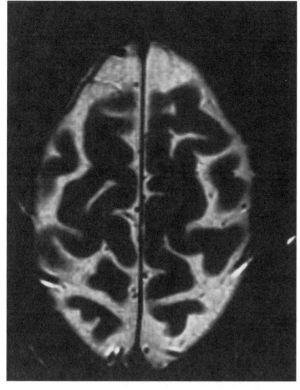

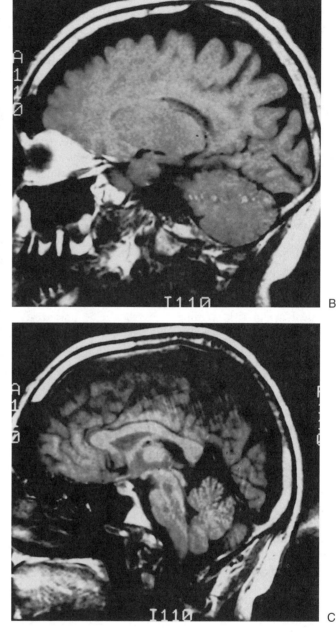

FIG. 11-10. Magnetic resonance image of a 49-year-old man 23 years after a single intense accidental exposure to industrial trichloroethylene vapors (Feldman and Lessell, 1969; Feldman et al., 1985). **A:** T2-weighted axial image showing prominent cortical sulci bilaterally. **B:** T1-weighted sagittal image showing diffuse severe atrophy, with marked atrophy in parietal and occipital cortices. **C:** T1-weighted sagittal image showing cerebellar vermis atrophy.

group; the myelin thickness in the smallest fibers in both groups had increased. Why this difference in effect should depend upon the size of the peripheral nerve fibers is unclear, but the variability seen in the effects of TCE on various brain myelin areas is similar (Haglid et al., 1980; Kyrklund, et al., 1983; Kyrklund et al., 1984).

The fatty acid composition of the total lipid extract of the trigeminal nerve of TCE- and DCA-treated rats as compared to controls showed altered proportions of some fatty acids (Barret et al., 1992). In the TCE-exposed groups, the fatty acids of the linoleate series were 46% lower ($p < 0.05$), while the fatty acids of the linolenate series showed only a tendency toward decrease (-22%). A fall in polyunsaturated fatty acids (PUFAs) of the linoleate series in the nerve total lipid extract accounted for an increase ($+40\%$)

in the linolenate/linoleate ratio. The effects of chronic DCA exposure on total lipid extract, however, were strikingly different. The pattern here was reversed, with a statistically significant ($p < 0.05$) decrease (-27%) in linolenate series fatty acids, with the only exception to this pattern seen in docosahexanoic acid. The level of total fatty acids was insignificantly lower (-32%), while the linolenate/linoleate ratio went unchanged.

In contrast to the trigeminal nerve preparations, TCE and DCA appear to have less effect on brain PUFAs, but the effect of chronic DCA exposure on total brain lipid fatty acid composition seems less in comparison to that of TCE exposure. These changes are compatible with demyelination, perhaps mediated by free-radical-induced lipid peroxidation.

Soluble protein content was significantly reduced in the hippocampus, posterior cerebellar vermis, and brain stem of gerbils exposed to TCE (Haglid et al., 1980). Bundles of neurofilaments were also noted in axons (Haglid et al., 1981), suggesting dysruption of axonal transport. Damage to the oligodendrogliocytes in the hippocampus has been shown to affect transmission of incoming impulses from the entorhinal cortex and to alter the synaptology of these cortical neurons making contact with the CA1 dendrites (Isaacson et al., 1990). Additional work is needed in this area to elucidate the possible relationship between the morphological changes seen in the hippocampus of these animals and the memory problems encountered in humans who have been exposed to TCE.

PREVENTIVE AND THERAPEUTIC MEASURES

Workplaces where TCE is used should be well-ventilated. The potential for neurotoxic effects resulting from exposure to TCE and its breakdown product DCA should be explained to all employees at the time of hiring. Occupational health risk warning signs should be posted at worksites where TCE is used. Bottles and other storage containers should have warning labels. Respirators should be available for those workers at risk of exposure to high concentrations of TCE vapor. Routine biological monitoring and neurological examination of workers at risk of exposure is essential in the prevention of injuries resulting from the acute narcotic effects of TCE and in the prevention of the development of chronic neurological manifestations (Vesterberg et al., 1976). Degreaser vats should be equipped with cooler cuffs (Sagawa et al., 1973; Feldman, 1994). Trichloroethylene which has spilled or leaked into the environment should not be heated or exposed to any alkali products because under these conditions TCE may break down to DCA, possibly potentiating the risk of neurotoxic effects (Greim et al., 1984).

Routine monitoring of drinking water supplies by town engineers is essential in the prevention of nonoccupational exposures. Drinking water wells found to be contaminated with TCE should be shut down and a safe water supply should be provided until the source of TCE contamination is identified and the condition is rectified. In addition, to prevent exposure to TCE vapors as well as dermal absorption the contaminated water should not be used for cooking or bathing (McKone and Knezovich, 1991). Detoxification of TCE-contaminated sites and drinking water sources may be necessary (Freedman and Gassett, 1989; McCarty and Wilson, 1992).

The first step in treating TCE intoxication is to recognize the condition and remove individuals from risk of further exposure. Since inhalation of vapors is the most likely route of intake, displacing the TCE-contaminated air in the lungs is essential in emergency care (Perbellini et al., 1991). Immediate measures include providing a vapor-free source of air and an oxygen tank while encouraging energetic deep breathing. Absorption from the gastrointestinal tract is slower than from the lungs; however, when liquid TCE has been swallowed, stomach gavage should be done

to empty it of the TCE-containing contents as soon as possible. Syrup of ipecac can be used in cases of poison ingestion, but the risk of further inhalation of TCE vapors from the oropharynx or by aspiration of vomitus containing TCE makes controlled stomach gavage a safer method of eliminating residual ingested TCE. In addition, appropriate general supportive measures as well as specific interventions may be needed for cardiac arrhythmia, pulmonary edema, and vasomotor instability in susceptible persons (Musclow and Awen, 1971; White and Carlson, 1981; King et al., 1985). Hemodialysis and blood transfusion for acute renal failure, myopathy, and hepatic involvement may be necessary (Olivares-Esquer et al., 1974; Sasdelli et al., 1986).

Recovery from acute intoxication depends upon the intensity and duration of the exposure. For example, acute encephalopathy related to the narcotic effects of TCE and its metabolites generally subside within hours to days following cessation of exposure (Feldman and Lessell, 1969; Buxton and Hayward, 1967; Martinelli et al., 1984; Szlatenyi and Wang, 1996). Long-term follow-up after a single severe toxic exposure revealed persistence of impairment in neuropsychological performance and emotional disturbances (Feldman et al., 1985; White et al., 1992). Chronic exposure may be accompanied by the gradual appearance of clinical indicators of neurotoxicity. In particular, when the ongoing body burden accumulates over time, symptoms may arise at times of peak reexposure or when tolerance to the burden is surpassed. For example, covert toxicological effects may be unmasked when alcohol, stress, or age interact singularly or in combination with each other and with trichloroethylene (Kjellstrand et al., 1980). In addition to acute neurological manifestations, cardiac dysrhythmias may occur in persons who have also taken or received adrenergic stimulating drugs such as epinephrine, amphetamines, and cocaine (White and Carlson, 1981; Szlatenyi and Wang, 1996). The risk of the patient developing cardiac arrhythmia may also be increased by conditions which inhibit metabolism of TCE such as hepatic failure (White and Carlson, 1981). Sensitization to TCE or its metabolites develops after exposure in some individuals, so that reexposure at a later time may result in symptoms at a lower concentration or duration of exposure. Low-grade fever, liver enzyme elevations, exfoliative dermatitis, and eosinophilia were observed in severe cases considered to have experienced delayed hypersensitivity to TCE, and to its metabolite trichloroethanol in particular. The use of skin tests for identifying these persons has been proposed (Bond, 1996).

Prognosis of patients with chronic TCE encephalopathy varies according to time of follow-up and type of neurological tests performed. For example, our long-term follow-up study of a worker's single toxic exposure to TCE revealed persistence of impairment of cognitive functioning as demonstrated by neuropsychological test performance (Feldman et al., 1985). Furthermore, this patient's neurobehavioral deficits actually interfered with his ability to perform multiple tasks and to concentrate on his job. In addition, the patient reported annoying residual paresthesia and myokymia following cranial and peripheral neuropathy. Lindstrom et al. (1982) studied the psychological prognosis of persons diagnosed with chronic TCE-exposure-associated organic encephalopathy and concluded that the overall prognosis of psychological test results was better with a longer follow-up period and in persons of younger age. Patients who had also used CNS-active drugs had a poorer overall psychological prognosis. Nevertheless, some improved in certain aspects and others remained unchanged or even deteriorated. This was further illustrated when Antti-Poika (1982) studied the prognosis of patients diagnosed 3 to 9 years earlier with chronic organic solvent intoxication. There were three groups of patients: those who got better, those who remained unchanged, and those who worsened. Antti-Poika concluded that there was no statistically significant correlation between the overall prognosis and age, sex, the duration and level of exposure, the termination of exposure after diagnosis, the presence of other diseases, or the use of alcohol. Effective management nevertheless requires that an individual suspected of TCE exposure be removed from further exposure to TCE, refrain from alcohol intake, and avoid future exposure to various volatile organic solvents. Once established, many of the effects of TCE exposure on the CNS are irreversible (Kjellstrand et al., 1980; Feldman et al., 1985; Feldman, 1994). The long-term affective disorders following toxic encephalopathies are particularly difficult to treat and adversely affect the patient's recovery and prognosis (Gregersen et al., 1984). To compensate for permanent impairments of behavior and cognitive functioning, treatment must include individualized recommendations for maintaining the patient's vocational and financial security. For example, a patient with a previously highly demanding and well-compensated job will require a vocational change and retraining to accommodate postexposure intellectual capabilities and to preserve his or her financial security (White et al., 1992).

CLINICAL EXPERIENCES

Group Studies

TCE in Drinking Water

Adverse health effects of TCE in drinking water have been reported by several communities (Ziglio et al., 1983; Logue et al., 1985; Lagakos et al., 1986; Landrigan et al., 1987; Bernad et al., 1987; Feldman et al., 1988, 1994; Barton et al., 1996; ATSDR, 1996). Various nonspecific complaints were found among the several cohorts, but common to them all were fatigue, dizziness, headache, mood changes, poor concentration, and memory disturbances (Burg et al., 1995; ATSDR, 1996). Low levels of exposure to TCE can produce changes in behavior that may be experienced by the exposed individual before any overt manifestation can be objectively documented by neurophysiological and neuropsychological testing. Several examples are summarized below.

Case 1. The residents of a neighborhood in the city of Woburn, Massachusetts were exposed to TCE when chemical waste contaminated their drinking water from 1964 to 1979. Drinking water was supplied to the city by eight municipal wells, two of which, designated as wells G and H, were found at initial testing to be contaminated with TCE at a concentration of 267 ppb, tetrachloroethylene at 21 ppb, chloroform at 12 ppb, dichloroethylene at 28 ppb, and trichlorotrifluoroethane at 23 ppb. Subsequent to testing, the wells were closed. The mean concentration of TCE in well G over a 2-year period after its closing was 256 ppb, with a maximum contamination level of 400 ppb; the mean concentration for well H was 111 ppb, with a maximum contamination of 188 ppb.

Many of the residents began to notice subjective symptoms of exposure including headache, dizziness, fatigue, irritability, insomnia, memory and concentration impairment, and paresthesias. Of the residents who shared the water source, 28 members of eight families were examined in detail (Feldman et al., 1994). Trichloroethylene concentrations in the well water supplied to the homes of these individuals ranged from 63 ppb to 400 ppb. Routine neurological examinations revealed tendon reflex abnormalities in 26 of the 28 patients, and there were sensory impairments in four of the 28 patients. Nerve conduction studies documented abnormalities in proximal motor amplitude, distal sensory amplitude, and distal motor and sensory latency, along with a significantly ($p < 0.0001$) prolonged R_1 component of the blink reflex (see Neurophysiological Diagnosis section). Neuropsychological tests revealed significant memory deficits in 24 of the 27 individuals tested. In addition, significant deficits were observed on tests of attention and executive function, visuospatial ability, and manual motor function. Twenty-four persons were diagnosed as having mild to moderate encephalopathy (see Neuropsychological Diagnosis section).

Case 2. From 1951 until 1981, a company manufacturing precision-formed tubular assemblies in Alpha, Ohio allowed an average of 50,000 gallons of waste water per day to flow into a surface drainage ditch, which then discharged its contents into Beaver Creek (Feldman, 1994). In 1986, a ground-water investigation found 13 area wells contaminated with 1,1,1-trichloroethane (up to 2,569 ppb) and TCE (up to 760 ppb). Twelve individuals with exposure levels ranging from 3.3 to 330 ppb were assessed. Subjective symptoms included headache, impaired concentration and memory, insomnia, and paresthesias. Neurological examinations showed signs of peripheral nerve involvement including sensory impairment in the extremities, facial numbness, and reflex abnormalities. Nerve conduction studies documented peripheral neuropathy in these patients. Neuropsychological performance deficits were found on tests of attention/executive function in 10 patients. Neuropsychological tests revealing decreases in cognitive functioning included the Wisconsin Card Sorting Test, Digit Spans, and Visual Spans. Tests of memory—in particular, Word Triads and Figural Memory—revealed impaired functioning in seven of the residents. Three individuals showed manual motor slowing on the Digit Symbol test, and two showed impairment on visuospatial tasks. Eight were diagnosed with mild to moderate encephalopathy (Feldman et al., 1994).

Case 3. Private wells used for drinking and bathing water and located near an army ammunition plant in Minnesota had TCE concentrations of 261 to 2,440 ppb. Subjective symptoms among the 14 exposed residents assessed included headache, fatigue, insomnia, concentration and memory impairment, depression, irritability, and paresthesia. Neurological signs included facial numbness and reflex abnormalities. Neurophysiological testing and formal neuropsychological assessment was performed on six of the 14 persons. These subjects included two adults and four children, all of whom had been exposed to TCE in water from their private well. Nerve conduction studies documented peripheral neuropathy in five patients. All six members of the family had memory function impairments, with performance on the Word Triad test the most significantly affected. The Digit Span and Wisconsin Card Sorting tests showed deficits in attention/executive function. Four individuals showed manual motor slowing as evidenced by difficulties with the Digital Symbol test. All four children performed below expectation on tests of language and verbal skills, and three of the children had difficulty with the Boston Naming Test. A diagnosis of TCE-induced encephalopathy was made in all six cases.

Individual Case Studies

Acute Intense Exposure: Immediate and Long-Term Effects

While working as a substitute manager in his father's absence, an inexperienced 26-year-old man attempted to repair a broken degreasing machine in a carburetor reconditioning shop during an emergency (Feldman et al., 1970). Ignorant of the risks and the precautions that should be taken when working with TCE, he wore no protective clothing and no respirator mask. He entered the room where the degreasing machine was located and began to make repairs but within 5 minutes he was overcome by the noxious vapors. Feeling lightheaded and dizzy, he left the room and donned an ill-fitting gas mask containing a potassium superoxide canister without a fresh-air supply. Wearing the mask, he returned to the room to work on the degreaser. After 1.5 hours in the room, he became lightheaded, confused, and stuporous. He was taken to the hospital, where he was described as somnolent, apathetic, and having difficulty following commands.

Over the first 10 to 12 hours after this person's removal from the exposure, additional symptoms appeared. These included nausea, vomiting, blurred vision, and numbness of the face, oral cavity, and pharynx. Articulation and chewing were difficult because of facial and jaw muscle weakness. During the first 60 hours after his admission to the hospital, the patient's neurological examinations showed weakness of facial muscles with an inability to crease his brow or deepen his nasolabial folds. In addition, he had anesthesia to pinprick over the entire trigeminal nerve distribution. He had difficulty concentrating on the tasks at hand and could not follow multiple-step commands. He was lethargic, and his speech was slow and labored. These clinical features gradually began to clear over the next 2 to 3 weeks.

Serial nerve conduction studies revealed delayed facial nerve latencies as well as slowed peripheral nerve conduction velocity. Facial nerve latency conduction improved and muscle function returned and was normal after 120 weeks. Neurophysiological studies demonstrated persistently delayed direct (R_1) blink reflexes, but visual evoked potentials were normal (Feldman et al., 1992). Facial muscle cramping recurred with cold weather or fatigue (Feldman, 1979) and remained as a permanent residual effect of the exposure (Feldman et al., 1985). In 12-, 16-, and 18-year follow-up neuropsychological examinations, the patient continued to exhibit impaired attention and short-term memory, as well as diminished visuospatial organization and sequencing abilities. These chronic findings are similar to those reported by Gregersen et al. (1984). The patient has also exhibited affective symptoms of chronic depression throughout the course of more than 25 years. He is disturbed by his inability to perform multiple tasks concurrently and to handle multiple-person conversations with his former adeptness; he becomes confused with too much concurrent input. Despite occasions of unexplainable depression, his affect is considerably improved over all these years. However, he has continued to experience chronic and recurrent episodes of dizziness and a sense of unsteadiness ever since his accident. In addition, he has continued to have distal as well as facial paresthesias, malar hypalgesia, and facial myokymia.

Although actual workplace air sampling for TCE was not done in this case, its description illustrates the effects of a single, intense, acute exposure to industrial TCE used as a degreaser under heated, poorly ventilated, and unprotected conditions. The patient developed encephalopathic, cranial, and peripheral neuropathic symptoms. The selective neurotoxic effects of TCE on the fifth and seventh cranial nerves observed in this patient, and as previously described by Buxton and Hayward (1967), have subsequently been reported by others (Barret et al., 1982, 1987; Perbellini et al., 1991; Leandri et al., 1995; Szlatenyi and Wang, 1996).

Acute Reexposures and the Development of Recurrent and Reversible TCE Encephalopathy

A 25-year-old man experienced dizziness and lightheadedness while at work (McCunney, 1988). On his way home, with his driving skill impaired, he had an automobile accident. In retrospect, he recalled that he had been having "blue flashes" and impaired memory at work for 2 weeks before the automobile accident. He reported experiencing blurred vision and lightheadedness while he was using TCE to clean a steel bar. His coworkers also commented that he was behaving in an unusual manner.

Upon initial presentation, the patient's carboxyhemoglobin level was normal, eliminating the possibility of carbon monoxide as a source of his symptoms. A 24-hour urine collection taken on the day of the symptoms revealed the presence of trichloroacetic acid, but he returned to his job because an air-level test reported a TCE level of less than 25 ppm which is considered "safe." Trichloroacetic acid concentration in the patient's urine measured after an additional 3 weeks on the job was 210 mg/L. He complained of a dazed, numb feeling in his head and exhibited severe anxiety. Examination revealed tremor, profound imbalance, and lack of coordination. His urine level of TCAA was 194 mg/L on that day. The World Health Organization (WHO) recommends that the average urinary concentration of TCAA not exceed 50 mg/L (WHO, 1981). As a result, he was removed from the job for several weeks.

When an air analysis of the atmosphere around the degreaser revealed TCE levels of 10, 7, and 12 ppm and his urine TCAA level had decreased to 15 mg/L, the worker was advised that he could return to work provided that he avoid submerging his hands in the degreasing tank. Once back on the job, however, he began to have symptoms of irritability, he "felt like punching something," and he had a sense that he might lose control. Sensation to pinprick was reduced over his face and on the dorsum of his hands. Tendon reflexes were hypoactive. Neuropsychological tests showed moderate cognitive impairments. He was again removed from the job. Results of a follow-up examination 6 weeks later showed that the patient had improved in mood and memory, no longer had a "spacey" feeling, and no longer had visual flashes. He was transferred to another area of the plant where he would have no further direct or indirect exposure to TCE.

Symptoms of inebriation were present both while this man worked with TCE and after he left the workplace. It is possible that impaired ability to operate his automobile led to the accident and that the mood changes observed by others were signs of mild to moderate toxic encephalopathy. The presence of TCAA in the urine coincided with the clinical symptoms that occurred while he was on the job being exposed to TCE.

This case demonstrates that removal from exposure may be accompanied by clinical improvement but that returning to work and reexposure to TCE is promptly followed by a return of symptoms, and that this may also occur at exposure levels which are lower than were previously encountered or were necessary to initiate the symptoms. Furthermore, these findings demonstrate that although tests of air concentration of TCE may fall within safety limits, an exposed person's body burden as reflected by biological exposure indices, as well as his or her subjective symptoms and clinical manifestations, must be considered to determine the individual's tolerable level of exposure and the need for exposure prevention.

Degreasers Chronically Exposed to TCE

Case 1. A 51-year-old man worked with TCE, degreasing finished electronic parts daily for 16.5 years (Feldman, 1994). While on the job, he experienced occasional symptoms of exhilaration, lightheadedness, decreased concentration, and memory problems. These feelings diminished on weekends and during vacations, and their severity varied with the degreasing workload. He also noted that he would have a "flush" in his face when he occasionally drank a beer after work.

Neurological examination performed while he remained on the job showed reduced sensation to pain, temperature, and vibration in the extremities. Mild decrease in malar sensitivity was detected when his face was touched with a cotton wisp or a pin. Tendon reflexes were reduced in the knees and ankles bilaterally. Neurophysiological testing showed that sensory and motor conduction latencies and velocities were consistent with a generalized peripheral neuropathy. The electrically induced (R_1) blink reflex latency response was prolonged, confirming impairment of trigeminal nerve function. A metabolite of TCE, trichloroacetic acid (TCAA), was found (356 mg/L) in a urine sample taken while the patient was on the job; serum at that time contained 18.9 mg/mL of trichloroethanol. Gas chromatographic and spectroscopic analysis of a gluteal fat biopsy revealed concentrations of 0.7 ppm TCE and 35 ppm 1,1,2-trichloroethane, respectively.

Symptoms of acute intoxication, such as exhilaration, dizziness, headache, and confusion, occurred while this man inhaled TCE vapors on his job. In addition, he experienced the vasomotor effect of facial flushing as a result of the interaction of alcohol with TCE metabolites. Ongoing exposure was indicated by the urine TCAA and serum trichloroethanol. Accumulation of the effects of TCE and its metabolites over the 16.5-year work history of exposure resulted in the neuropathy and encephalopathy.

Case 2. A 60-year-old degreaser cleaned various articles in an open tank containing TCE, for a short period several times each week over 15 years (Feldman, 1994). In this case, the tank was equipped with a cooling mechanism around its rim to reduce vaporization of the TCE. Over the duration of his employment, this individual occasionally complained of headaches, dizziness, and lethargy. For the 2 to 3 years prior to evaluation, he noted mood changes and gradual loss of sensation in the extremities. He became more depressed and had difficulties in comprehension and concentration.

A neurological exam confirmed findings of peripheral neuropathy, with decreased perception of pinprick and vibration sensation in the distal portions of the legs and in the fingers. Neurophysiological studies demonstrated slowing in nerve conduction velocity, and the electrophysiological measure of the blink reflex showed prolonged R_1 latency time. The most notable neuropsychological test results included difficulties in psychomotor speed, visuospatial organization, mental control, sequencing, storage of information, and cognitive flexibility. Diabetes, nutritional deficiency, and other potential sources of neurotoxicity were excluded, and the man's condition was attributed to the TCE known to be present in his workplace and used in his job.

Air sampling for TCE content was not available at the workplace, nor had blood or urine tests of TCE been done, but a fat biopsy performed 1 year after termination of employment indicated the presence of 0.28 ppm TCE and 0.56 ppm methylene chloride. The significance of these findings remains uncertain but raises the question of whether the TCE found in the fat of this patient was the result of long-term storage of TCE from his previous exposures or reflected more recent nonoccupational exposures. Although several studies have demonstrated the presence of TCE in adipose tissue after cessation of exposure (Savolainen et al., 1977; Bergman, 1983; Cohr, 1986), fat biopsies should not be used as a biological marker of body burden until further carefully controlled studies have been performed to establish relationships between previous exposure dose and individual body burden (Anderson, 1985).

REFERENCES

Agency for Toxic Substances and Disease Registry (ATSDR). *Toxicological profile for trichloroethylene.* Atlanta: US Department of Health and Human Services, Public Health Service, GA, 1993.

Agency for Toxic Substances and Disease Registry (ATSDR). *National exposure registry, trichloroethylene (TCE) subregistry followup 1 technical report.* Atlanta, GA: US Department of Health and Human Services, 1996.

Allemand H, Pessayre D, Descatoire V, Degott C, Feldmann G, Benhamou J-P. Metabolic activation of trichloroethylene into a chemically reactive metabolite toxic to the liver. *J Pharmacol Exp Ther* 1978;204:714–723.

American Conference of Governmental Industrial Hygienists (ACGIH). *Documentation of the threshold limit values and biological exposure indices,* 5th ed. Cincinnati: ACGIH, 1989:595–597.

American Conference of Governmental Industrial Hygienists (ACGIH). *Threshold Limit Values (TLVs) for chemical substances and physical agents and biological exposure indices (BEIs).* Cincinnati: ACGIH, 1995.

Amoore JE, Hautala E. Odor as an aid to chemical safety: odor thresholds compared with threshold limit values and volatilities for 214 industrial chemicals in air and water dilution. *J Appl Toxicol* 1983;3:272–290.

Anderson HA. Utilization of adipose tissue biopsy in characterizing human halogenated hydrocarbon exposure. *Environ Health Perspect* 1985;60:127–131.

Anger WK, Johnson BL. Chemicals affecting behavior. In: O'Donoghue JL, ed. *Neurotoxicity of industrial and commercial chemicals,* vol 1. Boca Raton, FL: CRC Press, 1985:51–148.

Antti-Poika M. Overall prognosis of patients with diagnosed chronic organic solvent intoxication. *Int Arch Occup Environ Health* 1982;51:27–138.

Arlien-Søborg P. *Solvent neurotoxicity.* Boca Raton, FL: CRC Press, 1992:259–289.

Åstrand I. Uptake of solvents in the blood and tissues of man. *Scand J Work Environ Health* 1975;1:199–218.

Baker AB. The nervous system in trichloroethylene intoxication: an experimental study. *J Neuropathol Exp Neurol* 1958;17:649–655.

Baker EL, White RF. The use of neuropsychological testing in the evaluation of neurotoxic effects of organic solvents. In: *Chronic effects of organic solvents on the central nervous system and diagnosis criteria: report on Joint WHO/Nordic Council of Ministers Working Group.* Copenhagen: WHO, 1985:224.

Barceloux DG. Metabolism of trichloroethylene. In: Sullivan JB Jr, Krieger GR, eds. *Hazardous materials toxicology: clinical principles of environmental health,* vol 64. Baltimore: Williams & Wilkins, 1992:739.

Bardodej Z, Vyskocil J. The problem of trichloroethylene in occupational medicine. *AMA Arch Ind Health* 1956;13:581–592.

Barret L, Arsac P, Vincent M, Faure J, Garrel S, Reymond F. Evoked trigeminal nerve potential in chronic trichloroethylene intoxication. *J Toxicol Clin Toxicol* 1982;19:419–423.

Barret L, Garrel S, Daniel V, Debru JL. Chronic trichloroethylene intoxication: a new approach by trigeminal evoked potentials? *Arch Environ Health* 1987;42:297–302.

Barret L, Torch S, Usson Y, Gonthier B, Saxod R. A morphometric evaluation of the effects of trichloroethylene and diachloroacetylene on the rat mental nerve. Preliminary results. *Neurosci Lett* 1991;131:141–144.

Barret L, Torch S, Leray C, Sarlieve L, Saxod R. Morphometric and biochemical studies in trigeminal nerve of rat after trichloroethylene or dichloracetylene oral administration. *Neurotoxicology* 1992;13:601–614.

Barton HA, Flemming CD, Lipscomb JC. Evaluating human variability in chemical risk assessment: hazard identification and dose-response assessment for noncancer oral toxicity trichloroethylene. *Toxicology* 1996;111:271–287.

Bartonicek V. The effect of some substances on elimination of trichloroethylene metabolites. *Arch Int Pharmacodyn Therap* 1963;144:69–85.

Bartonicek V, Teisinger J. Effect of tetraethyl thiram disulphide (disulfiram) on metabolism of trichloroethylene in man. *Br J Ind Med* 1962;19:216–221.

Bartonicek V, Brun A. Subacute and chronic trichloroethylene poisoning. A neuropathological study in rabbits. *Acta Pharmacol Toxicol* 1970;28:359–369.

Bergman K. Application and results of whole body autoradiography in distributions. Studies of organic solvents. *CRC Crit Rev Toxicol* 1983;12:59–118.

Bernad PG, Newell S, Spyker DA. Neurotoxicity and behavior abnormalities in a cohort chronically exposed to trichloroethylene. *Vet Hum Toxicol* 1987;29:475.

Bhakuni V, Roy R. Interaction of trichloroethylene with phosphatidylcholine and its localization in the phosphatidyl vesicles: a 1H-NMR study. *Biochem Pharmacol* 1994;47:1461–1464.

Blain L, Lachapelle P, Molotchnikoff S. Evoked potentials are modified by long term exposure to trichloroethylene. *Neurotoxicology* 1992;12:203–206.

Bolt HM, Laib RJ, Filser JG. Reactive metabolites and carcinogenicity of halogenated hydrocarbons. *Biochem Pharmacol* 1982;31:1–4.

Bond GR. Hepatitis, rash and eosinophilia following trichloroethylene exposure: a case report and speculation on mechanistic similarity to halothane induced hepatitis. *J Toxicol Clin Toxicol* 1996;34:461–466.

Bondy SC. Reactive oxygen species: relation to aging and neurotoxic damage. *Neurotoxicology* 1992;13:87–100.

Brodzinsky R, Singh HB. Volatile organic chemicals in the atmosphere: an assessment of available data. Menlo Park, CA: Atmospheric Science Center, SRI International. Contract no. 69-02-3452:107–108, 1982.

Brown HS, Bishop DR, Rowan CA. The role of skin absorption as a route of exposure for volatile organic compounds (VOCs) in drinking water. *Am J Public Health* 1984;74:479–484.

Bruckner JV, Davis DD, Blancato JN. Metabolism, toxicity and carcinogenicity of trichloroethylene. *CRC Crit Rev Toxicol* 1989;20:31–50.

Burg JR, Gist GL, Alldred SL, Radtke TM, Pallos L, Cusack CD. The National Exposure Registry—Morbidity analysis of noncancer outcomes from the trichloroethylene subregistry baseline data. *Int J Occup Med Toxicol* 1995;4:237–257.

Burmaster DE. The new pollution-groundwater contamination. *Environment* 1982;24:7–36.

Buxton PH, Hayward M. Polyneuritis cranialis associated with industrial trichloroethylene poisoning. *J Neurol Neurosurg Psychiatry* 1967;30:511–518.

Cavanagh JB, Buxton PH. Trichloroethylene cranial neuropathy: is it really a toxic neuropathy or does it activate latent herpes virus? *J Neurol Neurosurg Psychiatry* 1989;52:297–303.

Chalupa B, Synkova J, Sevcik M. The assessment of electroencephalographic changes and memory disturbances in acute intoxications with industrial poisons. *Br J Ind Med* 1960;17:238–241.

CMR. Chemical profile—trichloroethylene. *Chemical Marketing Reporter,* January 27, 1986.

Cohen HP, Cohen MM, Lin S, Baker AB. Tissue levels of trichloroethylene after acute and chronic exposure. *Anesthesiology* 1958;19:188–196.

Cohr K. Uptake and distribution of common industrial solvents. In: Riihimaki V, Ulfvarson U, eds. *Safety and health aspects of organic solvents: International course on safety and health aspects of organic solvents (Espoo, Finland, April 22–26, 1985).* New York: Alan R Liss, 1986:45–60.

Cojocel C, Beuter W, Müller W, Mayer D. Lipid peroxidation: a possible mechanism of trichloroethylene induced nephrotoxicity. *Toxicology* 1989;55:131–141.

Cooper JR, Friedman PJ. The enzymatic oxidation of chloral hydrate to trichloroacetic acid. *Biochem Pharmacol* 1958;1:76–82.

Cooper KW, Hickman KE. Refrigeration. In: Grayson M, Eckroth P, eds. *Kirk–Othmer encyclopedia of chemical technology,* vol 20, 3rd ed. New York: John Wiley & Sons, 1982:91–92.

Corcoran GB, Fix L, Jones DP, Moslen MT, Nicotera P, Oberhammer FA, Buttyan R. Contemporary issues in toxicology. Apoptosis: molecular control point in toxicity. *Toxicol Appl Pharmacol* 1994;128:169–181.

Costa AK, Katz D, Ivanetich KM. Trichloroethylene: its interactions with hepatic microsomal cytochrome P-450 *in vitro. Biochem Pharmacol* 1980;29:433–439.

Costa AK, Ivanetich KM. Trichloroethylene metabolism by the hepatic microsomal cytochrome P-450 system. *Biochem Pharmacol* 1980;29: 2863–2869.

Crawford JS, Davies P. A return to trichloroethylene for obstetrical anaesthesia. *Br J Anaesth* 1975;47:482–489.

Davidson IWF, Beliles RP. Consideration of the target organ toxicity of trichloroethylene in terms of metabolite toxicity and pharmacokinetics. *Drug Metab Rev* 1991;23:493–599.

Defalque RJ. Pharmacology and toxicology of trichloroethylene. A critical review of the world literature. *Clin Pharmacol Ther* 1961;2:665–688.

Dekant W, Henschler D. New pathways in trichloroethylene metabolism. In: Hayes AW, Schnell R, Mivaeds TS, eds. *Developments in the science and practice of toxicology.* Amsterdam: Elsevier, 1983:399–402.

Dekant W, Metzler M, Henschler D. Novel metabolites of trichloroethylene through dechlorination reactions in mice and humans. *Biochem Pharmacol* 1984;33:2021–2027.

Dillon JB. Trichloroethylene for the reduction of pain associated with malignant disease. *Anesthesiology* 1956;17:208–209.

Dogui M, Mrizak N, Yacoubi M, Ben Hadj Ali B, Paty J. Potentiels éoqués somesthésiques du trijumeau chez des travailleurs manipulant le trichloréthylène. *Neurophysiol Clin* 1991;21:95–103.

Ellenhorn MJ, Barceloux DG. *Medical toxicology: diagnosis and treatment of human poisoning.* New York: Elsevier, 1988:990–993.

Entz RC, Diachenko GW. Residues of volatile halocarbons in margarines. *Food Addit Contam* 1988;5:267–276.

Entz RC, Thomas KW, Diachenko GW. Residues of volatile halocarbons in foods using headspace chromatography. *J Agric Food Chem* 1982; 30:846–849.

Ertle T, Henschler D, Müller G, Spassowski M. Metabolism of trichloroethylene in man. I. The significance of trichloroethanol in long-term exposure conditions. *Arch Toxikol* 1972;29:171–188.

Fan AM. Trichloroethylene: water contamination and health risk assessment. *Rev Environ Contam Toxicol* 1988;101:55–92.

Federal Register. National primary drinking water regulation on volatile synthetic organic chemicals. *Fed Regist* 1985;50:46880–46933.

Federal Register. Trichloroethylene. Rules and regulations. *Fed Regist* 1989a;54(12):2432–2434.

Federal Register. Dichloroacetylene. Rules and regulations. *Fed Regist* 1989b;54:2410–2411.

Feldman RG, Mayer R, Taub A. Evidence for peripheral neurotoxic effect of trichloroethylene. *Neurology* 1970;20:599–606.

Feldman RG. Trichloroethylene: intoxications of the nervous system, part I. In: Vinken P, Bruyn G, eds. *Handbook of clinical neurology,* vol 36. Amsterdam: North-Holland, 1979:457–464.

Feldman RG. Occupational exposure to trichloroethylene: controversies concerning neurotoxicity. In: Mehlman MA, Upton A, eds. *The identification and control of environmental and occupational disease.* Princeton, NJ: Princeton Scientific Publishing Company, 1994.

Feldman RG, Lessell S. Neuro-ophthalmological aspects of trichloroethylene intoxication. In: Burnett J, Bardeau, eds. *Progress in neuro-ophthalmology,* vol 2. Amsterdam: Excerpta Medica, 1969:281–286.

Feldman RG, White RF, Currie JN, Travers PH, Lessell S. Long term follow up after single toxic exposure to trichloroethylene. *Am J Ind Med* 1985;8:119–126.

Feldman RG, Chirico-Post JA, Proctor SP. Blink reflex latency after exposure to trichloroethylene in well water. *Arch Environ Health* 1988;43:143–148.

Feldman RG, Niles C, Proctor SP, Jabre J. Blink reflex measurement of effects of trichloroethylene exposure on the trigeminal nerve. *Muscle Nerve* 1992;15:490–495.

Feldman RG, White RF, Eriator II, Jabre JF, Feldman ES, Niles CA. Neurotoxic effects of trichloroethylene in drinking water: approach to diag-

nosis. In: *The vulnerable brain and environmental risks,* vol 3: Isaacson RL, Jensen RF, eds. *Special hazards from air and water.* New York: Plenum Press, 1994:3–23.

Fernandez JG, Droz PD, Humbert BE. Trichloroethylene exposure simulation of uptake, excretion, and metabolism using mathematical model. *Br J Ind Med* 1977;34:43–55.

Freedman DL, Gassett JM. Biological reductive dechlorination of tetrachloroethylene and trichloroethylene to ethylene under methanogenic conditions. *Appl Environ Microbiol* 1989;55:144–151.

Gennaro AR, ed. *Remington's pharmaceutical sciences.* Easton, PA: Mack Publishing Company, 1985:1043.

Gevins AS: Quantitative aspects of EEG and evoked potentials. In: Aminoff MJ, ed. *Electrodiagnosis in clinical neurology,* 2nd ed. New York: Churchill Livingstone, 1986:149–203.

Gist GL, Burg JR. Trichloroethylene—a review of the literature from a health effects perspective. *Toxicol Ind Health* 1995;11:253–307.

Goeptar AR, Commandeur JNM, van Ommen B, van Bladeren PJ, Vermeulen PE. Metabolism and kinetics of trichloroethylene in relation to toxicity and carcinogenicity. Relevance of the mercapturic acid pathway. *Chem Res Toxicol* 1995;8:3–21.

Gonthier BP, Barret LG. *In vitro* spin trapping of free radicals produced during trichloroethylene and diethylether metabolism. *Toxicol Lett* 1989;47:225–234.

Graham DG, Amarath V, Valentine WM, Pyle SJ, Anthony DC. Pathogenic studies of hexane and carbon disulfide neurotoxicity. *Crit Rev Toxicol* 1995;25(2):91–112.

Grandjean E, Munchinger R, Turrian V, Hass PA, Knoepfel HK, Rosemund H. Investigations into the effects of exposure to trichloroethylene in mechanical engineering. *Br J Ind Med* 1955;12:131–142.

Green T, Prout MS. Species differences in response to trichloroethylene. II. Biotransformation in rats and mice. *Toxicol Appl Pharmacol* 1985; 79:401–411.

Gregersen P, Angelso B, Nielson TE, Norgaard B, Uldal C. Neurotoxic effects of organic solvents in exposed workers: an occupational, neuropsychological, and neurological investigation. *Am J Ind Med* 1984; 5:201–221.

Greim H, Wolff T, Höfler M, Lahaniatis E. Formation of dichloroacetylene from trichloroethylene in the presence of akaline material—possible cause of intoxication after abundant use of chloroethylene-containing solvents. *Arch Toxicol* 1984;56:74–77.

Gruener G, Bosch EP, Strauss RG, Klugman M, Kimura J. Predictions of early beneficial response to plasma exchange in Guillain–Barré syndrome. *Arch Neurol* 1987;44:295–298.

Haglid K, Kjellstrand P, Rosengren L, Wronski A, Briving C. Effects of trichloroethylene inhalation on proteins of the gerbil brain. *Arch Toxicol* 1980;43:187–199.

Haglid KG, Briving C, Hanson H-A, et al. Trichloroethylene: long-lasting changes in the brain after rehabilitation. *Neurotoxicology* 1981;2:659–673.

Halliwell B. Oxidants and the central nervous system: some fundamental questions. Is oxidant damage relevant to Parkinson's disease, Alzheimer's disease, traumatic injury and stroke? *Acta Neurol Scand* 1989; 126:23–33.

Hathway DE. Consideration of the evidence for mechanisms of 1,1,2-trichloroethylene metabolism, including new identification of its dichloroacetic acid and trichloroacetic acid metabolites in mice. *Cancer Lett* 1980;8:263–269.

Henschler D, Broser F, Hopf HG. Polyneuritis cranialis following poisoning with chlorinated acetylenes while handling vinylidene chloride copolymers. *Arch Toxicol* 1970;26:62–75.

Hess K, Kern S, Schiller HH. Blink reflex in trigeminal sensory neuropathy. *Electromyogr Clin Neurophysiol* 1984;24:185–190.

Hetzler BE, Heibronner RL, Griffin J, Griffin G. Acute effects of alcohol on evoked potentials in visual cortex and superior-colliculus of rats. *Electroencephalogr Clin Neurophysiol* 1981;51:69–79.

Humphrey JH, McClelland M. Cranial-nerve palsies with herpes following general anaesthesia. *Br Med J* 1944;1:315–318.

Ikeda M. Reciprocal metabolic inhibition of toluene and trichloroethylene *in vivo* and *in vitro. Int Arch Arbeitsmed* 1974;33:125–130.

Ikeda M, Ohtsuji H, Kawai H, Kuniyoshi M. Excretion kinetics of urinary metabolites in a patient addicted to trichloroethylene. *Br J Ind Med* 1971;28:203–206.

Ikeda M, Ohtsuji H, Imamura T, Komoike Y. Urinary excretion of total trichloro-compounds, trichloroethanol, and trichloroacetic acid as a measure of exposure to trichloroethylene and tetrachloroethylene. *Br J Ind Med* 1972;29:328–333.

Inoue O, Seiji K, Kawai T, et al. Relationship between vapor exposure and urinary metabolite excretion among workers exposed to trichloroethylene. *Am J Ind Med* 1989;15:103–110.

International Agency for Research on Cancer (IARC). *Some halogenated hydrocarbons. Monographs on the evaluation of the carcinogenic risk of chemicals to humans,* vol 20. Lyons, France: WHO, 1979:545–572.

Isaacson L, Spohler S, Taylor D. Trichloroethylene affects learning and decreases myelin in the rat hippocampus. *Neurotoxicol Teratol* 1990;12:375–381.

Jacobs JM. Permeability and neurotoxicity. *Environ Health Perspect* 1978;26:107–116.

Juntunen J. Occupational toxicology of trichloroethylene with special reference to neurotoxicity. In: Chambers PL, Gehring P, Sakai F, eds. *New concepts and developments in toxicology.* Amsterdam: Elsevier, 1986:189–200.

Kautiainen A, Vogel JS, Turteltaub KW. Dose-dependent binding or trichloroethylene to hepatic DNA and protein at low doses in mice. *Chemico Biol Interact* 1997;106:109–121.

Kelly JM, Brown BR. Biotransformation of trichloroethylene. *Intern Anesthesiol Clin* 1974;12:85–92.

Kiers L, Carrol WM. Blink reflexes and magnetic resonance imaging in focal unilateral central trigeminal pathway demyelination. *J Neurol Neurosurg Psychiatry* 1990;53:526–529.

Kimura J. Conduction abnormalities of the facial and trigeminal nerves in polyneuropathy. *Muscle Nerve* 1982;5:129–144.

King GS, Smialek JE, Troutman WG. Sudden death in adolescents resulting from inhalation of typewriter correction fluid. *JAMA* 1985;253:1604–1606.

Kjellstrand P, Lanke J, Bjerkemo M, Zelterqvist L, Mansson L. Irreversible effects of trichloroethylene exposure on the central nervous system. *Scand J Work Environ Health* 1980;6:40–47.

Koppel C, Lanz H-J, Ibe K. Acute trichloroethylene poisoning with additional ingestion of ethanol—concentrations of trichloroethylene and its metabolites during hyperventilation therapy. *Intensive Care Med* 1988;14:74–76.

Kuney JH. *Chemcyclopedia,* vol 5. Washington, DC: American Chemical Society, 1986:116.

Kyrklund T, Alling C, Haglid K, Kjellstrand P. Chronic exposure to trichloroethylene: lipid and acyl group composition in gerbil cerebral cortex and hippocampus. *Neurotoxicology* 1983;4:35–42.

Kyrklund T, Goracci G, Haglid KG, Rosengren L, Porcellatti G, Kjellstrand P. Chronic effects of trichloroethylene upon S-100 protein content and lipid composition in gerbil cerebellum. *Scand J Environ Health* 1984;10:89–93.

Lagakos S, Wessen B, Zelen M. An analysis of contaminated well water and health effects in Woburn, Massachusetts. *J Am Stat Assoc* 1986;81:583–596.

Landrigan PJ, Stein GF, Kominsky JR, Ruke RL, Watanabe AS: Common-source community and industrial exposure to trichloroethylene. *Arch Environ Health* 1987;42:327–332.

Lauwerys R. *Guidelines for biological monitoring.* Davis, CA: Biomedical Publications, 1983:87–91.

Lawrence WH, Partyka EK. Chronic dysphagia and trigeminal anesthesia after trichloroethylene exposure. *Ann Int Med* 1981;95:710.

Leandri M, Parodi CI, Favale E. Early evoked potentials detected from the scalp of a man following infraorbital nerve stimulation. *Electroencephalogr Clin Neurophysiol* 1985;62:99–107.

Leandri M, Schizzi R, Scielzo C, Favale E. Electrophysiological evidence of trigeminal root damage after trichloroethylene exposure. *Muscle Nerve* 1995;18:467–468.

Leibman KC. Metabolism of trichloroethylene in liver microsomes. I. Characteristics of the reaction. *Mol Pharmacol* 1965;1:239–246.

Ligocki MP, Leuenberger C, Pankow JF. Trace organic compounds in rain-II. Gas scavenging of neutral organic compounds. *Atmos Environ* 1985;19:1609–1617.

Lilis R, Stanescu D, Muica N, Roventa A. Chronic effects of trichloroethylene exposure. *Clin Occup Dis* 1969;60:595–601.

Lindstrom K, Antti-Poika M, Tola S, Hyytiainen A. Psychological prognosis of diagnosed chronic organic solvent intoxication. *Neurobehav Toxicol Teratol* 1982;4:581–588.

Liu YT, Jin C, Chen Z, Cai SX, Yin SN, Watanabe T, Nakatsuka H, Seiji K, Inoue O, Kawai T, Ukai H, Ikeda M. Increased subjected symptom prevalence among workers exposed to trichloroethylene at sub-OEL levels. *Tohuku J Exp Med* 1988;155:183–195.

Logue JN, Stroman RM, Hayes CW, Sivarjah K. Investigation of potential health effect associated with well water chemical contamination in Londonderry township, Pennsylvania, U.S.A. *Arch Environ Health* 1985;40:155–160.

Mannsville. *Chemical product synopsis: trichloroethylene.* Cortland, NY: Mannsville Chemical Products Corporation, 1992.

Martinelli P, Gulli MR, Gabellini AS. Acute intoxication of trichloroethylene with complete recovery: a case report. *Ital J Neurol Sci* 1984;5:469–470.

McCarty PL, Wilson JT. Natural anaerobic treatment of a TCE plume, St. Joseph, Michigan, NPL site. In *US EPA bioremediation of hazardous wastes.* EPA/600/R-92/126. Cincinnati: EPA, 1992:47–50.

McCunney R. Diverse manifestations of trichloroethylene. *Br J Ind Med* 1988;45:122–126.

McKone TE, Knezovich JP. The transfer of trichloroethylene (TCE) from a shower to indoor air: experimental measurements and their implications. *J Air Waste Manag Assoc* 1991;41:282–286.

Miller RE, Guengerich FP. Oxidation of trichloroethylene by lever microsomal cytochrome P-450: evidence for chlorine migration in transition state not involving trichloroethylene oxide. *Biochemistry* 1982;21:1090–1109.

Monster AC. Trichloroethylene. In: Aitio A, Riihimaki V, Vainio H, eds. *Biological monitoring and surveillance of workers exposed to chemicals.* New York: Hemisphere Publishing Corporation, 1984:111–130.

Monster AC, Boersma G, Duba WC. Pharmacokinetics of trichloroethylene in volunteers. Influence of workload and exposure concentration. *Int Arch Occup Environ Health* 1976;38:87–102.

Monster AC, Boersma G, Duba WC. Kinetics of trichloroethylene in repeated exposure of volunteers. *Int Arch Occup Environ Health* 1979;42:283–292.

Müller G, Spassovski M, Henschler D. Metabolism of trichloroethylene in man. II. Pharmacokinetics of metabolites. *Arch Toxicol* 1974;32:283–295.

Müller G, Spassovski M, Henschler D. Metabolism of trichloroethylene in man. III. Interaction of trichloroethylene and ethanol. *Arch Toxicol* 1975;33:173–189.

Musclow CE, Awen CF. Glue sniffing: report of a fatal case. *Can Med Assoc J* 1971;104:315–319.

National Institute for Occupational Safety and Health (NIOSH). *Pocket guide to chemical hazards.* Washington, DC: US Department of Health and Human Services, Centers for Disease Control and Prevention, 1997.

Nomiyama K, Nomiyama H. Dose response relationship for trichloroethylene in man. *Int Arch Occup Environ Health* 1977;39:237–248.

Noseworthy JH, Rice GP. Trichloroethylene poisoning mimicking multiple sclerosis. *Can J Neurol Sci* 1988;15:87–88.

Occupational Safety and Health Administration (OSHA). Code of Federal Regulations, 29, 1910.1000. Office of the Federal Register, National Archives and Records Administration, Washington, DC, 1995:18.

Office of Technology Assessment (OTA). *Coming clean: superfund's problems can be solved.* Washington, DC: US Government Printing Office, 1991.

Ohtahara K, Ogata M, Inoue T, et al. Studies on trichloroethylene poisoning in a dry-cleaning factory. *Okayama Med J* 1958;70:4081.

Olivares-Esquer J, Saldana-Arevalo M, Garcia-Torres R, Trevino-Becerra A. Treatment using hemodialysis and exsanguination transfusion of acute renal failure myopathy and toxic hepatitis, caused by trichloroacetylene. Report of a case and review of the literature. *Prensa Med Mexicana* 1974;39:461–467.

Parkinson A. Biotransformation of xenobiotics. In: Klaassen CD, ed. *Casarett and Doull's toxicology: The basic science of poisons.* New York: McGraw–Hill, 1996:113–186.

Peoples RW, Weight FF. Trichloroethanol potentiation of γ-aminobutyric acid-activated chloride current in mouse hippocampal neurones. *Br J Pharmacol* 1994;113:555–563.

Peoples RW, Lovinger DM, Weight FF. Inhibition of excitatory amino acid currents by general anesthetic agents. *Soc Neurosci Abstr* 1990;16:1017.

Perbellini L, Olivato D, Zedde A, Miglioranzi R. Acute trichloroethylene poisoning by ingestion: clinical and pharmacokinetic aspects. *Int Care Med* 1991;17:234–235.

Prout MS, Provan WM, Green T. Species differences in response to trichloroethylene. I. Pharmacokinetics in rats and mice. *Toxicol Appl Pharmacol* 1985;79:389–400.

Rall TW. Hypnotics and sedatives; ethanol. In: Goodman-Gilman A, Rall TW, Nies AS, Taylor P, eds. *Goodman and Gilman's The Pharmacological Basis of Therapeutics,* 8th ed. Elmsford, NY: Pergamon Press, 1990:345–382.

Rasmussen K, Arlien-Soberg P, Sabroe S. Clinical neurological findings among metal degreasers exposed to chlorinated solvents. *Acta Neurol Scand* 1993;87:200–204.

Reichert D, Liebaldt G, Henschler D. Neurotoxic effects of dichloro-acetylene. *Arch Toxicol* 1976;37:23–38.

Reichert D, Metzler M, Henschler D. Decomposition of the neuro- and nephrotoxic compound dichloroacetylene in the presence of oxygen: separation and identification of novel products. *J Environ Pathol Toxicol* 1980;4:525–532.

Ruijten MWMM, Verbeck MM, Sallé HJA. Nerve function in workers with long term exposure to trichloroethylene. *Br J Ind Med* 1991;48:87–92.

Sagawa K, Nishitani H, Kawai H, Kuge Y, Ikeda M. Transverse lesion of the spinal cord after accidental exposure to trichloroethylene. *Int Arch Arbeitsmed* 1973;31:247–264.

Sasdelli N, Vagnolli E, Duranti E, Imperiali P, Tilli G. Treatment of acute "triline" poisoning by plasmapheresis and hemoperfusion. *Int J Artif Organs* 1986;9(3):195–196.

Sato A, Nakajima T. Differences following skin or inhalation exposure in the absorption and excretion kinetics of trichloroethylene and toluene. *Br J Ind Med* 1978;35:43–49.

Sato A, Nakajima T, Fujiwara Y, Murayama N. A pharmacokinetic model to study the excretion of trichloroethylene and its metabolites after an inhalation exposure. *Br J Ind Med* 1977;34:55–63.

Sato A, Endoh K, Kaneko T, Johanson G. Effects of consumption of ethanol on the biological monitoring of exposure to organic solvent vapours: a simulation study with trichloroethylene. *Br J Ind Med* 1991;48:548–556.

Savolainen H. Pharmacokinetics, pharmacodynamics, and aspects of neurotoxic effects of inhaled aliphatic chlorohydrocarbon solvents as relevant in man. *Eur J Drug Metab Pharmacokinet* 1981;6:85–90.

Savolainen H, Pfäffli P, Tengen M, Vainio H. Trichloroethylene and 1,1,1 trichloroethane: effects on brain and liver after five days' intermittent inhalation. *Arch Toxicol* 1977;38:299–337.

Sax NI. *Dangerous properties of industrial materials,* 5th ed. New York: Van Nostrand Reinhold, 1979.

Schaumburg HH, Berger AR. Human toxic neuropathy due to industrial agents. In: Dyck PJ, Thomas PK, Griffin JW, Low PA, Poduslo JF, eds. *Peripheral neuropathy,* 3rd ed., Philadelphia: WB Saunders, 1993: 1533–1548.

Seiji K, Inoue O, Jin C, et al. Dose–excretion relationship in tetrachloroethylene-exposed workers and the effect of tetrachloroethylene co-exposure on trichloroethylene metabolism. *Am J Ind Med* 1989;16:675–684.

Sellers EM, Koch-Weser J. Potentiation of warfarin-induced hypoprothrombinemia by chloral hydrate. *N Engl J Med* 1970;283:827–831.

Sellers EM, Lang M, Koch-Weser J, LeBlanc E, Kalant H. Interaction of chloral hydrate and ethanol in man. I. Metabolism. *Clin Pharmacol Ther* 1972;13:37.

Seppäläinen AM, Raitta C, Huuskonen MS. *n*-Hexane induced changes in visual evoked potentials and electroretinogram of industrial workers. *Electroencephalogr Clin Neurophysiol* 1979;47:492–498.

Seppäläinen AM, Antti-Poika M. Time course of electrophysiological findings for patients with solvent poisoning. *Scand J Work Environ Health* 1983;9:15–24.

Siegel J, Jones RA, Coon RA, Lyon JP. Effects on experimental animals of acute, repeated and continuous inhalation exposures to dichloroacetylene mixtures. *Toxicol Appl Pharmacol* 1971;18:168–174.

Snyder R, Andrews LS. Toxic effects of solvents and vapors. In: Klaassen CD, ed. *Casarett and Doull's Toxicology. The basic science of poisons,* 5th ed. New York: McGraw-Hill, 1996:737–771.

SRI. *1987 Directory of chemical producers: United States of America.* SRI International, Menlo Park, CA: 1987:1055.

Steinberg W. Residual neuropsychological effects following exposure to trichloroethylene (TCE): a case study. *Clin Neuropsychol* 1981;3:1–4.

Stephens JA. Poisoning by accidental drinking of trichloroethylene. *Br Med J* 1945;2:218–219.

Stewart RD, Dodd HC. Absorption of carbon tetrachloride, trichloroethylene, tetrachloroethylene, methylene chloride, and 1,1,1-trichloroethane through human skin. *Am Ind Hyg Assoc J* 1964;25:439–446.

Stewart RD, Dodd HC, Gay HH, Erley DS. Experimental human exposure to trichloroethylene. *Arch Environ Health* 1970;20:64–71.

Stewart RD, Hake CL, Peterson, Forster HV, Newton PE, Soto RJ, Lebrun GJ. Development of biological standards for trichloroethylene. In: Xintaias C, Johnson B, eds. *Behavioral toxicology; early detection of occupational hazards,* vol 74(126). Washington, DC: USDHEW (NIOSH), 1974:81–91.

Stracciari A, Gallassi R, Ciardulli C, Coccagna G. Neuropsychological and EEG evaluation in exposure to trichloroethylene. *J Neurol* 1985; 232:120–122.

Subramonian A, Goel S, Pandya KP, Seth PK. Influence of trichloroethylene treatment on phosphoinositides in rat brain. *Toxicol Lett* 1989;49: 55–60.

Szlatenyi CS, Wang RY. Encephalopathy and cranial nerve palsies caused by intentional trichloroethylene inhalation. *Am J Emerg Med* 1996; 14:464–467.

Takeuchi Y, Iwata M, Hisanaga N, Ono Y, Shibata E, Huang J, Takegami T, Okamoto S, Koike Y. Polyneuropathy caused by chronic exposure to trichloroethylene. *Ind Health* 1986;24:243–247.

Tanaka S, Ikeda M. A method for determination of trichloroethylene and trichloroacetic acid in urine. *Br J Ind Med* 1968;25:214–219.

Töftgard R, Gustafsson J. Biotransformation of organic solvents. *Scand J Work Environ Health* 1980;6:1–18.

Triebig G, Trautner P, Weltle D, Saure E, Valentin H. Untersuchungen zur neurotoxiitat von arbeitsstofen; III. Messung der motorischen und sensorischen nervenleitgeschwindigkeit bei beruflich triclorathylen-belastenten personen. *Int Arch Occup Environ Health* 1982; 51:25–34.

Tucker AN, Sanders VM, Barnes DW, et al. Toxicology of trichloroethylene in the mouse. *Toxicol Appl Pharmacol* 1982;62:351–357.

United States Environmental Protection Agency (USEPA). *Drinking water regulations and health advisories.* EPA 822-R-96-001. Washington, DC: Office of Water, 1996.

Vernon RJ, Ferguson RK. Effects of trichloroethylene on visual motor performances. *Arch Environ Health* 1969;18:894–900.

Vesterberg O, Gorczak J, Krasts M. Exposure to trichloroethylene. II. Metabolites in blood and urine. *Scand J Work Environ Health* 1976;4: 212–219.

Wallace L, Pellizari E, Hartwell T, Zelon H, Sparacino C, Perritt R, Whitmore R. Concentrations of 20 volatile organic compounds in the air and drinking water of 350 residents of New Jersey compared with concentrations in their exhaled breath. *J Occup Med* 1986;28(8): 603–608.

Wallace LA, Pellizari ED, Hartwell TD, Whitmore R, Zelon H, Perritt R, Sheldon L. The California team study: breath concentrations and personal exposures to 26 volatile compounds in air and drinking water of 188 residents of Los Angeles, Antioch, and Pittsburg, CA. *Atmos Environ* 1988;22(10):2141–2163.

Waters EM, Gerstner HB, Huff JE. Trichloroethylene. 1. An overview. *J Toxicol Environ Health* 1977;2:671–707.

White RF. Clinical neuropsychological investigation of solvent neurotoxicity. In: Chang LW, Dyer RS, eds. *Handbook of neurotoxicology.* New York: Marcel Dekker, 1995:355–376.

White JF, Carlson GP. Epinephrine-induced cardiac arrhythmias in rabbits exposed to trichloroethylene: role of trichloroethylene metabolites. *Toxicol Appl Pharmacol* 1981;60:458–465.

White RF, Proctor S. Research and clinical criteria for the development of neurobehavioral test batteries. *J Occup Med* 1992;34:140–148.

White RF, Feldman RG, Proctor SP. Neurobehavioral effects of toxic exposure: Clinical syndromes in adult neuropsychology. In: White RF, ed. *The practitioners handbook.* Amsterdam: Elsevier, 1992:1–51.

White RF, Feldman RG, Eviator II, Jabre JF, Niles CA. Hazardous waste and neurobehavioral effects: a developmental perspective. *Environ Res* 1997;73:113–124.

Winneke G, Kastka J. Effects of trichloroethylene on signal detection and auditory evoked potentials in man. Presented at the 1st World Congress of Environmental Medicine and Biology held July 1–5 1974 in Paris.

Withey JR, Collins BT, Collins PG. Effect of vehicle on the pharmacokinetics and uptake of four halogenated hydrocarbons from the gastrointestinal tract of the rat. *J Appl Toxicol* 1983;3:249–253.

Wolff MS, Anderson HA, Selikoff IJ. Human tissue burdens of halogenated aromatic chemicals in Michigan *JAMA* 1982;247:2112–2116.

World Health Organization (WHO). *Recommended health based limits in occupational exposure to selected organic solvents.* Technical Report Series 664. Geneva: World Health Organization, 1981.

World Health Organization (WHO). *Trichloroethylene.* Environmental Health Criteria 50. Geneva: World Health Organization, 1985.

Ziglio G, Fara GM, Beltramelli G, Pregliasco F. Human environmental exposure to trichloro- and tetrachloroethylene in water and air in Milan, Italy. *Arch Environ Contam Toxicol* 1983;12:57–64.

CHAPTER 12

Tetrachloroethylene

Tetrachloroethylene (perchloroethylene, tetrachloroethene, PCE, perc, ethylene tetrachloride, carbon bichloride, carbon dichloride) is a colorless liquid with a sweet pungent odor at room temperature (Sax, 1979; Torkelson, 1994). Perchloroethylene (PCE) is the most commonly used name for this compound. The vapor pressure of PCE is 15.8 mm at 22°C (72°F), and therefore this solvent vaporizes at room temperature (Sax, 1979). Most PCE produced for commercial use is synthesized by reacting chlorine with hydrocarbons such as methane and ethane. PCE can also be produced by the reaction of ethylene dichloride with chloride (and/or hydrogen chloride) and oxygen; trichloroethylene (TCE) is also formed as a by-product of this reaction (Waters et al., 1977; ATSDR, 1995) (see Chapter 11). PCE is an intermediate in the synthesis of hexafluoroethane as well as many chlorinated fluorocarbons such as 1,1,2-trichloro-1,2,2-trifluoroethane (IARC, 1979; Torkelson, 1994). The double bond of PCE renders the compound prone to oxidation (Savolainen et al., 1977). PCE decomposes readily in the presence of hydroxyl ($\cdot$OH) radicals (Singh et al., 1982). Decomposition products of PCE include chloroacetylchlorides, chlorine, carbon monoxide, phosgene, and formic acid. Amines or mixtures of epoxides and esters are added as stabilizers to retard decomposition (IARC, 1979). Biotransformation by reductive dehalogenation of PCE in the environment results in the formation of TCE, dichloroethylene, and vinyl chloride (Vogel and McCarty, 1985).

PCE has been used commercially in the United States since 1925 (Hardie, 1964). It is used industrially to degrease metal and synthetic materials (Morse and Goldberg, 1943; Coler and Rossmiller, 1953; Lackore and Perkins, 1970), and it has been employed medicinally in humans as an anthelmintic and as a treatment for hookworm (Kendrick, 1929; Sandground, 1941; Haerer and Udelman, 1964) and as an anesthetic (Foot et al., 1943). PCE dissolves wax, grease, and oil without harming textiles, and therefore it finds widespread use as a dry-cleaning solvent. Because of its relatively low toxicity and better dry-cleaning efficiency, PCE has replaced other halogenated dry-cleaning solvents such as carbon tetrachloride and TCE

(Kaplan, 1980). As of 1986, 53% of the total PCE produced in the United States was used by the dry-cleaning industry (Solet, 1990). Individual dry-cleaning operations consume PCE in amounts ranging from 4 to 600 gallons per month (Earnest, 1993; Earnest and Spencer, 1993; Earnest et al., 1993). The *National Occupational Exposure Survey* (NOES), conducted by the National Institute for Occupational Safety and Health (NIOSH), reported that there are approximately 45,000 dry-cleaning plants in the United States and that these companies employ over 600,000 workers who are potentially at risk of exposure to PCE (NIOSH, 1990).

PCE produces neurological effects following inhalation of low as well as high vapor concentrations (Carpenter, 1937; Coler and Rossmiller, 1953; Seeber, 1989). Oral ingestion of PCE has also been associated with neurological manifestations including seizures and coma (Kendrick, 1929; Sandground, 1941; Haerer and Udelman, 1964; Köppel et al., 1985). Chronic exposure to PCE may lead to hepatic failure (Gehring, 1968), and has been implicated as a carcinogen (Coler and Rossmiller, 1953; Kaplan, 1980; Stemhagen et al., 1983; Aschengrau et al., 1993). Exposure to PCE occurs in both industrial and nonindustrial settings (Saland, 1967; Levine et al., 1981; Garnier et al., 1996). The importance of being aware of the neurotoxicant properties of this widely used volatile chlorinated hydrocarbon is based upon the need to avoid the acute neurotoxic effects of PCE exposure, which can impair the cognitive and motor performance of workers and cause accidents on the job, as well as to prevent long-term effects on the nervous and other organ systems (Rao et al., 1993).

SOURCES OF EXPOSURE

Professional dry cleaners are at risk of exposure both during the cleaning process and during maintenance of the dry-cleaning vats and equipment (Gold, 1969; MMWR, 1983; Materna, 1985; Solet et al., 1990). Dry-cleaning workers who transfer wet clothing from washers to dryers have relatively high rates of exposure to PCE. Individuals who use coin-operated dry-cleaning machines are at risk of exposure both during and after the process, particularly if the machines are overfilled by the unsuspecting user, thereby allowing large amounts of PCE to be retained in the dry-cleaned garments (Gaillard et al., 1995). Twenty-five cases of PCE intoxication were reported to the Paris Poison Center from May 1989 through June 1995. In eight cases, overloading of the machine or cleaning of bulky items was determined to be responsible for the exposure (Garnier et al., 1996). Measurement of PCE levels in residences in the immediate vicinity of dry-cleaning establishments revealed levels ranging from 0.1 to 55 mg/m³ (control range: 0.007 to 0.1 mg/m³) (Schreiber et al., 1993). Concentrations of PCE and its metabolites were elevated in the blood and urine of persons living near a dry-cleaning shop (Popp et al., 1992). Persons employed in the dry-cleaning industry passively transport PCE both in their body (from which it is released as a vapor in exhaled breath) and on their workclothes (from which condensed PCE vaporizes into the ambient air), thus exposing their family members to significantly higher levels than the general population (Thompson and Evans, 1993; Aggazzotti et al., 1994). Median PCE levels measured in the homes of dry cleaners were 0.3 mg/m³ and were significantly higher than those in the homes of controls (median: 0.006 mg/m³) (Aggazzotti et al., 1994). PCE has been detected in high-fat foods such as margarine, with higher levels found in foods obtained from supermarkets located near dry-cleaning establishments (Entz and Diachenko, 1988).

Superfund toxic waste sites have documented PCE contamination of ground water and soil (Evans, 1991). PCE has been detected in ground water in New Jersey (1,500 ppb), Connecticut (740 ppb), and New York (714 ppb) (Burmaster, 1982). Drinking water can be a source of PCE (Skender et al., 1993, 1994; Webler and Brown, 1993). For example, drinking water supplies in Massachusetts contained PCE which was believed to have leached form vinyl polymer (Piccotex)-lined water pipes (Aschengrau et al., 1993; Webler and Brown, 1993). Private and public water sources have also been contaminated by improper toxic waste disposal (ATSDR, 1995). Drinking water in Massachusetts, Los Angeles, Milan, and Croatia was found to contain PCE (Ziglio, 1983; Wallace et al., 1988; Webler and Brown, 1993; Skender et al., 1993). A significant correlation was found between PCE concentrations in drinking water and urine trichloroacetic acid and blood PCE levels among members of an urban population in Zagreb, Croatia (Skender et al., 1993, 1994). Increased PCE concentration in indoor ambient air can result from the vaporization of PCE-contaminated tap water (McKone, 1987). PCE levels of 0.09 to 0.66 ppb were found on their breath, and PCE levels of 0.35 to 260 ppb were found in the blood of residents of Love Canal (Barkley et al., 1980). PCE and its metabolites were detected in the blood and urine of persons without known occupational exposures (Hajimiragha et al., 1986; Skender et al., 1993, 1994; Webler and Brown, 1993).

The *United States Environmental Protection Agency* (USEPA) estimates the average individual daily intake of PCE through consumption of contaminated food and beverages ranges from 0 to 6 μg (USEPA, 1985). PCE has been detected in dairy products (0.3 to 13 μg/kg), meats (0.9 to 5 μg/kg), oils and fats (0.17 to 7 μg/kg), beverages (2 to 3 μg/kg), and fruits and vegetables (0.7 to 2 μg/kg) (McConnell et al., 1975). Following exposure, PCE can be detected in the breast milk of nursing mothers (Sheldon et al., 1985; Schreiber, 1993). In addition, PCE is used in lighter, cleaning, and typewriter correction fluids, and intentional inhalation of the vapors for the psychotropic effects of these products has been reported (ATSDR, 1995).

EXPOSURE LIMITS AND SAFETY REGULATIONS

The odor threshold for PCE vapor in air is 27 ppm (Amoore and Hautala, 1983). The ability to detect the odor of PCE, which initially alerts an individual to its presence, is diminished with chronic exposure, thus increasing the risk of unrecognized exposure (Stewart et al., 1970). The *Occupational Safety and Health Administration* (OSHA) has established an 8-hour time-weighted average (TWA) permissible exposure level (PEL) of 100 ppm for PCE (Table 12-1). The OSHA PEL ceiling for an 8-hour workday is a 15-minute TWA of 200

TABLE 12-1. *Established and recommended occupational and environmental exposure limits for perchloroethylene in air and water*

	Air (ppm)[a]	Water (mg/L)[a]
Odor threshold*	27	0.17
OSHA		
PEL (8-hr TWA)	100	—
PEL ceiling (15-min TWA)	200	—
PEL ceiling (5-min peak)	300	—
NIOSH		
REL (10-hr TWA)	Carcinogenic	—
STEL (15-min TWA)	—	—
IDLH	150	—
ACGIH		
TLV (8-hr TWA)	25	—
STEL (15-min TWA)	100	—
USEPA		
MCL	—	0.005
MCLG	—	0.0

[a]*Unit conversion:* 1 ppm = 6.89 mg/m³; 1 ppm = 1 mg/L.
OSHA, Occupational Safety and Health Administration; PEL, permissible exposure limit; TWA, time-weighted average; NIOSH, National Institute for Occupational Safety and Health; REL, recommended exposure limit; STEL, short-term exposure limit; IDLH, immediately dangerous to life and health; ACGIH, American Conference of Governmental Industrial Hygienists; TLV, threshold limit value; USEPA, United States Environmental Protection Agency; MCL, maximum contamination level; MCLG, maximum contamination level goal.
Data from *Amoore and Hautala, 1983; OSHA, 1995; ACGIH, 1996; USEPA, 1996; NIOSH, 1997.

ppm, with an acceptable 5-minute maximum peak concentration of 300 ppm within any 3-hour period of the day (OSHA, 1995). The *National Institute for Occupational Safety and Health* (NIOSH) considers PCE to be a human carcinogen and recommends that exposure be limited to the lowest possible concentration. The NIOSH immediately dangerous to life and health (IDLH) exposure level for PCE is 150 ppm (NIOSH, 1997). The *American Conference of Governmental Industrial Hygienists'* (ACGIH) recommended 8-hour TWA threshold limit value (TLV) for PCE is 25 ppm, below which no narcotic or neuropathic effects are expected to be observed. The ACGIH 15-minute short-term-exposure-limit (STEL) is 100 ppm (ACGIH, 1995). The ACGIH and NIOSH recommended STELs for the PCE decomposition product, dichloroacetylene (DCA), are both 0.1 ppm (NIOSH, 1994; ACGIH, 1995).

The odor threshold concentration for PCE in water is 0.17 mg/L (Amoore and Hautala, 1983). The USEPA has established a maximum contamination limit (MCL) of 0.005 mg/L for PCE in drinking water. The USEPA has recommended a maximum contamination limit goal (MCLG) of 0.0 mg/L for PCE in drinking water (USEPA, 1996). These values are based on studies of carcinogenicity rather than those of neurotoxicity.

METABOLISM

Tissue Absorption

The principal route of intake for PCE is via inhalation. PCE vapors are readily absorbed across the pulmonary alveoli into the systemic circulation (Fernandez et al., 1976; Hake and Stewart, 1977; Pegg et al., 1979; Monster, 1979; Monster et al., 1983). The initial efficient pulmonary absorption of PCE is explained by a relatively high blood/air partition coefficient (Monster, 1984). Uptake of PCE through the lungs is rapid at the beginning of an exposure and then decreases as the blood and body tissues become saturated (Guberan and Fernandez, 1974; Fernandez et al., 1976; Monster et al., 1979). Pulmonary uptake of PCE is influenced by variations in lean body mass; individuals with a higher percentage of lean body mass initially take up more of the solvent (Monster et al., 1979). Uptake of PCE is increased by physical activities that increase both the pulmonary ventilation rate and cardiac output (Fernandez et al., 1976; Monster et al., 1979). Individuals with a higher percentage of body fat can generally carry a higher body burden of PCE before any clinical effects of exposure are manifested. However, a sudden mobilization of fat, such as can occur during dieting, can increase blood PCE levels and depending on the amount released and other variables including concurrent exposures and excretion rates, biological effects including toxicity are possible (Rozman and Klaassen, 1996).

PCE is readily absorbed through the gastrointestinal mucosa following oral ingestion (Kendrick, 1929; Sandground, 1941; Pegg et al., 1979; Köppel et al., 1985; War-

ren et al., 1996). PCE can be detected in the blood and in the brain within 1 minute after oral intake in the rat. Blood and brain levels of PCE reach 94% and 80% of their respective maximums within 15 minutes after ingestion (Warren et al., 1996). Peak blood levels are reached within 60 to 90 minutes (Pegg et al., 1979; Warren et al., 1996). Oral intake of PCE can cause inebriation, seizures, coma, and death (Kendrick, 1929; Sandground, 1941; Chaudhuri and Mukerji, 1947; Rower et al., 1952; Haerer and Udelman, 1964; Köppel et al., 1985; Hayes et al., 1986). A 6-year-old boy was comatose 1 hour after ingesting 12 to 16 g of PCE, and his blood PCE level was 21.5 mg/L (Köppel et al., 1985). Absorption of PCE is slower, but more complete, when the solvent is ingested in a mixture with fats or oils (Lamson et al., 1929; Gold, 1969; Pegg et al., 1979; Withey et al., 1983; Warren et al., 1996).

PCE vapor is absorbed through the skin (Riihimäki and Pfaffli, 1978). Absorption of liquid PCE through the skin occurs in workers who have direct dermal contact with PCE. For example, a peak alveolar PCE concentration of 0.31 ppm was measured in the expired air of volunteers whose source of exposure was one thumb immersed in liquid PCE for 40 minutes. This alveolar concentration level corresponded with that resulting from a respiratory PCE exposure at a vapor concentration of 10 to 15 ppm for 40 minutes (Stewart and Dodd, 1964). Dermal absorption of PCE is influenced by the duration of exposure, the temperature of the solvent, and the type, surface area, and degree of hydration of the skin exposed and contributes to the total uptake of the exposed individual (Hake and Stewart, 1977; Brown et al., 1984; Bogen et al., 1992). PCE disrupts the integrity of the stratum corneum, thereby enhancing its absorption through the skin (ATSDR, 1995). Dermal absorption of PCE is slow relative to that of other halogenated hydrocarbons such as trichloroethylene (Reichert, 1983). However, because of its relatively long biological half-life, the contribution to total body burden resulting from dermal absorption of PCE during chronic exposures is of greater significance (Hake and Stewart, 1977).

Tissue Distribution

The rate and magnitude of blood flow through the tissues as well as the solubility of PCE in the specific tissue determines the distribution of PCE within the body (Guberan and Fernandez, 1974; Monster et al., 1979; Warren et al., 1996). PCE and its metabolites readily crosses the blood–brain barrier (BBB) and the placenta (Lukaszewski, 1979; Levine et al., 1981; Ghantous et al., 1986; Kyrklund and Haglid, 1991; Warren et al., 1996). PCE is a highly lipophilic compound, and therefore its distribution is influenced by the tissue's lipid content (Stewart et al., 1977; Lukaszewski, 1979; Levine et al., 1981; Dallas et al., 1994; Warren et al., 1996). PCE concentrations were greatest in the adipose tissue, with lower levels seen in the liver, brain,

and muscles, respectively, 90 minutes after oral ingestion of PCE by rats (Warren et al., 1996). PCE concentrations in the liver, kidney, brain, and lungs of a dry cleaner who died following exposure to high concentrations of PCE vapors were 240, 71, 69, and 30 mg/kg, respectively. An abnormally high lipid content and the high lipophilicity of the solvent account for the relatively higher PCE content in the liver of this patient (Levine et al., 1981). Existing tissue levels and total body burden determine further tissue distribution (Pegg et al., 1979). Well-perfused tissues such as the parenchymal organs, brain, and skeletal muscles quickly reach saturation, while saturation is reached more slowly in the poorly perfused adipose tissues (Guberan and Fernandez, 1974; Monster et al., 1979; Warren et al., 1996) (Fig. 12-1). Levels of PCE in adipose tissue continue to increase after cessation of exposure, due to redistribution of the solvent (Guberan and Fernandez, 1974). Elimination from adipose tissue is slow and accumulation occurs with repeated exposures (Monster et al., 1979). Total accumulation of PCE is related to the volume of adipose tissue within the body, which in turn proportionally alters the biological half-life of the compound (Guberan and Fernandez, 1974; Cohr, 1986). Thus, obese persons accumulate larger amounts and exhibit a longer biological half-life of the PCE body burden than do lean persons (Monster et al., 1983). Furthermore, after cessation of exposure, the release of PCE stored in adipose tissue becomes a continuing source of further exposure to the solvent (Stewart et al., 1970; Guberan and Fernandez, 1974; Monster et al., 1979; Cohr, 1986).

Tissue Biochemistry

Most (80% to 95%) of an absorbed dose of PCE remains unchanged and does not undergo biotransformation. Ap-

proximately 20% of an absorbed dose of PCE is oxidized (epoxidation) in the liver by the cytochrome P-450 metabolic pathway to the reactive intermediate PCE epoxide (Yllner, 1961; Daniel, 1963; Leibman and Ortiz, 1975, 1977; Savolainen et al., 1977; Moslen et al., 1977; Pegg et al., 1979; Costa and Ivanetich, 1980; Toftgard and Gustafsson, 1980). Metabolism of PCE is saturable in humans (Ohtsuki et al., 1983). PCE epoxide undergoes spontaneous intramolecular rearrangement to become trichloroacetyl chloride, which is rapidly hydrolyzed to trichloroacetic acid (TCAA) (Leibman and Ortiz, 1975, 1977; Lauwerys et al., 1983). Trichloroacetaldehyde (chloral) is formed from TCAA (Mutti and Franchini, 1987). Chloral is subsequently hydrated to chloral hydrate, which is converted to trichloroethanol (TCEtOH) and TCAA through the actions of alcohol dehydrogenase and chloral hydrate dehydrogenase, respectively (Lauwerys et al., 1983; Mutti and Franchini, 1987). Trichloroethanol and TCAA are conjugated with glucuronide before being excreted in the urine (Ogata et al., 1971; Monster et al., 1983; Lauwerys et al., 1983; Monster, 1984; Garnier et al., 1996). The urinary metabolites of PCE also include thioethers, which result from glutathione conjugation of PCE epoxide formed by the epoxidation of PCE (Yllner, 1961; Lafuente and Mallol, 1986) (Fig. 12-2). Urinary thioether levels of six female dry cleaners showed gradual increases throughout a workweek of exposure to PCE (Lafuente and Mallol, 1986). Other possible metabolites of PCE include oxalic acid, dichloroacetic acid, and inorganic chloride (Yllner 1961; Daniel, 1963; Lafuente and Mallol, 1986). Ethnic differences in PCE metabolism have been noted (Seiji et al., 1989).

The acute effects of PCE appear to be due to the metabolite trichloroethanol, which potentiates GABA-ergic activity and inhibits excitatory amino acid activity (Peoples and Weight, 1994). The chronic effects associated with exposure to PCE have been attributed to the metabolite PCE epoxide, which is an electrophilic alkylating agent (Moslen et al., 1977; Pegg et al., 1979; Buben and O'Flaherty, 1985). Increased blood ammonia levels associated with PCE-induced liver damage may also contribute to the neurotoxic effects of PCE (Moslen et al., 1977; Reynolds and Moslen, 1977).

PCE interacts with other chemicals, often affecting its metabolism and clinical effects. Chemicals (such as ethanol) which induce cytochrome P-450 activity enhance the metabolism and toxicity of PCE (Ikeda and Imamura, 1973; Moslen et al., 1977; Toftgard and Gustafsson, 1980). The metabolism of trichloroethylene is suppressed during coexposure to PCE, possibly due to competition for cytochrome P-450 monooxygenases which are involved in the epoxidation of both of these chemicals, suggesting that PCE metabolism may also be suppressed by coexposure to trichloroethylene (Ikeda, 1977; Seiji et al., 1989). A positive interaction resulting in enhanced toxicity has been demonstrated during simultaneous exposure to mixtures of

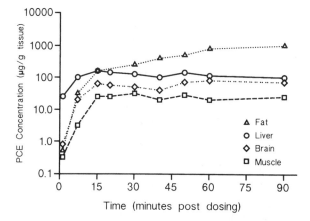

FIG. 12-1. Perchloroethylene concentrations in the brain, fat, liver, and skeletal muscle of rats at 0 to 90 minutes after exposure. This figure demonstrates uptake of PCE following oral ingestion of 160 mg/kg. (From the data of Warren et al., 1996, with permission.)

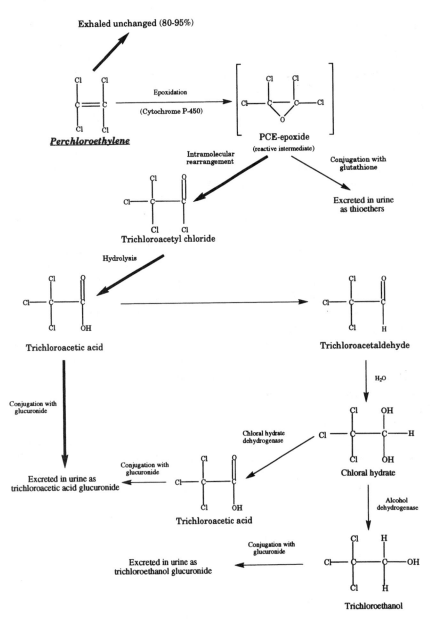

FIG. 12-2. Proposed metabolic pathway for perchloroethylene in humans (Yllner, 1961; Daniel, 1963; Ogata et al., 1971; Leibman and Ortiz, 1975, 1977; Savolainen et al., 1977; Moslen et al., 1977; Pegg et al., 1979; Costa and Ivanetich, 1980; Toftgård and Gustafsson, 1980; Lauwerys et al., 1983; Monster et al., 1983; Monster, 1984; Lafuente and Mallol, 1986; Mutti and Franchini, 1987; Garnier et al., 1996).

PCE, TCE, and 1,1,1,-trichloroethane both *in vitro* and *in vivo,* suggesting that the effects of coexposure are additive (Stacy, 1989). Concurrent consumption of ethanol also inhibits the metabolism of PCE, and intolerance to alcohol has been reported (Gold, 1969; Müller et al., 1975; Stewart et al., 1977). Liver alcohol dehydrogenase catalyzes the reduction of chloral hydrate to TCEtOH, and it also catalyzes the oxidation of ethanol to acetaldehyde. Thus, coexposure increases blood ethanol levels (Bartonicek, 1962; Müller et al., 1975; Köppel et al., 1988; Sato et al., 1991). The PCE metabolite TCAA increases the effects of anticoagulant drugs such as warfarin, which competes for the same protein sites as does TCAA (Sellers and Koch-Weser, 1970).

Ethanol and benzodiazepine anxiolytic prescription drugs, such as diazepam, are commonly used by workers who may be concurrently exposed to PCE (Rall, 1990). A controlled study of the effects of ethanol, diazepam, and PCE alone and in combination was done in 12 human volunteers (Stewart et al., 1977). PCE exposure was a low level of 25 ppm and a maximum of 100 ppm; ethanol doses were 0.75 and 1.50 mL of 100-proof vodka per kilogram body weight to achieve blood levels of 40 and 80 mg/dL; diazepam, 6 mg/day (low) and 10 mg/day (high), was administered in divided daily doses. Exposure to PCE at a concentration of 25 ppm with concurrent ethanol exposure significantly increased the PCE blood levels of the volunteers above the basal blood levels measured during exposure to PCE alone. In contrast, at the higher PCE exposure concentration of 100 ppm, ethanol consumption did not significantly increase the PCE blood levels of the volunteers, indicating that metabolism of PCE was saturated at this level of exposure. In contrast, diazepam did not have an effect on PCE blood levels at exposures of 25 ppm or 100 ppm. Behavioral effects of administered combinations of PCE and ethanol or diazepam were also assessed. Decrements in eye–hand coordination (which could impair the job performance), were found in subjects exposed to either PCE, ethanol, or diazepam alone. However, performance was not further decreased during simultaneous exposure at these levels. It was concluded that use of low doses of ethanol or diazepam during exposure to PCE at concentrations up to 100 ppm had no consistent additive effect on human performance of neurobehavioral tasks and therefore would not increase the risk of worker injury associated with exposure to ethanol or diazepam alone.

Excretion

The excretion characteristics of PCE are similar whether following either inhalation or oral ingestion, and they reflect this solvent's low degree of metabolism (Pegg et al., 1979). The solubility of PCE in the blood and body tissues is high, where it is retained; correspondingly, the ease of release and rate of elimination through exhalation is low (Monster et al., 1983). The biological half-life for the percentage of PCE excreted through the lungs is approximately 65 hours (Ikeda and Imamura, 1973). The majority (80% to 95%) of an absorbed dose of PCE is excreted unchanged through the lungs (Fernandez et al., 1976; Pegg et al., 1979; Köppel et al., 1985), and pulmonary elimination is enhanced by activities that increase the pulmonary ventilatory rate (Guberan and Fernandez, 1974; Köppel et al., 1985). That portion of an absorbed dose of PCE which is metabolized is excreted through the kidneys and is eliminated in the urine as TCAA and trichloroethanol (Yllner, 1961; Daniel, 1963; Fernandez et al., 1976; Leibman and Ortiz, 1977; Pegg et al., 1979; Ohtsuki et al., 1983; Köppel et al., 1985; Garnier et al., 1996). Unchanged PCE has been detected in the urine following oral ingestion (Köppel et al., 1985). It is also found in the breast milk of exposed women (Schreiber, 1993).

The relationship between PCE exposure and TCAA excretion is linear up to approximately 100 ppm; at concentrations above 100 ppm, metabolism begins to become saturated and the percent of the PCE excreted as TCAA is decreased (Ikeda et al., 1972; Pegg et al., 1979; Ohtsuki et al., 1983; Seiji et al., 1989). Maximum urinary excretion of TCAA occurs within 24 to 48 hours after cessation of exposure and reflects elimination of PCE from the well-perfused parenchymal organs and muscle tissue (Ogata et al., 1971; Guberan and Fernandez, 1974; Fernandez et al., 1976). The biological half-life for total trichloro compounds (TCAA + TCEtOH) excreted in the urine following exposure to PCE is 144 hours (Ikeda and Imamura, 1973). Because PCE accumulates in adipose tissue, its gradual release into blood and subsequent metabolism results in a corresponding increase in urinary TCAA concentration during chronic exposures (Stewart et al., 1970; Ikeda and Imamura, 1973; Guberan and Fernandez, 1974).

The urinary concentration of total trichloro compounds is decreased during concurrent exposures to PCE and trichloroethylene, reflecting the competitive inhibitions of metabolism that occur during coexposure to these two solvents (Seiji et al., 1989). Concurrent consumption of ethanol interferes with the metabolism of PCE and therefore decreases the concentration of TCAA in urine (Müller et al., 1975; Köppel et al., 1988; Sato et al., 1991). Chemicals (such as phenobarbital) which induce cytochrome P-450 enzyme activity enhance the urinary excretion of total trichloro compounds (Ikeda and Imamura, 1973).

CLINICAL MANIFESTATIONS AND DIAGNOSIS

Symptomatic Diagnosis

Exposure to PCE by oral intake or inhalation has been associated with acute and chronic neurological manifestations (Kendrick, 1929; Sandground, 1941; Rowe et al., 1952; Haerer and Udelman, 1964; Stewart et al., 1961; Stewart, 1969; Morgan, 1969; Gold, 1969; Lackore and Perkins, 1970; Patel et al., 1973; Hake and Stewart, 1977; Lukaszewski, 1979; Levine et al., 1981; Lauwerys et al., 1983; Köppel et al., 1985; Seeber, 1989; Garnier et al., 1996). Because many of the symptoms associated with exposure to PCE are nonspecific, information regarding the patient's potential for exposure to PCE and other neurotoxicants from either occupational and/or environmental sources should be obtained.

Acute Exposure

Acute oral ingestion results in reversible symptoms of nausea, vomiting, inebriation, dizziness, irritability, and amnesia (Kendrick, 1929; Sandground 1941; Haerer and Udelman, 1964; Köppel et al., 1985). Prolonged narcosis follows larger oral doses. For example, 1 hour after ingesting 5 mL of PCE as an anthelmintic, a 21-year-old army cadet officer became irrational and was extremely agitated. The patient remained in this state for approximately 1 hour, following which he was amnesic for the entire episode (Haerer and Udelman, 1964). A 6-year-old boy who ingested 8 to 10 mL of pure liquid PCE was comatose within 1 hour after ingestion. The child recovered and was discharged from the hospital in apparently good clinical health 9 days after the incident (Köppel et al., 1985).

Acute inhalation of PCE vapors produces irritation of mucous membranes, lacrimation, nausea, light-headedness, dizziness, floating sensation, sense of inebriation, ataxia, headache, fatigue, mood changes, impaired cognition, loss of consciousness, coma, and death (Rowe et al., 1952; Coler and Rossmiller, 1953; Stewart et al., 1961; Saland, 1967; Stewart, 1969; Morgan, 1969; Lackore and Perkins, 1970; Patel et al., 1973; Hake and Stewart, 1977; Lukaszewski, 1979; Garnier et al., 1996). Symptoms experienced at work by dry cleaners exposed to PCE at concentrations of up to 20 ppm included dizziness and a drunken feeling (Cai et al., 1991) (Table 12-2). In a study of 16 healthy volunteers acutely exposed to PCE vapors at a concentration of 100 ppm for 7 hours, 10 (63%) experienced mild eye, nose, and throat irritation (Stewart et al., 1970). Three subjects had difficulty performing a modified Romberg test within the first 3 hours of exposure; but with greater mental effort, these same subjects were able to perform a second Romberg's test normally. By the end of the 7-hour exposure period, 4 (25%) of the subjects reported frontal headache and some difficulty speaking. These findings suggest differences in individual susceptibility to the effects of PCE (Seiji et al., 1989). Although the central nervous system effects of PCE at this level of exposure appear clinically to be minor, an individual's ability to perform his or her job properly and safely may already be impaired, and performance on specific and selected tasks may reveal deficits.

Another group of volunteers were exposed to PCE at concentrations of up to 5,000 ppm. Subjects were initially exposed to PCE vapors at an average concentration of 935 ppm for 90 minutes. Effects experienced at this level included conjunctival and nasal irritation, frontal sinuses pressure, mental slowness, lethargy, and then a feeling of exhilaration. After 90 minutes the concentration in the chamber was raised to 1,500 ppm. At this level, all subjects were definitely inebriated, but after several minutes of exposure they began to experience feelings of dizziness and faintness prompting termination of the session. Following a brief exposure-free period, the subjects reentered the chamber and were exposed to a PCE concentration of 2,000 ppm. At this concentration, the narcotic effect was immediately significant and was accompanied by nausea, tinnitus, and vertigo. The PCE vapor concentration was then increased to 5,000 ppm. This level produced severe eye irritation, increased salivation, nausea, vertigo, depressed mental activ-

ity, and somnolence and could only be tolerated by the subjects for about 6 minutes before impelling their departure from the exposure chamber. These results illustrate the acute symptomatic effects of PCE exposure and demonstrate the relationship between these effects and the concentration of an acute exposure dose (Carpenter, 1937).

An example of a short but intense occupational exposure to PCE is a patient examined in our clinic (R. G. Feldman, personal observation). A 42-year-old woman worked in a dry-cleaning shop for 4 years. The room in which she worked was 5 feet by 15 feet and had no ventilation system and no windows, and the door was kept closed during the winter months. She reported that she never used personal protective equipment such as gloves, an apron, or a respirator. One day a down coat she was cleaning came apart and spread feathers all over the inside of the chamber of the dry-cleaning machine. She promptly turned off the machine and began to clean up all the feathers, which were soaked with PCE. She lost consciousness as a result of this unexpected high-level exposure and was sent to a local hospital for treatment. At the hospital she was given oxygen, but no other treatment for exposure to PCE was provided. When she regained consciousness she was "confused." She was released from the hospital and stayed home for 2 weeks. After 2 weeks she returned to her job at the dry-cleaning shop. Residual confusion and vertigo made it difficult for her to perform her job properly, and after only 2 months she left work permanently. She has also developed sensitivity to a variety of household chemicals including Lysol, Clorox, perfumes, and gasoline. The patient experiences dizziness whenever she smells these chemicals and has what can be described as multiple chemical sensitivity. She has not worked around PCE or other volatile chemicals since quitting her job at the dry cleaner.

Chronic Exposure

Chronic inhalation exposure to PCE results in persistent symptoms of altered mood, ethanol intolerance, fatigue, decreased attention, poor short-term memory, impaired intellectual functioning, perseveration, and disorientation (Coler and Rossmiller, 1953; Gold, 1969; Lauwerys et al., 1983; Seeber, 1989; Cai et al., 1991). A 47-year-old man developed persistent impairment of short-term memory, mood lability, and stammering speech following occupational exposure to unknown concentrations of PCE for 3 years (Gold, 1969). In an epidemiological study (Cai et al., 1991) the prevalence of subjective symptoms occurring during the immediate past 3-month period among 56 dry cleaners exposed to PCE at an 8-hour TWA ambient air concentration of 20 ppm for durations of 1 to 120 months were assessed using a questionnaire. The responses of the exposed dry cleaners were compared with those of 69 nonexposed age- and sex-matched controls. Forgetfulness and fainting after standing up were the most frequently experienced symptoms (Table 12-3). In a simi-

TABLE 12-2. *Prevalence of acute symptoms among dry cleaners (n = 56) exposed to PCE at an 8-hr TWA concentration of 20 ppm*

Symptom	Exposed, number (%)	Controls, number (%)
Dizziness	25 (44.6)[a]	8 (11.6)
Drunken feeling	10 (17.9)[c]	0 (0.0)
Heavy feeling in head	11 (19.6)[c]	1 (1.4)
Unusual smell	11 (19.6)[c]	0 (0.0)
Nasal irritation	16 (28.6)[b]	5 (7.2)
Floating sensation	13 (23.2)[b]	4 (5.8)
Face flushing	5 (8.9)[a]	0 (0.0)
Headache	13 (23.2)	8 (11.6)
Sore throat	11 (19.6)	6 (8.7)

Symptom prevalence among exposed workers is compared with that of nonexposed controls (*n* = 69).

[a]$p < 0.05$.
[b]$p < 0.01$.
[c]$p < 0.001$.

Modified from Cai et al., 1991, with permission.

TABLE 12-3. *Prevalence of chronic symptoms experienced during the past 3 months among dry cleaners (n = 56) exposed to PCE at an 8-hr TWA concentration of 20 ppm for up to 120 months*

Symptom	Exposed, number (%)	Controls, number (%)
Forgetfulness	22 (39.3)[b]	10 (14.5)
Fainting after standing up	20 (35.7)[b]	10 (14.5)
Poor appetite	15 (26.8)[b]	4 (5.8)
Heavy feeling in head	9 (16.1)[b]	1 (1.4)
Changes in perspiration	10 (17.9)[b]	1 (1.4)
Joint pain	8 (14.3)[b]	0 (0.0)
Drunken feeling	6 (10.3)[b]	8 (11.6)
Dullness in extremities	15 (26.8)[a]	8 (11.6)

Symptom prevalence among exposed workers is compared with that of nonexposed controls (*n* = 69).
[a]*p* < 0.05.
[b]*p* < 0.01.
Modified from Cai et al., 1991, with permission.

lar study, symptoms experienced among degreasers chronically exposed to PCE at vapor concentrations of 230 to 385 ppm include nausea, lightheadedness, dizziness, feelings of intoxication, laughing spells, ataxia, fainting spells, headache, fatigue, slowed ability to think, and impaired memory function (Coler and Rossmiller, 1953). Chmielewski et al. (1976) assessed workers exposed to PCE for periods ranging from 2 months to 27 years. The most frequently reported symptoms among these workers were dizziness, drowsiness, fatigue, and headache. In addition, the workers who had longer durations of exposure showed increased tolerance, suggesting that adaptation to the effects of PCE occurs among chronically exposed workers.

The clinical presentation of cognitive impairments associated with long-term exposure to PCE and/or mixed volatile organic solvents are similar to the dementia of the Alzheimer's type (Freed and Kandel, 1988). Careful differentiation of the symptoms of dementing syndromes (such as probable Alzheimer's disease or multiinfarct vascular disease) from those associated with solvent encephalopathy—although it is sometimes difficult without exposure data and serial clinical and neuropsychological test measures—is extremely important (Moss et al., 1986; White, 1987; White et al., 1992; Echeverria et al., 1995; Mikkelsen, 1995). In dementias associated with neurodegenerative diseases such as Alzheimer's disease, the dementia is persistent and progressive, whereas a solvent-induced dementia generally does not progress and may remit once the individual is removed from further toxic exposure (Mikkelsen, 1995). Furthermore, the results of neuropsychological testing which often demonstrate features which are more or less typical for cortical, white matter, diffuse, focal, or primarily affective disorders can assist in the differentiation of these dementias. Neuropsychological tests of language/verbal skills tend to demonstrate greater relative preservation of this functional domain in cases of solvent encephalopathy than is typically seen in Alzheimer's

disease (Moss and Albert, 1992; White et al., 1992) (see Neuropsychological Diagnosis section).

Neurophysiological Diagnosis

Electroencephalographic recordings of three male and four female volunteers acutely exposed to PCE at 100 ppm showed an overall slowing of the brain-wave frequency and an accompanying increase in amplitude, predominantly in the occipital leads. This pattern is similar to that seen when a patient is in the first stages of anesthesia (Stewart et al., 1981). Paroxysmal high-voltage slow waves and sharp waves were seen in four workers chronically exposed to PCE for 4 to 13 years (Chmielewski et al., 1976). In contrast, the electroencephalogram (EEG) of a 47-year-old man who developed persistent impairment of short-term memory, mood lability, and stammering speech after 3 years of exposure to unknown concentrations of PCE was symmetrical with well-regulated alpha activity and no abnormalities at rest, or during photic stimulation or hyperventilation (Gold, 1969) (see Clinical Experiences section). Thus, acute effects of PCE cause significant slowing in the EEG, while chronic exposure cases may also produce slow waves or may have no effect on the background electroencephalographic pattern. In comparison, the EEG of metabolic encephalopathy is slow and recovers with time as the chemical derangement associated with the metabolic disturbance is corrected; the EEG of Alzheimer's disease, on the other hand, remains normal until late in the course of the disease and then progresses as does the dementia (Aminoff, 1986).

Visual evoked potentials (VEPs), *visual contrast sensitivity* (VCS), and *brain-stem auditory evoked potentials* (BAEPs) were used to assess the subclinical acute CNS effects of PCE in 22 male volunteers (Altmann et al., 1990). The subjects were divided into high (50 ppm) and low (10 ppm) exposure groups and inhaled PCE vapor in a special chamber for 4 hours per day for 4 days. Blood concentrations of PCE were also determined daily. Peak latencies of the VEP components N75, P100, and N150 were measured on the four exposure days as well as on the day before exposure began and the day after cessation of exposure. Exposure to PCE at 50 ppm produced a significant prolongation of the peak VEP latencies of N75, P100, and N150. The average prolongation of latencies in the high-exposure group reached significance by the fifth day of exposure, and the effects of PCE on N150 latency persisted for at least 1 day after cessation of exposure, reflecting the longer half-life of the larger dose of PCE (Table 12-4). While the VEPs of the high-exposure group tended to increase during exposure, the VEP latencies of the low-exposure subjects showed a tendency to decrease, suggesting that the effects of PCE on visual system functioning are biphasic. VCS was impaired in the high-exposure group; this effect was most pronounced on the fourth day of exposure. Blood concentrations of PCE were highest on the last day of exposure, correlating with the greatest impairments in VCS. These results suggest that acute exposure to PCE affects the visual system, delays neuronal processing time, and alters visual contrast perception. Differences in BAEP peak latencies were not seen.

Neuropsychological Diagnosis

Neuropsychological assessment can be used to document the clinical presentation and to detect the subclinical effects of PCE exposure (White et al., 1990; Echeverria et al., 1995). Exposure to PCE has been associated with impaired performance on tests of attention and executive function, memory, psychomotor speed, and visuospatial functioning. Tests of personality and affect reveal emotional lability and irritability. Verbal and language functioning are spared (Seeber, 1989; Echeverria et al., 1995).

A computer-based performance system was used to assess the subclinical neurobehavioral effects of PCE in 60 female dry cleaners (mean age: 39.7 years) (Ferroni et al., 1992). These women had been exposed to PCE for a mean of 10 years at a media ambient air concentration of 15 ppm (range: 1 to 67 ppm). Median PCE blood level for the exposed workers was 145 mg/L (range: 12 to 846 mg/L). The performance of the dry cleaners was compared with that of 30 unexposed age- and sex-matched controls. Tests in-

cluded finger tapping (dominant and nondominant hands), simple reaction time, Digit Symbol, and two different shape comparison tests, one of vigilance and one of response to stress. The overall performances of the dry cleaners were impaired on simple reaction time, the shape comparison tests of vigilance, and response to stress, despite this, however, the performance scores did not significantly correlate with the duration of exposure, PCE concentrations in the ambient air, or individual PCE blood levels. The results of this study of dry cleaners at a median exposure level of 15 ppm can be compared with results in a group of 101 dry-cleaning-shop workers who were exposed to PCE at a higher level (TWA ambient air concentration of 30 ppm) (Seeber, 1989). The workers, divided into high-exposure (TWA: 52 ppm) and low-exposure (TWA: 12 ppm) groups, were compared with 84 unexposed controls. Differences in age, gender, and intelligence were controlled for by regression analysis. The subjects each completed a symptoms questionnaire and a personality inventory, and each received neuropsychological testing. Neurobehavioral domains assessed included perceptual speed, sensorimotor function and coordination, memory and attention, and intellectual functioning. Significant differences between the performance of the dry cleaners and the controls were found on tests of perceptual speed, memory, and intellectual functioning. Results of the symptoms questionnaire and personality assessment revealed increased incidence of nausea, unsteadiness of gait, emotional lability, tingling and numbness in the hands, and limb aches among the dry cleaners. Although this study also found a significant difference between the exposed workers and the controls, a dose–response relationship could not be established at these levels.

PCE and other chlorinated organic solvents affect specific neuropsychological domains, particularly functions mediated by the frontal and limbic systems of the brain (see Neuropathological Diagnosis section). For example, neuropsychological assessment of four individuals exposed to PCE revealed impaired motor skills in three patients, impaired performance on visuospatial tests in three patients, and memory was affected in all four patients (Echeverria et al., 1995). Tests of attention and executive function also revealed impairments and, the Wisconsin Card Sorting Test was the most sensitive measure of im-

TABLE 12-4. *Mean peak visual evoked potential latencies and standard deviations in one volunteer following acute exposure to PCE at 50 ppm for 4 days*[a]

Component	Day 1[b]	Day 2	Day 3	Day 4	Day 5	Day 6[b]
N75	82.0 ± 2.5	83.8 ± 2.5	84.1 ± 2.6	84.3 ± 2.2	85.7 ± 2.4	82.6 ± 1.9
P100	105.4 ± 1.9	106.8 ± 2.8	108.0 ± 2.8	107.4 ± 2.8	109.5 ± 1.4	105.8 ± 2.8
N150	143.5 ± 2.4	141.6 ± 3.5	147.1 ± 1.4	147.0 ± 0.7	149.4 ± 1.7	146.8 ± 2.0

[a]This table demonstrates prolongation of peak latencies of VEP components N75, P100, and N150 seen among all volunteers following acute exposure to PCE.
[b]Nonexposure control days.
Modified from Altmann et al., 1990, with permission.

pairments in this cognitive domain both during and after cessation of exposure. In contrast, performance on tests of language/verbal functions tended to be within expected limits both during and after cessation of exposure (Table 12-5).

Mood complaints were also common among these four PCE-exposed patients. Fatigue (four of four), tension (three of four), confusion (three of four), and anger (one of four) were reported on the Profile of Mood States (POMS). Two patients (1 and 2) reported an unusual number of somatic complaints on the Minnesota Multiphasic Personality Inventory (MMPI). However, the scores of these two subjects on the MMPI validity scales indicated a tendency to underreport symptoms, suggesting that these symptoms were not exaggerated or faked. Depression as assessed by the MMPI was not common among this group. Although affective and behavioral changes were reported, the symptoms were not consistent with clinical depression and appear to reflect an organic affective syndrome associated with solvent encephalopathy. In addition, the affective and behavioral changes in these patients do not explain the cognitive findings for the following reasons: (a) residual deficits in cognitive functioning remained when mood improved, and (b) deficits tended to cluster into specific

TABLE 12-5. *Neuropsychological findings in four persons exposed to PCE*

Neuropsychological test	1 38/F Exposure: 1 yr Test 1 (still exposed)	2 34/F Exposure: 10 yrs Test 1 (still exposed)	3 44/M Exposure: 16 yrs Test 1 (still exposed)	3 Retest 11 months after exposure	4 27/F Exposure: NR Test 1 (still exposed)	4 Retest 22 months after exposure	4 Retest 2 46 months after exposure
Intelligence quotient (WAIS-R)							
Verbal IQ	117	81	84[a]	99	107	115	105
Performance IQ	99	82	90[a]	107	84[a]	94	92
Full-scale IQ	109	80	86	101	97	106	99
Attention/executive function:							
Wechsler memory scale							
Digit spans	8/7	5/2[a]	5/4[a]	5/7	6/4	8/5	7/7
Mental control	6/6	7/9	4/6	4/6	6/9[a]	9/9	9/9
Wisconsin card sort (#sort/trials)	6/97[a]	—	5[a]/139[a]	2[a]/128[a]	—	—	1/64[a]
Continuous performance test	—	—	—	—	Slow	22 errors	—
Verbal language							
WAIS-R							
Information/vocabulary	13/10	6/7	—	13/7	11/12	14/12	11/10
Comprehension similarities	11/15	7/7	—	12/10	10/11	13/12	12/12
Boston Naming Test							
Total uncued	55/60	54/85	—	—	78/85	78/85	81/85
Total cued	3	18	—	—	4	4	3
Motor							
Santa Ana							
Right/left	17[a]/16[a]	—	19[a]/32	18[a]/20[a]	16.5/16.5[a]	19[a]/19[a]	—
Both	21[a]	—	24[a]	27	25[a]	23.5[a]	—
Visuospatial							
Picture completion/arrangement	10/11	6/8	9/8[a]	14/11	8/9	9/9	11/8
Block design/object assembly	10/8[a]	7/9	10/9	10/11	4[a]/6[a]	7[a]/1	8[a]/7
Sticks test: copy/reversed	—	—	8[a]/5[a]	10/5[a]	—	—	—
Memory							
WMS (R): MQ, GMQ	100	79	78[a]	93	84[a]	106	120
Log memory IR:score/%ile or ASS	29/64%	19/9.9	14[a]/9%	20/32	11[a]/7.1[a]	15/9.1	19/9.9
Log memory DR:score/%ile or ASS	22[a]/51%	18/—	11[a]/9%	19/45	6[a]/—	12/—	15/—
Verbal PAL IR:score/possible	19/24	20/30	12[a]/24	15[a]/24	25/30	28/30	29/30
Verbal PAL DR:score/possible	7/8	7[a]/10	5[a]/8	6[a]/8	9/10	10/10	10/10
Visual PAL:IR/DR	18/6	—	9[a]/3[a]	9[a]/3[a]	—	—	—
Visual reproduction IR/DR:(%ile or ASS)	20%/11%	4.8[a]/4	68%/18%	98%/98%	5.6[a]/0[a]	8.8[a]/8	9.3[a]/8
Benton Visual Retention: F/G (15 poss)	12[a]/14	11/12	11[a]/8[a]	13/15	—	13/15	—
Difficult PAL: IR/DR	28/9	—	—	—	3[a]/—	12[a]/5[a]	30/10
Milner recall (score/12)	10	12	6[a]	8[a]	10	8[a]	9

WAIS-R, Wechsler Adult Intelligence Scale–Revised; IQ, intelligence quotient; NR, not reported; [a], impaired performance; PAL, pair associates learning; IR, immediate recall; DR, delayed recall; ASS, age scaled score.
Modified from Echeverria et al., 1995, with permission.

behavioral domains rather than occurring sporadically or evenly across domains, as would be expected with depressed or distracted patients.

Postexposure retests were made in two of the four patients. Patient 3 (44-year-old man) showed marked improvement across all affected functional domains on follow-up testing 11 months after ending exposure. However, he continued to show performance deficits on the more difficult tasks in the affected domains, especially the Wisconsin Card Sorting Task (executive function); the Sticks Test, design reversal condition (visuospatial function); Visual and Verbal Paired Associate Learning Tests and Milner Recall (memory); and the Santa Ana Formboard test (motor coordination).

Patient 4 (27-year-old woman) was retested 2 years and again 4 years after cessation of exposure. At 2-year follow-up, improvement was seen across all functional domains. However, mild impairment of performance was still seen on the Continuous Performance Test (attention), on Block Designs (visuospatial), and on the Visual Reproductions, Difficult Paired Associate Learning, and Milner Recall tests (memory). At follow-up exam 4 years after exposure, the patient's husband reported that he did not feel that she was quite the same as she had been before the onset of her symptoms. Indeed, although the patient showed improvement on testing of some domains, marked impairment was still seen on the Wisconsin Card Sorting Test, and performance on Block Designs remained mildly below expectation. Although her score was within expected limits on Visual Reproductions, qualitative inspection of her drawing showed perseverative contamination of details from one drawing to another. These findings suggest that permanent

neuropathological changes resulting in impaired performance in specific functional domains occurs in persons exposed to PCE.

The effectiveness of a battery of neuropsychological tests in detecting subclinical effects of PCE neurotoxicity was studied epidemiologically in a group of 65 dry cleaners exposed to known levels ($\leq$40.8 ppm) of PCE (Echeverria et al., 1995) (see Clinical Experiences section). Neuropsychological assessment revealed impaired performance on tests of short-term visual memory including the Visual Reproductions Test, the Pattern Memory Test, and the Pattern Recognition Test (Table 12-6). These findings suggest that chronic low-level exposure to PCE produces subclinical effects on visually mediated functions, and they demonstrate that behavioral testing can be used to document the subclinical effects of PCE exposure.

The results of these neuropsychological tests have definite implications for the challenges of daily living. Impairment in nonverbal memory could produce tendencies to become lost or disoriented in unfamiliar places, diminish the exposed individual's safety when working with machines requiring good visuomotor coordination, or impair memory of new faces, as well as impair the ability to process nonverbal information, including facial expressions or emotional nuances in interpersonal interactions.

Color vision function following chronic low-level exposure to PCE has been investigated with equivocal results (Nakatsuka et al., 1992; Cavalleri et al., 1994). Workers exposed only to PCE (mean exposure: 13 ppm) were compared with workers exposed to a mixture of PCE (mean exposure: 12 ppm) and TCE (mean exposure: 7 ppm). Both groups were also compared with a group of unexposed

TABLE 12-6. *Neuropsychological findings in 65 dry cleaners exposed to PCE*

Neuropsychological test	Exposure level			Difference (low–high)	Percent difference	Statistical significance
	Low	Moderate	High			
Attention/executive function:						
Digit span: A/U	5.63/5.74	5.69/5.59	5.72/5.68	−0.09/0.06	1.5/1.0	NS/NS
Trails						
Test A: A/U	30.49/27.80	33.19/36.92	35.47/35.35	−4.97/−7.54	10.3/27.1	NS/NS
Test B: A/U	87.31/80.17	85.14/103.28	96.21/89.46	−8.90/−9.29	16.2/11.6	NS/NS
Psychomotor function						
Symbol digit						
Number correct: A/U	0.87/0.79	0.76/0.78	1.10/1.17	−0.24/−0.38	27.6/48.1	NS/NS
Response time: A/U	23.34/23.69	24.52/23.71	26.04/26.30	−2.70/−2.61	11.6/11.0	NS/NS
Visual function						
Visual reproduction: A/U	9.45/9.66	8.89/8.77	8.08/7.95	1.36/1.71	14.4/17.7	0.0/0.03
Pattern memory						
Number correct: A/U	10.51/10.67	10.36/10.50	9.70/9.43	0.70/1.23	6.7/11.5	0.00/0.02
Response time: A/U	5.79/5.69	5.78/5.99	6.37/6.32	−0.58/−0.63	10.0/11.0	0.00/NS
Pattern recognition						
Number correct: A/U	14.39/14.50	13.97/13.94	13.83/13.74	0.56/0.74	3.9/5.1	0.00/0.04
Response time: A/U	3.68/3.66	3.72/3.84	4.30/4.23	−0.61/−0.57	16.6/15.6	NS/NS

NS, not significant; NS > 0.10; A/U, adjusted/unadjusted scores.
Modified from Echeverria et al., 1995, with permission.

controls (Nakatsuka et al., 1992). No difference in color discrimination was found between the groups at these levels of exposure. In contrast, a subclinical dose-dependent loss of color discrimination in the blue–yellow range was detected in 35 workers from 12 small dry-cleaning shops (Cavalleri et al., 1994). The exposed group consisted of 33 women and two men who were exposed to PCE at vapor concentrations ranging from 0.38 to 31.19 ppm. The dry cleaners were compared with 35 unexposed controls matched for age, sex, alcohol consumption, and cigarette smoking habits. Color vision loss in this group of workers was assessed using the Lanthony D-15, (Mergler and Blain, 1987). Because acquired dyschromatopsia can be monocular, the test was performed on each eye separately. In addition, the test scores from this group of PCE-exposed workers were expressed as a color confusion index (CCI), which further increases the sensitivity of this test (Bowman, 1982). Only three of the 35 dry cleaners had a perfect CCI score, while this was achieved by 13 of the 35 unexposed control subjects. CCI scores were not related to duration of PCE exposure. Neurophysiological tests of the effect of PCE on color vision reveal definite effects, but the results are affected by the sensitivity of the tests used (Bowman, 1982).

Biochemical Diagnosis

Direct analysis of adipose tissue for its PCE content is the most specific method of biochemical diagnosis, especially for confirming of chronic exposures to low levels of PCE (Anderson, 1985). However, other preferred and less invasive methods are available for general monitoring of populations and individuals exposed to PCE. These include determination of PCE in exhaled air and the urinary concentration of the PCE metabolite TCAA. The ACGIH has determined and recommended *biological exposure indices* (BEIs) for TCAA in urine and for PCE in alveolar air and in blood (ACGIH, 1995) (Table 12-7). Because PCE accumulates in the body tissues of chronically exposed individuals, these BEIs correlate better with the TWA exposure for the preceding workweek than with that for the immediately preceding day. In addition, persons with a higher percentage of body fat can absorb more PCE and therefore may show an initial acute increase in their tolerance to its effects (Monster et al., 1983) (see Tissue Distribution section).

Measures of PCE and TCAA levels in blood can be used as a means of monitoring an individual's acute and chronic exposures to PCE (Monster et al., 1979, 1983; Monster, 1984). PCE concentration in blood reflects acute and the immediate past exposures better than does blood TCAA level (Monster et al., 1979). PCE is detectable in the blood of persons who have consumed drinking water containing a PCE concentration greater than 120 µg/L (Kido et al., 1989). Repeated exposures lead to accumulation of PCE in the body, and thus the daily basal blood level is usually increased over a totally unexposed basal state (Monster et al., 1983). Therefore, when monitoring chronically exposed workers, the blood samples should be taken at the beginning of the work shift on the last day of the workweek to obtain a measure of total exposure. The concentration of PCE in the blood should not exceed 1 mg/L (ACGIH, 1995). Recent dermal exposure to liquid PCE should also be considered when sampling the blood of workers because the skin source of PCE may contaminate and add to the PCE in the blood sample (Monster et al., 1983; Aitio et al., 1984). PCE concentrations in blood taken from the exposed arms of volunteers (the exposed arm had been immersed in PCE for 5 minutes) were markedly increased over those in the unexposed arm for up to 5 hours after cessation of exposure (Aitio et al., 1984).

ACGIH has not determined a BEI for blood TCAA, but Monster et al. (1983) showed that a blood TCAA level of 20 µmol/L would not be exceeded if the PCE exposure levels were kept under 50 ppm. Blood TCAA can be used to assess the TWA exposure over the preceding week (Müller et al., 1974; Monster et al., 1983; Monster, 1984). The TCAA concentration in the blood of volunteers continued to rise until 20 hours after the end of an exposure episode. From about 60 hours after cessation of exposure, the blood TCAA concentration of these volunteers decreased with a half-time of 75 to 80 hours. The half-life of TCAA in blood is greater than that of PCE because TCAA binds to plasma proteins and accumulates (Monster et al., 1979). Since TCAA is also a metabolite of other solvents such as TCE, exposure to other sources of this metabolite must be considered when using TCAA as a marker of exposure to PCE (Monster, 1988).

PCE concentration in alveolar air is the most accurate noninvasive method of ascertaining an individual's exposure level. The concentration of PCE in alveolar air is

TABLE 12-7. *Biological exposure indices for perchloroethylene*

	Urine	Blood	Alveolar air
Determinant:	TCAA	PCE	PCE
Start of shift:	Not established	Not established	Not established
During shift:	Not established	Not established	Not established
Prior to last shift of workweek:	3.5 mg/L	1 mg/L	10 ppm

Data from ACGIH, 1995.

related to total uptake; it is therefore an indication of the level and duration of exposure as well as that of an individual's workload during an exposure period (Fernandez et al., 1976; Monster et al., 1979; Monster, 1984). The PCE concentration in the alveolar air closely parallels that of the blood (Monster et al., 1983) (Fig. 12-3). The ACGIH BEI for PCE in end-exhaled air (alveolar air) prior to the last shift of the workweek is a maximum of 10 ppm. The concentration of PCE in the alveolar air is at equilibrium with the pulmonary capillary blood, which is at equilibrium with the other various tissues of the body. Therefore, alveolar air concentration of PCE reflects the total body burden (Fernandez et al., 1976). The composition of the ambient air in an individual's work environment can vary considerably during the course of the day, and a worker's breath ventilation rate can vary with his or her level of physical activity; because of this, the quantity of PCE absorbed by two individuals working in the same shop may be considerably different and therefore can be used to identify workers with increased risk of developing exposure-related effects.

Urinary concentrations of PCE, TCAA, and trichloroethanol (TCEtOH) can also be used to confirm and/or monitor for exposure to PCE (Ikeda et al., 1972; Monster et al., 1983; Imbriani et al., 1988). The ACGIH BEI for TCAA in urine at the end of a workweek of exposure is a concentration of 3.5 mg/L (ACGIH, 1995–1996). However, urinary concentrations of TCAA are only related to exposure levels up to a PCE vapor concentration of 100 ppm (Ikeda et al., 1972; Pegg et al., 1979; Ohtsuki et al., 1983; Seiji et al., 1989). Furthermore, PCE metabolism is saturable, and therefore there may be no relationship between the amount of TCAA excreted at a particular time and the degree of exposure, stored tissue PCE, or injury the person may have already suffered (Ikeda et al., 1972;

Pegg et al., 1979; Ohtsuki et al., 1983; Seiji et al., 1989; Fernandez et al., 1976). Urinary concentrations of TCAA increase gradually during chronic exposures, and therefore urine TCAA concentration is more suitable for monitoring cumulative exposure than for documenting the most recent exposure (Stewart et al., 1970; Ikeda et al., 1972; Ikeda and Imamura, 1973; Guberan and Fernandez, 1974; Müller et al., 1974). Although TCEtOH concentration in urine is not recommended as a BEI by ACGIH, Monster et al. (1983) suggest that TCEtOH may better reflect PCE exposure over the immediately previous 2 days than does urine TCAA because it has a shorter urinary half-life than TCAA; 10 to 12 hours versus 65 to 90 hours, respectively.

Concurrent exposures to other chemicals alters concentrations of total trichloro compounds in the urine. Urinary concentration of total trichloro compounds is decreased during concurrent exposures to PCE and TCE (Seiji et al., 1989). Concurrent consumption of ethanol decreases the concentration of TCAA in urine (Müller et al., 1975, Köppel et al., 1988; Sato et al., 1991). Chronic exposure to chemicals (such as ethanol and phenobarbital) which induce cytochrome P-450 enzyme activity enhances the urinary excretion of the total trichloro compounds (Ikeda and Imamura, 1973).

Neuroimaging

Magnetic resonance imaging (MRI) and *computer-assisted tomography* (CT scan) can be used to differentiate PCE encephalopathy from other structural neurological disorders. An individual's occupational and environmental exposure history, as well as the reversibility or persistence of clinical findings and results on neurophysiological and neuropsychological testing, must be considered when interpreting the MRI or CT scan (Freed and Kandel, 1988). The MRI and CT scan of dementing diseases of the Alzheimer's type in early stages are usually normal; as the disease progresses, however, cerebral atrophy can be detected on these image studies (Freed and Kandel, 1988; Braffman et al., 1991). Neuroimaging in some individuals with PCE encephalopathy may also reveal cerebral atrophy. However, while the neuropsychological test results of patients with Alzheimer's disease show a progressive dementia, the results of neuropsychological testing in cases of solvent encephalopathy generally stabilize or improve following cessation of exposure (Freed and Kandel, 1988). A pneumoencephalogram and a brain scan did not reveal any abnormalities in a 47-year-old man who developed persistent impairment of short-term memory, mood lability, and stammering speech following occupational exposure to unknown concentrations of PCE for 3 years (Gold, 1969) (see Clinical Experiences section). The MRI was normal in a 62-year-old dry cleaner with dementia related to chronic PCE exposure and in a 42-year-old dry-cleaner worker

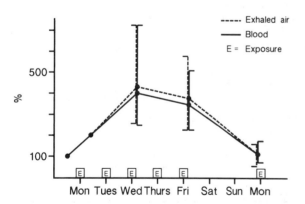

FIG. 12-3. Geometrical mean PCE concentrations in alveolar air and blood of workers from three dry-cleaning shops and one metal-cleaning shop exposed to PCE concentrations of 1.5 to 160 ppm. This figure demonstrates a close relationship between PCE concentrations in blood and alveolar air. (Modified from Monster et al., 1983, with permission.)

with subacute PCE-induced encephalopathy (R. G. Feldman, M.D., personal observation).

Neuropathological Diagnosis

Seldom does acute PCE exposure cause death, and there are virtually no reports of the histopathology in post-PCE encephalopathy. Chemical determinations of brain tissue PCE concentrations in postmortem samples from exposed individuals were found to be between 69 and 79 mg/kg, indicating that PCE crosses the BBB (Levine et al., 1981; Gaillard et al., 1995; Garnier et al., 1996). A PCE metabolite, PCE epoxide, reacts with membrane lipids, cytoskeletal proteins, and nucleic acids of DNA and RNA (Bonse et al., 1975; Moslen et al., 1977; Bolt and Filser, 1977; Pegg et al., 1979; Wang et al., 1993). Exposure to PCE has been associated with alterations in the fatty acid composition of phospholipids (Kyrklund et al., 1984, 1987). Decreased levels of cholesterol and monoenoic fatty acids are found in the brains of rats exposed to PCE, suggesting that exposure to this solvent produces a persisting loss of myelin (Kyrklund et al., 1990). A decrease in brain RNA content was seen following exposure of rats to 200 ppm PCE vapor for 6 hours per day for 4 days, suggesting that PCE also interferes with protein metabolism (Savolainen et al., 1977). Following exposure to 600 ppm of PCE vapor for 12 weeks, total brain tissue weights were reduced and brain weight ratios (brain area weight/total brain weight) were significantly lower in the frontal cerebral cortex and brain stems of rats. DNA content was also reduced in the frontal cortex and brain stem of these animals. In addition, the concentrations of glial and neuronal cytoskeletal proteins were reduced in the frontal cortex of these animals, indicating that PCE affects cytoskeletal proteins (Wang et al., 1993). These findings indicate that exposure to PCE reduces the number of brain cells and interferes with metabolism of cytoskeletal proteins in both glial and neuronal cells. Furthermore, these findings suggest that PCE affects specific brain regions (Renis et al., 1974; Savolainen et al., 1977; Wang et al., 1993).

Metabolites of PCE such as trichloroacetaldehyde react with dopamine *in vitro* and may be toxic to dopaminergic systems *in vivo,* resulting in dopamine depletion and central nervous system (CNS) dysfunction (Mutti and Franchini, 1987). PCE impairs dopaminergic control of prolactin, suggesting that PCE can affect the release of dopamine from dopaminergic neurons. In female dry cleaners exposed to PCE at a median concentration of 15 ppm (range: 1 to 67 ppm), serum prolactin levels were increased during the proliferative phase of their menstrual cycles (Ferroni et al., 1992). Exposure to PCE also alters brain levels of free amino acids (Honma et al., 1980; Briving et al., 1986). Following chronic exposure to PCE, taurine levels are significantly decreased in the cerebellar vermis and the hippocampus. Conversely, levels of glutamine are increased in the hippocampus. The PCE-induced increase in hippocampal glutamine levels may reflect astrocytic gliosis associated with the degeneration of neurons (Briving et al., 1986).

The chronic toxic effects of exposure to PCE have been attributed to its metabolite PCE epoxide (Moslen et al., 1977; Pegg et al., 1979; Buben and O'Flaherty, 1985). PCE epoxide is an electrophilic alkylating agent, and therefore it covalently binds to the nucleophilic centers of cellular macromolecules such as cytoskeletal proteins and to nucleic acids such as DNA (Bonse et al., 1975; Moslen et al., 1977; Bolt and Filser, 1977; Pegg et al., 1979). DNA altered by covalent binding of PCE epoxide may result in a decrease in cellular ATP content and an increase in intracellular free Ca^{2+}, possibly damaging neurons (Halliwell, 1989). Damage to the DNA of cells including neurons can induce apoptosis (Corcoran et al., 1994).

PREVENTIVE AND THERAPEUTIC MEASURES

Dry cleaning and degreasing shops should be properly ventilated, and ambient air levels of PCE should be determined regularly. Body burden of PCE in dry cleaners and other workers at risk of chronic exposure to PCE should be monitored. Handling of wet garments by dry cleaners should be kept to a minimum. Individuals using coin-operated dry-cleaning machines should line dry any damp items in a well-ventilated area.

The first step in treating PCE intoxication is to remove individuals from risk of further exposure and bring them into an area with fresh air. Since inhalation of vapors is the most likely route of intake, displacing the PCE-contaminated air in the lungs with oxygen and/or fresh air is essential in emergency care. Immediate measures include providing a vapor-free source of air and an oxygen tank while encouraging energetic, deep breathing. If oral ingestion of PCE has occurred, stomach gavage should be performed as soon as possible. Syrup of ipecac can be used in cases of PCE ingestion. However, the risk of further inhalation of PCE vapors from the oropharynx or by aspiration of vomitus containing PCE makes controlled stomach gavage a safer method of eliminating residual quantities of the ingested solvent. Because the elimination kinetics following oral and inhalation exposure are similar, hyperventilation of the patient is an effective method for increasing excretion of PCE that has been absorbed through the gastrointestinal tract (Köppel et al., 1985). In addition, appropriate general supportive measures as well as specific interventions may be needed for cardiac arrhythmia, pulmonary edema, and vasomotor instability in susceptible persons. Hemodialysis and blood transfusion for acute renal failure, myopathy, and hepatic involvement may be necessary (Olivares-Esquer et al., 1974; Sasdelli et al., 1986). Recovery from acute intoxication depends upon the intensity and duration of the exposure.

Chronic exposure may be accompanied by the gradual appearance of clinical indicators of neurotoxicity. In particular, when the ongoing body-burden accumulates over time, symptoms may arise at times of peak exposure or when the PCE body burden is mobilized (Rozman and Klaassen, 1996). Prognosis of patients with chronic perchloroethylene encephalopathy varies according to time of follow-up and type of neurological tests performed (Freed and Kandel, 1988; Echeverria et al., 1995). The long-term affective disorders following toxic encephalopathies are particularly difficult to treat and adversely affect recovery and prognosis of patients (Gregersen et al., 1988). To compensate for permanent impairments of behavior and cognitive functioning, treatment must include individualized vocational and psychosocial recommendations.

CLINICAL EXPERIENCES

Group Studies

Epidemiological Study of Neurobehavior in Dry-Cleaner Workers

Sixty-six workers from 23 different dry-cleaning shops were studied (Echeverria et al., 1995). All workers (mean age: 42 years; 35 male, 30 female) selected had no previous medical history of CNS health problems. One worker was eliminated from the study because of previous exposure to Stoddard solvent. The remaining 65 workers were divided into high ($n = 23$), moderate ($n = 18$), and low ($n = 24$), exposure groups based upon individual PCE breath concentrations, currently measured PCE vapor concentrations associated with a particular task, and lifetime cumulative exposure index (CI). The CI for each worker was estimated by the following criteria: (a) job description (for workers who did several jobs within a week, the percentage of time spent performing each job within a week was determined); (b) complete work histories; (c) industrial hygiene evaluations; and (d) hobbies. Neuropsychological testing of approximately 1 hour duration was performed in the afternoons after work on the first or second day of a workweek. Performance domains assessed and the tests performed included (a) attention (Digit Span), (b) visuospatial function (visual reproduction subtests of the Wechsler Memory Scale and the computer-based neurobehavioral evaluation system (NES) test of Pattern Memory, (c) perceptual recognition (NES Pattern Recognition Test), (d) complex cognitive tracking (Trailmaking Test), (e) psychomotor speed (NES Symbol-Digit Substitution Test), (f) verbal skills (vocabulary), and (g) mood (Profile of Mood States).

The concentration of PCE was sampled in 19 of the 23 dry-cleaning shops. PCE concentrations in the shops using the more common wet-transfer method were 11.2, 23.2, and 40.8 ppm in the breathing zones of clerks, pressers, and machine operators, respectively. The PCE concentrations in the shops using the dry-to-dry method were considerably lower. The PCE concentrations measured in these shops were in agreement with other industrial hygiene surveys (Materna, 1985; Solet et al., 1990). The as-

sociation between the mean concentration of PCE in breath and job category was statistically significant ($p < 0.001$). In general, the dry-cleaning machine operators were exposed to the highest levels of PCE for the longest duration. Transfer methodology (i.e., wet-transfer or dry-to-dry technique) was found to contribute to machine operator exposure. The wet-transfer processes required an operator to manually transfer cleaned, solvent-laden fabric into a cart every half-hour. The transfer of clothing requires about 5 minutes. In the dry-to-dry machines the manual transfer step is eliminated, since the cleaning and drying processes occur in the same machine. Therefore, operators in dry-to-dry shops receive considerably less exposure to PCE. The mean concentration in breath discriminated between low, moderate, and high PCE exposure within the wet-transfer processes, indicating differences in air levels for counter clerks, pressers, and operators. Within the dry-to-dry transfer shops, only the breath level between low and high exposure groups was significantly different. However, of the 23 shops participating in the study, only six used the dry-to-dry process. In addition, regardless of the type of transfer process used, the shop owners usually relied on general dilution or ventilation assisted only by stand-alone fans, located at open doors or windows to remove PCE vapors from the work environment. Protective clothing and masks were not used by the workers. There was on average one operator per shop with a mean employment duration of 20.2 years, and a mean duration of 14.8 years as an operator in the same shop. Pressers and counter clerks had been employed for shorter periods (3.9 and 2.1 years, respectively). Pressers generally had been exposed to moderate levels of PCE and were often exposed to higher levels by being placed in the same room with the sorting and hanging process. Age, education, vocabulary, and alcohol consumption were associated with a lifetime PCE exposure and performance. Age had the strongest association ($r = 0.51$) with lifetime PCE exposure. Although spot-remover solutions containing small quantities of various other solvents (i.e., trichloroethylene, 1,1,1-trichloroethane, isopropylacetate, and acetone) may also have been used by these workers, none of these solvents were detectable in breath measurements; therefore, the exposure to PCE is considered the only significant exposure for the study.

Performance by the workers on neuropsychological testing is summarized as follows:

Visual Reproductions: The CI was significantly associated ($p < 0.01$), with performance on these tests, as was education ($p < 0.04$), and vocabulary ($p < 0.03$). However, current exposure and exposure within the last 3 years was not associated with performance on these tests. The relationships between prior exposure to other solvents was marginally significant ($p < 0.06$). Performance of the workers from the high-exposure group was significantly ($p < 0.05$) impaired over that of workers from the low-exposure group. This difference was significant for the adjusted as well as the unadjusted scores.

Pattern Memory: The ability to recall patterns (visual memory) was scored by the number of correct responses and the subjects' response time. Multivariate regression for the number correct was significantly affected by a 3-year index of exposure to PCE ($p < 0.08$), the CI ($p < 0.03$), and education ($p < 0.02$). Number correct was not associated with current exposure. The multivariate regression for response time was significantly affected by current PCE exposures ($p < 0.03$), age ($p < 0.01$), and vocabulary ($p < 0.03$), but not by the CI of PCE exposure. Deficits in the number correct and response times of the high-exposure workers compared with low-exposure workers were significant ($p < 0.001$) for the adjusted scores.

Pattern Recognition: The ability to recognize patterns (visual memory) was scored by the number correct and the response time. The multivariate regression analysis for the number correct against CI was significant ($p < 0.02$), and it was marginally affected by vocabulary ($p < 0.08$). The multivariate regression for the response time was not affected by current PCE exposure, but was affected by age ($p < 0.01$) and vocabulary ($p < 0.02$). The high–low adjusted difference between means for the number correct was 3.9%.

Trailmaking Tests A and B: Cognitive tracking (executive functioning) was measured by the number of errors and the response time to connect alternate meaningful sequences on a spatial array. The number of errors was not affected by current exposure to PCE. The multivariant regression for test A was not affected by current exposure or CI of exposure to PCE, but was affected by age ($p < 0.02$), the frequency of alcohol consumption ($p < 0.02$), and possible prior pesticide exposure ($p < 0.1$). The multivariant regression for test B was also not affected by current or lifetime exposure to PCE, but was affected by age ($p < 0.02$) and vocabulary ($p < 0.01$). The differences in performance between the low- and high-exposure groups on tests A and B was in the direction of impairment, but the difference was not statistically significant.

Symbol-Digit Matching Task: Psychomotor skills were assessed by matching symbols with numbers and was scored by the number incorrect and the response time. The number incorrect and the response time were not associated with current exposure or CI of exposure to PCE. Age and vocabulary were associated with both variables ($p < 0.02$). Although the decrement in response time was in the direction of impairment, the difference was not statistically significant.

Digit Span: Tests of attention and short-term memory showed that the 50% maximum likelihood for memory of digit spans typed in to a computer in the correct order was not associated with CI or current PCE exposure in simple linear or multiple regression analysis. Vocabulary and education were associated with digit span (0.05 and 0.09). The

low–high (5% mean) decrement in digit span was in the wrong direction and was smaller than the minimum detectable effect level.

Among these PCE-exposed dry cleaners, the subclinical impairments of visually mediated function support available clinical evidence on a possible continuum of severity. The tests most sensitive to PCE exposure were those of short-term memory for visual designs (pattern memory and visual reproduction). Decrements in visual reproductions, pattern memory, and pattern recognition were consistently found in subjects employed as operators for an average of 14.6 (SD = 8.9 years) and exposed to an estimated TWA air concentration of 41 ppm, 16 ppm above the OSHA permissible exposure limit for PCE of 25 ppm.

Spray Painting Inside an Enclosed Area

Two workers were acutely exposed to PCE while spray painting the inside of a large water tank with a coal tar epoxy. The epoxy contained 29% PCE and 7% toluene. The entire job took 8 hours to complete. Although the PCE levels inside the tank were not measured, the air concentrations in this confined and poorly ventilated space most likely exceed established exposure limits in order to cause symptoms, since following exposure, both workers developed clinical peripheral neuropathy and persistent neuropsychological deficits (R. G. Feldman, M.D., personal observation).

Case 1. A 28-year-old painter with over 15 years of experience entered the tank at the beginning of the day with an air supply hood, but he wore no protective clothing. This worker's job was primarily spray painting the inside of the tank. He sprayed the compound for 4 to 5 hours and wore the air supply hood the entire time. When he finished painting, he removed the hood and began removing his scaffolding from inside the tank. During this process, which took 1 to 2 hours, he did not wear the air supply even though he felt lightheaded and "spacey."

Following the exposure, he was irritable and had episodes of rage during which he would throw things; this was a significant change in his personality. The patient complained of headaches, attentional difficulties, loss of memory, sleep disturbances, diplopia, blurred vision, loss of balance, impotence, mood changes, depression and apathy toward activities that formerly interested him. He also reported experiencing numbness, tingling, and muscle weakness in his extremities. Shortly after the incident, he began to experience periods of "blanking out" (seizures), for which he was given phenobarbital.

Neurological examination revealed sensory loss in the fingertips of both hands and in the toes and bottoms of both feet. The upper extremity, face, and corneal reflexes were preserved. Abdominal and cremasteric reflexes were also normal. Visual acuity and color vision were preserved and there was no optic neuropathy. Neuropsychological testing revealed mild constructional deficits, psychomotor slowing, and impairment of short-term memory, especially on visu-ospatial tasks. Electroencephalography showed slightly asymmetrical posterior slow rhythms. Nerve conduction velocity studies revealed slowing in the sensory fibers of the ulnar, superficial peroneal, posterior tibial, and sural nerves. Slowed motor conduction velocity was recorded in the right and left posterior tibial nerves. Amplitude of the sensory evoked potentials was reduced in the ulnar nerves. Muscles action potential amplitudes were reduced in both peroneal nerves. These findings indicate peripheral neuropathy of the axonal type (sensory).

Case 2. The second worker was a 30-year-old painter with 15 years of experience. He assisted his coworker (Case 1 above) by moving the scaffolding and keeping the hoses straight inside the tank. Although he had an air supply hood with him on the job site, he did not wear it because it was cumbersome and it was not functioning properly. He also did not wear protective clothing. He initially entered the tank intending only to move the scaffolding and then leave, but he ended up staying inside the tank for 6 to 8 hours. He remembered feeling high and believing that he was at the dentist's office shortly after entering the tank; he later reported having no memory for the remaining events of that day. Following this exposure, his family noticed a personality change and described him as having become irritable and short-tempered. The patient himself complained of having a poor short-term memory, dizziness, headache, blurred vision, confusion, anxiety, loss of manual dexterity, and decreased libido.

Memory disturbances persisted over the next 6 months. The patient also complained of numb feet and hands. At the time of follow-up, his neurological examination revealed intact facial sensation and corneal reflexes; facial symmetry was present. Coordination was normal. Abdominal and cremasteric reflexes were reduced. Sensation to pinprick was reduced in the fingertips and feet. Hyperventilation produced lightheadedness, unsteadiness of gait, and visual disturbances. Neuropsychological testing demonstrated impaired short-term memory, visuospatial disorientation, psychomotor slowing, and diminished attentional and mental control skills. MMPI results indicated that the patient was very depressed. EEG was normal. Nerve conduction velocity testing demonstrated evidence of mild to moderate motor and sensory neuropathy. Sensory conduction velocities (SCVs) were reduced in the left median and ulnar nerves. SCV was reduced in the left sural nerve; in the right sural nerve the velocities were at the lower limits of normal. There was a reduction in the SCV of the right superficial peroneal nerve, while in the left superficial peroneal the velocities were at the lower limits of normal. Motor conduction velocities (MCVs) were reduced in the right ulnar nerve distally and were at the lower limits of normal in the left ulnar nerve. For the right peroneal and left posterior tibial nerves, the MCVs were mildly reduced. Sensory action potential amplitudes were reduced in the ulnar nerves bilaterally and in the left median, superficial peroneal, and posterior tibial nerves.

The findings in the second case of PCE exposure during spray painting also indicates acute encephalopathy with residual memory and cognitive impairments, as well as neurophysiological evidence of peripheral neuropathy.

Individual Case Studies

Faulty Dry-Cleaning Equipment Resulting in Chronic PCE Exposure

A 27-year-old woman had worked for a dry-cleaning operation for 3 years and during this period she had complained to her employer several times about leakage of PCE fumes from faulty operating reclamation equipment. However, the equipment was never repaired. She reported that she experienced acute symptoms of dizziness and "feeling high" while at work. Over time, she began to experience other chronic symptoms away from her job including fatigue, mood changes, impaired memory, confusion, lack of coordination, and intolerance to alcohol. She left this job for a position at another dry cleaner where the employer was more conscientious about testing the workplace air. Although she occasionally experienced lightheadedness when the workplace had higher concentrations of PCE, the majority of her chronic symptoms seemed to improve at her new job. Nevertheless, her memory was poor and she found that it took her a very long time to learn the names of her new coworkers, although she reported that previously she had been able to learn names very easily and generally had no problems with memory (R. G. Feldman, personal observation).

Neuropsychological testing was performed 6 months after she left the site of the leaking equipment using the Wechsler Adult Intelligence Scale (WAIS) and revealed a full-scale IQ of 97. The patient's performance IQ of 84 was significantly lower than her verbal IQ, which was 107. Visuospatial skills were generally below average. Performances on replication of three-dimensional block design and puzzle assembly tests were significantly below average. Her psychomotor speed (Continuous Performance test) was also markedly below expectation. Memory function was significantly impaired compared to verbal skills. The Wechsler Memory Scale (WMS) showed the patient's memory quotient to be below expectation at 84. The WMS visual reproduction test showed her visual memory skills to be significantly impaired. Visual perseverative tendencies were also observed. Digit span was average at 6 forward and 5 backward. Retrograde memory as assessed by Albert's Famous Faces test was well preserved. Although the patient complained of irritability and a tendency to cry easily, the MMPI did not reveal signs of clinical depression.

The patient was advised to avoid working around organic solvents and to leave the dry-cleaning business, which she did. Follow-up neuropsychological assessment performed 21 months later showed marked improvements in memory, attention, visual organization, mood, and, to a lesser extent, reasoning. Peripheral nerve conduction studies revealed slowing of the right peroneal and sural nerves, indicating peripheral neuropathy.

Self-Employed Dry Cleaner with Chronic and Intense Exposure

A 44-year-old man developed persistent dizziness, irritability, impaired short-term memory and concentration, lassitude, intolerance to alcohol, and staggering gait over the course of a 3-year period during which he operated his own dry-cleaning business (Gold, 1969). The solvent he used for dry cleaning was PCE. He worked at his own business 6 days per week as the cleaner and clerk, and on the seventh day he cleaned the dry-cleaning vats, which were located in a small poorly ventilated room. Apparently the PCE levels in this room were extremely high, because each week he found himself confused and disoriented by the time he completed the job. He would then return home and sleep for 2 hours. After operating the business for approximately 2.5 years, he noted that he had become extremely forgetful, frequently leaving his cigarettes burning on the shop counter. This worried him enough to see a physician who prescribed a mild tranquilizer, but this provided no improvement in his mental status. His condition continued to deteriorate and he was admitted to the hospital 6 months later, at which time he was confused and agitated and stammered when he spoke.

On admission to the hospital, the patient's digit span was 7 forward and 4 backward, and he was unable to concentrate well enough to perform simple arithmetic, indicating impairment of attention and mental control. He stated that he had recently found himself needing to keep lists of things to do and that he had difficulty holding a conversation. His condition gradually improved and he was discharged 2 months later. At follow-up examinations 4, 7, and 10 months after his discharge, he continued to show impairment of his short-term memory, along with mood lability and stammering speech. In addition, he reported that his condition had made it necessary for him to stop driving a car. This clinical picture suggests cerebral cortical and basal ganglia involvement.

Dry-Cleaned Curtains and Fatal Off-Gassing of PCE Vapors in a 2-Year-Old

A 2-year-old boy was found dead in his bedroom 1.5 hours after laying down to take a nap on a winter day. There was a strong odor of solvent in the room at the time that he was discovered. Earlier that day, the three pairs of curtains in his bedroom had been taken down and cleaned at a nearby self-service coin-operated dry-cleaning shop. When the curtains were removed from the machine at the end of the cleaning cycle, they had a strong odor of solvent; nevertheless, they were placed in a plastic bag and taken home. At home, two pairs of the curtains were hung

in a well-ventilated room, while the remaining pair was hung back up in the child's bedroom with the window open until the odor of the solvent seem to have lessened. At this time, the window of the bedroom was closed. The child was then put into his bed for a nap and the door to his room was closed.

Police investigating the incident determined that PCE vapor had evolved from the damp cotton-lined chintz curtains that had been dry-cleaned early that day. Further investigation revealed that overloading of the dry-cleaning machine had resulted in inadequate extraction of the solvent at the end of the cleaning cycle; the three pairs of curtains which weighed 19 kg had been dry cleaned in a machine with a maximum load capacity of only 6 kg. The off-gassing presumably produced air levels of PCE that overwhelmed the small child.

At autopsy, no macroscopic abnormalities were noted. Blood PCE level was 66 mg/L. Analysis of the urine showed very low concentrations of PCE (0.4 mg/L), TCAA (0.9 mg/L) and TCEtOH (1.7 mg/L). Toxicological analysis of samples of brain, lung, and heart revealed PCE concentrations of 79, 46, and 31 mg/kg, respectively. The PCE concentration in the brain of this child closely resembles that reported by Levine et al. (1981), in a 53-year-old dry cleaner who died after being overcome by PCE vapor.

This case exemplifies the potential for nonoccupational exposure to PCE during unmonitored circumstances. The fatal outcome seen in this case is probably related to the overwhelming of the capacity of this small child's body to either store or metabolize and excrete the dose of PCE to which he was exposed; thus, the concentration of PCE in his brain and other vital organ systems reached toxic levels.

REFERENCES

Agency for Toxic Substances and Disease Registry (ATSDR). *Toxicological profile for tetrachloroethylene.* Atlanta: US Department of Health and Human Services, Public Health Service, 1995.

Aggazzotti G, Fantuzzi G, Righi E, et al. Occupational and environmental exposure to perchloroethylene (PCE) in dry cleaners and their family members. *Arch Environ Health* 1994;49:487–493.

Aitio A, Pekari K, Jarvisalo J. Skin absorption as a source of error in biological monitoring. *Scand J Work Environ Health* 1984;10:317–320.

Altmann L, Böttger A, Wiegand H. Neurophysiological and psychophysical measurements reveal effects of acute low-level organic solvent exposure in humans. *Arch Occup Env Health* 1990;62:493–499.

American Conference of Governmental Industrial Hygienists (ACGIH). *Threshold limit values (TLVs) for chemical substances and physical agents and biological exposure indices (BEIs).* Cincinnati: 1995.

Aminoff MJ. Electroencephalography: general principles and clinical applications. In: Aminoff MJ, ed. *Electrodiagnosis in clinical neurology,* 2nd ed. New York: Churchill Livingstone, 1986:21–75.

Amoore JE, Hautala E. Odor as an aid to chemical safety: odor thresholds compared with threshold limit values and volatilities for 214 industrial chemicals in air and water dilution. *J Appl Toxicol* 1983;3:272–290.

Anderson HA. Utilization of adipose tissue biopsy in characterizing human halogenated hydrocarbon exposure. *Environ Health Perspect* 1985;60:127–131.

Aschengrau A, Ozonoff D, Paula C, et al. Cancer risk and tetrachloroethylene-contaminated drinking water in Massachusetts. *Arch Environ Health* 1993;48:284–292.

Barkley J, Bunch J, Bursey JT, et al. Gas chromatography/mass spectrometry computer analysis of volatile halogenated hydrocarbons in man and his environment. A multimedia environmental study. *Biomed Mass Spectrom* 1980;7:139–147.

Bartonicek V. Metabolism and excretion of trichloroethylene after inhalation in human subjects. *Br J Ind Med* 1962;19:134.

Bogen KT, Colston BW Jr, Machicao LK. Dermal absorption of diluted aqueous chloroform, trichloroethylene, and tetrachloroethylene in hairless guinea pigs. *Fund Appl Toxicol* 1992;18:30–39.

Bolt HM, Filser JG. Irreversible binding of chlorinated ethylenes to macromolecules. *Environ Health Perspect* 1977;21:107–112.

Bonse G, Urban T, Reichert D, Henschler D. Chemical reactivity, metabolic oxirane formation and biological reactivity of chlorinated ethylenes in the isolated perfused rat liver preparation. *Biochem Pharmacol* 1975;24:1829–1834.

Bowman KJ. A method for quantitative scoring of the Farnsworth Panel D-15. *Acta Ophthalmol* 1982;60:907–916.

Braffman BH, Trojanowski JQ, Atlas SW. The aging brain and neurodegenerative disorders. In: Atlas SW, ed. *Magnetic resonance imaging of the brain and spine.* New York: Raven Press, 1991:567–624.

Briving C, Jacobson I, Hamberger A, Kjellstrand P, Haglid KG, Rosengren E. Chronic effects of perchloroethylene and trichloroethylene on gerbil brain amino acids and glutathione. *Neurotoxicology* 1986;7:101–108.

Brown HS, Bishop DR, Rowan CA. The role of skin absorption as a route of exposure for volatile organic compounds (VOCs) in drinking water. *Am J Public Health* 1984;74:479–484.

Buben JA, O'Flaherty EJ. Deliniation of the role of metabolism in the hepatotoxicity of trichloroethylene and perchloroethylene: a dose–effect study. *Toxicol Appl Pharmacol* 1985;78:105–122.

Burmaster DE. The new pollution-groundwater contamination. *Environment* 1982;24:7–13, 33–36.

Cai S-X, Huang M-Y, Chen Z, et al. Subjective symptom increase among dry-cleaning workers exposed to tetrachloroethylene vapor. *Ind Health* 1991;29:111–121.

Carpenter CP. The chronic toxicity of tetrachloroethylene. *J Ind Hyg Toxicol* 1937;19:323–336.

Cavalleri A, Gobba F, Paltrinieri M, Fantuzzi G, Righi E, Aggazzotti G. Perchloroethylene exposure can induce colour vision loss. *Neurosci Lett* 1994;179:162–166.

Chaudhuri RN, Mukerji AK. Death following administration of tetrachloroethylene. *Indian Med Gazette* 1947;82:115–116.

Chmielewski J, Tomaszewski R, Glombiowski P, et al. Clinical observations of the occupational exposure to tetrachloroethylene. *Bull Inst Maritime Trop Med Gdynia* 1976;27:197–205.

Cohr K. Uptake and distribution of common industrial solvents. In: Riihimäki V, Ulfvarson U, eds. *Safety and health aspects of organic solvents: International course on safety and health aspects of organic solvents (Espoo, Finland, April 22–26, 1985).* New York: Alan R Liss, 1986:45–60.

Coler HR, Rossmiller HR. Tetrachloroethylene exposure in a small industry. *AMA Arch Ind Hyg* 1953;8:277–233.

Corcoran GB, Fix L, Jones DP, Moslen MT, Nicotera P, Oberhammer FA, Buttyan R. Contemporary issues in toxicology. Apoptosis: molecular control point in toxicity. *Toxicol Appl Pharmacol* 1994;128:169–181.

Costa AK, Ivanetich KM. Trichloroethylene metabolism by the hepatic microsomal cytochrome P-450 system. *Biochem Pharmacol* 1980;29:2863–2869.

Dallas CE, Muralidhara S, Chen XM, et al. Use of a physiologically based model to predict systemic uptake and respiratory elimination of perchloroethylene. *Toxicol Appl Pharmacol* 1994;128:60–68.

Daniel JW. The metabolism of ^{36}Cl-labeled trichloroethylene and tetrachloroethylene in the rat. *Biochem Pharmacol* 1963;12:795–802.

Earnest GS. *Walk through survey report: perchloroethylene exposure in commercial dry cleaners at Springdale Cleaners.* Cincinnati: NIOSH, 1993:20.

Earnest GS, Spencer AB. *Walk through survey report: perchloroethylene exposure in commercial dry cleaners at Hyde Park "one hour" martinizing cleaners.* Cincinnati: NIOSH, 1993:20.

Earnest GS, Spencer AB, Smith SS. *Walk through survey report: perchloroethylene exposure and ergonomic hazards in commercial dry cleaners at Teasdale Fenton Cleaners.* Cincinnati: NIOSH, 1993:23.

Echeverria D, White RF, Sampaio C. A behavioral evaluation of PCE exposure in patients and dry cleaners: a possible relationship between clinical and preclinical effects. *JOEM* 1995;37:667–680.

Entz RC, Diachenko GW. Residues of volatile halocarbons in margarines. *Food Addit Contam* 1988;5:267–276.

Evans GM. The U.S. EPA SITE demonstration of AWD technologies' AguaDetox/SVE system. *J Air Waste Management Assoc* 1991;41:1519–1523.

Fernandez J, Guberan E, Caperos J. Experimental human exposures to tetrachloroethylene vapor and elimination in breath after inhalation. *Am Ind Hyg Assoc* 1976;37:143–150.

Ferroni C, Selis L, Mutti A, Folli D, Bergamaschi E, Franchini I. Neurobehavioral and neuroendocrine effects of occupational exposure to perchloroethylene. *Neurotoxicology* 1992;13:243–248.

Foot EB, Bishop K, Apgar V. Tetrachloroethylene as an anesthetic agent. *Anesthesiology* 1943;4:283–292.

Freed DM, Kandel E. Long-term occupational exposure and the diagnosis of dementia. *Neurotoxicology* 1988;9:391–400.

Gaillard Y, Billault F, Pépin G. Tetrachloroethylene fatality: case report and simple gas chromatographic determination in blood and tissues. *Forensic Sci Int* 1995;76:161–168.

Garnier R, Bédouin J, Pépin G, Gaillard Y. Coin-operated dry cleaning machines may be responsible for acute tetrachloroethylene poisoning: report of 26 cases including one death. *Clin Toxicol* 1996;34:191–197.

Gehring PJ. Hepatotoxic potency of various chlorinated hydrocarbon vapours relative to their narcotic and lethal potencies in mice. *Toxicol Appl Pharmacol* 1968;13:287–298.

Ghantous H, Danielsson BRG, Dencker L, et al. Trichloroacetic acid accumulates in murine amniotic fluid after tri- and tetrachloroethylene inhalation. *Acta Pharmacol Toxicol* 1986;58:105–114.

Gold JH. Chronic perchloroethylene poisoning. *Can Psychiatr Assoc J* 1969;14:627–630.

Gregersen P. Neurotoxic effects of organic solvents in exposed workers: two controlled follow-up studies after 5.5 and 10.6 years. *Am J Ind Med* 1988;14:681–701.

Guberan E, Fernandez J. Control of industrial exposure to tetrachloroethylene by measuring alveolar concentrations: theoretical approach using a mathematical model. *Br J Ind Med* 1974;31:159–167.

Haerer AF, Udelman HD. Acute brain syndrome secondary to tetrachloroethylene ingestion. *Am J Psychiatry* 1964;121:78–79.

Hajimiragha H, Ewers U, Jansen-Rosseck R, Brockhaus A. Human exposure to volatile halogenated hydrocarbons from the general environment. *Int Arch Occup Environ Health* 1986;58:141–150.

Hake CL, Stewart RD. Human exposure to tetrachloroethylene: inhalation and skin contact. *Environ Health Perspect* 1977;21:231–238.

Halliwell B. Oxidants and the central nervous system: some fundamental questions. Is oxidant damage relevant to Parkinson's disease, Alzheimer's disease, traumatic injury and stroke? *Acta Neurol Scand* 1989;126:23–33.

Hardie DWF. Chlorocarbons and chlorohydrocarbons: tetrachloroethylene. In: Kirk RE, Othmer DF, eds. *Encyclopedia of chemical technology,* vol 5, 2nd ed. New York: John Wiley and Sons, 1964:195–203.

Hayes JR, Condie LW, Borzelleca JF. The subchronic toxicity of tetrachloroethylene (perchloroethylene) administered in the drinking water of rats. *Fundam Appl Toxicol* 1986;7:119–125.

Honma T, Sudo A, Miyagawa M, Sto M, Gasegawa H. Effects of exposure to trichloroethylene and tetrachloroethylene on the contents of acetylcholine, dopamine, norepinephrine, and serotonin in the rat brain. *Ind Health* 1980;18:171–178.

IARC. *IARC monographs on the evaluation of the carcinogenic risk of chemicals in humans,* vol 20: *Tetrachloroethylene.* Lyons, France: World Health Organization, 1979:491–514.

Ikeda M, Ohtsuji H, Imamura T, Komoike Y. Urinary excretion of total trichloro-compounds, trichloroethanol, and trichloroacetic acid as a measure of exposure to trichloroethylene and tetrachloroethylene. *Br J Ind Med* 1972;29:328–333.

Ikeda M, Imamura T. Biological half-life of trichloroethylene and tetrachloroethylene in human subjects. *Int Arch Arbeitsmed* 1973;31:209–224.

Ikeda M. Metabolism of trichloroethylene and tetrachloroethylene in human subjects. *Environ Health Perspect* 1977;21:239–245.

Imbriani M, Ghittori S, Pezzagno G, Capodaglio E. Urinary excretion of tetrachloroethylene (perchloroethylene) in experimental and occupational exposure. *Arch Environ Health* 1988;43:292–298.

Kaplan SD. Dry cleaners workers exposed to perchloroethylene. A retrospective cohort mortality study. U.S. Department of Health Education and Welfare, Contract No. 210-77-0094. Cincinnati: National Institute for Occupational Safety and Health, 1980.

Kendrick JF. The treatment of hookworm disease with tetrachloroethylene. *Am J Trop Med* 1929;9:483–488.

Kido K, Shiratori T, Watanabe T, Nakatsuka H, Ohashi M, Ikeda M. Correlation of tetrachloroethylene in blood and in drinking water: a case of well water pollution. *Bull Environ Contam Toxicol* 1989;43:444–453.

Köppel C, Arndt I, Arendt U, Koeppe P. Acute tetrachloroethylene poisoning—blood elimination kinetics during therapy. *J Toxicol Clin Toxicol* 1985;23:103–115.

Köppel C, Lanz HJ, Ibe K. Acute trichloroethylene poisoning with additional ingestion of ethanol—concentrations of trichloroethylene and its metabolites during hyperventilation therapy. *Int Care Med* 1988;14:74–76.

Kyrklund T, Alling C, Kjellstrand P, Haglid KG. Chronic effects of perchloroethylene on the composition of lipid and acyl groups in cerebral cortex and hippocampus of the gerbil. *Toxicol Lett* 1984;22:343–349.

Kyrklund T, Kjellstrand P, Haglid K. Lipid composition and fatty acid pattern of the gerbil brain after exposure to perchloroethylene. *Arch Toxicol* 1987;60:397–400.

Kyrklund T, Kjellstrand P, Haglid KG. Long-term exposure of rats to perchloroethylene, with and without a post-exposure solvent-free recovery period: effects on brain lipids. *Toxicol Lett* 1990;52:279–285.

Kyrklund T, Haglid KG. Brain lipid composition in guinea pigs after intrauterine exposure to perchloroethylene. *Pharmacol Toxicol* 1991;68:146–148.

Lackore LK, Perkins HM. Accidental narcosis: contamination of compressed air system. *JAMA* 1970;211:1846.

Lafuente A, Mallol J. Thioethers in urine during occupational exposure to tetrachloroethylene. *Br J Ind Med* 1986;43:68–69.

Lamson PD, Robbins BH, Ward CB. The pharmacology and toxicology of tetrachloroethylene. *Am J Hyg* 1929;9:430.

Lanthony P. *Manual of new color test.* Lunseau, Paris: de Lanthony Selon Munsell, 1975.

Lauwerys R, Herbrand J, Buchet JP, Bernard A, Gaussin J. Health surveillance of workers exposed to tetrachloroethylene in dry cleaning shops. *Int Arch Occup Environ Health* 1983;52:69–77.

Leibman KC, Ortiz E. Microsomal metabolism of chlorinated ethylenes. Paper presented at the 6th International Congress on Pharmacology. Abstracts, 1975:257.

Leibman KC, Ortiz E. Metabolism of halogenated ethylenes. *Environ Health Persp* 1977;21:91–97.

Levine B, Fierro MF, Goza SW, Valentour JC. Case Report: A tetrachloroethylene fatality. *J Forensic Sci* 1981;26:206–209.

Lukaszewski T. Acute tetrachloroethylene fatality. *Clin Toxicol* 1979;15:411–415.

Materna BL. Occupational exposure to perchloroethylene in the dry cleaning industry. *Am Ind Hyg Assoc J* 1985;46:268–273.

McConnell G, Ferguson DM, Pearson CR. Chlorinated hydrocarbons and the environment. *Endeavor* 1975;34:13–18.

McKone TE. Human exposure to volatile organic compounds in household tap water: the indoor inhalation pathway. *Environ Sci Technol* 1987;21:1194–1201.

Mergler D, Blain L. Assessing color vision loss among solvent-exposed workers. *Am J Ind Med* 1987;12:195–203.

Mikkelsen S. Solvent encephalopathy: disability pension studies and other case studies. In: Chang LW, Dyer RS, eds. *Handbook of neurotoxicology.* New York: Marcel Dekker, 1995:323–338.

MMWR. Workers exposure to perchloroethylene in commercial dry-cleaning operations—United States. *MMWR* 1983;32:269–271.

Monster AC. Difference in uptake, elimination, and metabolism in exposure to trichloroethylene, 1,1,1-trichloroethane and tetrachloroethylene. *Int Arch Occup Environ Hlth* 1979;42:311–317.

Monster AC. Tetrachloroethylene. In: Aitio A, Riihimäki V, Vainio H, eds. *Biological monitoring and surveillance of workers exposed to chemicals.* New York: Hemisphere, 1984:131–139.

Monster AC. Biological markers of solvent exposure. *Arch Environ Health* 1988;43:90–93.

Monster AC, Boersma G, Steenweg H. Kinetics of tetrachloroethylene in volunteers; influence of exposure concentration and work load. *Int Arch Occup Environ Health* 1979;42:303–309.

Monster A, Regouin-Peeters W, van Schijndel A, van der Tuin J. Biological monitoring of occupational exposure to tetrachloroethylene. *Scand J Work Environ Health* 1983;9:273–281.

Morgan B. Dangers of perchloroethylene [Correspondence]. *Br Med J* 1969;2:513.

Morse KM, Goldberg L. Chlorinated solvent exposures at degreasing operations. *Ind Med* 1943;12:706–713.

Moslen MT, Reynolds ES, Szabo S. Enhancement of the metabolism and hepatotoxicity of trichloroethylene and perchloroethylene. *Biochem Pharmacol* 1977;26:369–375.

Moss MB, Albert MS. Neuropsychology of Alzheimer's disease. In: White RF, ed. *Clinical syndromes in adult neuropsychology: the practitioners handbook.* Amsterdam: Elsevier, 1992:305–343.

Moss MB, Albert MS, Bullers N, Payne M. Differential diagnosis of memory loss among patients with Alzheimer's disease, Huntington's disease, and alcoholic Korsakoff's syndrome. *Arch Neurol* 1986;4:239–246.

Müller G, Spassovski M, Henschler D. Metabolism of trichloroethylene in man. II. Pharmacokinetics of metabolites. *Arch Toxicol* 1974;32:283–295.

Müller G, Spassovski M, Henschler D. Metabolism of trichloroethylene in man. III. Interactions of trichloroethylene and ethanol. *Arch Toxicol* 1975;33:173–189.

Mutti A, Franchini I. Toxicity of metabolites to dopaminergic systems and the behavioral effects of organic solvents. *Br J Ind Med* 1987;44:721–723.

Nakatsuka H, Watanabe T, Takeuchi Y, et al. Absence of blue–yellow color vision loss among workers exposed to toluene or tetrachloroethylene, mostly at levels below occupational exposure limits. *Int Arch Occup Environ Health* 1992;64:113–117.

National Institute of Occupational Safety and Health (NIOSH): *National occupational exposure survey (1981–1983).* Washington, DC: US Department of Health and Human Services, Centers for Disease Control and Prevention, 1990.

National Institute for Occupational Safety and Health (NIOSH). *Pocket guide to chemical hazards.* Washington, DC: US Department of Health and Human Services, Centers for Disease Control and Prevention, 1997.

Occupational Safety and Health Administration (OSHA). Code of Federal Regulations: 29;1910.1000. Washington, DC: Office of the Federal Register, National Archives and Records Administration, 1995:18.

Ogata M, Takatsuka Y, Tomokuni K. Excretion of organic chlorine compounds in the urine of persons exposed to vapours of trichloroethylene and tetrachloroethylene. *Br J Ind Med* 1971;28:386–391.

Ohtsuki T, Sato K, Koizumi A, Kumai M, Ikeda M. Limited capacity of humans to metabolize tetrachloroethylene. *Int Arch Occup Environ Health* 1983;51:381–390.

Olivares-Esquer J, Saldana-Arevalo M, Garcia-Torres R, Trevino-Becerra A. Treatment using hemodialysis and exsanguination transfusion of acute renal failure myopathy and toxic hepatitis, caused by trichloro-acetylene. Report of a case and review of the literature. *Prensa Med Mexicana* 1974;39:461–467.

Patel R, Janakiraman N, Johnson R, Elman JB. Pulmonary edema and coma from perchloroethylene. *JAMA* 1973;223:1510.

Pegg DG, Zempel JA, Braun WH, Watanabe PG. Disposition of tetrachloro(^{14}C)ethylene following oral and inhalation exposure in rats. *Toxicol Appl Pharmacol* 1979;51:465–474.

Peoples RW, Weight FF. Trichloroethanol potentiation of γ-aminobutyric acid-activated chloride current in mouse hippocampal neurones. *Br J Pharmacol* 1994;113:555–563.

Popp W, Müller G, Baltes-Schmitz B, et al. Concentrations of tetrachloroethylene in blood and trichloroacetic acid in urine in workers and neighbors of dry-cleaning shops. *Int Arch Occup Environ Health* 1992;63:393–395.

Rall TW. Hypnotics and sedatives; ethanol. In: Goodman Gilman A, Rall TW, Nies AS, Taylor P, eds. *Goodman and Gilman's the pharmacological basis of therapeutics,* 8th Ed. Elmsford, NY: Pergamon Press, 1990:345–382.

Rao HV, Levy K, Lustik M. Logistic regression of inhalation toxicities of perchloroethylene—application in noncancer risk assessment. *Regul Toxicol Pharmacol* 1993;18:233–247.

Reichert D. Biological actions and interactions of tetrachloroethylene. *Mutat Res* 1983;123:411–429.

Renis M, Gioine A, Bertolino A. Protein synthesis in mitochondrial and microsomal fractions from the rat brain and liver after acute or chronic ethanol administration. *Life Sci* 1974;16:1447–1458.

Reynolds ES, Moslen MT. Damage to hepatic cellular membranes by chlorinated olefins with emphasis on synergism and antagonism. *Environ Health Perspect* 1977;21:137–147.

Riihimäki V, Pfäffli P. Percutaneous absorption of solvent vapors in man. *Scand J Work Environ Health* 1978;4:73–85.

234 / CHAPTER 12

Rowe VK, McCollister DD, Spencer HC, Adams EM, Irish DD. Vapor toxicity of tetrachloroethylene for laboratory animals and human subjects. *AMA Arch Ind Hyg Occup Med* 1952;5:566–579.

Rozman KK, Klaassen CD. Absorption, distribution, and excretion of toxicants. In: Klaassen CD, ed. *Casarett and Doull's toxicology the basic science of poisons*, 5th ed. New York: McGraw-Hill, 1996:91–112.

Saland G. Accidental exposure to perchloroethylene. *NY State J Med* 1967;67:2359–2361.

Sandground JH. Coma following medication with tetrachloroethylene. *JAMA* 1941;17(6):440–441.

Sasdelli N, Vagnolli E, Duranti E, Imperiali P, Tilli G. Treatment of acute "triline" poisoning by plasmapheresis and hemoperfusion. *Int J Artif Organs* 1986;9:195–196.

Sato A, Endoh K, Kaneko T, Johansen G. Effects of consumption of ethanol on the biological monitoring of exposure to organic solvent vapours: a simulation study with trichloroethylene. *Br J Ind Med* 1991; 48:548–556.

Savolainen H, Pfäffli P, Tengen M, Vainio H. Biochemical and behavioral effects of inhalation exposure to tetrachloroethylene and dichloromethane. *J Neuropathol Exp Neurol* 1977;36:941–949.

Sax NI. *Dangerous properties of industrial chemicals*, 5th ed. New York: Van Nostrand Reinhold, 1979.

Schreiber JS. Predicted infant exposure to tetrachloroethylene in human breastmilk. *Risk Anal* 1993;13:515–524.

Schreiber JS, House S, Prohonic E, Smead G, Hudson C, Styk M, Lauber J. An investigation of indoor air contamination in residences above dry cleaners. *Risk Anal* 1993;13:335–344.

Seeber A. Neurobehavioral toxicity of long-term exposure to tetrachloroethylene. *Neurotoxicol Teratol* 1989;11:579–583.

Seiji K, Inoue O, Jin C, et al. Dose–excretion relationship in tetrachloroethylene-exposed workers and the effect of tetrachloroethylene co-exposure on trichloroethylene workers and the effect of tetrachloroethylene co-exposure on trichloroethylene metabolism. *Am J Ind Med* 1989;16:675–684.

Sellers EM, Koch-Weser J, Sellers EM, Koch-Weser J. Potentiation of Warfarin-induced hypoprothrombinemia by chloral hydrate. *N Engl J Med* 1970;283:827–831.

Sheldon L, Handy RW, Hartwell TD, Zweidinger RA, Zelon H. Human exposure assessment to environmental chemicals—nursing mother's study. Final report. Research Triangle Park, NC: Research Triangle Institute, 1985.

Singh HB, Salas LJ, Stiles RE. Distribution of selected gaseous organic mutagens and suspect carcinogens in ambient air. *Environ Sci Technol* 1982;16:872–880.

Skender L, Karacic V, Bosner B, Prpic-Majic D. Assessment of exposure to trichloroethylene and tetrachloroethylene in population of Zagreb, Croatia. *Int Arch Occup Env Health* 1993;65:S163–S165.

Skender L, Karacic V, Bosner B, Prpic-Majic D. Assessment of urban populations exposure to trichloroethylene and tetrachloroethylene by means of biological monitoring. *Arch Environ Health* 1994;49:445–451.

Solet D, Robins TG, Sampaio C. Perchloroethylene exposure assessment among dry cleaning workers. *Am Ind Hyg Assoc J* 1990;51:566–574.

Stacey NH. Toxicity of mixtures of trichloroethylene, tetrachloroethylene, and 1,1,1-trichloroethane: similarity of in vitro to in vivo responses. *Toxicol Ind Health* 1989;5:441–450.

Stemhagen A, Slade J, Altman R, Bill J. Occupational risk factors and liver cancer. *Am J Epidemiol* 1983;117:443–454.

Stewart RD. Acute tetrachloroethylene intoxication. *JAMA* 1969;208:1490–1492.

Stewart RD, Dodd HC. Absorption of carbon tetrachloride, trichloroethylene, tetrachloroethylene, methylene chloride, and 1,1,1-trichloroethane through human skin. *Am Ind Hyg Assoc J* 1964;25:439–446.

Stewart RD, Erley DS, Schaffer AW, Gay HH. Accidental vapor exposure to anesthetic concentrations of solvent containing tetrachloroethylene. *Ind Med Surg* 1961;30:327–330.

Stewart RD, Baretta ED, Dodd HC, Torkelson TR. Experimental human exposure to tetrachloroethylene. *Arch Env Health* 1970;20:224–229.

Stewart RD, Hake CL, Wu A, et al. Effects of perchloroethylene/drug interaction on behavior and neurological function. Final report. Washington, DC: National Institute for Occupational Safety and Health, PB83-17460, 1977.

Stewart RD, Hake CL, Forster HV, Lebrun AJ, Peterson JE, Wu A, and Staff. Tetrachloroethylene: development of biologic standard for the industrial worker by breath analysis. Cincinnati: National Institute for Occupational Safety and Health, Contract No. HSM 99-72-84. PB82-152166, 1981.

Thompson KM, Evans JS. Worker's breath as a source of perchloroethylene (Perc) in the home. *J Expo Anal Environ Epidemiol* 1993;3:417–430.

Toftgård R, Gustafsson J-Å. Biotransformation of organic solvents: a review. *Scand J Work Environ Health* 1980;6:1–18.

Torkelson TR. Halogenated aliphatic hydrocarbons containing chlorine, bromine, and iodine. In: Clayton GD, Clayton FE, eds. *Patty's industrial hygiene and toxicology*, vol. II, Part E, 4th ed. 1994:4007–4251.

United States Environmental Protection Agency (USEPA): Drinking water criteria document for tetrachloroethylene. (Final). Washington, DC: Office of Water, NTIS PB86-118114, 1985.

United States Environmental Protection Agency (USEPA). Drinking water regulations and health advisories. EPA 822-R-96-001. Washington, DC: Office of Water, 1996.

Vogel TM, McCarty PL. Biotransformation of tetrachloroethylene to trichloroethylene, dichloroethylene, vinyl chloride and carbon dioxide under methanogenic conditions. *Appl Environ Microbiol* 1985;49:1080–1083.

Wallace LA, Pellizari ED, Hartwell TD, et al. The California team study: breath concentrations and personal exposure to 26 volatile compounds in air and drinking water of 188 residents of Los Angeles, Antioch, and Pittsburg, CA. *Atmos Environ* 1988;22:2141–2163.

Wang S, Karlsson J-E, Kyrklund T, Haglid K. Perchloroethylene-induced reduction in glial and neuronal cell marker proteins in rat brain. *Pharmacol Toxicol* 1993;72:273–278.

Warren DA, Reigle TG, Muralidhara S, Dallas CE. Schedule-controlled operant behavior of rats following oral administration of perchloroethylene: time course and relationship to blood and brain levels. *J Toxicol Environ Health* 1996;47:345–362.

Waters EM, Gerstner HB, Huff JE. Trichloroethylene. 1. An overview. *J Toxicol Environ Health* 1977;2:671–707.

Webler T, Brown HS. Exposure to tetrachloroethylene via contaminated drinking water pipes in Massachusetts: a predictive model. *Arch Environ Health* 1993;48:293–297.

White RF. Differential diagnosis of probable Alzheimer's disease and solvent encephalopathy in older workers. *Clin Neuropsychol* 1987;1:153–160.

White RF, Feldman RG, Travers PH. Neurobehavioral effects of toxicity due to metals, solvents, and insecticides. *Clin Neuropharmacol* 1990;5:392–412.

White RF, Feldman RG, Proctor SP. Neurobehavioral effects of toxic exposure: clinical syndromes in adult neuropsychology. In: White RF, ed. *The practitioner's handbook*. Amsterdam: Elsevier, 1992:1–51.

Withey JR, Collins BT, Collins PG. Effect of vehicle on the pharmacokinetics and uptake of four halogenated hydrocarbons from the gastrointestinal tract of the rat. *J Appl Toxicol* 1983;3:249–253.

Yllner S. Urinary metabolites of ^{14}C-tetrachloroethylene in mice. *Nature* 1961:191–820.

Ziglio G, Fara GM, Beltramelli G, Pregliasco F. Human environmental exposure to trichloro- and tetrachloroethylene from water and air in Milan, Italy. *Arch Environ Contam Toxicol* 1983;12:57–64.

CHAPTER 13

1,1,1-Trichloroethane

1,1,1-Trichloroethane (TCA, methyltrichloromethane, methylchloroform, α-trichloroethane), a saturated chlorinated hydrocarbon, is a volatile, nonflammable, colorless liquid with a mildly sweet, chloroform-like odor. TCA is very soluble in other organic solvents but is only slightly soluble in water (Sax, 1979; IARC, 1979; NIOSH, 1997). TCA is produced by chlorination of vinyl chloride, hydrochlorination of 1,1-dichloroethylene, or thermal chlorination of ethane (IARC, 1979). Commercial formulations commonly include stabilizers such as p-dioxane, nitromethane, N-methylpyrrole, and butylene oxide, which prevent TCA from oxidizing the various metal parts that are commonly degreased with this solvent (IARC, 1979). The effects of these stabilizer additives on the neurotoxicity of TCA is considered insignificant (Torkelson et al., 1958).

TCA is significantly less toxic than its isomer 1,1,2-trichloroethane, and therefore it is important to know to which isomer a patient has been exposed and which isomer is being discussed in case reports and other references. Because TCA is also relatively less toxic than other chlorinated hydrocarbons, such as perchloroethylene and trichloroethylene, it is used as an alternative to these and other more toxic industrial solvents (Hake et al., 1960; Stewart, 1968; ATSDR, 1990; NIOSH, 1997). Nevertheless, this volatile organic solvent has central and peripheral nervous system effects and affects cardiac, hepatic, and renal functions (Stewart et al., 1969; Herd and Martin, 1975; Halevy et al., 1980; Gresham and Treip, 1983; McLeod et al., 1987; Hodgson et al., 1989; Kelafant et al., 1994). Because of this solvent's documented ubiquity and neurotoxicity, the *Agency for Toxic Substances and Disease Registry* (ATSDR) has selected TCA as one of the ten primary environmental contaminants to be monitored by the *National Exposure Registry* (NER) (Burg and Gist, 1995).

SOURCES OF EXPOSURE

Occupational exposure to TCA can occur during the manufacture, formulation, and use of TCA-containing products such as glues, paints, lubricants, household clean-

ers, and degreasers (NIOSH, 1976; IARC, 1979; Liss, 1988). This solvent is found in fabric cleaners, in typewriter correction fluids, and in industrial degreasing agents (Hall and Hine, 1966; IARC, 1979; Ranson and Berry, 1986; Liss, 1988; House et al., 1994, 1996). TCA is also used as an aerosol propellant and a carrier for many of the active ingredients found in aerosol products (IARC, 1979). Degreaser-workers are exposed to TCA while cleaning parts in "cold baths" (i.e., tanks containing room-temperature TCA), and they are exposed to TCA vapors from "hot tanks" (i.e., tanks containing warm TCA) emitted into ambient air (Hodgson et al., 1989). In comparing exposure to TCA by occupation, Hajimiragha et al. (1989) found that 50% of dry cleaners, 33% of precision instrument makers, and 22% of motor vehicle mechanics had elevated blood levels of TCA. Ambient air TCA concentrations measured over a 2-year period at a yarn factory ranged from a low of 4 ppm in the shop's outer office, to a high of 838 ppm in the area adjacent to a machine that was being cleaned (Kramer et al., 1978). TCA is an ingredient in mixtures with other organic solvents, such as trichloroethylene, methylene chloride, toluene, and xylene in commercial solvents and household cleaners. Exposures occur when workers and hobbyists use mixed solvents. Microelectronics workers who are often involved in cleaning and degreasing operations are directly exposed to TCA, as well as to other organic solvents. TCA vapors are dispersed throughout the work area when compressed air is used to blow-dry degreased parts (Broadwell et al., 1995).

The general population is exposed to TCA through their use of spot removers, degreasing agents, typewriter correction fluids, adhesives, and certain household cleaning solutions (House et al., 1996). Vapors of TCA have been detected in the indoor air of New Jersey and California residences (Wallace et al., 1986, 1988). Exposure to neurotoxic levels of TCA is most likely to occur when the solvent is used in poorly ventilated areas (Stahl et al., 1969; Hatfield and Maykaski, 1970; McCarthy and Jones, 1983; Kelafant et al., 1994). Water contaminated with TCA may be ingested or may be used for cooking or bathing

(Burmaster, 1982; Wallace et al., 1988). Concentrations of TCA in drinking water samples from wells in New Jersey, Connecticut, New York, and Maine ranged from 965 to 5,440 ppb (Burmaster, 1982). This solvent has been detected in meats (3 to 6 μg/kg), fats and oils (5 and 10 μg/kg), teas (7 μg/kg), fruits and vegetables (1 and 4 μg/kg), and breads (2 μg/kg) (McConnell et al., 1975). TCA has been detected in breath and blood samples of nonoccupationally-exposed individuals, indicating environmental sources of exposure (Wallace et al., 1986, 1988). Sniffing TCA for its euphoric effects has also been reported (Hall and Hine, 1966; Travers, 1974; Ranson and Berry, 1986).

EXPOSURE LIMITS AND SAFETY REGULATIONS

The odor of TCA is usually detectable in air at 120 ppm (Amoore and Hautala, 1983). The *Occupational Safety and Health Administration* (OSHA) has established an 8-hour time-weighted average (TWA) permissible exposure level (PEL) for TCA of 350 ppm (OSHA, 1995). The *National Institute for Occupational Safety and Health* (NIOSH) has assigned a "ceiling" (C) designation to their recommended exposure limit (REL) for TCA. The NIOSH REL-C allows for a maximum 15-minute TWA exposure concentration of

TABLE 13-1. *Established and recommended occupational and environmental exposure limits for 1,1,1-trichloroethane in air and water*

	Air (ppm)[a]	Water (mg/L)[a]
Odor threshold*	120	0.97
OSHA		
PEL (8-hr TWA)	350	—
PEL ceiling (15-min TWA)	—	—
PEL ceiling (5-min peak)	—	—
NIOSH		
REL-C (10-hr TWA)	350	—
STEL (15-min TWA)	350	—
IDLH	700	—
ACGIH		
TLV (8-hr TWA)	350	—
STEL (15-min TWA)	450	—
USEPA		
MCL	—	0.2
MCLG	—	0.2

[a]*Unit conversion:* 1 ppm = 5.55 mg/m³; 1 ppm = 1 mg/L.
OSHA, Occupational Safety and Health Administration; PEL, permissible exposure limit; TWA, time-weighted average; NIOSH, National Institute for Occupational Safety and Health; REL-C, recommended exposure limit ceiling; STEL, short-term exposure limit; IDLH, immediately dangerous to life and health; ACGIH, American Conference of Governmental Industrial Hygienists; TLV, threshold limit value; USEPA, United States Environmental Protection Agency; MCL, maximum contamination level; MCLG, maximum contamination level goal.
Data from *Amoore and Hautala, 1983; OSHA, 1995; ACGIH, 1995; USEPA, 1996; NIOSH, 1997.

350 ppm; the ceiling value of 350 ppm should not be exceeded at anytime during a 10-hour work shift. An ambient air concentration of 700 ppm TCA is the exposure level considered by NIOSH to be immediately dangerous to life and health (IDLH) (NIOSH, 1997). The *American Conference of Governmental and Industrial Hygienists* (ACGIH) recommends an 8-hour TWA of 350 ppm for its threshold limit value (TLV). ACGIH recommends a 15-minute-TWA short-term exposure limit (STEL) of 450 ppm (ACGIH, 1995).

The maximum contaminant level (MCL) and the maximum contaminant level goal (MCLG) for drinking water set by the *United States Environmental Protection Agency* (USEPA) is 0.2 mg/L (USEPA, 1996). The odor threshold for TCA in water is 0.97 mg/L (Amoore and Hautala, 1983) (Table 13-1).

METABOLISM

Absorption

TCA enters the body primarily through inhalation of the solvent's vapors; it is readily absorbed across the pulmonary alveoli into the blood. Approximately 25% of an inhaled dose of TCA is retained (Nolan et al., 1984). Total pulmonary absorption of TCA is determined by the ambient air concentration and the blood air partition coefficient of the solvent (Imbriani et al., 1988). Because the blood/air partition coefficient of TCA is small and metabolism of TCA is relatively insignificant, the well-perfused tissues of the body rapidly approach saturation, and thus, the absorption rate declines during exposures to high concentrations. Pulmonary intake is enhanced by exercise. Although total pulmonary absorption is increased by physical activity, the percentage of the dose retained decreases because the accompanying increase in respiratory rate also allows for greater pulmonary elimination of the solvent (Astrand, 1973, 1979; Nolan et al., 1984; Imbriani et al., 1988).

TCA is rapidly absorbed through the gastrointestinal tract following oral ingestion (Stewart and Andrews, 1966; Stewart, 1968). It was detected on the breath of a 47-year-old man who accidentally ingested 1 ounce of TCA. The patient began vomiting and experiencing diarrhea 1 hour after ingesting the solvent. Six hours after the incident the patient's vomiting and diarrhea had subsided, although he continued to complain of lassitude (Stewart and Andrews, 1966).

Dermal absorption of liquid TCA in its pure form or in aqueous solutions contributes to the total uptake of the solvent, especially if dermal contact is prolonged, the TCA is warm, the size of the area of skin exposed is large, and the stratum corneum is damaged (Stewart and Dodd, 1964; Stewart, 1968; Brown et al., 1984). In addition, the greater the degree of hydration of the skin, either by perspiration or by immersion in water, the greater the rate of absorption. Dermal absorption of TCA is likely to occur when bathing or showering with TCA-contaminated water (Brown et al.,

1984). There is considerable interindividual variation in percutaneous absorption of TCA (Stewart and Dodd, 1964; Brown et al., 1984; Aitio et al., 1984). Peripheral sensory neuropathy has been reported with dermal exposure to liquid TCA, suggesting that percutaneous absorption may result in direct peripheral neurotoxicity and, thus, that direct dermal contact with this solvent should be avoided (Liss, 1988; Howse et al., 1989; House et al., 1994, 1996). Dermal absorption of TCA vapor is negligible (Riihimäki and Pfäffli, 1978).

Tissue Distribution

Tissue distribution of TCA is influenced by the concentration of the solvent in blood, the blood perfusion of the particular tissue, and the blood tissue partition coefficients of the solvent (Stewart et al., 1969; Monster, 1979). Because TCA is lipophilic, it readily crosses the human blood–brain barrier (BBB), as demonstrated by the markedly greater brain and liver TCA concentrations in seven fatal human cases (Stahl et al., 1969) (Table 13-2). The concentration of TCA in the brain reaches a steady state within 60 minutes in mice (You et al., 1994). In addition, because TCA is a lipophilic compound, it also has a high affinity for adipose tissue. However, because adipose tissue is not well-perfused with blood, during exposures the concentrations of TCA rise more rapidly in the more well-perfused tissues; TCA is initially distributed to the liver, kidneys, spleen, brain, and skeletal muscles. TCA is also readily released from the blood to these particularly well-perfused tissues. Because adipose tissue is not as well perfused with blood, as are the brain and parenchymal organs, the time required for adipose tissue to reach saturation is relatively long (half-time: 25 hours). The elimination half-life of the solvent is coincidentally long, and thus accumulation of TCA in adipose tissue occurs with continuing exposure.

Exposure to higher concentrations of TCA for shorter durations results in higher levels of TCA in the liver, kidneys, and brain than do longer-duration exposures to lower concentrations, reflecting that these tissues are well perfused and do not accumulate TCA and suggesting that during chronic exposure the body burden of TCA is redistributed to the lipid-rich adipose tissue (Holmberg et al., 1977). When a steady state between absorption and elimination is reached, the body will contain approximately 3.6 times more TCA than is found after a single 8-hour exposure, and 70% of the total body burden will be localized in fat (Nolan et al., 1984). After cessation of exposure, TCA is redistributed from the various tissues of the body back into the blood. The gradual release of the solvent from fat into the blood serves as a recycling internal source of exposure in those individuals who are chronically exposed to TCA (Stewart et al., 1969; Monster, 1979; Savolainen, 1981; Hodgson et al., 1989). TCA readily crosses the placenta and has been found in the fetus of mice (Danielson et al., 1986).

Tissue Biochemistry

TCA is a relatively stable compound compared to other chlorinated hydrocarbons (e.g., trichloroethylene). Unlike trichloroethylene, which contains a reactive double bond, the majority of TCA is not metabolized in the human body (Monster, 1979). The metabolism of the remaining TCA which does occur involves the cytochrome P-450 metabolic pathway and is independent of route of absorption (Ivanetich and van den Honert, 1981; Kaneko et al., 1994). The initial oxidative metabolite of TCA is trichloroethanol (TCEtOH), which is subsequently oxidized by alcohol dehydrogenase to trichloroacetic acid (TCAA) (Hake et al., 1960; Monster, 1979; Ivanetich and van den Honert, 1981; Imbriani et al., 1988). The blood and urine concentrations of TCAA are thus determined by the amount of TCEtOH formed (Monster, 1979) (Fig. 13-1). Other possible metabolites of TCA in humans include carbon dioxide, acetylene, chloride ion, and 1,1-dichloroethane (Hake et al., 1960; Dürk et al., 1992). In addition, experimental evidence *in vitro* and *in vivo* suggests that free radical intermediates are formed during the metabolism of TCA (Dürk et al., 1992).

Simultaneous exposure to TCA and other organic solvents alters the metabolism and the neurotoxic effects of each constituent compound (Ödkvist et al., 1980; Savolainen, 1981; Woolverton and Balster, 1981; Tham et al., 1984). Savolainen (1981) noted that simultaneous exposure to TCA and trichloroethylene decreased the neurotoxic effects of trichloroethylene. Ödkvist et al. (1980) reported that simultaneous exposure to TCA and trichloroethylene

TABLE 13-2. *Postmortem tissue distribution of TCA in humans following fatal acute intoxication*

Tissue	Case 1	Case 2	Case 3	Case 4	Case 5	Case 6	Case 7
Brain	0.32	2.7	9.3	36.0	50.0	56.0	59.0
Liver	0.49	9.8	13.2	5.0	12.0	11.0	22.0
Kidney	0.26	2.4	7.8	12.0			
Muscle	0.26	4.9					
Lung	0.18		2.2	1.0			
Blood	0.15			2.0	6.0	6.2	12.0
Urine	0.10						

Blood and urine TCA concentrations are reported in mg/L. TCA concentrations in brain, liver, kidney, muscle, and lung tissues are reported in mg/100 g. Data from Stahl et al., 1969 (Cases 1–3, 5–7) and Caplan et al., 1976 (Case 4).

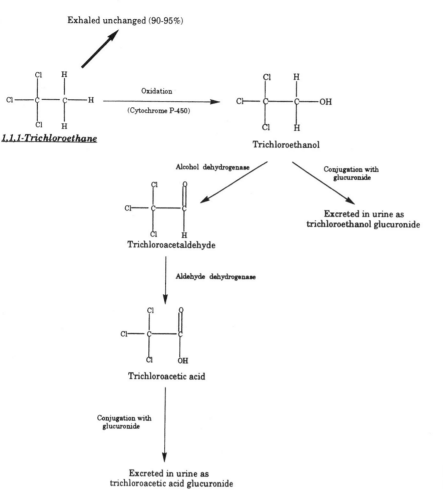

FIG. 13-1. Proposed metabolic pathways for 1,1,1-trichloroethane.

had an additive effect on impairment of the vestibulooculomotor functioning in rabbits (see Neurophysiological Diagnosis section). These findings suggest that TCA and trichloroethylene, both of which are metabolized to TCEtOH, an alcohol, may compete for cytochrome P-450 and alcohol dehydrogenase. Therefore, coexposure to these two solvents reduces the metabolism of trichloroethylene to trichloroethylene epoxide but also additively increases the total blood level of TCEtOH. The latter has been suggested as the metabolite responsible for the acute anesthetic effects of both TCA and trichloroethylene; a greater portion of an absorbed dose of trichloroethylene is metabolized to TCEtOH, and trichloroethylene induces anesthesia at much lower concentrations than does TCA (Siebecker et al., 1960; Savolainen, 1977, 1981; Peoples and Weight, 1994). A similar effect can be expected during simultaneous exposures to TCA and perchloroethylene, the latter of which is also metabolized to TCEtOH (Lauwerys et al., 1983; Mutti and Franchini, 1987). There is considerable evidence that alcohols react with specific hydrophobic sites on ligand-gated ion channels of cell membranes (Franks and Lieb, 1994). In addition, in vitro studies of ion current mediated by the 5-HT$_3$ receptors in NCB-20 neuroblastoma cell membranes indicate that the chemical structure of an alcohol determines which specific hydrophobic sites on the receptor a particular alcohol can interact with (Zhou and Lovinger, 1996). For example, concurrent exposure to TCA and a solvent such as xylene, which is metabolized to several different alcohols (methylbenzyl alcohols and xylenols) but is not metabolized to an epoxide intermediate or trichloroethanol, has not been shown to produce additive or synergistic effects (Savolainen et al., 1981). The effects of concurrent exposures to TCA and methylene chloride—which is primarily metabolized to carbon monoxide—is uncertain (Rall, 1990). Chronic exposure to chemicals such as ethanol and phenobarbital, which induce the production of cytochrome P-450 enzymes, enhances the metabolism of TCA and therefore may increase its toxicity by producing active metabolites (Savolainen, 1977; Ivanetich and van den Honert, 1981; Turina et al., 1986; Kaneko et al., 1994).

The acute neurotoxic effects of TCA have been attributed to the pharmacological activities of its metabolites. TCEtOH has been shown to potentiate neuronal γ-aminobutyric acid (GABA)-mediated responses in vitro (Peoples and Weight, 1994). In addition, TCEtOH has been shown to inhibit ion currents activated by excitatory amino acids (Peoples et al., 1990). These findings suggest that the TCA metabolite, TCEtOH, which induces potentiation of GABA-mediated synaptic responses and inhibition of excitatory amino acid-mediated responses, is involved in producing the acute sedative effects associated with exposure to TCA and other chlorinated hydrocarbons such as trichloroethylene and perchloroethylene. However, unlike other anesthetic agents such as ethanol and halothane, which interfere with mitochondrial energy production by altering the permeability of the mitochondrial membrane to calcium, potentiation of GABA-mediated responses by TCA does not depend on an increase in intracellular Ca^{2+} (Peoples and Weight, 1994).

The biochemical mechanisms by which TCA produces chronic effects are not known, but several interesting studies have been reported. Metabolism of TCA has also been shown to produce free radicals that can fragment DNA and induce apoptosis (Halliwell, 1989; Dürk et al., 1992; Corcoran et al., 1994). Cytochrome P-450 activates covalent binding of ^{14}C-labeled TCA metabolites, to DNA, RNA, and proteins *in vitro* and *in vivo*. In addition, this reaction was enhanced by phenobarbital, which then enhances the metabolism of TCA (Turina et al., 1986) (see Neuropathological Diagnosis section).

Excretion

The majority (~95%) of an absorbed dose of TCA is excreted unchanged from the lungs in humans (Stewart and Andrews, 1966; Stewart et al., 1969; Monster, 1979; Nolan et al., 1984). Following intraperitoneal injection of C^{14}-labeled TCA, approximately 98% of the absorbed dose was excreted unchanged via the respiratory system of rats (Hake et al., 1960). Due to the lower rate of metabolism and lower blood/air partition coefficient of TCA, it is excreted much faster via the lungs than are perchloroethylene or trichloroethylene (Monster, 1979). Five percent of an absorbed dose of TCA is metabolized to TCEtOH and TCAA, conjugated with glucuronic acid, and excreted in the urine as water-soluble metabolites (Stewart, 1968; Stewart et al., 1969; Monster, 1979, 1986) (see Fig. 13-1). Trace amounts (< 0.01%) of TCA are excreted unchanged in the urine (Stewart et al., 1961; Morgan et al., 1970; Imbriani et al., 1988) (see Bio-

chemical Diagnosis section). In addition, trace amounts (0.03%) of TCA and its metabolites are excreted in the feces (Hake et al., 1960). The elimination of TCA follows a three-compartment model, representing elimination from the parenchymal organs (i.e., liver, kidneys, and spleen), muscle, and adipose tissues, with half-lives of 44 minutes, 5.7 hours, and 53 hours, respectively (Nolan et al., 1984). The half-times for elimination of TCEtOH and TCAA from the blood are 10 to 12 hours and 80 to 100 hours, respectively (Monster, 1979).

CLINICAL MANIFESTATIONS AND DIAGNOSIS

Symptomatic Diagnosis

The concentration, duration, and circumstances of exposure determine the severity of the symptoms of TCA exposure (Tables 13-3 and 13-4). Although low concentrations of TCA are tolerated by most individuals (Kramer et al., 1978; Maroni et al., 1977; McCarthy et al., 1983), exposure to higher concentrations produces lightheadedness, headache, incoordination, drowsiness and anesthesia, cardiac arrhythmia, depression of respiration, coma and death (Krantz et al., 1959; Dornette and Jones, 1960; Stewart et al., 1961; Stewart, 1968; Gresham and Treip, 1983; Liss, 1988; Howse et al., 1989; House et al., 1994, 1996; Bowen and Balster, 1996). Cardiac irritability and arrhythmia are associated with cases of sudden death following acute exposures to TCA (Ranson and Berry, 1986; McLeod et al., 1987). While the short-term effects of acute low-level and nonfatal high-level exposures appear reversible, chronic occupational and environmental exposures are associated with permanent encephalopathy and, in some cases, sensory neuropathy (Rosengren et al., 1985; Karlsson et al., 1987; Liss, 1988; Kelafant et al., 1994; House et al., 1994, 1996).

Acute Exposure

Acute exposure to TCA causes oronasal pharynx and bronchial mucosal membrane irritation, dizziness, euphoria, headache, incoordination, ataxia, nausea, vomiting,

TABLE 13-3. *Acute symptoms of exposure in volunteers exposed to 1,1,1-trichloroethane*

Exposure level (ppm)	Duration	Acute symptoms	Reference
175–350	210 min	None	Torkelson et al., 1958
450–710	90 min	None	MacKay et al., 1987
415–590	450 min	None	Torkelson et al., 1958
890–1,190	30 min	None	
900–1,000	70–75 min	Lightheadedness, eye irritation, incoordination, loss of equilibrium	
1,740–2,180	5 min	Overt ataxia	
500[a]	6.5–7 h/day/5 days	Drowsiness and difficulty performing a postural maintenance test	Stewart et al., 1969
>10,000	min/hr	Anesthesia	Dornette and Jones, 1960

[a]The acute effects of repeated daily exposure to TCA in this study suggest that additional TCA and its metabolites accumulate in the tissues of subjects and thus contribute to the total exposure dose.

TABLE 13-4. *Chronic symptoms of exposure in volunteers exposed to 1,1,1-trichloroethane*

Exposure level (ppm)	Duration	Chronic symptoms	Reference
1–250	6.0 years	None	Kramer et al., 1978
110–345	6.7 years	None	Maroni et al., 1977
Not reported[a]	17.6 years	Headache, vertigo, concentration difficulties, memory problems, irritability, anxiety, sleep disturbances, fatigue	Kelafant et al., 1994

[a]See Clinical Experiences section of text for details of exposure history.

and diarrhea (Torkelson et al., 1958; Stewart et al., 1961, 1969). In addition, more prolonged or greater intensity acute exposures depress central nervous system (CNS) functioning, producing loss of consciousness, anesthesia, coma, and death (Dornette and Jones, 1960; Stahl et al., 1969; Halevy et al., 1980; Ranson and Berry, 1986). Fifty-two cases of severe occupational exposure to TCA were reported in the United Kingdom between 1961 and 1980. In 26 incidents the exposed worker lost consciousness, and in 18 situations the worker developed CNS symptoms and signs but did not lose consciousness (McCarthy and Jones, 1983). The autonomic nervous system is affected by TCA and it induces myocardial irritability with abnormal cardiac conduction associated with cardiac arrhythmia, resulting in sudden death (Herd et al., 1974; Herd and Martin, 1975; Kobayashi et al., 1987; McLeod et al., 1987). Exposure may also result in acute hepatic and renal dysfunction, presenting with abnormal liver function tests [serum bilirubin, serum glutamic oxaloacetic transaminase (SGOT), and alkaline phosphatase] and proteinuria, respectively (Stewart et al., 1961; Stewart, 1971; Halevy et al., 1980; Hodgson et al., 1989).

Acute exposure to relatively low concentrations of TCA may not produce subjective symptoms of exposure in some individuals. For example, no subjective complaints were reported in 12 volunteers exposed to ambient air TCA concentrations of 175 and 350 ppm for 3.5 hours (MacKay et al., 1987). However, interindividual differences in susceptibility to the effects of TCA lead to various rates and degrees of severity of symptoms of exposure in groups of workers who may have shared the same exposure levels of TCA (Stewart, 1968; Stewart et al., 1969; Halevy et al., 1980). Several studies reported the effects of TCA at various exposure levels. For example, only four of 11 human subjects experimentally exposed to 500 ppm TCA for 6.5 to 7 hours per day for 5 days consistently reported feeling sleepy, and only two consistently had difficulty performing postural maintenance tests during the exposure period (Stewart et al., 1969). Seven volunteers exposed to TCA experienced eye irritation, a sense of loss of equilibrium, and incoordination at concentrations of 900 to 1,000 ppm. At a concentration of 1,700 ppm the subjects were obviously ataxic. Not until reaching an exposure concentration of 2,650 ppm did three subjects experience lightheadedness and two subjects had difficulty maintaining an upright posture (Stewart et al., 1961). Torkelson et al. (1958) exposed groups of two to four individuals to TCA vapor con-

centrations ranging from 415 to 2,180 ppm (see Table 13-3). No subjective symptoms of exposure were noted at vapor concentrations of 415 to 590 ppm for a duration of 7.5 hours, or at vapor concentrations of 890 to 1,190 for a duration of 30 minutes. However, during exposure to TCA vapor concentrations of 900 to 1,000 ppm for 70 to 75 minutes the three of the four exposed individuals experienced lightheadedness, and tests of coordination and equilibrium revealed impairments in all four individuals. When the TCA vapor concentration was raised to 1,900 ppm, the subjects showed overt disturbances of equilibrium, which became apparent after only 5 minutes of exposure. Concentrations of greater than 10,000 ppm TCA produce anesthesia, bradycardia, hypotension, respiratory arrest, cardiac arrhythmia, and death (Krantz et al., 1959; Dornette and Jones, 1960).

Chronic Exposure

Chronic TCA exposure produces a myriad of nonspecific symptoms including headaches, vertigo, impairments of short-term memory, difficulty concentrating, increased irritability and moodiness, anxiety, sleep disturbances, and fatigue (Kelafant et al., 1994) (see Table 13-4). The symptoms associated with chronic exposure to TCA are often so mild that they may go unreported. If reported, they are often attributed to other causes or simply ascribed to depression, psychosomatic causes, or even malingering. For example, no differences in symptoms of exposure was determined when comparing workers chronically exposed to TCA at concentrations ranging from 1 to 250 ppm and a group of unexposed controls (Kramer et al., 1978). In another report, Maroni et al. (1977) found no significant increases in symptoms among 22 female workers chronically exposed to TCA at ambient air concentrations of 110 to 345 ppm for a mean duration of 6.7 years when compared to unexposed controls. One worker from this group was even frequently exposed to TCA at concentrations of 720 to 990 ppm. Nevertheless, these workers did report a greater frequency of subjective complaints including headache, anxiety, nervousness, irritability, insomnia, depression, and digestive disorders than did the control group. The contribution of TCA to the occurrence of these symptoms among the exposed workers cannot be disregarded (Kelafant et al., 1994).

Peripheral neuropathy has also been reported following chronic exposure to TCA and is frequently more marked in the upper extremities of those individuals who have had direct dermal contact with liquid TCA (Liss, 1988; Howse et al., 1989; House et al., 1994, 1996). Persistent findings that may develop following a nonfatal intense acute exposure in which cardiac arrest occurs are essentially those of tissue hypoxia (Gresham and Treip, 1983) (see Clinical Experiences section).

Neurophysiological Diagnosis

Electroencephalography (EEG) can be used to differentiate TCA exposure from metabolic encephalopathies. The EEG of volunteers acutely exposed to low levels of TCA reveals increased amplitude of alpha activity (Stewart et al., 1975). No specific changes are noted on the EEG of persons anesthetized with TCA until depression of circulatory system function produces hypotension and bradycardia with an associated generalized slowing of the dominant frequency (Siebecker et al., 1960). The EEG in rats exposed to TCA at concentration of 6,000 ppm for 1 hour also showed a generalized slowing of the dominant frequency (Hougaard et al., 1984). These animals were not anesthetized at this concentration, and therefore these findings suggest that it is possible that such EEG slowing may also be seen in humans exposed to subanesthetic concentrations of TCA. The EEG of a 35-year-old male machinist who had been chronically exposed to TCA for 10 years revealed normal alpha activity of 11 Hz and no spike discharges or paroxysmal activity were seen. No abnormalities were seen in response to hyperventilation and photic stimulation produced normal bilateral driving (R. G. Feldman, personal observation).

Visual evoked potentials (VEPs) documented the acute effects of TCA in nine male volunteers (age: 20 to 25 years) (Seppäläinen et al., 1983). The subjects were exposed to TCA at concentrations of 200 and 400 ppm for 4 hours per day. VEPs were measured before and after exposures as well as before and after an exposure-free control trial. The latencies of P150 were found to decrease during exposure to 400 ppm TCA. In addition, the decrease in P150 latency at 400 ppm seen in these subjects was correlated with increases in body sway and reaction times which were also documented at this level of exposure.

Nerve conduction velocity (NCV) studies can be used to document the peripheral nervous system effects associated with subacute and chronic exposure to TCA. No significant changes in ulnar and peroneal NCVs were found in a group of 22 female factory workers (mean age: 32.4 years) exposed to TCA at ambient air concentrations of 110 to 990 ppm for a mean duration of 6.7 years (SD ± 2.5 years) (Maroni et al., 1977). After 4 weeks of dermal and inhalation exposure to TCA, the NCV studies in a 40-year-old woman revealed prolongation of the distal sensory latency in the median nerves. Motor conduction velocity and distal sensory latencies were prolonged in the ulnar nerves. Results of sural nerve conduction studies were within normal limits (Liss, 1988). NCV studies in a 25-year-old woman who developed symptoms of peripheral neuropathy in all her extremities after 3 months of chronic dermal and inhalation exposure to TCA revealed low median and ulnar sensory action potentials. Motor conduction velocities and distal sensory latencies were within normal limits. No abnormalities were detected on sural nerve conduction studies. A 44-year-old woman developed peripheral neuropathy in her upper and lower extremities 18 months after she began working as a hydraulic pump dismantler. Her job required her to degrease the parts from the pumps she had dismantled, and it exposed her to TCA via dermal and inhalation routes. Sural NCV studies documented significantly decreased peak-to-peak sensory amplitudes bilaterally, suggesting axonal neuropathy. At follow-up 7 months after cessation of exposure, sensory amplitudes had improved to within normal limits in the left sural nerve but remained decreased in the right (House et al., 1994) (Table 13-5). Sensory conduction velocity was slowed in both sural nerves when she was removed from further exposure, reflecting secondary demyelinating changes. Seven months after absence from TCA, the right sural sensory CV increased significantly (see Neuropathology section).

Electronystagmography (ENG) can be used to document the acute subclinical effects of TCA on vestibulooculomotor functioning. Positional nystagmus was detected in rabbits with blood TCA levels of 75 ppm (Ödkvist et al., 1980). Simultaneous exposure to TCA and trichloroethylene had an additive effect on vestibulooculomotor functioning in these animals. Although blood trichloroethanol levels were not

TABLE 13-5. *Nerve conduction studies in a 44-year-old woman following chronic occupational exposure to TCA*

Examination	Nerve tested	Latency (msec)	Peak-to-peak amplitude (μV)	Conduction velocity (m/sec)
Initial	L-sural	2.9	4.4	48.3
	R-sural	3.0	3.7	46.7
Follow-up	L-sural	2.9	5.8	48.3
	R-sural	2.7	4.9	51.9

Reduced peak-to-peak amplitude (normal range: 10 μV ± 4.3 μV) of sensory nerve fibers in the left and right sural nerve. Conduction velocity in the right sural nerve was slowed although still within normal range (see Chapter 3). Improvement was recorded in the peak-to-peak amplitudes bilaterally and in the right sural nerve conduction velocity after 7 months without further exposure, suggesting that primary sensory axonal neuropathy was related to TCA exposure.
Data from House et al., 1994.

reported, these findings suggest that trichloroethanol (TCEtOH), a metabolite of TCA and TCE, may be involved in the acute neurotoxic effects produced by these two solvents (Peoples and Weight, 1994). In contrast, simultaneous exposure to trichloroethylene and styrene had a much-greater-than-expected (synergistic) effect on vestibulooculomotor functioning, suggesting that simultaneous exposure to those solvents that are metabolized to either two different alcohols and two different electrophilic intermediates significantly augments the neurotoxic effects of each of these xenobiotics (Savolainen, 1977; Ödkvist et al., 1980; Tham et al., 1984) (Fig. 13-2). These findings also suggest that neurons in the reticular formation and the cerebellum are particularly sensitive to the anesthetic effects of TCA (Ödkvist et al., 1980; Tham et al., 1984) (see Chapters 11 and 17).

Neuropsychological Diagnosis

Neuropsychological testing can be used to document the acute and chronic CNS effects of TCA exposures. The neuropsychological domain of attention and concentration appears to be particularly susceptible to the acute effects of TCA. The results of neuropsychological testing also suggest that the acute effects of TCA on the CNS are biphasic. Therefore, when assessing acute exposures using neuropsychological testing, findings should be interpreted not only with regard to the total exposure dose, but also with consideration of (a) the specific domain being assessed by a particular test instrument and (b) the rate of rise of blood and tissue concentrations of TCA and its metabolites (e.g., trichloroethanol) (Holmberg et al., 1977; Savolainen et al., 1981; Moser and Balster, 1986; MacKay et al., 1987; You et al., 1994; Bowen and Balster, 1996). Chronic exposure to TCA had been associated with attention and memory deficits (Kelafant et al., 1994) (see Clinical Experiences section).

Acute Exposure

The *acute effects of TCA* on performance of tests of simple and choice reaction times, manual dexterity, and perceptual speed were assessed in 14 healthy male subjects. Each subject served as his own control and was tested for 30 minutes while being exposed to 250, 350, 450, and 550 ppm of TCA as well as during nonexposed control conditions. Impairment was noted on the test of perceptual speed in these subjects at 350 ppm. Simple and choice reaction times and manual dexterity were impaired in 12 subjects during 30-minute exposures to 350, 450, and 550 ppm (Gamberale and Hultengren, 1973). Salvini et al. (1971) did not find significant functional impairments on neuropsychological tests of memory, complex reaction time, and manual dexterity among six male subjects acutely exposed to 450 ppm TCA for two consecutive 4-hour periods separated by a 1.5-hour exposure-free interval. However, performance on tests of perceptual ability was significantly impaired in this same group. In addition, the subjects' performance on the perceptual tests was positively correlated with mental stress. MacKay et al. (1987) assessed the acute neuropsychological effects of exposure to TCA at concentrations of 175 and 350 ppm for 3.5 hours in a group of 12 male volunteers. Tests used for the assessment included simple and choice reaction times (psychomotor speed), digital step-input tracking (visuomotor tracking), Stroop test (attention and concentration), syntactic reasoning (executive functioning), and stress-arousal checklist (mood). Simple and choice reaction times were significantly impaired, with the most marked performance deficits seen toward the end of exposure to 350 ppm. Performance on the digital step-input tracking task was also significantly impaired. No performance deficits were revealed by the syntactic reasoning test. In contrast, performance on the Stroop test improved with exposure in a dose-dependent manner, suggesting that TCA affects specific behavioral domains differently and that the domain of attention and concentration is particularly susceptible to the acute effects of TCA.

Neuropsychological testing of nine male volunteers exposed to concentrations of 200 and 400 ppm TCA revealed different acute effects at low and high concentrations (Savolainen et al., 1981). Simple reaction times and body sway were found to decrease in this group of subjects during exposure to 200 ppm TCA, whereas increased reaction times and body sway were seen during exposure to 400 ppm TCA. Exposure to 400 ppm TCA in combination with 200 ppm xylene tended to prolong the simple reaction times of these subjects. However, no significant difference was found on a test of finger tapping speed. These findings suggest that the acute effects of TCA on the CNS are biphasic and are similar to those of ethanol. Furthermore, these findings indicate that the subclinical acute effects of TCA are detected best by the

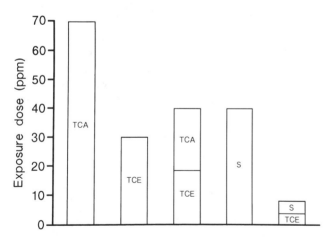

FIG. 13-2. Positional nystagmus in rabbits exposed to 1,1,1-trichloroethane (TCA), trichloroethylene (TCE), and styrene (S). This figure demonstrates differences in exposure levels necessary to induce acute effects on vestibulooculomotor functioning during exposure to: TCA alone; TCE alone; TCA and TCE; and TCE and styrene (see text for discussion of findings) (Data from Ödkvist et al., 1980.)

more complex psychomotor tasks which also measure attention and vigilance (Savolainen et al., 1981; Moser and Balster, 1986; MacKay et al., 1987; Bowen and Balster, 1996).

Chronic Exposure

The *effects of chronic exposure* to TCA on neuropsychological functioning was assessed in 22 female factory workers (mean age: 32.4) exposed to TCA at concentrations of 110 to 990 ppm for a mean exposure duration of 6.7 years (Maroni et al., 1977). Domains assessed included general intelligence (Raven PM 38), executive functioning (Picture Completion), visuospatial ability (Block Design), psychomotor function (Pauli Test and Symbol–Number Association), memory (Rey PRM), and personality and mood (Eysenck's Maudsley PI and Cattell's IPAT). No significant differences were found between the neuropsychological functioning of the exposed workers and the controls on these tests. Neuropsychological assessments were performed on a group of 28 workers with chronic exposure to TCA at levels which were high enough to induce acute dizziness and nausea; actual exposure concentrations were not reported (Kelafant et al., 1994) (see Clinical Experiences section). Tests administered included the Luria–Nebraska Psychological Battery (LNNB), Trails A and B, Symbol Digit, and the Personality Assessment Inventory (PAI). Findings were compared to published norms. Performance deficits were identified on the following LNNB subtests: rhythm ($p < 0.001$), memory ($p < 0.001$), intermediate memory ($p < 0.003$), and speed ($p < 0.009$). Mean performance time on Trails B was increased and approached significance ($p < 0.065$). Scores on the PAI were within the normal range. The group scores on Somatization and Depression scales approached significance ($p < 0.009$ and $p < 0.009$, respectively). These neuropsychological findings suggest that a long-term exposure to TCA decreases motor speed and impairs attention, concentration, and memory function. Although depression can also produce memory and attentional problems, these workers also experienced disequilibrium and olfactory disturbances, neither of which is characteristic of depression.

Biochemical Diagnosis

The initial CNS effects of exposure to TCA are subclinical and are not objectively evident. Exposures to and absorption of TCA, whether by oral, pulmonary, or dermal routes, can be documented by determining the concentrations of TCA and its metabolites in alveolar air, urine, and blood (Ghittori et al., 1987; Imbriani et al., 1988; Mizunuma et al., 1995; Tay et al., 1995; ACGIH, 1995). Blood TCA level is the most accurate method for documenting recent exposures to TCA (Monster, 1986; Tay et al., 1995). The baseline level of TCA in the blood of nonexposed subjects is 0.0002 mg/L (range: <0.0001 to 0.0034 mg/L) (Hajimiragha et al., 1989). Urine TCA concentration is a specific noninvasive method of documenting TCA exposures. Immediately following exposure to 50 ppm urine TCA levels are 4.9 mg/g creatinine (Monster, 1986).

The ACGIH has defined biological exposure indices (BEIs) which can be used to monitor and document exposure to TCA (ACGIH, 1995) (Table 13-6). Biological monitoring and early detection of exposure is important in protecting the health of individuals at risk (Mizunuma et al., 1995). The concentration of TCA in alveolar air serves as specific noninvasive BEI for monitoring TCA exposure and should be determined prior to the end of the last shift of the workweek and should not exceed 40 ppm (ACGIH, 1995). TCA is still detectable in the alveolar air of exposed individuals 64 hours after cessation of exposure.

Exposure to TCA can also be documented by determining blood levels of trichloroethanol (TCEtOH) and trichloroacetic acid (TCAA). The ACGIH (1995) recommended blood TCEtOH level as a BEI of exposure. Blood TCEtOH levels should not exceed 1 mg/L at the end of the last shift of the workweek. When using TCAA as a parameter of exposure, the blood sample should be taken at the end of the last shift of a full workweek to determine ongoing as well as previous day's accumulative exposures. For example, the blood TCAA levels in workers exposed to TCA at an ambient air concentration of 50 ppm, 8 hours/day for 5 days, had a mean of 2.3 mg/L when determined 5 to 15 minutes after cessation of exposure; the mean blood TCAA levels dropped to 1.6 mg/L by 64 hours after cessation of exposure (Monster, 1986).

Both TCEtOH and TCAA are the recommended urinary BEIs of TCA exposure and should be determined at the end of the workweek and should not exceed 30 mg/L and 10 mg/L, respectively (ACGIH, 1995). However, because blood and urinary TCEtOH and TCAA are not specific to the metabolism of TCA and because both compounds are also metabolites of other chlorinated hydrocarbon solvents such as trichloroethylene, these biochemical parameters cannot be relied upon for monitoring specifically for TCA

TABLE 13-6. *Biological exposure indices for 1,1,1-trichloroethane*

Determinant:	Urine		Blood	Alveolar air
	TCEtOH	TCAA	TCEtOH	TCA
Start of shift:	Not established	Not established	Not established	Not established
During shift:	Not established	Not established	Not established	Not established
Prior to last shift of workweek:	Not established	Not established	Not established	40 ppm
At end of last shift of workweek:	30 mg/L	10 mg/L	1 mg/L	Not established

Data from ACGIH, 1995.

in individuals who are simultaneously being exposed to more than one chlorinated hydrocarbon solvent (Stewart et al., 1969; Nolan et al., 1984). Although the ACGIH has not established BEIs for TCA levels in blood and urine, measurement of the levels of TCA in blood and urine are often useful to document the uptake of this compound in individuals who may be simultaneously exposed to other chlorinated hydrocarbons (Monster, 1986; Tay et al., 1995; ACGIH, 1995). However, recent dermal exposure to liquid TCA can increase blood levels in regions adjacent to the area of skin contact, and therefore this should be considered while taking blood samples from workers who have had direct dermal contact with the solvent. The blood concentrations of TCA in the exposed arms of volunteers were raised 35-fold immediately following exposure. In addition, a significant difference between the blood levels in the two arms was detectable up to 5 hours after cessation of exposure to TCA (Aitio et al., 1984).

Neuroimaging

Magnetic resonance imaging (MRI) and *computed tomography* (CT) scans can be used to differentiate the effects of TCA encephalopathy from other encephalopathies which result in cognitive deficits, behavioral abnormalities, and dementias. These may include vascular etiologies, Alzheimer's disease, neoplasms, or metabolic disturbances. The brain MRIs of 25 workers who developed symptoms of encephalopathy associated with chronic exposure to TCA revealed no morphological changes which could be attributed to the exposure circumstances (Kelafant et al., 1994). A brain CT scan performed in an 18-year-old man revealed cerebral atrophy 2 months after he was found unconscious in a degreasing bath of TCA (Gresham and Treip, 1983). However, by the time this patient was discovered, he had already suffered cardiac and respiratory arrest, and therefore the morphological changes seen on the CT scan in this patient may be partly, if not entirely, due to the effects of tissue hypoxia.

Positron emission tomography (PET) studies reveal changes in blood flow and glucose metabolism in the brains of six rats acutely exposed to TCA at concentrations of 3,500, 6,000 and 7,800 ppm for 30 minutes at each exposure level (Hougaard et al., 1984). No significant differences in cerebral blood flow was noted during exposure to 3,500 ppm. At 6,000 and 7,800 ppm a significant increase in blood flow was noted in all brain regions. Significant reductions in glucose metabolism were noted during exposure to 6,000 ppm TCA in 10 brain regions and were most marked ($p < 0.001$) in the red nucleus, thalamus, sensorimotor cortex, and inferior colliculus (Table 13-7). The changes in blood flow and glucose metabolism were related to decreases in motility and exploratory behavior of the animals. PET studies in humans exposed to TCA have not been found in the literature. However, Mullin and Krivanek (1982) noted that performance of rats on unconditioned reflex and conditioned avoidance response tests were not impaired until concentrations were at least twofold higher

TABLE 13-7. *Positron emission tomography in rat brains, demonstrating regional reductions in mean glucose metabolism (μmol/g/min) during exposure to 6,000 ppm TCA for 60 minutes*

Brain region	Exposed (*n* = 7)	Unexposed (*n* = 6)
Red nucleus	0.31	0.50
Substantia nigra	0.31	0.42
Sensorimotor cortex	0.51	0.72
Thalamus	0.51	0.66
Lateral thalamus	0.49	0.63
Inferior colliculus	0.62	1.11
Superior colliculus	0.44	0.56
Medial geniculate body	0.50	0.68
Septal nucleus	0.26	0.36
Cerebellum	0.31	0.39

Data from Hougaard et al., 1984.

than those reported to induce overt neurobehavioral effects in humans, suggesting that alterations in cerebral blood flow and glucose metabolism may begin at lower concentrations in humans, as well. Furthermore, areas with increased blood flow may be at greater risk for permanent damage as more TCA and its metabolites reach these areas.

Neuropathological Diagnosis

The neuropathological findings in the brains of persons after fatal acute TCA exposure are similar to those in persons who suffered hypoxia due to other causes (Hall and Hine, 1966; Hatfield and Maykoski, 1970). Gresham and Treip (1983) described the neuropathological findings in an 18-year-old man who died 39 months after he lost consciousness and collapsed with his head over a tank of TCA. The patient was in cardiac and respiratory arrest when he was discovered. The effects of hypoxia due to cardiac arrest also must be considered in this case. The brain was small (weight: 1,112 g), with generalized gyral atrophy, most marked in the occipital region. Coronal section through the mammillary bodies revealed moderate symmetrical ventricular dilation, shrinkage of both lenticular nuclei with a brownish discoloration to the globus pallidus, and bilateral cavitation of the putamen. The atrophy of the basal ganglia had resulted in a widening of the insular sulci. There was no visible atrophy of the cortex at this level. Coronal section at the level of the calcarine cortex revealed severe cortical atrophy. No macroscopic changes were noted in the brain stem or spinal cord. Microscopic examination of this brain revealed extensive damage in the calcarine cortex. Extensive cavitation with foamy and hemosiderin-filled macrophages was present in the lenticular nucleus. Astrocytic and capillary proliferation were prominent in the occipital cortex. Fibrillary gliosis was demonstrated in both areas by Holzer preparations. Fibrillary gliosis without necrosis was present in the thalamus. The lateral geniculate bodies appeared normal. All other areas of the cortex appeared normal in this case.

Specific neuropathological changes in the CNS have not been demonstrated in human cases following chronic exposure to TCA. However, animal studies suggest that chronic exposure to TCA does damage the CNS. The fatty acid pattern of ethanolamine phosphoglyceride was altered in the cerebral cortex of gerbils exposed to 1,200 ppm of TCA for 5 days (Kyrklund and Haglid, 1990). Histopatho-

logical studies of the brains of gerbils exposed to a concentration of 210 ppm of TCA for 4 months showed a significant and irreversible increase in the level of glial fibrillary acid (GFA) protein in the sensory motor cortex, indicating that the astroglial fibrils had formed in response to CNS damage (Rosengren et al., 1985). Savolainen et al. (1977) reported a slight decrease in RNA content in the brains of

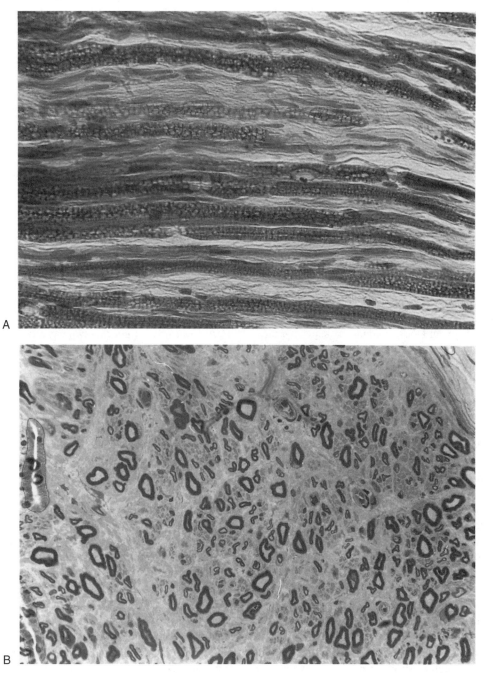

FIG. 13-3. Sural nerve biopsy of a 25-year-old woman occupationally exposed to TCA. **A:** Longitudinal section of sural nerve showing axon apathy with increased endoneurial connective tissue, fragmentation of myelin sheaths, and macrophage infiltration (stained with Luxol fats blue; original magnification, ×250). **B:** Cross section of sural nerve showing decrease in the number of myelinated fibers of all sizes (plastic embedded section stained with tetroxide and toluidine blue; original magnification, ×400). (Tissue provided by G. Liss and histology interpreted by Ann C. McKee.)

rats exposed to a TCA vapor concentration of 500 ppm for 6 hours per day for 4 days. In addition, decreases in DNA content have been reported in the posterior cerebellar hemisphere, the anterior cerebellar vermis, and the hippocampus of gerbils exposed to TCA, indicating cell loss in these areas (Karlsson et al., 1987).

The sural nerve biopsies of patients who have developed peripheral neuropathy after subchronic and chronic concomitant dermal and inhalation exposures to TCA reveal evidence of axonopathy and secondary myelinopathy (Liss, 1988; Howse et al., 1989). Specific neuropathological findings in the sural nerve biopsy of a 25-year-old woman who presented with paresthesia in all four extremities 3 months after she began using TCA as a degreasing solvent included a decrease in the number of myelinated fibers and fragmentation of myelin sheaths with ovoid formation; no evidence of neurofilament accumulation in the paranodal regions of the axons was seen (G. M. Liss; A.C. McKee, personal communications) (Fig. 13-3).

The chronic effects of TCA have been attributed to the parent compound and its metabolites. Rosengren et al. (1985) suggest that TCA, which is lipid-soluble, may induce cell death by altering membrane fluidity. Experimental evidence *in vitro* and *in vivo* suggests that dechlorination of TCA occurs and that free radicals are formed during its metabolism (Van Dyke and Wineman, 1971; Town and Leibman, 1984; Tomasi et al., 1984; Turina et al., 1986; Dürk et al., 1992). Free radicals can induce lipid peroxidation which subsequently alters membrane permeability to calcium and other ions, and they can fragment DNA; both mechanisms can induce cell death via apoptosis (Halliwell, 1989; Dürk et al., 1992; Corcoran et al., 1994; Wood and Youle, 1995). However, TCA is a stable saturated chlorinated hydrocarbon and has a correspondingly low rate of metabolism, resulting in relatively low chronic toxicity (Ivanetich and van den Honert, 1981; Turina et al., 1986; Dürk et al., 1992). In contrast, the unsaturated chlorinated hydrocarbons are readily metabolized and have greater toxicity. For example, trichloroethylene, which is readily metabolized to a reactive epoxide intermediate as well as a free radical, produces more persistent toxic effects than does TCA (Ivanetich and van den Honert, 1981; Gonthier and Barret, 1989; Dürk et al., 1992).

The tissue biochemical correlates of TCA exposure have been experimentally investigated in animals. Acute exposure of rats to 8,000 ppm TCA for 5 and 60 minutes did not alter blood levels of glucose, lactic acid, or pyruvate. However, assays of brain tissue from these animals revealed increased levels of lactate, pyruvate, and all citric acid cycle intermediates except succinate. In addition, brain tissue levels of glutamate and alanine were increased in these animals. All these levels returned to normal when exposure was terminated (Folbergrova et al., 1984).

PREVENTIVE AND THERAPEUTIC MEASURES

Workplace and household cleaning areas where TCA is used should be well-ventilated. Safety training programs and well-explained product warnings which include information about the toxicological risks of exposure to TCA should be available in occupational settings. Workers using liquid TCA for cleaning and degreasing operations should wear adequate protective gloves to prevent dermal absorption of the solvent. Respirators should be provided for workers at risk of exposure to TCA concentrations between 500 and 1,000 ppm, and self-contained air supplies should be provided for workers in areas where the potential for exposure to TCA concentrations greater than 1,000 ppm exists (NIOSH, 1976). Monitoring of workers' exposure in occupational settings by analysis of expired air, blood, and/or urine for TCA and its metabolites should be performed on a regular basis (see Biochemical Diagnosis section).

Prevention of recreational TCA abuse first requires identification of the problem. The hair, breath, and clothing of a person abusing TCA may reveal its presence by the subtle chemical aroma. Toxicological examination of tissue, blood, and urine samples can document the exposure postmortem confirming a diagnosis in those cases of sudden death in which TCA abuse is suspected (Flanagan and Ives, 1994).

Individuals suspected of being exposed to high concentrations of TCA should be moved to a well-ventilated area. Hyperventilation with fresh air or an oxygen supply increases displacement and elimination of the unchanged TCA vapors (Gerace, 1981). If liquid TCA has been ingested, gavage should be used to remove the stomach contents and the TCA. Controlled stomach gavage is a safer method of elimination than is administration of ipecac to induce vomiting because of the risk of further inhalation of solvent vapors or aspiration of vomitus containing TCA. Appropriate supportive measures as well as specific interventions to treat cardiac arrhythmia, pulmonary edema, and vasomotor instability may be necessary. Hemodialysis and blood transfusion for acute renal failure, myopathy, and hepatic involvement may be necessary following severe acute exposures. Recovery from acute intoxication depends upon the intensity and duration of the exposure.

Epinephrine should not be administered to persons exposed to TCA because of myocardial irritability. In addition, because both TCA and halothane interfere with mitochondrial respiration, the use of halothane as an anesthetic in persons with histories of recent acute or chronic exposures to TCA should be avoided (Herd and Martin, 1975; McLeod et al., 1987).

Chronic exposure may be accompanied by the gradual appearance of clinical indicators of neurotoxicity. In particular, when the ongoing body burden accumulates over time, symptoms may arise at times of peak reexposure or when tolerance to the burden is surpassed. The overall prognosis of persons exposed to TCA is better in younger patients (Lindstrom et al., 1982). Persistent behavioral deficits and peripheral neuropathy may interfere with the worker's ability to perform on the job (MacKay et al., 1987; Liss, 1988). Workers who develop behavioral manifestations or peripheral neuropathy following exposure to TCA may require re-training and/or transfer to another department where there is no potential for further exposure to organic solvents (Liss, 1988; House et al., 1994). To compensate for permanent impairments of behavior and cognitive functioning, treatment must include recommendations for maintaining the patient's vocational, social, and financial security (White et al., 1992).

CLINICAL EXPERIENCES

Group Studies

Chronic Occupational Exposure to TCA

A group of 28 degreaser workers (mean age: 42 years) worked for an average exposure duration of 17.6 years, using compressed air and TCA sprayers to clean parts (Kelafant et al., 1994). Work areas were poorly ventilated and the workers often washed grease off their arms and hands in liquid TCA. None of the workers had a history of seizures, head trauma, previous psychiatric problems, or chemical substance abuse. Actual workplace ambient air exposure levels were not determined.

The workers reported experiencing lightheadedness, vertigo, nausea, and fatigue; their remedy for these symptoms was "going outside to get some fresh air." Symptoms including headaches, increased irritability, impaired short-term memory, decreased ability to concentrate, disequilibrium, changes in olfaction, anxiety, and sleep disturbances were also reported. In addition, several other workers from the same work site, but who were not directly interviewed, had reportedly lost consciousness while working with the solvent.

Neurological examination revealed inability to maintain a monopedal stance for 5 seconds among the majority of the exposed workers. In addition, several workers had significant sway on Romberg's test and exhibited difficulty on tandem walking tests. Performance deficits were also noted on neuropsychological testing (see Neuropsychological Diagnosis section). The findings in these workers suggest that chronic exposure to TCA is associated with the occurrence of mild to moderate solvent encephalopathy.

A Matched-Pair Study of Workers Exposed to TCA

An epidemiological study of 151 workers exposed to TCA in concentrations ranging from 4 to 838 ppm was performed (Kramer et al., 1978). Exposure durations ranged from <1 year to a maximum of 6 years. The subjects were divided into five groups based on average daily exposure concentrations (<15; 15 to 49; 50 to 99; 100 to 149; and 150 to 249 ppm). Estimated cumulative exposure doses ranged from <2,000 ppm/month to 6,000 ppm/month. The subjects were compared with 151 workers from a control plant which did not use TCA. Subjects and controls were matched by job description, shift worked, socioeconomic status, age, sex, and race and were given complete health

examinations including electrocardiograms. Each person completed a past and current health history questionnaire. No clinically overt CNS effects were noted on examination. Electrocardiogram revealed no abnormalities. Enzyme studies revealed no evidence of hepatic dysfunction. These authors concluded that chronic exposure to TCA at levels less than 950 ppm is not associated with any clinical pattern of adverse effects.

Individual Case Studies

Peripheral Sensory Neuropathy Associated with Dermal TCA Exposure

Case 1. A 25-year-old woman developed numbness and paresthesias in her extremities approximately 3 months after she began working as a degreaser for a motor parts manufacturer (Liss, 1988). She repeatedly immersed her hands in TCA for several hours at a time each day. The patient had no history of previous toxic exposures. In addition, a search for systemic causes of the neuropathy such as diabetes mellitus, renal and/or liver disease, nutritional factors, vascular disease, and malignancies proved negative. Neurological examination revealed hypoactive reflexes and blunting of distal sensation in her hands. Nerve conduction studies documented sensory neuropathy in the median, ulnar, and sural nerves. She was transferred to a different department and no longer exposed to TCA, following which her symptoms began to improve and sensation in her extremities recovered. However, 3 years later, despite her removal from exposure to TCA, she was again experiencing subjective symptoms. A sural nerve biopsy was performed at that time and revealed evidence of ongoing axonopathy with secondary demyelination. (G. M. Liss; A. C. McKee, personal communications) (see Neuropathological Diagnosis section).

Case 2. A second female worker (age: 40 years) in the same company as Case 1 experienced dizziness and noted numbness in her cheeks 4 weeks after she started working as a parts degreaser (Liss, 1988). She continued to work for another 3 months during which time her symptoms progressively worsened. Neurological examination was performed 3 months after she began working with TCA and revealed impaired sensation to pinprick in her feet and hands in a stocking–glove distribution, which was more marked in the patient's hands. The sensory neuropathy was documented with nerve conduction studies. The patient had no history of metabolic disease or previous toxic exposure. Despite her symptoms the patient continued to work with TCA for another 2 years, during which time she continued to experience symptoms. A sural nerve biopsy performed after cessation of exposure revealed evidence of chronic axonopathy and myelinopathy.

Case 3. A 31-year-old male engineer used TCA in his home garage to degrease automobile parts (House et al., 1996). He used the TCA without safety precautions and reportedly had many hours of direct dermal contact with the solvent. Within several days he began to notice tingling and numbness in his hands, feet, and face. He stopped using the solvent after developing these symptoms. Nerve conduction studies at this time showed a mild reduction of the amplitude of the sensory evoked potentials in the median nerves consistent with axonal neuropathy. The patient continued to report mild numbness at a follow-up examination 6 months after cessation of exposure to TCA.

Chronic TCA Exposure and Sensory Neuropathy Confounded by Carpal Tunnel Syndrome: Long-Term Follow-Up

A 59-year-old woman presented in 1986 to an Occupational Health physician with a history of gradually worsening bilateral (left greater than right) hand and arm pain over a year's time. In addition, she complained of tingling in her fingers and her toes. She had a past history of liver problems in 1976 and a cholecystectomy in 1979.

The patient's work history revealed that she had worked on an assembly line from 1961 to 1968, applying velvet and plastic covers tightly over small gift boxes. It was during that time that she began to have localized wrist pain. In 1969 she underwent a surgical release procedure for a diagnosis of left carpal tunnel syndrome; relief was obtained from the operation. Fifteen years later, in 1984, the patient once again began experiencing hand and wrist discomfort. although it was "different" than that she had experienced preceding the earlier right carpal tunnel release. The upper extremity pain was episodic, burning, shooting, and tearing. Furthermore, the tingling and burning involved her feet as well. The pain was worse at night, but was often less when she was busy and distracted. Other than difficulty with sleep because of the peripheral discomfort, she did not complain of emotional or cognitive symptoms. A second release procedure was done on her right wrist, but this time the patient's pain persisted after surgery.

The patient had left the package covering job and worked as an electrical assembler from April 14, 1968 until October 4, 1984. Her tasks included inserting components into a circuit board, clipping extra wires of the component with a wire cutter, and marking the frames in serialization. She used TCA to clean off excess ink from the marking machine and to wash the circuit boards. This required putting the boards into a container of the hot solvent. An air hose was used to blow-dry the solvent-soaked circuit boards. She did not use gloves or masks, but each station had its own fan to diffuse the vapors into the room's atmosphere.

An extensive evaluation ruled out other causes of peripheral neuropathy, including normal test results for the following, antinuclear antibody (ANA); serum protein electrophoresis (SPEP); vitamin B-12 and folate levels; sedimentation rate; and heavy metal screen. Electrodiagnostic studies had not been done prior to her wrist surgeries but were performed by two different examiners within 10 months after the patient stopped her work, thereby stopping her exposure to TCA. Tests (August 29, 1985) of the right motor nerve distal latencies were reported as "normal": 2.7 milliseconds (median); 2.3 milliseconds (ulnar); 3.0 milliseconds (peroneal); and 4.6 milliseconds (tibial). Sensory nerve distal latencies were not reported but their amplitudes were: 15 μV (median); 10 μV (ulnar); and 6.0 μV (sural). The laboratory controls were not given with these test results. Therefore, to indicate that these amplitude values are reduced and abnormal, they can be compared with the values taken from a standard electrodiagnosis textbook. Normal values for sensory evoked potential amplitudes for the median, ulnar, and sural nerve are: 38.5 ± 15.6 μV; 35 ± 14.7 μV; and 23 ± 4.4 μV, respectively (Kimura, 1983). Follow-up neurophysiological testing performed in this patient after a total of 18 months without exposure to TCA (April 11, 1986) revealed prolonged left median motor nerve latencies (4.2 milliseconds; lab normal 3.7 ± 0.3); ulnar (3.8 milliseconds; lab normal 3.0 ± 0.25); and radial (4.1 milliseconds; lab normal 3.3 ± 0.4). Although no sensory studies were done, the report concluded as follows: "The only consistently abnormal result is the median motor distal latency. This is consistent with entrapment or residua from a carpal tunnel release." A sensory neuropathy was not recognized at that time.

Subsequent neurological evaluations were made by the author (R. G. Feldman, personal observations, February 5, 1987 and March 10, 1987). The patient continued to complain of paresthesias of burning and tingling in her feet and pain in her hands. The degree of discomfort was less severe in her hands as compared to 2 and 3 years earlier, but the paresthesias in her feet were "still as bad" as before. Patchy losses of pain sensation were noted in the palms and dorsum of the hands to the wrists and especially on the tips of the fingers. Sensation to pinprick was reduced over the bottoms of the feet and up the legs to the knees, bilaterally in a stocking–glove configuration. Vibration sense was reduced in the toes of both feet. Tendon reflexes were normal in the biceps and triceps and were reduced in the knees and ankles. Electrodiagnostic studies on February 24, 1987 (i.e., 2 years and 4 months after cessation of exposure to TCA) revealed a sural nerve amplitude of 20 μV (normal range) on the right and 15 μV (improved but still reduced) on the left; the medial sensory nerve amplitude was 35 μV on the right and 30 μV on the left. Motor and sensory conduction velocities were normal in median, ulnar, and peroneal nerves. A clinical diagnosis of peripheral neuropathy, primarily sensory, was made. The asymmetrical recovery of sural nerve amplitude response from 6 μV to normal range values is evidence of permanent left sural nerve damage, while the motor fibers had been spared throughout the course of this patient's illness.

Follow-up of this patient was made 9 years later (December 6, 1996). She did not return to any job involving exposure to organic solvents. Her feet and legs have continued to have painful paresthesias, especially when the extremities are cold.

Acute Hepatic Effects and Cognitive Impairment: Long-Term Follow-Up

A 41-year-old man had been in good health for most of his life, having worked between 1972 and 1978 as a mechanic and welder; and between 1978 and 1980, he worked as a production mechanic repairing equipment. From 1980 to 1982, he continued to work as a mechanic and welder, repairing trucks and buses. His hobbies included building and painting model railroads. Most of the models he constructed were of the "snap-together" type, although he did build the type requiring the use of model airplane glue for approximately 1 year (1965). In the past, he would drink two to three drinks per day once per week. On occasion he would drink up to five drinks in a sitting. He had stopped drinking in 1977. He had no symptoms nor problems at that time, although he had occasional contact with degreasing solutions. At work he wore earplugs when he worked around noises; and he wore goggles, a face mask, and gloves while welding.

In 1982 be began working as a knife-man in a textile factory, replacing large knives on looms and cleaning the equipment with TCA solution [75% TCA; 10% methylene chloride; and 15% petroleum distillates (naphtha and xylene)]. He had daily dermal and inhalation exposures to the solvent. During a 1-week plant shutdown in 1983 he worked full time completely cleaning the machines, washing all the parts in a bath of the TCA solution. Parts-washing was performed 8 to 12 times per day for approximately 15 minutes at a time; he did not use gloves or a respirator mask while performing this task. During this period he experienced headaches, dizziness, and nausea. Four weeks later, he continued to have headaches, balance problems, dizziness, fatigue, and general malaise. He did not complain of paresthesias, seizure activity, or loss of consciousness. The dizziness and imbalance problems resolved, but he continued to experience headaches and extreme fatigue. Nevertheless, he worked with the TCA solution for the next several months on the job.

In October of 1983 the patient was diagnosed with an enlarged underactive thyroid. In addition, his liver was enlarged. Liver function tests were abnormal: alkaline phosphatase ($n = 103$), LDH ($n = 239$), SGOT ($n = 53$), SGPT ($n = 132$). These tests were repeated on January 17, 1984 showing LDH ($n = 141$); SGOT ($n = 43$); SGPT ($n = 105$); and alkaline phosphatase ($n = 179$). A liver biopsy was not performed. A diagnosis of possible liver disease was made, and his physician removed him from his work in January 1984. After some improvement in liver function studies, he returned to work in March 1984. However, upon returning to work he soon began to complain of confusion, inability to concentrate, and difficulty contemplating ideas and thoughts. Other symptoms experienced during those times

at work included headaches, dizziness, and nausea. He found that he could not focus on the tasks required to manipulate the various tools and parts that he had to clean and work with. He lost confidence in what he was doing, and he was unable to perform functional requirements. Because of severe persistent fatigue and difficulties with maintaining attention, he had to leave the job and he did not work with TCA since then.

Since leaving his job, the patient pursued vocational rehabilitation. He subsequently worked as an office clerk, doing simple filing from May to October 1985. In October 1985, he began working as a campus security patrolman responsible for checking locks on gates and doors. At the time of his examination in 1986, he was still working as a security patrolman.

Neurological examination (R. G. Feldman, personal observation, August 1, 1986) revealed symptoms of fatigue and headache of a non-specific nature, but his primary impairment was that of memory disturbance. He reported that he was unable to focus his attention for sufficient periods of time on any particular subject or any conversation. Laboratory tests on August 27, 1986: normal bilirubin; glutamyl transpeptidase (35; normal: 5 to 60); SGOT (38; normal: 15 to 45); LDH (169; normal: 110 to 235); T3 uptake (30; normal: 23 to 34). His liver functions at that time were therefore normal as compared to the earlier tests of July 1983.

Neuropsychological testing on August 27, 1986 showed the patient to be well oriented to person, time, and place, and during the testing he had little difficulty understanding the demands of the tests and was enthusiastic. His intelligence quotient (IQ) was in the average range (FSIQ = 103; performance IQ = 106; verbal IQ = 102. Although his fund of general knowledge was within expectation, his performance on a vocabulary test was poor. His handwriting was legible but included several spelling and punctuation errors. Verbal fluency was impaired, but word retrieval was facilitated by a semantic strategy. Spontaneous speech was preserved, and his performance on a confrontation naming test was within expectation. A test of sequential thinking (picture arrangement test) was done relatively well, and the patient was able to self-correct. Tests of attention and mental control were done with some difficulty as he lost set while attempting to count by threes. Simple mental tracking (Trails A) was good, but performance on Trails B revealed difficulty with cognitive flexibility. His performance on the Wisconsin Card Sorting test (WCST) of executive function also revealed difficulty establishing, maintaining, and shifting set. Performance on the digit–symbol transcription tasks suggested slowed psychomotor speed (WAIS-R Digit Symbol = 25th percentile). Fine motor control (Grooved Pegboard) and motor speed (Finger Tapping) were slowed bilaterally. Visual spatial functioning (Object Assembly; Block Design; Hooper) was within expectation. His copies of the simple line drawings and a complex figure (Rey–Osterreith) were accurate except for some distortion of the figure. His performance on digit spans tests was relatively poor (WAIS-R: forward = 5; backward = 4). Recall of paragraph-length stories was fair to good, with no susceptibility to proactive interference. Performance on paired associates was within expectation; he was able to learn nine of ten unrelated pairs of words. Immediate and delayed recall of simple line drawings was also within expectation except for slight distortion of proportions. In contrast, his recognition of geometric forms (Benton Visual Retention Test) was poor on both immediate recall and delayed recall. Incidental learning of symbols on digit–symbol transcription was within expectation. His recognition of unfamiliar faces was impaired (Milner Faces = 7/12; 12/12 matching). He made good use of cues and performed within expectation on a test of retrograde memory (Albert's Famous Faces).

Although impaired performance was seen on several subtests sensitive to solvent exposure (e.g., Digit Spans; Trails B; and WCST), performance was normal on others (e.g., Block Design and Rey–Osterreith). This pattern of performance deficits is not consistent with Alzheimer's disease but is suggestive of long-term sequelae that may be related to TCA exposure.

In follow-up made December 5, 1996, the patient reported that his memory and attention had improved somewhat over the first 5 years after cessation of exposure (1984) but remained about the same for the next 8 years. The patient now works as a security guard, checking the property and buildings on a college campus. The routine of his job is structured, and he is able to perform his duties without difficulty. However, at home he often loses objects and forgets tasks he set out to perform, and occasionally he becomes lost when in previously familiar surroundings. His wife cues him, and together they have adapted to his long-term disability.

REFERENCES

Agency for Toxic Substances and Disease Registry (ATSDR). *Toxicological profile for 1,1,1-trichloroethane.* Washington, DC: US Public Health Service, 1990.

Aitio A, Pekari K, Järvisalo J. Skin absorption as a source of error in biological monitoring. *Scand J Work Environ Health* 1984;10:317–320.

American Conference of Governmental Industrial Hygienists (ACGIH). Threshold limit values (TLVs) for chemical substances and physical agents and biological exposure indices (BEIs). Cincinnati: ACGIH, 1995.

Amoore JE, Hautala E. Odor as an aid to chemical safety: odor thresholds compared with threshold limit values and volatilities for 214 industrial chemicals in air and water dilution. *J Appl Toxicol* 1983;3:272–290.

Åstrand I, Kilbom A, Wahlberg I, Ovrum P. Methylchloroform exposure. I. Concentration in alveolar air and blood at rest and during exercise. *Work Environ Health* 1973;10:69–81.

Bowen SE, Balster RL. Effects of inhaled 1,1,1-trichloroethane on locomotor activity in mice. *Neurotoxicol Teratol* 1996;18:77–81.

Broadwell DK, Darcey DJ, Hudnell HK, Otto DA, Boyes WK. Work-site clinical and neurobehavioral assessment of solvent-exposed microelectronics workers. *Am J Ind Health* 1995;27:677–698.

Brown HS, Bishop DR, Rowan CA. The role of skin absorption as a route of exposure for volatile organic compounds (VOCs) in drinking water. *Am J Public Health* 1984;74:479–484.

Burg JR, Gist GL. The National Exposure Registry: procedures for establishing a registry of persons environmentally exposed to hazardous substances. *Toxicol Ind Health* 1995;11:231–248.

Burmaster DE. The new pollution-groundwater contamination. *Environment* 1982;24:7–36.

Caplan YH, Backer RC, Whitacker JQ. 1,1,1-Trichloroethane: report of a fatal intoxication. *Clin Toxicol* 1976;9:69–74.

Corcoran GB, Fix L, Jones DP, et al. Contemporary issues in toxicology. Apoptosis: molecular control point in toxicity. *Toxicol Appl Pharmacol* 1994;128:169–181.

Danielson BRG, Ghantous H, Dencker L. Distribution of chloroform and methyl chloroform and their metabolites in pregnant mice. *Biol Res Preg Perinatol* 1986;7:77–83.

Dornette WHL, Jones JP. Clinical experiences with 1,1,1-trichloroethane: a preliminary report of 50 anesthetic administrations. *Anesth Analg* 1960;39:249–253.

Dürk H, Poyer JL, Klessen C, Frank H. Acetylene, a mammalian metabolite of 1,1,1-trichloroethane. *Biochem J* 1992;286:353–356.

Flanagan RJ, Ives RJ. Volatile substance abuse. Review. *Bull Narc* 1994; 46:49–78.

Folbergrova J, Hougaard K, Westerberg E, et al. Cerebral metabolic and circulatory effects of 1,1,1-trichloroethane, a neurotoxic industrial solvent. 2. Tissue concentrations of labile phosphates, glycolytic metabolites, citric acid cycle intermediates, amino acids, and cyclic nucleotides. *Neurochem Pathol* 1984;2:55–68.

Franks NP, Lieb WR. Molecular and cellular mechanisms of general anaesthesia. *Nature* 1994;367:607–614.

Gamberale F, Hultengren M. Methylchloroform exposure. II. Psychophysiological functions. *Work Environ Health* 1973;10:82–92.

Gerace RV. Near-fatal intoxication by 1,1,1-trichloroethane. *Ann Emerg Med* 1981;10:533.

Ghittori S, Imbriani M, Pezzagno G, Capodaglio E. The urinary concentration of solvents as a biological indicator of exposure: proposal for biological equivalent exposure limits for nine solvents. *Am Ind Hyg Assoc J* 1987;48:786–790.

Gonthier BP, Barret LG. *In vitro* spin trapping of free radicals produced during trichloroethylene and diethylether metabolism. *Toxicol Lett* 1989; 47:225–234.

Gresham GA, Treip CS. Fatal poisoning by 1,1,1-trichloroethane after prolonged survival. *Forens Sci Int* 1983;23:249–253.

Hajimiragha H, Ewers U, Brockhaus A, Biettger A. Levels of benzene and other volatile aromatic compounds in the blood of non-smokers and smokers. *Int Arch Occup Environ Health* 1989;61:513–518.

Hake CL, Waggoner TB, Robertson DN, Rowe VK. The metabolism of 1,1,1-trichloroethane by the rat. *Arch Environ Health* 1960;1:101–105.

Halevy J, Pitlik S, Rosenfeld J, Eitan B-D. 1,1,1-Trichloroethane intoxication: a case report with transient liver and renal damage. Review of the literature. *Clin Toxicol* 1980;16:467–472.

Hall FB, Hine CH. Trichloroethane intoxication: a report of two cases. *J Forens Sci* 1966;11:404–413.

Halliwell B. Oxidants and the central nervous system: some fundamental questions. Is oxidant damage relevant to Parkinson's disease, Alzheimer's disease, traumatic injury and stroke? *Acta Neurol Scand* 1989;126:23–33.

Hatfield TR, Maykoski RT. A fatal methyl chloroform (trichloroethane) poisoning. *Arch Environ Health* 1970;20:279–281.

Herd PA, Martin HF. Effects of 1,1,1-trichloroethane on mitochondrial metabolism. *Biochem Pharmacol* 1975;24:1179–1185.

Herd PA, Lipsky M, Martin HF. Cardiovascular effects of 1,1,1-trichloroethane. *Arch Environ Health* 1974;28:227–233.

Hodgson MJ, Heyl AE, Van Thiel DH. Liver disease associated with exposure to 1,1,1-trichloroethane. *Arch Intern Med* 1989;149:1793–1798.

Holmberg B, Jakobson I, Sigvardsson K. A study on the distribution of methylchloroform and *n*-octane in the mouse during and after inhalation. *Scand J Work Environ Health* 1977;3:43–52.

Hougaard K, Ingvar M, Wieloch T, Siesjö BK. Cerebral metabolic and circulatory effects of 1,1,1-trichloroethane, a neurotoxic industrial solvent: effects on local cerebral glucose consumption and blood flow during acute exposure. *Neurochem Pathol* 1984;2:39–53.

House RA, Liss GM, Wills MC. Peripheral sensory neuropathy associated with 1,1,1-trichloroethane. *Arch Environ Health* 1994;49:196–199.

House RA, Liss GM, Wills MC, Holness DL. Parethesias and sensory neuropathy due to 1,1,1-trichloroethane. *JOEM* 1996;38:123–124.

Howse DC, Shanks GL, Nag S. Peripheral neuropathy following prolonged exposure to methyl chloroform. *Neurology* 1989;39[Suppl 1]:242.

IARC. *Monographs on the evaluation of the carcinogenic risk of chemicals to humans,* vol 20: *1,1,1-Trichloroethane.* IARC, Lyons, France: World Health Organization, 1979:515–531.

Imbriani M, Ghittori S, Pezzagno G, Huang J, Capodaglio E. 1,1,1-trichloroethane (methylchloroform) in urine as biological index of exposure. *Am J Ind Med* 1988;13:211–222.

Ivanetich KM, van den Honert LH. Chloroethanes: their metabolism by hepatic cytochrome P-450 *in vitro. Carcinogenesis* 1981;2:697–702.

Kaneko T, Wang P-Y, Sato A. Enzymes induced by ethanol differently affect the pharmacokinetics of trichloroethylene and 1,1,1-trichloroethane. *Occup Environ Med* 1994;51:113–119.

Karlsson JE, Rosengren LE, Kjellstrand P, et al. Effects of low-dose inhalation of three chlorinated aliphatic organic solvents on deoxyribonucleic acid in gerbil brain. *Scand J Work Environ Health* 1987;13:453–458.

Kelafant GA, Berg RA, Schleenbaker R. Toxic encephalopathy due to 1,1,1-trichloroethane exposure. *Am J Ind Med* 1994;25:439–446.

Kimura J. *Electrodiagnosis in diseases of the nerve and muscle: principles and practice.* Philadelphia: FA Davis, 1983:198, 110, 133.

Kobayashi H, Hobara T, Satoh T, et al. Effect of 1,1,1-trichloroethane inhalation: a role of autonomic nervous system. *Arch Environ Health* 1987;42:140–143.

Kramer CG, Gerald Ott M, Fulkerson JE, Hicks N, Imbus HR. Health of workers exposed to 1,1,1-trichloroethane: a matched-pair study. *Arch Environ Health* 1978;33:331–342.

Krantz JC Jr, Park CS, Ling JSL. Anesthesia LX: the anesthetic properties of 1,1,1-trichloroethane. *Anesthesiology* 1959;20:635–640.

Kyrklund T, Haglid KG. Brain lipid changes after organic solvent exposure. *Upsala J Med Sci Suppl* 1990;48:267–277.

Lauwerys R, Herbrand J, Buchet JP, Bernard A, Gaussin J. Health surveillance of workers exposed to tetrachloroethylene in dry cleaning shops. *Int Arch Occup Environ Health* 1983;52:69–77.

Lindstrom K, Antti-Poika M, Tola S, Hyytiäinen A. Psychological prognosis of diagnosed chronic organic solvent intoxication. *Neurobehav Toxicol Teratol* 1982;4:581–588.

Liss GM. Peripheral neuropathy in two workers exposed to 1,1,1-trichloroethane. *JAMA* 1988;260:2217.

MacKay CJ, Campbell L, Samuel AM, et al. Behavioral changes during exposure to 1,1,1-trichloroethane: time-course and relationship to blood solvent levels. *Am J Ind Med* 1987;11:223–240.

Maroni M, Bulgheroni C, Cassitto MG, Merluzzi F, Gilioli R, Foa V. A clinical, neuropsychological, and behavioral study of female workers exposed to 1,1,1-trichloroethane. *Scand J Work Environ Health* 1977;3:16–22.

McCarthy TB, Jones RD. Industrial gassing poisonings due to trichloroethylene, perchloroethylene, and 1,1,1-trichloroethane, 1961–1980. *Br J Ind Med* 1983;40:450–455.

McConnell G, Ferguson DM, Pearson CR. Chlorinated hydrocarbons and the environment. *Endeavor* 1975;34:13–18.

McLeod AA, Marjot R, Monaghan MJ, Hugh-Jones P, Jackson G. Chronic cardiac toxicity after inhalation of 1,1,1-trichloroethane. *Br Med J* 1987;294:727–729.

Mizunuma K, Kawai T, Horiguchi S, Ikeda M. Urinary methylchloroform rather than urinary metabolites as an indicator of occupational exposure to methylchloroform. *Int Arch Environ Health* 1995;67:19–25.

Monster AC. Differences in uptake, elimination, and metabolism in exposure to trichloroethylene, 1,1,1-trichloroethane, and tetrachloroethylene. *Int Arch Occup Environ Health* 1979;42:311–317.

Monster AC. Biological monitoring of chlorinated hydrocarbon solvents. *J Occup Med* 1986;28:583–588.

Morgan A, Black A, Belcher DR. The excretion in breath of some aliphatic halogenated hydrocarbons following administration by inhalation. *Ann Occup Hyg* 1970;13:219–233.

Moser VC, Balster RL. The effects of inhaled toluene, halothane, 1,1,1-trichloroethane, and ethanol on fixed-interval responding in mice. *Neurobehav Toxicol Teratol* 1986;8:525–531.

Mullin LS, Krivanek ND. Comparison of unconditioned reflex and conditioned avoidance tests in rats exposed by inhalation to carbon monoxide, 1,1,1-trichloroethane, toluene or ethanol. *Neurotoxicology* 1982;3:126–137.

Mutti A, Franchini I. Toxicity of metabolites to dopaminergic systems and the behavioral effects of organic solvents. *Br J Ind Med* 1987;44:721–723.

National Institute of Occupational Safety and Health (NIOSH). *Criteria for a recommended standard . . . occupational exposure to 1,1,1-trichloroethane (methylchloroform).* Washington, DC: US Department of Health, Education and Welfare. Public Health Services, CDC, NIOSH, Publication No. 76-184, 1976.

National Institute of Occupational Safety and Health (NIOSH). *Pocket guide to chemical hazards.* Washington, DC: US Department of Health and Human Services, CDC, June 1997.

Nolan RJ, Freshour NL, Rick DL, McCarty LP, Saunders JH. Kinetics and metabolism of inhaled methyl chloroform (1,1,1-trichloroethane) in male volunteers. *Fundam Appl Toxicol* 1984;4:654–662.

Occupational Safety and Health Administration (OSHA). *Code of federal regulations,* 29, 1910.1000/.1047. Washington, DC: Office of the Federal Register, National Archives and Records Administration, 1995:411–431.

Ödkvist LM, Larsby B, Fredrickson MF, Liedgren SRC, Tham R. Vestibular and oculomotor disturbances caused by industrial solvents. *J Otolaryngol* 1980;9:53–59.

Peoples RW, Weight FF. Trichloroethanol potentiation of γ-aminobutyric acid-activated chloride current in mouse hippocampal neurones. *Br J Pharmacol* 1994;113:555–563.

Peoples RW, Lovinger DM, Weight FF. Inhibition of excitatory amino acid currents by general anesthetic agents. *Soc Neurosci Abstr* 1990;16:1017.

Rall TW. Hypnotics and sedatives; ethanol. In: Goodman Gilman A, Rall TW, Nies AS, Taylor P, eds. *Goodman and Gilman's The Pharmacological Basis of Therapeutics,* 8th ed. Elmsford, NY: Pergamon Press, 1990:345–382.

Ranson DL, Berry PJ. Death associated with the abuse of typewriter correction fluid. *Med Sci Law* 1986;26:308–310.

Riihimäki V, Pfäffli P. Percutaneous absorption of solvent vapors in man. *Scand J Work Environ Health* 1978;7:73–85.

Rosengren LE, Aurell A, Kjellstrand P, et al. Astrogliosis in the cerebral cortex of gerbils after long-term exposure to 1,1,1-trichloroethane. *Scand J Work Environ Health* 1985;11:447–456.

Salvini M, Binaschi S, Riva M. Evaluation of psychological functions in humans exposed to the 'threshold limit value' of 1,1,1-trichloroethane. *Br J Ind Med* 1971;28:286–292.

Savolainen H. Some aspects of the mechanisms by which industrial solvent produce neurotoxic effects. *Chem-Biol Interact* 1977;18:1–10.

Savolainen K. Pharmacokinetics, pharmacodynamics and aspects of neurotoxic effects of four inhaled aliphatic chlorohydrocarbon solvents as relevant to man. *Eur J Drug Metab Pharmacokinet* 1981;6:85–90.

Savolainen H, Pfaffli P, Tengen M, et al. Trichloroethylene and 1,1,1-trichloroethane: effects on brain and liver after five days intermittent inhalation. *Arch Toxicol* 1977;38:229–237.

Savolainen K, Riihimäki V, Laine A, Kekoni J. Short-term exposure of human subjects to *m*-xylene and 1,1,1-trichloroethane. *Int Arch Occup Environ Health* 1981;49:89–98.

Sax NI. *Dangerous properties of industrial chemicals,* 5th ed. New York: Van Nostrand Reinhold, 1979.

Seppäläinen AM, Salmi T, Savolainen K, Riihimäki V. Visual evoked potentials in short-term exposure of human subjects to *m*-xylene and 1,1,1-trichloroethane. In: Zbinden G, et al., eds. *Application of behavioral pharmacology in toxicology.* New York: Raven Press, 1983:349.

Siebecker KL, Bamforth BJ, Steinhaus JE, Orth OS. Clinical studies on new and old hydrocarbons. *Anesth Analg* 1960;39:180–188.

Stahl CJ, Fatteh AV, Dominguez AM. Trichloroethane poisoning: observations on the pathology and toxicology in six fatal cases. *J Forens Sci Soc* 1969;14:393–397.

Stewart RD. The toxicology of 1,1,1-trichloroethane. *Ann Occup Hyg* 1968;11:71–79.

Stewart RD. Methyl chloroform intoxication: diagnosis and treatment. *JAMA* 1971;215:1789–1792.

Stewart RD, Dodd HC. Absorption of carbon tetrachloride, trichloroethylene, tetrachloroethylene, methylene chloride, and 1,1,1-trichloroethane through human skin. *Am Ind Hyg Assoc J* 1964;25:439–446.

Stewart RD, Andrews JT. Acute intoxication with methyl chloroform. *JAMA* 1966;195:904–906.

Stewart RD, Gay HH, Erley DS, Hake CL, Schaffer AW. Human exposure to 1,1,1-trichloroethane vapor: relationship of expired air and blood concentrations to exposure and toxicity. *Am Ind Hyg Assoc J* 1961;22:252–262.

Stewart RD, Gay HH, Schaffer AW, Erley DS, Rowe VK. Experimental human exposure to methyl chloroform vapor. *Arch Environ Health* 1969;19:467–472.

Stewart RD, Hake CL, Wu A, et al. 1,1,1-Trichloroethane: Development of a biological standard for the industrial worker by breath analysis. Report No. NIOSH-MCOW-ENVM-1,1,1-T-75-4. Milwaukee, WI: The Medical College of Wisconsin, Department of Environmental Medicine, 1975.

Tay P, Pinnagoda J, Sam CT, et al. Environmental and biological monitoring of occupational exposure to 1,1,1-trichloroethane. *Occup Med* 1995;45:147–150.

Tham R, Bunnfors I, Eriksson B, Larsby B, Lindgren S, Ödkvist LM. Vestibulo-ocular disturbances in rats exposed to organic solvents. *Acta Pharmacol Toxicol* 1984;54:58–63.

Tomasi A, Albano E, Bini A, Botti B, Slater T, Vannini V. Free radical intermediates under hypoxic conditions in the metabolism of halogenated carcinogens. *Toxicol Pathol* 1984;12:240–246.

Torkelson TR, Oyen F, McCollister DD, Rowe VK. Toxicity of 1,1,1-trichloroethane as determined on laboratory animals and human subjects. *Am Ind Hyg Assoc J* 1958;19:353–362.

Town C, Leibman KC. The *in vitro* dechlorination of some polychlorinated ethanes. *Drug Metabol Dispos* 1984;12:4–8.

Travers H. Death from 1,1,1-trichloroethane abuse: case report. *Mil Med* 1974;139:889–890.

Turina MP, Colacci A, Grilli S, Mazzullo M, Prodi G, Lattanzi G. Short-term tests of genotoxicity for 1,1,1-trichloroethane. *Res Comm Chem Pathol Pharmacol* 1986;52:305–320.

United States Environmental Protection Agency (USEPA). *Drinking water regulations and health advisories.* EPA 822-R-96-001. Washington, DC: Office of Water, 1996.

Van Dyke RA, Wineman CG. ENzymatic dechlorination. Dechlorination of chloroethanes and propanes *in vitro. Biochem Pharmacol* 1971;20: 463–470.

Wallace L, Pellizari E, Hartwell T, Zelon H, Sparacino C, Perritt R, Whitmore R. Concentrations of 20 volatile organic compounds in the air and drinking water of 350 residents of New Jersey compared with concentrations in their exhaled breath. *J Occup Med* 1986;28:603–608.

Wallace LA, Pellizari ED, Hartwell TD, Whitmore R, Zelon H, Perritt R, Sheldon L. The California team study: breath concentrations and personal exposures to 26 volatile compounds in air and drinking water of 188 residents of Los Angeles, Antioch, and Pittsburg, CA. *Atmos Environ* 1988;22:2141–2163.

White RF, Feldman RG, Proctor SP. Neurobehavioral effects of toxic exposure: clinical syndromes in adult neuropsychology. In: White RF, ed. *The practitioner's handbook.* Amsterdam: Elsevier, 1992:1–51.

Wise MG, Fisher JG, de la Pena AM. Trichloroethane (TCE) and central sleep apnea: a case study. *J Toxicol Environ Health* 1983;11:101–104.

Wood KA, Youle RJ. The role of free radicals and p53 in neuron apoptosis *in vivo. J Neurosci* 1995;15:5851–5857.

Woolverton WL, Balster RL. Behavioral and lethal effects of combinations of oral ethanol and inhaled 1,1,1-trichloroethane in mice. *Toxicol Appl Pharmacol* 1981;59:1–7.

You L, Muralidhara S, Dallas CE. Comparisons between operant response and 1,1,1-trichloroethane toxicokinetics in mouse blood and brain. *Toxicology* 1994;93:151–163.

Zhou Q, Lovinger M. Pharmacologic characteristics of potentiation of 5-HT$_3$ receptors by alcohols and diethyl ether in NCB-20 neuroblastoma cells. *J Pharmacol Exp Ther* 1996;278:732–740.

CHAPTER 14

Toluene

Toluene (methyl benzene, phenyl methane, methyl benzol, toluol, toluen, methacide), a crude oil and coal tar derivative, is an alkylbenzene aromatic hydrocarbon compound with one methyl group attached to a benzene ring (EPA, 1983; ATSDR, 1994). Most toluene (96.5%) is produced during petroleum refining by catalytic reformation of petroleum fractions and by pyrolytic cracking; the remainder (4.5%) occurs as a byproduct of styrene production and coke oven operations (EPA, 1983). Purified (isolated) toluene is a clear, colorless, lipophilic, volatile, flammable liquid that usually contains less than 0.01% benzene. Pure toluene is used as an ingredient in paints, lacquers, urethanes, varnishes, resins, nail polish, trinitrotoluene (TNT), toluene diisocyanate, pesticides, inks, cosmetic products, solvents, paint thinners, and adhesives and in the production of other chemicals (ATSDR, 1994). Industrial grade toluene may contain up to 25% benzene and other organic compounds (WHO, 1985). Nearly 90% of the impure toluene produced is used in gasoline (EPA, 1983).

Reports of acute and chronic encephalopathy with cognitive changes and cerebellar ataxia began to appear soon after toluene was introduced to the rotogravure printing process (Fuhner and Pietrusky, 1934; Koelsch, 1935; Bumke and Foerster, 1936). To experience euphoria and psychotropic effects, the intentional sniffing and inhaling of toluene vapors released from glue, paint, and paint thinners has become a serious type of substance abuse and has been responsible for numerous cases of neurotoxicity (King et al., 1981; King, 1982; Lazar et al., 1983; Channer and Stanley, 1983; Ron, 1986). Descriptions of movement disorders (Bartolucci and Pellitier, 1984), and brainstem and cerebellar dysfunction (Lazar et al., 1983) among toluene-exposed persons promote interest in the possible site selectivity of this neurotoxicant. Toluene has been extensively studied under laboratory-controlled acute-exposure conditions for its neurobehavioral effects (Dick, 1995). Its importance in the differential diagnosis of occupational and environmental diseases relates to its unique effects as well as its interactions with other solvents, with which it is commonly used.

SOURCES OF EXPOSURE

Gasoline contains up to 7% toluene by weight and is the major nonoccupational source of toluene exposure (Verschueren, 1977; EPA, 1983; ATSDR, 1994). Toluene vaporizes from gasoline into the environment during refueling at the service station pump and is also a component of automobile exhaust. Toluene is the most prevalent aromatic hydrocarbon in the atmosphere, with average levels ranging from 0.53 to 200 $\mu g/m^3$ (EPA, 1983). Air concentrations of toluene in populated areas typically range from 5 to 25 $\mu g/m^3$; in remote areas, toluene air concentrations may be as low as 0.18 $\mu g/m^3$ (EPA, 1988; ATSDR, 1994). Indoor air can contain an average of 30 $\mu g/m^3$ toluene, derived mostly from cigarette smoke (80 to 160 μg of toluene per cigarette (Hajimiragha et al., 1989; ATSDR, 1994). The EPA has estimated that over 50 million people in the United States alone have been exposed to toluene through the inhalation of cigarette smoke, and this figure is probably an underestimate since it does not include passive inhalation by nonsmokers (EPA, 1983). The average person absorbs approximately 300 $\mu g/day$ from indoor sources of toluene such as cigarette smoke and off-gassing from common household products (ATSDR, 1994).

The unrestricted availability, relatively low cost, and rapid intense effect of toluene contribute to the popularity of this substance among its abusers. The euphoric effects of toluene appear at ambient air concentrations above 800 ppm (Hormes et al., 1986). Solvent vapor abusers are frequently exposed to toluene levels of 1,000 ppm or more, many times greater than the 100 ppm industrial threshold limiting value (TLV) (King, 1982; Hormes et al., 1986). Because the circumstances, intensity, frequency, and duration of each exposure episode among vapor abusers differ so much from the usually less direct, lower level, and more chronic exposures of workers, the severity of adverse health effects in abusers cannot be directly extrapolated to those seen after exposure to toluene in most industrial settings (von Oettingen et al., 1942; Bartolucci et al., 1986).

Industrial exposure to toluene occurs when it is used as a solvent, as it vaporizes out of mixtures containing toluene and other organic compounds, and during the degradation of toluene-containing chemical compounds. For example, large quantities of toluene diisocyanate are used during the manufacture of certain adhesives, urethane insulation, resins, lacquers, upholstery, and plastic materials, all of which provide opportunity for worker exposure (Wegman et al., 1982). As of 1977, nearly 5 million workers were reportedly exposed to toluene annually, and industrial use of toluene as a replacement for benzene has continued to increase over time (EPA, 1983; ATSDR, 1993). Individuals involved in the manufacture and distribution of gasoline, automobile mechanics, and painters are at greatest risk (ATSDR, 1994). Exposure levels as high as 30,000 ppm have resulted from industrial accidents involving toluene (Longley et al., 1967). Off-gassing of toluene and other chemicals occurs when materials containing toluene diisocyanate are burned, so that waste disposal workers, firefighters or fire victims may be at risk of exposure (LeQuesne et al., 1976). Since it has been regulated under the Resource Conservation and Recovery Act as a hazardous waste, there has been some reduction in the use of toluene; there have also been improvements in the methods by which it is handled and is disposed (ATSDR, 1994).

Ground water supplies can be polluted directly by hazardous waste spills and discharges containing toluene (Tardiff and Youngren, 1986). Although the intermedia transfer of toluene from soil to drinking water is relatively low, toluene is soluble in water, easily released from soils low in organic matter (e.g., sandy soil), and can contaminate domestic drinking water supplies following a spill or release of toluene into these soils (Wilson et al., 1981). Gasoline-contaminated ground water in Los Angeles contained 561 μg/L toluene (Karlson and Frankenberger, 1989). Toluene concentrations as high as 1.4 μg/L in surface water have been reported, but common drinking water usually contains less than 0.1 μg/L and thus, ordinary daily consumption of toluene is relatively small. The potential for inhalation or dermal absorption of toluene vapors, which are often volatized from heated shower water, exists around toxic waste disposal sites, and this type of exposure is more likely to occur than is oral intake from drinking contaminated water sources (National Research Council, 1991).

EXPOSURE LIMITS AND SAFETY REGULATIONS

The odor threshold for toluene in air is 2.9 ppm (Amoore and Hautala, 1983). Continuous exposure to toluene rapidly leads to olfactory fatigue, and the odor of the vapors are promptly tolerated, making the odor of little value as a warning signal of exposure (Patty, 1963; Mergler and Beauvais, 1992). The lowest concentration of toluene that

yields a measurable effect on tests of vigilance, visual acuity, color vision, and visual evoked potentials is 100 ppm (Dick, 1995). Acute or chronic central nervous system (CNS) effects have been observed after exposure to 50 to 200 ppm in workplace studies (Wilson, 1943). The permissible exposure level (PEL) established by the *Occupational Safety and Health Administration* (OSHA) is an 8-hour time-weighted average (TWA) of 200 ppm, with a 15-minute TWA ceiling of 300 ppm and a maximum exposure peak of 500 ppm that should not be exceeded for more than 10 minutes during an 8-hour work shift (OSHA, 1995). The *National Institute for Occupational Safety and Health* (NIOSH) has set its 10-hour TWA recommended exposure limit (REL) at 100 ppm. The NIOSH-recommended short-term exposure limit (STEL) is a maximum concentration of 150 ppm for 15 minutes. An ambient air concentration of 500 ppm toluene vapor is considered by NIOSH to be immediately dangerous to life and health (IDLH) (NIOSH, 1997). The *American Conference of Governmental Industrial Hygienists* (ACGIH) has set its 8-hour TWA TLV for toluene at 50 ppm (ACGIH, 1995) (Table 14-1).

Chronic ingestion of trace amounts of toluene in drinking water has been considered relatively unimportant. Regardless, a suggested no-adverse-response level (SNARL) has been set for potentially contaminated sources of drinking water (0.34 mg/L for continuous consumption; a 7-day

TABLE 14-1. *Established and recommended occupational and environmental exposure limits for toluene in air and water*

	Air (ppm)[a]	Water (mg/L)[a]
Odor threshold*	2.9	0.042
OSHA		
PEL (8 hr TWA)	200	—
PEL ceiling (15 min TWA)	300 (500 max.)	—
NIOSH		
REL (10 hr TWA)	100	—
STEL (15 min TWA)	150	—
IDLH	500	—
ACGIH		
TLV (8 hr TWA)	50	—
STEL (15 min TWA)	—	—
USEPA		
MCL	—	1.0
MCLG	—	1.0

[a]Unit conversion: 1.0 ppm = 3.83 mg/m³; 1 mg/L = 1 ppm
OSHA, Occupational Safety and Health Administration; PEL, permissible exposure limit; TWA, time-weighted average; NIOSH, National Institute of Occupational Safety and Health; REL, recommended exposure limit; STEL, short-term exposure limit; IDLH, immediately dangerous to life or health; ACGIH, American Conference of Governmental Industrial Hygienists; TLV, threshold limit value; USEPA, U.S. Environmental Protection Agency; MCL, maximum contamination level; MCLG, maximum contamination level goal.
Data from *Amoore and Hautala, 1983; OSHA, 1995; ACGIH, 1995; USEPA, 1996; NIOSH, 1997.

SNARL is 35 mg/L; a 1-day SNARL is 420 mg/L) (National Academy of Science, 1980). The *Environmental Protection Agency* (EPA) has set a maximum contamination level (MCL) for drinking water at 1.0 mg/L (EPA, 1996). Industrial waste containing more than 0.33 mg/L toluene or waste water containing more than 1.12 mg/L toluene may not be disposed of onto land sites (OTA, 1989).

METABOLISM

Tissue Absorption

The major route of body entry for toluene is by inhalation and absorption through the pulmonary alveoli. Tissue uptake is dependent on the concentration gradient across the alveolar membranes, the blood/air partition coefficient for toluene, and on the rate of blood circulation through the alveoli (Åstrand, 1975). Arterial blood concentrations closely correlate with alveolar air concentrations (Brugone et al., 1986). It is possible to detect toluene in the blood after only 10 seconds of inhalation exposure. Within 10 to 15 minutes of exposure to toluene in ambient air, blood levels reach 60% to 80% of maximum with saturation occurring after 25 minutes (Åstrand et al., 1972). The rate of absorption decreases to about 40% to 50% after 2 to 3 hours of exposure; the average retention for a 5-hour period of exposure is a 50% (Cohr and Stockholm, 1979). An increase in basal metabolic rate will increase pulmonary alveolar absorption (Åstrand, 1975; Carlsson, 1982). Löf et al. (1993) found total pulmonary uptake to be 50% in volunteers performing light exercise (50 W) during a 2-hour exposure to toluene at a concentration of 200 mg/m³; uptake at rest was not determined for comparison in this study. Moderate physical activity (100 W) was found to increase alveolar concentration by 47% (Baelum et al., 1987). In volunteers performing light exercise (50 W) while exposed to toluene at concentrations of 300 mg/g³ for 2 hours, total uptake of the solvent was approximately 2.5 times higher than it was at rest (Carlsson, 1982).

Following oral intake, toluene is absorbed through the gastrointestinal tract at a significantly slower rate than it is through the lungs (Cohr and Stockholm, 1979). Blood toluene concentration does not reach its peak until 2 hours after oral intake (Pyykkö et al., 1977). Nevertheless, cases of death following oral ingestion of toluene have been reported (Ameno et al., 1989).

Dermal absorption of toluene also contributes to the total body burden accumulated. Dermal uptake is related to temperature, hydration, surface area, type, and condition of the skin (Dutkiewisez and Tyras, 1968; Riihimäki and Pfäffli, 1978; Brown et al., 1984). Only a very small percentage of toluene vapor is absorbed through the skin (Riihimäki and Pfäffli, 1978). Sato and Nakajima (1978), demonstrated that dermal absorption of liquid toluene occurs at a significantly slower rate than absorption via in-

halation. In addition, the maximum blood concentration of toluene is maintained for a while after termination of exposure, indicating that the toluene in the skin continues to be absorbed. To simulate the widely practiced habit of painters who wash their hands with paint thinner at the end of the work day, volunteers were asked to immerse one hand in toluene for 5 minutes. Following the exposure, maximum blood levels in the subjects ranged from 2.0 to 5.4 μmol/L and were 7- to 20-fold higher in the subjects' exposed arms than in their unexposed arms (Aitio et al., 1984). Dermal absorption can be significant and should not be overlooked when monitoring exposure to toluene (Aitio et al., 1984).

Tissue Distribution

Distribution of toluene throughout lipid-containing tissues is similar, whether after inhalation, ingestion, or dermal exposure (Ameno et al., 1992). The rate of rise for toluene concentrations in various organs is proportional to their vascularity, the diffusion rate of toluene into tissues, and the organ's lipid content (Gospe and Calaban, 1988). With ongoing or repeated exposures, tissue levels of toluene are increased due to accumulation, particularly in adipose tissue and other organs with high lipid content (Carlsson and Ljungquist, 1982; Cohr and Stockholm, 1979; Ameno et al., 1989). The half-life for toluene in the adipose tissue of volunteers exposed to an inspiratory air concentration of 300 mg/m³ ranged from 0.5 to 2.7 days, with longer retention times seen in individuals with higher amounts of body fat (Fig. 14-1) (Carlsson and Ljungquist, 1982). In addition, the concentrations of toluene in the subcutaneous adipose tissue of these individuals were 10 to 14 times higher after 2 hours of exercise due to an increase in blood perfusion as well as an increased concentration of toluene in the arterial blood. The rate of accumulation in adipose tissue is slower than that in the more highly per-

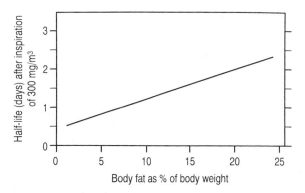

FIG. 14-1. Relationship between percent body fat and biological half-life for toluene in subcutaneous adipose tissue. Demonstrates increased half-time with increasing body fat in 12 male volunteers following exposure to 300 mg/m³ toluene. (Modified from Carlsson and Ljungquist, 1982, with permission.)

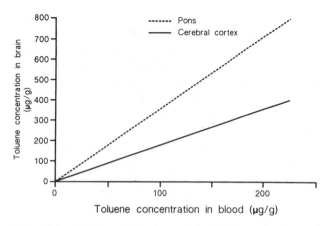

FIG. 14-2. Relationship between blood toluene levels and toluene tissue concentration in brain. Demonstrates affinity of toluene for lipid-rich tissues, with highest concentrations found in areas highest in myelin content (e.g., pons and medulla) and lowest in areas consisting mostly of neurons (e.g., cerebral cortex and hippocampus). (Modified from Ameno et al., 1992, with permission.)

fused lipid-rich nervous tissue, in which toluene quickly accumulates (Cohr and Stockholm, 1979). The brain shows a prompt rise in concentration, and toluene is still detectable in the human brain 10 days after inhalation (Fornazzari, 1990). A direct relationship exists between toluene concentrations in various brain regions and blood levels of toluene (Fig. 14-2) (Ameno et al., 1992).

The regional distribution of toluene after absorption is important because of its probable relationship to localization of the neurotoxic effects in these sites and the various resultant clinical manifestations and histopathological findings (Gospe and Calaban, 1988; Lazar et al., 1983; Fornazzari et al., 1983). Ameno et al. (1992) compared the regional brain distribution

of toluene measured in experimentally exposed rats with the postmortem levels found in a human case (Table 14-2). The toluene concentrations in the brain were expressed as the *brain region/blood toluene concentration ratio* (BBCR). In rats, following inhalation of 2,000 ppm or oral administration of 400 mg/kg for 0.5 hours, the BBCR for the various brain regions were as follows, ranking from lowest to highest: hippocampus, cerebral cortex, cerebellum, caudate–putamen, hypothalamus, thalamus, midbrain, medulla oblongata, and pons. The mean values for the BBCR were: *highest* (2.85 to 3.22) in the brainstem region (pons and medulla); *intermediate* (1.77 to 2.12) in the region of the midbrain, thalamus, hypothalamus, caudate–putamen, and cerebellum; and *lowest* (1.45 to 1.94) in the hippocampus and cerebral cortex. In the exposed human, the highest concentrations of toluene were found in the corpus callosum and cervical spinal cord; the lowest concentration was found in the hippocampus. Higher concentrations of toluene were found in areas with more white matter; the gray matter of the cerebral cortex and hippocampus had lower concentrations, reflecting the low molecular weight, high lipid solubility, and lack of protein binding capability of toluene that allow it to pass readily through the blood–brain barrier (BBB) and accumulate according to the lipid content of the various brain regions.

Tissue Biochemistry

Metabolism of toluene in the liver results in its detoxification and produces metabolites for excretion. Approximately 1% of absorbed toluene is hydroxylated at the benzene ring to *o*- and *p*-cresol at a ratio of 10 : 1 in favor of the latter compound (Bakke and Scheline, 1970). The remainder, via the microsomal mixed function oxidase system, is hydroxylated at the methyl group to form benzyl alcohol, which, through the actions of alcohol dehydrogenase, is ox-

TABLE 14-2. *Regional distribution of toluene in brains of human and rat*[a]

Brain region	Toluene levels in human brain (μg/g)	Human BBCR	Rat BBCR (range)
Hippocampus	6.86	1.47	1.45–1.64
Cerebral cortex	8.18	1.76	
Cerebellum	7.03	1.51	
Caudate–putamen	8.71	1.87	
Hypothalamus	9.51	2.04	1.77–2.12
Thalamus	8.93	1.91	
Midbrain	10.78	2.31	
Medulla	10.42	2.23	2.85–3.22
Pons	10.20	2.18	
Cervical spinal cord	11.00	2.35	
Corpus callosum	12.40	2.66	

[a]The toluene concentrations in the brain are expressed as the *brain region/blood toluene concentration ratio* (BBCR). In rats, following inhalation of 2,000 ppm or oral administration of 400 mg/kg for 0.5 hr, the mean values of BBCR for the various brain areas were (a) highest (2.85–3.22) in the brain-stem region (pons and medulla); (b) intermediate (1.77–2.12) in the region of the midbrain, thalamus, hypothalamus, caudate–putamen, and cerebellum; (c) lowest (1.45–1.94) in the hippocampus and cerebral cortex. In the human, the highest concentrations of toluene were found in the corpus callosum and cervical spinal cord; the lowest was found in the hippocampus.
Modified from Ameno et al., 1992, with permission.

idized to benzaldehyde. Benzaldehyde is oxidized via alde-hyde dehydrogenase to benzoic acid (Toftgard and Gustafsson, 1980), which is subsequently conjugated with glycine to form hippuric acid (about 80%) and with glucuronic acid to form benzoyl glucuronide (less than 20%) (Williams, 1959; Bakke and Scheline, 1970; Toftgard and Gustafsson, 1980) (Fig. 14-3). Both hippuric acid (HA) and benzoyl glucuronide are excreted in the urine.

Concurrent intake of various chemicals affects the rate of toluene metabolism in the liver, resulting in more or less formation and excretion of metabolites (Table 14-3) (Arlien-Soborg, 1992). Ethanol is of particular importance in its effects on toluene metabolism, because its common use by the general public provides ample opportunity for coexposure to these two chemicals. The consumption of ethanol during exposure to toluene interferes with the me-

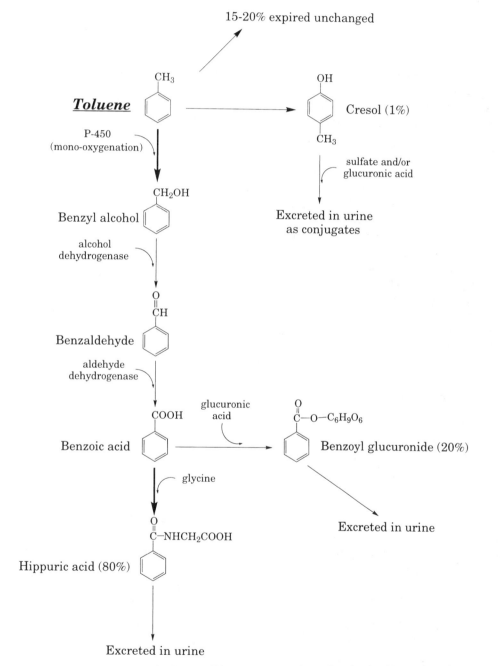

FIG. 14-3. Metabolic pathways of toluene. Fifteen to 20% of an absorbed toluene dose is excreted unchanged in the expired air (Cohr and Stokholm, 1979; Foo et al., 1991). The majority (about 80%) is excreted as hippuric acid, and the remainder is excreted as benzyol glucuronide (about 20%) and cresol (about 1.0%) (Williams, 1959; Bakke and Scheline, 1970; Ogata et al., 1970; Toftgard and Gustafsson, 1980; Cohr and Stokholm, 1979; Löf et al., 1993).

TABLE 14-3. *Effects of various chemicals on toluene metabolism*

Chemical	Metabolism	Reference
Ethanol		
Acute	Decreased	Sato and Nakajima, 1979
		Waldron et al., 1983
		Wallen et al., 1984
Chronic	Increased	Waldron et al., 1983
Benzene	Decreased	Inoue et al., 1988
Xylene	Increased	Wallen et al., 1984
Phenobarbital	Increased	Pyykkö, 1984

Modified from Arlien-Soborg, 1992, with permission.

tabolism of toluene, so that blood levels remain elevated and urinary output of toluene metabolites is decreased, increasing the risk of toxic effects (Waldron et al., 1983; Wallen et al., 1987; Echeverria et al., 1991; Kawamoto et al., 1995). Ingestion of ethanol concurrently with or immediately following exposure to toluene is associated with a decrease in the urinary excretion of HA and *o*-cresol, as well as an increase in alveolar toluene concentration (Waldron et al., 1983; Wallen et al., 1984; Dossing et al., 1984). Wallen et al. (1984) showed that after intake of ethanol the blood concentration of toluene increased from 7.4 to 12.5 μmol/L. The drinking of alcohol during exposure to toluene affects the oxidation of benzyl alcohol metabolite of toluene to benzoic acid. The decrease in metabolism following ethanol ingestion is most likely due to competition for alcohol dehydrogenase, which is required for the metabolism of both ethanol and benzyl alcohol (Waldron et al., 1983); as soon as the ethanol is eliminated, the disturbance of toluene metabolism is no longer evident.

In contrast, the venous toluene concentrations in habitual drinkers exposed to toluene were lower than in nondrinkers, suggesting increased metabolism. This effect appears to be "protective," as the blood toluene concentration is lower in those who chronically consume ethanol (Table 14-4) (Waldron et al., 1983). In addition, ethanol ingested

TABLE 14-4. *Effect of ethanol consumption on blood toluene concentration at exposure levels above and below 100 ppm[a]*

Ethanol: rate of consumption	Blood toluene concentrations (μmol/L) at two levels of exposure	
	< 100 ppm	100–200 ppm
Occasional	2.2 (n = 9)	5.2 (n = 4)
Frequent	1.5 (n = 22)	2.6 (n = 11)

[a]Workers were grouped according to weekly ethanol intake as follows: *occasional,* not more than once per week; *frequent,* several drinks per week. Exposure levels ranged from 50 to 200 ppm.
Modified from Waldron et al., 1983, with permission.

in the hours prior to inhalation of toluene in short-term animal experiments resulted in increased metabolism of toluene (Sato et al., 1980). Chronic ethanol consumption results in the induction of hepatic microsomal oxidizing enzymes. Because toluene is also metabolized by the cytochrome P-450 pathway, the induction of these enzymes by ethanol increases the metabolism of toluene as well (Waldron et al., 1983). Phenobarbital has been shown to increase induction of cytochrome P-450 and the enzyme side-chain hydroxylase in rats. Blood toluene levels in phenobarbital pretreated rats were significantly lower than levels in untreated controls, suggesting increased hydroxylation of toluene to benzyl alcohol. The benzyl alcohol formed in this reaction is subsequently oxidized to benzoic acid through the actions of alcohol dehydrogenase and aldehyde dehydrogenase (Fig. 14-3). Correspondingly, the pretreated rats excreted three times more hippuric acid than the untreated controls. In addition, the narcotic actions of toluene on the pretreated rats were decreased (Ikeda and Ohtsuji, 1971).

A survey of health effects from toluene exposure in 456 workers in China found that urine HA levels were significantly lower in this group when compared with previous reports in the literature, suggesting an ethnic difference in toluene metabolism and excretion (Liu et al., 1992). Individual susceptibility, determined by genetic factors, influences clinical response to exposure. Because of a point mutation on the low K_m aldehyde dehydrogenase (ALDH2) gene, approximately half of the Japanese population lacks ALDH2 activity, resulting in catalytic deficiency in alcohol and aldehyde metabolism. In a group of 92 Japanese males (mean age: 36.9 years) who were occupationally exposed to toluene, with personal exposure levels ranging from 74 to 94 mg/m³, the benzyl alcohol levels in blood were significantly higher, in nine of the workers with the ALDH2 mutation. In addition, the urinary hippuric acid levels were significantly lower, indicating a possible genetic basis for disruption in the oxidation of benzyl alcohol to benzoic acid (Kawamoto et al., 1995) (see Excretion section).

The acute anesthetic effects of toluene have been attributed to the parent compound and the metabolite benzyl alcohol (Hahn et al., 1983; Williams and Howe, 1994; Korpela and Tähti, 1988). The persistent effects of chronic toluene exposure have been attributed to the parent compound as well as the metabolites benzyl alcohol and benzaldehyde (Hahn et al., 1983; Korpela, 1989; Williams and Howe, 1994; Gregus and Klaassen, 1996). The generation of free radicals during the metabolism of toluene has also been proposed as a possible mechanism of neurotoxicity (Mattia et al., 1993) (see Neuropathological Diagnosis section).

Excretion

The decline in alveolar concentration is biphasic (Baelum et al., 1987). Phase I reflects the elimination of toluene from the blood, while phase II reflects its elimination from the parenchymal organs and muscle (Carlsson, 1982; Baelum et al., 1987). A third slow phase reflecting toluene released from adipose follows. Pulmonary excretion of unmetabolized toluene is complete within 24 hours after cessation of exposure (Baelum et al., 1987). About 15% to 20% of an absorbed toluene dose is excreted unchanged in the expired air (Williams, 1959; Cohr and Stokholm, 1979; Foo et al., 1991). Less than 2% of the absorbed dose of toluene is excreted in the bile (Abou-El-Marahem et al., 1967). A small quantity of toluene is excreted in urine unchanged, corresponding to the low solubility of toluene in water; most is excreted as HA, benzoyl glucuronide, and benzyl alcohol (Cohr and Stokholm, 1979). HA, the major metabolite of toluene that is excreted in the urine is completely eliminated by about 24 hours after the end of exposure; its half-life is 1 to 2 hours. The excretion of HA increases gradually during exposure, and the rate of excretion is increased during exercise (Baelum et al., 1987). Following exposure of volunteers to deuterium-labeled toluene, 78% of the inhaled dose was excreted as labeled HA (Lof et al., 1993). Other metabolites of toluene in urine include *p*-cresol, *o*-cresol, and phenol (Bakke and Scheline, 1970). The half life for *o*-cresol was found to be decreased by moderate exercise (Baelum et al., 1987). A minor metabolite of toluene, *S*-benzyl-*N*-acetyl-L-cysteine, has also been found in the urine of glue sniffers and printing workers (Takahashi et al., 1994).

CLINICAL MANIFESTATIONS AND DIAGNOSIS

Symptomatic Diagnosis

Acute effects of exposure to toluene include dimmed vision, headache, fatigue, confusion, lightheadedness, feeling of drunkenness, memory difficulties, disturbed equilibrium and coordination, and occasionally nausea, vomiting, or unconsciousness (Table 14-5) (Lee et al., 1988). Cognitive changes and incoordination are behaviors commonly observed following acute toluene exposure. Unrecognized acute effects of toluene exposure may be mistaken for mood and affective disorders, such as manic–depressive illness or schizophrenia (Goldblum and Chouinard, 1985). In addition, the occurrence of symptoms related to episodes of solvent abuse is similar to the exposure–effects time relationship, as with other types of substance abuse. An apparent dose-dependent relationship exists in the overall prevalence of symptoms of toluene exposure. Subjective symptoms in shoemakers were reported to increase during the workday, as well as cumulatively over time with recurrent exposures to toluene vapor (Fig. 14-4) (Lee et al., 1988). At low concentrations, exposure to toluene produces fatigue; at higher concentrations, exhilaration and euphoria are experienced (Boor and Hurtig, 1977). Higher concentrations are increasingly more dangerous, even with shorter durations of exposure (Gamberale and Hultengren, 1972). Impaired suppression of the vestibuloocular responses was demonstrated in

Table 14-5. *Subjective symptoms in shoemakers following exposure to toluene vapor*

Symptoms experienced during workday
  Drunken feeling
  Headache
  Dizziness
  Heavy feeling in head
  Unusual taste
  Unusual smell
  Dimmed vision
  Irritation in eyes
  Nasal irritation
  Sore throat
Cumulative symptoms during 6 months of exposure
  Nervousness
  Lightheadedness
  Loss of consciousness
  Forgetfulness
  Headache
  Dizziness
  Dimmed vision
  Eye strain
  Ringing in ears
  Hearing loss
  Reduced muscle power in extremities
  Dullness in extremities
  Tremor in extremities
  Cramp in extremities
  Joint pain
  Shortness of breath
  Frequent cough
  Unusual feeling in throat
  Weight loss
  Nausea
  Dry mouth

Modified from Lee et al., 1988, with permission.

15 subjects (mean age: 28) who were exposed to concentrations of 103 to 148 ppm for 130 minutes while doing light physical work (Hyden et al., 1983).

Chronic or episodic exposure to toluene produces a variety of acute symptoms that are experienced during the exposure, including dizziness, impaired handwriting, nystagmus on lateral gaze, mental confusion, inappropriate laughter, staring into space, and in some cases suicidal ideations. With accumulation of toluene in the CNS, neurological abnormalities occur and may persist beyond the end of exposure. These may involve cognitive impairments, as well as impairments of coordination, including disturbances in posture and fine motor control (Panse and Bender, 1934; Lazar et al., 1983). Intention tremor of both hands and feet, unsteady titubating gait, rebound of stretch reflexes and awkward rapid alternating hand movements (adiadochokinesis) are observed (Grabski, 1961; Knox and Nelson, 1966). For example, gross action tremor, head titubation, and truncal ataxia were observed in a 42-year-old man who was exposed to toluene vapors after he had worked in a photoengraving and silk screen manufacturing shop for

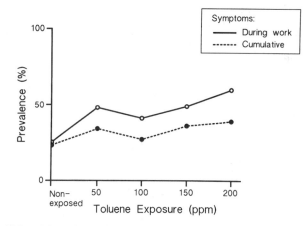

FIG. 14-4. Dose-dependent prevalence of subjective symptoms among 193 shoemakers, increased with increasing exposure dose both during work and cumulatively. (Modified from Lee et al., 1988, with permission.)

over 4 years (R. G. Feldman and R. S. Burns, personal observation, 1996) (see Clinical Experiences section).

The effects of intentionally inhaling toluene vapors have been reported in many individual cases as well as in groups of people (see Clinical Experiences section). Hormes et al. (1986) studied 16 men and four women who abused these vapors (primarily toluene) for psychotropic effects over a mean duration of 12 years. They experienced cognitive deficits (60%), most prominently in attention, memory, visuospatial, and complex executive functions; motor disorders (50%); and cerebellar dysfunction (primarily ataxic gait and postural tremor) (45%). Brain stem and cranial nerve symptoms occurred in 25%. Chronically inhaled volatile substances containing a mean amount of 425 ± 366 mg of toluene daily for 6.3 ± 3.9 years produced neurological effects in a group of 24 persons (mean age 23 ± 4.4 years), which included tremor and ataxia (45%), followed by memory impairment (20%). There was decreased olfaction, optic atrophy, hearing impairment, spasticity, and hyperreflexia in 8%. In addition, some of the older patients in the group, with longer histories of toluene vapor abuse, had evidence of mild peripheral neuropathy as well (Fornazzari et al., 1983). The most common features in 14 younger chronic toluene sniffers (aged 8 to 14 years), exposed to unknown concentrations in glue, included euphoria and hallucinations (seven cases); psychological impairment (five cases); coma (four cases); ataxia and convulsions (three cases); and diplopia (two cases) (King et al., 1981).

Chronic encephalopathy following long-term toluene abuse is characterized by apathy, inattention, poor memory, and impaired performance of complex cognitive function. Symptoms may appear following as few 1 year or as many as 20 years of exposure (Spencer et al., 1980). Anxiety, mood swings, and irritability occur early, followed by memory impairments and problem-solving difficulties. The absence of aphasia helps to differentiate a dementia due to the encephalopathy associated with toluene expo-

sure from other organic dementias, such as those seen in vascular or Alzheimer's disease (Hormes et al., 1986; White, 1987; Anger, 1990). Chronic toluene-induced encephalopathy is a primary white matter syndrome (Filley et al., 1990); in some cases, it may be difficult to distinguish from multiinfarct vascular disease with related dementia. These clinical manifestations must also be differentiated from the similar features of encephalopathies caused by other specific neurodegenerative diseases, drug effects, hypoglycemia, hyperglycemia, transient ischemic attacks, partial epilepsy (psychomotor), head injury, hysteria, or meningitis. Since increasing duration of exposure coincides with increasing age of exposed workers, a potential confounder in the diagnosis of toxic encephalopathy is the effect of aging. With continued exposure, cognitive function worsens, and motor signs progress to include frontal release signs and motor signs, including increased tone and postural disturbances. The clinical picture at this time is difficult to distinguish from the combination of extrapyramidal and pyramidal features, such as is seen in multisystem atrophy-related parkinsonism (Bartolucci and Pellitier, 1984; Ikeda and Tsukagoshi, 1990; Ameno et al., 1992; Fornazzari et al., 1983; M. Mimura et al., personal communication, 1995).

It is difficult to attribute to toluene alone all the manifestations of exposures to glues, gasoline, paints, and paint thinners, since other potentially neurotoxic organic substances are often present in such mixtures of solvents (OSHA, 1978). Paresthesias in the extremities occurred following toluene exposure (Korobkin et al., 1975). However, clinically obvious peripheral neuropathy due to pure toluene exposure has rarely been reported (Fornazzari et al., 1983), and the neuropathy when present is possibly related to concomitant exposure to other organic solvents, such as n-hexane (Goto et al., 1974; Shirabe et al., 1974; Ron, 1986). Cranial neuropathy affecting the optic and auditory nerves accompanies other features of toluene intoxication (Keane, 1978; Ehyai and Freemon, 1983; Hollo and Vargo, 1992). Pendular nystagmus with vertical and horizontal components has been observed in four patients who had chronically sniffed glue containing toluene (Maas et al., 1991). These effects are derived from combinations and the mutually enhancing effects of interacting compounds of different neurotoxicants (Winchester and Madjar, 1986). For example, in a study comparing the effects of the combined exposure to toluene and ethanol in humans, eight subjects (mean age: 33 years) were exposed to toluene at a concentration of 80 ppm for 4 hours and ethanol at 0.4 mL/kg body weight. No differences were found in either subjective or psychological performances between the subjects and a control group who had been exposed to only ethanol. However, performance and mood deteriorated more when the alcohol and toluene were administered acutely together than when toluene was administered alone (Cherry et al., 1983). Coexposures to toluene and p-xylene did not alter the effects of one or the other substance during a 4-hour exposure (Olson et al., 1985). However, neurotoxicity is augmented with exposure to mixtures of toluene and other solvents such as *n*-hexane (Escobar and Aruffo, 1980), trichloroethylene, methyl ethyl ketone (Grabski, 1961), and benzene (Inoue et al., 1988). *Single-photon emission computed tomography* (SPECT) studies in workers exposed to mixed solvents including toluene have revealed changes in regional cerebral blood flow consistent with neurological dysfunction (see Neuroimaging section) (Fincher et al., 1997).

Neurophysiological Diagnosis

Electroencephalographic (EEG) findings of diffuse 5- to 7-Hz slow waves were observed in toluene abusers. In addition, these individuals showed memory impairment and disturbances in motor control (Fornazzari et al., 1983). In another report, EEG and *electronystagmographic* abnormalities persisted for 6 months following accidental acute exposure to toluene vapors (Biscaldi et al., 1981). Visual hallucinations were experienced by a 16-year-old glue sniffer who had been abusing toluene for 3 months. His initial EEG and visual evoked responses were abnormal and remained so 4 months after cessation of exposure (Channer and Stanley, 1983). Although changes in the EEG observed after solvent abuse or passive exposure are consistent with general and nonspecific evidence of an effect, the recordings were performed at various times in relation to the exposure and thus reflect variable conditions and intensities of exposure to toluene and/or mixtures of solvents including toluene and must be interpreted accordingly.

Visual evoked potential (VEP) abnormalities correlate positively with the duration of toluene exposure and may be used as an electrophysiological marker of a neurotoxic effect of toluene. Keane (1978) described a 20-year-old

man who had inhaled the vapors of a mixture of toluene, xylene, isobutane propane, and methylene chloride for 3 years. The patient developed diminished visual acuity (4/200), poor color perception, and constricted visual fields; pupillary response to light was poor, but normal to convergence. VEPs were severely affected and showed decreased amplitude and delayed latencies, although the electroretinogram was normal, indicating intact outer retinal functions. With abstinence from further exposure, the visual acuity improved to 20/30, and the VEP latencies were less prolonged, although color vision was still mildly impaired. In contrast, color vision was not impaired in a study of workers and a referent population following low-level occupational exposure to toluene and tetrachloroethylene. These results may be due to low-exposure concentrations, insensitive measurement techniques, or simply no effect of these solvents alone on color vision (Nakatsuka et al., 1992).

VEPs were recorded in a group of 49 printing press workers (mean age: 42.3 years) in a print shop where toluene had been used exclusively as an organic solvent for the previous 30 years (mean duration of exposure: 21.4 years; Vrca et al., 1995). Toluene concentrations in the ambient air ranged from 40 to 60 ppm. Fifty-nine age-matched factory workers with no known exposure to any neurotoxic substance served as controls. No significant difference was found in the following parameters of waves N75, P100, and N145: time of onset, time of offset, total duration of each wave, and total duration of all three waves together. However, P100 wave latency was significantly longer in the exposed workers than in the controls. In addition, amplitude was significantly higher in all three waves in the exposed workers, suggesting increased excitation and hypersynchronization within the visual pathway (Table 14-6). In a similar study by Urban and Lukas (1990) of VEPs in a group of

TABLE 14-6. *Visual evoked potentials (VEPs) in toluene-exposed printers and nonexposed controls[a]*

	Printers (*n* = 47)		Controls (*n* = 59)		
	Range	Mean	Range	Mean	*p* value
VEP N75					
Onset (msec)	24.5–84.0	62.6	25.0–111.5	62.3	NS
Peak (msec)	47.5–92.0	77.8	46.9–98.5	77.3	NS
Offset (msec)	68.0–111.0	88.4	58.0–106.0	88.9	NS
Amplitude (μV)	2.16–11.75	5.7	1.19–16.8	4.6	< 0.01
VEP N100					
Onset (msec)	68.0–111.0	88.4	58.0–106.5	88.7	NS
Peak (msec)	98.0–125.5	11.3	99.5–135.0	109.0	< 0.05
Offset (msec)	105.0–169.0	133.4	113.5–167.0	135.4	NS
Amplitude (μV)	1.78–17.25	7.3	0.94–10.25	5.1	< 0.001
VEP N145					
Onset (msec)	105.0–169.0	133.4	113.5–167.0	135.4	NS
Peak (msec)	116.5–207.5	157.9	128.5–210.5	160.7	NS
Offset (msec)	144.5–265.6	190.5	140.5–259.5	187.7	NS
Amplitude (μV)	0.62–14.5	4.8	0.55–8.6	3.1	< 0.01

[a]A significant amplitude increase is seen in all three waves of the exposed workers, suggesting increased excitation and hypersynchronization within the visual pathway. In addition, P100 wave latency was significantly longer in the exposed workers than in the controls.
Modified from Vrca et al., 1995, with permission.

rotogravure printers exposed to toluene at concentrations at least two to three times higher, a decrease was seen in the amplitude of these same waves, suggesting a possible dose–response relationship; at low levels the effects of organic solvents can be excitatory rather than inhibiting (WHO, 1985). Follow-up examination revealed considerable stability of the VEP changes in the rotogravure printers, indicating that these manifestations are stable, perhaps reflecting permanent structural changes.

Brain-stem auditory evoked potential (BAEP) abnormalities were present in two patients who habitually sniffed the vapors of paint containing toluene. Findings included presence of waves I and II and absence of later waves, suggesting lower brainstem dysfunction. These findings were correlated with computed tomography (CT) evidence of pontomedullary atrophy (Metrick and Brenner, 1982). Prolongation of waves I and III interpeak latencies and abnormalities of waves III, IV, and V bilaterally have also been described (Hormes et al., 1986). The BAEPs from 5 of 11 persons with histories of chronic toluene abuse by spray paint inhalation for at least 1 year (but who had abstained for at least 1 month before being tested) showed significantly prolonged latencies of wave V ($p < 0.01$), and prolonged wave III–wave V interpeak latencies ($p < 0.01$) when compared as a group with control subjects. Of note was that two of the five with abnormal BAEPs showed normal neurological examinations and magnetic resonance images (MRI) (Rosenberg et al., 1988a).

Neuropsychological Diagnosis

The importance of recognizing and documenting neurobehavioral manifestations of solvent encephalopathies is well established (Anger, 1985; Anger and Johnson, 1985; White et al., 1992; Dick, 1995). Neurobehavioral assessments of exposed individuals by survey and by various self-reporting subjective testimonials about working conditions provide definite trends and indications of a relationship between their complaints of unwellness and a probable source of exposure (Paull, 1984). The acute and chronic neuropsychological effects of toluene have been tested for both in the laboratory and at work site research settings (Cherry et al., 1983; Hanninen et al., 1987). The clinical application of standardized neuropsychological test batteries to individuals and/or groups suspected of exposure has provided evidence in those affected of impairments in one or more of the following functional areas: attention, executive function, verbal fluency, psychomotor functioning, visuospatial skills, and short-term memory; changes in mood and affect were also seen (White et al., 1992). Psychomotor slowing and impaired attention and short-term memory function appear to be the neuropsychological deficits most consistently associated with acute and chronic toluene exposure.

Following exposure to toluene, selected tests have been used to assess function in various cognitive domains; these include (1) *attention:* Bourdon-Wiersma, continuous per-

formance tasks, dual task tests, pattern recognition/pattern comparison, and visual-search; (b) *short-term memory:* digit span; (c) *executive function:* symbol digit test, verbal arithmetic; (d) *psychomotor functioning:* simple and choice reaction time, Purdue Pegboard, finger tapping; (e) *sensory:* smell and color discrimination, critical flicker fusion, and visual acuity; and (f) *sensorimotor:* postural sway.

Toluene abuse has been associated with lower verbal IQ, suggesting that educationally, culturally, and emotionally deprived individuals are at greater risk for abusing this substance (Fornazzari et al., 1983). Therefore, identifying neuropsychological deficits in a patient who has a history of potentially significant exposure to toluene requires careful differentiation of the various possible etiologies. These include premorbid cognitive status and coexisting psychiatric or neurological disorders, as well as consideration of the neurotoxicity of toluene alone or in a mixture with other volatile organic solvents (Baelum et al., 1985; Goldblum and Chouinard, 1985; Juntunen et al., 1985; Ron, 1986; Nelson et al., 1994; White et al., 1995).

Effects of acute and chronic exposures to mixed solvents containing various proportions of toluene have been documented by neuropsychological testing of volunteers in controlled laboratory settings and in worker populations at the work site (Iregren, 1986; Anger, 1990; Dick, 1995; Echeverria et al., 1989; White et al., 1995). The digit symbol test is likely to detect psychomotor slowing associated with acute toluene exposure; prolonged toluene exposures are associated with poor performance on the incidental learning subtest of the digit symbol test, the imbedded figures test of distractibility, the block design test of spatial relations, the grooved pegboard tests of coordination, and simple reaction time tests of motor speed (Dick, 1995). Following acute exposure to toluene, volunteers have exhibited impairments on tests of attention including simple, choice, and compound reaction time; dual tasks; vigilance. Impairment on digit spans, identical number, and pattern recognition tests have also been reported. However, effects are not noted on testing with variants of the Benton Visual Retention test.

Acute exposure to toluene at 80 ppm for 4 hours in a controlled exposure chamber had no significant effect on performance of a computerized battery of tests given to spray painters (Iregren, 1986). Using the subject as his own control, at toluene exposure levels of 150 ppm, a 5% to 7% decrease in performance was detected in the following domains: (a) visual memory, on a pattern recognition test; (b) verbal short-term memory, on digit span; (c) visual perception, on pattern recognition latency; and (d) manual dexterity, on one-hole test and critical tracking (Echeverria et al., 1989).

Tests of simple attention, cognitive tracking, and cognitive flexibility are commonly affected in patients with exposure to a variety of neurotoxicants including toluene and frequently are the only manifestation of encephalopathy. Deficits in visuospatial functioning are also frequently seen. Patients sometimes show temporal gradients on formal retrograde tasks such as Albert's Famous Faces Tests;

however, it is unclear whether this is true forgetting of known information (retrograde memory loss) or simply the effect of anterograde memory deficits at the time of exposure resulting from the lack of encoding of information including facts about the exposure conditions (White and Proctor, 1995). Persons exposed to toluene and xylene during a varnishing process exhibited impairments in immediate and delayed memory, with visual memory most affected. Psychomotor abilities were significantly impaired among workers directly exposed to toluene, compared with occasionally exposed workers and nonexposed control subjects (Gupta et al., 1990). In a 2-year prospective study of a group of silk screen printers who were still fully employed and not complaining of any particular illness, those with higher acute exposures demonstrated significantly impaired test performance on tasks involving manual dexterity, visual memory, and mood (White et al., 1995). Furthermore, those with higher chronic exposure showed poorer performance on visual memory tasks and mood, indicating that the effects associated with acute exposure may persist following removal from exposure.

The neurobehavioral effects of occupational exposure were assessed in a group of 30 female workers (mean age: 25.6 years) exposed to toluene at 88 ppm in an electronic assembly factory, with a mean exposure duration of 5.7 years. All workers were nondrinkers and nonsmokers and were not taking any medication regularly or on the day of testing. The workers had no clinical symptoms or signs. A group of 30 age-, sex-, and ethnicity-matched workers from an area in the same factory where the toluene concentration in their work environment was only 13 ppm were used as controls. Averaged blood toluene concentrations at the time of testing were 1.25 mg/L in the exposed workers and 0.16 mg/L in the controls. Comparison of performance on neurobehavioral tests of manual dexterity (grooved pegboard), verbal memory (digit span), and visual scanning and executive functioning (trail making, Benton visual retention, digit symbol, and visual reproduction) revealed significant dose-dependent differences in the exposed workers. No effect was noted on tests of simple reaction time or finger tapping. Because of elevated blood toluene levels at the time of exposure, the question arises as to whether these results demonstrate acute or early chronic effects (Foo et al., 1990).

Results of a brief test battery designed to reveal neuropsychological impairment in solvent-exposed workers did not reveal a significant difference between 52 toluene-exposed workers at a factory making rubberized asbestos matting and a group of age-matched unexposed controls. From 1970 to 1976 work site air toluene concentrations frequently exceeded 300 ppm. At the time of testing, ambient air concentrations in all areas of the factory were below 200 ppm. Although a significant difference between the performance of the exposed workers and the controls was not found, the performance of the exposed workers was worse than the controls on the following: trail making, vi-

sual search, digit symbol, block design, grooved pegboard, and memory tests (Cherry et al., 1985).

The chronic effects of toluene exposure were assessed in a group of 43 rotogravure printers exposed to toluene concentrations of 68 to 185 ppm for 11 to 40 years. Testing was performed following 2 to 3 days without exposure to toluene. The workers were compared with a referent group comprised of 31 nonexposed offset printers of the same age. The two groups were further divided into subgroups according to toluene exposure and drinking habits. The exposed workers demonstrated significantly inferior performance than controls on block design and embedded figures tests of visual cognition, as well as impaired performance on neurobehavioral tests of visual memory and eye–hand coordination. Scores on tests of verbal memory were slightly higher among the exposed workers. The mean test performances in the subgroups according to drinking habits and toluene exposure indicate that a drinking habit did not explain the impairment in cognitive functions. Increased alcohol consumption seemed to have a protective effect on the workers, as the lowest scores were seen in nondrinking workers with the highest exposure, while heavy drinkers with high exposure tended to perform better than equally exposed workers with more moderate drinking habits (Hanninen et al., 1987).

Neuropsychological testing of 24 chronic toluene abusers revealed deficits in several domains including short-term verbal memory (Wechsler Memory Scale), verbal IQ, and performance IQ (Wechsler Adult Intelligence Scale). These deficits were significantly correlated with CT scan measurements of the cortical sulci, cerebellum, and ventricles (Fornazzari et al., 1983).

Olfactory perception tests have been used to measure the workers' capacity to identify odors in a printing plant following exposure to a variety of solvents, including toluene. A significantly higher olfactory perception threshold was observed among exposed subjects (Mergler, 1995). The results of an earlier study showed a sixfold increase in the olfactory perception threshold (OPT) for toluene following 7 hours of exposure; this threshold for a control substance (PM-carbinol) remained stable (Mergler and Beauvais, 1992).

Biochemical Diagnosis

The exhaled air toluene concentration closely parallels blood toluene levels (Brugone et al., 1986). Therefore, both can be used for confirming acute exposure and estimating absorption (Gamberale and Hultengren, 1972; Carlsson, 1982; Foo et al., 1991). However, the ACGIH (1995) has not established a biological exposure index (BEI) for toluene in end-exhaled air. In addition, analysis of the morning blood sample taken after a previous day's exposure is considered more reliable than just testing the expired air. Samples of alveolar air and blood, taken from a group of rotogravures, printers, and shoe workers during their work shifts and early in the morning of the next day, showed that whereas alveolar toluene concentration measured during the work shift correlated significantly with exposure, the blood toluene concentrations collected at the end of the shift correlated better with the simultaneously collected samples of environmental toluene concentration (Brugone et al., 1986).

The end of shift BEI for toluene in venous blood is 1 mg/L (ACGIH, 1995) (Table 14-7). Blood concentrations in 232 workers not occupationally exposed to toluene were found to be approximately 3,000 ng/L, which has been suggested as a reasonable reference limit (Wang et al., 1993). Detecting toluene in venous blood can be used to confirm absorption when acute exposure concentration is less than 50 ppm (Kawai et al., 1992). Morning blood concentrations of toluene in a group of printers exposed to toluene concentrations ranging from 40 to 60 ppm were found to be 30 times greater than those of a group of age-matched controls (Vrca et al., 1995). Immediately following dermal exposure, blood toluene levels may be elevated, especially in the arm with the greatest exposure, resulting in erroneous estimations of total exposure (Aitio et al., 1984). The concentration of toluene in blood increases after ingestion of acetylsalicylic acid (Löf et al., 1990). The elimination curve for toluene in blood consists of two fast components with biological half-lives of 9 minutes and 2 hours, respectively, and a slow component with a median half-life of 90 hours, due to the slow release of toluene that had been bound to tissue lipids (Nise et al., 1989; Löf et al., 1993). Furthermore, the apparent accumulation of toluene, as indicated by the higher levels after a day of exposure, suggests that two consecutive work shifts is insufficient for complete elimination of the toluene absorbed during a shift (Brugnone et al., 1986).

Measurement of end of shift urinary HA levels is the recommended BEI for monitoring groups of workers and for exposure levels above 100 ppm (DeRosa et al., 1985; Brugnone et al., 1995). The end of shift urinary HA concentration should not exceed 2.5 g/g creatinine if the 8-hour TWA exposure level has not exceeded 200 ppm (ACGIH, 1995) (Table 14-7). Urine specimens tested at the end of a work shift are useful if taken right before the end of the exposure period. End of work shift HA levels in the urine of exposed workers significantly correlated with the mean daily environmental concentrations (DeRosa et al., 1985). Four to 6 hours after the end of a shift, the concentration of HA in the urine may already be decreased to 30% of its original maximum value (Ron, 1986). By the following morning, when testing preshift urinary samples, the baseline HA level can represent dietary and other non-workplace sources of toluene. For example, HA measurements may be confounded by concurrent exposures to ethylbenzene, styrene, and benzoic acid, which are also metabolized to hippuric acid. The total contribution of these extraneous sources of HA was assessed in nine volunteers exposed to 200 mg/m³ of deuterium-labeled toluene for 2 hours while performing a workload of 50 W on a stationary bicycle. The total amount of HA (labeled plus unlabeled) excreted in the urine was found to exceed the exposure dose by four times, demonstrating the presence (in urine) of HA derived from other chemical sources (Fig. 14-5) (Lof et al., 1993). In addition, the metabolism of toluene can be inhibited by concurrent exposure to other chemicals such as benzene, which has been shown to suppress the metabolism of toluene to HA (Inoue et al., 1988). HA levels were found to be significantly reduced by cigarette smoking and consumption of ethanol (Inoue et al., 1993). Therefore, the use of HA has certain limitations as an indicator of toluene exposure, especially for assessing low-level exposures (Inoue et al., 1994; Kawamoto et al., 1995).

Determination of o-cresol concentrations in urine has been suggested as an alternative to HA as an indicator for toluene exposure; o-cresol is regarded as the only metabolite specific to toluene (Angerer, 1979; Baelum et al., 1987). However, a very small proportion (<1%) of toluene is excreted as o-cresol, and this correlates less well with daily exposure than does HA (DeRosa et al., 1987). Smokers have three to four times higher background levels of o-cresol (Dossing et al., 1983) due to the toluene in cigarette smoke, and thus smoking habits must be taken into consideration when monitoring low-level exposure to toluene (Nise, 1992). Concurrent exposure to toluene and benzene has been shown to reduce conversion of toluene to o-cresol (Inoue et al., 1988).

Although generally not used as indicators of exposure, other metabolites present in the urine of persons exposed to toluene include p-cresol (ACGIH, 1986) and S-benzyl-N-acetyl-L-cysteine (Takahashi et al., 1994). In addition, the possible modification of urinary metabolite excretion due to combined exposure to chemicals other than the target solvent (i.e., toluene) is an important factor in the bio-

TABLE 14-7. *Biological exposure indices for toluene*

	Urine	Blood	Alveolar air
Determinant	Hippuric acid	Toluene	Toluene
Start of shift	Not established	Not established	Not established
During shift	Not established	Not established	Not established
End of shift at end of workweek	2.5 g/g creatinine	1.0 mg/L	Not established

Data from ACGIH, 1995.

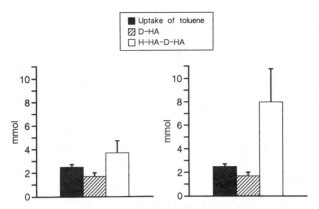

FIG. 14-5. Excretion of hippuric acid in nine volunteers, following exposure to deuterium-labeled toluene; mean values and standard deviations. Demonstrates the contribution from extraneous sources to the total urinary output of hippuric acid following exposure of volunteers to 200 mg/m³ of deuterium-labeled toluene. **Left:** Most (65%) of the deuterium-labeled toluene was excreted as deuterium-labeled hippuric within 4 hours of exposure. **Right:** Most of the hippuric acid excreted in the urine over the next 16 hours was unlabeled and derived from other sources. (Modified from Löf et al., 1993, with permission.)

chemical diagnosis of solvent exposure (Ikeda, 1990, 1995; Kawai et al., 1992).

Neuroimaging

Magnetic resonance imaging and *computed tomography* are useful and sensitive tools for evaluating the severity of neuropathological effects of toluene as well as estimating the prognosis for recovery. Toluene abuse has been associated with cerebral and cerebellar atrophy on CT scans (Boor and Hurtig, 1977; Metrick and Benner, 1982; Fornazzari et al., 1983; Hormes et al., 1986; Xiong et al., 1993). There appears to be no correlation between the severity of these radiological abnormalities and the frequencies and durations of episodes of toluene exposure (Fornazzari et al., 1983; Lazar et al., 1983; Hormes et al., 1986). The radiological findings on CT scans include widening of the cerebellar and cerebral sulci and basal cisterns, with enlargement of the ventricular system. Marked impairments on neurological and neuropsychological tests noted in heavy toluene abusers were significantly correlated with the presence of abnormalities on CT scan measurements of cerebellum, cerebral cortical sulci, and ventricles when compared with age-matched controls. In the more severe cases, there was also involvement of the brain stem (Fornazzari et al., 1983).

The MRI studies in toluene sniffers also reveal diffuse atrophy of the cerebellum, cerebrum, and brain stem, with decreased differentiation between the gray and white matter and increased periventricular white matter signal intensity on T_2-weighted images (Rosenberg et al., 1988a). The degree of white matter abnormalities significantly corre-

lated with neuropsychological deficits (Filley et al., 1990). Ikeda and Tsukagoshi (1990) reported atrophy of the cerebellum, corpus callosum, cerebrum, and brain stem, as well as abnormal intensity of the internal capsule on MRI examination of a 27-year-old man with a 10-year history of toluene abuse who presented with dementia, cerebellar ataxia, dysarthria, and pyramidal signs. The MRI of a 28-year-old man with a 1-year history of toluene abuse showed marked cerebellar atrophy with enlarged cerebellar sulci on the T_1-weighted images. In addition, T_1-weighted images revealed marked atrophy of the corpus callosum. Loss of gray–white matter discrimination in the parietooccipital region and the cerebellar region was seen on the T_2-weighted images (Fig. 14-6) (Xiong et al., 1993).

Both the MRI and the CT scan of a 19-year-old man with a 5-year history of abusing thinner (50% toluene and 20% aliphatic alcohols with small amounts of methanol and ethanol) showed mild diffuse widening of the cerebral sulci, ventricular dilation, and bilateral symmetrical lesions of the putamen, caudate nucleus, and cingulate gyrus (Figs. 14-7 and 14-8). There were no abnormalities of the cerebellum or pons. Bilateral lesions of the basal ganglia and the cingulate gyrus resulting from toluene abuse have not previously been reported. However, similar lesions of the putamen and the caudate nucleus are seen in methanol poisoning, suggesting that the combined effects of toluene and methanol—both of which were in the thinner this young man abused—may have been responsible for the abnormalities revealed by CT and MRI (Ashikaga et al., 1995).

Neuropathological Diagnosis

The region-specific neurotoxic effects of toluene are partly due to its high lipid solubility and associated distribution in various lipid-rich brain regions. Clinical studies of acute exposure to toluene and other solvents suggest that the effects may be transient and reversible; chronic and repeated exposures result in long-term and often permanent nervous system dysfunction. Most of the intense exposures have been reported in individuals intentionally inhaling toluene vapors from glues and paint thinners. Few pathological studies have been done on chronically exposed workers who have developed clinical manifestations of cortical, brain stem, and cerebellar involvement. Death occurred 30 minutes after a person swallowed approximately 60 mL of toluene. Although the heart, lungs, and kidneys showed congestion and hemorrhage, there were no remarkable changes seen in the brain. Apparently the short time from ingestion to death did not allow for observable pathological changes to develop in the brain (Ameno et al., 1989). In contrast, the autopsy findings in a 27-year-old man with a 12-year history of inhaling toluene vapors from glue and the mixed solvents contained in paint thinner, revealed diffuse cerebral and cerebellar cortical atrophy. Microscopic examination revealed decreased neuronal density in the cerebral cortex and basal ganglia, diffuse

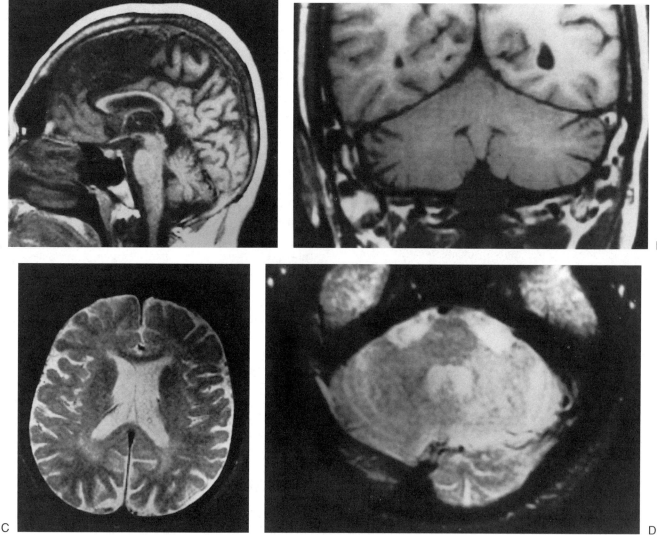

FIG. 14-6. MRI of 27-year-old man with a 1-year history of toluene abuse. **A:** T_1-weighted sagittal image demonstrating marked atrophy of corpus callosum. **B:** T_1-weighted coronal image showing frank cerebellar atrophy as indicated by enlarged cerebellar sulci. **C:** T_2-weighted axial image showing generalized atrophy, loss of gray–white matter discrimination, and irregular hyperintense areas in the parietooccipital white matter bilaterally. **D:** T_2-weighted axial image revealing a loss of gray–white matter discrimination in an asymmetrical slice through the cerebellar region. (From Xiong et al., 1993, with permission.)

subcortical demyelination, marked loss of Purkinje cells in the cerebellar cortex, and both central and peripheral axonopathy. Ballooning of Purkinje cells of the cerebellum was evident, and the corpus callosum was atrophied. Fragmentation of axons and vacuolization of myelin sheaths were evident in the subcortical white matter. Since the patient had also been exposed to *n*-hexane and other volatile organic solvent ingredients in the glue he sniffed, these agents probably contributed to the total pathological picture (Escobar et al., 1980).

The pathological findings in a 55-year-old man with a 29-year history of exposure to toluene and other solvents involved the same brain stem and subcortical areas, which were described in multisystem atrophy cases (Feldman and

McKee, 1993) as well as in other case reports of toluene intoxication (Ameno et al., 1992). There was diffuse loss of myelin and astrogliosis within the subcortical white matter. In the cerebellum, there was Purkinje cell loss with reactive gliosis and cell rarefaction within the granule cell layer. The inferior olivary and dentate nuclei showed increased astrogliosis with relative neuronal preservation. There was moderate gliosis within the tegmentum of the mesencephalic reticular formation, in the central gray surrounding the aqueduct, and within the inferior and superior colliculi. Throughout the pontine nuclei, particularly within the basis pontis, there was astrogliosis as well as demyelination and loss of neurons. Free pigment, neuronal loss, and gliosis were noted in the locus ceruleus. The cerebral peduncles

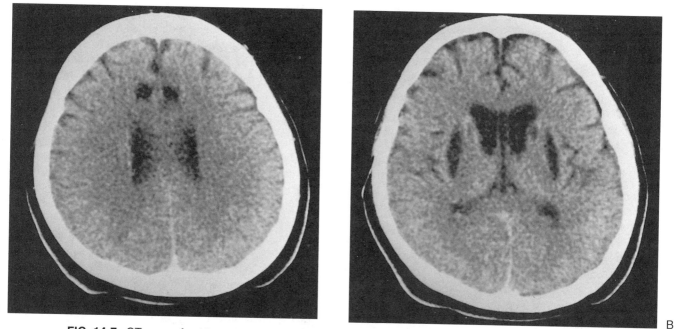

FIG. 14-7. CT scan of a 19-year-old man with a 5-year history of toluene abuse. **A:** Cerebral atrophy and bilateral symmetrical lesions of the cingulate gyri are shown. **B:** Bilateral lesions in the basal ganglia are shown. (From Ashikaga et al., 1995, with permission.)

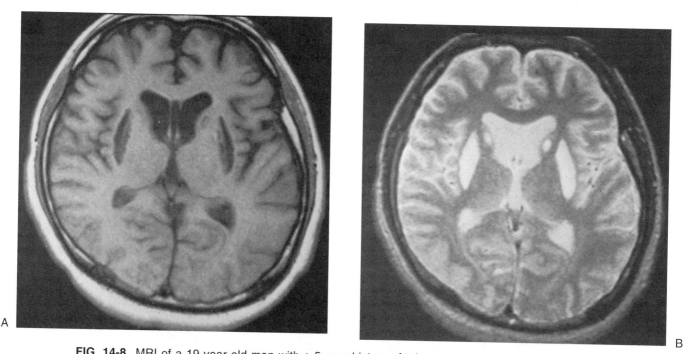

FIG. 14-8. MRI of a 19-year-old man with a 5-year history of toluene abuse. **A:** T_1-weighted image shows bilateral low-intensity signals in the lentiform nucleus, caudate nucleus, and cingulates gyrus. No abnormalities are seen in the pons or cerebellum. **B:** T_2-weighted image demonstrates the same lesions appearing bilaterally as high-intensity signals in the lentiform nucleus, caudate nucleus, and cingulates gyrus. (From Ashikaga et al., 1995, with permission.)

were uninvolved. There was destruction of the substantia nigra with marked neuronal loss, free pigment, extensive astrogliosis, and the presence of Lewy bodies within the substantia nigra pars compacta. Much less neuronal loss and gliosis were seen in the substantia nigra pars reticulata. The substantia nigra had a mediolateral gradient in severity of tissue involvement, with the lateral aspect more severely affected. Within the basal ganglia, the putamen and the globus pallidus were most severely involved, also with a mediolateral gradient of severity of tissue destruction. There was more severe gliosis and neuronal loss within the lateral putamen and the external globus pallidus. The dorsal–caudal putamen was more affected, as a dorsal–ventral and rostral–caudal gradient was noted. Gliosis and neuronal loss were seen within the gray–white matter bridges, with the dorsal–lateral caudate nucleus only slightly affected caudally from the level of the anterior commissure. Mild global cortical neuronal loss and atrophy were present, especially within the frontal cortex. Alzheimer's neurofibrillary tangles and plaques were not seen using silver strains. Demyelination and gliosis was prominent within the occipital-temporal, inferior–parietal, and frontal areas. The hippocampus was normal. Neuronal loss was also present within the lateral horns and pyramidal and the posterior spinocerebellar tracts of the spinal cord. Demyelination was also present in spinal nerve roots without signs of chronic neuropathy. These findings, which are similar to the atrophy of the cortex, cerebellum, and brain stem reported by others (Lazar et al., 1983; Fornazzi et al., 1983), can explain the changes seen with MRI and CT in individuals exposed to toluene and other solvents (Prockop, 1995; Caldemyer et al., 1983; Rosenberg et al., 1988b).

The acute and chronic effects of toluene have been attributed to the metabolites benzyl alcohol and benzaldehyde, to free radicals, and to the parent compound (Hahn et al., 1983; Williams and Howe, 1994). Benzyl alcohol has been shown to block neuronal action potentials reversibly *in vitro*. Chronic *in vitro* exposure of rat nerve roots to benzyl alcohol resulted in scattered demyelination and axonal degeneration (Hahn et al., 1983). Benzaldehyde is an electrophilic compound, and therefore it can react with cellular macromolecules such as cytoskeletal proteins, as well as DNA and RNA (Gregus and Klaassen, 1996). Mattia et al. (1993) have suggested that free radicals produced during the metabolism of toluene induce lipid peroxidation. These authors have demonstrated that toluene increases oxidative activity in the hippocampus, cerebellum, and the striatum of rats. In addition, pretreatment with phenobarbital further enhanced the production of free radicals. The highest levels of oxidative activity were seen in the hippocampus, suggesting that this brain region is particularly vulnerable and may explain the memory and cognitive deficits seen in persons chronically exposed to toluene.

Exposure to toluene has been shown to alter membrane composition, function, and fluidity. Toluene significantly decreases synaptosomal phosphatidylethanolamine, resulting in a decrease in synaptosomal phospholipid methylation (LeBel and Schatz, 1989). The methylation of phosphotidylethanolamine to phosphatidylcholine affect β-adrenergic receptor–adenylase cyclase coupling events (Hirata and Axelrod, 1980). Exposure to toluene results in an increase in the number of β-adrenergic receptors and a decreased affinity of these receptors for β-adrenergic antagonists (Fuxe et al., 1987). Changes observed in other synaptic functions including receptor binding, protein phosphorylation, monoamine turnover rates, and changes in hormonal levels may also be related to altered synaptosomal membrane composition (von Euler et al., 1988). The activity of synaptosomal membrane bond enzymes is also affected by toluene. Both acetylcholinesterase (AChE) and adenosine triphosphatase (ATPase) activity are significantly ($p < 0.001$) inhibited in rat synaptosomes exposed to toluene *in vitro* and *in vivo* (Korpela, 1989).

Toluene has been shown to affect the tissue levels selectively of various behaviorally significant neurotransmitters (Rea et al., 1984). Noradrenaline levels were reduced in the hypothalamus following long-term exposure to 80 ppm toluene (von Euler et al., 1988). Following acute exposure to 1,000 ppm toluene in rats, serotonin concentrations were significantly increased in the cerebellum, medulla, and striatum. In the same study, concentrations of dopamine in the striatum were significantly increased as well (Rea et al., 1984). Longer duration exposures to toluene at 400 ppm resulted in a decrease in dopamine levels in the striatum (Ikeda et al., 1986). Long-term low-level (more than 80 ppm) exposure to toluene can lead to persistent increases in the affinity of dopamine D_2 agonist binding in the caudate–putamen (Hellefors-Berglund et al., 1995). At low levels in rats, toluene alters dopaminergic transmission and affects dopamine-mediated behaviors under specific challenges (von Euler, 1994). Acute exposure to toluene results in disturbances of the vestibulo and optoocular motor system (VOOMS). The action of toluene on Purkinje cell function and the cerebellar control of this system is believed to be due to a change in γ-aminobutyric acid (GABA) transmission. Baclofen, a GABA agonist, is known to produce similar effects on the VOOMS, as toluene and intracerebroventricular injection of a GABA antagonist in rats has been shown to inhibit the effects of toluene on the VOOMS (Niklasson et al., 1995).

THERAPEUTIC AND PREVENTIVE MEASURES

All workers subject to toluene exposure should have comprehensive preplacement and biennial medical examinations, with particular attention given to the incidence of headache, nausea, and dizziness (NIOSH, 1977). Proper ventilation of work areas, monitoring of ambient air concentrations, and biological monitoring of employees at risk of increased exposure are necessary for prevention of toluene intoxication in occupationally exposed persons. If toluene intoxication is identified, appropriate procedures must be taken to remove persons at risk from further exposure, to improve ambient air quality, and to reduce alveolar air concentrations of the neurotoxicant. Brief inhalation of toluene vapors produces mild, transient, reversible symptoms, leaving no neurological sequelae. Repeated exposures, however, does cause more permanent disturbances. Acute neurological symptoms usually disappear after withdrawal from exposure, but cognitive impairments and emotional instabilities associated with chronic toxic effects may persist. Specific systemic features may be treated symptomatically, for example with antidepressants or soporifics.

Because of the possibility of contamination of toluene sources with mixtures of other organic compounds, such as benzene and *n*-hexane, careful assessment of hepatic or peripheral neuropathic effects may be required (Pryor and Rebert, 1992). After formal neuropsychological tests indicate affected functional domains, the remaining functional strengths can be used in techniques in compensating for deficits. This often requires specialized psychological rehabilitative therapies (White et al., 1992).

CLINICAL EXPERIENCES

Group Studies

Symptoms among Photographic Printers

A cross-sectional survey was taken (Mørck et al., 1988) among 262 male employees in two photographic printing plants with 6 to 30 years (median: 20 years) of exposure to toluene. Each employee was given an exposure score based on duration of employment (1 point for every 10 years), presence or lack of mechanical ventilation of work area, frequency of wearing protective clothing, and frequency of peak exposures above the TLV. All workers were given a complete physical examination including biochemical assays of urine and blood. In addition, each participant was required to complete a questionnaire, with specific questions on family history of chronic disease, previous hospitalizations, symptoms from all major organ systems. smoking and alcohol consumption habits, drug use, and one question on sexual disturbances.

Symptoms that significantly and positively correlated with exposure included nasal or eye irritation, dizziness, decreased concentration, decreased memory, fainting, abdominal pains, sexual disturbances, and muscle pains in legs and ankles. After adjusting for age, alcohol consumption, smoking, and body indices, the following symptoms were significantly correlated with exposure score: dizziness, poor concentration, subjective feeling of decreased memory, high systolic blood pressure, and sexual problems.

A few days after the initial investigation, a plant shutdown allowed for a follow-up study on the effects from acute toluene exposure. Among a 140-member cohort from the original group, significant changes included decreased plasma alanine aminotransferase (P-ALAT), decreased systolic blood pressure, and increased plasma testosterone level. Decreased blood pressure and P-ALAT levels were correlated with exposure intensity. A correlation between P-ALAT levels and toluene exposure has previously been demonstrated (Tahti et al., 1981).

Muscle Weakness, Encephalopathy, and Persistent Signs Following Inhalation of Toluene Vapors

Clinical and laboratory findings in 25 adults (age range: 18 to 40 years) with repeated hospitalizations for intentional inhalation of toluene vapors during a 9-year period revealed three different patterns of symptoms (Streicher et al., 1981). Nine in the group were hospitalized for muscular weakness, including two who were unable to walk without assistance and four who had quadriparesis, two of which were initially hospitalized with a diagnosis of Guillain-Barré syndrome. All nine in this subgroup had significantly lower serum potassium and phosphorus concentrations compared with the remaining 16 abusers. Muscle weakness resolved within 1 to 3 days following cessation of sniffing and correction of fluid and electrolyte balance. Ten of the 25 patients presented with neurological findings including headache, dizziness, hallucinations, lethargy, cerebellar signs, and peripheral neuropathy. The remaining six individuals were admitted for gastrointestinal complaints including abdominal pain and hematemesis. Generally, recovery was rapid and complete in all, except for the patients with signs of cerebellar or peripheral nerve dysfunction.

Individual Case Reports

Recovery of Cognitive Impairments after Abstinence from Toluene Vapors

Case 1

A 59-year-old optician used toluene regularly to clean eyeglasses and contact lenses in a small room. He was admitted to the hospital due to clumsiness of the left side and fatigue. Other features included staggering, slurred speech, hypersomnia, decreased concentration, and disturbed memory. Symptoms were mild at first but progressed. Examination on admission showed minimal dysarthria, gait and limb ataxia, normal mental function, normal eye movements, and normal strength, sensation, and tendon reflexes. The EEG, CT scan, and cerebrospinal fluid were all normal. Recovery was complete within 1 month of discharge without further exposure to toluene (Boor and Hurtig, 1977).

Case 2

An 18-year-old woman who had sniffed pure toluene for 6 years (Malm and Lying-Tunell, 1980) exhibited personality changes including irritability, apathy, emotional lability, carelessness, weight loss, vomiting, and loss of appetite. One week before presentation, she developed slurred speech, and increased difficulty with walking. Examination revealed unsteadiness, incoordination of arms and legs, broad-based ataxic gait, nystagmus, and a positive Babinski sign bilaterally. Muscle strength and tendon reflexes were normal. Mental state examination showed emotional instability, euphoria, and lack of insight. She also had poor concentration and impaired visual spatial and abstraction functioning. Her symptoms gradually disappeared over 8 months of abstinence from glue sniffing.

Severe Tremor, Head and Truncal Titubation, and Evoked Potential Abnormalities after Toluene Exposure

Case 1

A 23-year-old man with a 12-year history of intentionally inhaling paint vapors that contained toluene presented with tremor and clumsiness of all extremities for a 3-month period (Metrick and Brenner, 1982). Examination revealed bilateral optic atrophy, ocular dysmetria, head titubation, intention tremor of upper extremities, and clumsiness of rapid alternating movements, worse on the right side. Gait was ataxic and wide based. Deep tendon reflexes were hyperactive. However, tactile sensation was normal. EEG, BAEPs, and VEPs were abnormal, and a CT scan showed severe pontomedullary atrophy. Abuse continued after discharge, and 9 months later, the BAEPs and CT scan were unchanged. The patient was then lost to follow-up.

Case 2

A 25-year-old man with a 5-year history of daily toluene abuse (glue) experienced progressive tremor of the limbs, trunk and head, difficulty maintaining balance, slurred speech, hearing loss, and continuous jerking movements of the eyes (Lazar et al., 1983). Examination revealed a cerebellar gait, four-limb ataxia, scanning speech, head and truncal titubation, and opsoclonus. There was a significant delay in absolute latencies for waves II, III, IV, and V on BAEP. There was moderate atrophy of cerebral cortex, cerebellum, and brain stem on CT scan.

Case 3

High-amplitude excursion action tremor, head titubation, and truncal ataxia were observed in a 42-year-old man who worked in a photoengraving and silk screen manufacturing shop for 4 years. Over a period of 2 years before he stopped working, he gradually developed symptoms of episodic nausea, blurred vision, and dizziness, which were worse at the end of a work shift and less noticeable after being away from his job. He developed an insidiously progressive tremor in his right arm and hand, soon followed by a to-and-fro movement of his head. These movements were increased with excitement. Several months later his walking was unstable, and he had to hold onto rails, walls, and furniture to steady himself. At that time he stopped working. He also experienced paresthesias of his feet, legs, and hands. Over the next 12 to 18 months, even after he had left his job, the head titubation and truncal ataxia continued to progress, and both arms showed action tremor and ataxia of extension. These neurological signs stabilized; over the

next 15 years he showed some improvement in walking using a cane and often a wheelchair for greater distances, but he remained at essentially the same state of disability (R. G. Feldman and R. S. Burns, personal observations, 1995).

REFERENCES

Abou-El-Marahem MM, Millburn P, Smith RL, Williams RT. Biliary excretion of foreign compounds: benzene and its derivatives in the rat. *Biochem J* 1967;105:1269–1274.

Agency for Toxic Substances and Disease Registry (ATSDR). U.S. Public Health Service. *Toxicological profile for toluene.* Atlanta, GA: Clement Associates Inc. (contract no. 205-88-0608), 1993:1–8.

Agency for Toxic Substances and Disease Registry (ATSDR). U.S. Public Health Service. *Toxicological profile for toluene.* Atlanta, GA: Clement International Corp. (contract no. 205-88-0608), 1994.

Aitio A, Pekari K, Jarvisalo J. Skin absorption as a source of error in biological monitoring. *Scand J Work Environ Health* 1984;10:317–320.

Ameno K, Fuke C, Ameno S, et al. A fatal case of oral ingestion of toluene. *Forensic Sci Int* 1989;41:255–260.

Ameno K, Kirui T, Fuke C, et al. Regional brain distribution in rats and human autopsy. *Arch Toxicol* 1992;66:153–156.

American Conference of Governmental Industrial Hygienists (ACGIH). *Threshold limit values (TLVs) for chemical substances and physical agents and biological exposure indices (BEIs).* Cincinnati, OH: ACGIH, 1995.

Amoore JE, Hautala E. Odor as an aid to chemical safety: odor thresholds compared with threshold limit values and volatilities for 214 industrial chemicals in air and water dilution. *J Appl Toxicol* 1983;3:272–290.

Anger WK. Neurobehavioral testing of chemicals—impact on recommended standards. *Neurobehav Teratol Toxicol* 1985;6:147–153.

Anger WK. Worksite behavioral research; results, sensitive methods, test batteries and the transition from laboratory data to human health. *Neurotoxicology* 1990;11:629–720.

Anger WK, Johnson BL. Chemicals affecting behavior. In: O'Donohue JL, ed. *Neurotoxicity of industrial chemicals.* Boca Raton, FL: CRC Press, 1985:51–148.

Angerer J. Occupational chronic exposure to organic solvents. VII. Metabolism of toluene in man. *Int Arch Occup Environ Health* 1979;43:63–67.

Arlien-Soborg P. Toluene. In: Arlien-Soborg P, ed. *Solvent neurotoxicity.* Boca Raton, FL: CRC Press, 1992.

Ashikaga R, Araki Y, Miura K, Ishida O. Cranial MRI in chronic thinner intoxication. *Neuroradiology* 1995;37:443–444.

Åstrand I. Uptake of solvents in the blood and tissues of man: a review. *Scand J Work Environ Health* 1975;1:199–218.

Åstrand I, Ehrner-Samuel H, Kilbom A, Ovrum P. Toluene exposure: I. Concentration in alveolar air and blood at rest and during exercise. *Work Environ Health* 1972;9:119–130.

Baelum J, Andersen IB, Lundqvist GR, et al. Response of solvent-exposed printers and unexposed controls to six-hour toluene exposure. *Scand J Work Environ Health* 1985;11:271–280.

Baelum J, Dossing M, Hansen SH, Lundqvist GR, Andersen NT. Toluene metabolism during exposure to varying concentrations combined with exercise. *Int Arch Occup Environ Health* 1987;59:281–294.

Bakke OM, Scheline RR. Hydroxylation of aromatic hydrocarbons in the rat. *Toxicol Appl Pharmacol* 1970;16:691–700.

Bartolucci G, Pellettier J. Glue sniffing and movement disorder [Letter]. *J Neurol Neurosurg Psychiatry* 1984;47:1259.

Biscaldi GP, Mingardi M, Pollini G, Moglia A, Bossi MC. Acute toluene poisoning. Electroneurophysiological and vestibular investigations. *Toxicol Eur Res* 1981;3:271–273.

Boor W, Hurtig H. Persistent cerebellar ataxia after exposure to toluene. *Ann Neurol* 1977;2:440–442.

Brown HS, Bishop D, Rowan CA. The role of skin absorption as a route of exposure for volatile organic compounds (VOCs) in drinking water. *Am J Public Health* 1984;74:479–484.

Brugnone F, Rosa E, Perbellini L, Bartolucci GB. Toluene concentrations in the blood and alveolar air of workers during the workshift and the morning after. *Br J Ind Med* 1986;43:56–61.

Brugnone F, Gobbi M, Ayyad K, et al. Blood toluene as a biological index of environmental toluene exposure in the "normal" population and in occupationally exposed workers immediately after exposure and 16 hours later. *Int Arch Occup Environ Health* 1995;66:421–425.

Bumke O, Foerster O. *Handbuch der Neurologie.* Berlin: Verlag von J Springer, 1936.

Caldemyer KS, Pascuzzi RM, Moran CC, Smith RR. Toluene abuse causing reduced MR signal intensity in the brain. *AJR* 1993;161:1259–1261.

Carlsson A. Exposure to toluene uptake, distribution and elimination in man. *Scand J Work Environ Health* 1982;8:43–55.

Carlsson A, Ljungquist E. Exposure to toluene: concentration in subcutaneous adipose tissue. *Scand J Work Environ Health* 1982;8:56–62.

Channer K, Stanley S. Persistent visual hallucinations secondary to chronic solvent encephalopathy. Case report and review of the literature. *J Neurol Neurosurg Psychiatry* 1983;46:83–86.

Cherry N, Johnson J, Venables H, et al. The effects of toluene and alcohol on psychomotor performance. *Ergonometry* 1983;26:1081–1087.

Cherry N, Hutchins H, Pace T, Waldron HA. Neurobehavioral effects of repeated occupational exposure to toluene and paint solvents. *Br J Ind Med* 1985;42:291–300.

Cohr K, Stockholm J. Toluene: a toxicologic review. *Scand J Work Environ Health* 1979;5:71–90.

DeRosa E, Brugnone F, Bartolucci GB, et al. The validity of urinary metabolites as indicators of low exposure to toluene. *Int Arch Occup Environ Health* 1985;56:135–145.

DeRosa E, Bartolucci GB, Sigon M, et al. Hippuric acid and ortho-cresol as biological indicators of occupational exposure to toluene. *Am J Ind Med* 1987;11:529–537.

Dick RB. Neurobehavioral assessment of occupationally relevant solvents and chemicals in humans. In: Chang LW, Dyer RS, eds. *Handbook of neurotoxicology.* New York: Marcel Dekker, 1995:217–321.

Dossing M, Baelum J, Hansen SH, et al. Urinary hippuric acid and ortho-cresol excretion in man during experimental exposure to toluene. *Br J Ind Med* 1983;40:470–473.

Dossing M, Baelum J, Hansen SH, Lundqvist GR. Effect of ethanol, cimetidine and propranolol on toluene metabolism in man. *Int Arch Occup Environ Health* 1984;54:309–315.

Dutkiewiscz T, Tyras H. Skin absorption of toluene, styrene and xylene by man. *Br J Ind Med* 1968;25:243.

Echeverria D, Fine LJ, Langolf G, et al. Acute neurobehavioral effects of toluene. *Br J Ind Med* 1989;46:483–495.

Echeverria D, Fine L, Langolf T, et al. Acute behavioural comparisons of toluene and ethanol in human subjects. *Br J Ind Med* 1991;48:750–761.

Ehyai A, Freemon F. Progressive optic neuropathy and sensorineural hearing loss due to chronic glue sniffing. *J Neurol Neurosurg Psychiatry* 1983;46:349–351.

Environmental Protection Agency (EPA). *Health assessment document for toluene: final report.* Washington: EPA, 1983.

Environmental Protection Agency (EPA). *National ambient volatile organic compounds (VOCs) data base update.* Atmospheric Sciences Research Laboratory. EPA-600/3-88/010(a), Research Triangle Park, NC: EPA, 1988.

Environmental Protection Agency (EPA). *Drinking water regulations and health advisories.* EPA 822-R-96-001. Washington: United States Environmental Protection Agency Office of Water, 1996.

Escobar A, Aruffo C. Chronic thinner intoxication: clinico-pathological report of a human case. *J Neurol Neurosurg Psychiatry* 1980;43:986–994.

Feldman RG, McKee A. Case records of Massachusetts General Hospital: weekly clinicopathological exercises. *N Engl J Med* 1993;329:1560–1567.

Filley CM, Heaton RK, Rosenberg NL. White matter dementia in chronic toluene abuse. *Neurology* 1990;40:532–534.

Fincher CE, Chang T-S, Harrell EH, et al. Comparison of single photon emission computed tomography findings in cases of healthy adults and solvent-exposed adults. *Am J Ind Med* 1997;31:4–14.

Foo SC, Jeyaratnam J, Ong CN, Khoo NY, Koh D, Chia SE. Biological monitoring for occupational exposure to toluene. *Am Ind Hyg Assoc J* 1991;52:212–217.

Fornazzari L. The neurotoxicity of inhaled toluene. *Can J Psychiatry* 1990;35:723.

Fornazzari L, Wilkinson D, Kapur BM, Carlen PL. Cerebellar, cortical and functional impairment in toluene abusers. *Acta Neurol Scand* 1983;67:319–329.

Fuhner H, Pietrusky F. Butylazetat toluol vergifung, chronische, berufliche Spatfolgen? In: Fugner H, ed. *Samlung von Vergistungfallen.* Berlin: Verlag von FCW Vogel, 1934.

Fuxe K, Martire M, von Euler G, et al. Effects of subacute treatment with toluene on cerebrocortical alpha and beta adrenergic receptors in rats: evidence for an increased number and a reduced affinity of beta adrenergic receptors *Acta Physiol Scand* 1987;130:307–311.

Gamberale F, Hultengren M. Toluene exposure II. Psychophysiological functions. *Work Environ Health* 1972;9:131–139.

Goldblum D, Chouinard G. Schizophreniform psychosis associated with chronic industrial toluene exposure: Case report. *J Clin Psychiatry* 1985;46:350–351.

Gospe S, Calaban M. Central nervous system distribution of inhaled toluene. *Fund Appl Toxicol* 1988;11:540–545.

Goto I, Matsumura M, Inoue N, et al. Toxic polyneuropathy due to glue sniffing. *J Neurol Neurosurg Psychiatry* 1974;37:848–853.

Grabski D. Toluene sniffing producing cerebellar degeneration. *Am J Psychiatry* 1961;118:461–462.

Gregus Z, Klaassen CD. Mechanisms of toxicity. In: Klaassen KD, ed. *Casarett and Doull's toxicology: the basic science of poisons,* 5th ed. New York: McGraw-Hill, 1996:35–74.

Gupta BN, Kumar P, Strivastava AK. An investigation of the neurobehavioural effects on workers exposed to organic solvents. *J Soc Occup Med* 1990;40:94–96.

Hahn AF, Feasby TE, Gilbert JJ. Paraparesis following intrathecal chemotherapy. *Neurology* 1983;33:1032–1038.

Hajimiragha H, Ewers U, Brockhaus A, Biettger A. Levels of benzene and other volatile aromatic compounds in the blood of non-smokers and smokers. *Int Arch Occup Environ Health* 1989;61:513–518.

Hänninen H, Antii-Poika M, Savolainen P. Psychological performance, toluene exposure and alcohol consumption in rotogravure printers. *Int Arch Occup Environ Health* 1987;59:475–483.

Hellefors-Berglund M, Liu Y, von Euler G. Persistent, specific and dose-dependent effects of toluene exposure on dopamine D_2 agonist binding in the rat caudate-putamen. *Toxicology* 1995;100:185–194.

Hirata F, Axelrod J. Phospholipid methylation and biological signal transmission. *Science* 1980;209:1082–1090.

Hollo G, Vargo M. Toluene and visual loss. [Letter]. *Neurology* 1992;42:266.

Hormes J, Filey C, Rosenberg N. Neurologic sequelae of chronic solvent vapor abuse. *Neurology* 1986;36:698–702.

Hyden D, Larsby B, Anderson H, et al. Impairment of visuo-vestibular interaction in humans exposed to toluene. *Otorhinolaryngology* 1983;45:262–269.

Ikeda M. Exposure to complex mixtures: implications for biological monitoring. *Toxicol Lett* 1995;77:85–91.

Ikeda M, Ohtsuji H. Phenobarbitol-induced protection against toxicity of toluene and benzene in the rat. *Toxicol Appl Pharmacol* 1971;20:30.

Ikeda M, Tsukagoshi H. Encephalopathy due to toluene sniffing. *Eur Neurol* 1990;30:347–349.

Inoue O, Seiji K, Watanabe T, et al. Mutual metabolic suppression between benzene and toluene in man. *Int Arch Occup Environ Health* 1988;60:15–20.

Inoue O, Seiji K, Watanabe T, et al. Effects of smoking and drinking on excretion of hippuric acid among toluene-exposed workers. *Int Arch Occup Environ Health* 1993;64:425–430.

Inoue O, Seiji K, Watanabe T, et al. Effects of smoking and drinking habits on urinary o-cresol excretion after occupational exposure to toluene vapor among Chinese workers. *Am J Ind Med* 1994;25:697–708.

Iregren A. Subjective and objective signs of organic solvent toxicity among occupationally exposed workers. *Scand J Work Environ Health* 1986;12:469–475.

Juntunen J, Matikainen E, Antti-Poika M, et al. Nervous system effects of long-term occupational exposure to toluene. *Acta Neurol Scand* 1985;72:512–517.

Karlson U, Frankenberger WT. Microbial degradation of benzene and toluene in ground water. *Bull Environ Contam Toxicol* 1989;43:505–510.

Kawai T, Yasugi T, Mizunuma K, et al. Comparative evaluation of urinalysis and blood analysis as means of detecting exposure to organic solvents at low concentrations. *Int Arch Occup Environ Health* 1992;64:223–234.

Kawamoto T, Koga M, Murata K, et al. Effects of ALDH2, CYP1A1, and CYP2E1 genetic polymorphisms and smoking and drinking habits on toluene metabolism in humans. *Toxicol Appl Pharmacol* 1995;133: 295–304.

Keane JR. Toluene optic neuropathy. *Ann Neurol* 1978;4:390.

King M, Day E, Oliver J, Lush H, Watson JM. Solvent encephalopathy. *BMJ* 1981;283:663–665.

King MD. Neurological sequelae of toluene abuse. *Hum Toxicol* 1982;1: 281–287.

Knox W, Nelson J. Permanent encephalopathy from toluene inhalation. *N Engl J Med* 1966;275:1494–1496.

Koelsch F. *Handbuch der Berufskransheiten.* Jena: Fischer, 1935.

Korobkin R, Asbury AD, Summer AJ, Nielsen SL. Glue sniffing. *Arch Neurol* 1975;32:158–162.

Korpela M. Inhibition of synaptosome membrane-bound integral enzymes by organic solvents. *Scand J Work Environ Health* 1989;15: 64–68.

Korpela M, Tahti H. The effects of in vitro and in vivo toluene exposure on rat erythrocyte and synaptosome membrane integral enzymes. *Pharmacol Toxicol* 1988;63:30–32.

Lazar RB, Ho SU, Melen O, Daghestani AN. Multifocal central nervous system damage caused by toluene abuse. *Neurology* 1983;33:1337–1340.

LeBel C, Schatz R. Effect of toluene on rat synaptosomal phospholipid methylation and membrane fluidity. *Biochem Pharmacol* 1989;38: 4005–4011.

Lee B-K, Lee S-H, Lee K-M, et al. Dose-dependent increase in subjective symptom prevalence among toluene-exposed workers. *Ind Health* 1988;26:11–23.

Lequesne PM, Axford AT, McKerrow CB, Jone AP. Neurological complications after a single exposure to toluene di-isocyanante. *Br J Ind Med* 1976;33:72–78.

Liu S-J, Qu Q-S, Xu X-P, et al. Toluene vapor exposure and urinary excretion of hippuric acid among workers in China. *Am J Ind Med* 1992; 22:313–323.

Löf A, Wallen M, Hjelm EW. Influence of paracetamol and acetylsalicylic acid on the toxicokinetics of toluene. *Pharmacol Toxicol* 1990;66: 138–141.

Löf A, Hjelm EW, Colmsjo A, et al. Toxikinetics of toluene and urinary excretion of hippuric acid after human exposure to $^2H_8$-toluene. *Br J Ind Med* 1993;50:55–59.

Longley ED, Jones AT, Welch R, Lomaev O. Two acute toluene episodes in merchant ships *Arch Environ Health* 1967;14:481–487.

Maas EF, Ashe J, Spiegel P, Zee DS, Leigh RJ. Acquired pendular nystagmus in toluene addition. *Neurology* 1991;41:282–285.

Malm G, Lying Tunell U. Cerebellar dysfunction related to toluene sniffing. *Acta Neurol Scand* 1980;62:188–190

Mattia CJ, Adams JD Jr, Bondy SC. Free radical induction in the brain and liver by products of toluene metabolism. *Biochem Pharmacol* 1993;46:103–110.

Metrick SA, Brenner RP. Abnormal brain stem auditory evoked potentials in chronic paint sniffers. *Ann Neurol* 1982;12:553–556.

Mergler DZ. Behavioral neurophysiology: quantitative measures of sensory toxicity, In: L. Chang, W. Slikker JR, eds. *Neurotoxicology: approaches and methods.* San Diego: Academic Press, 1995:727–736.

Mergler D, Beauvais B. Olfactory threshold shift following controlled 7-hour exposure to toluene and/or xylene. *Neurotoxicology* 1992;13:211–216.

Mørck H, Winkel P, Gyntelberg F. Health effects of toluene exposure. *Dan Med Bull* 1988;35:196–200.

Nakatsuka H, Wanatabe T, Takeuchi Y, et al. Absence of blue-yellow color vision loss among workers exposed to toluene or tetrachlorethylene, mostly at levels below occupational exposure limits. *Int Arch Occup Environ Health* 1992;64:113–117.

National Academy of Science. *Drinking and health,* vol 3. Washington: National Academy Press, 1980.

National Institute for Occupational Safety and Health (NIOSH). *A recommended standard for occupational exposure to toluene.* 757-009/40, U.S. Department of Health, Education, and Welfare, Public Health Service, CDC, Washington: US Government Printing Office, 1977.

National Institute for Occupational Safety and Health (NIOSH). *Pocket guide to chemical hazards.* US Department of Health and Human Services, CDC. Washington: US Government Printing Office: 1997.

National Research Council (NRC). *Environmental epidemiology: dimensions of the problem: exposure assessment.* Washington: National Academy Press, 1991.

Nelson NA, Robins RG, White RF, Garrison RP. A case-control study of chronic neuropsychiatric disease and organic solvent exposure in automobile assembly plant workers. *Occup Environ Med* 1994;51:302–307.

Niklasson M, Stengard K, Tham R. Are the effects of toluene on the vestibulo and opto-ocular motor system inhibited by the action of $GABA_B$ antagonist CGP 35348? *Neurotoxicol Teratol* 1995;17:351–357.

Nise G. Urinary excretion of *o*-cresol and hippuric acid after toluene exposure in rotogravure printing. *Int Arch Occup Environ Health* 1992;63:377–381.

Nise G, Attewell R, Skerfving S, Orbaek P. Elimination of toluene from venous blood and adipose tissue after occupational exposure. *Br J Ind Med* 1989;46:407–411.

Occupational Safety and Health Administration (OSHA). *Occupational health guideline for toluene.* U.S. Department of Health and Human Service. Washington: Centers for Disease Control, 1978:1–5.

Occupational Safety and Health Administration (OSHA). Code of Federal Regulations, 29-1910.1000. U.S. Department of Health and Human Service Washington; Centers for Disease Control, 1995:18.

Office of Technology Assessment (OTA) U.S. Congress. *Coming clean: Superfund's problems can be solved.* OTA-ITE-433, Washington: US Government Printing Office, 1989.

Ogata M, Tomokuni K, Takatsuka Y. Urinary excretion of hippuric acid and m- and p-methylhippuric acid in the urine of persons exposed to vapours of toluene and m- and p-xylene as a test of exposure. *Br J Ind Med* 1970;27:43–50.

Olson LM, Gamberale F, Iregren A. Coexposure to toluene and p-xylene in man: central nervous functions. *Br J Ind Med* 1985;42:117–122.

Panse F, Bender W. Toluol-xylol-psychose bei einen tiefdruck-arbiteiter. *Monatsschr Psychiatr Neurol* 1934;89:249–259.

Paull JM. The origin and basis of threshold limit values. *Am J Ind Med* 1984;5:227–238.

Patty FA. Toxicology. In: Patty FA, ed. *Industrial hygiene and toxicology,* 2nd ed. rev., vol. II. New York: Interscience, 1963.

Prockop L. Multifocal nervous system damage from inhalation of volatile hydrocarbons. *J Occup Med* 1977;19:139–149.

Prockop L. Neuroimaging in neurotoxicology, In: L. Chang and W. Slikker Jr., eds. *Neurotoxicology: approaches and methods.* San Diego: Academic Press, 1995:753–763.

Pryor GT, Rebert CS. Interactive effects of toluene and hexane on behavior and neurophysiologic responses in Fischer-344 rats. *Neurotoxicology* 1992;13:225–234.

Pyykkö K, Tahti H, Vapaatalo H. Toluene concentrations in various tissues of rats after inhalation and oral administration. *Arch Toxicol* 1977;38:169–176.

Pyykkö K. Effects of pretreatment with toluene, phenobarbital and 3-methylcholantrene on the in vivo metabolism of toluene and on the concentration of hippuric acid in the rat. *Pharmacol Res Commun* 1984; 16:217.

Rea TM, Nash JF, Zabik JE, et al. Effects of toluene inhalation on brain biogenic amines in the rat. *Toxicology* 1984;31:143–150.

Riihimäki V, Pfäffli P. Percutaneous absorption of solvent vapors in man. *Scand J Work Environ Health* 1978;4:73–85.

Ron MA. Volatile substance abuse: a review of possible long-term neurological, intellectual and psychiatric sequelae. *Br J Psychiatry* 1986;148:235–246.

Rosenberg NL, Spitz MC, Filley CM, et al. Central nervous system effects of chronic toluene abuse—clinical, brain stem evoked response and magnetic resonance imaging studies *Neurotoxicol Teratol* 1988a; 10:489–495.

Rosenberg NL, Kleinschmidt-Demasters BK, Davis KA, et al. Toluene abuse causes diffuse CNS white matter changes. *Ann Neurol* 1988b;23: 611–614.

Sato A, Nakajima T. Differences following skin or inhalation exposure in the absorption and excretion kinetics of trichloroethylene and toluene. *Br J Ind Med* 1978;35:43–49.

Sato A, Nakajima T. Dose dependent metabolic interaction between benzene and toluene in vivo and in vitro. *Toxicol Appl Pharmacol* 1979;48: 249.

Sato A, Nakajima T, Koyama Y. Effects of chronic ethanol consumption on hepatic metabolism of aromatic and chlorinated hydrocarbons in rats. *Br J Ind Med* 1980;37:383–386.

Shirabe T, Tsuda T, Terao A, Araki S. Toxic polyneuropathy due to glue sniffing. *J Neurol Sci* 1974;21:101–113.

Spencer PS, Couri D, Schaumburg HH. *n*-Hexane and methyl *n*-butyl ketone. In: Spencer PS, Schaumburg HH, eds. *Experimental and clinical neurotoxicology.* Baltimore: Williams & Wilkins, 1980:456–475.

Streicher HZ, Gabow PA, Moss AH, Kono D, Kaehny WD. Syndromes of toluene sniffing in adults. *Ann Intern Med* 1981;94:758–762.

Tahti H, Karkkainen S, Pyykko K, et al. Chronic occupational exposure to toluene. *Int Arch Occup Environ Health* 1981;48:61–69.

Takahashi S, Kagawa M, Shiwaku K, Matsubara LK. Determination of S-benzyl-N-acetyl-L-cysteine by gas chromatography/mass spectrometry as a new marker of toluene exposure. *J Anal Toxicol* 1994;18:78–80.

Tardiff RG, Youngren SH. Public health significance of organic substances in drinking water. In: Ram NM, Calabrese EJ, Christman RF, eds. *Organic carcinogenesis in drinking water.* New York: John Wiley & Sons, 1986:405–436.

Toftgard R, Gustafsson J-A. Biotransformation of organic solvents: a review. *Scand J Work Environ Health* 1980;6:1–18.

Urban P, Lukas E. Visual evoked potentials in rotogravure printers exposed to toluene. *Br J Ind Med* 1990;47:819–823.

Verschueren K. *Handbook of environmental data on organic chemicals,* 1st ed. New York: Van Nostrand Reinhold, 1977.

von Euler G. Toluene and dopaminergic transmission. In: Isaacson RL, Jensen KF, eds. *The vulnerable brain and environmental risks,* vol. 3, *Toxins in air and water.* New York: Plenum Press, 1994:301–321.

von Euler G, Fuxe K, Hansson T, et al. Effects of chronic toluene exposure on central monoamine and peptide receptors and their interaction in the adult male rat. *Toxicology* 1988;52:103–126.

von Oettingen W, Neal P, Svirbely J, et al. *The toxicity and potential dangers of toluene, with special reference to its maximal permissible concentration.* Public Health Bulletin no. 279. Washington: US Public Health Service, 1942.

Vrca A, Bozicevic D, Karacic V, et al. Visual evoked potentials in individuals exposed to long-term low concentrations of toluene. *Arch Toxicol* 1995;69:337–340.

Waldron HA, Cherry N, Johnsberry JD. The effects of ethanol on blood toluene concentrations. *Int Arch Occup Environ Health* 1983;51:365–369.

Wallen M, Naslund H, Nordqvist B. The effects of ethanol on the kinetics of toluene in man. *Toxicol Appl Pharmacol* 1984;76:414–419.

Wang G, Maranelli G, Perbellini L, Guglielmi G, Brugnone F. Reference values for blood toluene in the occupationally nonexposed general population. *Int Arch Occup Environ Health* 1993;65:201–203.

Wegman DH, Musk W, Main D, Pagnotto LD. Accelerated loss of FEV-1 in polyurethane production workers: a four-year prospective study. *Am J Ind Med* 1982;3:209–215.

White RF. Differential diagnosis of probable Alzheimer's disease and solvent encephalopathy in older workers. *Clin Neuropsychol* 1987;1:153–160.

White RF, Feldman RG, Proctor SP. Neurobehavioral effects of toxic exposures. In: *Clinical syndromes in adult neuropsychology: the practitioner's handbook.* Amsterdam: Elsevier Science Publishers, 1992:1–51.

White RF, Proctor SF. Clinico-neuropsychological assessments in behavioral neurotoxicology. In: Chang L, Slikker W, eds. *Neurotoxicology: approaches and methods.* San Diego: Academic Pres, 1995:711–726.

White RF, Proctor SP, Echeverria D, Schweikert J, Feldman RG. Neurobehavioral effects of acute and chronic mixed solvent exposure in the screen printing industry. *Am J Ind Med* 1995;28:221–231.

Williams RT. *Detoxication mechanisms,* 2nd ed. London: Chapman and Hall, 1959:188–236.

Williams JM, Howe NR. Benzyl alcohol attenuates the pain of lidocaine injections and prolongs anesthesia. *J Dermatol Surg Oncol* 1994;20:730–733.

Wilson JT, Enfield CG, Dunlap WJ, et al. Transport and fate of selected organic pollutants in a sandy soil. *J Environ Qual* 1981;10:501–506.

Wilson RH. Toluene poisoning. *JAMA* 1943;123:1106–1108.

Winchester RV, Madjar VM. Solvent effects on workers in the paint, adhesive and printing industries. *Ann Occup Hyg* 1986;30:307–317.

World Health Organization (WHO). *Toluene; environmental health criteria.* Geneva: WHO, 1985.

Xiong L, Matthes JD, Jinkins JR. MR imaging of "spray heads": toluene abuse via aerosol paint inhalation. *AJNR* 1993;14:1195–1199.

CHAPTER 15

Xylene

Xylene (dimethylbenzene), is a volatile, flammable, aromatic alkylbenzene derivative of petroleum and coal tar (NIOSH, 1975). Xylene occurs in three isomeric forms, ortho-xylene, meta-xylene, and para-xylene; a mixture of all three isomers is called xylol. Most commercial xylene produced from petroleum contains a mixture of 20% ortho-, 44% meta-, and 20% para-xylene and 15% ethylbenzene (NIOSH), 1975; Fishbein, 1985). The physicochemical properties of the various isomeric forms are similar, and usually separation is unnecessary as well as impractical (Utidjian, 1976; Low et al., 1989). Commercial supplies of xylene and xylol often contain contaminants, such as ethylbenzene, benzene, toluene, butanol, ethylene glycol, and white spirits. Although xylene is a commonly found chemical in workplace air (NIOSH, 1976), it is frequently only a relatively minor ingredient of mixed solvent solutions. Thus, monitoring of exposure circumstances for specific effects of xylene is difficult without considering the possible effects of interactions with other organic compounds (Goldie, 1960; Kawai et al., 1991).

Valuable information about the effects of xylene have been derived from studies in animals; exposure conditions are controlled and are quite different from those in random occupational settings. Xylene's potential for impairing vigilance and for inducing neurobehavioral changes raises concern about its neurotoxicity. Acute exposure causes some individuals to experience only mild, transient dizziness and light-headedness; in others, diminished ability to react quickly hinders job performance and jeopardizes safety. Prolonged exposure has been associated with disturbances of mood and memory. These neurological effects, some subtle or others more pronounced, should not be overlooked in the assessment of persons who are at risk of exposure to xylene alone or in mixed solvents (Ducatman and Moyer, 1984; Bakinson and Jones, 1985; Roberts et al., 1988; ATSDR, 1995).

SOURCES OF EXPOSURE

Xylene is used in the manufacture of plastics, textile fabrics, epoxy resins, insect repellents, and perfumes and for coating and impregnating papers and fabrics (Riihimaki and Hanninen, 1978). It is an ingredient in solvents for spray paints, lacquers, inks, dyes, and glues (Low et al., 1989). Common household products such as paints, varnishes, and rust preventatives contain an average xylene concentration of 9.5% (Fishbein, 1985). Dental professionals are exposed during the coloring of dental prostheses (Engelmeier, 1985). Xylene and xylol are used by histology laboratory technologists in the preparation of tissues for pathological diagnosis (Langman, 1994). Intake from both inhalation and through the skin occurs when manual tasks make skin contact likely (Riihimaki and Hanninen, 1987). A large number of workers in machinery trades, fabricated metal production, and health services industries, as well as assemblers, janitors, cleaners, painters and paint-spraying machine operators, and automobile mechanics are exposed to xylol (mixed *o-*, *m-*, and *p*-xylenes). Many workers employed in the chemical and allied chemical industries (i.e., chemists, technicians, production inspectors, and machine operators) are specifically exposed to *o*-xylene. Most workers who are exposed specifically to *m*-xylene work in jobs related to cleaning electrical, gas, and business equipment. Clinical laboratory technologists and others in the health services industry are exposed primarily to *p*-xylene (NIOSH, 1984).

Xylene vapors are released into the environment during the production, processing, and transport of petroleum. Xylene vapor has been detected on the breath of individuals who recently visited a gasoline station or have been involved in automobile-related activities. Because it vaporizes easily and is flammable, it is a constituent of number 2 home heating fuel oil and automobile and aviation fuels; its combustion produces exhaust that contains xylene and its breakdown products (Wallace et al., 1986, 1988; ATSDR, 1995).

Xylene is highly soluble in alcohol and other organic solvents, but it is relatively insoluble in water. Xylene is introduced into ground water following gasoline, fuel oil, and mixed solvent spills as well as through inappropriate disposal of these chemicals. Migration of petroleum products and gasoline from leaking underground storage tanks and pipelines may lead to ground water contamination. One example occurred in Los Angeles, where a sample of gasoline contaminated ground water had a xylene level of at least 153 ppb (Karlson and Frankenberger, 1989). Due to rapid volatilization of xylene, typical surface water concentrations are usually less than 1 ppb (ATSDR, 1995).

Cigarette smoke contains xylene vapor (Hajimiragha et al., 1989). Breath levels of xylene are more than twofold higher in smokers, and the presence of a smoker on the premises is a nonoccupational source of *m*- and *p*-xylene (Wallace et al., 1988). Passive intake occurs in nonsmokers. The median 12-hour indoor air concentrations of xylenes in 350 New Jersey residences were 3 ppb for *m*- and *p*-xylene and 1 ppb for *o*-xylene. Median breath concentrations for the residents were 1.5 ppb for *m*- and *p*-xylene and 0.5 ppb for *o*-xylene (Wallace et al., 1986). Nonoccupationally exposed persons in the United States had blood concentrations of xylene ranging from 0.074 to 0.78 ppb (median: 0.19 ppb) for *m*- and *p*-xylene and from 0.044 to 0.30 ppb (median: 0.11 ppb) for *o*-xylene when tested during the Third National Health and Nutrition Examination Survey (Ashley et al., 1994).

Most people who encounter xylene vapors are initially affected with upper respiratory irritation and/or annoyed by its odor. Usually an exposed person is motivated by discomfort to seek better ventilation and to move away from the source of xylene exposure, thus preventing further risk of adverse effects. Some individuals become tolerant to these obnoxious effects and undergo continuous exposure (Amoore and Hautala, 1983; Mergler and Beauvais, 1992).

EXPOSURE LIMITS AND SAFETY REGULATIONS

The odor threshold for mixed xylenes in air is 1.0 ppm (Amoore and Hautala, 1983; Carpenter et al., 1975) (Table 15-1). At this level, a worker should be alerted to the presence of xylene vapors (Amoore and Hautala, 1983). The *Occupational Safety and Health Administration* (OSHA) has established an 8-hour time-weighted average (TWA) permissible exposure limit (PEL) for xylene of 100 ppm (OSHA, 1995). The *National Institute for Occupational Safety and Health's* (NIOSH) recommended 8-hour TWA exposure limit (REL) for xylene is 100 ppm (NIOSH, 1994). The NIOSH recommended 15-minute TWA short-term exposure limit (STEL) is 150 ppm (NIOSH, 1994). The *American Conference of Governmental Industrial Hygienists'* (ACGIH) 10-hour TWA threshold limit value (TLV) is 100 ppm; this level is intended to avoid upper respiratory irritant effects and to prevent central nervous system (CNS) effects of disturbed awareness (ACGIH, 1995). The ACGIH 15-minute TWA-STEL is 150 ppm (ACGIH, 1995). A workplace is considered contaminated if the industrial hygiene measurements exceed half (50 ppm) of the recommended TWA limit (Utidjian, 1976). All at-risk

TABLE 15-1. *Established and recommended occupational and environmental exposure limits for xylene in air and water*

	Air (ppm)[a]	Water (mg/L)[a]
Odor threshold*	1.0	0.017
OSHA		
PEL (8 hr TWA)	100	—
PEL ceiling (15 min TWA)	—	—
NIOSH		
REL (10 hr TWA)	100	—
STEL (15 min TWA)	150	—
IDLH	900	—
ACGIH		
TLV (8 hr TWA)	100	—
STEL (15 min TWA)	150	—
USEPA		
MCL	—	10
MCLG		10

[a]Unit conversion: 1.0 ppm = 4.41 mg/m³; 1 mg/L = 1 ppm
OSHA, Occupational Safety and Health Administration; PEL, permissible exposure limit; TWA, time-weighted average; NIOSH, National Institute of Occupational Safety and Health; REL, recommended exposure limit; STEL, short-term exposure limit; IDLH, immediately dangerous to life or health; ACGIH, American Conference of Governmental Industrial Hygienists; TLV, threshold limit value; USEPA, U.S. Environmental Protection Agency; MCL, maximum contamination level; MCLG, maximum contamination level goal.
Data from *Amoore and Hautala, 1983; OSHA, 1995; NIOSH, 1997.

workers, especially laboratory technologists and technicians, should be monitored frequently for hypersensitivity and adverse effects of exposure (Hippolito, 1980; Langman, 1994). Exposure to xylene becomes dangerous when the immediately dangerous to life and health (IDLH) concentration for xylene of 900 ppm is reached, and workers should immediately vacate the contaminated area (NIOSH, 1994).

The odor threshold for xylene in water is 0.017 ppm (Amoore and Hautala, 1983). The *United States Environmental Protection Agency* (USEPA), has established a maximum contamination level (MCL) for xylene in drinking water of 10 ppm; at this level there are no known or anticipated health risks from long-term use (USEPA, 1994; USEPA, 1996) (Table 15-1). Drinking water is considered safe when it contains a xylene concentration of less than 21 ppm and is consumed for no more than one day, or 11.2 ppm and is consumed for no more than 7 days; the *National Academy of Science* has set these as suggested no-adverse-response levels (NAS, 1980).

METABOLISM

Tissue Absorption

Xylene is absorbed through the pulmonary alveoli and enters the bloodstream. Uptake via the lungs depends on diffusion of the solvent through the alveolar–capillary membrane, the blood/air partition coefficient of xylene, the circulation rate of blood through the lungs, diffusion of the xylene through the tissue membranes, and the blood/tissue partition coefficient of xylene (Åstrand, 1975). Approximately 60% of inspired vapors are absorbed into the systemic circulation, where the xylenes are highly soluble in blood (Sedivec and Flek, 1976). Xylene levels in venous blood initially increases rapidly, leveling off after a few hours (Riihimäki et al., 1979a). Exercise increases respiratory rate, thereby increasing the amount of xylene vapor available for pulmonary absorption (Åstrand et al., 1978; Riihimäki et al., 1979b). In volunteers exposed to m-xylene (30 ppm), alveolar air concentrations immediately following exercise were increased 40% over resting baseline levels (Laparé et al., 1993).

Xylene causes severe acute oral and gastric mucosal irritation after ingestion, but it is promptly absorbed from the gastrointestinal tract. Urinary metabolites are found following oral ingestion of xylene (Ogata et al., 1980). The lowest lethal dose reported in a human after oral ingestion was 50 mg/kg (NIOSH, 1978).

The quantity of xylene vapor absorbed through the skin is relatively low compared with that following inhalation and only about 1.4% of the total xylene vapor absorbed at a given air concentration is taken up through the skin. However, percutaneous absorption of liquid xylene can be more similar in quantity to pulmonary xylene absorption, especially under conditions of prolonged immersion. Pure liquid m-xylene penetrates intact skin of the immersed hands at a rate of about 2 μg/cm²/min (Engström et al., 1977). Dermal uptake of xylene is affected by temperature, hydration, surface area, type, and condition of the skin (Riihimäki and Pfäffli, 1978; Brown et al., 1984). Xylene and its vapors are absorbed through diseased skin with altered permeability at a rate three times greater than that of healthy skin (Riihimäki and Pfäffli, 1978).

Tissue Distribution

Xylene is a nonpolar compound and is highly soluble in blood and lipids (Sato et al., 1974; Sherwood, 1976; Riihimäki et al., 1979a; Riihimäki and Hänninen, 1987). Xylene is mainly associated with plasma proteins in blood, and relatively small amounts are found in red cells (Riihimäki et al., 1979a). Tissue distribution of xylene is dependent on blood perfusion of the organs and the tissue/blood partition coefficient of xylene (Åstrand et al., 1978; Engström and Riihimäki, 1979). The blood is rapidly cleared of xylene, but not before most of it is distributed to highly perfused tissues such as muscle. Lesser amounts are distributed to the less well-perfused tissues, such as subcutaneous adipose, which receives only 4% to 8% of the total body uptake (Engström and Riihimäki, 1979). However, during periods of increased physical activity, blood flow and perfusion of the subcutaneous adipose tissue is in-

creased, thereby enhancing distribution and increasing accumulation of xylene in adipose tissue (Riihimäki et al., 1979b). The slow continuous uptake of xylene by adipose tissue, along with its faster uptake in the more well-perfused tissues such as muscles, parenchymal organs, and the nervous system, all of which contain neutral fat, leads to a proportionate balance between tissue xylene levels and blood xylene concentrations (Sato et al., 1974; Riihimäki et al., 1979a). Tissue concentrations of xylene reached a steady state within one workday in the more well-perfused lipid-containing tissues, whereas in adipose tissue, a steady state was not attained after a week, suggesting the potential for its accumulation in chronically exposed workers (Engström and Bjurstrom, 1978). In general, the efficient metabolism of xylene limits its rate of accumulation in adipose tissue.

Xylene levels in the brain closely follow the blood concentration (Engström and Riihimäki, 1979; Riihimäki and Savolainen, 1980; Riihimäki, 1984). The concentration of xylene and/or its metabolites in the cerebrum and cerebellum, as well as in skeletal muscles, was about 40% of that in the arterial blood immediately after inhalation by rats exposed to radioactive p-xylene for 1 to 8 hours at an ambient air concentration of 45 ppm (Carlsson, 1981). Since its solubility in brain phospholipids is less than it is in the neutral fat of other tissues, xylene does not accumulate at high concentrations in brain phospholipids. Xylene accumulation in the brain was found to be both time- and concentration-dependent in rats exposed to 50, 400, and 750 ppm for 1- and 2-week periods. The brain tissue concentrations at each of the dose levels increased by 33% to 44% after a week of exposure. There was a ninefold increase when the dose for 1 week was increased from 50 to 400 ppm and a tenfold increase with this incremental dose change for a duration of 2 weeks. The rate of increase in brain tissue m-xylene resulting from m-xylene exposure at 750 ppm was less than with the initial rise in exposure level, being fourfold after 1 week and only twofold after the second week (Table 15-2) (Savolainen and Pfäffli, 1980). This finding suggests that saturation was being reached with increased doses, whereas the rate of accumulation was fairly constant with continued exposure. Very brief periods of exposure are not likely to result in a brain tissue concentration level sufficient to produce symptoms, but when uptake is rapid (such as during periods of exercise), the rate of rise of blood xylene and the

TABLE 15-2. *Brain tissue* m-xylene concentration (nmol/g) as a function of exposure level and duration of exposure

Duration of exposure	Exposure level (ppm)		
	50	400	750
7 days	6.2 ± 0.8	54 ± 8	83 ± 17
14 days	9.6 ± 2.6	96 ± 16	124 ± 17

Modified from Savolainen and Pfäffli, 1980, with permission.

peak levels reached in the brain can be correlated with acute symptoms (see Clinical Manifestations section) (Riihimäki and Savolainen, 1980).

Tissue Biochemistry

Most of the absorbed xylene undergoes biotransformation in the liver through cytochrome P-450 microsomal enzyme oxidation of one of the methyl groups (Toftgård and Gustafsson, 1980) (Fig. 15-1). Metabolic products include the corresponding (i.e., *o*-, *m*-, and *p*-)methyl benzyl alcohols, methyl benzaldehydes, and methyl benzoic acids (toluic acids). The toluic acids are further conjugated with glycine, to form the corresponding methylhippuric acids (toluric acids), which are the principal urinary metabolites of xylene (Bray et al., 1949). A second minor metabolic pathway occurs to a lesser extent (less than 1% to 4%) and involves the aromatic hydroxylation of xylene at its benzene ring, generating the xylenols (dimethylphenols) (Bray et al., 1950; Bakke and Scheline, 1970; Sedivec and Flek, 1976; Toftgård and Gustafsson, 1980; Engström et al., 1984; Riihimäki et al., 1979a).

Xylene is frequently found in combination with other chemicals, which affect its metabolism and alter its clinical manifestations. Mutual inhibition of metabolism of *m*-xylene (150 ppm) and ethylbenzene (150 ppm) occurs with simultaneous exposure to both solvents (Engström et al., 1984). In human volunteers, ingestion of xylene together with ethanol, for example, results in inhibition of biotransformation of xylene. Ingestion of ethanol prior to exposure to xylene results in an increased blood xylene concentration (1.5 to 2.0-fold) and a decreased urinary excretion of methylhippuric acid (50%). In addition, blood acetaldehyde levels are increased in subjects who reported dose-dependent symptoms of nausea and dizziness during acute exposure to both xylene and ethanol (Riihimäki et al., 1982). Coexposure to methyl ethyl ketone (MEK) and *m*-xylene results in increased blood levels of *m*-xylene and decreased excretion of *m*-methylhippuric acid. This effect may be due to competition between xylene and MEK for cytochrome P-450 (Liira et al., 1988).

Chronic exposure to ethanol (10% solution in drinking water) and xylene (more than 2,700 ppm) had an additive inductive effect on hepatic microsomal monooxygenases in the rat, increasing the level of cytochrome P-450 by 70% (Wisniewska-Knypl et al., 1989; Elovaara et al., 1980; Raunio et al., 1990; David et al., 1979; Kaneko et al., 1993, 1995). Ethanol pretreatment of rats did not increase metabolism of xylene at low vapor concentrations (50 to 100 ppm), but it did increase the metabolism of xylene at a vapor concentration of 500 ppm (Kaneko et al., 1993). Experimental pretreatment of humans and rats with phenobarbital, a known

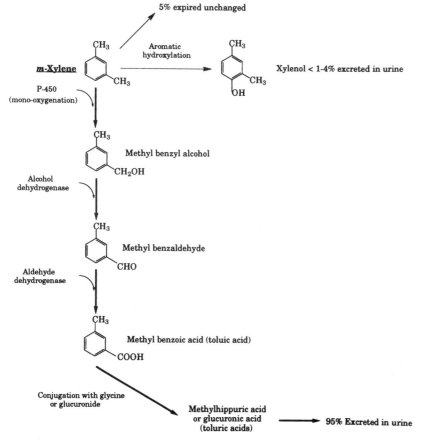

FIG. 15-1. Metabolic pathways of xylene. (Data from Bray, 1949; Bray et al., 1950; Bakke and Scheline, 1970; Sedivic and Flek, 1976; Riihimäki et al., 1979a; Toftgard and Gustafsson, 1980; Engromstrom et al., 1984.)

inducer of cytochrome P-450 enzymes, did not significantly affect methylhippuric acid excretion at low levels (90 to 180 ppm) of exposure to *m*-xylene. However, at higher concentrations of *m*-xylene (450 to 900 ppm), methylhippuric acid excretion in rats was increased fourfold, suggesting that the increased metabolic capacity afforded by enzyme induction is exploited only during exposure to high concentrations of xylene when normal biotransformation is surpassed (David et al., 1979; Kaneko et al., 1993, 1995). Methyl ethyl ketone and xylene had an additive effect on liver cytochrome P-450 induction (Raunio et al., 1990).

Since glycine conjugates with both xylene and aspirin (acetylsalicylic acid), formation of their respective metabolites, methylhippuric acid and salicyluric acid, is inhibited with simultaneous exposure (Fig. 15-2) (Campbell et al., 1988). A possible explanation is that there is competition between methylbenzoic acid and salicylic acid for the enzymes acyl CoA synthetase and acyl CoA-glycine *N*-acyl transferase, both of which are necessary for glycine conjugation. This finding is of particular importance in cases of occupational exposure, because persons who experience headaches resulting from chronic exposure to xylene may take analgesics containing aspirin for relief. Consequently, the metabolism and excretion of xylene will be delayed and urinary concentration of methylhippuric acid reduced, resulting in underestimation of exposure dose during biological monitoring of exposed populations (see Biochemical Diagnosis section).

Excretion

Elimination of xylene occurs in three phases. The first is rapid and corresponds to elimination from the blood and parenchymal organs; the second (half-time: 1 hour) represents elimination from highly perfused muscle tissue; the third (half-time: 20 hours) reflects slow elimination from adipose tissue (Riihimäki et al., 1979a).

Approximately 5% of the absorbed xylene dose is excreted unchanged in the exhaled air; most of the intake (about 95%) is metabolized and excreted in the urine as methylhippuric acid (Sedivec and Flek, 1976; Astrand et al., 1978; Engström et al., 1984; Hajimiragha et al., 1989). The amount of methylhippuric acid excreted increases as the absorption of xylene increases (Riihimäki et al., 1979b). Excretion of xylenes as xylenols accounts for less than 1% to 4% (Bray et al., 1950; Bakke and Scheline, 1970; Sedivec and Flek, 1976; Toftgård and Gustafsson, 1980; Engström et al., 1984; Riihimäki et al., 1979a). Excretion of unchanged xylene in the urine is negligible (about 0.001%) (Sedivec and Flek, 1976). No xylene or metabolites are detected in the feces (Bray et al., 1949).

Concurrent exposure to other chemicals affects the rate of excretion of xylene and its metabolites. Acute ingestion of moderate amounts of ethanol immediately prior to exposure to xylene decreases the clearance of *m*-xylene by approximately one-half (Riihimäki et al., 1982). Excretion of xylene metabolites was decreased in volunteers following coexposure to *m*-xylene (150 ppm), ethylbenzene (150 ppm) (Engström et al., 1984), and MEK (Raunio et al., 1990).

CLINICAL MANIFESTATIONS AND DIAGNOSIS

Symptomatic Diagnosis

Initial awareness of xylene vapor in the environment is related to an individual's ability to recognize its sweet odor, usually at the odor threshold level of 1.0 ppm (Carpenter et al., 1975). Perception of the odor of xylene vapor and irritation of the respiratory tract at higher concentrations annoy most exposed people sufficiently to cause their departure from the noxious conditions. Persons who become tolerant to the odor, no longer notice it and remain in its presence soon experience eye irritation, nasopharyngeal irritation, nausea and vomiting, anorexia, fatigue, vertigo, headache, mood irritability, insomnia, feeling of inebriation, impaired memory, confusion, loss of coordination, and staggering gait (Klaucke et al., 1982; Hipolito, 1980; Uchida et al., 1993). The most frequently reported symptom among workers exposed to low concentrations (21 ppm) was a floating sensation; at the higher concentrations (700 ppm), the most frequently reported symptom was headache (Table 15-3) (Uchida et al., 1993; Klaucke et al., 1982). Impaired work performance or a change in mood and interpersonal relations may be the first indications of adverse effects of exposure to xylene as observed by coworkers; the affected person may be unaware of these changes.

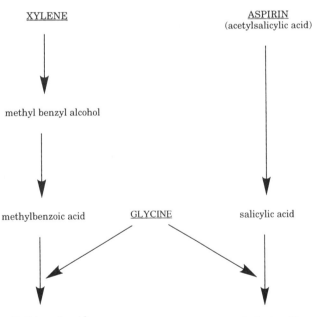

FIG. 15-2. Pathways of metabolic competition between xylene and aspirin (acetylsalicylic acid). (Modified from Cambell et al., 1988, with permission.)

TABLE 15-3. *Prevalence of acute subjective symptoms at low and high levels of exposure to xylene*

	Percent of workers reporting symptom	
Symptom	Low levels (21 ppm)[a]	High levels (700 ppm)[b]
Headache	23	80
Dizziness	14	47
Floating sensation	50	N/R
Heavy feeling in head	7	N/R
Nasal irritation	41	47
Throat irritation	31	47
Eye irritation	25	53
Unusual taste	14	N/R
Nausea	N/R	67
Vomiting	N/R	40

Modified from [a]Uchida et al., 1993; and [b]Klaucke et al., 1982.

CNS effects are initially excitatory, occurring during the early (absorption) phase of exposure; a soporific or depressant effect occurs during the later (elimination) phase (Schwarz et al., 1981; Seppäläinen et al., 1991; Laine et al., 1993). Severe intoxication can lead to unconsciousness and death (Browning 1937, 1953; Goldie, 1960; Morley et al., 1970). Thirty-eight cases of occupational exposure to xylene, severe enough to disable the worker for at least 3 days, were reported to Her Majesty's Factory Inspectorate of the United Kingdom from 1961 to 1980. In 24 of these cases, the individuals were working in a confined space; of these, 1 died, 16 were rendered unconscious, and in the remaining 21, xylene produced CNS effects including dizziness ($n = 6$), headache ($n = 5$), confusion ($n = 5$), drunkenness ($n = 3$), and incoordination ($n = 2$) (Bakinson and Jones, 1985). Chronic and repeated exposures have been associated with headache, fatigue, loss of sleep, stupor, giddiness, and irritability, as well as kidney, cardiac, and circulatory injury (Riihimäki and Hänninen, 1987).

Dose–effect relationships of exposure to xylene have been observed in controlled settings, in which known concentrations of xylene were administered to volunteers. Mild eye irritation was reported in four of six subjects exposed to 460 ppm of xylene vapor for 15 minutes. In addition, at an air xylene concentration of 690 ppm, four of these same subjects experienced dizziness and lightheadedness; in one subject, this was accompanied by a loss of balance (Carpenter et al., 1975). Exposure of eight volunteers to a constant concentration of 200 ppm m-xylene decreased body movements during the night and resulted in the subjects spending a longer time in bed (Laine et al., 1993). Concurrent exposure to other chemicals can alter the metabolism of xylene and thus enhance its effects. Symptoms were more easily produced by the combined exposure of volunteers to ethanol and xylene (Riihimäki et al., 1982).

Recordings of "body sway," which occurs while a subject attempts to maintain a steady upright posture, have been used as a test of balance impairment in volunteers exposed to xylene either when sedentary or following brief periods of exercise (Savolainen et al., 1980; Savolainen et al., 1985a,b; Laine et al., 1993). However, subjective responses and variability in reproducibility of testing techniques make the sway test difficult to evaluate as a measure of xylene's effect on vestibular functioning. Since exposed workers have complained of unsteady gait, it is nevertheless reasonable to consider some of the results of studies in which the sway test was used. Maximal body sway correlates positively with the rate of rise of (and) blood xylene levels reached during exposure (Savolainen et al., 1985b). Exposure to m-xylene vapor concentrations of 100 to 400 ppm significantly increased body sway over the previously recorded baseline values of eight volunteers (Savolainen et al., 1980; Riihimäki and Savolainen, 1980). A negative correlation between intensity of exposure and body sense of balance was seen at the beginning of exposure in volunteers exposed to xylene vapor while sedentary or exercising (100 W). In addition, although physical exercise during exposure generally improved body sway, the exercise-induced arousal was overcome at higher blood xylene levels such as 50 to 72 μmol/L (Savolainen et al., 1985a). Similarly, improvement rather than impairment of body sway with eyes closed was noted along both the anteroposterior and the lateral axes following peak exposures of 400 ppm m-xylene (basal concentration: 135 ppm), while sedentary and following exercise (Laine et al., 1993). Two-way analysis of variance showed that both exercise and exposure to m-xylene had a stabilizing effect on body balance. A conscious effort to maintain an erect posture may induce increased alertness and a subsequent heightened ability to compensate for any effects of xylene on posture (Seppäläinen et al., 1981). At low levels of exposure (145 ppm), simultaneous exposure to xylene and ethanol significantly increased body sway, although at higher concentrations (290 ppm), this effect was less pronounced. Nevertheless, these findings suggest that concurrent exposure to xylene and ethanol increases a worker's risk of incurring an occupational injury due to unstable balance (Savolainen, 1980).

Neurophysiological Diagnosis

Electroencephalographic (EEG) monitoring of brain activity of subjects during exposure to xylene reveals changes in the background rhythms and frequencies normally associated with states of arousal and drowsiness. No specific EEG changes were noted when the exposure concentrations of xylene were constant. However, during exposure to fluctuating concentrations of xylene, with peak exposures of 200 ppm, the incidence of slow-frequency (theta) wave transients recorded over the occipital regions was increased. Such changes were not seen under controlled conditions without exposure to xylene (Savolainen et al., 1980). The proportion of the dominant alpha waves significantly increased in subjects exposed to an average air xylene concentration of 200 ppm with peaks of 400 ppm, while performing moderate exercise (100 W) (Seppalainen et al., 1991).

Visual evoked potentials (VEPs) and *brain-stem auditory evoked potentials* (BAEPs) were studied in subjects exposed to various levels of *m*-xylene vapor (Seppalainen et al., 1989). VEPs were tested by stimulating both eyes using a pattern reversal stimulus (pattern-VEP) and a light flash (flash-VEP). For pattern-VEP the latencies of P50, N70, P100, N135, and P170, as well as the peak-to-peak amplitude of N70–P100, were measured. The latencies of P50, N70, P100, N150, and P200, as well as the peak-to-peak amplitude of N150–P200, were measured for flash-VEP. Healthy male volunteers were exposed (3 hours in the morning and 40 minutes in the afternoon) to *m*-xylene vapor at a stable concentration of 200 ppm or to a fluctuating dose ranging from 135 ppm (basal) to 400 ppm (peak); participants were either sedentary through the exposure or exercised briefly at 100 W for 10 minutes at the beginning of the exposure session. The latencies for all VEPs during exposure of the sedentary subjects were not related to exposure level and did not differ significantly from those recorded under control conditions. However, a decrease was found in the latency of N135 of the pattern-VEP following a 20-minute peak exposure to 400 ppm xylene in those subjects who exercised. In addition, a decrease in the latency of P210 in the flash-VEP was recorded at both the constant and fluctuating exposure levels with exercise. No significant changes in VEPs were found in the same subjects on exposure-free control days. The BAEPs were recorded in response to a click stimulus and were not significantly affected by exposure to xylene.

Chemosensory evoked potentials have been introduced as a novel approach for objective assessment of early neurophysiological changes through measurement of responses to chemical stimulations of the olfactory and/or trigeminal nerves, in persons occupationally exposed to volatile organic solvents (Otto and Hudnell, 1993). Mergler and Beauvais (1992) suggested receptor-specific saturation as the explanation for a sixfold increase in olfactory perception threshold seen during exposure to serially increasing concentrations of toluene, xylene, and a mixture of the two compared with a control substance (PM-carbinol). Olfactory fatigue or adaptation, which often occurs during prolonged or repeated exposures, increases the olfactory perception threshold of an exposed individual and hinders his or her ability to perceive and thus respond to xylene exposure (Mergler and Beauvais, 1992; Otto and Hudnell, 1993).

Nerve conduction studies (NCS) in workers exposed to xylene vapors must be evaluated critically because of the likelihood that other neurotoxic solvents capable of producing peripheral neuropathy may be present in the solvent mixture (Bleeker et al., 1991). Slight decreases in nerve conduction velocity (NCV) and reductions in amplitudes of sensory action potentials have been recorded in spray painters exposed to unknown amounts of xylene (Seppalainen et al., 1978, 1980; Elofsson et al., 1980).

NCV studies were made in 31 shipyard spray painters who were exposed to solvent-based paints containing more than 50% xylene; other organic solvents these workers were exposed to included trimethylbenzene, butanol, and small amounts of white spirit (Ruijten et al., 1994). Analysis of the test results was done on 28 exposed and 25 non-exposed subjects, after excluding those with alcohol consumption of more than 50 units per week or occupational exposures to other neurotoxicants. There was a significant decrease in motor NCVs in the peroneal and median nerves. No significant changes in sensory NCVs were found. Motor nerve refractory periods were increased in the painters as well. The changes in both motor NCVs and motor nerve refractory period were related to a cumulative exposure index (CEI) for xylene dose. The CEI was calculated for each worker using methylhippuric acid levels, task-specific exposure values, and duration of tasks during a typical workday as well as throughout the person's job history. The average CEI for the painter group in this study was determined to be one-third the biological exposure index (BEI) [1.5 g of methylhippuric acid per gram creatinine in urine at an exposure concentration of 100 ppm (ACGIH, 1995)], suggesting that low-level exposure to mixed solvents, of which xylene is the major component, affects the human peripheral nervous system. Although the occurrence of peripheral neuropathy in humans following exposure to pure xylene has rarely been proved, there are reports of the effects of xylene on axonal transport (Padilla et al., 1992; Ruijten et al., 1994).

Neuropsychological Diagnosis

Exposed persons may appear to be quite capable of working at constant levels of exposure and performing simpler psychomotor tasks despite depressive effects of the xylene. Decompensation and impaired performance may appear on more complicated tasks. Changes in cognitive functioning have been associated with the increases in vapor uptake, especially with increases in physical workload during exposure to xylene. The greatest impairments at these times are noted on the more complex cognitive tests; only slight changes in performance are seen on simpler psychomotor and perceptual tests (Gamberale et al., 1978). For example, tests of simple reaction time and choice reaction time revealed no significant differences during acute low-level exposure to xylene at 70 ppm (Olson et al., 1985), whereas acute exposure to an air concentration of 100 ppm significantly impaired the performance on tests of simple and choice reaction time in ten male volunteers (aged 22 to 35 years) (Dudek et al., 1990). Reaction-time-test performance is most impaired at peak exposure concentrations and with active exercising, especially in persons who have not had previous exposure to xylene (Laine et al., 1993; Savolainen et al., 1979; Savolainen et al., 1980). No significant impairment of simple or choice visual reaction times was found in sedentary volunteers exposed to xylene at a stable concentration of 200 ppm; however, following 20-minute peak concentrations of 400 ppm (basal concentration: 135 ppm), the simple visual reaction times of these subjects were significantly prolonged. In addition, auditory choice reaction times were significantly prolonged while subjects performed exercise at a workload of 100 W at this same level of exposure to xylene (basal: 135 ppm; peak: 400 ppm) (Laine et al., 1993). Simple and choice reaction times were also significantly impaired in sedentary volunteers exposed to xylene vapor 8 hr/day for 1 week, at concentrations that ranged between 100 and 400 ppm. In the same group of volunteers, no significant change in performance was observed on tests of manual dexterity or extraoccular muscle balance (Savolainen et al., 1979). A similar study included four brief periods of exercise during exposure to xylene vapor at either constant or fluctuating concentrations of 90 to 200 ppm for 5 consecutive days and then 1 day after an exposure-free weekend. This study revealed significant impairments in manual coordination as well as simple and choice reaction time at both levels of exposure. These findings were most marked during the beginning of each exposure week, during periods of exercise, and at those times when the concentration of xylene was temporarily increased (Savolainen et al., 1980). In both of the preceding studies by Savolainen et al. (1979, 1980), impairments were less pronounced by the fifth day of exposure than on the first, suggesting that either adaptation to the test stimuli or development of tolerance to xylene (possibly through induction of cytochrome P-450 enzymatic activity) had occurred.

Simple reaction time was more prolonged during exposures to a combination of xylene and ethanol than during exposure to xylene alone (Savolainen, 1980). Significant impairment in simple reaction time occurred during combined exposure to xylene (50 ppm) and toluene (50 ppm); this effect was surpassed when the exposure to xylene vapor alone was at a concentration of 100 ppm (Dudek et al., 1990). Concurrent use of xylene and 1,1,1-trichloroethane in the workplace is common, but short-term exposures to these agents did not produce the apparent additive effects as were observed during exposure to xylene and ethanol (Savolainen et al., 1982). These observations are of particular importance because some workers may consume ethanol on the job, while being exposed to xylene (and other solvents), thus increasing risk of injury through slowed reaction times.

Tests of short-term memory, numerical ability (addition reaction time), and simple and choice reaction times were assessed in male volunteers (aged 21 to 33 years) in a two-part experiment (Gamberale et al., 1978). Exposure periods for both parts of the study were 70 minutes long, and the subjects were required to remain sedentary for the entire period. In the first part, 15 subjects were studied individually on three separate occasions. On each occasion, they were exposed to xylene at concentrations of either 98 or 294 ppm, or to ordinary atmospheric air (control), via a breathing apparatus with the taste and smell of the inspired gas disguised by menthol crystals in the mouthpiece. Neuropsychological testing was performed during the second 35 minutes of the exposure period, while the subjects were still being exposed. No significant changes in performance as a function of xylene exposure were observed during this part of the experiment, when the average total uptake was estimated to be 180 mg at the low level (98 ppm) and 540 mg at the high level (294 ppm) exposure concentrations. These results were similar to those of Olson et al. (1985), who found no significant difference in performance on tests of short-term memory at low levels (70 ppm) of acute exposure to xylene.

In the second part, all conditions as described for part one remained the same, except that an eight-subject cohort from the original study group was exposed to xylene only at the higher concentration of 294 ppm while exercising at a workload of 100 W during the first 35 minutes of the exposure period. Testing was again performed during the second half of the exposure session, while the subject was sedentary. The results of the second part of this experiment revealed that the period of physical work had increased the average uptake to 1200 mg (at the higher exposure concentration of 294 ppm) and an impairment of performance in all areas tested with the greatest differences found on the following tests: numerical ability ($p < 0.05$); short-term memory ($p < 0.05$), and choice reaction time ($0.05 < p < 0.10$). These results indicate that the increase in uptake generated by a period of moderately heavy physical activity, as might be seen during occupational exposures, can significantly increase the effects of xylene on the CNS. They also suggest that monitoring individual uptake of this solvent may be a better predictor of the potential for neurotoxic effects than measurement of ambient air concentrations in the work environment (Gamberale et al., 1978).

Because xylene exposure frequently occurs concurrently with exposure to other neurotoxic solvents, the combined effects of chronic exposure to more than one chemical must be considered when assessing the neuropsychological effects of occupational exposures. Neuropsychological test performance was assessed in 45 workers exposed to xylene (mean level: 38 ppm; maximum level: 126 ppm) and toluene (mean level: 32 ppm; maximum level: 120 ppm) during a varnishing process in the electrical parts manufacturing industry (Gupta et al., 1990). Thirty of these workers were continuously exposed; the remaining 15 (mainly supervisors) were only occasionally exposed. Among the continuously exposed workers, significant deficits were seen in visual memory (Benton Visual Retention Test), visual ability (Koh's Block Test), and psychomotor functioning (Digit Symbol) and psychomotor ability (Mirror Drawing). Neuropsychological testing of the occasionally exposed workers revealed significant deficits in visual memory and visual ability. In addition, the results of this study suggest a dose–response relationship, as workers continuously exposed showed greater deficits than workers who were only occasionally exposed.

The effects of chronic exposure (average duration of exposure: 16.9 years) to paints that contained predominantly xylene (more than 50% of the total weight of the solvents) was studied with neuropsychological tests in 28 painters. They were compared with 25 unexposed age-matched control subjects. Deficits in attention (Color Word Vigilance Test), motor performance (Hand–Eye Coordination Test), and perceptual coding (Symbol Digit Substitution Test) were observed. In addition, there was a significant relationship between performance and duration of exposure on the Symbol Digit Substitution Test and Color Word Vigilance Test (Ruijten et al., 1994).

Biochemical Diagnosis

Xylene concentrations in alveolar air (end-exhaled air) can be used to estimate the severity of an immediate past exposure to xylene. However, because samples taken during or immediately after exposure reflect uptake during the previous hour rather than a TWA of work shift exposure, end-exhaled air is not recommended for use as a BEI for occupational exposure to xylene (ACGIH, 1989). A good correlation has been demonstrated between ambient and alveolar air concentrations of xylene at low levels (25 to 50 ppm) of exposure (Laparé et al., 1993). Concurrent exposure to other chemicals can affect alveolar concentration of xylene. For example, although exposure of five volunteers to low levels of toluene (50 ppm) and xylene (40 ppm) did not alter the concentrations in alveolar air, simultaneous exposure to higher concentrations of xylene (80 ppm) and toluene (95 ppm) increased end-exhaled air concentrations of both solvents (Tardif et al., 1991). In volunteers exposed to 200 ppm xylene, the concentrations of xylene in both alveolar air and arterial blood declined rapidly at the end of exposure. Xylene was still detectable in the blood of six volunteers 19 hours after exposure had ended (Åstrand et al., 1978).

Blood samples drawn in the morning before the day's work begins, preferably toward the end of the work week, will reflect the amount of xylene accumulated and stored in the body over several days of exposure (Riihimäki and Hänninen, 1987). For example, in volunteers exposed to xylene for 5 consecutive days, blood xylene levels measured before exposure began on the morning of the fifth day were 20% higher than corresponding levels on the first day (Riihimäki et al., 1979a). Although a BEI for blood has not been established by the ACGIH, an end of the work week morning blood xylene concentration of approximately 2 μmol/L has been shown to correspond to a TWA daily air sample exposure concentration of about 430 mg/m³ (100 ppm) of xylene vapor (Riihimäki and Hänninen, 1987). However, xylene concentrations in venous blood at the end of a work shift more closely reflect immediate past exposures and as such may not accurately reflect the TWA exposure over the entire work shift. Therefore, in cases of chronic occupational exposure, concentration of xylene in venous blood does not offer an advantage over determination of methylhippuric acid concentration in the urine (ACGIH, 1989).

Simultaneous exposure to other chemicals can affect blood levels of xylene. For example, exposure to toluene (95 ppm) and xylene (80 ppm) resulted in increased concentrations of both solvents in the blood of three nonsmoking male volunteers (Tardif et al., 1991). Coexposure to MEK caused the xylene concentration in the blood of eight volunteers to increase nearly twofold over exposure to xylene alone, indicating that MEK has an inhibitory effect on the metabolism of xylene (Liira et al., 1988). Blood levels of xylene are also raised by simultaneous ingestion of ethanol (Savolainen, 1980). Concurrent ingestion of ethanol (0.8 g/kg) increased blood xylene levels twofold in ten volunteers exposed to m-xylene (290 ppm). In addition, three of these individuals had elevated blood levels of acetaldehyde within the first hour after ethanol ingestion (Riihimäki et al., 1982).

Detection of methylhippuric acid in urine accurately reflects an 8-hour TWA exposure and is the recommended BEI for xylene; a urine concentration of 1.5 g/g creatinine should not be exceeded if daily exposure remains at or below 100 ppm (Table 15-4) (ACGIH, 1986, 1995). A sample collected at the end of the work shift is a reflection of the xylene uptake in the preceding hours. When it is possible to collect an accurately timed urine specimen during the last 4 hours of exposure, a rate of 2.0 mg methylhippuric acid excreted per minute (2 mg/min) reflects the TLV-TWA of 100 ppm (ACGIH, 1989). Exercise increases absorption of xylene and therefore excretion of metabolites. Excretion of methylhippuric acid was increased 24% by inclusion of four ten-minute periods of exercise (100 W) during a 6-hour experimental exposure to xylene (Riihimäki et al., 1979b).

Exposure to other chemicals can affect the excretion of methylhippuric acid, and this should be taken into account when evaluating results during biological monitoring of xylene exposure. Excretion of methylhippuric acid was delayed in volunteers simultaneously exposed to toluene (95 ppm) and xylene (80 ppm), suggesting that competitive inhibition is likely when the exposure concentrations of these two solvents is greater than 50 ppm each (Tardif et al., 1991). Combined exposure to m-xylene and ethylbenzene resulted in mutual inhibition, as indicated by decreased amounts of xylene and ethylbenzene metabolites in the urine (Engström et al., 1984). Aspirin administered simultaneously with exposure to xylene decreases excretion of methylhippuric acid (Campbell et al., 1988). Ingestion of ethanol immediately before or concurrently with exposure to xylene decreases urinary excretion of methylhippuric acid by about 50% (Riihimäki et al., 1982).

TABLE 15-4. *Biological exposure indices for xylene and xylene metabolites*

	Urine	Blood	Alveolar air
Determinant	Methylhippuric acid	Xylene	Xylene
Start of shift	Not established	Not established	Not established
During shift	Not established	Not established	Not established
End of shift	1.5 g/g creatinine	Not established	Not established

Data from ACGIH, 1995.

Neuroimaging

Specific changes in computed tomography or magnetic resonance imaging after xylene exposure have not yet been reported. Thus, when using these tests during the course of the differential diagnosis, abnormal images should be closely scrutinized, as these may be indicative of illnesses other than that caused by exposure to xylene. Although *single-photon emission computed tomography* (SPECT) studies in workers exposed to mixed solvents including xylene have revealed changes in regional cerebral blood flow consistent with neurological dysfunction, the contribution of the other solvents to these findings must be considered significant (Fincher et al., 1997).

Neuropathological Diagnosis

An autopsy was performed on a painter who died after being acutely overcome by xylene fumes, while working along with two other men in a double-bottomed tank in the engine room of a ship. The paint being used was known to contain in excess of 90% xylene by weight, with a trace of toluene. The estimated exposure level was as high as 10,000 ppm, and the estimated exposure duration was 19 hours. The two survivors became unconscious, but they recovered (see Clinical Experiences section) (Morley et al., 1970).

Postmortem examination in the fatal case showed acute pulmonary edema and intraalveolar hemorrhage. Liver cells were vacuolated and swollen, especially in the centrilobular area. So little time had elapsed between exposure and loss of consciousness and death that few neuropathological changes had occurred. Petechial hemorrhages were present in both gray and white matter, and blood was present in Virchow-Robin spaces. There was evidence of acute anoxic neuronal damage with swelling and loss of Nissl substance.

No decrease in brain weight such as that observed following toluene exposure was found after exposure to xylene (Kyrklund et al., 1987). Nevertheless, pathological evidence of the neurotoxic effect of xylene has also been reported in animals. Concentrations of glial fibrillary acidic protein were significantly increased in the anterior and posterior cerebellar vermis and in the frontal cortex following exposure of gerbils to xylene vapor at a concentration of 320 ppm. In addition, there were increased concentrations of the astroglial protein S-100 in the frontal cerebral cortex, and DNA concentrations were signifi-

cantly increased in the posterior cerebellar vermis. These changes are compatible with astrogliosis in these brain regions and indicate that xylene is neurotoxic to the gerbil brain (Rosengren et al., 1986).

Dopamine levels and turnover were increased in the caudate, median eminence, and hypothalamus following acute exposure of rats to high concentrations (2,000 ppm) of xylene (Andersson et al., 1981). In a similar study, no effect on striatal or tuberoinfundibular dopamine levels was observed in rabbits exposed to 750 ppm xylene for 12 hours a day for 7 days (Mutti et al., 1988). Other studies suggest that xylene-induced changes in the levels of dopamine and other neurotransmitters are not always dose dependent and are often region specific. Dopamine content in the striatum of the rat was decreased by exposure to xylene at 200 and 800 ppm but was conversely increased at 400 ppm (Honma et al., 1983). By contrast, concentrations of serotonin and norepinephrine in the cortex and hippocampus of these animals were increased by exposure to xylene at 200 and 800 ppm and decreased at 400 ppm. In addition, this study reported a dose-dependent decrease in acetylcholine content in the striatum and whole brain, as well as changes in midbrain amino acid content including a dose-dependent increase in glycine and an overall increase in γ-aminobutyric acid.

Region-specific changes in enkephalinergic neuromodulatory activity have been reported following acute intraperitoneal administration of xylene to rats. Significant reductions in met-enkephalin levels were seen in the globus pallidus and the medial preoptic area of the hypothalamus, whereas no changes were seen in the parietal cortex, caudate–putamen, and central amygdaloid nuclei (DeGandarias et al., 1995). These region-specific findings are in agreement with an early study by DeGandarias et al. (1993) in which a decrease in neutral aminopeptidase activity in the thalamus of the rat brain following acute intraperitoneal injection of xylene was found, and no changes were seen in the cortical regions. These findings suggest that changes in enkephalinergic neuromodulatory activity are involved in the acute neurotoxic effects of xylene.

Reversible effects on brain enzymes including NADPH-diaphorase, azoreductase, and superoxide dismutase follow xylene exposure (Savolainen and Pfäffli, 1980). Transient changes in brain ethanolamine phosphoglyceride fatty acid patterns have also been reported. Following a 30-day exposure of rats to xylene in air (320 ppm), a decrease in linoleic acid was observed in cerebral cortex ethanolamine phosphoglyceride; these changes were normalized after 90 days (Kyrklund et al., 1987).

Xylene can interact with membrane-bound integral proteins, and these interactions may be the critical factor in determining the anesthetic effects of xylene on the CNS. Xylene has been shown to decrease significantly acetylcholine esterase and adenosine triphosphatase activity dose dependently in rat synaptosomes (Korpela, 1989).

Exposure to xylene has been associated with the development of peripheral neuropathy in humans (Ruijten et al., 1994). Although the chemical mechanism by which xylene can induce peripheral neuropathy has not been established, animal studies indicate that xylene disrupts fast axonal transport; such disruption has been associated with peripheral neuropathy following exposure to other solvents and polymers (Padilla et al., 1992; Graham et al., 1995). In addition, chronic consumption of ethanol reduces the effects of xylene on axonal transport, indicating that induction of drug-metabolizing enzymes has a protective effect (Padilla et al., 1992). These findings do not provide evidence of whether xylene or a metabolite (e.g., methyl benzaldehyde) is the toxin responsible for the disruption of axonal transport. However, methyl benzaldehyde has been shown to bind covalently to cellular macromolecules and has been demonstrated to interfere with axonal transport (Patel et al., 1978; Graham et al., 1995).

PREVENTIVE AND THERAPEUTIC MEASURES

Comprehensive preplacement and biennial medical examinations should be performed on workers subject to xylene exposure (NIOSH, 1975). In addition to ongoing monitoring, safety education programs should be provided. Work areas should be properly ventilated, and protective clothing should be used to avoid prolonged skin contact. When not in use, containers of xylene should be kept closed (Engelmeier, 1985).

During emergency situations such as following a spill, appropriate eye protection, clothing, and respirators should be provided as necessary. Nonessential employees should be evacuated from the contaminated area during an emergency (NIOSH, 1975). Any clothing that becomes wet with xylene should be removed, and the skin should be washed with soap and water (see Exposure Limits and Safety Regulations section).

Possible effects of xylene on the skin, blood, nervous system, and gastrointestinal tract as well as liver and kidney should be monitored. Results obtained from simultaneous measurements of ambient air levels and testing of blood and urine content for xylene and its metabolites can serve as a means of early detection of unusual peaks in exposure and thus aid in identifying instances of increased potential for human intoxication from exposure to xylene vapor.

Because xylene causes severe aspiration pneumonitis, gastric lavage should be used to remove ingested xylene. In this way, the risks of aspiration associated with induced emesis can be avoided. (Ellenhorn and Barceloux, 1988; Goldfrank et al., 1990). Oral administration of activated charcoal has not been shown to reduce the body burden effectively (Goldfrank et al., 1990). Hemoperfusion has been used to speed removal of xylene from the body of an individual following accidental ingestion (Recchia et al., 1985).

CLINICAL EXPERIENCES

Group Studies

An Outbreak of Xylene Poisoning among Hospital Workers

An employee presented to the emergency room because of headache, nausea, vomiting, dizziness, burning eyes, and throat irritation, which had started after he arrived at work (Klauke et al., 1982). By the end of that same morning 14 other employees had become ill. They all reported onset of symptoms between 8:45 and 9:45 AM and shared the same complaints to varying degrees. Twelve of the 15 had headache, 10 had nausea, eight had eye irritation, and seven had dizziness or vertigo, or vomiting (Table 15-3). Of the 15 exposed workers, 14 reported smelling an unusual odor prior to the onset of their symptoms, and five of these described it as smelling like model airplane glue. Four other hospital employees noticed the odor but did not develop symptoms. None of the other 180 employees in the hospital detected the odor or developed symptoms requiring medical attention. In total 22 employees and four patients had been exposed, all of whom were either in the operating room, recovery room, intensive care unit, central supply, pharmacy, or housekeeping office at the time of the incident. All of the exposed persons were interviewed and nine were examined.

The areas of the hospital where the exposures occurred were found to be served by a common ventilation system. The ventilation system was found to have an open inspection door on the fan unit to allow some warm air to be drawn into the system and mix with the colder air from the outdoors. This was done to prevent freezing air from damaging the system. It was further established that a backflow of air from the sewer system was occurring. As a result, vapors from approximately 1 L of xylene that had been discarded down a sink drain in the pathology laboratory at 8:30 AM on the morning of the outbreak had apparently been drawn up through a dry floor drain trap in the fan room of the hospital's central ventilation system. This xylene-vapor-contaminated air was then drawn through the open inspection door on the central ventilation fan and subsequently pumped into the affected areas.

The median duration of illness was 36 hours (range: 2 to 48 hours); headache was the only symptom to last more than 12 hours. A carboxyhemoglobin blood test (used to screen for carbon monoxide poisoning) performed on one of the workers was normal; as a result, this test was not done on the other employees. Blood samples drawn 2 weeks after the incident revealed elevated serum glutamic oxaloacetic transaminase (SGOT) in two of the exposed workers. At follow-up testing 5 weeks later, their SGOT levels had dropped from 25 and 26 IU (normal range: 0 to 23 IU) to 9 and 11 IU, respectively.

A simulated spill was conducted to test the system for a source of the suspected xylene contamination. With the fan-unit inspection door tied open, the hallway doors closed, and 500 mL of xylene poured down the sink drain in the pathology laboratory, an odor of xylene was detected in the fan room in less than 2 minutes. The air measured over the floor drain contained 400 ppm of xylene vapor, an increase from the baseline reading of 0.6 ppm. It was concluded that the illness was related to exposure to xylene vapors. The hospital established preventive practices to avoid a recurrence of this unfortunate event and set forth safety rules for handling toxic chemicals.

Urinary Methylhippuric Acid Levels to Monitor Exposure

A survey was conducted on 175 workers employed either in a rubber boot factory, a plant manufacturing plastic-coated wire, or a printing plant (Uchida et al., 1993). At least 70% of these workers were exposed to xylene. A group of 241 nonexposed workers from the same or similar factories in the same region served as controls. Average duration of employment was about 7 years in both groups. Air content monitoring was by personal diffusive sampling. Measures of air concentration of xylene in the space near the exposed group were as high as 175 ppm. Other chemicals to which these workers were exposed included ethyl benzene, toluene, and (rarely) n-hexane.

Members of the exposed group had significantly more symptoms than the controls, including floating sensation, anxiety, forgetfulness, anorexia, weakness in extremities, and nightmares. There was a correlation between the intensity of exposure to xylene and the urinary concentration of methylhippuric acid, but there was no dose-dependent increase in the prevalence of symptoms, possibly because the intensity of exposure was low.

Individual Case Reports

Hazards of Warm Xylene Vapor in Paint-Mixing Pots

The job of an employee at a paint factory included cleaning paint mixing pots (Glass, 1961). After he had been doing this job for about 2 months, he began to feel giddy and unsteady on his feet. One day he became severely ataxic and vomited. He felt unwell and was anorexic for a week after the episode, although he had stayed away from his job. This man was required to soak the mixing pot in a hot caustic wash, after which it was rinsed in cold water. Once cooled, the pot was mopped out with a 1-gallon mixture of solvents containing 75% xylene and 25% ethyl benzene, methyl ethyl benzene, and trimethyl benzene. The process usually took 15 minutes for each pot.

This patient's symptoms were attributed to mopping out the pots while they were still warm. This was a common practice among the workers despite a company ruling that the pots be mopped out only when cold to avoid additional vaporization of any residual solvent. Xylene vapor levels over a warm paint pot were determined to be 270 to 350 ppm, more than double the concentration over a cold pot (60 to 100 ppm). The worker recovered and returned to work; he was reminded to wait until the pots cooled down before he cleaned them.

Chronic Xylene Poisoning in Unsuspecting Laboratory Workers

Many exposed workers accept their subjective symptoms as a part of their work experience and therefore do not seek medical attention. Hipolito (1980), reported several cases of xylene poisoning among laboratory technologists.

Case 1

A female laboratory technologist worked for 15 years in a small room without a fan or ventilation hood; her employer did not consider xylene to be toxic. The woman stained slides at a rate of 50,000 a year. At age 52, she began to experience headaches while at work. Initially, the headaches were relieved by temporarily leaving the room; later they became more severe and were accompanied by vertigo, nausea, dyspnea, flushes, and a low-grade fever. At age 56, she collapsed with severe chest pain. Her electrocardiogram was abnormal. After several medical consultations, a diagnosis of xylene poisoning was made. She subsequently left her job and remained disabled.

Case 2

Approximately 5 years after beginning work as a cytotechnologist, a woman began to experience chronic headaches, intellectual dullness, fatigue, and chest pain. She initially accepted her symptoms as being common among people in her profession. However, as they worsened, and since another histotechnologist in her laboratory had experienced similar symptoms several years before, she suspected that solvent fumes might be responsible for her condition as well. She saw a physician who found that her pulmonary function was impaired. Her leukocyte count was below normal at 3,800/mm³; it had previously been 7,200 mm³. A diagnosis of xylene poisoning was made. She then left the laboratory, and her symptoms cleared. She has subsequently retrained for work in another paramedical field, with no further exposures.

Severe but Reversible Personality Change in a Boat Repairman

A 58-year-old catamaran hull mold repairman used 99.7% pure xylene for 1.5 years (Roberts et al., 1988). For approximately 4 hours a day he used a brush dipped into an open bucket of xylene to clean the molds, during which time exposure to xylene was assessed to be at several hundred ppm; readings over a half-filled bucket registered 7,000 ppm. Throughout the first year, he experienced work-related headaches that were worse toward the end of the week but improved over the weekend. His workload increased, and 6 months later his headaches were worse, he complained of irritability and dizziness, and he felt unsafe driving himself home from work. He was admitted to the hospital because of agitation, breathlessness, extreme tiredness, lightheadedness, headache, confusion, and impairment of concentration and short-term memory. In addition, he complained of a sensation of shaking in his limbs when lying or sitting. Neurological examination revealed a fine tremor of his outstretched hands, hyperreflexia, unstable gait, and dysphasia. Peripheral nerve conduction velocity studies were normal.

He gradually improved, but after 7 months he still had imbalance on walking or turning. Neurobehavioral testing showed impaired concentration and attention, but no intellectual or memory impairment. Over the next 6 to 8 months, away from exposure to xylene, the patient experienced gradual improvement. The excessive tiredness, irritability, lassitude, and impaired concentration and attention had lessened. At approximately 1 year after initial presentation, the patient still had variable concentration, noise sensitivity, increased sleep requirement, and lack of initiative.

Seizures in a Painter Exposed to Xylene in a Confined Space

Eight men were spray painting gun towers with paint containing 80% xylene and 20% methylglycolacetate (Goldie, 1960). The men were told to use masks during spraying, which was apparently sufficient protection while painting out of doors in the fresh air as the workers complained of no discomfort. However, while painting the inside of the towers, they noticed a strong smell, identified as xylene. A ventilation system in the tower caused such a draft that it rendered work impossible and thus was never switched on. Within about half an hour after beginning work inside the tower, the men began to experience symptoms including headache, vertigo, gastric discomfort, dryness of throat, and a drunken feeling. These symptoms reportedly vanished after a few minutes in the fresh air, and the workers were sub-sequently told to go outside for 10 minutes every half hour to avoid further discomfort.

While cycling home from work one afternoon, one of the workers, a young man of 18 who had been working with the paints for about 2 months, began to feel weak and dizzy. By the time he arrived at his home, he had difficulty comprehending speech, and his own speech was incoherent. Shortly thereafter, he became aphonic, with a staring gaze and dyspnea. This was followed by complete loss of consciousness, during which there were short sharp jerks of the upper and lower limbs; his eyes were rotated to one side, and chewing behavior was observed. There was no incontinence of the bladder or bowel. The patient regained consciousness after about 20 minutes and was subsequently admitted to the hospital, where he had another episode of much shorter duration. Physical and neurological examinations were performed. Blood pressure was 120/75, and complete blood count was normal. Pupillary response and reflexes were normal. Skull radiograph and EEG revealed no pathological changes. When the patient regained consciousness, he felt quite well and was discharged a week later.

This young man had previously (at age 14) experienced a fit of cramps preceded by sensations that might be regarded a simple partial seizure although he reportedly did not lose consciousness. Stocke (1928) reported on a patient with latent epilepsy who complained of increased seizures when exposed to xylene vapors.

Seizures while Building Model Aircraft

The mother of an adolescent boy with a 2-year history of seizures noticed that his brief absences, which had previously been abolished with ethosuximide, reappeared after the young man had spent an evening making model aircraft (Arthur and Curnock, 1982). This disparity was noted on several occasions and prompted the parents to investigate its cause. It was subsequently discovered that the glue the boy was using contained xylene as its principal solvent, prompting a change to a glue with a lower xylene content.

One evening the boy reverted to the old glue. Twenty-four hours later he had a generalized grand mal seizure and was taken to the hospital. The EEG showed occasional sharp wave bursts in the parietal leads consistent with epilepsy. One month later, the boy once more used the old glue and again experienced a series of absences within 24 hours after the exposure. This incident was followed by another series of absences 1 month later, although this time they were not associated with exposure to glue. The boy's anticonvulsant therapy was subsequently changed to sodium valproate; he has remained well since. He has avoided the culprit glue and its vapors.

Xylene Poisoning and Prolonged Unconsciousness

Morley et al. (1970), described three workers who were overcome by xylene fumes while painting a double-bottomed tank in the engine room of a ship. Xylene was the principal solvent in the paint (90%), which also included trace amounts of toluene. About 1.5 gallons of paint had been applied, representing about 1 hour of work for three men. Ventilation was minimal, and none of the workers were wearing a respirator. Estimated exposure levels were as high as 10,000 ppm, and exposure duration was approximately 19 hours. One painter died and the other two recovered after a period of unconsciousness (see Pathological Diagnosis section). One worker recovered after 5 hours of unconsciousness but was confused and had amnesia for all events during the previous 24 hours; the other survivor was fully alert after 24 hours but also did not recall events preceding his collapse. In addition, he had slurred speech and ataxia, both of which cleared over the next 48 hours.

Case 1

On admission to the hospital, the victim was unconscious, his face was flushed, there was peripheral cyanosis, and his expired air smelled strongly of solvent fumes. In addition, he was shivering (temperature 90°F) and showed only a slight response to painful stimuli. His pulse was regular (90/min), and blood pressure was 100/80. SGOT was 64 IU (normal range: 4 to 20 IU). Five hours after arrival at the hospital, he regained consciousness but was confused and amnesic for the events that had occurred during the previous 24 hours. By the third day after admission, the patient's confusion had disappeared, but the amnesia persisted. The worker remembered leaving the premises to eat lunch at approximately 1:15 PM but did not remember anything else until he regained consciousness in the hospital.

Case 2

On arrival at the hospital, a worker was unconscious and his breath smelled strongly of solvent. He began to regain consciousness in the emergency room, at which time he was confused and had a retrograde amnesia for the events of the preceding 24 hours. In addition, his speech was slurred, and he was ataxic on walking. His temperature was normal, his pulse was 88/min, and his blood pressure was 120/90. SGOT was 36 IU (normal range: 4 to 20 IU). His recovery was uneventful, and within 24 hours after admission he was fully conscious and alert. The ataxia reportedly disappeared with 48 hours of admission. The patient continued to be unable to recall anything that had occurred between 10:30 AM and the time he regained consciousness in the hospital.

REFERENCES

Agency for Toxic Substances and Disease Registry (ATSDR). Toxicological profile for xylenes. Atlanta, GA: US Department of Health and Human Services, 1995.

American Conference of Governmental and Industrial Hygienists (ACGIH). Documentation of the threshold limit values and biological exposure indices, 5th ed., Cincinnati, OH: ACGIH, 1989.

American Conference of Governmental and Industrial Hygienists (ACGIH). Threshold limit values (TLVs) for chemical substances and physical agents and biological exposure indices (BEIs). Cincinnati, OH: ACGIH, 1995.

Amoore JE, Hautala E. Odor as an aid to chemical safety: odor threshold compared with threshold limit values and volatilities for 214 industrial chemicals in air and water dilution. *J Appl Toxicol* 1983;3:272–290.

Andersson K, Fuxe K, Nilson OG, Toftgard R, Enerot P, Gustafsson JA. Production of discrete changes in dopamine and noradrenaline levels and turnover in various parts of the rat brain following exposure to xylene, ortho-, meta-, and para-xylene, and ethyl benzene. *Toxicol Appl Pharmacol* 1981;60:535–548.

Arthur LJH, Curnock DA. Xylene-induced epilepsy following innocent glue sniffing. *BMJ* 1982;284:1787.

Ashley DL, Bonin MA, Cardinali FL, McCraw JM, Wooten JV. Blood concentrations of volatile organic compounds in a nonoccupationally exposed US population and in groups of suspected exposure. *Clin Chem* 1994;40:1401–1404.

Åstrand I. Uptake of solvents in the blood and tissues of man: a review. *Scand J Work Environ Health* 1975;1:199–218.

Åstrand E, Engström J, Ovrum P. Exposure to xylene and ethylbenzene I: Uptake, distribution and elimination in man. *Scand J Work Environ Health* 1978;4:185–194.

Bakke OM, Scheline RR. Hydroxylation of aromatic hydrocarbons in the rat. *Toxicol Appl Pharmacol* 1970;16:691–700.

Bakinson MA, Jones RD. Gassings due to methylene chloride, xylene, toluene, and styrene reported to Her Majesty's Factory Inspectorate 1961–1980. *Br J Ind Med* 1985;42:181–190.

Bleeker ML, Bolla KI, Agnew J, Schwartz BS, Ford DP. Dose-related subclinical neurobehavioral effects of chronic exposure to low levels of organic solvents. *Am J Ind Med* 1991;19:715–728.

Bray HG, Humphris BG, Thorpe WV. Metabolism of derivatives of toluene. 3. *o-, m-,* and *p*-xylenes. *Biochem J* 1949;45:241–244.

Bray HG, Humphris BG, Thorpe WV. Metabolism of derivatives of toluene. 5. The fate of the xylenols in the rabbit, further observations on the metabolism of the xylenes. *Biochem J* 1950;47:395–399.

Brown HS, Bishop D, Rowan CA. The role of skin absorption as a route of exposure for volatile organic compounds (VOCs) in drinking water. *Am J Public Health* 1984;74:479–484.

Browning E. *Toxicity of industrial solvents: Summaries of published work.* Compiled by Ethel Browning under the direction of the Committee on the Toxicity of Industrial Organic Solvents, Report No. 80. London: Her Majesty's Stationery Office, 1937:73–82.

Browning E. *Toxicity of industrial solvents.* Revised in consultation with the Toxicology Committee by Ethel Browning. New York: Chemical Publishing, 1953:73–82.

Campbell L, Wilson HK, Samuel AM, Gompertz D. Interactions of *m*-xylene and aspirin metabolism in man. *Br J Ind Med* 1988;45:127–132.

Carpenter CP, Kinkead ER, Geary DL Jr, Sullivan LJ, King JM. Petroleum hydrocarbon toxicity studies. V: Animal and human response to vapors of mixed xylenes. *Toxicol Appl Pharmacol* 1975;33:543–558.

Carlsson A. Distribution and elimination of 14C-xylene in rat. *Scand J Work Environ Health* 1981;78:51–55.

David A, Flek J, Frantik E, Gut I, Sedivec V. Influence of phenobarbital on xylene metabolism in man and rats. *Int Arch Occup Environ Health* 1979;44:117–125.

DeGandarias JM, Echeverria E, Irazusta J, Gil J, Casis L. Brain amino peptidase activity after subacute xylene exposure. *Neurotoxicol Teratol* 1993;15:51–53.

DeGandarias JM, Echeverria E, Casis E, Martinez-Millan L, Casis L. Effects of acute xylene exposure on the enkephalineric neuromodulatory system in rats. *Ind Health* 1995;33:1–6.

Ducatman AM, Moyer TP. Environmental exposure to common industrial solvents. *Am Assoc Clin Chem* 1984;5:1–18.

Dudek B, Gralewicz K, Jakubowski M, Kostrzewski P, Sokal J. Neurobehavioral effects of experimental exposure to toluene, xylene and their mixture. *Pol J Occup Med* 1990;3:109–116.

Ellenhorn MJ, Barceloux DG. *Medical toxicology: diagnosis and treatment of human poisoning.* New York: Elsevier, 1988:962–964.

Elofsson SA, Gamberale F, Hindmarsh T, et al. Exposure to organic solvents. A cross-sectional epidemiologic investigation on occupational exposed car and industrial painters with special reference to the nervous system. *Scand J Work Environ Health* 1980;6:239–273.

Elovaara E, Collan Y, Pfäffli P, Vainio H. The combined toxicity of technical grade xylene and ethanol in the rat. *Xenobiotica* 1980;10:435–445.

Engelmeier RL. Effective measures to reduce xylene exposure. *J Prost Dent* 1985;53:564–565.

Engström K, Bjurstrom R. Exposure to xylene and ethylbenzene. II. Concentration in subcutaneous adipose tissue. *Scand J Work Environ Health* 1978;4:195–203.

Engström K, Husman K, Riihimäki V. Percutaneous absorption of *m* xylene in man. *Int Arch Occup Environ Health* 1977;39:181–189.

Engström J, Riihimäki V. Distribution of *m*-xylene to subcutaneous adipose tissue in short term experimental human exposure. *Scand J Work Environ Health* 1979;5:126–134.

Engström K, Riihimäki V, Laine A. Urinary disposition of ethylbenzene and *m*-xylene in man following separate and combined exposure *Int Arch Occup Environ Health* 1984;54:355–363.

Fincher CE, Chang T-S, Harrell EH, et al. Comparison of single photon emission computed tomography findings in cases of healthy adults and solvent-exposed adults. *Amer J Ind Med* 1997;31:4–14.

Fishbein L. An overview of environmental and toxicological aspects of aromatic hydrocarbons. III. Xylene. *Sci Tot Environ* 1985;43:165–183.

Gamberale F, Anwall G, Hultengren M. Exposure to xylene and ethyl benzene. III. Effects on central nervous functions. *Scand J Work Environ Health* 1978;4:204–211.

Glass WI. Annotation: a case of suspected xylol poisoning. *NZ Med* 1961;60:113.

Goldfrank LR, Kulberg AG, Bresnitz EA. Hydrocarbons. In: Goldfrank LR, ed. *Goldfrank's toxicologic emergencies.* Norwalk, CT: Appleton Lange, 1990:759–768.

Goldie I. Can xylene (xylol) provoke convulsive seizures? *Ind Med Surg* 1960;29:33–35.

Graham DG, Amarath V, Valentine WM, et al. Pathogenic studies of hexane and carbon disulfide neurotoxicity. *Crit Rev Toxicol* 1995;25:91–112.

Gupta B, Kumar P, Srivastava A. An investigation of the neurobehavioral effects on workers exposed to organic solvents. *J Soc Occup Med* 1990;40:94–96.

Hajimiragha H, Ewers U, Brockhaus A, Biettger A. Levels of benzene and other volatile aromatic compounds in the blood of non-smokers and smokers. *Int Arch Occup Environ Health* 1989;61:513–518.

Hipolito RN. Xylene poisoning in laboratory workers: case reports and discussion. *Lab Med* 1980;11:593–595.

Honma T, Sudo A, Miyagawa M, Sato M, Hasegawa H. Significant changes in the amounts of neurotransmitter and related substances in the rat brain induced by subacute exposure to low levels of toluene and xylene. *Ind Health* 1983;21:143–151.

Kaneko T, Wang P-Y, Sato A. Enzyme induction by ethanol consumption affects: the pharmacokinetics of inhaled *m*-xylene only at high levels of exposure. *Arch Toxicol* 1993;67:473–477.

Kaneko T, Wang P-Y, Tsukada H, Sato A. *m*-Xylene toxicokinetics in phenobarbital-treated rats: comparison among inhalation exposure, oral administration, and intraperitoneal administration. *Toxicol Appl Pharmacol* 1995;131:13–20.

Karlson U, Frankenberger WT. Microbial degradation of benzene and toluene in ground water. *Bull Environ Contam Toxicol* 1989;43:505–510.

Kawai T, Mizunuma K, Yasugi T, et al. Urinary methylhippuric acid isomer levels after occupational exposure to a xylene mixture. *Int Arch Occup Environ Health* 1991;63:69–75.

Klaucke DN, Johansen M, Vogt RL. An outbreak of xylene intoxication in a hospital. *Am J Ind Med* 1982;3:173–178.

Korpela M. Inhibition of synaptosome membrane-bound integral enzymes by organic solvents. *Scand J Work Environ Health* 1989;15:64–68.

Kyrklund T, Kjellstrand P, Haglid K. Brain lipid changes in rats exposed to xylene and toluene. *Toxicology* 1987;45:123–133.

Laine A, Savolainen K, Riihimäki V, Matikainen E, Salmi T, Juntunen J. Acute effects of *m*-xylene inhalation on body sway, reaction times, and sleep in man. *Int Arch Occup Environ Health* 1993;65:179–188.

Langman JM. Xylene: its toxicity, measurement of exposure levels, absorption, metabolism, and clearance. *Pathology* 1994;26:301–309.

Laparé S, Tardif R, Brodeur J. Effects of various exposure scenarios on the biological monitoring of organic solvents in alveolar air. *Int Arch Occup Environ Health* 1993;64:569–580.

Liira J, Riihimäki V, Enström K, Pfäffli P. Coexposure of man to *m*-xylene and methyl ethyl ketone: kinetics and metabolism. *Scand J Work Environ Health* 1988;14:322–327.

Low L, Meeks JR, Mackerer CR. Health effects of the alkylbenzenes. II. Xylenes. *Toxicol Ind Health* 1989;5:85–105.

Mergler D, Beauvais B. Olfactory threshold shift following controlled 7-hour exposure to toluene and/or xylene. *Neurotoxicology* 1992;13:211–216.

Morley R, Eccleston DW, Douglas CP, Greville WE, Scott DJ, Anderson J. Xylene poisoning: a report on one fatal case and two cases of recovery after prolonged unconsciousness. *BMJ* 1970;3:442–443.

Mutti A, Falzoi M, Romanelli A, Bocchi MC, Ferroni C, Franchini I. Brain dopamine as a target for solvent toxicity: effects of some monocyclic aromatic hydrocarbons. *Toxicology* 1988;49:77–82.

National Academy of Science (NAS). *Drinking water and health,* vol. 3. Washington: National Academy of Sciences Press, 1980.

National Institute for Occupational Safety and Health (NIOSH). U.S. Department of Health Education and Welfare. *Criteria for a recommended standard for occupational exposure to xylene,* HEW Publication No. (NIOSH) 75-168, GPO No. 017-033-00075, Washington: US Government Printing Office, 1975.

National Institute for Occupational Safety and Health (NIOSH). National occupational hazard survey (1970). Cincinnati, OH: US Department of Health and Human Services, 1976. National Institute for Occupational Safety and Health (NIOSH). Registry of toxic effects of chemical substances. Washington: US Department of Health, Education and Welfare, 1978; 79–100.

National Institute for Occupational Safety and Health (NIOSH). National occupational hazard survey (1970). Cincinnati, OH: US Department of Health and Human Services, 1984.

National Institute for Occupational Safety and Health (NIOSH). Pocket guide to chemical hazards. Washington: US Department of Health and Human Services, CDC, 1994.

Occupational Safety and Health Administration (OSHA). Code of Federal Regulations (1910.1000). Washington: US Department of Health and Human Services, CDC, 1995.

Ogata M, Yamazaki Y, Sugihara R, et al. Quantitation of urinary *o*-xylene metabolites of rats and human beings by high performance liquid chromatography. *Int Arch Occup Environ Health* 1980;46:127–139.

Olson A, Gamberale F, Iregren A. Coexposure to toluene and *p*-xylene in man: central nervous functions. *Br J Ind Med* 1985;42:117–122.

Otto DA, Hudnell HK. The use of visual and chemosensory evoked potentials in environmental and occupational health. *Environ Res* 1993;62:159–171.

Padilla S, Lyerly DL, Pope CN. Subacute ethanol consumption reverses *p*-xylene-induced decreases in axonal transport. *Toxicology* 1992;75:159–167.

Patel JM, Harper C, Drew RT. The biotransformation of *p*-xylene to a toxic aldehyde. *Drug Metab Dispos* 1978;6:368.

Raunio H, Liira J, Elovaara E, Riihimäki V, Pelkonen O. Cytochrome P-450 isozyme induction by methyl ethyl ketone and *m*-xylene in rat liver. *Toxicol Appl Pharmacol* 1990;103:175–179.

Recchia G, Perbellini L, Prati GF, Dean P, Ancona G. Coma da probabile ingestione accidentale di xilene: trattamento mediante emoperfusione con carbone attivato. *Med Lav* 1985;76:67–73.

Riihimäki V. Xylene. In: Aittio A, Riihimäki V, Vainio H, eds. *Biological monitoring and surveillance of workers exposed to chemicals.* Washington: Hemisphere Publishing, 1984:83–97.

Riihimäki V, Hänninen O. Xylenes. In: Snyder R, ed. *Ethel Browning's toxicity and metabolism of industrial solvents.* vol. 1. Hydrocarbons. Amsterdam: Elsevier Science Publishers, 1978:64–84.

Riihimäki V, Pfäffli P. Percutaneous absorption of solvent vapors in man. *Scand J Work Environ Health* 1978;4:73–85.

Riihimäki V, Savolainen K. Human exposure to *m*-xylene. Kinetics and acute effects on the CNS. *Ann Occup Hyg* 1980;23:411–422.

Riihimäki V, Hänninen O. In: Snyder R, ed. *Ethel Browning's toxicity and metabolism of industrial solvents,* 2nd ed., vol. 1: Hydrocarbons. Amsterdam: Elsevier Science Publishers, 1987:64–84.

Riihimäki V, Pfäffli P, Savolainen K, Pekari K. Kinetics of *m*-xylene in man: general features of absorption, distribution, biotransformation and excretion in repetitive inhalation exposure. *Scand J Work Environ Health* 1979a;5:217–231.

Riihimäki V, Pfäffli P, Savolainen K. Kinetics of *m*-xylene in man: influence of intermittent physical exercise and changing environmental concentrations on kinetics. *Scand J Work Environ Health* 1979b;5:232–248.

Riihimäki V, Savolainen K, Pfäffli P, Pekari K, Sippel HW, Laine A. Metabolic interaction between *m*-xylene and ethanol. *Arch Toxicol* 1982;49:253–263.

Roberts F, Lucas E, Marsden CD, Trauer T. Near pure xylene causing irreversible neuropsychiatric disturbance. *Lancet* 1988;2:273.

Rosengren LE, Kjellstrand P, Aurell A, Haglid KG. Irreversible effects of xylene on the brain after long term exposure: a quantitative study of DNA and glial cell marker proteins S-100 and GFA. *Neurotoxicology* 1986;7:121–136.

Ruijten MWMM, Hooisma J, Brons JT, Habets CEP, Emmen HH, Muijser H. Neurobehavioral effects of long-term exposure to xylene and mixed organic solvents in shipyard painters. *Neurotoxicology* 1994;15:613–620.

Sato A, Fujiwara Y, Nakajima T. Solubility of benzene, toluene and *m*-xylene in various body fluids and tissues of rabbits. *Jpn J Ind Health* 1974;16:30–31.

Savolainen K. Combined effects of xylene and alcohol on the central nervous system. *Acta Pharmacol Toxicol* 1980;46:366–372.

Savolainen K, Pfäffli P. Dose dependent neurochemical changes during short term inhalation exposure to m-xylene. *Arch Toxicol* 1980;45:117–122.

Savolainen K, Riihimäki V, Linnoila M. Effects of short-term xylene exposure on psychophysiological functions in man. *Int Arch Occup Environ Health* 1979;44:201–211.

Savolainen K, Riihimäki V, Seppalainen A, Linnoila M. Effects of short term *m*-xylene exposure and physical exercise on central nervous system. *Int Arch Occup Environ Health* 1980;45:105–121.

Savolainen K, Riihimäki V, Laine A, Kekoni J. Short term exposure of human subjects to m-xylene and 1,1,1-trichloroethane. New toxicology for old. *Arch Toxicol* 1982;Suppl 5:96–99.

Savolainen K, Riihimäki V, Mouna O, Kekoni J, Luukkonen R, Laine A. Conversely exposure-related effects between atmospheric *m*-xylene concentrations and human body sense of balance. *Acta Pharmacol Toxicol* 1985a;57:67–71.

Savolainen K, Riihimäki V, Luukkonen R, Mouna O. Changes in the sense of balance correlate with concentrations of *m*-xylene in venous blood. *Br J Ind Med* 1985b;42:765–769.

Schwarz E, Kielholz P, Hobi V, et al. Alcohol-induced biphasic background and stimulus-elicited EEG changes in relation to blood alcohol levels. *Int J Clin Pharmacol Ther Toxicol* 1981;19:102–111.

Sedivec V, Flek J. The absorption, metabolism, and excretion of xylenes in man. *Int Arch Occup Env Health* 1976;37:205–217.

Seppäläinen AM, Husman K, Martenson C. Neurophysiological effects of long-term exposure to a mixture of organic solvents. *Scand J Work Environ Health* 1978;4:304–314.

Seppäläinen AM, Lindstrom K, Martelin T. Neurological and psychological picture of solvent poisoning. *Am J Ind Med* 1980;1:31–42.

Seppäläinen AM, Savolainen MK, Kovala T. Changes induced by xylene and alcohol in human evoked potentials. *Electroencephalogr Clin Neurophysiol* 1981;51:148–155.

Seppäläinen AM, Laine A, Salmi T. Changes induced by short term xylene exposure in human evoked potentials. *Int Arch Occup Environ Health* 1989;61:443–449.

Seppäläinen AM, Laine A, Salmi T, Verkkala E, Riihimäki V, Luukkonen R. Electroencephalographic findings during experimental human exposure to *m*-xylene. *Arch Environ Health* 1991;46:16–24.

Sherwood RJ. Ostwald solubility coefficients of some industrially important substances. *Br J Ind Med* 1976;33:106–107.

Stocke A. *Zentralb gewerbe Hyg.* 1928;5–6:355.

Tardif R, Laparé S, Plaa GL, Brodeur J. Effect of simultaneous exposure to toluene and xylene on their respective biological exposure indices in humans. *Int Arch Occup Environ Health* 1991;63:279–284.

Toftgård R, Gustafsson J-A. Biotransformation of organic solvents: a review. *Scand J Work Environ Health* 1980;6:1–18.

Uchida Y, Nakatsuka H, Ukai H, et al. Symptoms and signs in workers exposed predominantly to xylenes. *Int Arch Occup Environ Health* 1993;64:597–605.

United States Environmental Protection Agency (USEPA). National primary drinking water standards. EPA, 810-F-94-001, Office of Water, 4601. Washington: EPA, 1994.

United States Environmental Protection Agency (USEPA). Drinking water regulations and health advisories. EPA, 822-R-96-001, Office of Water, 4304. Washington: EPA, 1996.

Utidjian HM. Criteria documents: recommendations for a xylene standard. *J Occup Med* 1976;18:567–570.

Wallace L, Pellizzari E, Hartwell T, et al. Concentrations of 20 volatile organic compounds in the air and drinking water of 350 residents of New Jersey compared with concentrations in their exhaled breath. *J Occup Med* 1986;28:603–608.

Wallace L, Pellizzari E, Hartwell T, et al. The California team study: breath concentrations and personal exposures to 26 volatile compounds in air and drinking water of 188 residents of Los Angeles, Antioch, and Pittsburg, CA. *Atmos Environ* 1988;22:2141–2163.

Wisniewska-Knypl JM, Wronska-Nofer T, Jajte J, Jedlinska U. The effect of combined exposures to ethanol and xylene on rat hepatic microsomal monooxygenase activities. *Alcohol* 1989;6:347–352.

CHAPTER 16

n-Hexane and Methyl *n*-Butyl Ketone

Aliphatic alkanes (e.g., *n*-hexane) and ketones (e.g., methyl *n*-butyl ketone and methyl *iso*-butyl ketone) occur naturally in the environment as constituents of the earth's natural gases and they are products derived from refined crude petroleum (Sandmeyer, 1981). Of the aliphatic hexacarbons, *n*-hexane and methyl *n*-butyl ketone are among the most commonly used and the most highly neurotoxic (Ducatman and Moyer, 1984). Since these compounds have a common toxic metabolite (i.e., 2,5-hexanedione) it is reasonable to consider them together in one chapter.

n-Hexane

n-Hexane (normal-hexane; hexane; hexyl hydride) is a volatile colorless lipophilic liquid with a gasolinelike odor (Sax, 1979; NIOSH, 1997). Commercial supplies of *n*-hexane are produced by petroleum cracking or by isolation of *n*-hexane from natural gas (Sandmeyer, 1981). Industrial-grade hexane is a mixture of varying quantities of *n*-hexane and its isomers (2-methylpentane; 3-methylpentane; and 2,3-dimethylbutane), plus small amounts of methylcyclopentane, cyclohexane, and heptane (Yamamura, 1969; Perbellini et al., 1981a; Low et al., 1987). Although acute inhalation of *n*-hexane was known to affect central nervous system (CNS) functioning, the transient effects of acute exposure to *n*-hexane were not considered a problem; thus *n*-hexane was introduced to industry as a low-hazard replacement for more toxic solvents (Nelson et al., 1943). It soon became apparent that chronic and/or repeated exposures to *n*-hexane were neurotoxic. Reports of severe peripheral neuropathy soon began to appear in the literature along with warnings that the solvent and its vapors must be contained and/or used under well-ventilated conditions (Oishi et al., 1964; Yamada, 1967; Yamamura, 1969; Herskowitz et al., 1971; Oryshkevich et al., 1986; Altenkirch et al., 1977). The risk of encountering neurotoxic effects from *n*-hexane exposures is widespread because it is an ingredient in common household and hobby materials as well as an important chemical with many industrial uses.

Methyl *n*-Butyl Ketone

Methyl *n*-butyl ketone (M*n*BK; *n*-hexanone; 2-hexanone; *n*-butyl methyl ketone), a monoketone, is a clear, colorless, volatile liquid with an acetonelike odor (Sax, 1979). Commercial supplies of M*n*BK are produced by a catalytic reaction between acetic acid and ethylene (Couri and Milks, 1982). M*n*BK is also a metabolite of the enzymatic oxidation of *n*-hexane (see Tissue Biochemistry section). Chronic exposure to M*n*BK has been associated with peripheral neuropathy (Billmaier et al., 1974; Allen et al., 1975; Saida et al., 1976; Mallov, 1976; Davenport et al., 1976).

The neurotoxic properties of *n*-hexane have been known since 1964 when an outbreak of peripheral neuropathy occurred in a Japanese printing plant (Oishi et al., 1964; Yamada, 1964). Approximately 10 years later a similar outbreak of neuropathy occurred in a factory in Ohio where M*n*BK was used as a solvent in the production of plastic-coated and color-printed fabrics (Billmaier et al., 1974; Mendell et al., 1974; Allen et al., 1975). The similarity between the axonopathy associated with exposures to *n*-hexane and M*n*BK led to investigations demonstrating that both *n*-hexane and M*n*BK are metabolized to 2,5-hexanedione, a γ-diketone (O'Donoghue and Krasavage, 1979; Allen, 1980; DiVincenzo et al., 1980; Graham et al., 1995). Additional studies indicated that the neurotoxicity of 2,5-hexanedione is directly related to the γ-spacing of its functional groups (i.e., the second ketone group is located on the third carbon atom away (γ-position) from the first ketone group of the alkane). It was noted that aliphatic alkanes and ketones such as propane, butane, pentane, methyl ethyl ketone (MEK), and methyl *iso*-butyl ketone (M*i*BK) cannot form γ-diketones, due to their chemical structures (i.e., the longest parent alkane chain contains only five carbon atoms), are less neurotoxic, and do not produce neuropathies characterized by axonal swelling with paranodal accumulation of neurofilaments (Spencer and Schaumburg, 1976; Saida et al., 1976; Granvil et al., 1994; Graham et al., 1995). Thus, the ability of an aliphatic alkane or monoketone to produce the type of peripheral neuropathy characteristic of *n*-hexane and/or

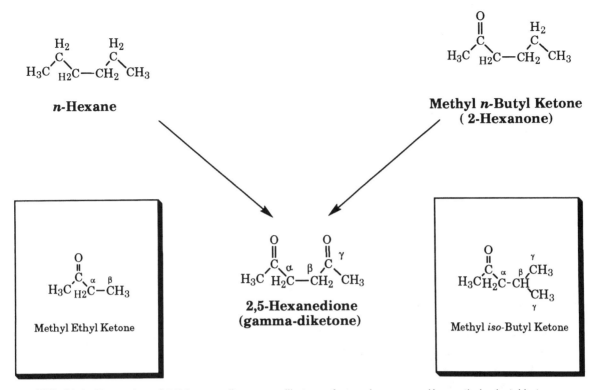

FIG. 16-1. Formation of 2,5-hexanedione, a γ-diketone, from *n*-hexane and/or methyl *n*-butyl ketone. The integral importance of a chemical's structure to the formation of a γ-diketone is shown. Methyl ethyl ketone is prevented from forming a γ-diketone because it does not have a third (γ) carbon atom. Methyl *iso*-butyl ketone has two carbon atoms in the γ position, but both are terminal; the carbonyl group of a ketone must be bound to two carbon atoms. Thus, because neither γ carbon of methyl *iso*-butyl ketone is bound to a second carbon atom, it too cannot form a γ-diketone; the principal metabolites of methyl *iso*-butyl ketone include 4-methyl-2-pentanol and 4-hydroxy-4-methyl-2-pentanone. These structural features are responsible for the relative differences in neurotoxicity of these four common industrial solvents.

M*n*BK exposure requires (a) that the longest continuous (parent) alkane chain contain at least six carbon atoms; and (b) that there is *in vivo* formation of a γ-diketone from the parent alkane or ketone (Spencer and Schaumburg, 1975; O'Donoghue and Krasavage, 1979; Sickles, 1989; Graham et al., 1995) (Fig. 16-1).

Low levels of 2,5-hexanedione have been detected in the urine and blood of unexposed persons; they appear to be partly derived from an endogenous metabolic source such as lipid peroxidation and partly from micropollution of ambient air (Perbellini et al., 1993). Monitoring of ambient air levels of *n*-hexane and M*n*BK can indicate risk of exposure and urinary levels of 2,5-hexanedione in persons at risk of exposure to exogenous sources of *n*-hexane and M*n*BK can reveal increases in body burden before the cumulative effects of continuing exposure leads to the development of clinically overt and persistent neurotoxic effects (Aiello et al., 1980; Barregård et al., 1991; Cardona et al., 1996).

SOURCES OF EXPOSURE

Occupational exposures to *n*-hexane and M*n*BK occur during petroleum production and refining; commercial production of *n*-hexane in 1992 was approximately 150 million kg (USITC, 1994). Once produced, *n*-hexane and M*n*BK are often mixed with other chemicals (e.g., MEK, methyl *iso*-butyl ketone, acetone, benzene, and toluene) for various uses (Altenkirch et al., 1977). Workers are exposed to *n*-hexane and M*n*BK during the manufacture and use of glues, inks, paints, paint thinners, plastics, rubber products, and polyethylene laminate (Yamada, 1964; Wickersham and Fredericks, 1976; Mallov, 1976; Saida et al., 1976; Jørgensen and Cohr, 1981; Pryor and Rebert, 1992). Cabinet makers are at risk of simultaneous exposure to multiple sources of *n*-hexane including glues, polyethylene laminates, and cleaning solvents (Yamada, 1964; Herskowitz et al., 1971; Oryshkevich et al., 1986). Exposure to M*n*BK occurs among workers involved in the manufacture of plastic-coated and color-printed fabrics (Billmaier et al., 1974; Allen et al., 1975). *n*-Hexane-containing glues are used during the manufacture and repairing of genuine and artificial leather goods such as shoes, boots, handbags, and luggage (Yamamura, 1969; Cianchetti et al., 1976; Cavalleri and Cosi, 1978; Bravaccio et al., 1981; Mutti et al., 1984; Murata et al., 1994). The water-resistant seams of some raincoats are created by bonding the fabric together with n-hexane-containing glues (Scelsi et al., 1980). Adhesives containing n-hexane are also used on adhesive tapes and bandages (Ruff et al., 1981; Jørgensen and Cohr, 1981). n-Hexane is used in the food industry to extract vegetable oils from seeds (Seppäläinen et al., 1979). Printers are exposed to solvents and inks that contain n-hexane (Wang et al., 1986; Chang, 1991). n-Hexane is commonly used as an ingredient in degreasing solutions (Takeuchi et al., 1975; Ono et al., 1982; Yokoyama et al., 1990). Gasoline typically contains 1.5% n-hexane (McDermott and Killiany, 1978). Petroleum benzine is a widely variable mixture of C_5 to C_9 hydrocarbons, paraffins, cycloparaffins, and aromatic hydrocarbons and contains at least 10% n-hexane (Takeuchi et al., 1975; Ono et al., 1982). Naphtha solutions contain n-hexane (Tenebein et al., 1984). Exposure to various mixed solvents has been associated with peripheral neuropathy, which often can be traced to their n-hexane content (Takeuchi et al., 1975; Vallat et al., 1981).

Hobbyists and repair-it-yourself persons are exposed to n-hexane and MnBK in glues, paints, solvents, and polyethylene laminates. Recreational inhalation of n-hexane-containing glues for the acute euphoric effects continues to be a problem among workers as well as others including young adults and children (Gonzalez and Downey, 1972; Goto et al., 1974; Shirabe et al., 1974; Altenkirch et al., 1977). Additional nonoccupational exposure to n-hexane occurs through consumption and use of contaminated water supplies (Beavers et al., 1996; EPA, 1996).

EXPOSURE LIMITS AND SAFETY REGULATIONS

n-Hexane

The odor detection threshold for n-hexane is 130 ppm, and therefore an individual detecting the odor of this solvent has already been exposed to significant ambient air concentrations (Amoore and Hautala, 1983). The *Occupational Safety and Health Administration's* (OSHA) permissible exposure limit (PEL) for n-hexane is an 8-hour time-weighted average (TWA) of 500 ppm (OSHA, 1995). The *National Institute for Occupational Safety and Health's* (NIOSH) recommended exposure limit (REL) for n-hexane is a 10-hour TWA exposure concentration of 50 ppm. NIOSH has recommended an immediately dangerous to life and health (IDLH) exposure limit for n-hexane of 1,100 ppm; this limit is based on the solvent's explosive properties (NIOSH, 1997). The *American Conference of Governmental Industrial Hygienists'* (ACGIH) recommended threshold limit value (TLV) for n-hexane is an 8-hour TWA of 50 ppm (ACGIH, 1995). Neither the OSHA, NIOSH, nor ACGIH has established short-term exposure limits for n-hexane (OSHA, 1995; NIOSH, 1997; ACGIH, 1995) (Table 16-1).

The *United States Environmental Protection Agency* (USEPA) has not established a maximum contamination level (MCL) for n-hexane in drinking water (EPA, 1996) (Table 16-1).

TABLE 16-1. *Established and recommended occupational and environmental exposure limits for n-hexanea in the air and water*

	Air (ppm)[a]	Water (mg/L)[a]
Odor threshold*	130	—
OSHA		
PEL (8-hr TWA)	500	—
STEL ceiling (15-min TWA)	—	—
NIOSH		
REL (10-hr TWA)	50	—
STEL (15-min TWA)	—	—
IDLH	1,100	—
ACGIH		
TLV (8-hr TWA)	50	—
USEPA		
MCL	—	—
MCLG	—	—
SMCL	—	—

[a]Unit conversion: 1 ppm = 3.53 mg/m³. 1 ppm = 1 mg/L.
OSHA, Occupational Safety and Health Administration; PEL, permissible exposure limit; TWA, time-weighted average; NIOSH, National Institute of Occupational Safety and Health; REL, recommended exposure limit; STEL, short-term exposure limit; IDLH, immediately dangerous to life or health; ACGIH, American Conference of Governmental Industrial Hygienists; TLV, threshold limit value; USEPA, U.S. Environmental Protection Agency; MCL, maximum contamination level; MCLG, maximum contamination level goal; SMCL, secondary MCL.
Data from *Amoore and Hautala, 1983; OSHA, 1995; ACGIH, 1995; USEPA, 1996; NIOSH, 1997.

TABLE 16-2. *Established and recommended occupational and environmental exposure limits for methyl n-butyl ketone in the air and water*

	Air (ppm)[a]	Water (mg/L)[a]
Odor threshold*	0.076	—
OSHA		
PEL (8-hr TWA)	100	—
STEL ceiling (15-min TWA)	—	—
NIOSH		
REL (10-hr TWA)	1	—
STEL (15-min TWA)	—	—
IDLH	1,600	—
ACGIH		
TLV (8-hr TWA)	5	—
USEPA		
MCL	—	—
MCLG	—	—
SMCL	—	—

Unit conversion: 1 ppm = 4.10 mg/m3; 1 ppm = 1 mg/L.
For abbreviations and unit conversion, see footnotes to Table 16-1.
Data from *Amoore and Hautala, 1983; OSHA, 1995;

Methyl *n*-Butyl Ketone

The odor detection threshold for M*n*BK is 0.076 ppm and therefore serves as an adequate warning of this solvent's presence in air (Amoore and Hautala, 1983). OSHA's PEL for M*n*BK is an 8-hour TWA of 100 ppm (OSHA, 1995). NIOSH's REL for M*n*BK is a 10-hour TWA exposure concentration of 1 ppm. NIOSH has recommended an IDLH exposure limit for M*n*BK of 1,600 ppm (NIOSH, 1997). The ACGIH's recommended TLV for M*n*BK is an 8-hour TWA of 5 ppm (ACGIH, 1995). Neither the OSHA, NIOSH, nor ACGIH has established short-term exposure limits for M*n*BK (OSHA, 1995; NIOSH, 1997; ACGIH, 1995) (Table 16-2).

The USEPA has not established an MCL for M*n*BK in drinking water (EPA, 1996) (Table 16-2).

METABOLISM

Tissue Absorption

Inhalation is the primary route of entry for *n*-hexane and M*n*BK vapors. Due to the relatively low blood/air partition coefficient of *n*-hexane, only about 20% of an inhaled dose of *n*-hexane vapor is absorbed across the pulmonary alveoli and into the systemic circulation; because of its low solubility in the blood, 80% of an inhaled dose of *n*-hexane is immediately exhaled unchanged (Brugnone et al., 1978; Jørgensen and Cohr, 1981; Veulemans et al., 1982; Mutti et al., 1984; Perbellini et al., 1985; Filser et al., 1996). In contrast, approximately 85% of an inhaled dose of M*n*BK is retained in humans (DiVincenzo et al., 1978). Total pulmonary absorption of *n*-hexane and M*n*BK is related to the ambient air concentration of the particular solvent, the duration of exposure and the individual's pulmonary ventilation rate. The proportion retained of an inhaled dose of both solvents decreases as the pulmonary ventilation rate increases and as body tissue absorption approaches saturation (Böhlen et al., 1973; Baker and Rickert, 1981; Veulemans et al., 1982).

n-Hexane and M*n*BK are both liquids at room temperature. Following oral intake, *n*-hexane and M*n*BK are readily absorbed through the gastrointestinal mucosa (Krasavage et al., 1980). The pharmacokinetics of gastrointestinal absorption were studied in two human volunteers who ingested ¹⁴C-labeled M*n*BK dissolved in corn oil. Approximately 40% of the radioactive material was exhaled as carbon dioxide, and 25% was excreted in the urine; specific urinary metabolites were not reported in this study (DiVincenzo et al., 1978) (see Excretion section). A single oral dose (2,000 mg/kg) of *n*-hexane produced mild weakness, which persisted for 2 to 4 days in hens (Abou-Donia et al., 1982). Peripheral neuropathy was reported in a 28-year-old man following the ingestion of petroleum benzine solution, which also contained *n*-hexane. The patient thought that the solution would cure gonorrhea, and he had been swallowing a mouthful twice a day for 5 weeks, when he began to notice weakness of his legs and arms. The leg weakness

progressed, and muscle atrophy due to denervation became evident several weeks later, despite discontinuation of exposure. His condition stabilized, and gradual improvement was seen over the ensuing months, leaving a slight permanent weakness in his legs (Schwarz, 1933).

Dermal absorption of liquid *n*-hexane and M*n*BK is affected by the duration of exposure, as well as the size and condition of any exposed areas of skin, and it contributes to the individual's total exposure dose (DiVincenzo et al., 1978; Jakobson et al., 1982; Tsuruta, 1982; Lodén, 1986; Cardona et al., 1993). The rate of dermal absorption for M*n*BK in two volunteers ranged from 4.8 to 8.0 $\mu g/cm^2/hr$, indicating that significant dermal absorption of M*n*BK occurs in humans (DiVincenzo et al., 1978). The use of protective clothing such as gloves significantly decreases dermal absorption of these two solvents and thus reduces the individual's total exposure dose. For example, biological monitoring of shoe factory workers exposed to *n*-hexane revealed significantly higher levels of 2,5-hexanedione in those workers who did not wear gloves, indicating that additional absorption of *n*-hexane occurred through the skin of those without gloves (Cardona et al., 1993) (Fig. 16-2).

Tissue Distribution

n-Hexane and M*n*BK are both lipophilic aliphatic hydrocarbon compounds. Their distribution in the various tissues of the body correlates closely with the lipid content as well as the extent of the blood perfusion of the particular tissue (Böhlen et al., 1973). Both solvents readily cross the blood–brain barrier (Böhlen et al., 1973; Granvil et al.,

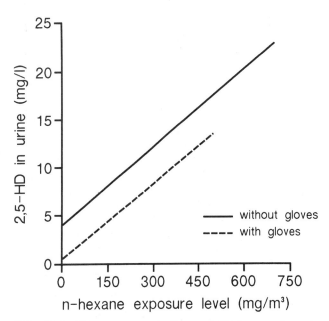

FIG. 16-2. Urinary concentrations of 2,5-hexanedione in workers with and without direct dermal exposure to *n*-hexane. (Data from Cardona et al., 1993, with permission.)

1994; Masotto et al., 1995). Equilibrium is reached most rapidly in well-perfused and lipid-rich tissues such as the kidneys, spleen, brain, and muscles; the less well-perfused tissues such as adipose tissue require significantly more time to reach saturation (Böhlen et al., 1973; Baker and Rickert, 1981; Veulemans et al., 1982). The concentration of hexane (i.e., *n*-hexane plus its isomers) in the liver increases throughout the exposure period and reflects a consequent increase in the lipid content of this particular tissue (Böhlen et al., 1973) (Fig. 16-3). Following exposure, *n*-hexane is redistributed to the less well-perfused adipose tissue (Böhlen et al., 1973; Baker and Rickert, 1981). Elimination is also slower from adipose tissue; the half-life for *n*-hexane in adipose tissue is approximately 64 hours (Perbellini et al., 1986). During chronic exposures, *n*-hexane and MnBK as well as their metabolites accumulate in adipose tissue, from which they are then gradually released (DiVincenzo et al., 1978; Iwata et al., 1983; Ahonen and Schimberg, 1988; Cardona et al., 1993) (see Excretion section). That *n*-hexane and its metabolites accumulate in the body during chronic exposures was demonstrated by serial biological monitoring studies of *n*-hexane-exposed workers (Cardona et al., 1993). The ratio of urinary excretion of 2,5-hexanedione to *n*-hexane exposure concentration gradually increased during the workweek as *n*-hexane

and its metabolites accumulated in the exposed workers; the increase in the ratio was less marked in those workers who wore gloves to prevent dermal absorption (Fig. 16-4). The 2,5-hexanedione in human blood and other tissues is not conjugated and thus can react with cellular macromolecules (Perbellini et al., 1993; Graham et al., 1995).

n-Hexane levels increase rapidly within peripheral nerve fibers (Baker and Rickert, 1981). Levels of 2-hexanol were higher in the brain than in the blood of mice exposed to MnBK, suggesting that MnBK is metabolized to 2-hexanol in the brain (Granvil et al., 1994). The metabolite 2,5-hexanedione is electrophilic and thus can covalently bind to the nucleophilic centers of neurofilaments in the axoplasm (Graham et al., 1995). A consistent increase of 2,5-hexanedione was found in the striatum and cerebellum of mice at 0.5 and 2 hours following intraperitoneal injection of *n*-hexane and 2,5-hexanedione. A decline to baseline was observed after 24 hours (Masotto et al., 1995).

Although few reports have described the quantitative distribution of *n*-hexane and MnBK or their metabolites in the CNS, certain findings do provide evidence of alterations in neurochemical activity and thus indicate the presence of these compounds in particular CNS areas. For example, the finding in mice of increased striatal dopamine and homovanillic acid levels, along with a significant increase of striatal synaptosomal dopamine uptake after intraperitoneal injection of *n*-hexane and 2,5-hexanedione suggests a dopamine-releasing effect on dopaminergic terminals in this area (Masotto et al., 1995). The distribution of *n*-hexane within the brain can also be deduced from various clinical manifestations and experimental results including (a) indirect evidence of cortical and limbic system involvement derived from reports of inebriation, sedation, and euphoria, associated with acute *n*-hexane exposure; (b) the occurrence of parkinsonism, as well as positron emission tomography scan evidence of a reduction of D_2 dopamine receptors in the caudate nucleus and putamen, and also glucose metabolism abnormalities indicative of a possible postsynaptic dopaminergic effect of *n*-hexane exposure, suggesting an effect in the basal ganglia (Pezzoli et al., 1995); (c) an increase in glutamine content of the midbrain of the rat following short-term exposure to *n*-hexane (Honma et al., 1982); (d) a significant decrease in the integrated amplitudes of brainstem auditory evoked potentials after *n*-hexane exposure, indicating a central site of action (Pryor and Rebert, 1992); and (e) involvement of hypothalamic and brainstem centers of autonomic nervous system function, suggested by reports of changes in the electrocardiogram and R-R interval variability in humans exposed to *n*-hexane (Murata et al., 1994) (see Neuropathological Diagnosis section).

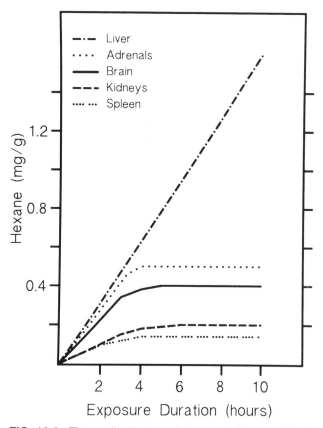

FIG. 16-3. Tissue distribution of hexane (*n*-hexane plus its isomers) in rats. (Data from Böhlen et al., 1973, with permission.)

Tissue Biochemistry

After absorption, the metabolism of *n*-hexane and MnBK is primarily hepatic; metabolism also occurs in other tissues including the brain (Baker and Rickert, 1981;

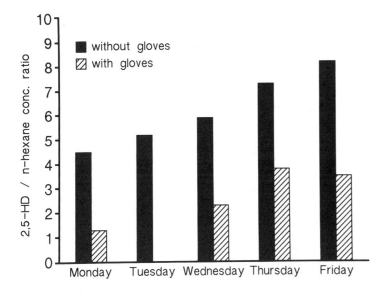

FIG. 16-4. Ratio between 2,5-hexanedione in urine and *n*-hexane exposure concentration, showing proportionate accumulation increases over a workweek of exposure. (From Cardona et al., 1993, with permission.)

Granvil et al., 1994). Approximately 90% of an absorbed dose of *n*-hexane is oxidized to 2-hexanol via the cytochrome P-450 metabolic pathway in humans; the high yield of 2-hexanol may account for the acute narcotic effects of *n*-hexane (Kramer et al., 1974) (Fig. 16-5). 2-Hexanol is further oxidized by cytochrome P-450 to 2,5-hexanediol. An alternative, but less significant, biochemical pathway involving alcohol dehydrogenase-mediated oxidation (i.e., the loss of a hydrogen atom) of the OH group of 2-hexanol also exists and leads to the formation of 2-hexanone, also known as M*n*BK; the reverse reaction (i.e., reduction of M*n*BK) also occurs, and thus 2-hexanol is principally a metabolite of M*n*BK (Sharkawi et al., 1994; Granvil et al., 1994). 2,5-Hexanediol and M*n*BK are both metabolized to 5-hydroxy-2-hexanone, which is metabolized primarily to 4,5-dihydroxy-2-hexanone and to a lesser extent to 2,5-hexanedione (Kramer et al., 1974; DiVincenzo et al., 1976; Abdel-Rahman et al., 1976; Granvil et al., 1994). 4,5-Dihydroxy-2-hexanone is subsequently conjugated with glucuronic acid and is the major urinary metabolite of *n*-hexane and M*n*BK in humans (DiVincenzo et al., 1977, 1978; Fedtke and Bolt, 1987; Perbellini et al., 1993) (see Excretion and Biochemical Diagnosis sections).

The acute narcotic effects of *n*-hexane and M*n*BK are most likely due to the action of their common metabolite, 2-hexanol, which is an aliphatic alcohol with demonstrated general anesthetic properties (Alifimoff et al., 1987; Arakawa et al., 1992; Granvil et al., 1994; Sharkawi et al., 1994; Forman et al., 1995). The more persistent neurological effects of *n*-hexane and M*n*BK are related to the ability of their mutual metabolite, 2,5-hexanedione, a γ-diketone, to cross-link axonal neurofilaments chemically and to interrupt axonal transport mechanisms (Schaumburg and Spencer, 1978; Sickles, 1989; St. Clair et al., 1989; Pyle et al., 1992, 1993; Granvil et al., 1994; Graham et al., 1995; Filser et al., 1996). How-

ever, due to the structure of the parent compound and the associated pharmacokinetics, M*n*BK produces less acute narcotic effects and is significantly more neurotoxic than *n*-hexane (Krasavage et al., 1980; Spencer et al., 1980) (see Clinical Manifestations and Diagnosis and Neuropathological Diagnosis sections).

Simultaneous exposures to other chemicals can enhance or inhibit the metabolism of *n*-hexane and/or M*n*BK. Exposure to ethanol and M*n*BK has been shown to have an additive acute depressant effect on CNS functioning, possibly due to competition between 2-hexanol and ethanol for alcohol dehydrogenase (Sharkawi et al., 1994). Chronic exposure to chemicals that induce cytochrome P-450 activity, such as ethanol, phenobarbital, and MEK, enhances the metabolism of *n*-hexane and M*n*BK, thus increasing the production of 2,5-hexanedione (Abdel-Rahman et al., 1976; Couri et al., 1977; Robertson et al., 1989). MEK also appears to interfere with the formation of 4,5-dihydroxy-2-hexanone, thereby further increasing blood and tissue levels of 2,5-hexanedione and consequently potentiating the neurotoxic effects of *n*-hexane and M*n*BK (Ralston et al., 1985; Fedtke and Bolt, 1987) (Fig. 16-5). Benzene derivatives such as toluene and xylene inhibit the metabolism of *n*-hexane and thus reduce the production of 2,5-hexanedione and decrease the neurotoxic effects of *n*-hexane (Takeuchi et al., 1981; Perbellini et al., 1982; Iwata et al., 1984; Pryor and Rebert, 1992; Cardona et al., 1993; Nylén et al., 1994; Nylén and Hagman, 1994).

Additive neurological effects occur following simultaneous exposures to two or more γ-diketones. The effects of simultaneous exposures to *n*-hexane and M*n*BK are additive. Furthermore, although chemically dissimilar, compounds such as carbon disulfide also react with the nucleophilic centers of cellular proteins, resulting in adduct formation and the chemical cross-linking of axonal neurofilaments. The formation of neurofilament-filled axonal

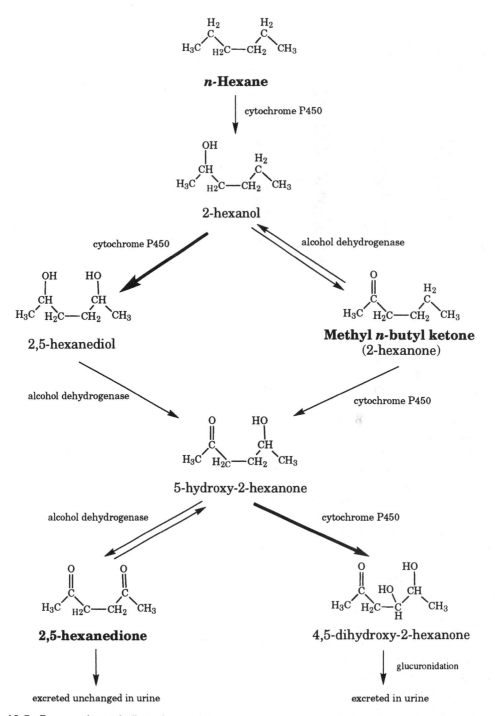

FIG. 16-5. Proposed metabolic pathways for *n*-hexane and methyl *n*-butyl ketone. (Data from Kramer et al., 1974, DiVincenzo et al., 1976, Abdel-Rahman et al., 1976, Perbellini et al., 1981b, 1993, Fedtke and Bolt, 1987, and Granvil et al., 1994.)

swellings occurs following exposure to either carbon disulfide or 2,5-hexanedione; this similar outcome of exposure with accumulation of cross-linked neurofilaments and associated axonal transport abnormalities makes concurrent exposures to carbon disulfide and *n*-hexane and/or M*n*BK synergistic in their neurotoxic effects (Anthony et al., 1983; Graham et al., 1995).

Excretion

n-*Hexane*

Approximately 10% of an absorbed dose of *n*-hexane is exhaled unchanged (Mutti et al., 1984; Periago et al., 1993). Elimination of unchanged *n*-hexane from the lungs in humans is biphasic, with median half-times for the fast and slow components of approximately 10 and 100 minutes, respectively (Veulemans et al., 1982; Mutti et al., 1984).

Approximately 90% of an absorbed dose of *n*-hexane is metabolized and excreted in the urine as 4,5-dihydroxy-2-hexanone glucuronide; 2,5-dimethylfuran and γ-valerolactone, which have been reported as metabolites in previous studies, appear to be artifacts of urine sample analysis (Perbellini et al., 1981b; Governa et al., 1987; Fedtke and Bolt, 1987; Perbellini et al., 1993). Less than 5% is excreted as 2,5-hexanedione (unconjugated), and only 1% is excreted as 2-hexanol glucuronide in humans (Baker and Rickert, 1981; Mutti et al., 1984; Fedtke and Bolt, 1987; Perbellini et al., 1981b, 1993; Periago et al., 1993; van Engelen et al., 1995; Filser et al., 1996). Other minor urinary metabolites of *n*-hexane in humans include unchanged *n*-hexane, 1- and 3-hexanol, and M*n*BK (Perbellini et al., 1981a,b; Baker and Rickert, 1981; Imbriani et al., 1984; Mutti et al., 1984; Fedtke and Bolt, 1987; Cardona et al., 1993).

The half-life for *n*-hexane in adipose tissue was estimated by a physiologically based pharmacokinetic model to be 64 hours, indicating that at least 10 days without exposure is required for complete elimination of the body burden (Perbellini et al., 1986). Biological monitoring of shoe factory workers exposed to *n*-hexane documented increased urinary excretion of 2,5-hexanedione at the end of the workweek compared with the beginning, suggesting that chronic exposure results in accumulation of *n*-hexane and its metabolites (Cardona et al.,1993) (Fig. 16-4).

Simultaneous acute and chronic exposures to various chemicals, such as ethanol, MEK, and toluene, can increase or decrease excretion of 2,5-hexanedione as well as other urinary metabolites of *n*-hexane, depending on how they affect *n*-hexane metabolism (Ralston et al., 1985; Robertson et al., 1989; Shibata et al., 1990; Sharkawi et al., 1994; Nylén et al., 1994; Nylén and Hagman, 1994). For example, exposure to MEK induces microsomal enzyme activity and thus enhances the *in vivo* formation of 2,5 hexanedione. Furthermore, MEK has also been shown to inhibit the formation of 4,5-dihydroxy-2-hexanone, thereby decreasing urinary excretion of 4,5-dihydroxy-2-hexanone while further increasing blood and urine levels of 2,5-hexanedione (Ralston et al., 1985; Fedtke and Bolt, 1987) (see Tissue Biochemistry section).

Methyl n-Butyl Ketone

Approximately 5% of an oral dose is exhaled by rats unchanged (DiVincenzo et al., 1977). After oral ingestion of ^{14}C-labeled M*n*BK by human volunteers, approximately 40% was metabolized and exhaled as radioactive carbon dioxide. Pulmonary elimination of radioactive carbon dioxide reached a peak 4 hours after ingestion, after which it slowly decreased. Maximum urinary excretion of M*n*BK occurred from 24 to 48 hours after ingestion of radioactive

liquid M*n*BK in human volunteers. Approximately 25% of the oral dose was excreted in the urine during the first 8 days after exposure. Thus, only 65% of the radioactivity, as radioactive metabolites derived from the ingested ^{14}C-labeled M*n*BK, was excreted 8 days after ingestion. This suggests that chronic exposure to this solvent may lead to accumulation of M*n*BK and increased blood levels of its neurotoxic metabolite 2,5-hexanedione (DiVincenzo et al., 1978). The urinary metabolites of M*n*BK in humans include 2-hexanol, 5-hydroxy-2-hexanone, 4,5-dihydroxy-2-hexanone, and 2,5-hexanedione (Abdel-Rahman et al., 1976; DiVincenzo et al., 1978; Fedtke and Bolt, 1987; Bos et al., 1991; Perbellini et al., 1993). Rats exposed to M*n*BK excreted 22% as 2-hexanol, 21% as 5-hydroxy-2-hexanone, and 14% as 2,5-hexanedione (De Rosa et al., 1977).

Simultaneous acute and chronic exposures to other chemicals, such as phenobarbital and MEK, will increase urinary excretion of 2,5-hexanedione. Phenobarbital enhances the metabolism of M*n*BK by induction of cytochrome P-450 enzymes, resulting in increased urinary excretion of 5-hydroxy-2-hexanone, 4,5-dihydroxy-2-hexanone, and 2,5-hexanedione. MEK also induces microsomal enzyme activity and thus enhances the in vivo formation of 2,5-hexanedione, but MEK also inhibits the next step in the metabolic pathway, which is the formation of 4,5-dihydroxy-2-hexanone, thereby decreasing urinary excretion of 4,5-dihydroxy-2-hexanone and further increasing blood and urine levels of the toxic metabolite 2,5-hexanedione (Abdel-Rahman et al., 1976; Couri et al., 1977; Ralston et al., 1985; Fedtke and Bolt, 1987) (see Tissue Biochemistry section).

CLINICAL MANIFESTATIONS AND DIAGNOSIS

Symptomatic Diagnosis

n-*Hexane*

Acute Exposure

Acute inhalation of *n*-hexane produces transient dizziness, euphoria, and anesthetic effects, which are probably due to 2-hexanol, an aliphatic alcohol and a principal metabolite of *n*-hexane (Nelson et al., 1943; Korobkin et al., 1975; Haydon et al., 1977a,b). Acute experimental exposure of human volunteers to 1,500 ppm of *n*-hexane produced irritation of the ocular, nasal, and pharyngeal mucous membranes, and then headache and nausea (Drinker et al., 1943). Dizziness and euphoria were reported by volunteers exposed to 5,000 ppm of *n*-hexane vapor for 10 minutes (Patty and Yant, 1929). The euphoric, exhilarating, and (rarely) hallucinogenic effects of *n*-hexane exposure are transient, developing rapidly during inhalation and quickly subsiding following cessation of exposure. The apparent promptness of reversibility of the acute effects of *n*-hexane may lead an exposed person to believe that brief exposure to high levels are harmless. For this reason, abuse of *n*-

hexane for recreational purposes is a common problem; unfortunately, these recurrent episodes of inhalation often produce neurological damage. The acute encephalopathic effects associated with glue and/or lacquer sniffing ("huffing") may also be partly due to the other volatile organic compounds such as toluene and acetone, which are frequently constituents of the solvent mixtures used in these products; therefore clinicians treating solvent abusers should make an effort to identify the constituents of the solvent(s) used in the various brands of glue, thinner, or paint most frequently abused by the patient (Prockop et al., 1974; Channer, 1983; Cardona et al., 1996) (see Toluene chapter).

Chronic Exposure

Sensorimotor polyneuropathy is a common result of prolonged and/or repeated exposure to n-hexane and MnBK (Yamada, 1964; Allen et al., 1975; Yamamura, 1969; Iida et al., 1969; Herskowitz et al., 1971; Spencer et al., 1980; Passero et al., 1983; Oryshkevich et al., 1986; Yokoyama et al., 1990). Following a sufficient level of exposure to these chemicals, an exposed individual gradually experiences weakness and/or numbness and paresthesias in the distal extremities (Iida et al., 1969; Ruff et al., 1981; Wang et al., 1986; Chang, 1990). The severity of the peripheral neuropathy and the accompanying clinical signs and symptoms are related to the intensity, duration, and frequency of recurrence of exposure (see Neurophysiological Diagnosis section). Motor symptoms appear with continuing low-level exposure or recurrent episodic exposures to higher concentrations (Allen et al., 1975; Shirabe et al., 1974; Yokoyama et al., 1990). Inability to walk on heels due to extensor weakness results in bilateral footdrop and an awkward, slapping gait. Neurogenic atrophy of affected muscles becomes apparent more distally than proximally in the extremities, initially in the feet and then in the hands (Wang et al., 1986; Chang, 1990; Yokoyama et al., 1990).

Cessation of exposure is followed by a period of continued worsening of symptoms before stabilization and the beginning of a long course of clinical improvement (Yamada, 1964; Yamamura, 1969; Chang, 1990; Yokoyama et al., 1990). The progression of symptoms following cessation of exposure to n-hexane and/or MnBK reflects the continued "dying back" of axons associated with the covalent binding of 2,5-hexanedione to neurofilaments and the concomitant impairment of axonal transport mechanisms responsible for maintenance of normal cellular functioning (Spencer et al., 1980; Graham et al., 1995). Complete recovery from profound peripheral neuropathy is unlikely (see Neuropathological Diagnosis and Clinical Experiences sections).

Employees in shoe factories and home-based shoe workers ($n = 654$), who were known to be using n-hexane-containing glue, were surveyed for symptoms and signs of the effects of exposure to n-hexane (Passero et al., 1983). Ninety-eight symptomatic workers were identified from the total of 654 exposed persons. Recurrent acute symptoms included headache, nausea or vomiting, epigastric pain, insomnia, irritability, and dizziness preceding the emergence of numbness, tingling, and weakness of the extremities that developed in those workers with more prolonged exposures. Initial neurological manifestations included slowly developing weakness and/or paresthesia of feet and then hands. Painful cramps were reported before overt weakness of muscles became obvious. The weakness and atrophy of distal muscles in the limbs extended proximally in the more severe cases. Some patients experienced truncal weakness with involvement of respiratory muscles. Sensory findings on examination were bilaterally symmetrical and were limited to feet and hands. Rarely numbness extended to the forearms, although numbness extended to the level of the head of the fibula in the legs when the distal upper extremities were affected. Loss of sensation of touch and painful stimulation by pinprick was usually present; vibratory and position sense was impaired only when the patient had been severely affected by exposure. All workers were subjected to motor nerve conduction velocity and electromyographic studies. The results of the various clinical and electrophysiological tests were scored and divided into three groups according to the severity of neuropathy. Group I, moderately to severely affected, consisted of 16 of 98 workers, all of whom had extensive clinical and electrodiagnostic evidence of peripheral neuropathy; group II, mildly affected, included 45 of 98 who had a lower score but still showed clinical signs and had electrodiagnostic confirmation of peripheral neuropathy; and group III, minimally affected, included those 37 remaining workers who had no clinical neurological signs but did exhibit characteristic electrodiagnostic evidence of peripheral neuropathy.

Blurred vision was among the initial symptoms reported by 12 of 39 patients diagnosed with peripheral neuropathy following exposure to n-hexane (Yamamura, 1969). Ophthalmological studies in these patients revealed seven with constricted visual fields, two with optic nerve atrophy, and one with retrobulbar neuritis. Maculopathy and color discrimination deficits have also been reported in workers chronically exposed to n-hexane (Raitta et al., 1978; Seppäläinen et al., 1979; Wang et al., 1986).

The CNS may also be damaged by chronic exposure to n-hexane (Spencer et al., 1980). Muscle cramps, residual spasticity, and hyperactive deep tendon reflexes are often seen in patients after chronic exposure, suggesting that irreversible damage to the long tracts of the spinal cord has occurred in these patients (Chang, 1990). However, Chang (1990) and Dimitrijevic (1985) have suggested that some of these phenomena, particularly the spasticity, may also reflect increased peripheral stimulation related to recovery of peripheral nervous system function. Parkinsonism has also been reported following exposure to n-hexane (Pezzoli et al., 1995) (see Clinical Experiences section).

Methyl n-Butyl Ketone

Acute Exposure

Acute symptoms are difficult to blame on a single ingredient associated with exposure to spray paint because of the various pigments and thinners found in the commonly used paints (Dick, 1995). Methyl *n*-butyl ketone is a common solvent found in spray paints and plasticizers. Symptoms associated with acute exposure to pure M*n*BK are less marked than those seen following exposure to pure *n*-hexane; a possible explanation is that 2-hexanol is not an obligatory metabolite of M*n*BK biotransformation and thus less 2-hexanol is formed during exposure to M*n*BK (Fig. 16-5). Nevertheless, exposure to high concentrations of M*n*BK does produce acute narcosis (Spencer et al., 1975). When spray painting is done out of doors, in well-ventilated areas, or while wearing a respirator, inhalation of vapors and the occurrence of acute effects should be minimal. However, under conditions of poor ventilation, acute symptoms do occur and include mucous membrane irritation, headache, and dizziness. The effects of acute exposure by inhalation are typically not sufficiently noxious or narcotic for workers to heed them as early warning signs of a possibly hazardous situation. It is often not until after recurrent inhalation exposures to M*n*BK and/or multiple episodes of dermal absorption related to its use to remove paint from skin produces clinical effects that workers become aware of the potential toxicity of the materials. Symptoms usually appear 2 to 3 months after initial contact and include emerging signs of peripheral neuropathy, essentially the features of chronic neurotoxicity (Billmaier et al., 1974; Allen et al., 1975; Saida et al., 1976).

Chronic Exposure

Chronic exposure to M*n*BK produces neuropathy sooner and at lower exposure levels than does *n*-hexane (Krasavage et al., 1980). An outbreak of peripheral neuropathy in a color-printed plastic fabric factory brought attention to the danger (Billmaier et al., 1974; Allen et al., 1975). The clinical manifestations in workers appeared insidiously over weeks and months, causing progressive weakness of the hands and feet and resulting in significant impairment of fine motor control and walking. Loss of sensation in the distal limbs accompanies the motor involvement but progresses at a slower rate. Sensation of crude touch, pain, and temperature are usually more affected than vibration and position senses. Severe fatigue, weight loss, and muscle atrophy follow, progressing after cessation of exposure. Recovery with minimal deficit follows in most cases, but in others residual disabilities due to the effects of severe denervation atrophy and associated muscle weakness persist indefinitely; in some severe cases signs of spasticity are also seen.

The clinical pictures of the neuropathy as well as the histopathology of M*n*BK and *n*-hexane are identical. Histological evidence of peripheral neuropathy in animals experimentally exposed to M*n*BK includes a gradual accumulation of neurofilaments in the proximal paranodal region, which causes axonal swelling and secondary localized thinning of the myelin sheath (Krasavage et al., 1980). Similar changes were identified in the sural nerve biopsy from a patient with prolonged occupational exposure to M*n*BK (Saida et al., 1976) (see Neuropathological Diagnosis section).

Histopathological studies also show accumulation of neurofilamentous axonal masses in humans (i.e., giant axonal neuropathy) exposed to acrylamide and carbon disulfide (Davenport et al., 1976; Graham et al., 1995). Thus, the similar clinical appearance of the effects of chronic exposure to several industrial chemicals (*n*-hexane, M*n*BK, carbon disulfide, and acrylamide) makes it necessary for the clinician to consider the chronological pattern derived from a time line of materials usage, the specific contents of each product, and the approximate point in time of emergence of symptoms in relation to documented exposure to suspected neurotoxicants. In addition, elimination of other confounding illnesses and/or concomitant nonoccupational exposures must be identified before a specific causal diagnosis such as exposure to M*n*BK can be made. For example, Saida et al. (1976) reported on a case of M*n*BK-induced neuropathy in a spray painter who also had a history of lead exposure and an increased body burden of lead. The diagnosis of M*n*BK versus lead neuropathy was established by a sural nerve biopsy that showed the typical accumulation of neurofilaments associated with exposure to a γ-diketone. A subsequent review of materials data sheets and the chronological relationship between the patient's exposure history and his development of symptoms allowed identification of the neurotoxicant, confirming that in this case M*n*BK was responsible for the patient's neurologic illness (see Clinical Experiences section).

Neurophysiological Diagnosis

Electrodiagnostic studies have been used to document the central and peripheral nervous system effects of *n*-hexane and M*n*BK.

n-Hexane

Electroencephalography (EEG) did not reveal abnormalities in volunteers acutely exposed to *n*-hexane at concentrations of 2,000 to 3,000 ppm for durations of 10 to 30 minutes (Seppäläinen et al., 1979, 1980). However, EEG studies in seven boot workers who developed peripheral neuropathy following chronic exposure to *n*-hexane revealed abnormalities in six of the seven workers (Battistini et al., 1975). Follow-up electrophysiological studies showed marked improvements in peripheral and central nervous system functioning in three workers. The EEGs had worsened in the three workers who had shown the most severe clinical and electrophysiological evidence of peripheral neuropathy at the initial examination; the electromyography and nerve conduction studies in these workers showed marked improvements. These findings suggest that chronic exposure to n-hexane damages the CNS and the PNS.

Visual evoked potentials (VEPs) were measured in a group of 15 workers aged 30 to 65 years (mean: 46 years) who had been exposed to n-hexane for durations of 5 to 21 years (mean: 12 years) and were compared with those of 10 unexposed control subjects (Sepäläinen et al., 1979). This study revealed an overall decrease in VEP amplitude among the exposed subjects. However, an augmentation of the early phase of the evoked potentials was also seen, possibly due to a release from inhibition. In addition, the latencies of the P1 and N1 components were prolonged. In a similar study, Chang (1987) measured VEPs in 22 workers exposed to n-hexane for less than 1 to 25 years (mean: 5.8 years) and found prolonged N1, P1, and N2 latencies and prolonged N1–N2 interpeak latencies. Significant decreases in N1–P1 and P1–N2 interpeak amplitudes were also found. Other potential causes of these findings such as idiopathic maculopathy and optic neuritis were excluded. The findings of these two studies suggest that n-hexane exposure produces a conduction block in the visual system possibly due to lesions located before the geniculate bodies, possibly in the intracerebral axons (Seppäläinen et al., 1979; Chang, 1987).

Sensory evoked potentials (SEP) have also been used to document subclinical CNS effects of n-hexane. Mutti et al. (1982) performed SEP studies in n-hexane-exposed workers and found lower amplitude SEP peaks, which were attributed to central blocks within spinal cord tracts. Increased P-15 latencies in these workers were attributed to peripheral neuropathy. These SEP findings suggest that exposure to n-hexane may produce spinal cord pathology as well as peripheral neuropathy (Schaumburg and Spencer 1976; Chang, 1987).

Bravaccio et al. (1981) demonstrated an increased excitability of α-motor neurons by studying the *H-reflex*, confirming that n-hexane affects the pyramidal system as well as the peripheral nerves. Similar findings were reported by Battistini et al. (1975), and neuropathological evidence of the effects of n-hexane on the spinal cord has been demonstrated by Schaumburg and Spencer (1976) (see Neuropathological Diagnosis section).

Nerve conduction velocity (NCS) *studies* can be used to document cases of overt peripheral neuropathy and to detect subclinical damage to nerve fibers early in the course of exposure before the exposed individual develops clinical symptoms and signs that may not be entirely reversible (Pastore et al., 1994). Nerve conduction studies reveal diminished amplitude of sensory nerve action potentials and slowed sensory and motor nerve conduction velocities

(NCV) in the distal extremities of n-hexane-exposed individuals (Korobkin et al., 1975; Mutti et al., 1982; Yokoyama et al., 1990; Chang, 1991; Pastore et al.,1994). Pastore et al. (1994) used NCV studies to detect subclinical neuropathy in a group of 20 asymptomatic workers with chronic exposure to n-hexane documented by elevated urine levels of 2,5-hexanedione. Significant reductions in the amplitude of sensory nerve action potentials were found in the sural, ulnar, and median nerves in five (25%) of these workers, indicating axonal damage. In addition, the reductions in sensory nerve action potential amplitude correlated significantly with the duration of exposure to n-hexane.

Motor distal latencies frequently stabilize soon after removal from exposure and often return to normal before the more proximal NCV. The recovery of distal latencies reflect preservation of the more distal portions of the motor nerve fibers (Chang, 1990). Slowing of NCVs and prolongation of distal latencies reflect secondary demyelination-associated swelling of the paranodal regions (Chang, 1991). Wang et al. (1986) performed sensory and motor NCV studies on 54 printshop workers (mean age: 25.8 years) exposed to n-hexane at ambient air vapor concentrations of up to 190 ppm for a mean duration of 5.8 years (range: less than 1 to 25 years). The mean length of exposure among these workers was only 1.5 years (range: less than 1 to 5 years), and the mean age was only 19 years (range: 16 to 29 years); none of these workers had a history of diabetes mellitus or alcoholism. Seventeen of the 54 workers had significant slowing of motor and sensory NCVs in the median, ulnar, tibial, and peroneal nerves. Fifteen of these 17 workers also had clinically overt signs and symptoms of peripheral neuropathy. Serial NCV studies were made in 11 of these same workers, after their removal from exposure (Chang, 1991). A further reduction in sensory and motor nerve NCVs was seen in 5 of the 11 workers at 5 and 10 months after cessation of exposure, indicating that the neuropathy had continued to progress after removal from further exposure. By contrast, distal latencies did not worsen during this time. Motor NCVs in the median, ulnar, peroneal, and sural nerves were improved but remained significantly reduced below laboratory normal values at the final follow-up examination performed 4 years after cessation of exposure. Distal motor latencies and sensory NCV studies were normal at this time. These findings indicate that motor fibers are more vulnerable to the effects of n-hexane and that damage to these fibers persists at least 4 years after cessation of exposure. This author has observed persistence of weakness and sensory loss in a patient as long as 12 years after the end of exposure (see Clinical Experiences section).

A computer model capable of estimating the proportion of fast and slow fibers responsible for an electrically evoked compound nerve action potential has been used to determine noninvasively which populations of fibers have been affected by exposures to neurotoxicants (Sax et al.,

1981). Yokoyama et al. (1990) applied this method to model the distribution of nerve conduction velocities in three young (age range: 23 to 27 years) male precision grinders who worked in a jet engine factory. These men had developed symptoms and signs of peripheral neuropathy over six months while they were exposed to a degreasing solvent containing 95% n-hexane. A sample of the ambient air in the work area showed an n-hexane concentration of 195 ppm (687 mg/m³), but exposure to higher concentrations during specific job tasks was common (see Clinical Experiences section). The distribution of conduction velocities (DCVs) was determined in the sural nerves of the three exposed workers and compared with an unexposed control group of 11 men aged 23 to 40 years. In each case, comparison of the initial DCV studies with follow-up studies performed several months after cessation of exposure showed a relative improvement in the DCV. In one patient, a 27-year-old man, a computer-generated histogram of the DCVs was made 2 months after cessation of exposure and revealed a shift in the DCV reflecting a change in the fiber distribution, with smaller slower fibers contributing more to the conduction velocity (Fig. 16-6). In addition, DCV studies indicated a loss of nerve fibers with conduction velocities greater than 50 m/sec. The DCV was also calculated from the actual nerve fiber diameters following a sural nerve biopsy. The computerized DCV studies correlated significantly with the predicted DCV calculated from the morphological changes seen in the sural nerve biopsy, which showed a marked loss of large myelinated fibers and a mild decrease in the number of smaller myelinated fibers (see Fig. 16-6 and Neuropathological Diagnosis section). These findings indicate that the loss of large myelinated fibers contributed significantly to the slowing of conduction velocities. DCV was again per-

formed on this patient 36 months after he had been removed from exposure to n-hexane; the histogram showed a shift back toward a more normal distribution. The DCV studies also indicated that conduction velocities had returned to normal limits in those fibers with conduction velocities less than 80 m/sec but that conduction velocity in the fastest fibers (i.e., those with conduction velocities of 90 m/sec) remained reduced, indicating that regeneration of the fastest fibers had not occurred at that time (see Fig. 16-6).

Electromyography (EMG) can be used for the detection and documentation of muscle denervation resulting from n-hexane-induced motor neuropathy. In an n-hexane-poisoned precision grinder with clinical and electrophysiological evidence of peripheral neuropathy, needle EMG examination of the right anterior tibialis, extensor digitorum brevis, and gluteus medius muscles showed increased insertional activity, positive waves, and spontaneous fibrillations at rest (Yokoyama et al., 1990). With maximal voluntary contraction, the interference pattern showed reduced numbers of motor unit potentials. EMG studies of proximal muscles (right vastas lateralis and gluteus medius muscles) did not show a reduced number of motor unit potentials. The H-reflex was unobtainable, and the F-wave latency was prolonged in the posterior tibial nerve (68 milliseconds) but was unobtainable from the superficial peroneal nerve. Repeat electrophysiological studies were done 5 years after the n-hexane exposure ended and showed mild improvement in sural sensory amplitude and conduction velocity on the contralateral leg (the original nerve was biopsied). Slowed left peroneal motor conduction velocity (35.1 m/sec) persisted. Single-fiber EMG studies were also done at the 5-year follow-up and revealed jitter in the tibialis anterior muscle and an increase in fiber density compatible with reinervated muscle and stabilized

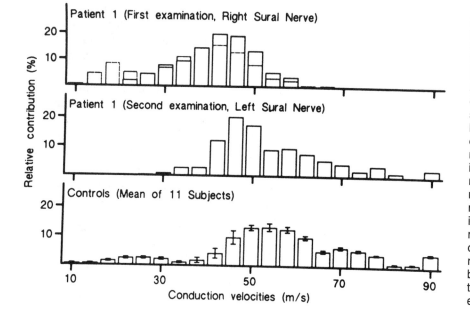

FIG. 16-6. Histograms of the distribution of nerve conduction velocities (DCV) in a worker exposed to n-hexane. First examination showed an initial shift of the DCV in favor of slower fibers (i.e., those with a conduction velocity less than 50 m/sec), is seen reflecting a loss of the faster large myelinated fibers. The DCV calculated from fiber diameter measurement is presented with a computerized estimation of DCV and is represented by broken lines. A more normal DCV was seen at follow-up 36 months after cessation of exposure, indicating that regeneration and remyelination of the affected axons had occurred. DCVs were recorded in the right at the first examination, prior to biopsy of the right sural nerve, and in the left at follow-up. (From Yokoyama et al., 1990, with permission.)

neuromuscular transmission despite the persistence of slowed conduction velocity in peripheral nerves. Blink reflex latency studies done at this time showed R_1 values of 12.1 milliseconds (left) and 11.9 milliseconds (right), which were at the upper limit of the laboratory normal range of 8.25 to 12.5 milliseconds.

Among other reports of EMG studies, Iida et al. (1969) studied 44 sandal makers with chronic exposure to *n*-hexane at vapor concentrations of 500 to 2,500 ppm. The workers were divided into three groups based on clinical presentation: group I—sensory neuropathy; group II—sensorimotor neuropathy; and group III—sensorimotor neuropathy with amyotrophy. Evidence of muscle denervation including fibrillation potentials and positive sharp waves was seen in 70% of the patients in groups I and II and 100% of the patients in group III. The EMG studies of Korobkin et al. (1975) revealed evidence of muscle denervation including fibrillations and sharp waves, which were most prominent in the distal extremities of *n*-hexane exposed workers. EMG studies in a 58-year-old man who developed a marked gait disturbance after he had been exposed to *n*-hexane at relatively low concentrations (average exposure: 325 ppm with peaks up to 450 ppm, for 2 hr/day, 5 days/week, for 6 years) also showed evidence of muscle denervation in the lower extremities, suggesting that peripheral neuropathy can occur during exposure to concentrations below the current OSHA PEL of 500 ppm (Ruff et al., 1981; OSHA, 1995).

Methyl n-Butyl Ketone

Nerve conduction studies (NCS) in an 18-year-old man who developed peripheral neuropathy following occupational exposure to MnBK revealed slowing of motor conduction velocities and increased distal latencies in the peroneal, tibial, median, and ulnar nerves (Wickersham and Fredericks, 1976). Sensory nerve conduction studies in the median and ulnar nerves revealed reduced amplitudes of evoked potentials and increased latencies of the action potentials. Follow-up NCS documented further deterioration of motor and sensory nerve function during the first 2 months after cessation of exposure to MnBK. NCS still showed abnormalities at a follow-up examination 1.5 years after exposure. These findings indicate that the prognosis of patients exposed to MnBK depends on both the intensity and the duration of exposure and that permanent damage to the peripheral nervous system occurs in individuals chronically exposed to high levels of this organic solvent.

NCS documented peripheral neuropathy in a group of 86 workers exposed to MnBK (Allen et al., 1975). The workers were grouped according to the severity of their clinical manifestations; group 1 (*moderate to severely* affected) had overt and often disabling signs and symptoms of peripheral neuropathy (*n* = 11); group 2 (*mildly* affected) had objective findings on clinical examination as well as electrophysiological evidence of neuropathy (*n* = 38); and group 3 (*mini-*

mally affected) had no objective clinical signs but did have electrophysiological evidence of peripheral neuropathy. Slowing of NCV was frequently found in the ulnar, peroneal, tibial, and sural nerves of these patients. Peroneal NCVs were less than 40 m/sec in 36 of the 86 patients (laboratory normal: 44 to 56 m/sec). Of the 11 patients from group 1 (moderate to severe neuropathy) only 1 had a peroneal NCV within normal limits. In addition, the EMG studies of these 11 patients showed positive waves, fibrillations, and fasciculations, most pronounced in the distal muscles. Furthermore, motor unit potentials were abnormal in eight of the 11. The findings on NCV and EMG studies in these patients correlated with the severity of their clinical symptoms (see Clinical Experiences section).

Neuropsychological Diagnosis

Transient lethargy, depression, and confusion are common effects of acute *n*-hexane exposure. These are probably due to the effects of the *n*-hexane metabolite 2-hexanol. Abnormal EEGs suggest CNS effects, but no comprehensive neuropsychological studies on the effects of *n*-hexane and/or MnBK exposure have been reported (Bleeker, 1994). Patients exposed to *n*-hexane and MnBK frequently develop peripheral neuropathy and thus may show impaired performance on finger tapping and other neuropsychological tests of motor function. Hold tests of language and verbal functioning can be used to predict premorbid intelligence and to differentiate solvent encephalopathy from dementias of the Alzheimer's type in adults exposed to *n*-hexane and MnBK (White et al., 1992).

n-Hexane

Performance on tests of visual system functioning show impairments after exposure to *n*-hexane (Yamamura 1969; Raitta, 1978). Raitta (1978) assessed color discrimination in 15 workers, 4 female and 11 male, aged 30 to 65 years (mean: 45.8 years) exposed to *n*-hexane for a mean duration of 12 years (range: 5 to 21 years). Ambient air concentrations of *n*-hexane averaged less than 500 ppm, with peak exposures up to 3,000 ppm. Color vision was assessed in these exposed workers using both the Lanthony D-15 and the Farnsworth-Munsell 100-Hue tests. Color discrimination was found to be impaired in 11 of the 15 workers. Of the four female workers, only one had normal color discrimination. One of the three women had normal color discrimination on the Lathony D-15 test but was found to have an acquired color vision deficit when tested with the more sensitive Farnsworth-Munsell 100-Hue test. The Lathony D-15 test revealed color discrimination deficits in six of the male workers. Three of the male workers had normal color vision, and one had a congenital deuteranopia. Color discrimination deficits in the 11 affected workers were of the acquired type and thus were mainly in the blue-yellow spectrum, as revealed by the Farnsworth–Munsell 100-Hue test. Visual acuity was normal in these workers. Ophthalmoscopy and fluorescein angiography revealed maculopathy in these workers, suggesting that *n*-hexane or a metabolite may have a direct toxic effect on photoreceptor cells. Bäckström and Collins (1992) found a significant loss of rods and cones in the retinae of rats exposed to 2,5-hexanedione. Dyschromatopsia has also been reported following exposure to carbon disulfide and thus, exposure to carbon disulfide should be considered in the differential diagnosis of visual disturbances associated with neurotoxicant exposures (Raitta et al., 1981; Vanhoorne et al., 1996) (see Chapter 21; Carbon Disulfide).

Methyl **n-***Butyl Ketone*

The mental status of a 22-year-old man who developed peripheral neuropathy following occupational exposure to M*n*BK was reported as "normal," but the specifics of the neuropsychological assessment of this patient were not given (Allen et al., 1975).

Biochemical Diagnosis

Biochemical diagnosis of exposure to neurotoxicants is important for confirmation of exposure and estimation of the intensity of a possible toxic hazard. Detecting elevated blood and urine levels of *n*-hexane, M*n*BK, or their common metabolite 2,5-hexanedione early in the course of chronic exposure will prevent the development of neurotoxic effects related to an ongoing increased body burden. Because 2,5-hexanedione is formed following exposure to both *n*-hexane and M*n*BK, determination of the ambient air levels of these two solvents is a useful adjunct to biological monitoring of exposed individuals and for determining the probable source of the 2,5-hexanedione found in the patient's urine or blood.

n-*Hexane*

The biochemical diagnosis of *n*-hexane exposure can be made by determining the concentrations of *n*-hexane and/or its metabolites in the breath, blood, and urine of an exposed individual (Perbellini et al., 1993; Periago et al., 1993). Determination of *n*-hexane in an end-exhaled air sample at the end of the work shift is a solvent-specific and noninvasive indicator of *n*-hexane exposure (Periago et al., 1993). Blood levels, and to a lesser extent urine levels, of *n*-hexane correlate well with exposure dose (Kawai et al., 1993). Blood levels of 2,5-hexanedione can also be used to monitor exposed populations. Nonexposed persons have been found to have blood concentrations of 2,5-hexanedione ranging from 6 to 30 μg/L and urine levels of 0.17 to 0.98 mg/L; this background level reflects unidentified environmental sources as well as endogenous sources such as lipid peroxidation (Perbellini et al., 1993). Quantitative relationships can be made between *n*-hexane found in breathing zone air and amounts of unchanged *n*-hexane in exhaled air and both of these with urinary excretion of 2,5-hexanedione (Fig. 16-7).

The biological monitoring of workers with chronic exposure to *n*-hexane is best achieved by measuring 2,5-hexanedione concentrations in end of shift urine samples (Perbellini et al., 1981a,b; Iwata et al., 1983; Mutti et al., 1984; Ahonen and Schimberg, 1988; Takeuchi, 1993). 2,5-Hexanedione urine concentrations ranged from 1.5 to 4.4 mg/L in workers exposed to *n*-hexane vapor concentrations of 25 ppm (Perbellini et al., 1981b). The ACGIH-recommended BEI for *n*-hexane is determination of 2,5-hexanedione concentration in an end of shift urine sample; the concentration should not exceed 5 mg/g creatinine in workers exposed to *n*-hexane vapor concentrations up to 50 ppm (ACGIH, 1995) (Table 16-3). Acid hydrolysis treatment must be used during this analysis to optimize detection of 2,5-hexanedione by converting the other

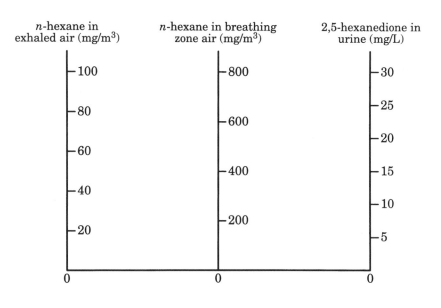

FIG. 16-7. Relationship of biological markers of *n*-hexane exposure to breathing zone air levels. (Data from Pergiago et al., 1993.)

TABLE 16-3. *Biological exposure indices for* n-*hexane and methyl* n-*butyl ketone*

	Urine	Blood	Alveolar air
n-Hexane			
Determinant	2,5-Hexanedione	*n*-Hexane or 2,5-hexanedione	*n*-Hexane
Start of shift	Not established	Not established	Not established
During shift	Not established	Not established	Not established
End of work shift	5 mg/g creatinine	Not established	Not established
Methyl *n*-butyl ketone			
Determinant	2,5-Hexanedione	2,5-Hexanedione	Methyl *n*-butyl ketone
Start of shift	Not established	Not established	Not established
During shift	Not established	Not established	Not established
End of work shift	Not established	Not established	Not established

Data from ACGIH, 1995.

n-hexane metabolite, conjugated 4,5-dihydroxy-2-hexanone, to 2,5-hexanedione (Fedtke and Bolt, 1987; Perbellini et al., 1993; ACGIH, 1995). Any samples that are not treated in this way, with strong acid, will show a lower level of exposure than has actually occurred (Fedtke and Bolt, 1987; Perbellini et al., 1993; ACGIH, 1995). The relationship between exposure dose and total urine 2,5-hexanedione is linear ($r = 0.8553$; $p < 0.001$), and therefore this method can be used to predict the health risks accurately in exposed populations (Perbellini et al., 1993).

Simultaneous exposure to *n*-hexane and MEK significantly reduces the amount of total 2,5-hexanedione detected in the urine sample; thus, to avoid underestimations of exposure dose and risk of neurotoxicity, coexposures to these two solvents must be identified (Iwata et al., 1984; Shibata et al., 1990).

Methyl n-Butyl Ketone

The biochemical diagnosis of exposure to M*n*BK can be made by analysis of blood and urine samples. 2,5-Hexanedione was detected in the serum of human volunteers following exposures to M*n*BK vapor at concentrations greater than 50 ppm, indicating that blood levels of 2,5-hexanedione are suitable for biological monitoring of workers exposed to M*n*BK; blood levels should be determined at the end of the work shift. Humans exposed to an oral dose of ^{14}C-labeled M*n*BK excreted approximately 25% of the radioactivity in the urine within 8 days after dosing; 40% was exhaled as ^{14}C-labeled CO_2. Maximum urinary excretion of radioactivity occurred 48 hours after ingestion (DiVincenzo et al., 1978). Exposure of human volunteers to M*n*BK vapor at concentrations of 100 ppm (i.e., the current OSHA PEL) for 4 hours did not result in detectable levels of urinary metabolites including 2,5-hexanedione, indicating that although this method is noninvasive, urinalysis may not be suitable for biological monitoring of occupational exposures to M*n*BK (DiVincenzo et al., 1978; OSHA, 1995). The ACGIH has not determined a BEI for M*n*BK (ACGIH, 1995) (Table 16-4).

2,5-Hexanedione Adducts as Markers of Exposure

2,5-Hexanedione is an electrophilic compound that can bind to the nucleophilic centers of hemoglobin. Hemoglobin adduct formation has been suggested as a novel method of monitoring and documenting exposures to *n*-hexane and M*n*BK (Graham et al., 1995). Graham et al. (1995) suggest that the rate of hemoglobin adduct formation may correlate with neurofilament cross-link formation and thus may be useful in predicting an exposed individual's risk of developing neuropathy. Because human erythrocytes have a life span of 120 days, this test may also be useful for documenting remote exposures after blood and urine levels have returned to within normal limits.

Neuroimaging

Neuroimaging studies are useful in the differential diagnosis of *n*-hexane and M*n*BK exposure and can be used to reveal other underlying pathologies as well as any possible CNS pathology resulting from exposures to these two organic solvents.

n-Hexane

Magnetic resonance imaging (MRI) and positron emission tomography (PET) studies were performed in a 53-year-old self-employed male leather worker who developed peripheral neuropathy and parkinsonism after working with *n*-hexane in a poorly ventilated room for 30 years (Pezzoli et al., 1995). His 24-hour urine 2,5-hexanedione level was 785 μg/L (normal: 450 μg/L). His MRI was normal. However, the PET studies in this patient, which were made using 6-L[18F]fluorodopa, revealed a bilateral reduction in dopamine metabolism in the caudate and putamen, a finding similar to that seen in patients with idiopathic Parkinson's disease (IPD) and in patients exposed to 1-methyl-4-phenyl-1,2,3,6-tetrahydropyridine (MPTP). By contrast, studies using [18F]fluorodeoxyglucose as a tracer in this same patient showed bilateral decreases in glucose metabolism in the caudate nucleus and putamen, a finding not typically seen in patients with IPD. Symptoms and neuropathological evidence of extrapyramidal system involvement have also been reported following exposure to carbon disulfide, which has also been shown to produce a giant axonal peripheral neuropathy in humans (Abe, 1933; Alpers, 1939; Richter, 1945; Vigliani, 1950, 1954; Peters et al., 1988; Chu et al., 1995; Graham et al., 1995). Although the findings in the basal ganglia in this study are not conclusive with regard to the role of *n*-hexane in the etiology of this patient's clinical picture of Parkinson's disease, they do demonstrate the potential clinical utility of isotope ligand neuroimaging studies as a tool in the differential diagnosis of persons exposed to *n*-hexane and possibly other neurotoxicants.

Methyl n-Butyl Ketone

No neuroimaging studies have been reported on persons exposed to M*n*BK.

Neuropathological Diagnosis

n-Hexane

Exposure to *n*-hexane has been associated with neuropathological changes in the central and the peripheral nervous systems which Spencer and Schaumburg (1976) referred to as *central–peripheral distal dying back neuropathy* to describe these morphological changes. Lesions in the ventromedial and ventrolateral tracts of the spinal cords of rats experimentally exposed to *n*-hexane were noted and neuropathological evidence of the peripheral nervous system damage has been reported following human exposure, as well as following experimental exposure

of laboratory animals (Schaumburg and Spencer, 1976; Yokoyama et al., 1990).

Light microscopy studies were made on the sural nerve biopsy of a 26-year-old man who developed muscle weakness, numbness, and tingling in his lower extremities after he was occupationally exposed to *n*-hexane at an ambient air concentration of at least 195 ppm for 6 months (Yokoyama et al., 1990). A cross section revealed a marked decrease in large myelinated fibers and a mild reduction in smaller myelinated fibers. Teased fibers showed paranodal swelling, due to accumulation of neurofilaments, with corresponding retraction of the myelin sheath. Areas of focal demyelination were also seen. These findings are consistent with previous reports of *n*-hexane peripheral neuropathy (Herskowitz et al., 1971; Shirabe et al., 1974; Scelsi et al., 1980) (Fig. 16-8A–C).

Electron microscopic studies of the morphological changes in the peripheral nerves reveal accumulation of neurofilaments within the proximal paranodal region of the axon (Herskowitz et al., 1971; Schaumburg and Spencer, 1976; Scelsi et al., 1980). Clumping and degeneration of mitochondria as well as dense bodies are seen in the axon terminal (Herskowitz et al., 1971; Gonzalez et al., 1972; Scelsi et al., 1980). Electron micrographs of the motor end plates of anterior tibialis muscle biopsied from a 27-year-old woman who was exposed to *n*-hexane at a TWA of 650 ppm revealed swelling of the terminal axoplasmic expansions with many glycogen granules, as well as an increased number of mitochondria, some of which were degenerating and an increased number of dense bodies (Herskowitz et al., 1971). Large osmiophilic bodies composed of concentrically arranged membranes were also seen. Synaptic folds and vesicles were increased. These findings are in-

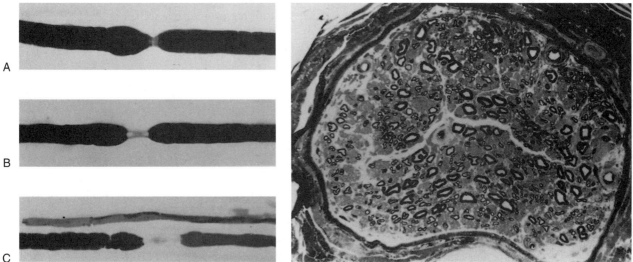

FIG. 16-8. Sural nerve biopsy of a patient occupationally exposed to *n*-hexane. Teased sural fibers showing; **A:** paranodal enlargement. **B:** Retraction of myelin sheath. **C:** Focal demyelination. **D:** Cross section showing marked decrease in the number of large myelinated fibers as well as mild reduction in the number of small myelinated fibers. (From Yokoyama et al., 1990, with permission.)

dicative of interruption of anterograde and retrograde axonal transport mechanisms (Thomas et al., 1993).

Muscle biopsy studies reveal evidence of denervation marked by neurogenic atrophy (Herskowitz et al., 1971; Goto et al., 1974; Shirabe et al., 1974; Gonzalez et al., 1972; Scelsi et al., 1980). Light microscopy of the muscle biopsy of an 18-year-old woman who had been exposed to unreported levels of n-hexane for 6 months showed numerous groups of small angulated atrophic fibers (Scelsi et al., 1980). Targetoid fibers with a pale central area containing a large number of dense bands, separated by irregular bundles of myofilaments and a peripheral concentric area with irregularities of the Z-lines were seen on transverse sections, as well as true target fibers characterized by three concentric areas of different morphology.

Electron microscopic studies of muscle biopsies were made in two glue sniffers who developed peripheral neuropathy shortly after the n-hexane content of the glue they had been using was increased (Shirabe et al., 1974). In both cases the widths of the muscle fibers and myofibrils were occasionally reduced. The myofilaments were disorganized, with distorted, shortened, and thickened Z-lines. Mitochondria were swollen and had lost their cristae. Vacuoles and lipid bodies were seen among the myofibrils. Many nuclei had lost their nucleoli. The sarcoplasmic membranes of atrophied muscle fibers were indented. Fibroblasts and collagen fibers were increased in the interstices.

Visual system pathological changes following n-hexane exposure have been described. Ophthalmoscopy and fluorescein angiography revealed maculopathy in 11 of 15 workers exposed to n-hexane at concentrations up to 3,000 ppm, suggesting that n-hexane may have a direct toxic effect on photoreceptor cells (Raitta et al., 1978). VEP studies in these same patients suggested that damage had also occurred in the cerebral part of the visual pathway (Seppäläinen et al., 1979) (see Symptomatic Diagnosis, Neurophysiological Diagnosis, and Neuropsychological Diagnosis sections). Axonal swelling was noted in the distal optic tracts, lateral geniculate bodies, and superior colliculi of

cats administered water containing 0.5% 2,5-hexanedione for 136 days (Schaumburg and Spencer, 1978). Pathological studies in monkeys that had developed decreased visual contrast sensitivity following oral intake of 2,5-hexanedione also revealed axonal swelling in the distal optic tracts (Lynch et al., 1989).

Experimental studies of levels of neuron-specific enolase (NSE) and the glial cell marker proteins creatine kinase-B and beta-S100 reveal that n-hexane significantly reduces the amount of these marker proteins in the distal segments of the sciatic nerves of rats exposed to 2,000 ppm of n-hexane vapor for 12 hr/day, 6 days/week, for 24 weeks (Huang et al., 1992). In addition, levels of NSE were reduced in the spinal cord of these same animals. These changes in levels of nerve marker proteins indicate that exposure to n-hexane disrupts axonal transport mechanisms and/or energy metabolism.

Methyl n-Butyl Ketone

Nerve biopsy studies of humans exposed to MnBK reveal neuropathological changes identical to those seen following exposures to n-hexane (Davenport et al., 1976; Saida et al., 1976). The sural biopsy of a 41-year-old male spray painter who developed peripheral neuropathy after he had been exposed to MnBK for 11 months revealed a decrease in the number of myelinated fiber; denuded swollen axons showed an accumulation of neurofilaments in the proximal paranodal regions (Fig. 16-9). Ongoing wallerian-type degeneration with myelin debris was seen. Evidence of axonal regeneration (i.e., axonal sprouting in the residual basement membrane) and remyelination was also noted.

Experimental studies in laboratory animals have also shown that MnBK produces a neuropathy morphologically identical to that of n-hexane (Allen et al., 1975; Saida et al., 1976; Spencer and Schaumburg, 1976). Microscopic examination of teased fibers of the sciatic nerve of rats ex-

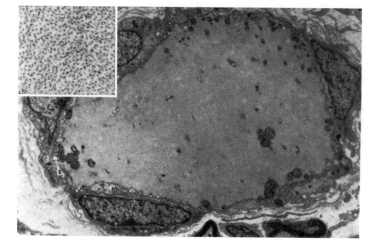

FIG. 16-9. Sural nerve biopsy of a patient occupationally exposed to methyl n-butyl ketone showing swollen denuded axon (original magnification, ×4,000). Inset is an electron micrograph of a paranodal portion of the axon showing accumulation of neurofilaments (original magnification, ×20,000). (From Saida et al., 1976, with permission.)

posed to M*n*BK revealed marked axonal swelling with associated thinning of the myelin sheath proximal to the node of Ranvier. Electron micrographs of these axons demonstrated densely packed masses of neurofilaments at the proximal paranodal region (Saida et al., 1976). Schwann cells are relatively well preserved but often contain myelin breakdown products (Allen et al., 1975; Saida et al., 1976).

The neurotoxic properties of both *n*-hexane and M*n*BK have been attributed to their common metabolite 2,5-hexanedione, which is a γ-diketone (Sickles, 1989; St. Clair et al., 1989; Stoltenburg-Didinger et al., 1992; Graham et al., 1995; Filser et al., 1996). M*n*BK is more toxic than *n*-hexane because more 2,5-hexanedione is formed after exposure (DiVincenzo et al., 1978; O'Donoghue and Krasavage, 1979; Filser et al., 1996). Experimental studies have demonstrated that 2,5-hexanedione slows fast antero- and retrograde axonal transport (Sahenk and Mendell, 1981; Sickles, 1989). In addition, slow axonal transport of neurofilaments is accelerated both during and after exposure to 2,5-hexanedione (Pyle et al., 1992). Abnormal nerve function due to alterations in fast axonal transport followed exposure of rats to M*n*BK (Mendell et al., 1977). Sickles (1989) demonstrated that 2,5-hexanedione reduces the rate of fast anterograde transport in the sciatic nerve of the rat; similar effects were not seen after exposure to the γ-diketone, 2,3-hexanedione. These findings indicate that γ-spacing of the ketone groups is critical to the development of neuropathy (Sickles, 1989; Graham et al., 1995).

That 2,5-hexanedione can disrupt axonal transport and induce a distal–central dying back axonal neuropathy appears to result from the formation of chemical cross-links between axonal neurofilaments (Schaumburg and Spencer, 1978; Sickles, 1989; St. Clair et al.,1989; Graham et al., 1995). The formation of chemical cross-links occurs through several steps beginning with the reaction of one of the carbonyl carbon atoms of 2,5-hexanedione with the nitrogen atom of an amino group (Filser et al., 1996). This reaction is followed by cyclization to pyrrolidine, which subsequently loses two water molecules to yield a pyrrole. The subsequent oxidation of the pyrrole to an electrophile, which can subsequently react with the nucleophilic centers of proteins, is probably the essential final step in the chemical cross-linking of neurofilaments (Graham et al., 1995). The progression of the neuropathy following cessation of exposure to γ-diketones appears to be related to the subsequent oxidation of pyrroles formed during exposure (St. Clair et al., 1989; Graham et al., 1995).

The location along the axon at which cross-linked neurofilaments accumulate appears to be related to the neurotoxicity of the γ-diketone, which further appears to be related to the rate of formation of neurofilamentous cross-links. For example, exposure to the more potent neurotoxic analogue of 2,5-hexanedione, 3,4-dimethyl-2,5-hexanedione, results in both a significantly faster formation of neurofilament cross-links and a more proximal accumulation of neurofilaments along the length of the

axon than does exposure to 2,5-hexanedione (Graham et al., 1995).

The changes in the structure of neurofilaments that occur following exposure to γ-diketones results in a concomitant disruption of their transport along the axon and thus their accumulation within the more distal segments of the axon. In addition, these findings suggest that the axonal transport of cellular organelles such as mitochondria, which are necessary to the viability of distal segments of the cell, as well as the transport of proteins and neurotransmitters required for the transmission of information between neurons and/or muscles may be disrupted and/or blocked by exposure to γ-diketones. Thus, the disruption of axonal transport mechanisms induced by γ-diketones such as *n*-hexane and M*n*BK produces serious acute and chronic neurological effects.

PREVENTIVE AND THERAPEUTIC MEASURES

Safety training to inform workers about the acute and chronic effects of *n*-hexane and M*n*BK exposure should be available in all occupational settings where these solvents are used. Material data sheets explaining solvent mixtures that may include *n*-hexane and/or M*n*BK must be offered to those who use these solvents. Complaints of transient and reversible lightheadedness, dizziness, mucous membrane irritation, drowsiness, and fatigue experienced among workers at risk are often accepted as "just part of the job." Drowsiness, poor attention, and impaired judgment resulting from the effects of acute exposure may cause accidents when operating equipment at work and when driving home immediately after acute exposures to high concentrations. Workers who cannot tolerate the acute effects often leave the job. Prolonged exposure by workers who are seemingly unbothered by the mild acute reversible effects must be routinely monitored to prevent the development of more serious peripheral and central nervous system toxicity.

Employees as well as employers must be alerted to the potential hazards associated with exposure to liquid *n*-hexane and/or M*n*BK as well as the vapors of these two solvents. Protective clothing and gloves should be worn by all workers with potential for dermal contact with *n*-hexane and/or M*n*BK, to prevent dermal absorption (DiVincenzo et al., 1978; Cardona et al., 1993). Work areas where *n*-hexane- and/or M*n*BK-based products such as glues and solvents are used should be well ventilated (Wang et al., 1986). Respirators should be provided for those workers at risk of exposure to high concentrations of *n*-hexane and/or M*n*BK. Ambient air concentrations of *n*-hexane and/or M*n*BK in the workplace should be measured periodically, and urine samples for biological monitoring of exposed individuals should be examined on a regular basis. Urinary 2,5-hexanedione is a good indicator of exposure to *n*-hexane and M*n*BK (Takeuchi, 1993; Cardona et al., 1993; Granvil et al., 1994) (see Biochemical Diagnosis section).

The first step in treating the effects of acute exposure to *n*-hexane and/or M*n*BK is to recognize that the condition exists and to remove the individual(s) from further exposure. Hyperventilation with fresh air or supplemental oxygen should be encouraged to displace the contaminated air from the lungs and to enhance respiratory elimination of the unmetabolized solvent. If the individual is unconscious, intubation and administration of oxygen are necessary. If liquid *n*-hexane and/or M*n*BK has been swallowed, stomach gavage should be done immediately to empty the stomach of the solvent-containing contents, thus preventing further absorption. Hemodialysis and blood transfusion for acute renal and/or hepatic failure may also be necessary following acute oral intake. In addition, hypotension must be treated with appropriate fluid and vasopressor medications. Cardiac complications from changes in autonomic nervous system function following exposure to *n*-hexane and/or M*n*BK, as well as other ingredients in the culprit solvent solution, must be assessed in the setting of acute toxicity (Murata et al., 1994).

The acute narcotic effects of both *n*-hexane and M*n*BK disappear rapidly with no residual sequelae, but subacute and subchronic exposures to these solvents is associated with the insidious development of central and peripheral nervous system dysfunction (Yokoyama et al., 1990). It is impractical to overlook early clinical symptoms and not remove the worker from further exposure until more overt manifestations of peripheral neuropathy such as muscle weakness and atrophy become so severe as to interfere with his or her ability to perform job tasks. Chronic exposures to low concentrations, like subchronic exposures at higher levels, are accompanied by the gradual appearance of signs of peripheral neuropathy and other effects of exposure (Ruff et al., 1981; Barregård et al., 1991). As the body burden accumulates over time with chronic exposure, acute symptoms may occur at times of peak exposures, resolving with cessation of exposure. These episodes of acute symptoms occur at lower levels of exposure in those workers who have already been accumulating a body burden of *n*-hexane and/or M*n*BK. Effective case management of individuals chronically exposed to *n*-hexane and/or M*n*BK requires immediate removal from further exposure when clinical signs first manifest (Wang et al., 1986). Permanent removal from exposure to *n*-hexane, M*n*BK, and other organic solvents is usually necessary in susceptible individuals.

Significant economic losses are associated with subsequent disability, loss of work, and the very long time needed for rehabilitation. Recovery from acute and subacute exposures to *n*-hexane and/or M*n*BK depends on the intensity and duration of the exposure (Herskowitz et al., 1971; Shirabe et al., 1974; Yokoyama et al., 1990). Even after several years of absence from further exposure, return of function may be incomplete, and performing activities of daily living may be difficult (Herskowitz et al., 1971;

Shirabe et al., 1974; Wang et al., 1986; Chang, 1990; Yokoyama et al., 1990). The prognosis of patients with clinical evidence of chronic effects of *n*-hexane and/or M*n*BK exposure varies according to time of follow-up and type of neurological tests performed. Chang (1990, 1991) evaluated the clinical and neurophysiological prognosis of patients exposed to *n*-hexane and concluded that prognosis was better with a longer follow-up period. In cases of severe exposure, residual gait disturbances and other signs of peripheral neuropathy may persist indefinitely (Oryshkevich et al., 1986; Chang, 1990, 1991). Damage to the CNS fibers associated with exposure to *n*-hexane and/or M*n*BK exposure may be irreversible (Chang, 1990, 1991). Persistent CNS effects may interfere with a worker's ability to perform job tasks and to concentrate on the job. Patients with permanent neurological impairments may require vocational retraining. A 12-year follow-up of the worker studied by Yokoyama et al. (1990) found that he still had mild bilateral footdrop but no longer required short leg braces. He has avoided exposure to solvents and has not returned to his previous job as a precision grinder. He was retrained to drive a truck and operate a backhoe and is now a worker for the state highway department (R. G. Feldman, personal observation).

CLINICAL EXPERIENCES

n-Hexane

Group Studies

Sentinel Cases that Led to the Detection of Other Affected Workers

Two Chinese printing press workers who had been using an *n*-hexane-based solvent to clean printing molds developed progressive muscle weakness and numbness in their upper and lower extremities (Wang et al., 1986). Neurological examination revealed muscle wasting and decreased deep tendon reflexes in both patients. These two sentinel cases prompted a larger industrial hygiene survey. Fifty-nine workers (57 males and 2 female clerks) from four factories were examined. The mean age was 25.8 years, and the mean exposure duration was 5.8 years (range: less than 1 to 25 years). Ambient air concentrations of *n*-hexane vapor measured during the survey ranged from 21 to 190 ppm.

Of the 59 workers, 15 (25%) had clinical signs and symptoms of peripheral neuropathy including paresthesia, muscle weakness, decreased vibration, pain, and temperature sensation in the extremities, gait disturbances, muscle wasting, and hyperreflexia or absence of deep tendon reflexes. Two patients had mild impairment of color discrimination. Fifteen of the symptomatic patients as well as two asymptomatic workers had abnormalities on NCS. All 17 cases of peripheral neuropathy were associated with exposure to solvents containing at least 65% *n*-

hexane. Among these 17 cases of peripheral neuropathy were all ($n = 6$) the employees from the factory at which air samples had revealed the highest ambient air concentrations of *n*-hexane vapor (190 ppm). The practice of sleeping in the factory, which significantly prolonged exposure, was also associated with the incidence of peripheral neuropathy. The incidence of peripheral neuropathy among 13 workers who frequently slept in the factory was 92% (12 of 13), compared with an incidence of only 7% (three of 46) among those workers who did not sleep in the factory.

It was concluded that the outbreak of peripheral neuropathy seen in these Chinese printing shop workers was related to four factors: (a) the principal solvent used in the press proofing process had recently been changed from toluene to *n*-hexane; (b) poor air quality was made worse by the recent installation of air conditioning units, which had prompted the shutting down of ventilation fans as well as the closing of doors and windows to improve cooling of the work areas; (c) production volume had been increased, which led to longer working hours; and (d) workers slept in the factories. Factors c and d significantly prolonged exposure. Improvements in safety measures included (a) cessation of the use of *n*-hexane as a solvent; (b) improvement of shop ventilation systems; and (c) restriction of the number of hours the employees could spend at the factory between work shifts.

Follow-up studies of 11 of the workers reported by Wang et al. (1986) were conducted by Chang (1990, 1991). Delayed worsening of motor symptoms during the first 2 to 3 months following cessation of exposure was seen in five patients. By contrast, sensory symptoms did not show worsening following removal from exposure. Eight workers left the printing industry, recuperated at home for several months, and then began working in jobs that did not require contact with organic solvents. The other three workers returned to work at a printing factory where *n*-hexane was no longer used and significant improvements had been made to the shop's ventilation system. Sensory disturbances disappeared much sooner than motor symptoms and were usually ameliorated within 3 to 4 months after removal from exposure. Six patients complained of tightness in their legs that was most prominent in the morning or after sitting and improved after walking or exercise. Leg tightness appeared approximately 10 months after cessation of exposure and disappeared 6 to 20 months later. Muscle cramps were experienced by the six patients who experienced leg tightness. In contrast to the leg tightness, the muscle cramps worsened with exercise, were still present in all affected patients 4 years after cessation of exposure, and may be indicative of spinal cord damage. Deep tendon reflexes gradually improved in all patients, with ankle jerks reappearing last. Ten patients showed good clinical recovery within 30 months after cessation of exposure. The most severely affected patient continued to have mild gait disturbances at follow-up 4

years after removal from exposure (Chang, 1990). NCV studies of all 11 patients still showed evidence of peripheral nerve dysfunction 4 years after removal from exposure (Chang, 1991).

Outbreak of Neuropathy: Underestimate of Solvent Toxicity and Corrective Measures

A machine shop involved in the manufacture of close tolerance machine parts for the oil drilling, aerospace, and defense industries employed expert precision grinders who performed a manual grinding operation known as "lapping" by using a diamond paste and a rubbing block to remove small amounts of metal from machine parts such as vanes, rotors, and cams. Each worker had his own bench at which he performed the lapping operation. Following the lapping procedure, the machinists would clean the parts in a degreasing solvent; small parts were dipped into an open bucket of degreasing solvent kept on each workbench, and larger parts were dipped into a large vat of solvent. The part was subsequently checked for tolerance using an electronic calibrator; if necessary, the lapping operation and degreasing process were repeated until the part was within the specified tolerance range.

The large vat of degreasing solvent was kept on top of a heavy table near the door to the lapping room and diagonally across from the air intake source of the lapping room. Fresh air entering the room through the air intake was drawn across the work areas to the open door. Ventilation in the room was poor since this was the only source. Inhalation of solvent vapors and dermal contact with the liquid solvent was commonplace and was accepted as part of the job. The company had been successfully and apparently "safely" precision grinding metal parts for 8 years using this manual lapping procedure; Shell Sol B, which at that time contained less than 25% *n*-hexane, was the degreasing solvent. No neurological problems had been reported by any of the precision grinders working in the lapping room during that time.

A change in the company's materials supplier in early 1983 led to a consequent change in the degreasing solution used in the lapping room. Shell Sol B was replaced by a new product called Hexasol, which contained only 2% to 5% *n*-hexane and was therefore considered "safer." The workers used this new solvent, and no medical problems were encountered (Fig. 16-10).

In April of 1983, a young man (aged 27 years) began working in the lapping room as a precision grinder. Like the other workers, he too kept a bucket of Hexasol on his bench to clean smaller parts before checking them for tolerance. However, unlike the other workers, the workbench of this machinist was situated immediately adjacent to the large vat of Hexasol used for cleaning large parts.

In June of 1983 a new drum of degreasing solvent labeled 95% *n*-hexane arrived at the machine shop instead of

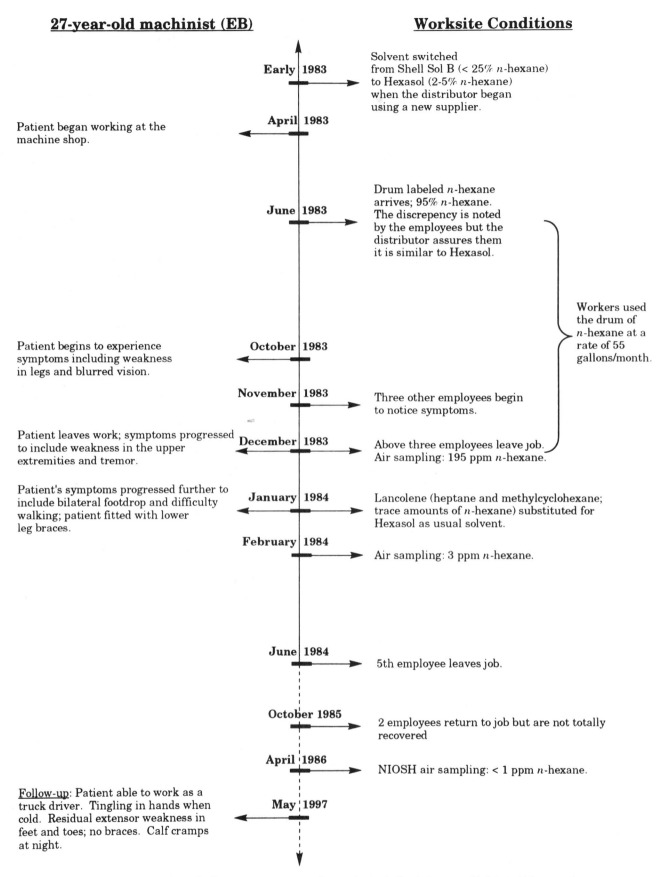

FIG. 16-10. Time line of *n*-hexane exposure and neurological effects in a machinist and his coworkers.

the Hexasol ordered. The employer questioned the supplier and was assured that it was similar to Hexasol; workers began to use it in the usual manner at a rate of 55 gallons a month. After 4 months (early November, 1983) of using the *n*-hexane solution, four grinders began to experience weakness in their hands and feet. These symptoms progressed throughout November until early December, when the inability to walk properly due to weakness in the lower extremities motivated them to seek medical attention. The outbreak prompted an industrial hygiene survey (Arnold Green Testing Labs, Springfield, MA). Air sampling results obtained in December 1983 showed *n*-hexane levels of 195 ppm. However, because the air sampling pump was located 12 feet from the main dipping vat, and because most of the benches were less than 12 feet from the vat and most machinists kept a small bucket of solvent on their bench, it was estimated that individual inhalation exposure exceeded this level.

All four affected workers had similar job tasks and were involved in the lapping of rotors and vanes. Unaware that the new solvent was more hazardous, the workers had used it for 6 months with no additional hygienic precautions. After approximately 3 months, the workers began to experience symptoms of peripheral neuropathy that included paresthesias and decreased muscle strength. The symptoms progressed rapidly over the next 3 months until all four workers had difficulty walking and were unable to hold their tools properly because of decreased muscle strength. Neurological examinations of these patients revealed distal muscle weakness and decreased sensation to pinprick and vibration (sensorimotor neuropathy). In each case the clinical signs of sensorimotor neuropathy were more manifest distally in the upper and lower but especially in the lower extremities. Extensor muscles were more severely affected than flexors. NCS documented peripheral neuropathy. The most severely affected was the 27-year-old man who began working in the lapping room in April of 1983 and whose workbench was next to the drum of *n*-hexane (Fig. 16-10). By contrast, a fifth employee who occasionally worked on rotors and vanes and who frequently worked at a machine situated in the path of vapor travel experienced less marked symptoms of peripheral neuropathy. Those employees who were not involved in this process and/or who worked upstream from the path of vapors did not develop overt evidence of peripheral neuropathy. Follow-up NCS reflected the course of clinical recovery seen in these patients. The clinical prognosis and improvement in NCVs seen in all four affected workers following their removal from exposure to *n*-hexane indicate that their subacute exposure to *n*-hexane, at an ambient air concentration of at least 195 ppm, produced a distal sensorimotor neuropathy.

An air filtering system was installed, and the 95% hexane solution was replaced with Lacolene, a solvent that contained mostly heptane and methylcyclohexane, but only trace amounts of *n*-hexane. Repeat air sampling in February 1984 showed a decrease in ambient air *n*-hexane to 3 ppm.

A NIOSH Health Hazard Evaluation was performed in April of 1986 (NIOSH, 1986), subsequent to installation of the air filtering system and substitution of Lacolene for *n*-hexane, and found that two of the four workers were physically able to return to work in the lapping room and had done so 6 months earlier, although their neurological symptoms had still not completely resolved at the time of the study. The most severely affected worker, the 27-year-old man who began working as a precision grinder in April 1983, was unable to return to work at his previous position as a precision grinder due to the severity of his neurological condition and the physical demands of the job. As a result, he required vocational retraining and now works as a truck driver for the state. The fourth worker was lost to follow-up.

Air sampling performed by NIOSH at that time found the *n*-hexane concentration to be less than 1 ppm, indicating minimal exposure to *n*-hexane; the concentration of total C_5 to C_8 alkanes was above the action level of 200 mg/m^3 (57 ppm) but below the NIOSH 10-hour TWA REL of 350 mg/m^3 (100 ppm) (NIOSH, 1977, 1986). NIOSH recommended the use of impervious gloves when parts were dipped into the degreasing solution and also suggested that employee exposure to *n*-hexane as well as other C_5 to C_8 alkanes could be further reduced by the installation of exhaust hoods over those areas where cleaning of parts took place. NIOSH also recommended that employees receive preplacement and annual physical examinations with specific attention given to neurological functioning.

Individual Case Studies

Subacute Exposure to High Concentrations of n-*Hexane in the Cabinet Making Industry*

Herskowitz et al. (1971) reported on three female cabinet finishers who began to experience symptoms of peripheral neuropathy following 2 to 4 months of daily exposure to *n*-hexane. The job required the women to dip a rag frequently into a drum of *n*-hexane, after which they would use the solvent-soaked rag to wipe excess glue from the cabinets. These women worked in an enclosed, small (13 m^2), and poorly ventilated area where ambient air vapor concentrations of *n*-hexane averaged 650 ppm and frequently reached peak concentrations of 1,300 ppm.

Case 1. A 27-year-old woman began to experience symptoms 2 months after beginning work as a cabinet finisher. She complained of headaches, abdominal cramps, and numbness and weakness in her distal extremities but continued to work for an additional 6 months. Neurological examination 6 months after the onset of symptoms revealed moderate distal symmetrical weakness and bilateral footdrop. Absent ankle tendon reflexes, mild decreases in vibration and position sense, and moderate reductions in sensation to pinprick and touch in her lower extremities were also noted on the clinical examination. Complete blood count, blood urea nitrogen, liver function tests, serum thyroxine, blood sugar, and electrolytes were normal. EMG, NCS, and nerve biopsy studies documented peripheral neuropathy (see Neurophysiological and Neuropathological Diagnosis sections).

Case 2. A second cabinet finisher, a 47-year-old woman, began to experience abdominal cramps, paresthesias, and distal weakness in her extremities 2 months after she was employed in the same work area of the factory. Neurological examination revealed bilateral foot and wrist drop; reduced sensation to touch, position, and vibration was noted distally and symmetrically in all four extremities, and ankle tendon reflexes were absent bilaterally. Laboratory tests were normal. EMG, NCS, and nerve biopsy studies documented peripheral neuropathy.

Case 3. The third worker in the cabinet finishing department, a 46-year-old woman who began to notice weakness in her extremities 4 months after she began to work in the department, continued to work for another 6 months before she sought medical attention for her symptoms. Moderate weakness and decreased sensation to touch, position, and vibration distally were present in all four extremities. Patellar and Achilles tendon reflexes were absent bilaterally. Urinalysis, complete blood count, blood urea nitrogen, liver function tests, transaminases, and serum thyroxine were normal. Cerebrospinal fluid protein was normal (34 mg/100 mL). Electromyography and NCS documented peripheral neuropathy.

Glue Sniffer's Neuropathy

Two young Japanese men who worked together as house painters also had in common the daily habit of sniffing glue (Shirabe et al., 1974). In addition to exposure to various types of paints, the two had been huffing (i.e., sniffing) glue together for at least 2 years without experiencing any persistent adverse effects. However, shortly after they changed from their usual brand of glue, which used toluene as its primary solvent, to one that contained 45% *n*-hexane, both young men began to experience symptoms of peripheral neuropathy.

Case 1. The most severely affected was a 20-year-old man with a history of sniffing glue who began to experience weakness in the lower extremities shortly after changing his brand of glue. Unaware of the possible relationship between his symptoms and the new glue, he continued to sniff. His symptoms progressed and he soon developed mild numbness and tingling paresthesia in both feet and a gait disturbance associated with muscle weakness. Despite a progressively worsening condition, he continued to sniff the new glue. After 2 more weeks, he was unable to walk without assistance. Several days later, he began to experience weakness in his upper extremities;

realizing that his symptoms might be related to the new glue, he stopped sniffing it.

Despite cessation of exposure, the patient's symptoms continued to progress for another 2 to 3 weeks, when he had become bedridden. At that time he experienced paresthesia in his hands, feet, and lower legs. He was also incontinent, dysphagic, and dysarthric. Unable to stand or even support himself to sit up, he was admitted to the hospital.

Neurological examination revealed an alert individual. His pupils were equal and reacted briskly to light. Visual acuity was normal and optic fundi were unremarkable. Muscle tone in all four extremities was flaccid and there was overt evidence of atrophy. The patient was unable to move his toes, feet, and wrists. Deep tendon reflexes were absent bilaterally. Touch, pain, and temperature sensations were profoundly impaired, more distally than proximally, in all four extremities, but vibration sensation and joint position sense were impaired only in the lower extremities. NCS, EMG, and a sural nerve biopsy documented the peripheral neuropathy in this patient. The patient showed gradual clinical improvement and was able to be discharged 3 months later, with slow but incomplete recovery over 6 months.

Case 2. A 19-year-old man who was a coworker and the huffing partner of the patient described above began to experience heaviness in his legs at about the same time as his friend. He also noticed numbness in his feet. His symptoms continued to progress over the next month and soon he could not climb stairs without pulling himself along by the banister. Despite his symptoms, like his friend he too continued to sniff the glue for 2 more weeks, at which time his symptoms had progressed to include reduced strength in the upper extremities.

On neurological examination the patient was alert and cooperative. His pupils were equal and reacted briskly to light. Visual acuity and hearing were normal. Muscle tone was normal, but strength was reduced in the upper extremities. The lower extremities were moderately atrophic, muscle tone was flaccid, and strength was markedly reduced distally. Sweating was profuse in both feet. Deep tendon reflexes were absent bilaterally. Touch, pain, and temperature sensations were decreased below the knees bilaterally. Vibration and position sense were intact. He walked with a steppage gait and was unable to walk on his toes or heels. NCS and EMG documented the peripheral axonal neuropathy in this patient. He improved gradually but had not returned to normal after 6 months.

Gloves Alone Did Not Protect against Chronic Exposure to n-Hexane

A 52-year-old male janitor at an adhesive manufacturing plant used *n*-hexane to clean glue from worktable tops (Ruff et al., 1981). He always wore gloves to prevent dermal contact with the solvent. He was exposed to the solvent for approximately 2 hours a work shift 5 days a week

for 6 years. Average air concentrations of *n*-hexane in the man's work zone were 325 ppm, with occasional peaks of up to 450 ppm.

After he had been using the *n*-hexane for approximately 3 years, the patient began to notice numbness and weakness in his lower extremities. He continued to use the solvent despite these early symptoms of peripheral neuropathy. His symptoms continued to progress and eventually included gait disturbances. He was forced to retire 6 years after he began using *n*-hexane because, at only 58 years old, he could no longer walk without assistance.

A neurological examination performed at the time of his retirement revealed marked weakness in the lower extremities and sensory loss in the distal upper and lower extremities. NCS documented sensorimotor neuropathy in the upper and lower extremities, and EMG demonstrated denervation in the distal muscles of the lower extremities.

At a follow-up examination 2 years later, the patient reported subjective sensory improvement in his lower extremities but he still had a severe gait disturbance. The neurological examination showed a stocking-glove sensory loss in the distal extremities. Ankle jerks were absent. NCVs were improved over the earlier studies but still not within normal range. A sural nerve biopsy revealed pathological evidence of neuropathy.

Methyl n-Butyl Ketone

Group Studies

A Switch from Methyl iso-Butyl Ketone to Methyl n-Butyl Ketone and the Emergence of Neurotoxicity

An outbreak of peripheral neuropathy occurred at a factory manufacturing plastic-coated and color-printed fabrics after the principal solvent used was changed from methyl *iso*-butyl ketone to M*n*BK (Billmaier et al.,1974; Mendell et al., 1974; Allen et al., 1975). The recognition of M*n*BK as a neurotoxicant began when an employee of the factory presented at Ohio State University Hospital with symptoms and signs of peripheral neuropathy. The etiology of the neuropathy was not identified until several months later when the patient produced a list of five coworkers who had had similar symptoms. The Ohio Department of Health was notified, prompting an industrial hygiene survey of the factory.

All workers (*n* = 1,157) were asked to complete a neurological symptoms questionnaire and to undergo a clinical neurological examination, an EMG, and NCS; 194 workers were suspected of having peripheral neuropathy related to their occupation. Twenty-seven had other neurological disorders, and 81 were found to be normal or had minimal findings. In total, 86 cases of toxic neuropathy were identified. Of these, 11 were classified as moderately to severely affected and had overt and often disabling clinical evidence of peripheral neuropathy; 38 were classified as mildly affected and had objective findings on clinical examination and electrophysiological evidence of neuropa-

thy; and 37 were classified as minimally affected and were without objective signs but had electrodiagnostic findings characteristic of peripheral neuropathy. The latter cases might be referred to as "subclinically" affected.

The clinical neurological manifestations included a distal sensorimotor neuropathy with depressed ankle and finger tendon reflexes. Motor symptoms were more common among the 11 most severely affected patients, whereas sensory symptoms predominated in the 38 mild cases. When present, muscle weakness typically began in the intrinsic muscles of the feet and hands and subsequently extended proximally and bilaterally to involve the ankles and wrists. In the most severe cases muscle weakness extended proximally to involve the hamstrings, thigh adductors, gluteus maximus, iliopsoas, and shoulder rotators. Muscle atrophy and bilateral footdrop was seen in the more severely affected patients. Sensory loss was typically bilateral, initially involving the feet and hands and extending proximally to as high as the knee in the more severely affected patients. In no case was sensory ataxia or Romberg's sign found. Cranial nerves were normal.

Follow-up clinical neurological examinations of the 86 affected workers at 6 months after cessation of exposure showed marked clinical improvement in all 11 of the moderate to severely affected patients; muscle strength was improved and atrophy was disappearing. Among the 38 mildly affected patients, 33 improved, 4 showed no change, and 1 showed slight worsening. Improvement was seen in 26 of the minimally affected workers, whereas the remainder of the workers in this group showed no change or were slightly worse. In total, one-sixth of the patients showed clinical as well as electrophysiological evidence of progression of the neuropathy following cessation of exposure, in most cases reaching maximum severity by 5 months after cessation of exposure.

Possible causative agents among the 275 chemicals used at that factory included tetrahydrofuran and methacrylate, but these were only used at two printer machines. Analysis of ambient air samples revealed MEK concentrations of 331 to 516 ppm and M*n*BK concentrations of 9.2 to 36.0 ppm; trace amounts of xylene, toluene, methyl alcohol, acetone, and methyl *iso*-butyl ketone were also detected. The solvent used as an ink thinner had in the past contained MEK and methyl *iso*-butyl ketone, but immediately prior to the outbreak it had been replaced with a solvent that contained M*n*BK. Thus, the circumstances pointed to M*n*BK as the most likely causative agent. To verify the hypothesis, an epidemiological study was conducted at another factory that used MEK but had never used M*n*BK. Although mild neurological abnormalities were found in this second group, the pattern of sensorimotor neuropathy seen in the affected workers from the plant using M*n*BK was not observed.

Following this outbreak, the use of M*n*BK as an ink thinner was discontinued. In addition, ventilation of the work area was improved, and better hygienic practices including avoidance of dermal contact with solvents were instituted. A follow-up industrial hygiene survey 4 months after the use of M*n*BK was discontinued and revealed no new cases of peripheral neuropathy (Allen et al., 1975).

Individual Studies

Toxic Neuropathy due to MnBK or Lead: Differential Diagnosis

A 41-year-old man had been a painter for 15 years when he began to use a paint thinner containing M*n*BK for a period of 10 months (Saida et al., 1976). He worked 8 hours a day, 5 days a week. He not only mixed and thinned the paint with these solutions but also used it to remove paint from his hands and face when he finished painting each day. Most of his work was done through a spray-type applicator in a closed environment. This man's past medical history revealed no excessive alcohol intake and no history of diabetes or any other illnesses. Previous exposure to lead was detected by blood lead levels of 85, 55, 65, and 66 mg/dL; urine content of lead was 196, 158, 192 µg in 24-hour volumes of 740, 2,360, and 1,165 mL respectively. Following chelation (with ethylenediamine tetraacetic acid) 1,885 µg of lead was mobilized and excreted in 24 hours. Because of his known exposure to lead paint and the blood and urine evidence of increased body burden of lead, a diagnosis of lead neuropathy was considered when this painter complained of weak legs when climbing stairs toward the end of 10 months of exposure.

Although he stopped painting, his leg weakness continued to progress for another 3 months, reaching a state of disability due to inability to walk or hold objects in his hands. He also had a tight feeling in his legs and feet from below the knees. The symptoms remained at this level for another 3 months before beginning to improve. Two other painters with whom he had worked also complained of similar problems.

Neurological examination, performed 1 month after the leg weakness began, showed that the patient could walk only with assistance; he had bilateral footdrop as well as proximal weakness in the quadriceps and hamstring muscles. Upper extremity weakness involved the wrist flexors and extensors, as well as the biceps and triceps muscles. Tendon reflexes were hypoactive in the upper extremities and absent in the ankles and knees, bilaterally. Sensory examination revealed normal position sense, minimal vibratory loss in the toes, decreased pinprick sensation to the head of the fibula, and mild loss of pain perception in the hands to the wrists.

Laboratory tests revealed evidence of anemia (hemoglobin of 10.8 and hematocrit 34.2) and basophilic stippling of red cells. Cerebrospinal fluid was normal. Electromyography showed evidence of denervation (fibrillation) and reinnervation (polyphasic motor unit potentials with incomplete interference pattern). NCV was reduced (left median nerve motor conduction velocity was 36 m/sec with a distal

motor latency of 6.5 msec). A sural nerve biopsy revealed neurofilamentous accumulations in the proximal paranodal regions of the axons, providing neuropathological evidence of an M*n*BK-induced neuropathy (see Neuropathological Diagnosis section).

Although the lead levels reported in blood (55 to 85 µg/dL) and significant amounts of lead were mobilized by chelation, the clinicians at that time (1976) considered the values "atypical" for lead neuropathy. Their skepticism about lead poisoning led to a better history of intake, which revealed the possible exposure to M*n*BK. The sural nerve biopsy findings of an enormous increase in neurofilaments, degenerating mitochondria, and active wallerian degeneration with myelin debris in the Schwann cell cytoplasm and axonal degeneration were, however, more consistent with exposure to M*n*BK. Many small myelinated fibers were noted and considered evidence of regeneration. Although the biopsy in this patient with current M*n*BK exposure exhibited axonal degeneration with accumulation of neurofilaments, the presence of moderately diminished myelinated fibers with increased amounts of connective tissue and proliferation of Schwann cells around denuded fibers can also be attributed to the chronic effects of lead on peripheral nerves (Lampert and Schochet, 1968).

It is likely that this patient had been exposed to both lead and M*n*BK. The findings of the sural biopsy in this patient were similar to those of experimentally induced M*n*BK neuropathy in rats. A differential diagnosis could not be made by biochemical means, as a specific diagnostic test of recent M*n*BK exposure, such as the concentrations of 2,5-hexanedione in urine, or tests reflecting more remote exposures such as hemoglobin adducts had not yet been validated when this patient was being evaluated.

REFERENCES

Abdel-Rahman MS, Hetland LB, Couri D. Toxicity and metabolism of methyl *n*-butyl ketone *Am Ind Hyg Assoc J* 1976;37:95–102.
Abe M. Beitrag zur pathologischen Anatomie der chronischen Schwefelkohlenstoffvergiftung. *Jpn J Med Sci* 1933;3:1.
Abou-Donia MB, Makkaway H-AM, Graham DG. The relative neurotoxicity of *n*-hexane, methyl *n*-butyl ketone, 2,5-hexanediol, and 2,5-hexanedione following oral or intraperitoneal administration in hens. *Toxicol Appl Pharmacol* 1982;62:369–389.
Ahonen I, Schimberg RW. 2,5-Hexanedione excretion after occupational exposure to *n*-hexane. *Br J Ind Med* 1988;45:133–136.
Aiello I, Rosati G, Serra G, Manca M. Subclinical neuropathic disorders and precautionary measures in the shoe industry. *Acta Neurol* 1980;35:285–291.
Alifimoff JK, Firestone LL, Miller KW. Anesthetic potencies of secondary alcohol enantiomers. *Anesthesiology* 1987;66:55–59.
Allen N. Identification of methyl *n*-butyl ketone as the causative agent. In: Spencer PS, Schaumburg HH, eds. *Experimental and clinical neurotoxicology*. Baltimore: Williams & Wilkins, 1980:846–855.
Allen N, Mendell JR, Billmaier DJ, Fontaine RE, O'Neil J. Toxic polyneuropathy due to methyl *n*-butyl ketone. *Arch Neurol* 1975;32:209–218.
Alpers BJ. Changes in the nervous system in carbon disulfide poisoning. *Neurol Psychiatry* 1939;42:1173.
Altenkirch H, Mager J, Stoltenburg G, Helmbrecht H. Toxic polyneuropathies after sniffing glue thinner. *J Neurol* 1977;214:137–152.
American Conference of Governmental Industrial Hygienists (ACGIH). *Threshold limit values (TLVs) for chemical substances and physical*

agents and Biological Exposure Indices (BEIs). Cincinnati, OH: ACGIH, 1995.

Amoore JE, Hautala E. Odor as an aid to chemical safety: odor thresholds compared with threshold limit values and volatilities for 214 industrial chemicals in air and water dilution. *J Appl Toxicol* 1983;3:272–290.

Anthony DC, Boekelheide K, Graham DG. The effects of 3,4-dimethyl substitution on the neurotoxicity of 2,5-hexanedione. *Toxicol Appl Pharmacol* 1983;71:362–371.

Arakawa O, Nakahiro M, Narahashi T. Chloride current induced by alcohols in rat dorsal rat ganglion neurons. *Brain Res* 1992;578:275–281.

Bäckström B, Collins VP. The effects of 2,5-hexanedione on rods and cones of the retina of albino rats. *Neurotoxicology* 1992;13:199–202.

Baker TS, Rickert DE. Dose-dependent uptake, distribution and elimination of inhaled *n*-hexane in the Fischer-344 rat. *Toxicol Appl Pharmacol* 1981;61:414–422.

Barregård L, Sällsten G, Nordberg C, Gieth W. Polyneuropathy possibly caused by 30 years of low exposure to *n*-hexane. *Scand J Work Environ Health* 1991;17:205–207.

Battistini N, Lenzi GL. EEG observations in the polyneuropathy of boot workers. *Elecroencephalog Clin Neurophysiol* 1975;39:531–538.

Beavers JD, Himmelstein JS, Hammond SK, Smith TJ, Kenyon EM, Sweet CP. Exposure in a household using gasoline contaminated water. *J Occup Environ Med* 1996;38:35–38.

Billmaier D, Yee HT, Allen N, Craft B, Williams N, Epstein S, Fontaine R. Peripheral neuropathy in a coated fabrics plant. *J Occup Med* 1974;16:665–671.

Bleeker ML. Clinical presentation of selected neurotoxic compounds. In: Bleeker ML, ed. *Occupational neurology and clinical neurotoxicology.* Baltimore, MD: Williams & Wilkins, 1994:207–234.

Böhlen P, Schlunegger UP, Läuppi E. Uptake and distribution of hexane in rat tissues. *Toxicol Appl Pharmacol* 1973;25:242–249.

Bos PMJ, de Mik G, Bragt PC. Critical review of the toxicity of methyl *n*-butyl ketone: risk from occupational exposure. *Am J Ind Med* 1991;20:175–194.

Bravaccio and Ammendola A, Barruffo L, Carlomagno S. H-reflex behavior in glue (*n*-hexane) neuropathy. *Clin Toxicol* 1981;18:1369–1375.

Brugnone F, Perbellini L, Grigolini L, Apostoli P. Solvent exposure in a shoe-upper factory. *Int Arch Occup Environ Health* 1978;42:51–62.

Cardona A, Marhuenda D, Marti J, Brugnone F, Roel J, Perbellini L. Biological monitoring of occupational exposure to *n*-hexane by measurement of urinary 2,5-hexanedione. *Int Arch Occup Environ Health* 1993;65:71–74.

Cardona, Marhuenda D, Prieto MJ, Marti J, Periago JF, Sanchez JM. Behaviour of urinary 2,5-hexanedione in occupational co-exposure to *n*-hexane and acetone. *Int Arch Occup Environ Health* 1996;68:88–93.

Cavalleri A, Cosi V. Polyneuritis incidence in shoe factory workers: case report and etiological considerations. *Arch Environ Health* 1978;33:192–197,.

Chang Y-C. Neurotoxic effects of *n*-hexane on the human central nervous system: evoked potential abnormalities in *n*-hexane polyneuropathy. *J Neurol Neurosurg Psychiatry* 1987;50:269–274.

Chang Y-C. Patients with *n*-hexane induced polyneuropathy: a clinical follow-up. *Br J Ind Med* 1990;47:485–489.

Chang Y-C. An electrophysiological follow up of patients with *n*-hexane polyneuropathy. *Br J Ind Med* 1991;48:12–17.

Channer S. Persistent visual hallucinations secondary to chronic solvent encephalopathy: case report and review of the literature. *J Neurol Neurosurg Psychiatry* 1983;46:83–86.

Chu C-C, Huang C-C, Chen R-S, Shih T-S. Polyneuropathy induced by carbon disulfide in viscose rayon workers. *Occup Environ Med* 1995;52:404–407.

Cianchetti C, Abbritti G, Perticoni G, Siracusa A, Curradi F. Toxic polyneuropathy of shoe-industry workers: a study of 122 cases. *J Neurol Neurosurg Psychiatry* 1976;39:1151–1161.

Couri D, Hetland LB, Abdel-Rahman MS, Weiss H. The influence of inhaled ketone vapors on hepatic microsomal biotransformation activities. *Toxicol Appl Pharmacol* 1977;41:285–289.

Couri D, Milks M. Toxicity and metabolism of the neurotoxic hexacarbons *n*-hexane, 2-hexanone, and 2,5-hexanedione. *Annu Rev Pharmacol Toxicol* 1982;22:145–166.

Davenport JG, Farrell DF, Sumi SM. 'Giant axonal neuropathy' caused by industrial chemicals: neurofilamentous axonal masses in man. *Neurology* 1976;26:919–923.

De Rosa E, Bartolucci GB, Cocheo V, Manno M. Ambiente de lavoro calzaturiero inquinamento da solventi. *Riv Infort Mal Prof* 1977;64:215–222.

Dick RB. Neurobehavioral assessment of occupationally relevant solvents and chemicals in humans. In: Chang LW, Dyer RS, eds. *Handbook of neurotoxicology.* New York: Marcel Dekker, 1995:217–322.

Dimitrijevic MR. Spasticity. In: Swash M, Kennard C, eds. *Scientific basis of clinical neurology.* Edinburgh: Churchill Livingstone 1985:108–115.

DiVincenzo GD, Kaplan CJ, Dedinas J. Characterization of the metabolites of methyl *n*-butyl ketone, methyl *iso*-butyl ketone, and methyl ethyl ketone in guinea pig serum and their clearance. *Toxicol Appl Pharmacol* 1976;36:511–522.

DiVincenzo GD, Hamilton ML, Kaplan CJ, Dedinas J. Metabolic fate and distribution of ^{14}C-labeled methyl *n*-butyl ketone in the rat. *Toxicol Appl Pharmacol* 1977;41:547–560.

DiVincenzo GD, Hamilton ML, Kaplan CJ, Krasavage WJ, O'Donoghue JL. Studies on the respiratory uptake and excretion of and the skin absorption of methyl *n*-butyl ketone in humans and dogs. *Toxicol Appl Pharmacol* 1978;44:593–604.

DiVincenzo GD, Hamilton ML, Kaplan CJ, Dedinas J. Characterization of the metabolites of methyl *n*-butyl ketone. In: Spencer PS, Schaumburg HH, eds. *Experimental and clinical neurotoxicology.* Baltimore: Williams & Wilkins, 1980:846–855.

Drinker P, Yaglou CP, Warren MF. Threshold toxicity of gasoline vapors. *J Ind Hyg Toxicol* 1943;25:225–232.

Ducatman AM, Moyer TP. Environmental exposure to common industrial solvents. *Am Assoc Clin Chem* 1984;5:1–18.

Environmental Protection Agency (EPA). *Drinking water regulations and health advisories.* Washington: Office of Water, 1996.

Fedtke N, Bolt HM. The relevance of 4,5-dihydroxy-2-hexanone in the excretion kinetics of *n*-hexane metabolites in rat and man. *Arch Toxicol* 1987;61:131–137.

Filser JG, Csanády GA, Dietz W, et al. Comparative estimation of the neurotoxic risks of *n*-hexane and *n*-heptane in rats and humans based on the metabolites 2,5-hexanedione and 2,5-heptanedione. *Adv Exp Med Biol* 1996;387:411–427.

Forman ST, Miller KW, Yellen G. A discrete site for general anesthetics on a postsynaptic receptor. *Mol Pharmacol* 1995;48:574–581.

Gonzalez EG, Downey JA. Polyneuropathy in a glue sniffer. *Arch Phys Med Rehab* 1972;53:333–337.

Goto I, Matsumura M, Inoue N, et al. Toxic polyneuropathy due to glue sniffing. *J Neurol Neurosurg Psychiatry* 1974;37:848–853.

Governa M, Calisti R, Coppa G, Tagliavento G, Colombi A, Troni W. Urinary excretion of 2,5-hexanedione and peripheral polyneuropathies in workers exposed to hexane. *J Toxicol Environ Health* 1987;20:219–228.

Graham DG, Amarath V, Valentine WM, Pyle SJ, Anthony DC. Pathogenic studies of hexane and carbon disulfide neurotoxicity. *Crit Rev Toxicol* 1995;25:91–112.

Granvil CP, Sharkawi M, Plaa GL. Metabolic fate of methyl *n*-butyl ketone, methyl ethyl ketone and their metabolites. *Toxicol Lett* 1994;70:263–267.

Haydon DA, Hendry BM, Levinson SR, Requena J. The molecular mechanisms of anæsthesia. *Nature* 1977a;268:356–358.

Haydon DA, Hendry BM, Levinson SR, Requena J. Anæsthesia by the *n*-alkanes. A comparative study of nerve impulse blockage and the properties of black lipid bilayer membranes. *Biochem Biophsys Acta* 1977b;470:17–34.

Herskowitz A, Ishii N, Schaumburg H. *n*-Hexane neuropathy: a syndrome occurring as a result of industrial exposure. *N Engl J Med* 1971;285:82–85.

Honma T, Miyagawa M, Sato M, Hasegawa H. Increase in glutamine content of rat brain induced by short-term exposure to toluene and hexane. *Ind Health* 1982;20:109–115.

Huang J, Shibata E, Kata K, Asaeda N, Takeuchi Y. Chronic exposure to *n*-hexane induces changes in nerve-specific marker proteins in the distal peripheral nerve on the rats. *Human Exp Toxicol* 1992;11:323–327.

Iida M, Yamamura Y, Sobue I. Electromyographic findings and conduction velocity on *n*-hexane polyneuropathy. *Electromyography* 1969;9:247–261.

Imbriani M, Ghittori S, Pezzagno G, Capodglio E. *n*-Hexane urine elimination and weighted exposure concentration. *Int Arch Occup Environ Health* 1984;55:33–41.

Iwata M, Takeuchi Y, Hisanaga N, Ono Y. A study on biological monitoring of *n*-hexane exposure. *Int Arch Occup Environ Health* 1983;51:253–260.

Iwata M, Takeuchi Y, Hisanaga N, Ono Y. Changes in *n*-hexane neurotoxicity and its urinary metabolites by long-term co-exposure with MEK or toluene. *Int Arch Occup Environ Health* 1984;54:273–281.

Jakobson I, Wahlberg JE, Holberg B, Johansson G. Uptake via the blood and elimination of 10 organic solvents following epicutaneous exposure of anesthetized guinea pigs. *Toxicol Appl Pharmacol* 1982;63:181–187.

Jørgenson NK, Cohr K-H. *n*-Hexane and its toxicological effects. A review. *Scand J Work Environ Health* 1981;7:157–168.

Kawai T, Yasugi T, Mizunuma K, Horiuchi S, Ikeda M. Comparative evaluation of blood and urine analysis as a tool for biological monitoring of *n*-hexane and toluene. *Int Arch Occup Environ Health* 1993;65:S123–S126.

Korobkin R, Asbury AK, Sumner AJ, Nielsen SL. Glue-sniffing neuropathy. *Arch Neurol* 1975;32:158–162.

Kramer A, Staudiner H, Ullrich V. Effect of *n*-hexane inhalation on the monooxygenase system in mice liver microsomes. *Chem Biol Interact* 1974;8:11–18.

Krasavage WJ, O'Donoghue JL, DiVincenzo GD, Terhaar CJ. The relative neurotoxicity of methyl *n*-butyl ketone, *n*-hexane and their metabolites. *Toxicol Appl Pharmacol* 1980;52:433–441.

Lampert PW, Schochet SS. Demyelination and remyelination in lead neuropathy: electron microscopic studies. *J Neuropathol Exp Neurol* 1968;27:527–545.

Lodén M. The in vitro permeability of human skin to benzene, ethylene glycol, formaldehyde, and *n*-hexane. *Acta Pharmacol Toxicol* 1986;58:382–389.

Low LK, Meeks JR, Mackerer CR. Hexane isomers. In: Snyder R, ed. *Ethel Browning's toxicity and Metabolism of industrial solvents*, 2nd ed., vol. 1: *Hydrocarbons*. London: Elsevier Science Publishers, 1987:291–296.

Lynch JJ 3rd, Merigan WH, Eskin TA. Subchronic dosing of macaques with 2,5-hexanedione causes long-lasting motor dysfunction but reversible visual loss. *Toxicol Appl Pharmacol* 1989;98:166–180.

Mallov JS. MBK neuropathy among spray painters. *JAMA* 1976;235:1455–1457.

Masotto C, Bisiani C, Camisasca C, et al. Effects of acute *n*-hexane and 2,5-hexanedione treatment on the striatal dopaminergic system in mice. *J Neural Transm Suppl* 1995;45:281–285.

McDermott HJ, Killiany SE Jr. Quest for a gasoline TLV. *Am Ind Hyg Assoc J* 1978;39:110–117.

Mendell JR, Saida K, Ganasia MF. Toxic polyneuropathy produced experimentally by methyl *n*-butyl ketone. *Science* 1974;185:787–789.

Mendell JR, Sahenk Z, Saida K, Weiss HS, Savage R, Couri D. Alterations of fast axoplasmic transport in experimental methyl *n*-butyl ketone neuropathy. *Brain Res* 1977;133:107–118.

Murata K, Araki S, Yokoyama K, Yamashita K, Okajima F, Nakaaki K. Changes in autonomic function as determined by ECG R-R interval variability in sandal, shoe and leather workers exposed to *n*-hexane, xylene and toluene. *Neurotoxicology* 1994;15:867–876.

Mutti JR, Ferri F, Lommi G, Lotta S, Lucertini S, Franchini I. *n*-Hexane-induced changes in nerve conduction velocities and somatosensory evoked potentials. *Int Arch Occup Environ Health* 1982;51:45–54.

Mutti A, Falzoi M, Lucertini S, et al. *n*-Hexane metabolism in occupationally exposed workers. *Br J Ind Med* 1984;41:533–538.

National Institute for Occupational Safety and Health (NIOSH). *Criteria for a recommended standard: occupational exposure to alkanes.* Publication No. 77-151. DHEW, Cincinnati, OH: DHEW, 1977.

National Institute for Occupational Safety and Health (NIOSH). *Health hazard evaluation report.* Publication No. HETA 86-004-1740. Washington: US Department of Health and Human Services, CDC, 1986.

National Institute for Occupational Safety and Health (NIOSH). *Pocket guide to chemical hazards.* Washington: US Department of Health and Human Services, CDC, 1997.

Nelson KW, Ege JF Jr, Ross M, Woodman LE, Silverman L. Sensory response to certain industrial solvent vapors. *J Ind Hyg Toxicol* 1943;25:282.

Nylén P, Hagman M. Function of the auditory and visual system, and of peripheral nerve, in rats after long-term combined exposure to *n*-hexane and methylated benzene derivatives. II. Xylene. *Pharmacol Toxicol* 1994;74:124–129.

Nylén P, Hagman M, Johnson A-C. Function of the auditory and visual system, and of peripheral nerve, in rats after long-term combined exposure to *n*-hexane and methylated benzene derivatives. I. Toluene. *Pharmacol Toxicol* 1994;74:116–123.

Occupational Safety and Health Administration (OSHA). Code of Federal Regulations, 29, 1910.1000/.1047. Washington: Office of the Federal Register, National Archives and Records Administration, 1995:411–431.

O'Donoghue JL, Krasavage WJ. Hexacarbon neuropathy: a γ-diketone neuropathy? *J Neuropathol Exp Neurol* 1979;38:333 (abstract).

Oishi H, Mineno K, Yamada M, Chiba K, Shibata K. Polyneuropathy caused by an organic solvent (*n*-hexane). *Saigai Igaku* 1964;7:218.

Ono Y, Takeuchi Y, Hisanaga N, Iwata M, Kitoh J, Sugiura Y. Neurotoxicity of petroleum benzine compared with *n*-hexane. *Int Arch Occup Environ Health* 1982;50:219–229.

Oryshkevich RS, Wilcox R, Jhee WH. Polyneuropathy due to glue exposure: case report and 16-year follow-up. *Arch Phys Med Rehabil* 1986;67:827–828.

Passero S, Battistini N, Cioni R, et al. Toxic encephalopathy of shoe workers in Italy. A clinical, neurophysiological, and follow-up study. *Ital J Neurol Sci* 1983;4:463–472.

Pastore C, Marhuenda D, Marti J, Cardona A. Early diagnosis of *n*-hexane-caused neuropathy. *Muscle Nerve* 1994;17:981–986.

Patty FA, Yant WP. *U.S. Bureau of Mines Report, Investigation No. 2979.* Washington: US Bureau of Mines, 1929.

Perbellini L, Brugnone F, Gaffuri E. Neurotoxic metabolites of "commercial hexane" in the urine of shoe factory workers. *Clin Toxicol* 1981a;18:1377–1385.

Perbellini L, Brugnone F, Faggionato G. Urinary excretion of the metabolites of *n*-hexane and its isomers during occupational exposure. *Br J Ind Med* 1981b;38:20–26.

Perbellini L, Amantini MC, Brugnone F, Frontali N. Urinary excretion on *n*-hexane metabolites. A comparative study in rat, rabbit and monkey. *Arch Toxicol* 1982;50:203–215.

Perbellini L, Brugnone F, Caretta D, Maranelli G. Partition coefficients of some industrial aliphatic hydrocarbons (C5–C7) in blood and human tissues. *Br J Ind Med* 1985;42:162–167.

Perbellini L, Mozzo P, Brugnone F, Zedde A. Physiologicomathematical model for studying human exposure to organic solvents: kinetics of blood/tissue *n*-hexane concentrations and 2,5-hexanedione in urine. *Br J Ind Med* 1986;443:760–768.

Perbellini L, Pezzoli G, Brugnone F, Canesi M. Biochemical and physiological aspects of 2,5-hexanedione: endogenous or exogenous product? *Int Arch Occup Environ Health* 1993;65:49–52.

Periago JF, Cardona A, Marhuenda D, et al. Biological monitoring of occupational exposure to *n*-hexane by exhaled air and urinalysis. *Int Arch Occup Environ Health* 1993;65:275–278.

Peters HA, Levine RL, Matthews CG, Chapman LJ. Extrapyramidal and other neurological manifestations associated with carbon disulfide fumigant exposure. *Arch Neurol* 1988;45:537–540.

Pezzoli G, Antonini A, Barbieri S, et al. *n*-Hexane-induced parkinsonism: pathogenetic hypotheses. *Mov Disord* 1995;10:279–282.

Prockop LD, Alt M, Tison J. "Huffer's" neuropathy. *JAMA* 1974;229:1083–1084.

Pryor GT, Rebert CS. Interactive effects of toluene and hexane on behavior and neurophysiologic responses in Fischer 344 rats. *Neurotoxicology* 1992;13:225–234.

Pyle SJ, Amarnath V, Graham DG, Anthony DC. The role of pyrrole formation in the alteration of neurofilament transport induced during exposure to 2,5-hexanedione. *J Neuropathol Exp Neurol* 1992;51:451–458.

Pyle SJ, Amarnath V, Graham DG, Anthony DC. Decreased levels of the high molecular weight subunit of neurofilaments and accelerated neurofilament transport during the recovery phase of 2,5-hexanedione exposure. *Cell Motil Cytoskel* 1993;26:133–143.

Raitta C, Seppäläinen A-M, Huuskonen MS. *n*-Hexane maculopathy in industrial workers. *Aldr Graefes Arch Klin Ophthalmol* 1978;209:99–110.

Raitta C. Tier H, Tolonen M, Nurminen M, Helpiö E, Malmström S. Impaired color discrimination among viscose rayon workers exposed to carbon disulfide. *J Occup Med* 1981;23:189–192.

Ralston WH, Hilderbrand RL, Uddin DE, Andersen ME, Gardier RW. Potentiation of 2,5-hexanedione neurotoxicity by methyl ethyl ketone. *Toxicol Appl Pharmacol* 1985;81:319–327.

Richter R. Degeneration of the basal ganglia in monkey from carbon disulfide poisoning. *J Neuropathol Exp Neurol* 1945;4:324–353.

Robertson P Jr, White EL, Bus JS. Effects of methyl ethyl ketone pretreatment on hepatic mixed-function oxidase activity and on in vivo metabolism of *n*-hexane. *Xenobiotica* 1989;19:721–729.

Ruff RL, Petito CK, Acheson LS. Neuropathy associated with chronic low level exposure to *n*-hexane. *Clin Toxicol* 1981;18:515–519.

Sahenk Z, Mendell JR. Acrylamide and 2,5-hexanedione neuropathies: abnormal bidirection transport rate in distal axons. *Brain Res* 1981; 219:397–405.

Saida K, Mendell JR, Weiss HS. Peripheral nerve changes induced by methyl *n*-butyl ketone and potentiation by methyl ethyl ketone. *J Neuropathol Exp Neurol* 1976;35:207–225.

Sandmeyer EE. Aliphatic hydrocarbons. In: Clayton GD, Clayton FE, eds. *Patty's industrial hygiene and toxicology,* 3rd ed. New York: 1981: 3175–3200.

Sax NI. *Dangerous properties of industrial chemicals,* 5th ed. New York: Van Nostrand Reinhold, 1979.

Sax DS, Kovacs ZL, Johnson TL, Feldman RG. Clinical applications of the estimation of nerve conduction velocity distributions. *Progr Clin Biol Res* 1981;52:113–136.

Scelsi R, Poggi P, Fera L, Gonella G. Toxic polyneuropathy due to *n*-hexane. A light- and electron-microscopic study of the peripheral nerve and muscle from three cases. *J Neurol Sci* 1980;47:7–19.

Schaumburg HH, Spencer PS. Degeneration in central and peripheral nervous system produced by pure *n*-hexane—an experimental study. *Brain* 1976;99:183–192.

Schaumburg HH, Spencer PS. Environmental hydrocarbons produce degeneration in cat hypothalamus and optic tract. *Science* 1978;199:199–200.

Schwarz HG. Benzin-Vergiftung, chronische, medizinale. *Samml Vergiftungsf* 1933:4:247–248.

Seppäläinen AM, Raitta C, Huuskonen MS. *n*-Hexane-induced changes in visual evoked potentials and electroretinograms of industrial workers. *Electroencephalogr Clin Neurophysiol* 1979;47:492–498.

Seppäläinen AM, Raitta C, Huuskonen MS. Nervous and visual effects of occupational *n*-hexane exposure. In: Lechner H, Aranibar A, eds. *EEG and clinical neurophysiology.* Amsterdam: Exerpta Medica, 1980: 656–661.

Sharkawi M, Granvil C, Faci A, Plaa GL. Pharmacodynamic and metabolic interactions between ethanol and two industrial solvents (methyl *n*-butyl ketone and methyl isobutyl ketone) and the principal metabolites in mice. *Toxicology* 1994;94:187–195.

Shibata E, Huang J, Ono Y, Hisanaga N, Iwata M, Saito I, Takeuchi Y. Changes in urinary *n*-hexane metabolites by co-exposure to various concentrations of methyl ethyl ketone and fixed *n*-hexane levels. *Arch Toxicol* 1990;64:165–168.

Shirabe T, Tsuda T, Terao A, Araki S. Toxic polyneuropathy due to glue-sniffing. Report of two cases with a light and electron microscopic study of the peripheral nerves and muscles. *J Neurol Sci* 1974;21: 101–113.

Sickles DW. Toxic neurofilamentous axonopathies and fast anterograde axonal transport. II. The effects of single doses of neurotoxic and non-neurotoxic diketones and β,β′-iminodipropionitrile (IDPN) on the rate and capacity of transport. *Neurotoxicology* 1989;10:103–112.

Spencer PS, Schaumburg HH, Raleigh RL, Terhaar CJ. Nervous system degeneration produced by methyl *n*-butyl ketone. *Arch Neurol* 1975; 32:219–222.

Spencer PS, Schaumburg HH. Experimental neuropathy produced by 2,5-hexanedione—a major metabolite of the industrial solvent methyl *n*-butyl ketone. *J Neurol Neurosurg Psychiatry* 1975;8:771–775.

Spencer PS, Schaumburg HH. Feline nervous system response to chronic intoxication with commercial grades of methyl *n*-butyl ketone, methyl *iso*-butyl ketone and methyl ethyl ketone. *Toxicol Appl Pharmacol* 1976;37:301–311.

Spencer PS, Couri D, Schaumburg HH. *n*-Hexane and methyl *n*-butyl ketone. In: Spencer PS, Schaumburg HH, eds. *Experimental and clinical neurotoxicology.* Baltimore: Williams & Wilkins, 1980:456–475.

St. Clair MBG, Anthony DC, Wikstrand CJ, Graham DG. Neurofilament protein crosslinking in γ-diketone neuropathy: in vitro and in vivo studies using the seaworm *Myxicola infundibulum. Neurotoxicology* 1989;10:743–756.

Stoltenburg-Didinger G, Boegner F, Grüning W, Wagner M, Marx P, Altenkirch H. Specific neurotoxic effects of different organic solvents on dissociated cultures of the nervous system. *Neurotoxicology* 1992;13: 161–164.

Takeuchi Y. *n*-Hexane polyneuropathy in Japan: a review of *n*-hexane poisoning and its preventive measures. *Environ Res* 1993;62:76–80.

Takeuchi Y, Mabuchi C, Takagi S. Polyneuropathy caused by petroleum benzine. *Int Arch Arbeitsmed* 1975;34:185–197.

Takeuchi Y, Ono Y, Hisanaga N. An experimental study on the combined effect of hexane and toluene on the peripheral nerve of the rat. *Br J Ind Med* 1981;38:14–19.

Tenebein M, de Groot W, Rajani KR. Peripheral neuropathy following intentional inhalation of naphtha fumes. *Can Med Assoc J* 1984;131: 1077–1079.

Thomas PK, Berthold C-H, Ochoa J. Microscopic anatomy of the peripheral nervous system. In: Dyck PJ, Thomas PK, eds. *Peripheral neuropathy,* 3rd ed. Philadelphia: WB Saunders, 1993:28–91.

Tsuruta H. Percutaneous absorption of organic solvents. III. On the penetration rates of hydrophobic solvents through the excised rat skin. *Ind Health* 1982;20:335–345.

United States International Trade Commission (USITC). *Synthetic organic chemicals: United States production and sales, 1992.* USITC Pub #2720. Washington: USITC, 1994.

Vallat JM, Leboulet A, Loubet C, Piva C, Dumas M. *n*-Hexane- and methylethylketone-induced polyneuropathy abnormal accumulation of glycogen in unmyelinated axons. *Acta Neuropathol* 1981;55:275–279.

van Engelen JG, Kezix S, de Haan W, Opdam JJ, de Wolff FA. Determination of 2,5-hexanedione, a metabolite of *n*-hexane, in urine: evaluation and application of three analytical methods. *J Chromatogr* 1995;667: 233–240.

Vanhoorne M, de Douck A, Bacquer D. Epidemiological study of the systemic ophthalmological effects of carbon disulfide. *Arch Environ Health* 1996;51:181–188.

Vigliani EC. Clinical observations on carbon disulfide intoxication in Italy. *Ind Med Surg* 1950;19:240–242.

Vigliani EC. Carbon disulphide poisoning in viscose rayon factories. *Br J Ind Med* 1954;11:235–244.

Veulemans H, Van Vlem E, Jansses H, Masschelein R, Leplat A. Experimental human exposure to *n*-hexane: study of the respiratory uptake and elimination, and of *n*-hexane concentrations in peripheral venous blood. *Int Arch Occup Environ Health* 1982;49:251–263.

Wang J-D, Chang Y-C, Kao K-P, Huang C-C, Lin C-C, and Yeh W-Y. An outbreak of *n*-hexane induced polyneuropathy among press proofing workers in Taipei. *Am J Ind Med* 1986;10:111–118.

White RF, Feldman RG, Proctor SP. Neurobehavioral effects of toxic exposure: clinical syndromes in adult neuropsychology. In: White RF, ed. *The practitioners handbook.* Amsterdam: Elsevier Science Publishers, 1992:1–51.

Wickersham CW, Fredericks EJ. Toxic polyneuropathy secondary to methyl *n*-butyl ketone. *Conn Med* 1976;40:311–312.

Yamada S. An occurrence of polyneuritis by *n*-hexane in the polyethylene laminating plants. *Jpn J Ind Health* 1964;6:192.

Yamada S. Intoxication polyneuritis in workers exposed to *n*-hexane. *Jpn J Ind Health* 1967;9:651–659.

Yamamura Y. *n*-Hexane polyneuropathy. *Folia Psychiatr Neurol Jpn* 1969;23:45–57.

Yokoyama K, Feldman RG, Sax DS, Salzsider BT, Kucera J. Relation of distribution of conduction velocities to nerve biopsy findings in *n*-hexane poisoning. *Muscle Nerve* 1990;13:314–320.

CHAPTER 17

Styrene

Styrene (vinyl benzene, ethenylbenzene, phenylethylene, phenylethene, cinnamene, cinnamol, cinnamenol, styrole, styrolene, styrene monomer, inhibited styrene) is an alkenylbenzene compound structurally similar to toluene and xylene. Styrene monomer is a colorless to yellow, flammable, oily liquid with a pleasant odor at low concentration and a disagreeable odor at higher concentrations (e.g., >200 ppm) (Sax, 1979; Stewart et al., 1968). It is naturally formed in the sap of the styracaceous tree (Patty, 1963). Organic chemical synthesis of styrene proceeds via an initial alkylation of benzene with ethylene, followed by catalytic dehydrogenation of the resultant ethylbenzene (Guthrie, 1960; Tossavainen, 1978). An oxidative process in which styrene is produced as a coproduct with propylene oxide is also used (Tossavainen, 1978).

Styrene is highly reactive and polymerizes in the presence of light and air; polymerization occurs more readily at elevated temperatures than at room temperature (*Chemical Review,* 1988). Polymerization inhibitors are usually added to it for stabilization to prevent the possibility of violent explosions (Sandmeyer, 1981; CSD, 1971; *Chemical Review,* 1988).

The odor of styrene usually alerts an exposed individual to its presence (Pratt-Johnson, 1964). However, a person's ability to perceive the odor begins to diminish within minutes (Stewart et al., 1968). Styrene irritates the eyes, mucous membranes, and respiratory system (Hayes et al., 1991; NIOSH, 1994) and causes nausea, vomiting, loss of appetite, and general weakness (Rogers and Hooper, 1957). Neurobehavioral and neurophysiological effects following exposure to styrene have been reported, reflecting changes in the central and peripheral nervous systems (Letz et al., 1990; Jegaden et al., 1993; Cherry and Gautrin, 1990; Lilis et al., 1978; Härkönen et al., 1978; Seppäläinen and Härkönen, 1976).

SOURCES OF EXPOSURE

Estimates of styrene exposure among workers in the United States range from 50,000 (directly exposed) to 300,000 (indirectly exposed) (Tossavainen, 1978; Fishbein, 1992; Brown, 1991). When heated to 200°F, styrene is polymerized to polystyrene, a clear plastic with good insulating properties (*Merck Index,* 1989). Other compounds containing styrene include: styrene–butadiene–rubber; acrylonitrile–butadiene–styrene terpolymers and styrene acrylonitrile copolymer resins; and styrenated polyester (*Chemical Review,* 1988). Occupational exposure to styrene occurs at sites of monomer production and polymerization, during the transportation and handling of liquid styrene monomer, and during the fabrication of styrene plastics. High levels of occupational exposure occur in the production of fiberglass-reinforced plastics, while lower levels of exposure occur during the use of latex paints and polyester putties and around the thermal decomposition of styrene plastics (Tossavainen, 1978).

Styrene is widely used in the boat building industry and in the manufacture of styrene modified polyester products, such as swimming pools and steeping baths (Gotell, 1972). The production of fiberglass-reinforced plastic boats or other products involves covering a wooden form having the converse shape of the hull or other component with fiberglass and styrene polyester resin, either by a hand lay-up technique or by a combination hand lay-up and spray-up procedure (Gotell, 1972; Crandall and Hartle, 1985). Occupational exposure potential varies depending on the size and configuration of the object under construction. Exposure to styrene in the boat-building industry frequently exceeds established exposure limits (Crandall and Hartle, 1985).

Styrene has been detected in the blood of nonoccupationally exposed persons (Ashley et al., 1994). Exposures occur among unsuspecting consumers in the home through use of floor waxes, polishes, paints, adhesives, auto body fillers, metal cleaners, putty, and varnishes. Residual styrene monomers leach into foods packaged in general-purpose and high-impact polystyrenes (Murphy et al., 1992). Tobacco smoke and automobile exhaust constitute additional sources of exposure among the general population. Styrene concentrations on the breath of smokers were found to be sixfold higher than those of nonsmokers (Wallace et al., 1988).

EXPOSURE LIMITS AND SAFETY REGULATIONS

The odor of styrene is detectable in air at 0.32 ppm (Amoore and Hautala, 1983) (Table 17-1). The *Occupational Safety and Health Administration*'s (OSHA) permissible exposure level (PEL) for styrene is an 8-hour time-weighted average (TWA) exposure of 100 ppm. OSHA PEL for brief periods of exposure is a 15-minute TWA ceiling concentration of 200 ppm, with a 5-minute maximum permissible peak exposure of 600 ppm within any 3-hour period of a workday (OSHA, 1995). *The National Institute for Occupational Safety and Health* (NIOSH) has set its recommended exposure limit (REL) at a 10-hour TWA concentration of 50 ppm. The NIOSH-recommended short-term exposure limit (STEL) is a 15-minute TWA exposure of 100 ppm. The NIOSH-recommended immediately dangerous to life and health (IDLH) level for styrene is an ambient air concentration of 700 ppm (NIOSH, 1997). The *American Conference of Governmental and Industrial Hygienists* (ACGIH) recommends an 8-hour TWA of 50 ppm for its threshold limit value (TLV). ACGIH recommends a 15-minute TWA STEL of 100 ppm (ACGIH, 1995).

TABLE 17-1. *Established and recommended occupational and environmental exposure limits for styrene in air and water*

	Air (ppm)[a]	Water (mg/L)[a]
Odor threshold*	0.32	0.011
OSHA		
PEL (8-hr TWA)	100	—
PEL ceiling (15-min TWA)	200 (600 max)	—
NIOSH		
REL (10-hr TWA)	50	—
STEL (15-min TWA)	100	—
IDLH	700	—
ACGIH		
TLV (8-hr TWA)	50	—
STEL (15-min TWA)	100	—
USEPA		
MCL	—	0.1
MCLG	—	0.1

[a]Unit conversion: 1.0 ppm = 4.33 mg/m^3; 1 ppm = 1 mg/L. OSHA, Occupational Safety and Health Administration; PEL, permissible exposure limit; TWA, time-weighted average; NIOSH, National Institute for Occupational Safety and Health; REL, recommended exposure limit; STEL, short-term exposure limit; IDLH, immediately dangerous to life and health; ACGIH, American Conference of Industrial Hygienists; TLV, threshold limit value; USEPA, United States Environmental Protection Agency; MCL, maximum contamination level; MCLG, maximum contamination level goal.
Data from *Amoore and Hautala, 1983; OSHA, 1995; ACGIH, 1995; USEPA, 1996; NIOSH, 1997.

The odor threshold for styrene in water is 0.011 mg/L (Amoore and Hautala, 1983). The maximum contaminant level (MCL) for drinking water set by the *United States Environmental Protection Agency* (USEPA) is 0.1 mg/L (USEPA, 1996) (see Table 17-1).

METABOLISM

Absorption

Styrene can be absorbed by pulmonary, percutaneous, and gastrointestinal routes (Leibman, 1975). Pulmonary absorption is dependent on respiratory rate, the solubility of styrene in blood, and the rate of blood circulation (Astrand, 1975). Reported pulmonary retention of styrene following exposure of volunteers to low (4.6 to 46 ppm) and high (70 to 206 ppm) concentrations has ranged from 60% to 95%, respectively (Petreas et al., 1995; Fernandez and Caperos, 1977; Bardodej and Bardodejova, 1970; Fiserova-Bergerova and Teisinger, 1965). Several studies indicate that retention is independent of inspired styrene concentration (Wieczorek and Piotrowski, 1985) or duration of exposure (Fernandez and Caperos, 1977), and therefore the reported differences in retention are most likely due to differences in experimental methodology (Petreas et al., 1995). Uptake is increased by physical exertion (Astrand, 1975). Engstrom et al. (1978a) determined that uptake is five to six times greater during periods of heavy work (150 W) than during exposure at rest; total uptake rose from an average of 40 mg at rest to 210 mg during the 150-W exercise period. Cherry and Gautrin (1990) noted that jobs requiring much physical exertion resulted in much higher retention than expected from the ambient air measurements. In humans and rats, uptake of styrene vapor continues throughout the exposure period and is proportional to the air styrene concentration, suggesting that limiting or plateau concentrations will take longer to reach at higher exposure levels (Astrand et al., 1974; Withey, 1978).

Styrene liquid is absorbed from the alimentary tract (Leibman, 1975). In rats, styrene in aqueous solution is readily absorbed with peak concentrations observed in less than 4 minutes after oral ingestion. Absorption of styrene in solution with vegetable oil is more complete but much slower, with peak concentration in blood reached approximately 2 hours after exposure (Withey, 1978).

Dermal absorption of styrene is related to temperature, hydration, surface area, type, and condition of the skin, as well as duration of exposure (Riihimaki and Pfaffli, 1978; Brown et al., 1984; Berode et al., 1985). Dermal absorption of styrene vapor is considered negligible, with a dermal vapor absorption coefficient of 0.022 m^3/hr (Wieczorek, 1985). The dermal absorption rate for pure liquid styrene through the skin of an immersed hand is 0.06 mg/cm^2/hr. Thus, the amount of styrene absorbed per hour through the skin of an immersed hand would be approximately 15 mg or 4% of the dose retained in the body following an 8-hour exposure to 50 ppm styrene vapor in air (Berode et al., 1985). These findings suggest that in most occupational situations, dermal absorption of styrene may also play a role in total uptake.

Tissue Distribution

Styrene is very soluble in blood and is mainly present in the serum fraction (Mizunuma et al., 1993). However, the blood contains only about 4% of a total absorbed dose following a 2-hour exposure to fluctuating concentrations of styrene, indicating that the remainder is readily released into organs and tissues (Astrand, 1975). Distribution to all major organs including the brain is rapid (Trenga et al., 1991; Lof et al., 1983; Withey, 1978; Withey and Collins, 1977; 1979). Due to its lipid solubility, styrene readily crosses the blood–brain barrier (BBB) and may reach high concentrations in the central nervous system (CNS) following exposure (Withey, 1978). The concentration of styrene and its metabolites in the brain increases exponentially with the exposure dose (Fig. 17-1) (Lof et al., 1983). Thus, with increasing exposure dose, styrene concentration in the well-perfused lipid-rich brain tissue is significantly higher than that in the blood (Withey, 1978). A linear relationship exists between the styrene content in the brain and that of the subcutaneous adipose tissue immediately following exposure (Savolainen and Pfaffli, 1978). Whole-body radiography of pregnant mice exposed to ^{14}C-labeled styrene revealed high concentrations of unmetabolized styrene in the lungs, kidney, liver, and adipose tissue, as well as in the brain (Kishi et al., 1989). In addition, considerable amounts of radioactivity were seen in the brains of the fetuses, indicating that styrene crosses the placenta. Furthermore, Holmberg (1977; 1980) noted a significant

increase in the incidence of anencephaly and hydrocephalus among children exposed to styrene in utero. This finding may be of particular importance in cases of maternal exposure to styrene.

The highest styrene concentrations are found in subcutaneous adipose, with successively lower concentrations seen in the kidneys, liver, lungs, and brain (Lof et al., 1983). Needle biopsy specimens of subcutaneous adipose tissue taken from human subjects at 2, 4, and 21 hours after cessation of exposure to styrene vapor at a concentration of 50 ppm for 30 minutes while either at rest or in conjunction with exercise at 50, 100, and 150 W had a mean styrene concentration of 3.6 mg/kg. Retention of styrene in adipose tissue was noted as late as 13 days after cessation of exposure (Engstrom, 1978). Because of the slow elimination from adipose tissue, chronically exposed workers carry a greater body burden. Styrene concentrations in the fat biopsies taken from two styrene workers on a Monday morning ranged from 2.8 to 8.1 mg/kg, while at the end of the week the concentrations were 4.7 to 11.6 mg/kg; these workers were exposed to styrene vapor at a time-weighted average concentration of 7.6 to 20.2 ppm (Engstrom, 1978). These findings indicate that chronically exposed individuals are at increased risk of neurotoxic effects.

Tissue Biochemistry

Styrene metabolism rapidly follows administration by any route. Biotransformation of styrene occurs in the liver by the microsomal cytochrome P-450 oxidizing system through the catalyzed oxidation of styrene to styrene-7,8-oxide (Fig. 17-2). Styrene-7,8-oxide is hydrated to phenylethylene glycol by microsomal epoxide hydrolase and is subsequently oxidized to the two major metabolites, mandelic acid (MA) (85%) and phenylglyoxylic acid (PGA) (10%), (Bardodej and Bardodejova, 1970; Oesch et al., 1971; Leibman and Ortiz, 1968, 1970; Leibman, 1975). The oxidation of phenylethylene glycol and MA to benzoic acid, followed by conjugation with glycine to form hippuric acid, occurs to a lesser extent (Toftgård and Gustafsson, 1980; Leibman, 1975; Bakke and Scheline, 1970; Bardodej and Bardodejova, 1970). Styrene metabolism is complex and involves multiple competing pathways including conjugations with glucuronide, glutathione, glycine, or sulfate. Minor metabolites include 4-vinylphenol (Pfaffli et al., 1981; Leibman, 1975; Guillemin and Berode, 1988). The presence of 4-vinylphenol in the urine of individuals exposed to styrene suggests that in humans styrene is also metabolized via arene oxidation and that styrene-3,4-oxide is formed as an intermediate in this reaction (Pfaffli et al., 1981).

The biotransformation of styrene to styrene-7,8-oxide occurs in the brain as well as in the liver (Marietta et al., 1979). The toxicity of styrene appears to be related to its biotransformation to styrene-7,8-oxide, the toxicity of which is approximately four times that of styrene (Ohtsuji

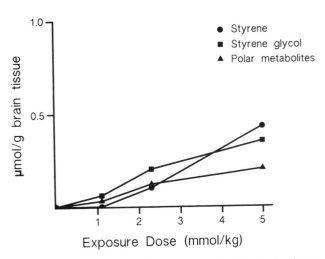

FIG. 17-1. Dose dependent increase in the brain tissue concentrations of styrene, styrene glycol and the polar metabolites of styrene. (Modified from Löf et al., 1983, with permission.)

and Ikeda, 1971). Styrene-7,8-oxide can react with cellular macromolecules including neurofilaments, DNA, and RNA, resulting in the disruption of axonal transport and protein synthesis, formation of neoantigens, mutations, cancer, and cell death (Parke, 1987). Styrene-7,8-oxide, because of its reactive electrophilic nature, is an alkylating agent and reacts mostly with deoxyguanosine, giving 7-alkylguanine, and also with deoxycytidine, giving *N*-3-alkylcytosine (Lilis, 1992).

Conjugation of styrene-7,8-oxide with glutathione provides a protective alternative to the covalent binding of styrene-7,8-oxide with cell structures (Parkki, 1978; Srivastava et al., 1983). Oral administration of styrene results in significant inhibition of glutathione-*S*-transferase and aryl hydrocarbon hydroxylase activity, followed by decreased levels of glutathione in the brains of rats (Dixit et al., 1982). Oral administration of styrene oxide decreased glutathione content significantly in medulla-pons of rats (Trenga et al., 1991). The brain and nervous system are especially prone to the effects of electrophilic alkylating agents, and decreased levels of brain glutathione contribute to injury of neuronal and glial cells by allowing cellular interactions with the styrene-7,8-oxide (Trenga et al., 1991) (see Neuropathological Diagnosis section).

Concurrent exposures to other chemicals alter the metabolism of styrene. For example, in humans, acute ingestion of ethanol inhibits cytochrome P-450–mediated oxidation of styrene (Wilson et al., 1983), and inhibits the oxidation of styrene glycol to mandelic acid (Cerny et al., 1990). Conversely, individuals who consume ethanol on a regular basis have an increased metabolic conversion rate, due to induction of hepatic microsomal oxidizing enzymes, leading to more efficient metabolism of both styrene and ethanol; but also increased formation of styrene-7,8-oxide (Cerny et al., 1990). Concurrent exposure to trichloroethylene and/or toluene has been shown to suppress the metabolism of styrene, while this effect is diminished after pretreatment with phenobarbital (Ikeda and Hirayama,

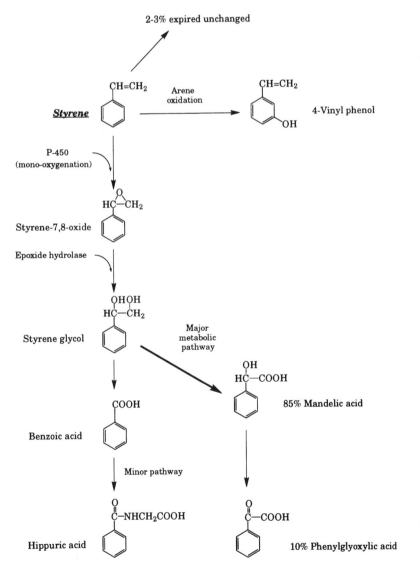

FIG. 17-2. Metabolic pathways of styrene (Leibman and Ortiz, 1968, 1970; Bakke and Scheline, 1970; Bardodej and Bardodejova, 1970; Oesch et al., 1971; Leibman, 1975; Toftgård and Gustafsson, 1980; Pfäffli et al., 1981; Guillemin and Berode, 1988).

1978; Ikeda et al., 1972). Phenobarbital, a known inducer of cytochrome P-450 microsomal enzymes, increases the oxidative conversion of styrene to styrene oxide (Ohtsuji and Ikeda, 1971). Exposure of rats to styrene and ethanol decreased levels of nonprotein sulfhydryls (including glutathione) by 60% (Coccini et al., 1996). These results are of clinical importance because of the potential for concurrent exposure among styrene workers who are at increased risk for neurotoxic effects.

Excretion

Clearance of styrene from the blood of humans exposed to styrene vapor at a steady concentration of 80 ppm follows a linear two-compartment pharmacokinetic model, with the second (slow) compartment representing clearance from adipose tissue (see Fig. 17-3) (Ramsey and Young, 1978). Studies of the dose-dependent kinetics of styrene elimination in rats reveal a similar biphasic pattern of elimination. However, while the elimination rate coefficient in the initial phase remains relatively constant with increasing exposure dose, it decreases in the second phase, reflecting the potential for accumulation of styrene in tissues at high levels of exposure (Withey, 1978). Styrene is slowly eliminated from adipose tissue, and there is a good correlation between skin-fold thickness and time required to reach maximum excretion of mandelic acid (Cherry and Gautrin, 1990). The half-life of styrene in the adipose tissue of workers with chronic exposure to styrene vapor at concentrations of 8 to 20 ppm, was determined to be 2.8 to 5.2 days (Engstrom, 1978).

Approximately 2% to 3% of the absorbed dose of styrene is exhaled unchanged, independent of concentra-

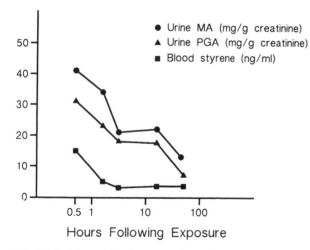

FIG. 17-3. Mean blood styrene levels in workers exposed to styrene at concentrations of 8 to 35 ppm. In addition, this figure shows the biphasic pattern of styrene excretion, with the prolonged second phase representing elimination from adipose tissue. (Modified from Wolff et al., 1978, with permission.)

tion or duration of exposure (Fernandez and Caperos, 1977; Ramsey and Young, 1978) or whether the uptake has been percutaneous or pulmonary (Riihimaki and Pfaffli, 1978). The main metabolites excreted in the urine of humans following exposure to styrene are mandelic acid (MA), phenylglyoxylic acid (PGA), and, to a lesser extent, hippuric acid (Leibman, 1975; Engstrom et al., 1978b). Minor urinary metabolites include 4-vinylphenol and phenylethylene glycol (Fig. 17-3) (Leibman, 1975; Pfaffli et al., 1981; Guillemin and Berode, 1988). Peak excretion of MA occurs at about 4 to 8 hours after cessation of exposure, and the patterns of excretion for MA and PGA are similar (Wilson et al., 1979). The half-life for MA in urine following exposure to styrene at vapor concentrations of 50 to 200 ppm is 7.8 hours; the half-life for phenylglyoxylic acid is 8.5 hours (Ikeda et al., 1974). However, because the proportion of these two metabolites varies from day to day, the sum of MA and PGA more accurately reflects the exposure dose (see Biochemical Diagnosis section).

CLINICAL MANIFESTATIONS AND DIAGNOSIS

Symptomatic Diagnosis

Acute symptoms of styrene exposure include mucous membrane irritation, headache, dizziness, drowsiness, impaired attention and memory, nausea, vomiting, and fatigue (Carpenter et al., 1944; Rogers and Hooper, 1957; Cherry et al., 1980; Shoenhuber and Gentilini, 1989; Geuskens et al., 1992; Matikainen et al., 1993). Stewart et al. (1968) studied nine human volunteers who were exposed to styrene vapors at the following durations and levels: 1 hour at 50, 215, and 375 ppm; 2 hours at 115 ppm; and 7 hours at 100 ppm. During the 1- and 2-hour exposures, at styrene vapor concentrations of 50 and 115 ppm, respectively, the subjects reported a moderately strong odor upon entering the chamber; however, this effect diminished with time spent in the chamber. There were no reported symptoms or objective signs of illness at these levels and lengths of exposure. At a concentration of 215 ppm, one subject reportedly began experiencing nasal irritation 20 minutes into the exposure. There were no other neurological symptoms or signs seen in any of the subjects at this level. At 375 ppm, the odor was reported to be perceptible throughout the exposure period; within 15 minutes after entering the chamber, four of the subjects reported eye and nasal irritation, and one subject reported a burning sensation in the skin of the face that began after about 20 minutes of exposure. Performance of a modified Romberg's sign was impaired in one subject after 25 minutes. After 45 minutes, one subject reported feeling nauseous. Performance of the Crawford test of manual dexterity, as well as the Flannagan coordination test, revealed performance deficits in two of the subjects after 50 minutes of exposure at this level; and two subjects reported feeling inebriated after 60 minutes. The 7-hour exposure period (styrene vapor concentration 100 ppm) was divided into two successive 3.5-hour periods, with a 30-minute break in an uncontaminated area in between each session. Three subjects had intermittent difficulty performing the modified Romberg test, and three subjects complained of mild eye irritation. Scores of the Flannagan Coordination test and the Crawford Manual Dexterity tests were unchanged from preexposure scores. No other objective signs of neurological impairments were reported at this level. Inhalation of higher concentrations results in transitory CNS depression, with prenarcotic symptoms of increasingly more severe drowsiness. Two volunteers exposed to 800 ppm of styrene vapor experienced immediate eye and throat irritation, increased nasal mucus secretion, metallic taste, listlessness, drowsiness, and vertigo during the exposure session, while slight muscular weakness, unsteadiness, and depression were reported even after cessation of exposure (Carpenter et al., 1944).

Individuals occupationally exposed to styrene report an increase in the occurrence of acute symptoms with increasing exposure dose (Edling et al., 1993; Rosen et al., 1978). Mild complaints, sometimes called "styrene sickness," may occur acutely and disappear after a few hours. These include mucous membrane irritation, headache, nausea, vomiting, loss of appetite, vertigo, and fatigue (Rogers and Hooper, 1957; Geuskens et al., 1992). Significantly more complaints of headache, depression, tinnitus, and eye and skin irritation, as well as nausea and dizziness, were reported among 68 fiberglass-reinforced plastic workers exposed to TWA styrene concentrations of 4 to 165 ppm, when compared to a group of 111 unexposed controls (Geuskens et al., 1992). However, there were no differences in the frequency of subjective complaints of cognitive or locomotor disabilities between the two groups. Workers exposed to styrene reported feeling more tired than nonexposed controls at the end of the workweek, suggesting that the effects of styrene are cumulative (Cherry et al., 1980).

Chronic symptoms of styrene exposure include impairment of attention and memory functioning, fatigue, excessive sweating, paresthesia, and muscle weakness (Table 17-2) (Rosen et al., 1978; Cherry et al., 1980; Behari et al., 1986; Triebig et al., 1989; Matikainen et al., 1993). Acute and chronic effects of styrene were assessed in a group of

36 polyester resin workers (age: 24 to 59 years) exposed to styrene vapor concentrations between 3 and 251 ppm (median: 18 ppm) with a median duration of 7 years (Triebig et al., 1989). The workers were compared with unexposed controls. Median sum concentrations of MA plus PGA in the urine of the exposed workers was 360 mg/L. Neurological examination found no evidence of peripheral neuropathy or encephalopathy. Neurobehavioral assessment including tests of intelligence, simple and complex reaction time, short-term memory, and personality revealed no significant differences between the exposed workers and the unexposed controls. Although eight workers who had been exposed to concentrations above 100 ppm for their entire work shift complained of experiencing dizziness, nausea, and headache both during and after work, it was concluded that no acute or chronic neurotoxic effects were detected in the workers if the TWA exposure concentrations did not exceed 100 ppm.

A group of 99 reinforced plastics workers were divided into three groups based on an exposure index (EI) derived from individual work environment styrene levels (range: <20 to >150), urinary MA concentrations (range: <3.2 to >15 mmol/L), and duration of exposure (range: <5 to >20 years) (Matikainen et al., 1993). The calculated EIs were 0 to 2.5, 2.6 to 3.5, and >3.5 for the low, medium, and high exposure groups, respectively. The most commonly reported acute symptoms among all the workers were excessive tiredness (49%), difficulty concentrating (20%), and nausea (14%). Acute memory disturbance and dizziness was reported with greater frequency among those workers with an EI greater than 3.0. The most frequently reported chronic symptoms among all exposed workers were tiredness (28%), forgetfulness (28%), tension in the neck (27%), memory disturbances (24%), headache (24%), and excessive sweating (20%). Clinical neurological exam revealed slight abnormalities in 26% of the workers, but these were not correlated with exposure.

Neurophysiological Diagnosis

Neurophysiological studies of styrene-exposed workers suggest that styrene is toxic to the central and peripheral nervous systems (Table 17-3). However, these results should be interpreted with caution, because workers

TABLE 17-2. *Percentage of workers reporting symptoms at low, medium, and high levels of exposure to styrene*

Symptom	Control (unexposed)	Low (< 5 ppm)	Medium (45 ppm)	High (> 125 ppm)
Unusual tiredness	17	20	40	85
Reduced short-term memory	17	30	40	62
Giddiness	0	10	40	54
Headache	33	30	40	46
Paresthesia in extremities	23	0	10	30
Limb weakness	8	0	20	0

Modified from Rosen et al., 1978, with permission.

TABLE 17-3. *Neurophysiological findings in styrene-exposed workers*

Exposure Level (ppm)	Duration	Urinary mandelic acid (as reported)	Number exposed	Job description	Manifestations	Reference
Not reported	5.1 yr (median)	808 mg/L	96 (cohort)	Laminating workers.	Dose-dependent EEG abnormalities including: excessive diffuse theta activity, local slow waves and bilateral spike and wave discharge.	Seppäläinen and Härkönen, 1976
≤ 5–175	1–21 yr	Not reported	33	Polystyrene production; fiberglass-boat builders; and manufacturing of styrene polyester cisterns.	EEG abnormalities including increased beta (fast) activity in the rostral and central parts of both hemispheres and increased theta (slow) activity in both hemispheres; no change in the dominant occipital alpha activity. Mild sensory neuropathy.	Rosen et al., 1978
< 50 to > 100	< 1 to > 20 yr	Not reported	70	Manufacturing boats and vehicle panels.	Decreased sensory conduction velocities in the median, ulnar, and sural nerves.	Cherry and Gautrin, 1990
22	0.5–9 yr	446 mg/g creatinine (MA + PGA)	11	Laminating workers.	Significant slowing of sensory nerve conduction velocities.	Murata et al., 1991
30–130	5–22 yr	200–1,400 μmol/mmol creatinine	20	Glass laminate manufacturing.	Prolonged latency of somatosensory evoked potentials in median nerves and decreased peripheral conduction velocities in median and tibial nerves.	Stetkarova et al., 1993

EEG, electroencephalographic; MA, mandelic acid; PGA, phenylglyoxylic acid.

exposed to styrene are frequently exposed to other chemicals capable of producing similar manifestations.

Electroencephalogram (EEG) is a useful tool that can aid in detecting the effects of styrene exposure, often revealing subclinical changes before overt clinical manifestations are noted. For example, the EEG revealed theta waves that were either diffuse or predominantly localized to the frontal area in nine of 14 styrene-exposed workers (Roth and Klimkova-Deutschova, 1963), and 105 subjects exposed to styrene in the polyester resin industry who reported headache, sleepiness, peripheral neuropathy, nystagmus, and facial palsy also exhibited acute and chronic changes in their EEGs (Klimkova-Deutschova et al., 1973). Because of the sensitivity of EEG, discretion must be used when interpreting the results of such population studies, since other conditions that can cause nonspecific slowing and/or activations in the EEG must not be erroneously attributed to styrene exposure (Rebert and Hall, 1994).

Quantitative electroencephalographic analyses on 99 reinforced plastic industry workers (mean age: 38 years) (Matikainen et al., 1993) were correlated with the mean styrene vapor concentration (32 ppm) and the average length of exposure (12.8 years). The workers were divided into three groups based on calculated exposure indices derived from duration of exposure, personal work environment styrene levels, and urine MA concentrations. Increased total power in all electrode regions in the alpha and beta bands was recorded in the workers with higher average styrene exposures. This was most obvious in the frontal and temporal regions of the brain. No significant change was noted in the total power of the theta and delta bands. Quantitative EEG was considered to be abnormal in 12 of total 20 workers tested from the high-exposure group, suggesting that exposure to styrene at high concentrations produces measurable acute effects on the CNS. While these results indicate that exposure to high levels of styrene does produce changes in the quantitative EEG that can be used to aid in the differential diagnosis, they do not necessarily represent neurologic dysfunction (Rebert and Hall, 1994).

Evoked potentials can also be used to assess CNS functioning. In a study by Stetkarova et al. (1993), 20 workers (5 men and 15 women) exposed to styrene at concentrations ranging from 32 to 132 ppm for 5 to 22 years (mean 11 years) were compared to 36 men occupationally exposed to toluene (522 ppm; mean exposure duration 12 years) and 30 healthy male controls. Neurasthenic symptoms were noted in 30% of the styrene exposed group (35% in toluene group). Neurobehavioral features, such as forgetfulness, irritability, and emotional lability, were noted in 10% of the styrene exposed group (5% in toluene exposed workers). Somatosensory evoked potentials (SEPs) were measured by stimulation of the median nerve at the wrist and the tibial nerve at the ankle. Significantly prolonged latencies of peripheral and cortical SEPs to median nerve stimulation as well as cortical SEPs to tibial nerve stimulation were found in the styrene exposed workers. The major SEP abnormalities found during median nerve stimulation were prolonged latencies of N10, P13, and cortical components of N20, P22, and P27. Significant abnormalities found in tibial nerves included prolonged latencies of N33 and late cortical components. Peripheral conduction velocities in both extremities and central conduction time after tibial nerve stimulation were significantly decreased in the workers exposed to either styrene or toluene. These findings show evidence of functional impairment at all somatosensory pathways indicative of potential toxic polyneuropathy, myelopathy, or encephalopathy, although gender or alcohol consumption must be considered to have played a part in the findings in this study.

Short-latency somatosensory evoked potentials (SSEPs), sensory conduction velocities (SCVs), motor conduction velocities (MCVs), and the distribution of nerve conduction velocities (DCVs)—to determine whether the fast or slow fibers are principally involved—were investigated in 11 male laminating workers exposed to styrene in the fiber-reinforced plastic boat industry (Murata et al., 1991; Araki et al., 1993). Age range was 22 to 61 (mean 40), duration of exposure was 0.5 to 9 years, and TWA concentration of styrene vapor was estimated to be 22 ppm (range: 3 to 63 ppm). Thus, the sum of MA + PGA in urine ranged from 60 to 1,274 mg/g creatinine (mean: 446). In comparison to age- and sex-matched controls, the styrene-exposed workers had significantly slower SCV and V80 velocities on the DCVs (i.e., the conduction velocity below which 80% of the nerve fibers lie). The distribution of conduction velocities among the exposed workers was shifted toward the slower nerve fibers, suggesting that styrene affects the faster myelinated fibers of the peripheral sensory nerves. There was no significant difference in the MCVs or the SSEPs.

Nerve conduction studies have been used to confirm the presence of sensory and motor neuropathy following known exposure to styrene and other neurotoxicants. Nerve conduction studies of 11 workers (age: 24 to 54 years) exposed to average styrene vapor concentrations of 100 ppm in the boat industry did not reveal any significant changes, suggesting that exposure to styrene at ambient air concentrations at or below 100 ppm has no adverse effects on the peripheral nerves (Triebig et al., 1985). However, mild sensory neuropathy was found in older workers who

were more heavily exposed (range: 74 to 175 ppm), suggesting that the effects of aging and chronic styrene exposure on the peripheral nervous system may be synergistic (see Clinical Experiences section, Table 17-5) (Rosen et al., 1978). Lilis et al. (1978) also found a greater frequency of peripheral neuropathic changes on nerve conduction studies of the radial and peroneal nerves in those workers in a monomer manufacturing and polymerization plant who had longer durations of styrene exposure. Exposures were judged to be low for 306 workers and high for 182. Durations of the exposures were classified as <7, 7 to 20, or >20 years. Out of 80 eligible workers who had radial nerve conduction velocities done, 15 (18.8%) had velocities less than 55 m/sec, but there was no definite correlation with duration or level of exposure. Out of 73 eligible workers who had peroneal nerve conduction velocities done, 12 (16.4%) had values less than 40 m/sec. Although there was no relationship to exposure levels, there was a consistent decrement with duration of exposure. Mean ages were higher in the workers who exhibited reduced conduction velocities in both radial and peroneal nerves.

In a report on 70 male workers (mean age 28.9) from the boat and vehicle panel manufacturing industry, whose exposure duration ranged from a few weeks to 20 years, Cherry and Gautrin (1990) noted mild sensory conduction deficits, which increased with regard to the number of workers affected as the exposure level increased. Seven men among the 30 (23%) exposed to concentrations less than 50 ppm had some deficit on sensory conduction velocity. The proportion doubled to 46% (7 of 15) at vapor concentrations between 51 and 100 ppm and increased to 71% (10 of 14) at styrene concentrations above 100 ppm. Follow-up of two workers with exposures to levels over 100 ppm and who initially showed deficits in sensory conduction velocities revealed improvement in conduction velocity after cessation of exposure because of a 67-day lay-off at the plant. A similar comparison of reaction times before and after cessation of exposure also revealed improvements. In both cases the more highly exposed workers showed the greatest improvement. These findings offer evidence of both central and peripheral recovery following removal from exposure.

Exposure to styrene affects the auditory and equilibrium systems (Ledin et al., 1989; Möller et al., 1990; Rebert et al., 1993). However, because exposure to excessive noise frequently occurs in industrial environments, workplace noise levels must be considered when assessing hearing loss in a styrene-exposed individual. An investigation into the association between exposure to styrene and hearing loss among 299 workers from the glass-fiber-reinforced plastic products industry, with average exposures of 8 to 25 ppm, did not reveal a significant relationship between styrene exposure and hearing loss after adjusting for noise exposure. In addition, a strong correlation was found between noise levels and styrene exposure, illustrating the importance of considering all associated variables in analysis of such data (Sass-Kortsak et al., 1995).

An otoneurologic test battery and posturography was administered to 18 workers occupationally exposed to styrene at a plant manufacturing reinforced polyester boats (Ledin et al., 1989; Möller et al., 1990). The mean age of the workers was 40 years (range: 28 to 61 years). Styrene levels in the shop ranged from less than 6 ppm to 23 ppm, and duration of exposure was 6 to 15 years (mean: 10.8 years). A referent group comprised of 18 unexposed industrial workers was also tested. Abnormal results on distorted speech and cortical response audiometry tests were noted in seven of the 18 workers, suggesting disturbances in the central auditory pathways. Central processing of impulses from different sensory equilibrium organs were abnormal in 16 workers. The styrene-exposed group had a significantly larger sway on posturography and a significantly poorer ability to suppress nystagmus than did the referent group. The latency time on the saccade test was significantly ($p <0.01$) higher in the exposed group. However, there were no differences in the maximum velocity of the saccades between the two groups. Romberg's sign and caloric tests were normal for all workers.

The influence of acute exposure to styrene on the vestibulooculomotor reflex was assessed in 10 volunteers (mean age: 24 years) exposed for 1 hour to concentrations of 90 to 140 ppm, more than two to three times the Swedish occupational exposure threshold limit of 40 ppm (Ödkvist et al., 1982). The solvents were inhaled through a breathing valve, and the subjects performed light exercise (50 W) during the exposure period. The mean styrene blood concentration following the exposure was 2.7 ppm (0.012 mg/L); these blood levels are often reached during longer periods of exposure at lower concentrations. The vestibulooculomotor system was assessed by electronystagmograph of eye movements during sinusoidal oscillations in the darkness and while fixating on a stationary target. Visual–vestibular interaction was tested by recording suppression of the vestibulooculomotor reflex in response to sinusoidal oscillations. In addition, the optomotor system was tested by recording the subjects' voluntary saccades, smooth pursuit movements, and optokinetic nystagmus that occur in response to rotation of the visual field. Exposure to styrene had no effect on the sinusoidal tests of eye movements in the dark or while fixating on a stable target. While no significant change in eye movement was seen at an amplitude of 60 degrees on visual suppression test, at 112 degrees eight of the 10 subjects had a significant ($p < 0.05$) increase in eye movement. The maximum speed of the saccade was significantly ($p < 0.05$) increased in eight of the 10 subjects as well. The latency and accuracy of the saccade were not significantly changed by exposure to styrene, although there was a tendency for the subjects to overshoot the target after exposure. Styrene had no effect on performance of the rotatory optokinetic test. These results suggest that styrene blocks cerebellar inhibition of the vestibulooculomotor system.

Kohn (1978) carried out ophthalmological assessment of 345 workers in a styrene plant and documented conjunctival irritation in 22% of the work force, but no instances of retrobulbar neuritis or retinal vein thrombosis were found in this study. However, testing for impairment of color vision among exposed workers was reported to reveal the subclinical effects of styrene (Gobba et al., 1991; Fallas et al., 1992). Solvent-induced color vision loss seems to reflect changes in neural functioning along the optic pathway, and it can be detected before overt symptoms or major abnormalities in ocular structures are evident (Mergler and Blain, 1987). The pathogenesis of styrene-induced color vision loss is not clear, and both demyelination of optic fibers and interference of styrene with the dopaminergic mechanism of retinal cells have been suggested (Gobba et al., 1991). In most subjects exposed to styrene, blue–yellow color range is affected; however, red–green loss has also been reported (Gobba et al., 1991; Fallas et al., 1992; Eguchi et al., 1995) (see Neuropsychological Diagnosis section).

Neuropsychological Diagnosis

Determination of subtle changes in neuropsychological performance is useful in assessing the effects of styrene exposure (Anger and Johnson, 1985). Studies in occupational settings and under controlled experimental conditions demonstrate a variety of CNS effects. Delayed simple and choice reaction times are related to exposure intensity and appear to be the most commonly reported neuropsychological effect of styrene (Dick, 1995). Work-site research has identified performance changes in attention, short-term memory, vigilance, and coordination (Schoenhuber and Gentilini, 1989; Lindstrom et al., 1976; Jegaden et al., 1993; Letz et al., 1990; Cherry et al., 1980).

Schoenhuber and Gentilini (1989) assessed neuropsychological functions in 55 styrene-exposed workers from factories where previous biological monitoring had shown levels of urinary metabolites, MA plus PGA, above 700 mg/L in at least 5% of the workers. Thirty-eight men and 17 women (mean age: 28 ± 10 years) were examined after four continuous workdays and again after 2 days away from the work site. Based on urinary (MA + PGA) measurements, the subjects were divided into high (MA + PGA > 700 mg/L) and low (MA + PGA < 700 mg/L) styrene-exposed groups; 14 and 41 subjects, respectively. Tests administered included digit forward test, symbol digit, selective attention, and divided attention. Comparison of the two groups revealed a significant ($p < 0.006$) impairment of short-term memory as measured by the digit forward test in the workers from the high-exposure group. The changes in performance were not significant on retesting after 2 days without exposure.

Similar results were found in 30 molders (mean age: 28 ± 6 years) exposed to a mean styrene level of 30 ppm, for a mean duration of 5 years (range: 1 to 14 years) (Jegaden et al., 1993). The mean for the urinary metabolites MA + PGA, measured at the end of the work shift, was determined to be 575 mg/g creatinine. Neurobehavioral tests administered included simple reaction time, choice reaction time, and digit span. Worker performance on these tests was compared with that of 30 age- and sex-matched controls. The molders performed significantly less well on the digit span test of short-term memory as well as on the tests of simple and choice reaction time, suggesting the existence of minor but significant effects of styrene at the levels reflected by the workers' urinary metabolite levels and the reported durations of the exposure.

One hundred and five fiberglass-boat builders from six different boat-building companies in New England were assessed using a computerized neurobehavioral evaluation system (Letz et al., 1990). Average duration of exposure was 2.9 years. The 8-hour TWA exposure was 30 ppm and the urinary MA averaged 347 mg/g creatinine. Worker performance was assessed before work, at midshift, and at the end of the work shift. Neurobehavioral domains tested included psychomotor speed, manual dexterity and eye–hand coordination, attention, and coding skills. Postshift performance on the digit symbol test of coding skills was statistically related to the styrene exposure and the urinary MA. In addition, workers exposed to levels above 50 ppm had significantly poorer performance on the digit symbol test than those workers exposed to levels below 50 ppm. There was no relationship found between styrene exposure and eye–hand coordination or reaction times.

Twenty-one workers in the reinforced-polyester boat-building industry were examined for subjective and neurobehavioral effects with a follow-up examination 7 months after cessation of exposure due to closing of the company (Flodin et al., 1989). Duration of exposure was between 6 and 21 years, and the mean age was 37 years (range: 28 to 61). Although the level of styrene exposure was much less than the other studies cited above, in this study the workers were divided into low- and high-exposure groups, with an average exposure of 6 and 12 ppm, respectively (short-term peak exposures rarely exceeded 70 ppm). Neurobehavioral domains assessed included verbal skills, cognitive reasoning, visuospatial, perceptual speed and accuracy, memory, and eye–hand coordination. There were no reported differences between the two groups in performance on most neurobehavioral tests, although eye–hand coordination was significantly impaired in the high-exposure group. Predominant subjective symptoms among workers in the low-exposure group included excessive tiredness and forgetfulness; while the workers in the high-exposure group reported both these symptoms, plus headache, irritability, difficulty concentrating, and problems with comprehension of written material. Clinical laboratory tests were normal. Five workers were diagnosed as having a neurasthenic syndrome due to styrene exposure, with excessive fatigue as the predominant symptom. In a follow-up examination 7 months after cessation of exposure, the number of subjective complaints reported in both groups were minimal.

The occurrence of dyschromatopsia among styrene exposed workers was investigated by Gobba et al. (1991). Seventy-three workers from the fiberglass-reinforced plastic industry were compared with 53 referents; the styrene-exposed workers were significantly younger than the referents (mean of 32 years compared to 37.6 years, respectively). Exposure duration of the fiberglass workers ranged from 1 month to 27 years (average: 7 years). Styrene air levels averaged 16 ppm (range: <1 to 127 ppm). Subjects were divided into three groups according to age: group 1, ≤29; group 2, 30 to 39; group 3, ≥40 years. Color vision was assessed using the Lanthony 15 Hue Desaturated Panel (Lanthony D-15), which is based on the ability to recombine a set of 15 desaturated colored "caps" (i.e., wooden buttons colored on the top with desaturated colors) according to a definite chromatic sequence. The results obtained are expressed as a Color Confusion Index (CCI). CCI was always higher in the styrene-exposed workers when compared to the age-matched referents, and this difference was significant ($p < 0.05$) for the subjects in group 3. There was also a significant correlation between environmental and urinary measures of styrene exposure and the CCI, indicating the possibility of a dose–response relationship. Subjects exposed to average concentrations above 50 ppm showed significantly higher CCI values than did workers with lower exposure. Blue–yellow range of colors was affected most, and only in a few workers was red–green discrimination affected. Multiple regression analysis showed that both age and exposure levels were related to color vision loss; however, duration of exposure was not demonstrated to influence CCI, suggesting that impairment of color vision resulting from styrene exposure may be synergistic with that due to normal aging. No sex-related differences in CCI were seen. In a follow-up of a 20-worker cohort performed after a 1-month summer holiday, CCI values were still elevated compared to controls, and no tendency toward a restoration of color vision was observed.

A similar assessment using the Lanthony D-15 was performed on 64 workers (mean age: 38 years) from a bathtub factory (Eguchi et al., 1995). Average atmospheric styrene vapor concentration was 20 ppm and mean urinary mandelic acid concentrations of the exposed workers was 220 mg/L. Sixty-nine unexposed age-matched workers served as controls. The exposed workers were divided into high-exposure (MA >420 mg/L) and low-exposure (MA <420 mg/L) groups; a urinary MA concentration of 420 mg/L is equivalent to an atmospheric styrene concentration of 30 ppm. Raw total color difference scores (TCDSs) revealed a significant linear correlation with age in both the exposed workers and the control groups. Analysis of CCI scores (derived by dividing the raw TCDS of the subject by the TCDSs for a perfect arrangement), after controlling for age, revealed a significant ($p <0.01$) difference between workers in the high-exposure group and controls. In addition, CCI scores were significantly and positively correlated with MA, suggesting that there is a dose–effect relation between styrene exposure and impairment of color vision. Duration of exposure did not have a significant relation with CCI scores. In most subjects the blue–yellow range of color vision was affected. These effects were not considered acute since the workers were tested on a Monday morning.

A study of color vision loss using the more sensitive Farnsworth-Munsell 100 Hue (FM-100) was conducted on a group of 60 styrene-exposed workers from the shipbuilding industry with a median exposure duration of 3.75 years (Fallas et al., 1992). Mean air styrene concentration during the 3-month testing period was 25 ppm, with occasional peaks as high as 469 ppm; mean urinary MA + PGA concentrations for the entire test period were 287 mg/g creatinine. Sixty unexposed workers matched according to age, intellectual level, and ethnic origin served as controls. The FM-100 requires the subject to place 85 caps of saturated colors in chromatic order (Mergler and Blain, 1987). The error scores revealed no significant difference between the two groups. However, the difference between the number of exposed subjects and controls with abnormal ranges for blue–yellow and red–green color discrimination was significant suggesting that exposure to styrene at moderate concentrations can lead to impairment of color vision.

Biochemical Diagnosis

Monitoring of ongoing occupational exposure can be done by measuring styrene in an end exhaled air sample either before or during a work shift, or by measuring urinary concentrations of MA or PGA at the end of the shift, or by measuring styrene level in venous blood at either the end of a shift or just before the next shift (ACGIH, 1993). The styrene concentration in end exhaled air during a shift should not exceed 2 ppm, if a TWA exposure concentration of 50 ppm is maintained (ACGIH, 1989) (Table 17-4).

Styrene and its metabolites can be detected in blood and urine up to 96 hours following exposure to levels as low as 8 ppm (Fig. 17-3) (Wolff et al., 1978). The American Conference of Governmental and Industrial Hygienists' recommended biological exposure index (BEI) for styrene in the venous blood of an exposed worker is 0.02 mg/L at the start of a shift and 0.55 mg/L at the end of a shift (see Table 17-4) (ACGIH, 1995). However, with increasing exposure dose, styrene concentration in the brain and liver is significantly higher than that in the blood, suggesting that blood levels may not accurately reflect the potential toxicological insult (Withey, 1978).

Determination of MA in the urine is the most convenient biological exposure index. Urinary MA excretion is correlated with exposure for concentrations up to 150 ppm at the end of an 8-hour shift (ACGIH, 1989). The summation of both MA and PGA in the urine correlates better with total exposure (WHO, 1983). The concentration of MA in the urine should not exceed 300 mg/g creatinine at the start of a work shift or 800 mg/g creatinine at the end of a shift. Preshift PGA concentrations should not exceed 100 mg/g creatinine, while the end of shift level for PGA in urine is 240 mg/g creatinine (see Table 17-4) (ACGIH, 1995). Unless the urine samples are frozen immediately, the levels of PGA will decrease due to spontaneous decarboxylation, thus affecting the measured output. At the end of the work shift, the sum of MA and PGA should not be greater than 1,000 mg/g creatinine.

The ratio of MA to PGA excreted in the urine is the same following both inhalation and dermal exposure (Riihimaki and Pfaffli, 1978). However, elimination is delayed following dermal exposure; therefore, in cases of simultaneous dermal and pulmonary exposure, measurement of urinary MA may not accurately reflect the total exposure (Dutkiewicz and Tyras, 1968; Riihimaki and Pfaffli, 1978). The influence of both acute and chronic ingestion of ethanol as well as exposure to other xenobiotics such as toluene and xylene on the urinary excretion of MA and PGA must be considered during the monitoring of occupationally exposed persons (Cerny et al., 1990). Concurrent acute exposure to toluene and xylene and/or ethanol can result in inhibition of metabolism and decreased excretion of the urinary metabolites of styrene. Chronic exposure to ethanol or other xenobiotics which induce cytochrome P-450 enzymatic activity enhances excretion of urinary metabolites. Biological monitoring of MA in workers simultaneously exposed to styrene and ethylbenzene should include the use of an enantioselective assay (Drummond et al., 1989). The enantiomorphic composition of MA produced by the metabolism of styrene is racemic. This is in contrast to the MA produced following exposure to ethylbenzene, which leads only to formation of only the R-enantiomer. The separate determination of these enantiomers of MA provides a way to determine whether the source of the MA is styrene, or ethylbenzene.

Adipose tissue concentration of styrene measured by fat biopsy is a sensitive indicator of exposure. Pierce and Tozer

TABLE 17-4. *Biological exposure indices for styrene*

	Urine		Blood	Alveolar Air
Determinant:	Mandelic acid	Phenylglyoxylic acid	Styrene	Styrene
Start of shift:	300 mg/g creatinine	100 mg/g creatinine	0.02 mg/L	Not established
During shift:	Not established	Not established	Not established	2 ppm
End of shift:	800 mg/g creatinine	240 mg/g creatinine	0.55 mg/L	Not established

Data from ACGIH, 1995.

(1992) indicated that in view of the tissue/blood partition coefficient of 39 and the longer tissue half-life, adipose tissue provides a useful physiologically damped internal measure of dose. Their measurement of styrene levels in adipose tissue of seven non-occupationally exposed human samples showed a mean of 1.12 ± 1.06 ppm (range: 0.053 to 2.92 ppm). They estimated daily environmental intake to be about 476 ppb.

A cross-sectional study correlated monoamine oxidase type B (MAO-B) activity as a marker of styrene neurotoxicity in peripheral blood cells and subjective symptoms among 60 reinforced-plastics workers exposed to styrene and 18 reference workers not exposed to styrene at three plants. An increase in the prevalence of headache, irritability, memory loss, dizziness, and lightheadedness was significantly positively correlated with increased blood styrene levels and decreased MAO-B activity (Checkoway et al., 1992). A slight relationship between increased serotonin uptake and increased blood levels of styrene was also found. However, there was no relationship between subjective symptoms and serotonin uptake or sigma receptor binding. Exposure to styrene has been associated with an increase in serum prolactin (Mutti and Smargiassi, 1998). However, the reliability of this marker of exposure for predicting risk of toxic effects has not yet been established. Hemoglobin adduct formation has also been proposed as a sensitive and consistent method of determining styrene exposure (Severi et al., 1994; Hemminki and Vodicka, 1995).

Neuroimaging

Melgaard et al. (1979) used computer-assisted tomography (CT) to assess six workers exposed to styrene vapor for a mean of 15 years (range: 6 to 27) with an estimated average exposure of 160 ppm. CT and pneumoencephalogram (PEG) revealed cerebral atrophy in five of the six workers. The atrophy was central and cortical in two of the workers, cortical only in two, and central only in one. In addition, a neurobehavioral assessment was performed on all six workers. The individual without cerebral atrophy also showed no impairment on tests of neuropsychological performance. Neuropsychological assessment of the workers with cerebral atrophy revealed general intellectual impairment, with short-term memory disturbances being most prominent. All six workers reported initial acute subjective symptoms including dizziness, headaches, and a feeling of drunkenness that improved over the weekends. Chronic subjective symptoms reported by these workers included excessive fatigue, impaired memory, headaches, and difficulty concentrating.

Neuropathological Diagnosis

The occurrence of astrogliosis in the hippocampus and in the sensory motor cortex indicates that exposure to styrene at moderate levels induces region-specific damage to brain tissues. In addition, the persistence of these astroglial alterations 4 months after cessation of exposure indicates that the changes induced by styrene are permanent (Rosengren and Haglid, 1989). Increased concentrations of glial cell marker proteins such as glial fibrillary acidic protein (GFA) and S-100 serve as an indicator of preceding brain injuries (Haglid et al., 1981; Rosengren et al., 1986). No significant changes were seen in concentrations of GFA or S-100 following exposure of rats to 90 ppm styrene vapor for 3 months followed by a 4-month postexposure solvent-free period. However, concentrations of GFA were significantly increased in the sensory motor cortex and the hippocampus of rats exposed to 320 ppm under the same conditions.

The mechanism by which styrene exerts its neurotoxicity still remains unclear. In addition, whether styrene directly interferes with neuronal membrane function, or whether metabolic transformation to toxic intermediates, such as the electrophylic alkylating agent styrene-7,8-oxide or free radicals, are responsible, has yet to be determined. Exposure of Pc-12 cells to nonlethal concentrations of styrene oxide *in vitro* increased cytosolic free Ca^{2+} concentrations and decreased intracellular concentrations of ATP and glutathione. In addition, these cells lost their ability to differentiate in response to nerve growth factor. Decreased levels of glutathione are most likely due to interactions with styrene-7,8-oxide and may increase vulnerability of neurons to damage by other neurotoxicants. Though styrene oxide is generally thought to be the ultimate toxicant, free radicals may also be responsible for the neurotoxicity of styrene (Rosen et al., 1978; Dypbukt et al., 1992). MAO-B activity is reduced in a dose-dependent manner in workers exposed to styrene, suggesting that changes in MAO-B activity may be involved as an intermediate step in styrene neurotoxicity (Checkoway et al., 1992). This observation raises the possibility that workers who are receiving MAO-B inhibitors (e.g., selegiline) may exhibit greater sensitivity to styrene exposure. No change in lipid peroxidation was found in the brains of rats following intraperitoneal administration of styrene at 300 to 500 mg/kg and styrene oxide at 200 and 300 mg/kg (Katoh et al., 1989). However, lipid peroxidation is not the only manifestation of free radical damage (Halliwell, 1989). Other early manifestations of oxidative stress that might be damaging to neurons include increases in levels of intracellular free calcium, decreased levels of ATP, and DNA damage.

Animal studies have shown increased sensitivity of dopamine receptors, as well as depletion of dopamine within the corpus striatum following styrene exposure (Agrawal et al., 1982; Mutti et al., 1985). Styrene significantly increases the binding of [³H]spiroperidol to dopamine receptors in the corpus striatum of the rat (Agrawal et al., 1982). The increase in binding may be due to the destruction of dopamine neurons in the nigrostriatal pathway. Styrene interferes with the activity of the tuberoinfundibular dopaminergic system. Styrene induced a marked decrease in dopamine levels and a significant increase in homovanillic acid concentration in the striatum and tuberoinfundibular systems of rabbits exposed to styrene vapor at 750 ppm (Romanelli et al., 1986). In addition, these same effects were found following administration of PGA and MA. Increased levels of the neuroendocrine hormones prolactin (PRL), human growth hormone (HGH), and thyroid-stimulating hormone (TSH) were found in workers exposed to styrene vapor at 65 to 300 ppm. These findings are consistent with depletion of dopamine in the tuberoinfundibular dopaminergic system (Mutti et al., 1984). Chronic exposure to styrene vapor concentrations of 1,000 ppm was found to decrease the affinity of neostriatal D-2 agonist binding sites in rats (von Euler and Bjornaes, 1990). These changes may be mediated by structural damage to the striatal nerve cell membrane, which may lead to changes in membrane fluidity. No effect on the number of binding sites was noted at this concentration. Thus, biotransformation of styrene to an active metabolite such as phenylglycine may compete with dopamine for vesicular storage capacity or may affect dopaminergic activity by destroying dopaminergic neurons (Mutti et al., 1984; Pahwa and Kalra, 1993).

It has been suggested (Halliwell, 1989) that free radicals act as mediators of endogenous cell damage and that it is possible that styrene or styrene oxide acts to initiate increased production of free radicals, resulting in damage to the PNS and CNS. The idea that the combination of increased production of free radicals and decreased scavenger capacity might lead to a styrene-induced acceleration of the normal aging process is speculative. However, data obtained in a group of older workers does show that among those with the highest degree of exposure for 10 years or more, five out of six persons who were 50 years of age or more at the time of testing had signs of peripheral neuropathy. Only one of five persons under the age of 41 years showed such signs (Rosen et al., 1978).

Light microscopic examination of a sural nerve biopsy taken from a 45-year-old man occupationally exposed to monomeric styrene daily for 5 years revealed many demyelinated nerve fibers (Behari et al., 1986). Further examination by electron microscopy revealed ultrastructural changes including occasional evidence of active myelin degeneration. In addition, a few fibers showed one or two laminae formed by Schwann cell processes, indicating remyelination. Axis cylinders were better preserved. Because there was no documentation of styrene levels either in air or in biological specimens in this report and the possibility exists that other neurotoxicants may have played a role in producing the neuropathy, these findings should be interpreted with caution because they do not conclusively indicate that styrene causes peripheral neuropathy (Rebert and Hall, 1994).

PREVENTIVE AND THERAPEUTIC MEASURES

Preemployment and periodic medical examinations should focus on neurological function in addition to hepatic, renal, and hematological assessment (NIOSH, 1983).

Employee education, including a comprehensive approach to motivating changes in work practices and provision of information on the toxicity of styrene, is essential to worker safety and health (Brigham and Landrigan, 1985). Precautionary measures to avoid undue uptake, while working in environments which contain styrene, should include the use of impervious clothing, including gloves, as well as eye protection, and masks which prevent inhalation of styrene droplets or vapor. Air levels should be constantly monitored for styrene. Proper ventilation of the workplace via exhaust fans is paramount to reducing worker exposure. Respirators should be available for air concentrations above the recommended levels. Biological monitoring of workers at risk for styrene exposure should be performed regularly. Measurements are best taken to reflect the time weighted average of an 8-hour exposure. Measurements to determine the employee ceiling exposure should be taken during anticipated periods of maximum exposure. Air samples more closely reflect individual exposure levels when taken in the employees' breathing zone (NIOSH, 1983).

An individual suspected of having been acutely exposed to styrene should be immediately removed from the source of exposure. Supplemental oxygen by mask should be administered. If breathing has stopped, artificial respiration should be instituted. The individual should be kept warm and in a resting position. If styrene has been ingested, do not induce vomiting; this is to avoid risk of pulmonary aspiration of styrene. Any nonimpervious clothing that becomes wet with liquid styrene should be immediately removed, and the skin that has become contaminated with styrene should be promptly washed with soap or mild detergent. There is no known antidote for acute styrene poisoning, so that immediate action is necessary in order to maintain respiratory, circulatory, and renal functions until metabolism can clear the increased body burden of the neurotoxicant (Weiss, 1980).

In cases of chronic exposures, where the specific toxic diagnosis is difficult to ascertain, determination of current urinary metabolites of styrene as well as the average exposure duration and intensity, along with documentation of the time course of the patient's symptoms, may be the only approach to take when making the differential diagnosis (Cherry and Gautrin, 1990). In addition, whether a worker has been exposed to other substances capable of producing similar symptoms should be determined (Lorimer et al., 1976). Neurobehavioral test performance can be used to reveal subclinical effects related to chronic exposure as well as in determination of the specific domains affected (Lindstrom et al., 1976). An EEG should be performed in cases of chronic exposure to styrene, particularly if exposure has exceeded the recommended limits (Seppäläinen and Härkönen, 1976). The goal of therapy for chronic exposure to styrene is to end further exposure and to provide supportive measures for the patient. Such measures may include sedation for sleep disturbances, antianxiety drugs, and behavioral approaches to assist in compensatory techniques in patients with cognitive impairments.

CLINICAL EXPERIENCES

Group Studies

Clinical Assessments in Polyester Plastic Workers

The relationship between occupational styrene exposure and the incidence of subjective symptoms was studied among 98 male workers, who made laminated and reinforced polyester plastic products in 24 different manufacturing plants (Härkönen, 1977). The median age of the study population was 28 years (range: 16 to 54) and the median duration of exposure was 5.1 years (range: 0.5 to 14). Styrene exposure levels were documented by measuring urinary MA in weekly samples for 5 weeks. The mean concentration of MA in the urine of the exposed workers was 808 mg/L (range: 7 to 4,715 mg/L). Reference groups with no occupational exposure to styrene served as controls.

The subjects were administered a two-part survey concerning (a) acute specific symptoms experienced only during the workday and (b) ongoing general symptoms. Acute specific symptoms included irritation of the nose and eyes, nausea, dizziness, and a drunken feeling. General symptoms included fatigue, forgetfulness, irritation of the skin and eyes, loss of appetite, and difficulty in concentrating among the exposed workers when compared to the controls. No correlation was found between the frequency of occurrence of any symptom and the mean concentration of MA in urine.

Neurophysiological effects of styrene were investigated in 96 of the original 98 workers (Seppäläinen and Härkönen, 1976). Twenty-three (24%) of the 96 workers displayed some abnormality in the EEG, while the other 73 had normal EEGs. Two workers had bilateral spike and wave discharge, eight had excessive diffuse theta activity, and 14 had local slow waves. The prevalence of abnormal EEG was higher among those workers with average MA concentrations exceeding 700 mg/L, about 30%, while the prevalence in those with levels of urinary MA less than 700 mg/L did not exceed that of the general population (average about 10%). The duration of exposure among the workers with abnormal EEG was similar to that of subjects whose EEGs were normal, suggesting differences in individual susceptibility.

Forty subjects with the highest number of previously reported subjective complaints among the 96-member cohort were given nerve conduction studies to determine maximum motor conduction velocities of the median, ulnar, deep peroneal, and posterior tibial nerves, as well as measurement of sensory conduction velocities in the median and ulnar nerves. As a group the conduction velocities did not differ from that of laboratory controls.

The relationship between styrene exposure and psychological functioning was also assessed in these plastics workers (Lindstrom et al., 1976). Forty-three concrete reinforcement workers served as controls (mean age: 33 years). The neurobehavioral domains assessed were intelligence, visuomotor speed, visuomotor accuracy, memory, vigilance, psychomotor performance, and personality. Compared to the controls, the exposed workers had decreased visuomotor accuracy, as indicated by an increased number of symmetry reversals on the symmetry drawing test. In addition, exposed workers had impaired psychomotor performance, interpreted as a high level of inhibition, as indicated by increased latencies of response times on the Rorschach inkblot test. These differences were significant at $p < 0.05$. An intragroup comparative analysis of the neurobehavioral performance of these workers based on high (urinary MA > 1,762 mg/L corresponding to an 8-hour TWA >75 ppm) and low (urinary MA <674 mg/L corresponding to an 8-hour TWA <25 ppm) average exposure was also performed. The workers in the high-exposure group performed significantly better on the form level section of the Rorschach inkblot test. However, they performed significantly less well on tests of visuomotor accuracy and psychomotor performance. A relationship between worker exposure duration and neurobehavioral performance was revealed by a significant decrease in visuomotor speed as assessed by latency on the Kuhnburg figure-matching time test and a significant impairment of visual memory as measured with the Kuhnburg figure recognition test. Multiple regression analysis of the worker's psychological functions with regard to intensity of exposure revealed a significant relationship between decreased visuomotor accuracy and increased urinary MA concentrations. In addition, decreased psychomotor performance, as measured by the Mira distance between straight lines test and decreased vigilance (Bourdon–Wiersma estimation of performance time test), was also found to be related to urinary MA concentration. Analysis of cumulative exposure (intensity and duration) revealed significant relationships between (a) increased latency times on the Rorschach inkblot test that were interpreted as a high level of inhibition and (b) decreased visuomotor accuracy as measured by symmetry drawing tests. These findings indicate that the subclinical/subacute effects of styrene at these levels are slight and affect a narrower range of psychological functions.

Workers Exposed to Three Differing Styrene Exposure Levels

Thirty-three exposed workers from three different industrial sites were examined using both motor and sensory nerve conduction and electroencephalography (Rosen et al., 1978). Styrene vapor concentrations in the three shops were: 74 to 175 ppm (mean: 125 ppm) in shop A; 21 to 67 ppm (mean: 50 ppm) in shop B; and less than 5 ppm in shop C. Findings were compared with an unexposed reference group of six hospital employees and with a group of 17 male patients with known neurologic sequelae resulting from long-term exposure to mixed organic solvents.

EEG revealed no changes in the dominant occipital alpha activity of the styrene-exposed workers. However, an increased occurrence of fast activity in the central and precentral areas was found in nine of the styrene exposed workers and in ten members of the mixed solvent group. In addition, an increase in slow activity was seen in six of the styrene-exposed workers and in ten members of the mixed solvent group. MCVs of the fast fibers were determined for the median, ulnar, fibular, and posterior tibial nerves by surface recording from the thenar, hypothenar, extensor digitorum brevis, and abductor hallucis muscles, respectively. Sensory action potentials (SAPs) were recorded from the median and ulnar nerves. No significant changes in MCV were found in the styrene-exposed workers. However, the latencies of the SAPs among the styrene-exposed workers and the mixed solvent group were significantly longer than those of the controls. In addition, SAP amplitudes tended to be lower among the styrene-exposed workers and among the mixed solvent group, although this difference was only significant for the styrene workers from shop B. The SCV were lower for the styrene-exposed workers and for the mixed solvent group. Further analysis demonstrated a significantly longer duration of exposure and heavier time-weighted exposure for the styrene workers with polyneuropathy. Five out of six styrene workers with the highest degree of exposure and who were over 50 years of age showed signs of neuropathy, while only one out of five workers with high exposure under 41 years of age showed such evidence of neuropathy, suggesting that the effects of aging and exposure to styrene may be synergistic (Table 17-5).

These results suggest that the neurophysiological changes seen among workers exposed to styrene are similar to those seen after chronic exposure to mixed solvents, and in both cases the neurophysiological profile includes sensory nerve evoked responses with low amplitude and long duration; slow SCV; near-normal motor conduction velocities; and EEG changes including an increased amount of fast activity in the central and precentral regions. This finding is of particular importance because individuals exposed to styrene are frequently exposed to other organic solvents, and therefore it stresses the importance of knowing an individual's complete exposure history when making a causative diagnosis.

Individual Studies

Neuropsychological Tests in a Fiberglass Worker with Exposure to Mixed Solvents, Including Styrene

White et al. (1990) examined the neuropsychological sequelae of a 27-year-old man with recurrent styrene exposure and who presented with psychosis. The clinical picture was confounded by multiple substance abuse (including alcohol and recreational drugs) as well as exposure to other solvents. Two years after beginning to work with limited protective equipment in a poorly ventilated fiberglass laminating factory, he sought psychiatric treatment for depression. Styrene blood level was 0.20 mg/L (see Table 17-4) when measured more than 24 hours after the end of his work shift. The urine sample also contained "minute amounts of toluene and trichloroethylene."

One month later, he became increasingly confused over the course of several days and experienced feelings of intoxication while at work. He was described as disoriented and paranoid and had reported that he had experienced both auditory and visual hallucinations. EEG was normal. Formal neuropsychological testing showed a verbal IQ of 96 (performance IQ: 79). The poorest performance was on the Wechsler Adult Intelligence Scale–Revised (WAIS-R) picture completion test (subtest score of 5). Academic skills (measured with the Wide Range Achievement Test–Revised) were consistent with his 11 years of education. Impairments were also noted in visual memory, complex problem-solving, and fine motor dexterity. The Minnesota Multiphasic Personality Index (MMPI) profile was similar to that of individuals with characteriological and somatic concerns. Repeat neuropsychological examination 10 months after the initial episode of psychosis showed significant improvement in cognitive function, memory, and complex problem-solving. The MMPI showed substantial reduction in somatic concerns, depression, agitation, and unusual sensory experience, though some characteriological problems remained. Just before this second testing, the patient had quit work and had been through an alcohol rehabilitation program for 1 month.

Peripheral Neuropathy After Styrene Exposure in a Photostat Shop

A 45-year-old self-employed man with his own photostat business was exposed to monomeric styrene while preparing the ink used for the photostats (Behari et al., 1986). The duration of exposure was 4 to 10 hours per day, 7 days per week, for 5 years; air styrene concentrations in the shop were not reported. The patient presented with a burning sensation in the feet and ankles. The sensation was most marked on the soles of the feet and was accompanied by a peculiar feeling, described to be as if he were walking on inflated balloons or cotton wool.

Clinical examination revealed a graded sensation loss up to 50% for pain and touch below the ankles. Vibration and position sense were preserved. Tendon reflexes were brisk with flexor plantar responses. Romberg's sign was negative. His gait was normal and there was no history of weakness, footdrop, or ataxia. He had no symptoms pertaining to the cranial nerves. Higher mental functions including speech were normal. General physical examination was unremarkable. Urine analysis, blood urea, blood sugar, serum electrolytes, plasma proteins, and immunoglobulins were normal. Medical history included hypertension treated with α-methyldopa (Aldomet) and depression for which he was

TABLE 17-5. *Motor and sensory nerve conduction studies in workers exposed to styrene at low (< 5 ppm), medium (50 ppm), and high (125 ppm) concentrations*

Parameter	Control	Low	Medium	High
Motor conduction velocity (m/sec)				
Median nerve	61.8 ± 7.4	58.9 ± 3.5	59.8 ± 3.9	61.0 ± 5.3
Ulnar nerve	62.8 ± 6.4	56.1 ± 4.1	61.0 ± 2.6	60.7 ± 6.7
Fibular nerve	48.5 ± 3.4	46.9 ± 4.3	50.6 ± 3.8	48.2 ± 3.2
Tibial nerve	46.8 ± 2.4	46.0 ± 4.7	49.6 ± 3.4	44.7 ± 2.9
Sensory conduction velocity (m/sec)				
First finger (distal)	49.0 ± 2.3	44.0 ± 3.7	48.2 ± 6.2	44.6 ± 6.6
Third finger (distal)	52.3 ± 3.2	47.1 ± 5.1	50.2 ± 6.1	48.5 ± 7.9
Wrist to elbow (proximal)	58.7 ± 4.4	58.2 ± 4.1	60.3 ± 3.2	62.9 ± 9.1
Sensory amplitude (μV)				
First finger	26.7 ± 11.3	20.2 ± 9.0	18.1 ± 6.3	18.3 ± 9.7
Third finger	16.0 ± 10.6	13.4 ± 10.1	11.2 ± 4.7	12.7 ± 7.4
Sensory duration (msec)				
First finger	1.8 ± 0.2	2.2 ± 0.5	2.4 ± 1.1	2.7 ± 1.2
Third finger	2.0 ± 0.1	2.5 ± 0.8	2.2 ± 0.7	2.5 ± 1.0

See text for significance of findings. Modified from Rosen et al., 1978, with permission.

administered imipramine (Depsonil). He did not drink and had smoked eight to ten cigarettes a day for the past 35 years.

Motor-nerve conduction velocities were normal in the upper extremities, but were slow in the lower limbs. The optic nerve was spared both clinically and electrophysiologically; visual evoked responses were measured as normal using checkerboard pattern reversal. Sural nerve biopsy examined by light microscopy revealed many demyelinated nerve fibers. Electron microscopy revealed ultrastructural changes including occasional evidence of active myelin degeneration (see Pathological Diagnosis section). A few fibers showed one or two laminae formed by Schwann cell processes, indicating remyelination. Axis cylinders were better preserved.

Optic Neuropathy in a Styrene Exposed Person

While monitoring of air levels prevents extreme exposures of industrial styrene workers, self-employed workers are unmonitored and therefore may be exposed to levels much higher than are found in the styrene polyester plastic industry. The worker reported here was most likely exposed to extremely high levels since no protective measures were employed and he frequently handled the styrene with his bare hands (Rebert and Hall, 1994).

A 48-year-old man experienced a sudden painless deterioration of his vision over the course of a week, by the end of which his vision had decreased to the point that he was unable to read (Pratt-Johnson, 1964; Grant and Schuman, 1993). For the past 5 years he had reportedly been a self-employed fiberglass worker with repeated exposure to styrene. He worked building fiberglass boats in a small room and admitted that he handled the styrene carelessly, frequently allowing it to come into contact with his bare

hands. He smoked 20 cigarettes a day and consumed about one beer a week. He had not previously experienced any problems with his vision and there was no familial history of any defects of vision. Examination revealed his vision to be 20/400 in each eye. Pupils were equal in size, and response to light and near objects was normal. The central visual fields in both eyes demonstrated centrocecal scotoma. The optic nerve heads and fundi were normal. There were no other abnormalities, and thorough medical examination revealed none of the known causes of retrobulbar neuritis or centrocecal scotoma. A provisional diagnosis of toxic bilateral retrobulbar neuritis due to repeated styrene exposure was made.

The patient was administered daily intramuscular injections of vitamin B compound and nicotinic acid. Prednisolone was administered initially but was discontinued after 1 week because it did not seem to affect his condition. He was discharged after 10 days, at which time there was no significant improvement in his condition. His medication was changed to an oral dose of vitamin B compound and nicotinic acid. He was advised to avoid any further contact with styrene.

Initial follow-up 10 days after discharge revealed that the scotoma in both eyes had decreased in size and that the vision in the left eye had improved to 20/40; however, there was no improvement of vision in the right eye. One week later, vision in both eyes had improved to 20/30. Vision further improved to 20/20 in both eyes after 6 months, but a small scotoma remained between the fixation point and the blind spot in both visual fields. After 1 year, vision was normal and no scotoma was demonstrable in either eye.

The previously described case report of retrobulbar neuritis provides only circumstantial evidence of styrene exposure and as such must be interpreted cautiously (Rebert and Hall, 1994). Ophthalmological assessment of 345 workers in a styrene plant did not find any instances of retrobulbar neuritis (Kohn, 1978). Other causes of central scotomas such as Leber's optic atrophy should not be overlooked when making the differential diagnosis (Grant and Schuman, 1993).

REFERENCES

Agrawal K, Srivastava S, Seth P. Effect of styrene on dopamine receptors. Bulletin of Environ. *Contam Toxicol* 1982;29:400–403.

American Conference of Governmental and Industrial Hygienists (ACGIH). *Documentation of the threshold limit values and biological exposure indices,* 5th ed. Cincinnati: ACGIH, 1989:BEI29–33.

American Conference of Governmental and Industrial Hygienists (ACGIH). *Threshold limit values and biological exposure indices for 1993–49.* Cincinnati: ACGIH, 1993.

American Conference of Governmental and Industrial Hygienists (ACGIH). *Threshold limit values (TLVs) for chemical substances and physical agents and biological exposure indices (BEIs).* Cincinnati: ACGIH, 1995.

Amoore JE, Hautala E. Odor as an aid to chemical safety: odor thresholds compared with threshold limit values and volatilities for 214 industrial chemicals in air and water dilution. *J Appl Toxicol* 1983;3:272–290.

Anger WK, Johnson BL. Chemicals affecting behavior. In: O'Donoghue JL, ed. *Neurotoxicity of industrial and commercial chemicals,* vol 1. Boca Raton, FL: CRC Press, 1985:52–148.

Araki S, Yokoyama K, Murata K. Assessment of the effects of occupational and environmental factors on all faster and slower large myelinated nerve fibers: a study of the distribution of conduction velocities. *Environ Res* 1993;62:325–332.

Ashley DL, Bonin MA, Cardinali FL, McCraw JM, Wooten JV. Blood concentrations of volatile organic compounds in a nonoccupationally exposed US population and in groups with suspected exposure. *Clin Chem* 1994;40:1401–1404.

Åstrand I. Uptake of solvents in the blood and tissues of man. *Scand J Work Environ Health* 1975;1:199–218.

Åstrand I, Kilbom A, Wahlberg I, et al. Exposure to styrene: I. Concentration in alveolar air and blood at rest and during exercise and metabolism. *Work Environ Health* 1974;11:69–85.

Bakke OM, Scheline RR. Hydroxylation of aromatic hydrocarbons in the rat. *Toxicol Appl Pharmacol* 1970;16:691–700.

Bardodej Z, Bardodejova E. Biotransformation of ethyl benzene, styrene, and alpha methyl styrene in man. *Am Ind Hyg Assoc J* 1970;31:206–209.

Behari M, Choudhary C, Roy S, Meheshwari M. Styrene induced peripheral neuropathy; a case report. *Eur Neurol* 1986;25:424–427.

Berode M, Droz PO, Guillemin M. Human exposure to styrene VI. Percutaneous absorption in human volunteers. *Int Arch Occup Environ Health* 1985;55:331–336.

Bond J. Review of the toxicology of styrene. *Crit Rev Toxicol* 1989;19:227–249.

Brigham CR, Landrigan PJ. Safety and health in boatbuilding and repair. *Am J Ind Med* 1985;8:169–182.

Brown HS, Bishop DR, Rowan CA. The role of skin absorption as a route of exposure for volatile organic compounds (VOCs) in drinking water *Am J Public Health* 1984;74:479–484.

Brown NA. Reproductive and developmental toxicity of styrene. *Reprod Toxicol* 1991;5:3–29.

Carpenter CP, Shaffer CB, Weil CS, Smyth HF. Studies on the inhalation of 1:3-butadiene; with a comparison of its narcotic effect with benzol, toluol, and styrene, and a note on the elimination of styrene by the human. *J Ind Hyg Toxicol* 1944;26:69–78.

Cerny S, Mraz J, Flek J, Tichy M. Effect of ethanol on the urinary excretion of mandelic and phenylglyoxylic acids after human exposure to styrene. *Int Arch Occup Environ Health* 1990;62:243–247.

Checkoway H, Costa LG, Camp J, Coccini T, Daniell WE, Dills RL. Peripheral markers of neurochemical function among workers exposed to styrene. *Br J Ind Med* 1992;49:560–565.

Chemical Review. Styrene. Dangerous properties of industrial materials report, 1988;8:10–44.

Chemical Safety Data SD-37(CSD), Properties and Essential Information for Safe Handling and Use of Styrene. Washington, DC: Manufacturing Chemists Association, 1971.

Cherry N, Gautrin D. Neurotoxic effects of styrene: further evidence. *Br J Ind Med* 1990;47:29–37.

Cherry N, Rodgers B, Venables H, Waldron HA, Wells GG. Acute behavioral effects of styrene exposure: a further analysis. *Br J Ind Med* 1980;38:346–350.

Coccini T, Di Nucci A, Tonini M, et al. Effects of ethanol administration on cerebral non-protein sulfhydryl content in rats exposed to styrene vapour. *Toxicology* 1996;106:115–122.

Crandall MS, Hartle RW. An analysis of exposure to styrene in the reinforced plastic boat-making industry. *Am J Ind Med* 1985;8:183–192.

Dick RB. Neurobehavioral assessment of occupationally relevant solvents and chemicals in humans. In: Chang LW, Dyer RS, eds. *Handbook of Neurotoxicology.* New York: Marcel Dekker, Inc., 1995:217–322.

Dixit R, Das M, Mushtaq M, Srivastava P, Seth PK. Depletion of glutathione content and inhibition of glutathione-*S*-transferase and aryl hydrocarbon hydroxylase activity of rat brain following exposure to styrene. *Neurotoxicology* 1982;3:142–145.

Drummond L, Caldwell J, Wilson HK. The metabolism of ethylbenzene and styrene to mandelic acid: stereochemical considerations. *Xenobiotica* 1989;19:199–207.

Dutkiewicz T, Tyras H. Skin absorption of toluene, styrene, and xylene by man. *Brit J Ind Med* 1968;25:243.

Dypbukt JM, Costa LG, Manzo L, Orrenius S, Nicotera P. Cytotoxic and genotoxic effects of styrene-7,8-oxide in neuradrenergic Pc 12 cells. *Carcinogenesis* 1992;13:417–424.

Edling C, Anundi H, Johanson G, Nilsson K. Increase in neuropsychiatric symptoms after occupational exposure to low levels of styrene. *Brit J Ind Med* 1993;50:843–850.

Eguchi T, Kishi R, Harabuchi I, et al. Impaired colour discrimination among workers exposed to styrene: relevance of a urinary metabolite. *Occup Environ Med* 1995;52:534–538.

Engström J. Styrene in subcutaneous adipose after experimental and industrial exposure. *Scand J Work Environ Health* 1978;4:119–120.

Engström J, Bjurstrom R, Astrand I, Ovrum P. Uptake, distribution and elimination of styrene in man: concentration in subcutaneous adipose tissue. *Scand J Work Environ Health* 1978a;4:315–323.

Engström K, Härkönen H, Pekari K, Rantanen J. Evaluation of occupational styrene exposure by ambient air and urine analysis. *Scand J Work Environ Health* 1978b;4:121–123.

Fallas C, Fallas J, Maslard P, Dally S. Subclinical impairment of color vision among workers exposed to styrene. *Br J Ind Med* 1992;49:679–682.

Fernandez J, Caperos J. Styrene exposure: 1. Experimental study of the pulmonary absorption and excretion on human volunteers. *Int Arch Occup Environ Health* 1977;40:1–12.

Fiserova-Bergerova V, Teisinger J. Pulmonary styrene vapor retention. *Ind Med Surg* 1965;34:620–622.

Fishbein L. Exposure from occupational versus other sources. *Scand J Work Environ Health* 1992;18:5–16.

Flodin U, Ekberg K, Angersson L. Neuropsychiatric effects of low exposure to styrene. *Br J Ind Med* 1989;46:805–808.

Geuskens RB, van der Klaauw M, van der Tuin J, van Hemmen J. Exposure to styrene and health complaints in the Dutch glass-reinforced plastic industry. *Ann Occup Hyg* 1992;36:47–57.

Gobba F, Galassi C, Imbriani M, Ghittori S, Candela S, Cavalleri A. Acquired dyschromatopsia among styrene-exposed workers. *J Occup Med* 1991;33:761–765.

Gotell P. Field studies on human styrene exposure. *Work Environ Health* 1972;9:76–83.

Grant WM, Schuman JS. *Toxicology of the eye: effects on the eyes and visual system from chemicals, drugs, metals and minerals, plants, toxins, and venoms: also, systemic side effects from eye medications.* 4th ed., Springfield, IL: Thomas, 1993:1333–1334.

Guillemin MP, Berode M. Biological monitoring of styrene: a review. *Am Ind Hyg J* 1988;49:497–505.

Guthrie VB. In: Guthrie VB, ed. *Petroleum products handbook.* New York: McGraw-Hill, 1960.

Haglid KG, Briving C, Hansson H-A, Rosengren L, Kjellstrand P, Stavron D, Swedin U, Wronski A. Trichloroethylene: long-lasting changes in the brain after rehabilitation. *Neurotoxicology* 1981;2:659–673.

Halliwell B. Oxidants and the central nervous system: some fundamental questions. Is oxidant damage relevant to Parkinson's disease, Alzheimer's disease, traumatic injury and stroke? *Acta Neurol Scand* 1989;126: 23–33.

Härkönen H. Relationship of symptoms to occupational styrene exposure and to findings of electroencephalographic and psychological examinations. *Int Arch Occup Environ Health* 1977;40:231.

Härkönen H, Lindstrom K, Seppäläinen AM, Asp S, Hernberg S. Exposure response relationship between styrene exposure and central nervous functions. *Scand J Work Environ Health* 1978;4:53–59.

Hayes JP, Lambourn L, Hopkirk JAC, Durham SR, Newman Taylor AJ. Occupational asthma due to styrene. *Thorax* 1991;46:396–397.

Hemminki K, Vodicka P. Styrene: from characterization of DNA adducts to application in styrene-exposed lamination workers. *Toxicol Lett* 1995;77:153–161.

Holmberg PC, Nurminen M. Congenital defects to the central nervous system and occupational factors during pregnancy; a case-referent study. *Am J Ind Med* 1980;1:167–176.

Holmberg PC. Central nervous system defects in two children of mothers exposed to chemicals in the reinforced plastic industry: chance or causal relationship. *Scand J Work Environ Health* 1977;3:212–221.

Ikeda M, Ohtsuji H, Imamura T. *In vivo* suppression of benzene and styrene oxidation by co-administered toluene in rats and effects of phenobarbital. *Xenobiotica* 1972;2:101–106.

Ikeda M, Imamura T, Hayashi M, Tabuchi T, Hara I. Evaluation of hippuric, phenylglyoxylic and mandelic acids in urine as indices of styrene exposure. *Int Arch Arbeitsmed* 1974;32:93–101.

Ikeda M, Hirayama T. Possible metabolic interaction of styrene with organic solvents. *Scand J Work Environ Health* 1978;4:41–46.

Jegaden D, Amann D, Simon JF, Habault M, Legoux B, Galopin P. Study of the neurobehavioral toxicity of styrene at low levels of exposure. *Int Arch Occup Environ Health* 1993;64:527–531.

Katoh T, Higashi K, Inoue N. Sub-chronic effects of styrene and styrene oxide on lipid peroxidation and the metabolism of glutathione in rat liver and brain. *J Toxicol Sci* 1989;14:1–9.

Kishi R, Katakura Y, Okui T, Ogawa H, Ikeda T, Miyake H. Placental transfer and adipose distribution of ^{14}C-styrene: an autoradiographic study in mice. *Brit J Ind Med* 1989;46:376–383.

Klimkova-Deutschova E, Jandova D, Salcmanova Z, Schwartzova K, Titman O. Recent advances concerning the clinical picture of professional styrene exposure [English summary]. *Cesk Neurol Neurochir* 1973;36: 20–25.

Kohn AN. Ocular toxicity of styrene. *Am J Ophthalmol* 1978;85:569–570.

Ledin T, Ödkvist L, Möller C. Posturography findings in workers exposed to industrial solvents. *Acta Otolaryngol (Stockh)* 1989;107:357–361.

Leibman KC. Metabolism and toxicity of styrene. *Environ Health Perspect* 1975;11:115–119.

Leibman KC, Ortiz E. Microsomal hydration of epoxides. *Fed Proc* 1968;27:302.

Leibman KC, Ortiz E. Epoxide intermediates in microsomal oxidation of olefins to glycols. *J Pharmacol* 1970;173:242–246.

Letz R, Mahoney FC, Hershman DL, Woskie S, Smith TJ. Neurobehavioral effects of acute styrene exposure in fiberglass boat builders. *Neurotoxicol Teratol* 1990;12:665–668.

Lilis R. Diseases associated with exposure to chemical substances. In: Last J, Wallace R, eds. *Maxcy–Rosenau–Last public health and preventive medicine*. New York: Appleton & Lange, 1992:410.

Lilis R, Lorimer W, Diamond S, Selikoff I. Neurotoxicity of styrene in production and polymerization workers. *Environ Res* 1978;15:133–138.

Lindstrom K, Härkönen H, Harnberg S. Disturbances in psychological functions of workers occupationally exposed to styrene. *Scand J Work Environ Health* 1976;2:129–139.

Löf A, Gullstrand E, Nordquist MB. Tissue distribution of styrene, styrene glycol and more polar styrene metabolites in the mouse. *Scand J Work Environ Health* 1983;9:419–430.

Lorimer W, Lilis R, Nicholson W, et al. Clinical studies of styrene workers: initial findings. *Environ Hlth Perspect* 1976;17:171–181.

Marietta M, Vessel E, Hartman R, Weisz J, Dvorchik BH. Characterization of cytochrome P-450-dependent aminopyrine *N*-demethylase in rat brain: comparison with hepatic aminopyrine *N*-demethylation. *J Pharmacol Exp Ther* 1979;208:271–279.

Matikainen E, Forsman-Gronholm L, Pfaffli P, Juntunen J. Nervous system effects of occupational exposure to styrene. A clinical and neurophysiological study. *Environ Res* 1993;61:84–92.

Melgaard B, Arlien-Søborg P, Bruhn P. Chronic toxic encephalopathy in styrene exposed workers. In: *3rd Industrial and Environmental Neurology Congress*. Prague, 1979.

Merck Index: An encyclopedia of chemicals, drugs and biologicals. Budavaris S, O'Niel MJ, Smith A, Heckleman PE, eds. Rahway, NJ: Merck & Co, 1989:1397.

Mergler D, Blain L. Assessing color vision loss among solvent-exposed workers. *Am J Ind Med* 1987;12:195–203.

Möller C, Ödkvist L, Larsby B, et al. Otoneurological findings in workers exposed to styrene. *Scand J Work Environ Health* 1990;16:189–194.

Mizunuma K, Yasugi T, Kawai T, Horiguchi S, Ikeda M. Exposure–excretion relationship of styrene and acetone in factory workers: a comparison of lipophilic solvent and a hydrophilic solvent. *Arch Environ Contam Toxicol* 1993;25:129–133.

Murata K, Araki S, Yokoyama K. Assessment of the peripheral, central, and autonomic nervous system function in styrene workers. *Am J Ind Med* 1991;20:775–784.

Murphy PG, MacDonald DA, Lickly TD. Styrene migration from general-purpose and high-impact polystyrene into food-simulating solvents. *Food Chem Toxicol* 1992;30:225–232.

Mutti A, Smargiassi A. Selective vulnerability of dopaminergic systems to industrial chemicals: risk assessment of related neuroendocrine changes. *Toxicology & Industrial Health* 1998;14:311–323.

Mutti A, Vescovi PP, Falzoi M, Arfini G, Valenti G, Franchini I. Neuroendocrine effects of styrene on occupationally exposed workers. *Scand J Work Environ Health* 1984;10:225–228.

Mutti A, Falzoi M, Romanelli A, Franchini I. Regional alterations of brain catecholamines by styrene exposure in rabbits. *Arch Toxicol* 1985;55: 173–177.

National Institute for Occupational Safety and Health (NIOSH). *Styrene: Criteria for a recommended standard*. Washington, DC: NIOSH, 1983:83–119.

National Institute for Occupational Safety and Health (NIOSH). *Recommendations for occupational safety and health compendium of policy documents and statements*. Cincinnati: US Department of Health and Human Services, Public Health Service Centers for Disease Control DHHS, NIOSH Publications, 1992.

National Institute for Occupational Safety and Health (NIOSH). *Pocket guide to chemical hazards*. Cincinnati: US Department of Health and Human Services, Centers for Disease Control and Prevention, NIOSH Publications, 1997.

Occupational Safety and Health Administration (OSHA). *Code of federal regulations* (1910.1000). Cincinnati: US Department of Health and Human Services, Centers for Disease Control, 1995.

Ödkvist LM, Larsby B, Tham R, Ahlfeldt H, Andersson B, Eriksson B, Liedgren SRC. Vestibulo-oculomotor interactions in humans exposed to styrene. *Acta Otolaryngol* 1982;94:487–493.

Oesch E, Jerina DM, Daly J. A radiometric assay for hepatic epoxide hydrase activity with [7-3H]styrene oxide. *Biochimica Biophysica Acta* 1971;227:685–691.

Ohtsuji H, Ikeda M. The metabolism of styrene in the rat and the stimulatory effect of phenobarbital. *Toxicol Appl Pharmacol* 1971;18:321–328.

Pahwa R, Kalra J. A critical review of the neurotoxicity of styrene in humans. *Vet Hum Toxicol* 1993;35:516–520.

Parke DV. Activation mechanisms to chemical toxicity. *Arch Toxicol* 1987;60:5–15.

Parkki MG. The role of glutathione in the toxicity of styrene. *Scand J Work Environ Health* 1978;4:53–59.

Patty FA. In: Patty FA, ed. *Industrial hygiene and toxicology*, vol II. New York: Wiley-Interscience, 1963.

Petreas MX, Woodlee J, Becker CE, Rappaport SM. Retention of styrene following exposure to constant and fluctuating air concentrations. *Int Arch Occup Environ Health* 1995;67:27–34.

Pfäffli P, Hesso A, Vainio H, Hyvonen M. 4-Vinylphenol excretion suggestive of arene oxide formation in workers occupationally exposed to styrene. *Toxicol Appl Pharmacol* 1981;60:85–90.

Pierce C, Tozer T. Styrene in adipose tissue of non-occupationally exposed persons. *Environ Res* 1992;58:230–235.

Pratt-Johnson J. Retrobulbar neuritis following exposure to vinyl benzene (styrene). *Can Med Assoc J* 1964;90:975–977.

Ramsey JC, Young JD. Pharmacokinetics of inhaled styrene in rats and humans. *Scand J Work Environ Health* 1978;4:84–91.

Rebert CS, Hall TA. The neuroepidemiology of styrene: a critical review of representative literature. *Crit Rev Toxicol* 1994;24(S1):S57–S106.

Rebert CS, Boyes WK, Pryor GT, et al. Combined effects of solvents on the rat's auditory system: styrene and trichloroethylene. *Int J Psychophysiol* 1993;14:49–59.

Riihimäki V, Pfäffli P. Percutaneous absorption of solvent vapors in man. *Scand J Work Environ Health* 1978;4:73–85.

Rogers JC, Hooper CC. M.A.C. for styrene. *Ind Med Surg* 1957;26:32.

Romanelli A, Falzoi M, Mutti A, Bergamaschi E, Franchini I. Effects of some monocyclic aromatic solvents and their metabolites on brain dopamine in rabbits. *J Appl Toxicol* 1986;6:431–436.

Rosen I, Haeger-Aronsen B, Rehnstrom S, Welinder H. Neurophysiological observations after chronic styrene exposure. *Scand J Work Environ Health* 1978;4:184–194.

Rosengren LE, Haglid KG. Long-term neurotoxicity of styrene. a quantitative of glial fibrillary acidic protein (GFA) and S-100. *Brit J Ind Med* 1989;46:316.

Rosengren LE, Kjellstrand P, Aurell A, Haglid KG. Irreversible effects of xylene on the brain after long term exposure: a quantitative study of DNA and the glial cell marker proteins S-100 and GFA. *Neurotoxicology* 1986;7:121–135.

Roth B, Klimkova-Deutschova E. The effect of the chronic action of industrial poisons on the electroencephalogram of man. *Rev Czech Med* 1963;9:217–227.

Sandmeyer EE. Aromatic hydrocarbons. In: Clayton GD, Clayton FE, eds. *Patty's industrial hygiene and toxicology,* vol IIB, third revised edition. John Wiley and Sons, New York, 1981:3253–3431.

Sass-Kortsak AM, Corey PN, Robertson JM. An investigation of the association between exposure to styrene and hearing loss. *Ann Epidemiol* 1995;5:15–24.

Savolainen H, Pfaffli P. Accumulation of styrene monomer and neurochemical effects of long-term inhalation exposure in rats. *Scand J Work Environ Health* 1978;4(2):78–83.

Sax NI. *Dangerous properties of industrial materials.* New York: Van Nostrand Reinhold, 1979:902–903.

Schoenhuber R, Gentilini M. Influence of occupational styrene exposure on memory and attention. *Neurotoxicol Teratol* 1989;11:585–586.

Seppäläinen AM, Härkönen H. Neurophysiological findings among workers occupationally exposed to styrene. *Scand J Work Environ Health* 1976;2:140–146.

Severi M, Pauwels W, Van Hummelen P, et al. Urinary mandelic acid and hemoglobin adducts in fiberglass-reinforced plastics workers exposed to styrene. *Scand J Work Environ Health* 1994;20:451–458.

Sorsa M, Anttila A, Jarventaus H, et al. Styrene revisited—exposure assessment and risk estimation in the reinforced plastic industry. *Prog Clin Biol Res* 1991;372:187–195.

Srivastava SP, Das M, Seth PK. Enhancement of lipid peroxidation in rat liver on acute exposure to styrene and acrylamide a consequence of glutathione depletion. *Chem Biol Interact* 1983;45:373–380.

Stetkarova I, Urban P, Prochazka B, Lukas E. Somatosensory evoked potentials in workers exposed to toluene and styrene. *Br J Ind Med* 1993;50:520–527.

Stewart RD, Dodd HC, Baretta ED, Schaffer AW. Human exposure to styrene vapor. *Arch Environ Hlth* 1968;16:656–662.

Tossavainen A. Styrene use and occupational exposure in the plastics industry. *Scand J Work Environ Health* 1978;4:7–13.

Toftgård R, Gustafsson JA. Biotransformation of organic solvents: a review. *Scand J Work Environ Health* 1980;6:1–18.

Trenga CA, Kunkel DD, Eaton DL, Costa LG. Effect of styrene oxide on rat brain glutathione. *Neurotoxicology* 1991;12:165–178.

Triebig G, Schaller KH, Valentin H. Investigations on neurotoxicity of chemical substances at the work place. *Int Arch Occup Environ Health* 1985;56:239–247.

Triebig G, Lehrl S, Weltle D, Schaller KH, Valentin H. Clinical and neurobehavioral study of the acute and chronic neurotoxicity of styrene. *Br J Ind Med* 1989;46:799–804.

United States Environmental Protection Agency (USEPA). *Drinking water regulations and health advisories.* EPA, 822-r-96-001, Washington, DC: Office of Water, 4304, February, 1996.

von Euler G, Bjornaes S. Persistent effects of chronic exposure to styrene on the affinity of neostriatal dopamine D-2 receptors. *Toxicol Lett* 1990;54:101–106.

Wallace L, Pellizzari E, Hartwell T, et al. The California team study: breath concentrations and personal exposures to 26 volatile compounds in air and drinking water of 188 residents of Los Angeles, Antioch, and Pittsburg, CA. *Atmos Environ* 1988;22:2141–2163.

Weiss G. In: Weiss G, ed. *Hazardous chemicals data book.* NJ: Noyes Data Corp, 1980.

White D, Daniell W, Maxwell J, Townes B. Psychosis following styrene exposure: a case report of neuropsychological sequelae. *J Clin Exp Neuropsychol* 1990;12:798–806.

Wieczorek H. Evaluation of low exposure to styrene II. Dermal absorption of styrene vapours in humans under experimental conditions. *Int Arch Occup Environ Hlth* 1985;57:71–75.

Wieczorek H, Piotrowski JK. Evaluation of low exposure to styrene I. Absorption of styrene vapours by inhalation under experimental conditions. *Int Arch Occup Environ Hlth* 1985;57:57–69.

Wilson HK, Cocker J, Purnell CJ, Brown RH, Gompertz D. The time course of mandelic and phenyloxyglyoxylic acid excretion in workers exposed to styrene under model conditions. *Brit J Ind Med* 1979;36:235–237.

Wilson HK, Robertson SM, Waldron HA, Gompertz D. Effect of alcohol on the kinetics of mandelic acid excretion in volunteers exposed to styrene vapor. *Br J Ind Med* 1983;40:75–80.

Withey JR. The toxicology of styrene monomer and its pharmacokinetics and distribution in the rat. *Scand J Work Environ Health* 1978;4:31–40.

Withey JR, Collins PG. Pharmacokinetics and distribution of styrene monomers in rats after intravenous administration. *J Toxicol Environ Health* 1977;3:1011.

Withey JR, Collins PG. The distribution and pharmacokinetics of styrene monomers in rats by the pulmonary route. *J Environ Pathol Toxicol* 1979;2:1329.

Wolff MS, Lorimer WV, Lilis R, Selikoff IJ. Biological indicators of exposure in styrene polymerization workers: styrene in blood and adipose tissue and mandelic and phenylglyoxylic acids in urine. *Scand J Work Environ Health* 1978;4:114–118.

World Health Organization (WHO). *Styrene. Environmental health criteria,* 26. Geneva: WHO, 1983.

CHAPTER 18

Acrylamide

Acrylamide (propenamide; 2-propenamide; acrylic amide) is a white crystalline vinyl monomer (alpha–beta unsaturated carbonyl), produced from acrylonitrile by various methods of hydration. Residues of acrylonitrile are found as a contaminant of commercial-grade acrylamide (Kuperman, 1958; Kirk–Othmer, 1978; WHO, 1985). Acrylamide may sublimate at room temperature and is odorless. It is highly soluble in water and, in order of decreasing solubility, acrylamide also dissolves in ethanol, acetone, and methanol (Sax, 1979; ACGIH, 1988; NIOSH, 1997).

Acrylamide monomer is stable in solution and does not spontaneously polymerize at room temperature. However, when heated above 120°F it polymerizes into polyacrylamide, an insoluble gel. Sodium bromate/sodium sulfite and potassium persulfate/sodium metasulfite are usually added to initiate polymerization of acrylamide monomer at lower temperatures, and dimethylaminoproprionitrile (DMAPN) and ammonium persulfate are used as catalysts to facilitate the polymerization process (Bikales and Kolodny, 1963; Spencer and Schaumburg, 1974; Kreiss et al., 1980; *Merck Index,* 1996). Commercial acrylamide monomer is also stabilized by additives (Windholz et al., 1976). Residual amounts of acrylamide and acrylonitrile often contaminate the polyacrylamide product (Auld and Bedwell, 1967; ACC, 1979; WHO, 1985). Acrylamide monomer content in polyacrylamide products ranges from less than 0.05% to 0.3% (Kirk–Othmer, 1978). Polyacrylamide can be degraded by heat and light, but changes in pH do not result in depolymerization (Smith et al., 1996). In addition to polymerization, acrylamide monomer is readily hydrolyzed under basic or acidic conditions to acrylate and acrylic acid, respectively (ACC, 1969). Acrylamide also forms copolymers with various organic compounds including styrene (Bale Oenick et al., 1990).

The distal axonopathy produced in animals by acrylamide poisoning has become a frequently used experimental model with which to study axonal disease processes, such as "distal dying back axonopathy" (Cavanagh, 1964; Schaumburg et al., 1974; Sickles and Goldstein, 1986), axoplasmic transport (Miller and Spencer, 1984; Gold et al., 1985), and axonal accumulations of neurofilaments

(Prineas, 1969; Schaumburg et al., 1989), as well as central nervous system (CNS) pathologies (Abou-Donia et al., 1993). Although acrylamide monomer is highly neurotoxic, its polymers and copolymers are generally not. The structural variations at the vinyl and/or at the carbonyl group of acrylamide analogs reduce or abolish their neurotoxicity (Spencer and Schaumburg, 1974). Unless there is exposure to the acrylamide monomer itself, adverse health effects are unlikely to occur. Occupational and nonoccupational exposures to acrylamide monomer have been associated with peripheral and central nervous system effects (Fujita et al., 1960; Garland and Patterson, 1967; Igisu et al., 1975; Davenport et al., 1976; Le Quesne, 1980; He et al., 1989; Myers and Macun, 1991; Calleman et al., 1994). Such mishaps can arise when relatively small amounts of the monomer contaminate a supply of otherwise nontoxic acrylamide polymer (McCollister et al., 1964; Igisu et al., 1975). With many workers at risk of exposure to acrylamide monomer and the possibility that continued exposures may lead to genetic, reproductive, developmental, and carcinogenic toxicities, the early detection of the neurotoxicity of this monomer has important health and economic significance (Dearfield et al., 1988, 1995; WHO, 1985; EPA, 1988; NIOSH, 1991; Calleman, 1996).

SOURCES OF EXPOSURE

Occupational exposures to acrylamide monomer occur during the manufacture of acrylamide from acrylonitrile and in the production of polyacrylamide from acrylamide. Acrylamide monomer is used in soil grouting to stabilize and prevent sliding and/or cave-ins during excavations in mines; the monomer in solution along with a polymerization initiator is pumped into the soil, where it polymerizes and hardens (Auld and Bedwell, 1967; EPA, 1991). Acrylamide grout is also used to form waterproof seals for sewers, tunnels, and other underground conducting systems. Although production of acrylamide grout in the United States ceased in 1978, companies using this type of grout continue to obtain it from foreign sources. Approximately

337

650,000 pounds of acrylamide grout were consumed in the United States in 1989. A derivative of acrylamide grout, *N*-methylolacrylamide, is also commonly used in the United States. The health effects associated with exposure to *N*-methylolacrylamide are similar to those seen following exposures to acrylamide grout (EPA, 1991).

Exposure to dust and solutions of acrylamide affects handlers during the production of polyacrylamide and the various products derived from the polymer, including adhesive tape, ceramics, metal coating, paint, paper, synthetic fibers, and textiles (He et al., 1989; Smith and Oehme, 1991; Cloeren, 1992; Calleman et al., 1994; Calleman, 1996). Gelatinous polyacrylamide flocculant is used to separate solid waste from liquid sewage and to deemulsify oil-in-water mixtures. Releases of acrylamide monomer residues from polyacrylamide flocculants used in sewage treatment and water purification processes often leach into potable water supplies. Variable quantities of acrylamide remain in solution after sewage treatment and can be found downstream from industrial effluent discharges (EPA, 1996). Migration and leaching from soil grouted with acrylamide monomer may contaminate well water sources as well as lakes, streams, rivers, and estuaries (Igisu et al., 1975; EPA, 1988; Myers and Macun, 1991; WHO, 1985). Consumption of animal products from livestock exposed to acrylamide through drinking from contaminated water sources can also contribute to an individual's total environmental intake (Brown et al., 1980). Although microbial biodegradation removes acrylamide from water sources within several days, it may take months to significantly decrease acrylamide levels in water bodies when bacterial counts are low (WHO, 1985).

In addition to consumption of acrylamide in contaminated drinking water, traces of polyacrylamides and acrylamide monomer can be ingested along with foodstuffs which have been washed and/or packaged with materials made of these chemicals. Workers involved in these processes are at risk, as are those exposed to acrylamide during the production of permanent press fabrics, paper products, and contact lenses (Takahashi et al., 1971; Kirk–Othmer, 1978; Bohnert et al., 1988; *Merck Index,* 1996).

Exposure to acrylamide monomer occurs in research laboratories where polyacrylamide gels are used for electrophoresis (EPA, 1988). The incidence of neurotoxic illness is rare among the very large number of molecular biologists who are potentially exposed to acrylamide in this way. However, it is possible that additional risk is encountered with long-term use because of the carcinogenic as well as neurotoxic effects of the acrylamide and its metabolite, glycidamide (Calleman, 1996).

EXPOSURE LIMITS AND SAFETY REGULATIONS

Education about the risks associated with exposure to acrylamide and proper precautions for preventing in-

creased absorption via dermal routes can prevent the adverse effects of exposure (see Preventive and Therapeutic Measures section). There are currently no widely used and/or accepted methods for the biological monitoring of workers exposed to acrylamide, and thus ambient air concentrations must be closely monitored to reduce risk of exposure and the resultant toxic effects (see Biochemical Diagnosis section). Air threshold concentrations estimated to cause neurotoxic effects in humans have been calculated from a dose–time–response model, using data from animal experiments and human case reports (Hattis and Shapiro, 1990). The World Health Organization (WHO) has estimated that a daily dose of 0.12 mg/kg can produce neurotoxic effects in humans (WHO, 1985). A no observable effect level (NOEL) has been estimated for acrylamide intake at 0.05 mg/kg per day (Burek et al., 1980). The *American Conference of Governmental Industrial Hygienists* (ACGIH) has calculated that this level will not be exceeded during an 8-hour exposure when the ambient air acrylamide concentration is 0.3 mg/m^3 and the respiratory exchange rate is 10 m^3/day (ACGIH, 1988). However, the contribution of dermal absorption to total daily intake is not considered in the derivation of this estimate, and thus the risk of neurotoxicity is significantly greater among workers who do not practice proper dermal hygienic procedures.

The *Occupational Safety and Health Administration* (OSHA) has established an 8-hour time-weighted average (TWA) permissible exposure level (PEL) of 0.3 mg/m^3 for acrylamide (OSHA, 1995). The *National Institute for Occupational Safety and Health's* (NIOSH) recommended exposure limit (REL) for acrylamide is a 10-hour TWA exposure at a concentration of 0.03 mg/m^3. NIOSH has also recommended an immediately dangerous to life and health (IDLH) exposure limit for acrylamide of 60 mg/m^3 (NIOSH, 1997). The ACGIH's recommended threshold limiting value (TLV) for acrylamide is an 8-hour TWA of 0.03 mg/m^3; this limit is based in part on the potential carcinogenic effects of acrylamide (ACGIH, 1995). The NIOSH also considers acrylamide to have carcinogenic potential (NIOSH, 1997) (Table 18-1).

Contact with acrylamide solutions as dilute as 10% can induce severe local skin reactions of erythema and subsequent dermal peeling (McCollister et al., 1964). The OSHA, NIOSH, and ACGIH have all assigned acrylamide a "skin" designation, indicating that dermal absorption contributes significantly to the toxic effects of this chemical (OSHA, 1995; NIOSH, 1994; ACGIH, 1995).

The *Environmental Protection Agency* (EPA) has not established a maximum contamination level (MCL) for acrylamide in drinking water but does recommend the monitoring and treatment of water supplies to remove excess residues (EPA, 1996). The EPA has recommended a maximum contamination level goal (MCLG) of 0.00 mg/L for acrylamide concentration in drinking water (see Clinical Experiences section).

TABLE 18-1. *Established and recommended occupational and environmental exposure limits for acrylamide in air and water*

	Air (mg/m³)[a]	Water (mg/L)[a]
Odor threshold*	—	0.017
OSHA		
PEL (8-hr TWA)	0.3	—
PEL ceiling (15-min TWA)	—	—
NIOSH		
REL (10-hr TWA)	0.3	—
STEL (15-min TWA)	—	—
IDLH	60	—
ACGIH		
TLV (8-hr TWA)	0.03	—
USEPA		
MCL	—	—
MCLG	—	0.0

[a]*Unit conversion:* 1 ppm = 1 mg/L.

OSHA, Occupational Safety and Health Administration; PEL, permissible exposure limit; TWA, time-weighted average; STEL, short-term exposure limit; NIOSH, National Institute for Occupational Safety and Health; REL, recommended exposure limit; IDLH, immediately dangerous to life and health; ACGIH, American Conference of Industrial Hygienists; TLV, threshold limit value; USEPA, United States Environmental Protection Agency; MCL, maximum contamination level; MCLG, maximum contamination level goal.

Data from *Amoore and Hautala, 1983; OSHA, 1995; ACGIH, 1995; EPA, 1996; NIOSH, 1997.

METABOLISM

Tissue Absorption

Exposures to acrylamide, whether as the dry monomer, in aqueous solutions, or in aerosols of acrylamide solutions, result in uptake by inhalation, dermal absorption, and/or oral absorption (Allen, 1979; Hills and Greife, 1986; He et al., 1989). Environmental levels are related to the nature of the acrylamide-related tasks being performed. The risk of inhalation, ingestion, and dermal absorption to individual workers depends upon their job task and the effectiveness of the protective measures taken during possible exposure (Table 18-2). Oral and/or dermal intake accounts for most of the adverse health effects following

exposure to acrylamide monomer (Hills and Greife, 1986) (see Clinical Experiences section).

Inhalation of particles of acrylamide monomer, smaller than 5 μm or as an aerosol mist of acrylamide solution, results in alveolar deposition, from which it readily enters the systemic circulation (Abou-Donia, 1995; Dearfield et al., 1995). Total pulmonary absorption of acrylamide is related to the ambient air concentration, the duration of exposure, the pulmonary ventilation rate, and the solubility of acrylamide in blood and other tissues. Quantitative differences in levels of acrylamide monomer exist among the various circumstances in which it is encountered, making it difficult to estimate the total uptake of the compound through the measurements of its ambient air concentration alone (Calleman, 1996).

Absorption through the gastrointestinal mucosa is more complete than is dermal absorption (Miller et al., 1982; Marlowe et al., 1986). Rats exposed orally to aqueous acrylamide begin to show evidence of neurotoxic effects at a dose of 1.0 mg/kg/day (Burek et al., 1980). Neurotoxic effects were seen in a family who drank well water containing an acrylamide monomer concentration of 400 ppm (Igisu et al., 1975).

A significant contribution is made by dermal absorption to the body burden of an exposed individual. For example, Calleman et al. (1994) noted an increased incidence of peripheral neuropathy among acrylamide workers who did not use satisfactory methods of protection against dermal contact and absorption. Furthermore, the neuropathy seen in these workers was more severe than that seen in workers from the same factory who were exposed to higher air concentrations of acrylamide but also used adequate protection against dermal absorption.

Overall dermal uptake is determined by the concentration of the acrylamide monomer solution, the size and condition of the exposed skin, and the duration of contact with the skin (McCollister et al., 1964; Carlson and Weaver, 1985; Frantz et al., 1985). Twenty-five percent of a topically applied dose of acrylamide monomer was absorbed through the intact skin of the rat in 24 hours (Frantz et al., 1985). Washing the skin removed most of the applied acrylamide; but an additional 35% remained in the skin, to be further absorbed into the systemic circulation later. Similar results were found *in vitro* using excised rat skin and acryl-

TABLE 18-2. *Relation of job task to ambient air acrylamide levels in a polyacrylamide flocculant factory*

Ambient air levels (mg/m³)	Job task
0.021 to 0.12	Closed reactor operators, warehouse workers, and laboratory personnel who do not handle acrylamide monomer.
0.21 to 0.36	Laboratory workers and closed reactor operators who handle acrylamide monomer.
0.48 to 0.51	Polymerizers (add catalysts to aqueous solutions of acrylamide monomer).
0.51 to 0.75	Makers (dissolve acrylamide monomer crystals in water).

Higher acrylamide exposure levels are found with job tasks involving handling of acrylamide monomer. Data from Myers and Macun, 1991.

amide monomers. Absorption of acrylamide monomer was 67% in 24 hours when a 1% aqueous solution of polyacrylamide was applied to a piece of excised rat skin. These results indicate that dilute aqueous solutions of acrylamide monomer derived from acrylamide polymers are readily absorbed through the intact skin of the rat and suggests that the same way be true for exposed humans. Neurotoxic effects were seen in a family following the combined oral and dermal absorption through drinking and bathing in well water containing acrylamide monomer (Igisu et al., 1975) (see Clinical Experiences section).

Tissue Distribution

Acrylamide is found both free and bound to sulfhydryl groups of hemoglobin in the blood (Hashimoto and Aldridge, 1970). Free acrylamide is a relatively polar compound with high water solubility; thus, in contrast to the relatively nonpolar organic solvents that are distributed according to tissue lipid content, tissue distribution of acrylamide is more reflective of tissue water content (Edwards, 1975). Acrylamide crosses the blood–brain barrier (BBB) and the placenta (Ikeda et al., 1985; Marlowe et al., 1986). All tissues, including the reproductive organs, receive some acrylamide, but the majority of an absorbed dose of acrylamide is found in the muscles (48%), with lower concentrations in the skin, heart, liver, kidneys, lungs, and brain (Miller et al., 1982; Ikeda et al., 1985; Marlowe et al., 1986). The widespread distribution of acrylamide brings with it the distribution of its neurotoxic *in vivo* metabolite, glycidamide. Glycidamide produces neurotoxic effects in those areas of the nervous system within which it is distributed, including the cerebral cortex, hippocampus, cerebellum, and brain stem (Schaumburg and Spencer, 1979; Abou-Donia et al., 1993; Calleman, 1996).

Hashimoto and Aldridge (1970) demonstrated in mice that 1 day after a single intraperitoneal injection of labeled ([14]C-)acrylamide, the highest levels of labeled free soluble and protein-bound acrylamide are found in the blood, with progressively lesser amounts detected in kidney, liver, brain, spinal cord, and sciatic nerve. By 14 days after the injection, the majority of free soluble acrylamide disappeared from the blood but the protein-bound labeled acrylamide remained at a level of about 25% of the first day's level. Radioactive labeled acrylamide content was 2.5 times greater in the distal half of the sciatic nerve of a mouse than it was in the proximal portion of the nerve; it was four times less in the brain than in the distal peripheral nerve (Ando and Hashimoto, 1972; cited by Spencer and Schaumburg, 1974). The localization in the distal portions of the nerve is of particular interest because most damage is found in this site after acrylamide exposure. Mice exposed to ^{14}C-labeled acrylamide showed relatively high levels of radioactivity in the cerebellar cortex (Marlowe et al., 1986).

Tissue distribution of acrylamide in the peripheral and central nervous systems can be inferred from the clinical manifestations and pathological findings observed following exposure (Spencer and Schaumburg, 1974; Abou-Donia et al., 1993; LoPachin and Lehning, 1994; Reagan et al., 1995) (see Neuropathological Diagnosis section). Morphological evidence of acrylamide's effects are found in the cerebellum, hippocampus, and striatum. A decreased population of Purkinje cells in the cerebellum reported following exposure to acrylamide can account for the cerebellar signs of truncal ataxia and nystagmus seen in humans and cats exposed to acrylamide (Kuperman, 1958; Garland and Patterson, 1967; Schaumburg et al., 1974; Igisu et al., 1975; Cavanagh, 1982; Abou-Donia et al., 1993). Hippocampal neurons (CA1 layer) of rats are particularly vulnerable to acrylamide (Chauhan et al., 1993; Kohriyama et al., 1994). Memory disturbances seen in humans exposed to acrylamide can be attributed to such damage to hippocampal neurons (Igisu et al., 1975; Chauhan et al., 1993). The presence of acrylamide increases the density and affinity of postsynaptic dopamine receptors in the striatum (Agrawal et al., 1981; Hong et al., 1982; Tilson and Squibb, 1982). Excitatory effects of acrylamide on subcortical brain structures may play a role in the induction of convulsions and behavior that is suggestive of hallucinations in cats and in patients' reports of hallucinations (Kuperman, 1958; Igisu et al., 1975; Tilson and Squibb, 1982).

Tissue Biochemistry

Acrylamide monomer is an electrophilic compound; its carbon–carbon double bond is a readily reactive site for thiol, hydroxyl, and amino groups, with which important metabolites, conjugates, and adducts are formed. These products reflect the biochemical pathways of metabolism and may also serve as biological markers for monitoring body burden levels following exposure to acrylamide monomer (Fig. 18-1).

After absorption into the blood, approximately 12% of a dose of radio-labeled acrylamide is bonded to the cysteine residues of hemoglobin for several days in the rat (Hashimoto and Aldridge, 1970; Miller et al., 1982). Another portion of the dose of acrylamide is oxidized to an epoxide (glycidamide), by the actions of cytochrome P-450 monoxygenases (Kaplan et al., 1973; Hashimoto et al., 1981; Srivastava et al., 1985; Calleman et al., 1990; Costa et al., 1992; Abou-Donia et al., 1993; Bergmark et al., 1993). Glycidamide also reacts with hemoglobin cysteine residues. Some toxic effects of chronic exposure to acrylamide have been attributed to its ability and that of its metabolite, glycidamide, to form adducts at the nucleophilic centers of cellular proteins and DNA (Calleman et al., 1994; Calleman, 1996; Dearfield et al., 1995) (see Neuropathological Diagnosis section).

Conjugation with glutathione at the carbon–carbon double bond of acrylamide is the major detoxification pathway for this chemical (Edwards, 1975; Dixit et al., 1980). Acrylamide conjugates with glutathione to yield S-β-proprionamide-glutathione which is further metabolized to the mercapturic acid derivative N-acetyl-S-(propionamide)-cysteine (Wu et al., 1993; Calleman et al., 1994) (see Biochemical Diagnosis section). Glycidamide is also conjugated with glutathione, forming several different metabolites which are also excreted in the urine as mercapturic acid derivatives. These include 3-dihydroxypropionamide and N-acetyl-S-(1-carbamoyl-2-hydroxyethyl)-cysteine (Sumner et al., 1992). A minor pathway results in approximately 5% of an absorbed dose of acrylamide being cleaved at the carbonyl carbon to yield carbon dioxide. It is likely that this results from hydrolysis of glycidamide to form glyceramide, which is subsequently oxidized to a compound with a labile 1–2 carbon–carbon bond (Hashimoto and Aldridge, 1970; Miller et al., 1982; Calleman, 1996).

Chronic exposure to acrylamide depletes glutathione levels and reduces the activity of glutathione-S-transferase in the brain and liver (Dixit et al., 1980; Mukhtar et al., 1981; Srivastava et al., 1983; Beiswanger et al., 1993).

Dixit et al. (1981) found that a decrease in glutathione-S-transferase activity occurred concurrently with the onset of neuropathy in rats exposed to acrylamide. Thus, an individual's risk of toxic effects from acrylamide increases with prolonged exposure. Furthermore, exposure to other neurotoxicants such as styrene, which are also detoxified by conjugation with glutathione, can increase the neurotoxicity of acrylamide (Dixit et al., 1980; Mukhtar et al., 1981; Parkki, 1978; Dixit et al., 1982; Trenga et al., 1991; Beiswanger et al., 1993). Exposure to other chemicals that can induce cytochrome P-450 activity (e.g., phenobarbital and ethanol) enhance the metabolism of acrylamide to glycidamide and thus increase the toxic effects associated with exposures to acrylamide (Kaplan et al., 1973; Hashimoto et al., 1981; Srivastava et al., 1985; Stetkiewicz et al., 1988; Costa et al., 1992).

Excretion

Elimination of free acrylamide is monophasic. Elimination of the conjugated metabolites of acrylamide is biphasic. The rate of elimination of acrylamide is slower in humans than it is in the rat (Miller et al., 1982; Calleman, 1996). Therefore, excretion data from animal studies as to

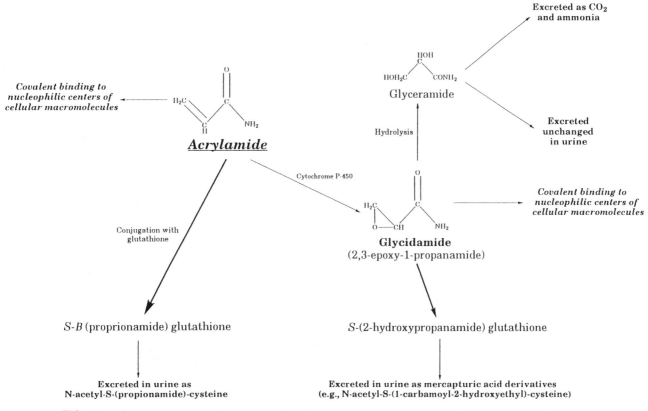

FIG. 18-1. Proposed metabolic pathways for acrylamide. (Data from Hashimoto and Aldridge, 1970; Kaplan et al., 1973; Edwards, 1975; Dixit et al., 1980; Hashimoto et al., 1981; Miller et al., 1982; Srivastava et al., 1985; Calleman et al., 1990, 1994; Costa et al., 1992; Sumner et al., 1992; Abou-Donia et al., 1993; Bergmark et al., 1993; Wu et al., 1993; Dearfield et al., 1995; Calleman, 1996.)

the relative speed of reducing the body burden of acrylamide may be misleading. These data may lead to underestimation of the continuing risk of toxicity in humans even after removal from exposure.

Less than 3% of an absorbed dose is excreted unchanged in the urine and feces of rats (Miller et al., 1982). Another 4% to 6% of an absorbed dose of acrylamide is metabolized through glycidamide to glyceramide, cleaved at the carbonyl group, and eliminated as CO_2 (Hashimoto and Aldridge, 1970). The majority (70%) of an absorbed dose of acrylamide is conjugated with glutathione and excreted in the urine as thioethers (mercapturic acid and cysteine conjugates) (Edwards, 1975; Miller et al., 1982; Rakesh et al., 1982; Wu et al., 1993; Calleman et al., 1994; Hashimoto et al., 1995). The principal urinary metabolite of acrylamide in humans is the glutathione conjugate, *N*-acetyl-*S*-(propionamide)-cysteine (Wu et al., 1993; Calleman et al., 1994). Less than 10% of an absorbed dose of acrylamide is excreted in the feces as mercapturic acids and cysteine derivatives (Hashimoto and Aldridge, 1970; Miller et al., 1982). The remainder of the dose is metabolized to glycidamide, the majority of which is conjugated with glutathione before being excreted in the urine as 2,3-dihydroxypropionamide and *N*-acetyl-*S*-(1-carbamoyl-2-hydroxyethyl)-cysteine (Sumner et al., 1992). Free glycidamide is also excreted in the urine following exposure to acrylamide (Miller et al., 1982; Sumner et al., 1992) (see Fig. 18-1).

Acrylamide is also excreted in the breast milk of lactating rats (Walden and Schiller, 1981). This finding suggests that excretion via this route may also occur in humans, with the result that nursing infants may be exposed to acrylamide.

CLINICAL MANIFESTATIONS AND DIAGNOSIS

Symptomatic Diagnosis

Toxic effects of acrylamide exposure are dose-dependent and cumulative. Clinical neurological manifestations will reflect the extent of reversible or irreversible damage to central and peripheral nervous tissue targets. Relatively short duration exposures result in acute and quickly resolving symptoms; but with chronic or repeated contacts, symptoms appear subsequently at progressively lower concentrations. Exposure to acrylamide for hours and/or days initially causes mucous membrane and dermal irritation and flaking. More prolonged exposure is followed by disturbances of behavior and feelings of malaise and unwellness. These early effects may be transient and clear soon after removal from exposure. In some cases, mild early symptoms are disregarded by exposed persons who may remain on the job until more serious and disabling symptoms appear. Loss of sensation, depressed reflexes, muscle weakness, unsteadiness of gait, and clumsiness of fine motor control as well as other signs of peripheral neuropathy develop over weeks (subacute) to months (chronic) of ex-

posure (Table 18-3). Adverse effects of low-level acrylamide exposure may be limited to the initial irritating symptoms with or without the insidious development of peripheral neuropathy. Heavy exposures induce initial central nervous system dysfunction that subsides soon after removal from exposure but is typically followed by peripheral neuropathy. Thus, the CNS may be the initial or critical organ of acrylamide exposure, but the PNS is the principal target of prolonged exposure. Progression of the neurotoxic process continues for a time after removal from the source of acrylamide exposure, the so-called "coasting effect" (Berger et al., 1992), results in subsequent increases in numbers of affected peripheral nerve fibers. Greater and clinically overt disability may be observed sometime after the at-risk person is removed from exposure and may seem unrelated to the exposure circumstances, causing an unsuspecting examiner to contribute these findings to nonneurotoxic causes, such as a viral illness followed by Guillain–Barré syndrome.

Acute Exposure

Overt dermal effects are common among workers who handle acrylamide. Skin irritation, erythema, drying, and desquamation are acute effects of contact with aqueous solutions of acrylamide and are early indicators that these workers are at increased risk for additional subsequently developing adverse health effects (Calleman et al., 1994). Autonomic nervous system dysfunction, such as reflex responses of heart rate and blood pressure, excessive palmar and sole sweating, and vasomotor changes with coldness and discoloration of fingers and toes, occur with acute exposure in humans and experimental animals (Navarro et al., 1993). Monitoring for autonomic nervous system responses in persons at risk may be a means of detecting early effects of acrylamide exposure (Auld and Bedwell, 1967; Sterman et al., 1980, 1983). Urinary retention with bladder distension has been associated with acute acrylamide toxicity, which is attributable to parasympathetic nervous system disturbances. However, this symptom has

TABLE 18-3. *Acute and chronic symptoms and signs of acrylamide poisoning*

Acute	Chronic
Dizziness	Excessive palmar sweating
Drowsiness	Fatigue
Disorientation	Muscle weakness in extremities
Hallucinations	Decreased sensation in extremities
Memory impairment	Ataxia of gait
Nystagmus	Myalgia
Dysarthria	Hypoactive reflexes
Truncal ataxia	Memory and cognitive impairment
Dysautonomia	

Data from Igisu et al., 1975; He et al., 1989; Bachman et al., 1992; and Calleman et al., 1994.

also been reported for dimethylaminoprionitrile, a catalyst often used in the production of polyacrylamide from acrylamide, and may either serve as a confounder by producing additive effects on urinary retention through its action on sacral nerves or may be the ultimate neurotoxicant responsible for this symptom (Kreiss et al., 1980).

Workers experience nonspecific effects including headache, anorexia, dizziness, lassitude, and fatigue during acute exposure; these symptoms are cleared by leaving the source of acrylamide exposure. Behavioral effects are often unrecognized by the affected person, but they may be apparent to others who observe a change in the subject's interpersonal relations and job task performance. Decreased alertness and slowed reaction time are indications of CNS effects. Mood and behavioral changes including irritability, impaired memory, delirium, and hallucinations occur and may persist between repeated episodes of peak exposure (Auld and Bedwell, 1967; Igisu et al., 1975; Schaumburg et al., 1989; Myers and Macun, 1991; Bachman et al., 1992; Calleman et al., 1994; Calleman, 1996). In addition to actual muscle fatigability and inefficiency, a sense of poor postural and gait stability arises from acrylamide's effect on muscle kinesthetics through the impairment of cerebellar, spinal cord, or peripheral nerve function. Diminished vibration sensation in addition to weakness in the extremities affects an exposed person's ability to manipulate tools and to lift weighty objects. Tremulousness of limbs and ataxia of the trunk are also experienced (Kuperman, 1958; McCollister et al., 1964; Fullerton and Barnes, 1966; Garland and Patterson, 1967; Auld and Bedwell, 1967; Fullerton, 1969; Spencer and Schaumburg, 1974; Igisu et al., 1975; Davenport et al., 1976; He et al., 1989). Subclinical neuropathy is detectable using neurophysiological techniques (Takahashi et al., 1971; Deng et al., 1993) (see Neurophysiological Diagnosis section).

The time to onset and the severity of the neuropathy are determined by the intensity and duration of the exposure as well as differences in individual susceptibility (Hopkins, 1970; Igisu et al., 1975; He et al., 1989). He et al. (1989) reported acute and persistent effects among 71 (45 men and 26 women) workers after 4 months of exposure to acrylamide at ambient air concentrations ranging from 5.56 to 9.02 mg/m³ for 8 hours per day, 6 days per week. Peripheral neuropathy develops more rapidly during exposure to high concentrations (Auld and Bedwell, 1967). The development of peripheral neuropathy is usually preceded by the dermal effects even when attempts to protect the skin have been made (Kuperman, 1958; Fullerton and Barnes, 1966; Garland and Patterson, 1967; Auld and Bedwell, 1967; Spencer and Schaumburg, 1974; Igisu et al., 1975). Vibration sensation is reduced early in the course of emerging peripheral neuropathy. Decreased sensation to touch, pain, and temperature become evident after several weeks to months of exposure. After cessation of exposure recovery of peripheral nerve function is incomplete as measured by

electrophysiological methods, although the patient may no longer report symptoms (see Clinical Experiences section).

Chronic Exposure

The principal sign of chronic acrylamide exposure is peripheral neuropathy, which develops insidiously over months or years of chronic exposure. The symptoms of acute poisoning, such as dizziness, anorexia, nausea, headache, insomnia, fatigue, numbness in extremities, ataxic gait disturbances, excessive sweating, urinary retention, and peeling skin, continue and possibly worsen with repeated exposures (Auld and Bedwell, 1967; Fullerton, 1969; Takahashi et al., 1971; Deng et al., 1993; Calleman et al., 1994) (see Table 18-3). Decreased perception of vibration sensation is an early clinical sign of peripheral neuropathy associated with exposure to acrylamide (He et al., 1989; Deng et al., 1993). Decreased muscle strength, loss of sensory perception, and decreased deep tendon reflexes develop, particularly in the distal portion of the lower extremities, with continuing exposure (Calleman et al., 1994). These symptoms and signs of peripheral neuropathy can be related to neurotoxic effects on the distal-most segments of the nerves to the extremities of the limbs (Spencer and Schaumburg, 1974; Calleman et al., 1994). With continuing exposure the neuropathy progresses proximally. Gait disturbance, bilateral footdrop, and neurogenic atrophy develop in severe cases (Myers and Macun, 1991; Calleman et al., 1994). Calleman et al. (1994) studied workers exposed to acrylamide at average air concentrations of up to 3.3 mg/m³ for periods of 0.1 to 11.5 years and

TABLE 18-4. *Prevalence (%) of symptoms and signs among workers currently exposed to acrylamide*

Symptom or sign	Acrylamide exposed	Controls
Numbness in extremities	71[a]	0
Fatigue	71[a]	0
Sweating hands	68[a]	0
Peeling of skin of hands	59[a]	0
Loss of sensation		
Pain	54[a]	0
Touch	46[b]	0
Vibration	41[b]	0
Dizziness	44[b]	0
Anorexia	41[b]	0
Nausea	39[b]	10
Insomnia	29	0
Headache	27	0
Unsteady gait	22	0
Loss of tendon reflexes		
Romberg sign	20	0
Triceps reflex	10	0
Biceps reflex	10	0

[a]Significant at $p < 0.01$.
[b]Significant at $p < 0.5$.
Data from Calleman et al., 1994.

found the prevalence rate of symptoms (numbness, fatigue, sweating hands, peeling skin) among these workers ranged from 59% to 71% (Table 18-4). Other frequently reported symptoms included decreased sensation to touch and vibration, predominantly in the hands and distal half of the lower limbs. Clinical improvement occurs within several months after removal from exposure, but subclinical evidence of peripheral neuropathy may persist indefinitely (Auld and Bedwell, 1967; Igisu et al., 1975; He et al., 1989; R. G. Feldman, personal observation) (see Neurophysiological Diagnosis section).

Neurophysiological Diagnosis

Electroencephalography records concurrent electrical cerebral responses and can be used to document dysrhythmias associated with acute toxic encephalopathies and/or possible residual pathological damage, as well as diffuse or focal dysrhythmias due to nontoxic causes. The electroencephalograms (EEGs) of three of 15 workers who had been occupationally exposed to acrylamide for at least 6 years showed nonspecific bursts of theta (6 to 7 Hz) activity, which were increased by hyperventilation (Takahashi et al., 1971). However, because such slow wave changes can also be attributed to normal drowsiness, vascular disease, and increasing age of the subjects, they cannot be uniquely related to persistent CNS effects of toxic exposure to acrylamide. In addition, findings in other cases suggest that the EEG following acrylamide exposure may be normal. For example, no specific abnormalities were found on the electroencephalographic studies of persons who developed acute clinical signs of CNS involvement following a brief (1 week) intense exposure to acrylamide-contaminated drinking water (Igisu et al., 1975). Another example is that of a 35-year-old man who used acrylamide in his grouting work intermittently for 1.5 years and daily for 2 months before he developed memory problems and numb hands and feet. His clinical recovery was slow and neuropsychological deficits persisted, although his EEGs recorded immediately after cessation of exposure and again 5 years after his removal from exposure were both normal (R. G. Feldman, personal observation) (see Clinical Experiences section). It is important to note the time, relative to the exposure, at which the initial EEG is made and, if abnormalities are noted, to follow up with subsequent EEGs to identify any relationship that may exist between the EEG recording and exposure to acrylamide. Except for the report by Takahashi et al. (1971), the EEG in cases of acrylamide does not appear to reflect pathological abnormalities and cannot be relied upon to substantiate the effects of exposure.

Evoked potentials (EPs) are useful measures of peripheral–central somatosensory function. This technique may detect deficits before there is other electrophysiological evidence of impaired peripheral nerve conduction following neurotoxicant exposure (Arezzo et al., 1985). Somatosensory evoked potentials (SSEPs) recorded in acrylamide-exposed rats suggested that impaired conduction occurred throughout the ascending somatosensory pathway but did not affect the cortical areas (Boyes and Cooper, 1981). Serial recording of SSEPs in acrylamide-exposed rats showed changes over segments of central and peripheral axons, which indicated that abnormalities of central conduction persisted even after peripheral conduction and clinical manifestations of neuropathy had recovered. Recovery from the central–peripheral distal axonopathy following exposure to acrylamide begins in the largest peripheral axons and occurs while the central conduction remains abnormal. Evidence from morphometric studies of nerve fibers revealed that there was regeneration of the largest diameter fibers. This finding coincided with the clinical recovery in the area innervated by the particular peripheral nerve. Persistent and even more severe loss of large- and medium-size fibers was observed in the cervical gracile tract (Kaji et al., 1989).

The clinical application of short-latency somatosensory evoked potentials (SLSEPs) in humans may be technically difficult because of problems with the interpretation of results, one of which is that aging affects vibratory sensation perception (Schaumburg et al., 1989). Studies of SLSEPs have been recorded in monkeys using surface electrodes placed over the spinal medullary junction (Schaumburg et al., 1982). Latencies were prolonged after low-level (below the no-effect dose of 3.0 mg/kg) subcutaneous injections of 3.0, 2.0, and 1.0 mg/kg of 99% pure acrylamide for 1.0, 1.2, and 2.6 years, respectively. Changes in latency were not closely associated with a reduction in the compound sensory amplitude. With continued exposure to acrylamide, a change in the rise-phase of the P2 component and a reduction in the peak amplitude were apparent.

A monkey that received only 0.5 mg/kg throughout the experiment did not exhibit electrophysiological or behavioral changes. The abnormal physiological responses in the animals affected by 1.0 and 2.0 mg/kg were attributed to the process seen on the postmortem examination of axons at the caudal level of the dorsal column nuclei in these animals when sacrificed at the peak of intoxication. Preterminal accumulation of axonal neurofilaments without synaptic disruption in the gracile nucleus was found. Functional impairment was seen in the animal that received 3.0 mg/kg and showed some clinical recovery after discontinuation of the acrylamide injections and before being sacrificed for postmortem histological examination. Induced alterations in the latency of the SLSEP and the changes in the axonal morphology were reversible in these animals after 7 months free of exposure; these findings did not return to a pretreatment baseline. Postmortem examination of one monkey after such clinical recovery showed little abnormality. Similarly, little abnormality was seen in tissues of the monkey which had received only 0.5 mg/kg and had served as a longitudinal (940 days) control subject. These experimental neurophysiological and histological findings suggest that functional recovery occurs after a period of dysfunction following chronic exposure to a relatively high dose, as indicated by delayed latency of the SLSEP (see Neuropathological Diagnosis section).

Reports of clinical studies of visual evoked potentials (VEPs) in humans after exposure to acrylamide have not been found. Merigan et al. (1982) reported abnormal VEPs in the macaque monkey after 20 days of exposure to acrylamide at a daily dose of 10 mg/kg. These evoked potentials were measured at a time well before overt clinical manifestations were seen. The probability that there would be abnormalities in VEPs might also be predicted from the findings that in rats a single dose of acrylamide in high concentrations (200 to 300 mg/kg) altered the distribution of fast axonally transported materials in optic nerves and tracts; while repeated doses (30 mg/kg for 5 days per week for 4 weeks) caused slowing of both fast and slow axonal transport in optic nerves and tracts, without evidence of axonal degeneration (Sabri and Spencer, 1990). Such impairment in both fast and slow axonal transport rate, in the absence of overt morphological damage, may explain the reversible impairment of visual as well as other nervous system functions after acrylamide exposure.

Nerve conduction studies can document the signs of peripheral neuropathy at subclinical and clinical stages of impairment. Larger-diameter sensory fibers are affected early in toxic exposure to acrylamide. These sensory nerves supply pacinian corpuscles, which detect touch and vibration; muscle spindle primary afferents that respond to stretch; and adjacent nerve terminals that transmit impulses for muscle contraction. Degeneration is seen first in pacinian corpuscle axons, often before muscle spindle axons degenerate or adjacent motor nerve terminals are affected. Thus sensory nerve terminals are apparently more vulnerable to acrylamide than are adjacent motor nerve terminals, a finding that explains why clinical sensory deficits and impairments of electrical conduction in sensory nerves are present in the early stages of acrylamide intoxication (Spencer and Schaumburg, 1974; Schaumburg et al., 1983). Sensory nerve action potentials in acrylamide-exposed workers were either absent or reduced in amplitude, whereas in the same group only slightly reduced or normal maximal motor nerve conduction velocities were found (Fullerton, 1969). In addition, this study showed a significantly ($p < 0.01$) greater prolongation of distal motor latencies in median, ulnar, and peroneal nerves suggesting disruption of the myelin sheath. Calleman et al. (1994) reported a relative slowing in mean motor nerve conduction velocity of the peroneal nerve in a group of acrylamide workers ($n = 41$) compared to the results of tests performed in a group of unexposed control subjects ($n = 10$) (Table 18-5). In addition, prolonged sensory distal latencies and reduced amplitudes of sensory action potentials were found in the median, ulnar, and sural nerves. The sensory conduction velocity of the sural nerve was also slowed in these currently exposed acrylamide workers. An earlier report by Takahashi et al. (1971) described nerve conduction studies in 15 workers exposed to acrylamide in a paper-coating factory. Individual durations of exposure ranged from 2 months to 8 years. Of the 15 workers, 11 had clinical peripheral neuropathy. Sensory nerve conduction velocities were reduced in six of the 15 cases. Sensory action potentials were unobtainable in the tibial nerves of nine of the 15 cases. Motor conduction velocities were normal.

Serial electrodiagnostic studies were performed in a worker who had been exposed to acrylamide grouting material, intermittently for 1.5 years and continuously for the last 2 months of his employment, until he had to stop working because of numbness and clumsiness in his extremities

TABLE 18-5. *Nerve conduction and electromyographic studies in workers currently exposed to acrylamide*

Parameter	Reference group ($n = 10$)	Acrylamide workers ($n = 41$)
Motor conduction velocity (m/sec)		
Median	59.6 ± 5.0	56.8 ± 7.2
Ulnar	62.5 ± 5.4	60.0 ± 9.2
Peroneal	48.1 ± 3.5	43.8 ± 8.5[a]
Motor distal latency (msec)		
Median	3.5 ± 0.4	4.6 ± 1.3[a]
Ulnar	2.3 ± 0.3	3.1 ± 1.1[a]
Peroneal	3.9 ± 0.5	6.0 ± 1.9[a]
Sensory conduction velocity (m/sec)		
Median	60.3 ± 4.1	61.6 ± 5.8
Ulnar	66.9 ± 4.3	61.9 ± 6.4
Sural	56.8 ± 4.0	46.6 ± 6.6[a]
Sensory distal latency (msec)		
Median	1.8 ± 0.4	2.8 ± 0.4[a]
Ulnar	1.6 ± 0.2	3.1 ± 0.8
Sural	2.4 ± 0.7	6.0 ± 0.8
Electromyography	No abnormalities	No denervation potentials; 20 of 94 sampled muscles showed variable recruitment pattern; abnormal recruitment pattern seen in 9 of 12 samples of anterior tibialis

[a]$p < 0.01$ by Student's test. See text.
Data from Calleman et al., 1994.

(R. G. Feldman, personal observation). Nerve conduction studies over the first 4 months after ending exposure revealed sensory and motor neuropathy, possibly reflecting coasting of the effects of the recent exposure. Follow-up nerve conduction studies 5 years later were within normal limits, although electromyography revealed evidence of denervation and reinnervation of motor units. For example, testing performed shortly after the patient was removed from exposure, showed positive sharp waves (PSWs) and/or fibrillation potentials (FPs) at rest whereas, upon maximal voluntary contraction, the motor unit interference pattern (MUIP) and action potential amplitudes (MUAPAs) were reduced and polyphasic potentials (PPs) were evident, indicating recent and ongoing denervation with partial reinnervation of motor units. Recovery took place to such a significant degree that by the 5th year after removal from exposure the EMG showed no spontaneous activity (i.e., fibrillations and positive sharp waves) but the interference pattern on contraction was still reduced with some polyphasic and giant potentials (Table 18-6). These EMG findings indicate partial chronic denervation and reinnervation of distal muscles of the extremities (see below).

Electromyography (EMG) is used to assess motor unit function. The time of EMG examination in relation to acrylamide exposure is important in interpreting the results of the tests. Initial EMG evidence of denervation does not appear until 14 to 20 days after damage of the motor units has occurred. Reversible or irreversible changes in neuromuscular function correlate with the duration of the exposure as well as its intensity. The appearance of the pattern of muscle action potentials recorded from a muscle upon full volitional contraction will reveal the dropout of motor units when there has been denervation and, therefore, loss of the connection between the motor neuron, its axon, and the muscle fiber it supplies. Acutely denervated muscle fibers exhibit spontaneous bioelectric discharges, called fibrillations, which can be recorded from a needle electrode inserted into the muscle when it is at rest. Polyphasic potentials are recorded from a previously denervated muscle which has become reinnervated; fibrillations may or may not be present depending upon whether or not active

denervation is occurring and on how much regeneration has taken place. Following a brief exposure there may be no abnormality in peripheral nerve function and time for denervation to occur may be insufficient. At such times, the EMG will not detect dropout of motor units as evidence of denervation. As neuropathy progresses clinical neuromuscular signs also emerge; EMG correlates are recordable.

EMG studies were made in 44 (37 men; seven women) workers exposed to acrylamide at mean air concentrations of 1.07 to 3.27 m/m³ for an average duration of 3 years (range: <1 to 11.5 years) (Calleman et al., 1994). No abnormalities were noted on EMG studies made at rest or during mild contraction. However, the EMG studies made during maximal contraction brought out mixed patterns of recruitment, with dropout of motor units, suggesting incomplete innervation but apparently no active denervation (see Table 18-5). EMG studies in another group of workers ($n = 15$) exposed to acrylamide while working in a paper-coating factory revealed a slight decrease in the number of motor unit potentials, polyphasic potentials, and occasional giant spikes in 7 of 15 cases. These results indicate evidence of denervated and reinnervated motor units following acrylamide neurotoxicity (Takahashi et al., 1971; Davenport et al., 1976).

EMG studies were performed in 69 acrylamide workers who developed symptoms of peripheral neuropathy within 4 months following increased ambient air levels (up to 9.02 mg/m³; 30 times the OSHA PEL) (He et al., 1989). Twenty-nine of the 69 workers showed polyphasic potentials on EMG, indicating reinnervation of motor units. Three of the 29 acrylamide workers showed evidence of ongoing denervation: polyphasic potentials and fibrillations (two); positive waves (one). Twenty-five of the 29 workers were overtly asymptomatic; twenty-three of these had clinically diminished or absent ankle tendon reflexes and had no detectable H-reflex (the electrically elicited spinal monosynaptic reflex which is equivalent to the monosynaptic reflex elicited by a tap to the tendon (i.e., the T-reflex). Prolongation of H-reflex latency was seen only among those workers who had clinical evidence of neu-

TABLE 18-6. *Serial electromyographic studies in an acrylamide grout worker*

Electromyographic findings	Time after ending exposure				
	3 weeks	2 months	3 months	4 months	5 years
Fibs	–	+	+	+	–
PSWs	+	+	+	+	–
PPs	+	+	+	+	+
MUAPAs	Reduced	Reduced	Reduced	Reduced	Reduced
MUIPs	Reduced	Reduced	Reduced	Reduced	Reduced

This table demonstrates evidence of chronic partial denervation and reinnervation. See text for case report. (EMG performed by Clyde M. Niles, M.D. on 4/4/80, personal communication.)

Fibs, fibrillations; PSWs, positive sharp waves; PPs, polyphasic potentials; MUAPAs, motor unit action potential amplitudes; MUIPs, motor unit interference pattern.

ropathy. Prolonged duration of motor unit potentials and abnormal H-reflexes following acrylamide exposure in the remaining 40 workers were attributed to (a) impairment of nerve conduction at more proximal locations, such as at the spinal dorsal root ganglion, (b) impairment of sensory processing in the dorsal horn, involving primary afferent terminals as well as anterior horn cells (Prineas, 1969; Takahashi et al., 1971; Goldstein and Lowndes, 1979; DeRojas and Goldstein, 1987).

Vibrotactile sensory threshold is tested clinically by using a tuning fork (128 Hz) placed on a toe or finger pad, or over the bony joints of the foot, ankle, tibia, finger, or wrist. The subject is asked to respond by telling if and when he or she first perceives the sensation of vibration and when it is no longer perceptible. The results of this test can be affected by the alertness and attentiveness of the subject; the response time (latency) may also be inaccurately reported. A more objective standardized electronic method, referred to as Quantitative Sensory Testing (QST), was developed to assess the function of the large sensory fibers of a peripheral nerve which carry the sensations of position and vibration (Arezzo et al., 1983; Gerr and Letz, 1988; Berger et al., 1989). These devices deliver various amplitudes of vibrating stimuli through two probe posts applied to the skin surface over a toe or finger pad, or an extremity joint. The frequency of vibration remains constant at 100 Hz, while the amplitude is varied. By forced choice method the subject is required to report when he or she perceives one or both poles vibrating. Alternatively, the vibration amplitude is initially set high and then is gradually reduced at a constant rate until the subject reports that he or she no longer can feel the vibration. The vibration amplitude is then set very low and gradually increased until the subject reports that he or she feels the vibrating sensation. After a series of five to six repeated ascending and descending tests of threshold (method of limits) an average is calculated from the values of the thresholds detected for the final four trials of each test series. The test results from groups of exposed individuals must be compared for statistical significance with those of unexposed control subjects. Testing is performed at the time of exposure, or soon afterwards, followed by serial tests after the exposed individual(s) have been removed from exposure. This is done to provide evidence of developing impairment and then recovery of vibrotactile sensation perception. A deficit in perception may be detected in a given individual with above-average exposure due to poor hygienic habits for instance; however, when such results are combined with the results of testing from many other individuals and analyzed as a group, abnormal threshold levels may be averaged with normal or less abnormal ones, thus becoming statistically insignificant and considered normal.

For example, workers in a factory which produced polyacrylamide flocculants were exposed to acrylamide monomer in the air at concentrations 0.07 to 2.5 times the NIOSH recommended exposure level of 0.3 mg/m³. In-

significant differences in their vibration sensation perception threshold, tested by clinical tuning-fork tests, were found when compared with the results of these tests in a group of unexposed control subjects (Myers and Macun, 1991). A follow-up exam of the workers in this factory using an electronic vibrotactile threshold measuring device was performed at atmospheric acrylamide monomer levels similar to those in the earlier study. The mean vibratory sensory perception thresholds of the exposed and the nonexposed groups were very similar (Bachman et al., 1992). The lack of significant differences between the groups may be attributed to design of these studies, which appear flawed in several ways: First, in this plant even "nonexposed" jobs provided some limited exposure to acrylamide, resulting in exposure among the "controls." Second, the two groups of subjects, exposed and nonexposed, were not controlled for age, a fact that could affect the results of the analysis because increasing age has been shown to affect vibration perception (Moody et al., 1986). Finally, individual exposure histories were not considered among the exposed persons, allowing for wide variations in exposure dosage. Therefore, it must be concluded that vibrotactile threshold testing, using either a tuning fork or a calibrated electronic device, failed to demonstrate differences between exposed and nonexposed subjects because the selected groups were not sufficiently different.

Deng et al. (1993) showed that with proper selection of subjects and analysis of results according to age group, statistically significant differences between acrylamide exposed and nonexposed subjects can be detected. These examiners used an electronic calibrated instrument to measure the sensory responses in acrylamide workers who were exposed to ambient air acrylamide levels ranging from 0.20 to 1.58 mg/m³ and who had durations of exposure ranging from 0.5 to 8 years. In their study, 24 of 41 (58.5%) workers had an increase in vibration thresholds to above the upper limits of that recorded from nonexposed subjects. In addition, only 15 of 41 (36.6%) workers showed decreases in perception of vibration sensation when tested with a tuning fork, demonstrating the increased sensitivity of the electronic test method.

These findings demonstrate the clinical utility of neurophysiological diagnostics in the early diagnosis of acrylamide poisoning. They also indicate that existing subclinical neuropathy can go unrecognized among acutely exposed workers and in others with prolonged exposure to acrylamide.

Neuropsychological Diagnosis

Neuropsychological testing has not been used extensively in cases of acrylamide poisoning. Reports of increased irritability as well as decreased attention span and disturbed memory following acrylamide exposure indicate CNS effects (Fujita et al., 1960; Igisu et al., 1975; R. G. Feldman, personal observation). The usually transient feelings of intoxication (e.g., drowsiness, difficulty concentrating, forgetfulness, and sometimes delirium and even hallucinations) associated with acrylamide exposure can account, in retrospect, for poor on-the-job performance and/or careless accidents. Reduced worker efficiency may be a manifestation of reduced alertness and poor attention span, resulting in difficulty with multiple tasks and slowed reaction times.

Formal neuropsychological testing may be necessary for documenting acute CNS effects in some patients (see Clinical Experiences section). The Profile of Mood States (POMS) and the Minnesota Multiphasic Personality Inventory (MMPI) can be used to assess changes in personality and affect associated with acrylamide exposure. Neuropsychological tests such as Trails A and B and the Wisconsin Card Sorting Test can be used to assess for deficits in attention and executive functioning. Digit Spans (forward and backward), the California Verbal Learning Test (CVLT), and the Rey–Osterreith Complex Figure can be used to assess for deficits in verbal and visual memory function (White et al., 1992). Motor and sensory deficits of the hands due to peripheral neuropathy may impair manual dexterity and, thus, performance on tests of psychomotor functioning and on timed tests with a motor component such as Digit Symbol. Thus, peripheral neuropathy in the upper extremities must be considered as a factor when evaluating test performance, and the practitioner should not simply consider the raw score in the evaluation of findings in such cases. Removal from exposure is typically followed by clearing of the behavioral symptoms associated with peripheral neuropathy, but CNS effects may persist. Neuropsychological testing performed within 1 year after removal from exposure provided documentation of enduring cognitive dysfunction in a 35-year-old man, who developed memory problems while he was being exposed to acrylamide. The Wechsler Adult Intelligence Scale (WAIS), the Bender Gestalt, a figure drawing test, a thematic perception test, and the Rorschach test revealed neuropsychological performance deficits (R. G. Feldman, personal observation). Serial testing following cessation of exposure can be used to document a patient's prognosis. Reports of comprehensive serial neuropsychological evaluations to determine the persistence of cognitive deficits resulting from acrylamide poisoning are not available.

Biochemical Diagnosis

A specific method for the biological monitoring of acrylamide-exposed workers has not yet been established by either the World Health Organization or the American Conference of Governmental Industrial Hygienists (WHO, 1985; ACGIH, 1995) (Table 18-7). Nevertheless, several methods have been developed for monitoring recent and remote exposures to acrylamide. For example, plasma levels of free acrylamide can be used to detect an immediate or very recent exposure to acrylamide in humans; plasma levels are not well correlated with the rate of development or the severity of acrylamide neurotoxicity (Calleman et al., 1994). The difficulty in obtaining a sample immediately following exposure renders this technique virtually impractical. Therefore, workplace ambient air sampling for acrylamide monomer levels has been relied upon for estimating exposure dose for those at risk.

Urinary levels of the acrylamide-derived mercapturic acid N-acetyl-S-(propionamide)-cysteine can also be used to monitor for recent exposures to acrylamide and reflect exposure levels encountered during the past 1 to 2 days; this is the least invasive method for occupational monitoring (Wu et al., 1993; Calleman et al., 1994) (see Fig. 18-1). Urine levels of S-(2-carboxyethyl)-cysteine, the product of N-acetyl-S-(propionamide)-cysteine hydrolysis, have also been used to monitor worker exposure to acrylamide. Studies indicate that urine S-(2-carboxyethyl)-cysteine levels are related to recent exposure dose (Calleman et al., 1994). High-performance liquid chromatography is required to identify and quantify the levels of N-acetyl-S-(propionamide)-cysteine and/or S-(2-carboxyethyl)-cysteine in the urine of acrylamide exposed workers (Wu et al., 1993; Calleman et al., 1994).

Hemoglobin adducts reflect recent and remote exposures to acrylamide and correlate best with the incidence and severity of neurotoxicity among acrylamide-exposed workers (Calleman et al., 1994; Hashimoto et al., 1995). This method of monitoring is also more convenient than is the determination of blood levels of free acrylamide since measurement need not be made immediately after exposure. The N-terminal valine (AAVal) adduct for acrylamide shows the best correlation with neurotoxicity. A no-observable effect level (NOEL), the lowest observable effect level (LOEL), and the level resulting in an effect in 50%

TABLE 18-7. *Biological exposure indices for acrylamide*

	Urine	Blood	Alveolar Air
Determinant:	N-acetyl-S-(propionamide)-cysteine	Acrylamide	Acrylamide
Start of shift:	Not established	Not established	Not established
During shift:	Not established	Not established	Not established
End of work shift:	Not established	Not established	Not established

See text for use of hemoglobin adducts.
Data from ACGIH, 1995.

(EL_{50}) of exposed persons developing peripheral neuropathy were determined to be 2, 6, and 7.9 nmol (g Hb)$^{-1}$, respectively, using AAVal hemoglobin adducts (Calleman, 1996). Increased hemoglobin adducts and higher urine S-(2-carboxyethyl)cysteine levels were detected in workers who did not use adequate protection against dermal absorption of acrylamide and who developed more severe neuropathy than did workers who used proper gloves (Calleman et al., 1994). These results demonstrate the contribution of dermal absorption to an exposed individual's total body burden of acrylamide and indicate that employer compliance with the current OSHA PEL for ambient air acrylamide levels may not provide all workers with adequate protection against exposure to neurotoxic levels of acrylamide. Furthermore, workers may ignore safety practices designed to prevent dermal absorption because of factors such as the awkwardness of performing tasks that demand a high level of fine motor control while wearing protective gloves or when the need arises for an acrylamide worker to perform a "brief" task immediately after having removed his or her gloves (see Clinical Experiences section). The use of biological monitoring would reduce the risk of acrylamide poisoning among exposed workers and is suggested as an adjunct to current safety precautions. The need for a biochemical marker of exposure has been stressed previously by the World Health Organization (WHO, 1985).

Neuroimaging

No neuroimaging studies of the CNS effects of acrylamide have been found. However, computer tomography (CT) scan and magnetic resonance imaging (MRI) studies must be used to differentiate the CNS effects of acrylamide poisoning from those due to acute disseminating encephalomyelopathy, multiple sclerosis, cerebellar tumors, and other CNS disorders associated with truncal ataxia and nystagmus.

Neuropathological Diagnosis

Results from animal experiments and from nerve biopsy material of human cases provide information about the pathological effects seen after exposure to acrylamide and its metabolite, glycidamide. Acrylamide selectively affects the longest and largest-diameter myelinated nerve fibers before it affects shorter, smaller, and unmyelinated fibers. Sensory nerve fibers are affected before motor fibers (Fullerton and Barnes, 1966; Schaumburg et al., 1974). Acrylamide also damages fibers of the autonomic nervous system (Ralevic et al., 1991). The principal pathological findings associated with acrylamide toxicity are those of distal axonal neuropathy with secondary myelin degeneration (Cavanaugh, 1964; Fullerton and Barnes, 1966; Spencer and Schaumburg, 1974; Abou-Donia et al., 1993) (Table 18-8). These changes are demonstrated in a 59-year-old man who exhibited clinical features of peripheral neuropathy within 18 months after he began working with acrylamide. His sural nerve biopsy revealed evidence of ongoing wallerian-type degeneration and signs of nerve sprout regeneration. Histograms of the distribution of the diameter sizes of the nerve fibers counted in the biopsy specimen revealed a reduction in the number of large myelinated fibers (Fullerton, 1969) (Fig. 18-2). A similar reduction in large-diameter fiber count was found in cats after exposure to acrylamide. The histogram of the fiber size distribution in the cats correlated well with the histogram distribution of conduction velocities of the fibers, using computerized electrophysiological estimates of nerve fiber distribution which had been done before the histological

TABLE 18-8. *Neuropathological findings in humans exposed to acrylamide*

Duration of exposure	Time at which sural nerve biopsy was performed	Neuropathological findings	Reference
6 months	Immediately after removal from exposure	Ongoing wallerian-type degeneration; loss of nerve fibers; many remaining axons were swollen with accumulation of neurofilaments, mitochondria, and other organelles visible in electron micrographs.	Davenport et al., 1976
3–4 months	Immediately after removal from exposure	Mild loss of nerve fibers and swelling of axons with relatively well-preserved myelin sheaths.	Satoyoshi et al., 1971
1 month	2.5 months after removal from exposure	Significant loss of large-diameter fibers; ongoing wallerian-type degeneration; shortened internodal length indicative of degeneration, regeneration, and remyelination.	Fullerton, 1969
1.5 months	8 months after removal from exposure	No evidence of active degeneration; shortened internodal length indicative of degeneration, regeneration, and remyelination.	Fullerton, 1969

This table demonstrates the relationship between the time, relative to cessation of exposure, at which the biopsy was performed and the morphological evidence of ongoing degeneration and/or regeneration. The data are listed in order of length of time between end of exposure and pathological studies.

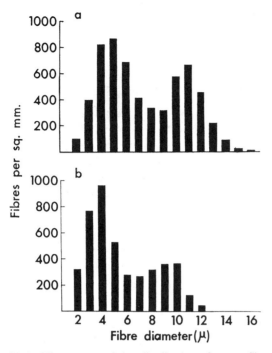

FIG. 18-2. Histograms of the distribution of nerve fiber diameters from a sural nerve biopsy of an unexposed control subject **(a)** a 59-year-old acrylamide-exposed patient **(b)**. (From Fullerton, 1969, with permission.)

studies of the nerve fiber sizes. Comparative serial studies in these acrylamide-intoxicated and control cats revealed a gradual loss of large fibers associated with decreased mean conduction velocities and amplitudes (71.6 to 46.2 m/sec; 32.4 to 4.3 µV) (Sax et al., 1984) (see Neurophysiological Diagnosis section). Studies in nonhuman primates exposed to acrylamide showed wallerian-type degeneration in the distal ends of the largest myelinated fibers in the sural nerve. In addition, decreases in the number of large myelinated fibers were proportional to increases in the duration of exposure (Hopkins, 1970).

The distal ends of the rostral projections of neurons in lumbar dorsal root ganglia terminating in the gracile nucleus are very vulnerable to the toxic effects of acrylamide (Schaumburg et al., 1989). In a monkey treated with acrylamide at a daily dose of 2.0 mg/kg for 2.5 years, pathological features in the gracile tract and nuclei included swollen dark-staining axons, with thinned myelin sheaths, and containing masses of whirled (10 nm) neurofilaments, occasional dense bodies, and clumps of mitochondria and neurotubules. Light microscopic studies of a longitudinal section of the tibial nerve of a cat exposed to acrylamide revealed paranodal axonal swelling with associated retraction of the myelin sheath. Electron micrograph (EM) of a cross section of these tibial nerves revealed swollen demyelinated axons containing increased numbers of neurofilaments, mitochondria, and dense bodies (Schaumburg et al., 1974).

Similar findings have been reported in tissues from exposed workers. After 6 months of occupational exposure to acrylamide, a 25-year-old man developed paresthesias and muscle weakness in his upper and lower extremities; he also exhibited dysarthria, ataxia, and intention tremor. A sural nerve biopsy of this man revealed an overall loss of nerve fibers; teased fiber preparation showed swollen axons and paranodal swelling. Some fibers showed loss of myelin, while others did not. Focal dilation of myelin sheaths was seen at random nodal and internodal areas (Fig. 18-3). Electron micrographs demonstrated accumulation of neurofilaments, mitochondria, and dense bodies in numerous axons. Some axons showing accumulation of neurofilaments and organelles were more swollen than others. Evidence of ongoing wallerian-type degeneration was also seen on *EM* (Davenport et al., 1976) (Fig. 18-4).

Neuropathological findings in the CNS of animals experimentally exposed to acrylamide include (a) decreased density of Purkinje cells in the cerebellum (Cavanagh, 1982), (b) axonal changes in neurons of the hypothalamus, optic tracts, and cerebellar vermis (Schaumburg and Spencer, 1979), (c) changes in the distribution of microtubule-associated proteins in the hippocampus, cerebellum, and cortex (these changes were most marked in the hippocampus and cerebellum) (Chauhan et al., 1993), and (d) altered neurofilament gene expression (Endo et al., 1994).

Abnormalities in axonal transport are involved in the pathogenesis of acrylamide neurotoxicity. Studies have demonstrated that exposure to acrylamide disrupts fast anterograde and retrograde axonal transport as well as slow anterograde transport (Pleasure et al., 1969; Souyri et al., 1981; Sahenk and Mendell, 1981; Gold et al., 1985; Moretto and Sabri, 1988; Schaumberg et al., 1989; Sickles, 1989, 1992; Sabri and Spencer, 1990; Chauhan et al., 1993; Harris et al., 1994). Studies in the sciatic nerves of rats exposed to acrylamide showed that the accumulation of neurofilaments and organelles within the axon is correlated with the severity of the axonal transport abnormalities (Sahenk and Mendell, 1981). Neurofilaments are transported to the distal-most portions of the axon via slow anterograde axonal transport, suggesting that disruption of this particular component of axonal transport would result in the accumulation of neurofilaments within the axon (Gold et al., 1985). Disruption of fast and slow axonal transport was seen in the absence of any morphological changes in the optic nerves of the rat (Sabri and Spencer, 1990). Together these findings indicate that disruption of axonal transport precedes axonal degeneration and is directly related to the severity of the neuropathological findings associated with exposure to acrylamide.

Interruption of axonal transport may account not only for paranodal swelling but also for the secondary demyelination associated with exposure to acrylamide. Droz et al. (1981) showed that fast axonal transport was involved in the delivery of neurotropic substances to Schwann cells. Disruptions of fast axonal transport have been shown to induce the process of wallerian-type degeneration and to ini-

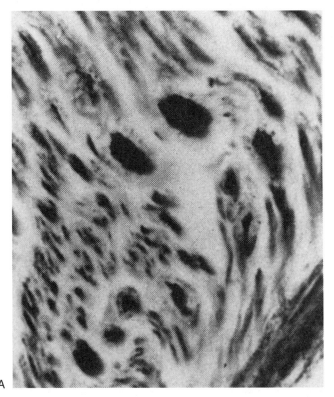

A

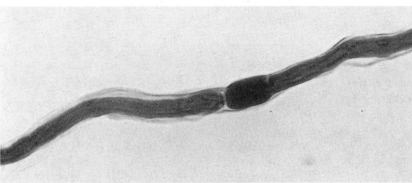

B

FIG. 18-3. A: Transverse section through sural nerve biopsy, from a 25-year-old man who was occupationally exposed to acrylamide, showing swollen axons (original magnification, ×420). **B:** Teased fiber, from the same patient, demonstrating paranodal axonal swelling. (From Davenport et al., 1976, with permission.)

tiate proliferation of Schwann cells, possibly by impeding the transport of neurotropic substances (e.g., nerve growth factor) (Csillik et al., 1977; Griffin et al., 1987; Oaklander and Spencer, 1988; Gold et al., 1993). Disruption of the delivery of neurotropic substances induces alterations in gene expression (e.g., protooncogenes such as *c-jun*), leading to morphological changes in response to cellular injury (Endo et al., 1993; Gold et al., 1993, 1994; Wu et al., 1994). Furthermore, disruptions of retrograde transport have been implicated in the induction of somatofugal axonal atrophy, which has been shown to precede axonal degeneration in the dorsal root of acrylamide exposed rats (Gold et al., 1992). The selective degeneration of cerebellar Purkinje cells seen after acrylamide exposure may be related to the long axonal processes and elaborate dendritic arborization seen in these cells, both of which are vulnerable to disruption of axonal transport (Chauhan et al., 1993). Differences in the dose–time relationships of exposure are reflected not

only as differences in the severity of clinical manifestations but also in the results of neuropathological findings, which are correlated with the degree of axonal transport disruption (Gold et al., 1992).

Proposed biochemical mechanisms of acrylamide neuropathy include (a) direct toxic effects on the perikaryon, (b) inhibition of glycolysis, (c) interference with synthesis of microtubule-associated proteins (MAPs), (d) an alteration in calcium homeostasis, (e) alteration of phosphorylation of neurofilament proteins by acrylamide and/or glycidamide, a metabolite of acrylamide, and (f) depletion of glutathione stores with a concomitant increase in lipid peroxidation (Schaumburg et al., 1974; Sterman, 1982; Cavanagh and Gysbers, 1983; Srivastava et al., 1983; Howland and Alli, 1986; Gold et al., 1988; Xiwen et al., 1992; Chauhan et al., 1993; Harris et al., 1994; Reagan et al., 1995). Concentrations of phosphocreatine, creatine, ATP, ADP, AMP, glucose, and lactate in the whole brain did not

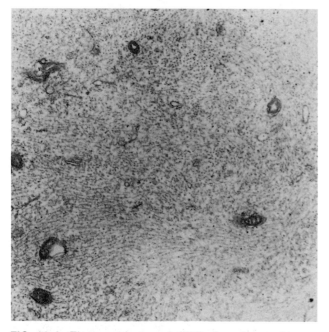

FIG. 18-4. Electron micrograph (EM) of sural nerve biopsy, from a 25-year-old man who was occupationally exposed to acrylamide, showing accumulation of neurofilaments within axon (original magnification, ×19,500). (From Davenport et al., 1976, with permission.)

differ among mice exposed to acrylamide and unexposed control animals. These findings indicate that acrylamide does not alter cellular energy metabolism in the brain (Matsuoka and Igisu, 1992). Although studies indicate that acrylamide does inhibit the activity of specific glycolytic enzymes (e.g., glyceraldehyde-3-phosphate dehydrogenase), inhibition of glycolysis does not appear to be responsible for acrylamide neuropathy (Brimijoin and Hammond, 1985; Matsuoka et al., 1990; Kohriyama et al., 1994).

Cell bodies in the dorsal root ganglion, sural nerves, and tibial nerves of rats exposed to acrylamide at a dose of 50 mg/kg for 6 days showed nuclear eccentricities, cytoplasmic reorganization with an outer mantle of Nissl, and an inner perinuclear zone of pigmented bodies; whereas distal axons showed little changes, suggesting that the cell body is affected early in the pathogenesis of acrylamide neuropathy (Sterman, 1982). Immunocytochemical localization of MAP1 and MAP2 following exposure to acrylamide revealed decreased immunoreactivity in dendrites and axons in the hippocampus, cerebellum, and cortex of rats, suggesting that acrylamide either interferes with the synthesis of MAPS1 and 2 or disrupts their transport within the axons (Chauhan et al., 1993). Acrylamide has been shown to disrupt calcium homeostasis in the rat brain, possibly by interfering with the activity of Ca^{2+},Mg^{2+}-ATPase. Alteration in Ca^{2+},Mg^{2+}-ATPase activity can interfere with the activity of cyclic-AMP and, thus, phosphorylation of cellular proteins (Xiwen et al., 1992).

The neurotoxic properties of acrylamide have been attributed to the parent compound and to its metabolite glycidamide (Abou-Donia et al., 1993; Harris et al., 1994; Costa et al., 1995; Reagan et al., 1995). Glycidamide as well as acrylamide has been shown to reduce antero- and retrograde axonal transport (Harris et al., 1994). Acrylamide and glycidamide have also been shown to increase calcium/calmodulin-dependent protein kinase phosphorylation of cytoskeletal proteins (Howland and Alli, 1986; Reagan et al., 1995). The presence of highly phosphorylated neurofilaments in the axon could disrupt axonal transport and thereby contribute to the axonal swelling seen in acrylamide neuropathy and induce cellular injury responses such as Wallerian-type generation (Howland and Alli, 1986; Reagan et al., 1995).

A dose-dependent decrease in glutathione content and an increase in lipid peroxidation were found in the livers of rats exposed to either acrylamide or styrene at doses of up to 100 and 600 mg/kg, respectively (Srivastava et al., 1983). However, these investigators did not find a significant dose-dependent increase in lipid peroxidation in the brains of these animals. Nevertheless, these findings and those of Dixit et al. (1981), who found that a decrease in glutathione-*S*-transferase activity occurred concurrently with the onset of neuropathy in rats exposed to acrylamide, indicate that acrylamide decreases glutathione stores and, thus, that an exposed individual's risks may be increased during chronic exposures (see Tissue Biochemistry section).

PREVENTIVE AND THERAPEUTIC MEASURES

Programs that educate workers about the risk of injury following exposure to acrylamide should be available in all occupational settings where acrylamide monomer is used. Workplace ambient air concentrations of acrylamide should be measured periodically; however, this documentation will not provide adequate protection against neurotoxicity unless dermal protection and proper ventilation are provided and used. Self-contained positive-pressure respirators with a full facepiece should be provided for workers at risk of exposure to high concentrations of acrylamide monomer dust and aqueous vapor. Proper precautions regarding the risk of dermal absorption and the use of appropriate impervious gloves and protective clothing should be taught to everyone involved in the manufacturing of acrylamide monomer as well as its polymers and copolymers (WHO, 1985; He et al., 1989). When properly used, personal dermal protection is generally effective (Bachman et al., 1992; Calleman et al., 1994). Ordinary surgical-type latex gloves do not provide protection against dermal absorption of acrylamide. The most recently hired and least experienced employees are at the greatest risk for hazardous contact and toxic exposure.

The first step in treating the effects of acute exposure to acrylamide is to remove improperly protected at-risk individuals from further exposure. If acrylamide monomer has been swallowed, stomach gavage should be done immediately to empty the stomach of the acrylamide-containing contents. Hemodialysis and blood transfusion for acute renal and/or hepatic failure may be necessary.

Prognosis for recovery from intoxication depends upon the intensity and duration of the exposure. For example, all five members of a family who ingested drinking water contaminated with acrylamide initially showed signs of CNS dysfunction, including irrational behavior, hallucinations, and truncal ataxia that persisted for 2 days to 1 month after ending further intake or exposure. Signs and symptoms of peripheral neuropathy appeared 2 to 4 weeks after exposure in those patients with the most intense exposures and the most severe initial symptoms (Igisu et al., 1975). Similar findings were reported by He et al. (1989) among three acrylamide workers exposed via dermal and inhalation routes. All three workers showed a marked reduction in cerebellar signs and symptoms 1 month after removal from exposure. Marked improvement in signs and symptoms of polyneuropathy was seen 5 months after exposure. In one of our patients, persistent electrodiagnostic evidence of neuropathy was seen at follow-up 5 years after exposure, indicating that permanent neurological damage can occur following exposure to acrylamide and that such cases may require vocational retraining (R. G. Feldman, personal observation).

CLINICAL EXPERIENCES

Group Studies

Polyneuropathy and Acrylamide Production

He et al. (1989) reported the acute and persistent effects seen among 71 (45 men and 26 women) workers after 4 months of exposure to acrylamide at ambient air concentrations ranging from 5.56 to 9.02 mg/m³ for 8 hours per day, 6 days per week. Dermal exposure was common in this plant due to an unawareness of acrylamide toxicity and poor personal hygiene. Symptoms were first seen among nine workers involved in the polymerization process during which they handled an aqueous solution of 30% acrylamide for only 3 months. Three of these nine workers had horizontal nystagmus, truncal ataxia, and incoordination. No disturbance of consciousness was reported among these workers. The cerebellar symptoms seen in these three acrylamide polymerization workers disappeared within 1 month after removal from exposure as polyneuropathy emerged. Symptoms and signs of polyneuropathy seen among these three workers, as well as among the other six workers from this department of the factory, included decreased muscle strength in the upper and lower extremities. This was clinically manifested by an inability to hold objects tightly and by difficulty in climbing stairs. Symptoms reported among these nine and the other 62 acrylamide-exposed workers included skin peeling from hands ($n = 38$), excessive sweating of hands ($n = 27$), numb-

ness in hands and feet ($n = 15$), lassitude ($n = 14$), sleepiness ($n = 12$), anorexia ($n = 8$), dizziness ($n = 7$), muscle cramps ($n = 6$), coldness of the hands and feet ($n = 6$), and unsteady gait ($n = 6$). Other signs of acrylamide poisoning included reduced vibration sensation, diminution of tendon reflexes, a positive Romberg's sign, and intention tremor. Visual acuity and visual fields were normal. Neurophysiological tests documented polyneuropathy in 52 (73.2%) of the 71 workers studied (see Neurophysiological Diagnosis section).

Based on these clinical and neurophysiological findings, these authors diagnosed three cases as severe acrylamide poisoning, six as having moderate poisoning, and 43 with mild poisoning; 25 members of the mild poisoning group had only neurophysiological evidence of neuropathy, illustrating the importance of electrodiagnostic testing for early detection of the effects of acrylamide and possible prevention of more severe and permanent neurologic effects. A follow-up examination of the nine workers with severe poisoning showed significant clinical improvement 5 months after removal from exposure to acrylamide.

Domestic Use of Acrylamide-Contaminated Well Water

Five members of a Japanese family were subacutely exposed to acrylamide monomer when their well water was contaminated following acrylamide grouting of a sewer adjacent to their property. The concentration of acrylamide in the well water was found to be 400 ppm (see Exposure Limits and Safety Regulations section). Approximately 4 weeks after completion of the sewer grouting operation, all five persons began to develop CNS symptoms (Igisu et al., 1975).

Patient 1. A 40-year-old housewife spent most of the day in the home doing cooking and laundry and drinking water as needed. She began to notice dizziness and rhinorrhea. She was admitted to the hospital 7 days later when she had become irrational, hallucinatory (visual, auditory, and tactile), and unable to urinate or defecate. She also had severe truncal ataxia. On examination she was disoriented, with poor memory, and had dysarthria. The cranial nerve exam was normal. Strength was normal. Deep tendon reflexes were mildly hyperactive. An EEG was normal. Nerve conduction velocity studies performed at that time showed borderline slowing of sensory conduction velocity in the sural nerve (patient: 37.1 m/sec; lab normal: >38 m/sec).

Two weeks after admission to the hospital the patient began to complain of numbness in her feet and hands. Examination at that time revealed decreased sensation to pain, touch, and vibration in the extremities, more notable distally. Ankle tendon reflexes were then absent. Nerve conduction studies revealed more slowing of sensory conduction velocity in the sural nerve (35.9 m/sec), while motor conduction velocities remained normal.

After having no further exposure for 1 month, the patient recovered, exhibiting no dysarthria or ataxia. Her mental status was normal. Dysuria subsided and bowel function was improved. Four months after cessation of exposure, she continued to complain of mild dysesthesia of her feet, although her sural sensory conduction velocity was reported as normal.

Patient 2. Patient 1's 65-year-old mother-in-law lived with her and her family. Her symptoms appeared at the same time as her daughter-in-law's, with whom she spent most of the day. Her initial symptoms were a cough and a sore throat followed in several days by the onset of unusual drowsiness and a mild disturbance of gait. At about the same time she also began to experience visual hallucinations. She was admitted to the hospital on the same day as her daughter-in-law.

On admission she was dysarthric and disoriented and showed poor memory functioning. She had bilateral horizontal nystagmus. Muscle strength and sensation were normal. Deep tendon reflexes were slightly hyperactive in the right lower extremity, where a Babinski sign was also noted. Truncal ataxia was so marked that she could not maintain standing posture nor perform tandem gait. Nerve conduction studies and EEG were normal.

Ten days after removal from exposure to acrylamide, her mental status had returned to normal. Over the next four weeks, however, this patient developed progressively greater sensory disturbances in her distal extremities. At that time, nerve conduction studies revealed slowing of the sensory conduction velocity in the sural nerve (34.9 m/sec). Motor nerve conduction velocities were normal.

At follow-up 2 months after exposure ended the patient was no longer experiencing dysesthesia, and sensory conduction velocity in the sural nerve had returned to within normal limits. The right Babinski sign was still noted and may have been unrelated to acrylamide exposure in this older woman.

Patient 3. A 42-year-old man, the husband of patient 1, began to experience rhinorrhea, coughing, and an unsteadiness of gait at the time other family members became ill; one week later he began to experience visual hallucinations. However, he was not admitted to the hospital for 3 days, at which time he was ataxic, dysarthric, and disoriented with impaired memory function. He also had horizontal nystagmus bilaterally. Deep tendon reflexes, muscle strength, and sensation of pain, touch, and vibration were normal. Sphincter function was intact. Nerve conduction studies and an EEG performed at that time were both normal. The hallucinations disappeared and the patient's mental status improved within 1 week after his removal from the acrylamide source.

However, 20 days after removal from exposure the patient experienced dysesthesia in his hands and feet. A neurological examination performed at that time revealed decreased sensation to vibration and touch, more prominent in the distal most portions of the upper and lower extremities. At this time his sensory sural nerve conduction velocity was slowed (35.7 m/sec). Neurological examination

and neurophysiological tests were normal at follow-up 2 months after exposure.

Patient 4. The 13-year-old son of this family experienced a gait disturbance and sleepiness at the same time the others became clinically affected. He was admitted to the hospital the day after his mother and grandmother—about 7 days after the onset of his illness. A moderate truncal ataxia was noted on admission. This patient's condition improved rapidly, and 2 weeks after exposure he was discharged from the hospital. His clinical and neurophysiological examinations at that time revealed no abnormalities.

Patient 5. The least affected of the family members, the 10-year-old daughter of patient 1, began to exhibit unusual behavior (e.g., asking silly questions) 2 days before her mother was admitted to the hospital. The patient recovered very rapidly, and her clinical examination 24 hours after she stopped using the water revealed no abnormalities.

The difference in severity of the five cases of acrylamide poisoning presented above reflects differences in total exposure dose. The two women (patients 1 and 2) were at home most of the day and consumed well water only. The father was away from the house during the day, but during the evening he would use the well water to mix himself alcoholic beverages. The children were both in school during the day and thus had less intake of drinking water. The striking similarities in the affected persons, however, are the two phases of effect of exposure to the acrylamide in their well water which they used for bathing, cooking, and drinking. The first phase involved acute CNS findings which appeared after about 4 weeks of exposure in the adults and their 13-year-old son and cleared within days of removal from exposure. Then, approximately 2 to 4 weeks after cessation of exposure, signs of peripheral neuropathy appeared, with slowed sural nerve sensory conduction velocities.

Individual Case Studies

Dermal Effects and Neuropathy Related to Inadequate Skin Protection

Davenport et al. (1976) described a 25-year-old man who developed numbness of his extremities and unsteadiness of gait after working in a factory where he handled acrylamide for 6 months, mixing raw acrylamide powder with other dry and liquid solvents in a sealed reactor vessel. He strictly followed the company's safety procedures concerning his skin, wearing coveralls, clear plastic gloves, and a filtering face mask. Nevertheless, he soon developed intense erythema on the skin of his palms and soles, with ulcerations and sloughing of the skin after beginning the job. Over the first 3 months of his employment he noted increasing fatigue, and he became anorexic and lost 40 pounds. He stopped working and was admitted to the hospital because of progressively worsening ataxia. Two weeks after having left the source of exposure, he began to experience severe tingling paresthesias of the hands and feet and clumsiness of fine motor control. Slurred speech and dysarthria soon followed. His examination at this time, more than 2 weeks since any additional exposure, revealed hyperhidrosis of the skin of the palms and soles, weakness of the extensor muscles of the wrists and ankles, decreased muscle tone, terminal dysmetria and intention tremor of the upper extremities, and a moderate truncal and gait ataxia. Fine sustained nystagmus was also noted. Objective testing for sensation to pinprick and temperature showed deficits bilaterally below the knees and mid-forearms. Position and vibration senses were absent, and tendon reflexes could not be elicited. Nerve conduction velocity was slowed, consistent with evidence found on a sural nerve biopsy of an axonal neuropathy (see Neurophysiological Diagnosis and Neuropathological Diagnosis sections).

Acrylamide Poisoning Following Disregard for Industrial Hygiene Practices

A 21-year-old man developed overt symptoms of peripheral neuropathy 6 weeks after he began working full-time as an acrylamide grouter in a mine (Auld and Bedwell, 1967). His job required him to first drill holes in the soil, after which he would load a hopper with a 10% aqueous solution of acrylamide, add a catalyst (β-dimethyl-amino-propionitrile), and then pour the mixture into the holes. He handled the acrylamide carelessly, frequently allowing it to come into contact with his forearms and face because "no one had ever gotten sick with it."

Approximately 2 weeks after the patient began working as a grouter, he developed a rash on his forearms. After about 6 weeks on the job, he began to experience weakness in his legs. His symptoms continued to progress and 2 weeks later he was experiencing difficulty walking and weakness in his hands. Despite these symptoms, which were so severe that they became obvious to his friends and coworkers, he continued to handle the acrylamide carelessly.

The patient was admitted to the hospital approximately 9 weeks after he began working as a grouter, at which time he was ataxic and had profuse sweating, coldness, paresthesias, and cyanosis in his hands and feet. The patient's medical history revealed that he was not diabetic and that he had not had a "flu" immediately before the onset of his symptoms. The patient reported that he "occasionally" drank a beer but that he did not consume hard liquor. Neurological examination revealed a mild impairment of sensations of temperature, position, and vibration. Muscle strength was decreased in the distal extremities, particularly in the legs. Deep tendon reflexes were absent. Cerebrospinal fluid was normal.

Six weeks after his admission to the hospital and his removal from acrylamide exposure the patient had regained normal sensation of touch and temperature but excessive sweating from the palms and soles of his feet persisted. Knee jerks returned on week 10. The patient was discharged 14 weeks after cessation of exposure, at which time he was reported to be clinically normal. The patient was advised to avoid further contact with acrylamide and to seek vocational retraining.

Residual Effects Five Years After Prolonged Acrylamide Exposure

A 28-year-old male construction worker had been using acrylamide as a grouting material intermittently for 1.5 years. Then, he used it daily for 2 months during the waterproofing of a tunnel. Within several days after beginning the project, he noticed that his hands were dry and the skin of his fingers began to peel. He continued working without any protective gloves or respiratory equipment. After 1 month on the job, he noticed cramping pains in his legs and hands and difficulty with his balance. He experienced numbness and stiffness of his fingers and legs. When he suddenly could not urinate, he sought medical attention. He also complained that he could not ejaculate and he felt very fatigued. He stopped working at that time and had no further exposure to acrylamide grouting solution.

At neurological examination (R. G. Feldman, personal observation) 1 week after ceasing exposure, he walked with a wide-based gait and stated that he felt as though he would stub his toes unless he was careful. Tendon reflexes were trace in biceps and absent at triceps, knees, and ankles. Abdominal and cremastic reflexes were present and brisk. Muscle strength was slightly reduced, considering this young man's muscular build. His grip was 25 to 30 pounds less than the examiner would have predicted the patient to be capable of. The sensory exam was intact for pain sensation, but he could not perceive position and vibration sensation in the feet and up to above the ankles. Slight appreciation for vibration and position sensation was present at the wrist.

Nerve conduction studies showed slowing of distal latencies for both sensory and motor nerves. Sensory potential amplitudes were also reduced. Sensory conduction velocity was not determined in this case. Subsequent examinations over the next several months showed gradual improvement in hand grip strength and gait stability. He continued to have difficulty with fine finger movements at 2 months after cessation of exposure. By 4 months after exposure, he showed slight improvement in fine motor control in his hands but continued to have numbness in his toes bilaterally. Serial nerve conduction studies were done over the 4 months and were repeated again 5 years after removal from exposure (see Neurophysiological Diagnosis section).

He was also examined 5 years after exposure, at which time he was well oriented with no gross difficulties with recall or language; comprehensive neuropsychological testing was not performed at that time. A cranial nerve exam revealed no evidence of defect in vision, and extraocular movements were intact as was facial sensation. Test of coordination with outstretched hands showed mild tremor slightly more marked on the left. Finger-to-nose testing was done with slight clumsiness and terminal tremor was noted. In addition, awkwardness with finger-to-nose testing was seen more on the left than on the right. When walking he had a broad-based gait and he was unable to walk tandem without some stagger. He did not have a marked Romberg sign, but there was some sway to his trunk without falling. Deep tendon reflexes were hypoactive. Positional sense was intact in his lower extremities, although vibration sensation was reduced in his toes and feet. Sensation to pinprick was in a shoe distribution bilaterally but was more noticeable on the right. Patchy sensation loss was present in his thighs and forearms.

REFERENCES

Abou-Donia MB. Metabolism and toxicokinetics of xenobiotics. In: Derelanko MJ, Hollinger MA (eds): *CRC handbook of toxicology.* New York: CRC Press, 1995:539–589.

Abou-Donia MB, Ibrahim SM, Corcoran JJ, Lack L, et al. Neurotoxicity of glycidamide, an acrylamide metabolite, following intraperitoneal injections in rats. *J Toxicol Environ Health* 1993;39:447–464.

Agrawal AK, Squibb RE, Bondy SC. The effects of acrylamide treatment upon the dopamine receptor. *Toxicol Appl Pharmacol* 1981;58:89–99.

Allen N. Solvents and other industrial compounds. In: Vinken PJ, Bruyn GW, series editors. *Handbook of clinical neurology,* vol 36; Vinken PJ, Bruyn GW, Cohen MM, Klawans HL, volume eds. *Intoxications of the nervous system,* part I. New York: North-Holland, 1979:361–389.

American Conference of Governmental Industrial Hygienists (ACGIH). *Documentation of the threshold limit values (TLVs) and biological exposure indices,* 5th Ed. Cincinnati: ACGIH, 1988.

American Conference of Governmental Industrial Hygienists (ACGIH). *Threshold limit values (TLVs) for chemical substances and physical agents and biological exposure indices (BEIs).* Cincinnati: ACGIH, 1995.

American Cyanamid Company (ACC). *Chemistry of acrylamide.* Bulletin PRC 109. Wayne, NJ: Process Chemicals Department, American Cyanamid Co., 1969.

American Cyanamid Company (ACC). *Safety instructions for handling AM-9 chemical grout.* Wayne, NJ: Industrial Chemicals Division, Engineering Chemicals, 1979.

Ando K, Hashimoto K. Accumulation of (^{14}C)-acrylamide in mouse nerve tissue. In: *Proceedings of the Osaka Prefectural Institute of Public Health,* vol 10, 1972:7–12. Cited by Spencer and Schaumburg, 1974.

Arezzo JC, Schaumburg HH, Petersen CA. Rapid screening for peripheral neuropathy: a field study with the Optacon. *Neurology* 1983;33:626–629.

Arezzo JC, Simson R, Brennan NE. Evoked potentials in the assessment of neurotoxicity in humans. *Neurobehav Toxicol Teratol* 1985;7:299–304.

Auld RB, Bedwell SF. Peripheral neuropathy with sympathetic overactivity from industrial contact with acrylamide. *Can Med Assoc J* 1967;96:652–654.

Bachman M, Myers JE, Bezuidenhout BN. Acrylamide monomer and peripheral neuropathy in chemical workers. *Am J Ind Med* 1992;21:217–222.

Bale Oenick MD, Danielson SJ, Daiss JL, Saundberg MW, Sutton RC. Antigen-binding activity of antibodies immobilized on styrene copolymer beads. *Ann Biol Clin* 1990;48:651–654.

Beiswanger CM, Mandella RD, Graessle TR, Reuhl KR, Lowndes HE. Synergistic neurotoxic effects of styrene oxide and acrylamide: glutathione-independent necrosis of cerebellar granule cells. *Toxicol Appl Pharmacol* 1993;118:233–244.

Berger AR, Schaumburg HH, Schroeder C, Apfel S, Reynolds R. Dose response, coasting, and differential fiber vulnerability in human toxic neuropathy: a prospective study of pyridoxine neurotoxicity. *Neurology* 1992;42:1367–1370.

Bergmark E, Calleman C, He F, Costa L. Determination of hemoglobin adducts in humans occupationally exposed to acrylamide. *Toxicol Appl Pharmacol* 1993;120:45–54.

Bikales NM, Kolodny ER. Acrylamide. In: Standon A, ed. *Encyclopedia of chemical technology,* 2nd ed. New York: Interscience 1963:274–284.

Bohnert JL, Horbett TA, Ratner BD, Royce FH. Absorption of proteins from artificial tear solutions to contact lens material. *Invest Ophthalmol Vis Sci* 1988;29:362–373.

Boyes WK, Cooper GP. Acrylamide neurotoxicity: effects on far field somatosensory evoked potentials in rats. *Neurobehav Toxicol Teratol* 1981;3:487–490.

Brimijoin WS, Hammond PI. Acrylamide neuropathy in the rat: effects on energy metabolism in sciatic nerve. *Mayo Clin Proc* 1985;60:3–8.

Brown L, Rhead MM, Bancroft KCC. Case studies of acrylamide pollution resulting from industrial use of polyacrylamides. *Water Pollut Control* 1980;79:507–510.

Burek JD, Albee RR, Beyer JE, et al. Subchronic toxicity of acrylamide administered to rats in the drinking water followed up to 144 days of recovery. *J Environ Pathol Toxicol* 1980;4:157–182.

Calleman CJ. The metabolism and pharmacokinetics of acrylamide: implications for mechanisms of toxicity and human risk estimation. *Drug Metab Rev* 1996;28:527–590.

Calleman CJ, Bergmark E, Costa LG. Acrylamide is metabolized to glycidamide in the rat: evidence from hemoglobin adduct formation. *Chem Res Toxicol* 1990;3:406–412.

Calleman CJ, Wu Y, He F, et al. Relationship between biomarkers of exposure and neurological effects in a group of workers exposed to acrylamide. *Toxicol Appl Pharmacol* 1994;126:361–371.

Carlson GP, Weaver PM. Distribution and binding of ^{14}C-acrylamide to macromolecules in SENCAR and BALB/c mice following oral and topical administration. *Toxicol Appl Pharmacol* 1985;79:307–313.

Cavanagh JB. The significance of the "dying-back" process in experimental and human neurological disease. *Int Rev Exp Pathol* 1964;3:219–267.

Cavanagh JB. The pathokinetics of acrylamide: a reappraisal of the problem. *Neuropathol Appl Neurobiol* 1982;8:315–336.

Cavanaugh JB, Gysbers MF. Ultrastructural features of Purkinje cell damage caused by acrylamide in the rat: a new phenomenon in cellular neuropathology. *J Neurocytol* 1983;12:413–437.

Chauhan NB, Spencer PS, Sabri MI. Effect of acrylamide on the distribution of microtubule-associated proteins (MAP1 and MAP2) in selected regions of rat brain. *Mol Chem Neuropathol* 1993;18:225–245.

Cloeren M. Acrylamide. In: Sullivan JB Jr, Krieger GR, eds. *Hazardous materials toxicology. Clinical principles of environmental health.* Baltimore: Williams & Wilkins, 1992:940–945.

Costa LG, Deng H, Gregotti C, Manzo L, et al. Comparative studies on the neuro- and reproductive toxicity of acrylamide and its epoxide glycidamide in the rat. *Neurotoxicology* 1992;13:219–224.

Costa LG, Deng H, Calleman CJ, Bergmark E. Evaluation of the neurotoxicity of glycidamide, an epoxide metabolite of acrylamide: behavioral, neurochemical and morphological studies. *Toxicology* 1995;98:151–161.

Csillik B, Knyihar E, Elshiekh AA. Degenerative atrophy of cantral terminals of primary sensory neurons induced by blockade of axoplasmic transport in peripheral nerves. *Experientia* 1977;33:656–657.

Davenport JG, Farrell DF, Sumi SM. 'Giant axonal neuropathy' caused by industrial chemicals: neurofilamentous axonal masses in man. *Neurology* 1976;26:919–923.

Dearfield KL, Abernathy CO, Ottley MS, Brantner JH, Hayes PF. Acrylamide: its metabolism, developmental and reproductive effects, genotoxicity, and carcinogenicity. *Mutat Res* 1988;195:45–77.

Dearfield KL, Douglas GR, Ehling UH, Moore MM, Sega GA, Brusick DJ. Acrylamide: a review of its genotoxicity and an assessment of heritable risk. *Mutat Res* 1995;330:71–99.

Deng H, He F, Zhang S, Calleman CJ, Costa LG. Quantitative measurements of vibration threshold in healthy adults and acrylamide workers. *Int Arch Occup Environ Health* 1993;65:53–56.

DeRojas TC, Goldstein BD. Primary afferent terminal function following acrylamide: alterations in the dorsal root potential and reflex. *Toxicol Appl Pharmacol* 1987;88:175–182.

Dixit R, Husain H, Seth PK, Mukhtar H. Effect of diethyl maleate on acrylamide induced neuropathy in rats. *Toxicol Lett* 1980;6:417–421.

Dixit R, Mukhtar H, Seth PK, Krishna Murti CR. Conjugation of acrylamide with glutathione catalyzed by glutathione-*S*-transferases in rat liver and brain. *Biochem Pharmacol* 1981;30:1739–1744.

Dixit R, Das M, Mushtaq M, Srivastava P, Seth PK. Depletion of glutathione content and inhibition of glutathione-*S*-transferase and aryl hydrocarbon hydroxylase activity of rat brain following exposure to styrene. *Neurotoxicology* 1982;3:142–145.

Droz B, Di Giamberardino L, Koenig HL. Contribution of axonal transport to the renewal of myelin phospholipids in peripheral nerves. I. Quantitative radiographic study. *Brain Res* 1981;219:57–71.

Edwards PM. The distribution and metabolism of acrylamide and its neurotoxic analogues in rats. *Biochem Pharmacol* 1975;24:1277–1282.

Endo H, Sabri MI, Stephens JM, Pekala PH, Kittur S. Acrylamide induces immediate-early gene expression in rat brain. *Brain Res* 1993;609: 231–236.

Endo H, Kuttur S, Sabri MI. Acrylamide alters neurofilament protein gene expression in rat brain. *Neurochem Res* 1994;19:815–820.

Environmental Protection Agency (EPA). *Preliminary assessment of health risks from exposure to acrylamide.* Washington, DC: US Environmental Protection Agency, Office of Toxic Substances, 1988.

Environmental Protection Agency (EPA). Proposed ban on acrylamide and *N*-methylolacrylamide grouts. *Federal Register,* 40 CFR, Vol. 56, No. 191, Part 764, 1991:49863–49874.

Environmental Protection Agency (EPA). *Drinking water regulations and health advisories.* EPA 822-R-96-001. Washington, DC: Office of Water, 1996.

Frantz SW, Dryzga MD, Freshour NL, Watanabe PG. *In vivo/in vitro* determination of cutaneous penetration of residual monomer of polyacrylamides (abstr). *Toxicologist* 1985;5:39.

Fujita A, Shibata J, Kato H, et al. Clinical observations of three cases of acrylamide poisoning. *Nippon Ijo Shimpo* 1960;1869:37–40.

Fullerton PM, Barnes JM. Peripheral neuropathy in rats produced by acrylamide. *Br J Ind Med* 1966;23:210–221.

Fullerton PM. Electrophysiological and histological observations on the peripheral nerves in acrylamide poisoning. *J Neurol Neurosurg Psychiatry* 1969;32:186–192.

Garland GT, Patterson MWH. Six cases of acrylamide poisoning. *Br Med J* 1967;4:134–138.

Gerr FE, Letz R. Reliability of a widely used test of peripheral cutaneous vibration sensitivity and a comparison of two testing protocols. *Brit J Ind Med* 1988;45:635–639.

Gerr F, Hershman D, Letz R. Vibrotactile threshold measurement for detecting neuropathy: reliability and determination of age- and height-standard normative values. *Arch Environ Health* 1990;45:148–154.

Gold BG, Griffin JW, Price DL. Slow axonal transport in acrylamide neuropathy: different abnormalities produced by single dose and continuous administration. *J Neurosci* 1985;5:1755–1768.

Gold BG, Price DL, Griffin JW, et al. Neurofilament antigens in acrylamide neuropathy. *J Neuropathol Exp Neurol* 1988;47:145–157.

Gold BG, Griffin JW, Price DL. Somatofugal axonal atrophy precedes development of axonal degeneration in acrylamide neuropathy. *Arch Toxicol* 1992;66:57–66.

Gold BG, Strom-Dickerson T, Austin DR. Regulation of the transcription factor c-JUN by nerve growth factor in adult sensory neurons. *Neurosci Lett* 1993;154:129–133.

Gold BG, Austin DR, Strom-Dickerson T. Multiple signals underlie the axotomy-induced up-regulation of c-JUN in adult sensory neurons. *Neurosci Lett* 1994;176:123–127.

Goldstein BR, Lowndes HE. Spinal cord defect in the peripheral neuropathy resulting from acrylamide. *Neurotoxicology* 1979;1:75–87.

Griffin JW, Drucker N, Gold BG, et al. Schwann cell proliferation and migration during paranodal demyelination. *J Neurosci* 1987;7:682–699.

Harris CH, Gulati AK, Friedman MA, Sickles DW. Toxic neurofilamentous axonopathies and fast axonal transport. V. Reduced bidirectional vesicle transport in cultured neurons by acrylamide and glycidamide. *J Toxicol Environ Health* 1994;42:343–356.

Hashimoto K, Aldridge WN. Biochemical studies on acrylamide, a neurotoxic agent. *Biochem Pharmacol* 1970;19:2591–2604.

Hashimoto K, Sakamoto J, Tanii H. Neurotoxicity of acrylamide and related compounds and their effects on male gonads in mice. *Arch Toxicol* 1981;47:179–189.

Hashimoto K, Ivano VV, Inomata K, et al. Biological monitoring of exposure to alkylating xenobiotics by determining them using new analytical approach in complexes with hemoglobin, plasma proteins, and mercapturic acids in urine. II. Acrylamide. *Vopr Med Khim* 1995;41:22–25.

Hattis D, Shapiro K. Analysis of dose/time/response relationships for chronic toxic effects: the case of acrylamide. *Neurotoxicology* 1990;11: 219–236.

He F, Zhang S, Wang H, et al. Neurological and electroneuromyographic assessment of the adverse effects of acrylamide on occupationally exposed workers. *Scand J Work Environ Health* 1989;15:125–129.

Hills BW, Greife AL. Evaluation of occupational acrylamide exposures. *Appl Ind Hyg* 1986;13:148–152.

Hong JS, Tilson HA, Agrawal AK, Karoum F, Bondy SC. Postsynaptic location of acrylamide-induced modulation of striatal ^{3}H-spiroperidol binding. *Neurotoxicology* 1982;3:108–112.

Hopkins AP. The effects of acrylamide on the peripheral nervous system of the baboon. *J Neurol Neurosurg Psychiatry* 1970;33:805–816.

Howland RD, Alli P. Altered phosphorylation of rat neuronal cytoskeletal proteins in acrylamide induced neuropathy. *Brain Res* 1986;363: 333–339.

Igisu H, Goto I, Kawamura Y, Kato M, Izumi K, Kuroiwa Y. Acrylamide encephaloneuropathy due to well water pollution. *J Neurol Neurosurg Psychiatry* 1975;38:581–584.

Ikeda GJ, Miller E, Sapienza PP, Michel TC, King MT, Sager AO. Maternal–foetal distribution studies in the late pregnancy. II. Distribution of [1-^{14}C]acrylamide in tissues of beagle dogs and miniature pigs. *Food Chem Toxicol* 1985;23:757–761.

Kaji R, Liu Y, Duckett S, Summer AJ. Slow recovery of central axons in acrylamide neuropathy. *Muscle Nerve* 1989;12:816–826.

Kaplan ML, Murphy SD, Gilles FH. Modification of acrylamide neuropathy in rats by selected factors. *Toxicol Appl Pharmacol* 1973;24: 564–579.

Kirk–Othmer Encyclopedia of Chemical Technology, vol 1: *A to alkanolamines,* 3rd ed. Mark HF, Othmer DF, Overberger CG, Seaborg GT, eds. New York: John Wiley and Sons, 1978.

Kohriyama K, Matsuoka M, Igisu H. Effects of acrylamide and acrylic acid on creatine kinase activity in the rat brain. *Arch Toxicol* 1994; 68:67–70.

Kreiss K, Wegman DH, Niles CA, Siroky MB, Krane RJ, Feldman RG. Neurological dysfunction of the bladder in workers exposed to dimethylaminopropionitrile. *JAMA* 1980;243:22–29.

Kuperman AS. Effects of acrylamide on the central nervous system of the cat. *J Pharmacol Exp Ther* 1958;123:180–192.

Le Quesne PM. Acrylamide. In: Spencer PS, Schaumburg HH, eds. *Experimental and clinical neurotoxicology.* Baltimore: Williams & Wilkins, 1980:309–325.

LoPachin RM, Lehning EJ. Acrylamide-induced distal axon degeneration: a proposed mechanism of action. *Neurotoxicology* 1994;15:247–260.

Marlowe C, Clark MJ, Mast RW, Friedman MA, Waddell WJ. The distribution of [^{14}C]acrylamide in male and pregnant Swiss–Webster mice studied by whole-body autoradiography. *Toxicol Appl Pharmacol* 1986;86:457–465.

Matsuoka M, Igisu H. Brain energy metabolites in mice intoxicated with acrylamide: effects of ischemia. *Toxicol Lett* 1992;62:39–43.

Matsuoka M, Igisu H, Lin J, Inoue N. Effects of acrylamide and *N,N'*-methylene-bis-acrylamide on creatine kinase activity. *Brain Res* 1990; 507:351–353.

McCollister DD, Oyen F, Rowe VK. Toxicology of acrylamide. *Toxicol Appl Pharmacol* 1964;6:172–181.

Merck Index, 12th ed. Rahway, NJ: Merck, 1996:23.

Merigan WH, Barkdoll E, Maurissen JP. Acrylamide-induced visual impairment in primates. *Toxicol Appl Pharmacol* 1982;62:342–345.

Miller MJ, Spencer PS. Single doses of acrylamide reduce retrograde transport velocity. *J Neurochem* 1984;43:1401–1408.

Miller MJ, Carter D, Sipes I. Pharmacokinetics of acrylamide in Fischer 344 rats. *Toxicol Appl Pharmacol* 1982;63:36–44.

Moody L, Arezo J, Otto D. Screening occupational populations for asymptomatic or early peripheral neuropathy. *J Occup Med* 1986;28:975–986.

Moretto A, Sabri MI. Progressive deficits in retrograde axon transport precede degeneration of motor axons in acrylamide neuropathy. *Brain Res* 1988;44:18–24.

Mukhtar H, Dixit R, Seth PK. Reduction in cutaneous and hepatic glutathione contents, glutathione-*S*-transferase and aryl hydrocarbon hydroxylase activities following topical application of acrylamide to mouse. *Toxicol Lett* 1981;9:153–156.

Myers JE, Macun I. Acrylamide neuropathy in a South African factory: an epidemiologic investigation. *Am J Ind Med* 1991;19:487–493.

National Institute for Occupational Safety and Health (NIOSH). NIOH and NIOSH basis for an occupational health standard. *Acrylamide: a review of the literature.* Cincinnati: US Department of Health and Human Services, CDC, Publication No. 91-115, 1991.

National Institute for Occupational Safety and Health (NIOSH). *Pocket guide to chemical hazards.* Cincinnati: US Department of Health and Human Services, CDC, June 1994.

Navarro X, Verdui E, Guerro J, Buti M, Gonalons E. Abnormalities of sympathetic sudomotor function in experimental acrylamide neuropathy. *J Neurol Sci* 1993;114:56–61.

Oaklander AL, Spencer PS. Cold blockade of axonal transport activates premitotic activity of Schwann cells and wallerian degeneration. *J Neurochem* 1988;50:490–496.

Occupational Safety and Health Administration (OSHA). Code of Federal Regulations, 29, 1910.1000/.1047. Washington, DC: Office of the Federal Register, National Archives and Records Administration, 1995:411–431.

Parkki MG. The role of glutathione in the toxicity of styrene. *Scand J Work Environ Health* 1978;4(2):53–59.

Pleasure DE, Mishler KC, Engel WK. Axonal transport of proteins in experimental neuropathies. *Science* 1969;166:524–525.

Prineas J. The pathogenesis of dying back polyneuropathies. Part II. An ultrastructural study of experimental acrylamide intoxication in the cat. *J Neuropath Exp Neurol* 1969;28:598–621.

Rakesh D, Prahlad KS, Hasan M. Metabolism of acrylamide into urinary mercapturic acid and cysteine conjugates in rats. *Drug Metab Dispos Biol Fate Chem* 1982;10:196–197.

Ralevic V, Aberdeen JA, Burnstock G. Acrylamide-induced autonomic neuropathy of rat mesenteric vessels: histological and pharmacological studies. *J Autonomic Nervous System* 1991;34:77–87.

Reagan KE, Wilmarth KR, Friedman MA, Adou-Donia MB. *In vitro* calcium and calmodulin-dependent kinase-mediated phosphorylation of rat brain and spinal cord neurofilament proteins is increased by glydamide administration. *Brain Res* 1995;671:12–20.

Sabri MI, Spencer PS. Acrylamide impairs fast and slow axonal transport in rat optic system. *Neurochem Res* 1990;15:603–608.

Sahenk Z, Mendell JR. Acrylamide and 2,5-hexanedione neuropathies: abnormal bidirectional transport rate in distal axons. *Brain Res* 1981;219:397–405.

Satoyoshi E, Kinoshita M, Yano H, Suzuki Y. Three cases of peripheral neuropathy due to acrylamide. *Clin Neurol (Tokyo)* 1971;11:667–672.

Sax DS, Johnson T, Salzieder B, et al. Electrophysiological estimate of nerve fiber diameter distribution and histogram of nerve fibers in toxic neuropathies. *Ann Neurol* 1984;16:148 (abst).

Sax NI. *Dangerous properties of industrial chemicals,* 5th ed. New York: Van Nostrand Reinhold, 1979.

Schaumburg HH, Wisniewski HM, Spencer PS. Ultrastructural studies of the dying-back process. 1. Peripheral nerve terminal and axon degeneration in systemic acrylamide intoxication. *J Neuropathol Exp Neurol* 1974;33:260–284.

Schaumburg HH, Spencer PS. Clinical experimental studies of distal neuropathy—a frequent form of brain and nerve damage produced by environmental chemical hazards. Bronx, NY: Departments of Neurology, Neuroscience, and Pathology (Neuropathology), Albert Einstein College of Medicine. Grant No. R01-OH-00535, NIOSHTIC, RN 00091771, 1979.

Schaumburg HH, Arezzo J, Spencer PS. Short-latency somatosensory evoked potentials in primates intoxicated with acrylamide: implications for toxic neuropathies in man. Abstract No. 490, presented at the Society of Toxicology, Boston, MA. *Toxicologist* 1982;2:139.

Schaumburg HH, Spencer PS, Thomas PK. *Disorders of peripheral nerves.* Philadelphia: FA Davis, 1983:131–133.

Schaumburg HH, Arezzo JC, Spencer PS. Delayed onset of distal axonal neuropathy after prolonged low-level administration of a neurotoxin. *Ann Neurol* 1989;26:576–579.

Sickles DW. Toxic neurofilamentous axonopathies and fast anterograde axonal transport. I. The effects of single doses of acrylamide on the rate and capacity of transport. *Neurotoxicology* 1989;10:91–102.

Sickles DW. Toxic neurofilamentous axonopathies and fast anterograde axonal transport. IV. *In vitro* analysis of transport following acrylamide and 2,5-hexanedione. *Toxicol Lett* 1992;61:199–204.

Sickles D, Goldstein BD. Acrylamide produces a direct, dose-dependent and specific inhibition of oxidative metabolism in motorneurons. *Neurotoxicology* 1986;7:187–196.

Smith EA, Oehme FW. Acrylamide and polyacrylamide: a review of production, use, environmental fate and neurotoxicity. *Rev Environ Health* 1991;9:215–228.

Smith EA, Prues SL, Oehme FW. Environmental degradation of polyacrylamides. 1. Effects of artificial environmental conditions: temperature, light, and pH. *Ecotoxicol Environ Safety* 1996;35:121–135.

Souyri F, Chretien M, Droz B. 'Acrylamide-induced' neuropathy and impairment of axonal transport of proteins. I. Multifocal retention of fast transported proteins at the periphery of axons as revealed by light microscope radioautography. *Brain Res* 1981;205:1–13.

Spencer P, Schaumburg HH. A review of acrylamide neurotoxicity, part I. Properties, uses, and human exposure. *Can J Neurol Sci* 1974;1: 143–150.

Srivastava SP, Das M, Seth PK. Enhancement of lipid peroxidation in rat liver on acute exposure to styrene and acrylamide a consequence of glutathione depletion. *Chem-Biol Interact* 1983;45:373–380.

Srivastava SP, Seth PK, Das M, Mukhtar H. Effects of mixed function oxidase modifiers on the neurotoxicity of acrylamide in rats. *Biochem Pharmacol* 1985; 34:1099–1102.

Sterman AB. Acrylamide induces early morphologic reorganization of neuronal cell body. *Neurology* 1982;32:1023–1026.

Sterman AB, Schaumburg HH. The neurological examination. In: Spencer PS, Schaumburg HH, eds. *Experimental and clinical neurotoxicology.* Baltimore: Williams & Wilkins, 1980:675–681.

Sterman AB, Panasci DJ, Sheppard RC. Autonomic-cardiovascular dysfunction accompanies sensory impairment during acrylamide intoxication. *Neurotoxicology* 1983;4:45–52.

Stetkiewicz J, Wronska-Nofer T, Klimczak J, Stetkiewicz I. Metabolic interaction and neurological effect of combined exposure to acrylamide and ethanol. *Pol J Occup Med* 1988;1:127–136.

Sumner SCJ, MacNeela JP, Finnell TR. Characterization and quantitation of urinary metabolites of [1, 2, 3-^{13}C]acrylamide in rats and mice using ^{13}C nuclear magnetic resonance spectroscopy. *Chem Res Toxicol* 1992; 5:81–89.

Takahashi M, Ohara T, Hashimoto K. Electrophysiological study of nerve injuries in workers handling acrylamide. *Int Arch Arbeitsmed* 1971;28:1–11.

Tilson HA, Squibb RE. The effects of acrylamide on the behavioral suppression produced by psychoactive agents. *Neurotoxicology* 1982;3: 113–120.

Trenga CA, Kunkel DD, Eaton DL, Costa LG. Effect of styrene oxide on rat brain glutathione. *Neurotoxicology* 1991;12:165–178.

Walden R, Schiller CM. Quantitative analysis of acrylamide in the milk of lactating rats following oral *in vivo* exposure. *Environ Toxicol* 1981; II:678.

White RF, Feldman RG, Proctor SP. Neurobehavioral effects of toxic exposure: clinical syndromes in adult neuropsychology. In: White RF, ed. *The practitioners handbook.* Amsterdam: Elsevier, 1992:1–51.

Windholz M, Budvari S, Stroumtoss LY, Fertig MN. In: *Merck Index,* 9th ed. Rahway, NJ: Merck & Co, 1976:127.

World Health Organization (WHO). *Acrylamide: environmental health criteria,* no. 49. Geneva: World Health Organization. 1985:121.

Wu YQ, Yu AR, Tang XY, Zhang J, Cui T. Determination of acrylamide metabolite, mercapturic acid by high performance liquid chromatography. *Biochem Environ Sci* 1993;6:273–280.

Wu W, Toma JG, Cahn H, Smith R, Miller RD. Disruption of fast axonal transport *in vivo* leads to alterations in Schwann cell gene expression. *Dev Biol* 1994;163:423–439.

Xiwen H, Jing L, Tao C, Ke Y. Studies on biochemical mechanism of neurotoxicity induced by acrylamide in rats. *Biomed Environ Sci* 1992; 5:276–281.

CHAPTER 19

Ethylene Oxide

Ethylene oxide (EtO) has a simple epoxide structure consisting of an oxygen atom linked to the two carbon atoms of an ethylene molecule (Fig. 19-1). Synonyms used for EtO include 1,2-epoxyethane, epoxyethane, ethene oxide, oxirane, dimethylene oxide, dihydrooxirene, oxane, oxidoethane, oxacyclopropane, and oxiran (Lewis, 1993). EtO is produced by the oxidation of ethylene in the presence of a silver catalyst at 10 to 30 atmospheres of pressure and at temperatures of 200°C to 300°C (WHO, 1994; Gardiner et al., 1994). Approximately 2,500 tons of EtO were produced in the United States in 1992 (WHO, 1994).

At room temperature, EtO is a colorless, flammable gas with a sweet ether-like odor (NIOSH, 1994; Gardiner et al., 1994). It is highly reactive and will react violently when exposed to heat, acids, or alkalis (Sax, 1979). Mixing EtO with water or an inert gas such as carbon dioxide or freon decreases its explosivity. The majority of EtO produced for commercial use is distributed in mixtures of low concentration—for example, 10% EtO with 90% CO_2 or 12% EtO with 88% halocarbon (OSHA, 1984).

Although occupational exposure limits have been established for EtO, the potential for exposure to levels capable of producing adverse effects exists where EtO is manufactured or used. An estimated 250,000 workers in the United States are exposed to EtO (WHO, 1994). In biological systems, EtO reacts with amines, alcohols, and sulfhydryl compounds such as glutathione (Gardiner et al., 1994). In addition, EtO reacts with molecules that have an active hydrogen atom to yield a substituted ethanol (Hollingsworth et al., 1956). Neurophysiological and neurobehavioral effects have been associated with exposure to EtO (Gross et al., 1979; Jay et al., 1982; Finelli et al., 1983; Kuzuhara et al., 1983; Zampollo et al., 1984; Landrigan et al., 1984; Schröder et al., 1985; Fukushima et al., 1986; Estrin et al., 1987, 1990; Crystal et al., 1988; Bryant et al., 1989; Klees et al., 1990).

SOURCES OF EXPOSURE

Occupational exposures to EtO can occur during its production, in industries where EtO is used in the processes of synthesizing other chemicals, during dry gas sterilization, and in fumigation activities. Approximately 70% of commercial grade EtO produced in the United States is used in the manufacture of ethylene glycol, a major component of automotive antifreeze products. EtO is also used in the synthesis of other organic chemicals that include: ethoxylated surfactants; ethanolamines, used in sweetening natural gas, specialty chemicals, detergents, and cosmetics; glycol ethers, utilized as jet fuel additive and in the formulation of coatings, cleaners, automotive brake fluids, and inks; diethylene and triethylene glycol, used in drying natural gas and in the production of polyester resins, plasticizers, emulsifiers, and lubricants; tetraethylene glycol, used to extract aromatic hydrocarbons; polyethylene glycol, used in the production of plasticizers, lubricants, dispersants, cosmetics, and water-soluble packaging; and crown ethers, used for extraction of liquids (OSHA, 1984). A relatively large quantity of EtO is used to produce polyester fiber and polyethylene film (Sheikh, 1984), while a smaller quantity is used as a fungicide, fumigant, and sterilizing agent for soils, plants, foodstuffs, textiles, cosmetics, and pharmaceutical/medical devices (OSHA, 1984). It is also used to fumigate books, leather, motor oil, paper, spices, animal bedding, clothing, furs, and furniture (WHO, 1994; Sheikh, 1984; Dellarco et al., 1990). EtO penetrates paper, cellophane, fabrics, rubber, polyethylene and polyvinyl chloride, making it very useful in the sterilization of products packaged in these materials (Landrigan et al., 1984).

The use of closed systems during EtO production generally keeps exposure levels below the OSHA PEL. However, workers are exposed at relatively high levels during product sampling and while loading and unloading EtO into transport tanks (NIOSH, 1981). The greatest risk of occupational exposure to EtO exists during materials sterilization, especially while unloading EtO treated supplies after sterilization (OSHA, 1984; Brugnone et al., 1986; Estrin et al., 1987, 1990), and during changing of EtO-containing gas cylinders, replacement of leaking valves, fittings, and piping, and as a result of improper ventilation of aerators and the aeration areas (Mortimer and Kercher, 1989).

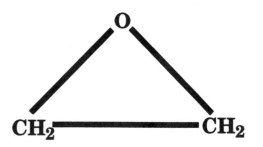

FIG. 19-1. Structure of ethylene oxide, the simplest epoxide.

Ethylene oxide vapor continues to be released from sterilized plastic and rubber articles; therefore, sterilized items must be aerated to allow residual EtO gas to diffuse from the article. This is particularly critical for articles that are being used to administer materials to the human body—for example, catheters, face masks, and tubing used in heart lung machines and artificial kidneys and syringes (O'Leary and Guess, 1968; Fishbein, 1969; OSHA, 1984). Thus, significant exposure is possible when EtO-treated materials are not fully aerated. Therefore, a sufficient aeration time must elapse before instruments sterilized with EtO are safe to use (Windebank and Blexrud, 1989).

Oxidation of ethylene in the ambient air serves as an environmental source of EtO. In addition, EtO is a by-product of ethylene metabolism in animals and humans (Ehrenberg et al., 1977; Filser and Bolt, 1983; Segerbäck, 1983; Filser et al., 1992; Törnqvist, 1994). Approximately 5% of an inhaled dose of ethylene is metabolized to EtO, while the remaining 95% of the ethylene inhaled is exhaled unchanged (Filser et al., 1992; Törnqvist, 1994). Ethylene from exogenous (e.g., auto exhaust and cigarette smoke) and endogenous (e.g., lipid peroxidation) sources is oxidized to EtO in the liver by monoxygenases (Ehrenberg et al., 1977; Harrison, 1981; Schmiedel et al., 1983; Filser and Bolt, 1983; Filser et al., 1992). Exhaled smoke from one cigarette contains approximately 55 μg of EtO, which is derived after inhalation from the metabolic oxidation of ethylene (Törnqvist et al., 1986; Törnqvist, 1994). Levels of hemoglobin adducts, a biomarker of EtO exposure, are increased in cigarette smokers (Törnqvist et al., 1989), and smokers have also been shown to have elevated levels of urinary thioethers (Törnqvist et al., 1986; Burgaz et al., 1992). Fruit store workers using ethylene for controlling the ripening of bananas were also found to have significantly elevated levels of hemoglobin adducts (Törnqvist et al., 1989) (see Biochemical Diagnosis section).

Because EtO is a chemically reactive compound, the fumigation of foodstuffs with EtO results in the formation of other toxic chemicals. For example, EtO combines with the moisture and natural inorganic chloride content of foodstuffs to form chlorohydrins (Fishbein, 1969). Ethylene chlorohydrin (chloroethanol), a highly toxic substance, was found at concentrations above 1,000 ppm in spices fumigated with EtO (Wesley et al., 1965).

EXPOSURE LIMITS AND SAFETY REGULATION

EtO has a notable odor, pleasant to sickeningly sweet and fruity in character. This odor is usually not recognizable in the environment until reaching an air concentration of 430 ppm, a level several hundred times above the established and recommended safe exposure limits for EtO (Amoore and Hautala, 1983). Therefore, dependence upon olfactory perception alone is inadequate for detection of significant releases of EtO into the workplace environment (see Preventative and Therapeutic Measures section).

The *Occupational Safety and Health Administration's* (OSHA) permissible exposure limit (PEL) for EtO is an 8-hour time-weighted average (8-hour TWA) concentration of 1 ppm, with a 15-minute excursion limit (i.e., short-term exposure limit) of 5 ppm (OSHA, 1995) (Table 19-1). OSHA considers EtO to be potentially carcinogenic in humans; on this basis, and not based on neurotoxicity, OSHA has established an 8-hour TWA exposure action level (EAL) of 0.5 ppm. According to this regulation, if initial monitoring reveals that levels are below the EAL, periodic monitoring must be performed only to ensure that this level of exposure is not exceeded. If monitoring reveals that the EAL is exceeded, an employer is required to institute measures to lower the ambient air concentration of EtO and also

TABLE 19-1. *Established and recommended occupational and environmental exposure limits for ethylene oxide in air and water*

	Air (ppm)[a]	Water (ppm)[a]
Odor threshold*	430	140
OSHA		
PEL (8-hr TWA)	1	—
PEL ceiling (15-min TWA)	15	—
Action level	0.5	
NIOSH		
REL (10-hr TWA)	<0.1	—
STEL (15-min TWA)	5	—
IDLH	800	—
ACGIH		
TLV (8-hr TWA)	1	—
STEL (15-min TWA)	—	—
USEPA		
MCL	—	—
MCLG	—	—

[a]*Unit conversion:* 1 ppm = 1.83 mg/m³; 1 ppm = 1 mg/L.
OSHA, Occupational Safety and Health Administration; PEL, permissible exposure limit; TWA, time-weighted average; NIOSH, National Institute for Occupational Safety and Health; REL, recommended exposure limit; STEL, short-term exposure limit; IDLH, immediately dangerous to life and health; ACGIH, American Conference of Governmental Industrial Hygienists; TLV, threshold limit value; USEPA, United States Environmental Protection Agency; MCL, maximum contamination level; MCLG, maximum contamination level goal.
Data from *Amoore and Hautala, 1983; OSHA, 1995; ACGIH, 1995; USEPA, 1996; NIOSH, 1997.

to increase the frequency of monitoring until successive measurements indicate that EtO levels are consistently below the EAL (OSHA, 1984, 1995). The *National Institute for Occupational Safety and Health* (NIOSH) also considers EtO to be a human carcinogen. The NIOSH 10-hour TWA recommended exposure limit (REL) for EtO is a concentration of <0.1 ppm, with a 10-minute exposure ceiling of 5 ppm that should not be exceeded at any time. The NIOSH also recommends an immediately dangerous to life or health (IDLH) concentration of 800 ppm for EtO (NIOSH, 1994). The *American Conference of Governmental Industrial Hygienists* (ACGIH), recommends an 8-hour TWA threshold limit value (TLV) for EtO of 1 ppm. ACGIH also considers EtO to be a potential human carcinogen (ACGIH, 1995).

The *United States Food and Drug Administration* (USFDA) permits the use of EtO in products that come into contact with food (USFDA, 1993), but the *United States Environmental Protection Agency* (USEPA) has established a 50-mg/kg limit for EtO residue following its use as a fumigant (USEPA, 1992). The USEPA has not established regulations or health advisories for EtO concentration in drinking water (USEPA, 1996).

METABOLISM

Tissue Absorption

Once inhaled, EtO passes through the pulmonary alveoli and enters into the systemic circulation (Filser and Bolt, 1983; Brugnone et al., 1986; Krishnan et al., 1992). Pulmonary uptake of gaseous EtO is influenced by the alveolar ventilation rate and the cardiac output (Fiserova-Bergerova, 1983). The amount of EtO absorbed during an 8-hour period of exposure to 1 ppm is estimated to be 7 to 8 mg (Brugnone et al., 1986). Seventy-five to eighty percent of an inhaled dose of EtO is retained in humans.

Ethylene oxide is a liquid at 10°C (51°F); therefore, oral intake is possible in humans and animals. A single 0.2-g/kg oral dose of liquid EtO in solution with vegetable oil was lethal to rats (Hollingsworth et al., 1956). Fifteen repeated oral doses of EtO (0.1 g/kg each) administered over 3 weeks to rats caused gastric irritation, a marked decrease in body weight, and slight liver damage. Chronic ingestion of EtO in solution with vegetable oil, administered twice weekly for approximately 3 years at doses of 0.03 and 0.0075 g/kg, increased the incidence of forestomach tumors in rats (Dunkelberg, 1982). Because EtO is a gas at room temperature, the opportunity for oral intake and subsequent gastrointestinal absorption is less likely than is pulmonary absorption following inhalation.

The percentage of EtO monomer that permeates through the skin during the routine use of substances containing and releasing EtO depends upon the specific formulation of the product. The permeation rate for EtO in an aqueous solution at 30°C through an excised sample of skin is 0.125 mg/cm^2/hr (Baumbach et al., 1987). The maximal permeation of EtO in water-in-oil emulsion is 14%, whereas the maximal permeation of EtO in oil-in-water emulsion is only 7.8%. The contribution of EtO from skin care products to total body burden is negligible (Filser et al., 1994). Dermal exposure to gaseous EtO released from sterilized materials can cause local injury and hypersensitivity reactions at the point of contact with the skin (Alomar et al., 1981; Biro et al., 1974; Poothullil et al., 1975).

Tissue Distribution

Ethylene oxide is very soluble in blood and is rapidly distributed to various body tissues following absorption (Brugnone et al., 1986; Walker et al., 1990; Brown et al., 1996). During a work shift, the average blood concentration of EtO is approximately three times the environmental air EtO concentration, reflecting the high solubility of EtO in blood (Brugnone et al., 1986). Tissue distribution of EtO is primarily influenced by the blood/tissue partition coefficient of the gas and tissue blood perfusion (Osterman-Golkar and Bergmark, 1988).

Ethylene oxide crosses the blood–brain barrier (BBB). Whole-body autoradiography, using ^{14}C-labeled EtO, showed that tissue distribution of EtO is similar after administration to mice by inhalation or by injection. Tissue levels of EtO and its metabolites were three to four times that of the blood as early as 2 minutes after injection. Levels continued to be higher in the cerebellum, liver, pancreas, kidney, intestinal mucosa, lungs, epididymis, and testicles than in blood for 20 minutes to 4 hours after injection. Twenty-four hours after injection, radioactivity was still present in these tissues as well as in the bronchi and in bone marrow (Applegren et al., 1977).

EtO retained in tissue after a prior exposure can be detected by the quantity of EtO-DNA adducts formed (see Chapter 3). For example, the reaction of EtO with DNA yields the adduct, 7-hydroxyethyl guanine (7-HEG). Following a single inhalation exposure to EtO, 7-HEG adducts were found on DNA of cells taken from the brain, liver, lungs, spleen, kidneys, and testes of rats. Concentrations of the 7-HEG adducts continued to increase up to 5 days after cessation of exposure. The 7-HEG adducts disappeared with a half-life of 7 days, reflecting repair of the damaged DNA (Walker et al., 1990).

Tissue Biochemistry

Two possible pathways (Fig. 19-2) responsible for metabolism of EtO in humans are (a) hydrolysis by reaction with water and chloride ions to yield ethylene glycol and (b) conjugation with glutathione to yield thioethers (Jones and Wells, 1981; Martis et al., 1982; Gérin and Tardif, 1986; Tardif et al., 1987; Burgaz et al., 1992). In the first of these two pathways, ethylene glycol is the major metabolic

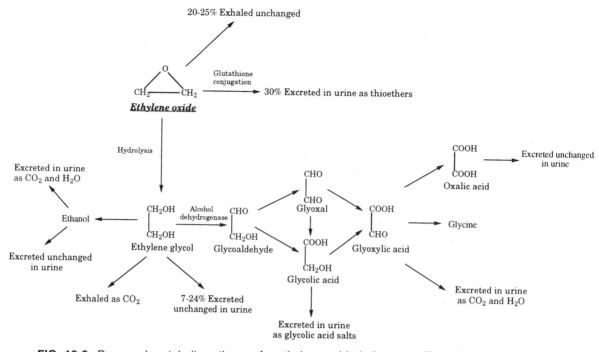

FIG. 19-2. Proposed metabolic pathways for ethylene oxide in humans. (Data from Gessner et al., 1961; Coen and Weiss, 1966; Parry and Wallach, 1974; Clay and Murphy, 1977; Jones and Wells, 1981; Rowe and Wolf, 1982; Martis et al., 1982; Wolfs et al., 1983; Endo et al., 1984; Gérin and Tardif, 1986; McKelvey and Zemantis, 1986; Tardif et al., 1987; Walker et al., 1990; Burgaz et al., 1992; Parkinson, 1996).

product of EtO hydrolysis (Martis et al., 1982; Wolfs et al., 1983; Tardif et al., 1987). The mean concentration of ethylene glycol in the blood of EtO-exposed workers was twice as high as that in unexposed controls (Wolfs et al., 1983). Ethylene glycol is oxidized by alcohol dehydrogenase to glycoaldehyde (Coen and Weiss, 1966). The actions of aldehyde oxidase promote the oxidation of glycoaldehyde to yield glycolic acid and glyoxal. Glycolic acid and glyoxal are subsequently oxidized to glyoxylic acid, which is toxic (Parry and Wallach, 1974; Rowe and Wolf, 1982). Metabolic detoxification of glyoxylic acid proceeds via several pathways, the metabolites of which include glycine, oxylic acid, carbon dioxide, and water (Parry and Wallach, 1974). Ethanol may also be formed from ethylene glycol (Endo et al., 1984). The affinity of alcohol dehydrogenase for ethylene glycol is 100 times less than it is for ethanol. Therefore, ethanol competitively binds to alcohol dehydrogenase and diminishes the metabolism of ethylene glycol. Accumulation of lipolytic metabolites such as ethylene glycol and ethanol may be involved in the neurotoxicity of EtO (Endo et al., 1984).

In the second proposed pathway, conjugation of EtO with glutathione is the major metabolic mechanism. Conjugation with glutathione prevents EtO from covalently binding to cellular proteins and nucleic acids (McKelvey and Zemantis, 1986; Parkinson, 1996). Approximately two-thirds of the human population possesses the ability to enzymatically conjugate EtO with glutathione, and the lack of this ability may increase an individual's susceptibility to the toxic effects of EtO

(Schröder et al., 1992; Hallier et al., 1993). EtO reacts with glutathione via the formation of chloroethanol through the action of glutathione transferase to form hydroxyethyl cysteine derivatives (thioethers) which are subsequently excreted in the urine (Jones and Wells, 1981; Gérin and Tardif, 1986; Tardif et al., 1987). Tissue levels of glutathione are decreased in rats and mice exposed to EtO for 4 hours at concentrations ranging from 100 to 1,200 ppm. These results suggest that high-level or repeated exposures to EtO result in a depletion of glutathione stores, thereby enhancing EtO toxicity (McKelvey and Zemantis, 1986; Katoh et al., 1990). Furthermore, concurrent exposure to other electrophilic xenobiotics [such as methylmercury (CH^3Hg^+)] or to electrophilic metabolites of xenobiotics (such as styrene-7,8-epoxide), which are also metabolically detoxified by conjugation with glutathione, may increase the toxic effects of EtO or vice versa (McKelvey and Zemantis, 1986; Gregus and Klaassen, 1996; Parkinson, 1996). Since glutathione is also important for protecting tissues from oxidative stress, it is possible that depletion of this protective enzyme may lead to neuronal damage by free radicals (see Neuropathological Diagnosis section).

Excretion

Pharmacokinetic studies in animals show that elimination of EtO can be represented by a one-compartment model and follows first-order kinetics (Martis et al., 1982; Brown et al., 1996). The elimination rates for EtO from the blood, brain, and muscle tissues are identical in the mouse. Clearance half-life for EtO is dependent upon the size of the exposed animal (Brown et al., 1996). The half-life for EtO in humans is approximately 45 minutes (Filser et al., 1992). Twenty to twenty-five percent of an inhaled dose of EtO is exhaled unchanged (Brugnone et al., 1986). Ethylene glycol is a major urinary metabolite of EtO in mammals. Between 7% and 24% of liquid EtO intravenously administered to dogs was eliminated in the urine as ethylene glycol within 24 hours (Martis et al., 1982). A small proportion of EtO which is metabolized to ethylene glycol is further metabolized to carbon dioxide before being exhaled or excreted in the urine (Rowe and Wolf, 1982; Katoh et al., 1989; Gardiner et al., 1994). In addition, the ethylene glycol metabolites glycolic acid and oxalic acid can be detected in the urine following exposure to EtO (Gessner et al., 1961; Clay and Murphy, 1977).

Conjugation of EtO with glutathione leads to urinary excretion of thioethers. Significantly elevated levels of total urinary thioethers were measured in a group of 31 hospital sterilization workers exposed to EtO at levels up to 200 ppm (Burgaz et al., 1992). Following exposure to EtO, rats excreted *N*-acetyl *S*-(2-hydroxyethyl)-L-cysteine (i.e., 2-hydroxyethylmercapturic acid) and *S*-(2-hydroxyethyl)-L-cysteine in urine, comprising about 30% of the administered dose of the epoxide (Jones and Wells, 1981; Gérin and Tardif, 1986; Tardif et al., 1987). The relationship between urinary levels of 2-hydroxyethylmercapturic acid and exposure dose is linear up to an ambient air EtO concentration of 200 ppm in rats (Gérin and Tardif, 1986). The thioether *S*-carboxymethyl-L-cysteine can also be detected in the urine of mammals (Tardif et al., 1987). Ethylene oxide is eliminated more slowly when glutathione levels are depleted by high or repeated exposure to EtO (Tardif et al., 1987; Katoh et al., 1989, 1990; Brown et al., 1996).

CLINICAL MANIFESTATIONS AND DIAGNOSIS

Symptomatic Diagnosis

Acute Exposure

Acute exposure to EtO for hours to weeks has been associated with (a) minor symptoms such as mucous membrane and respiratory tract irritation, asthma, nausea, vomiting, anorexia, headache, lightheadedness and dizziness, and fatigue and (b) more serious side effects such as somnolence, dysarthria, nystagmus, delirium, and seizures. Numbness and distal weakness in the extremities, incoordination, and ataxia may appear after 1 or more months of exposure to EtO (Gross et al., 1979; Salinas et al., 1981; Endo et al., 1984; Laurent, 1988; Bryant et al., 1989; Deschamps et al., 1992) (Table 19-2). A survey assessed personal and environmental exposure levels, the use of protective devices, and the occurrence of short-term health complaints among 165 health care workers who were exposed to EtO gas from sterilizers in 27 different hospitals in Alberta, Canada (Bryant et al., 1989). Personal exposure levels were positively correlated with acute

TABLE 19-2. *Acute and chronic symptoms reported after ethylene oxide exposure*

Acute (hours to weeks)	Chronic (months to years)
Mucous membrane irritation	Headache
Blunting of the senses of smell and taste	Dizziness
Nausea	Fatigue
Vomiting	Nausea
Lethargy	Anorexia
Headache	Memory loss
Lightheadedness	Cognitive impairment
Seizures	Delirium
	Nystagmus
	Difficulty swallowing
	Dysarthria
	Paresthesia and/or weakness in extremities
	Decreased sensation to touch and vibration
	Gait disturbance (steppage gait)
	Incoordination

Data from Joyner, 1964; Gross et al., 1979; Garry et al., 1979; Salinas et al., 1981; Endo et al., 1984; Schröder et al., 1985; Fukushima et al., 1986.

symptoms. Seventy-one percent of the workers reported the use of protective clothing; however, this apparently had only a slight effect on the incidence of short-term symptoms, because conjunctival and pharyngeal irritation and shortness of breath were reported at levels below 3.4 ppm and significantly ($p = 0.001$) more complaints of this nature at concentrations greater than 3.4 ppm despite the use of protective clothing. Eighty percent of the workers complained of one or more acute symptoms, with headaches, dry mouth, and drowsiness reported in 20% to 40% of these cases.

Gross et al. (1979) described a 28-year-old man who had worked as an EtO sterilizer operator for up to 70 hours per week for only 3 weeks during which he experienced conjunctival and mucous membrane irritation, transient blunting of his senses of smell and taste, headaches, nausea, vomiting, and lethargy. His exposure ended after 3 weeks because the patient began to have recurrent major motor seizures at 20- to 30-minute intervals requiring hospitalization. Interictally, he responded to pain with semipurposeful movements, but had neither nuchal rigidity nor focal neurologic signs. The seizures continued for 2 days before being controlled by medication; within 1 week he was discharged, apparently having recovered.

Chronic Exposure

Subacute and chronic exposures to EtO for months to years affect the central and the peripheral nervous systems. Central nervous system (CNS) symptoms include agitation, insomnia, dysarthria, impaired memory, and poor concentration and increased muscle tone, in some cases, suggesting parkinsonism. Signs of peripheral neuropathy—such as paresthesias, hand and leg cramps, decreased vibration, and pinprick sensation in the extremities; and, in more severely affected cases, incoordination, ataxia, distal muscle weaknesses—are seen (Gross et al., 1979; Finelli et al., 1983; Kuzuhara et al., 1983; Endo et al., 1984; Zampollo et al., 1984; Schröder et al., 1985; Fukushima et al., 1986; Crystal et al., 1988; Bryant et al., 1989; Estrin et al., 1990; Barbosa et al., 1992). Peripheral neuropathy follows longer-duration, low-level exposures to EtO as well as shorter-duration, higher-concentration exposures to EtO (Kuzuhara et al., 1983; Schröder et al., 1985; Ohnishi and Murai, 1993).

In an epidemiological study by Garry et al. (1979), 12 individuals who worked in an instrument and materials sterilization unit for 5 months were assessed for the chronic effects of occupational exposure to EtO. The TWA ambient concentration of EtO in the sterilization room was 36 ppm, a level which was below the OSHA PEL at the time (50 ppm). The symptom prevalence reported by these workers was as follows: headache 50% ($n = 6$), nausea 42% ($n = 5$), speech difficulties 42% ($n = 5$), memory loss 42% ($n = 5$), muscle weakness 33% ($n = 4$), dizziness 25% ($n = 3$), and incoordination 17% ($n = 2$). A decrease in reported symptoms occurred after routine safety checks of the sterilizing equipment.

Following 2 years of chronic exposure to EtO, four of 12 female sterilization center workers exposed to EtO at personal air concentrations which ranged from 10 to 400 ppm developed paresthesias and fatigue. Two of these individuals developed signs of peripheral neuropathy including lower limb weakness and distal paresthesia; the diagnosis of peripheral neuropathy was ascertained by nerve conduction studies (Zampollo et al., 1984) (Table 19-3).

TABLE 19-3. *Neurophysiological effects of ethylene oxide*

Patient profile: age and sex	Exposure level (ppm)	Neurophysiological findings	Reference
23-yr-old man	0–500	Reversible slowing of SCV in the sural nerve and reversible slowing of MCV in the tibial nerve. Reversible reduction of the amplitude of the motor evoked potentials in the tibial nerve.	Schröder et al., 1985
38-yr-old woman	10–400	NCS showed diffuse motor and sensory neuritic damage in the lower extremities. MEP amplitude was reduced in the distal muscles of the legs. Slowing of SCVs and MCVs was seen in the ulnar, peroneal, and posterior tibial nerves. Follow-up at 6 months after exposure was normal.	Zampollo et al., 1984
32-yr-old woman		NCS showed sensory impairment of the upper limbs. Slowing of SCVs and MCVs was seen in the ulnar, peroneal, and posterior tibial nerves. Reduction of the MEP amplitude in the peroneal and tibial nerves. Follow-up at 6 months after exposure was normal.	
28-yr-old man	NR	NCS were within normal limits.	Gross et al., 1979
27-yr-old man		Reversible slowing of the SCVs and MCVs and reversible decreased MEP amplitude.	
31-yr-old man		Reversible slowing of the SCVs and MCVs and reversible decreased MEP amplitude.	
30-yr-old man		Reversible slowing of the SCVs and MCVs and reversible decreased MEP amplitude.	
23-yr-old man	NR	No response to stimulation of the left peroneal nerve. Slowing of the MCV of the right peroneal and posterior tibial nerves. Absence of the right sural nerve SEP and right tibial H-reflex. Follow-up NCS at 7 months were normal except for the right tibial H-reflex, which remained suppressed.	Finelli et al., 1983
17-yr-old man		MCVs and SCVs were within normal limits. EMG showed scattered positive sharp waves, fibrillation potentials, and small-amplitude motor unit potentials in the leg and foot muscles. Follow-up EMG 4 months later was normal.	
19-yr-old man		Absent MEP in the extensor digitorum brevis muscle on stimulation of the right peroneal nerve. The right sural nerve SEP amplitude was normal but delayed. Right tibial MCV was slowed and the tibial H-reflex was absent on the right and delayed on the left. EMG of leg and foot muscles showed denervation potentials. At 7 months follow-up, EMG showed active denervation with some polyphasic and polyphasic giant potentials. Follow-up NCS continued to show mild slowing in the lower limbs.	

NCS, nerve conduction studies; EMG, electromyogram; SCV, sensory nerve conduction velocity; MCV, motor nerve conduction velocity; SEP, sensory evoked potentials; MEP, motor evoked potentials; NR, exposure levels not reported.

Clinical improvement is generally seen within 1 year after removing a person from exposure to EtO (Gross et al., 1979; Fukushima et al., 1986; Schröder et al., 1985; Finelli et al., 1983; Zampollo et al., 1984). For example, a 23-year-old man exposed to EtO at concentrations up to 500 ppm reported experiencing difficulty with his memory and concentration as well as paresthesia in both legs after only 2 months of exposure (Schröder et al., 1985). Despite his symptoms, this individual continued to work and 3 months later he was admitted to the hospital with weakness in his lower extremities and unsteadiness of gait. He was unable to walk on his heels, and sensations to pinprick and vibration were diminished in his lower extremities. Deep tendon reflexes were normal, except ankle jerks were absent. Biopsy of the sural nerve of this patient provided histological evidence of peripheral neuropathy (see Neuropathological Diagnosis section). At follow-up 1 year after removal from EtO exposure the patient was markedly improved.

Kuzuhara et al. (1983) reported the clinical courses of two young male workers who presented with gait disturbances following chronic exposure to EtO at a TWA concentration of 50 ppm and peak exposures of up to 700 ppm. One of these cases, a 33-year-old man, began to experience paresthesias and weakness in his distal limbs after working as a sterilizer operator for only 3 months. He continued to work, although his symptoms continued to progress, until he had to be admitted to the hospital 3 months later because of weakness. He was discharged after 1 month without any exposure, having clinically recovered. He returned to his job as a sterilizer worker for about 1 month, and then was readmitted to the hospital with the return of paresthesias and weakness in the lower extremities. His symptoms cleared entirely after 2 months away from exposure. The second worker, a 21-year-old man, developed paresthesias in his feet 6 months after he had started to load and unload medical supplies from sterilizers. His symptoms of peripheral neuropathy progressed over the course of the next month, at which time he was admitted to the hospital with increased paresthesias, weakness in the extremities, and staggering gait. Sensation was diminished in the lower extremities, and peripheral neuropathy was confirmed by neurophysiological studies and nerve biopsy (see Neuropathological Diagnosis section). His symptoms improved markedly within 1 month after his removal from EtO exposure.

A 26-year-old woman employed in a medical supply sterilization department, but not actually involved in the sterilization process, began to experience headaches, excessive fatigue, dizziness, memory loss, and difficulty concentrating after 7 years of exposure to EtO at levels of 2.4 to 4.2 ppm (Crystal et al., 1988). She continued working at the same job; 1 year later she began to stumble while descending the stairs at night. Her symptoms were worse by the end of a workday and they were improved after weekends or holidays. Her memory continued to deteriorate, necessitating her to compile lists in order to remember her

daily tasks; she soon after stopped working. One year after cessation of exposure, her symptoms had improved; however, she still exhibited diminished vibratory and thermal sensations in her distal extremities and her memory and concentration were still impaired. Follow-up examination 4 years after cessation of exposure revealed that there was further progression of her sensory neuropathy. Dretchen et al. (1992) questioned that EtO was the cause for the progression of the symptoms seen in this patient and suggested an alternative or accompanying etiology, such as an underlying psychiatric disorder or a thiamine deficiency. The original authors, however, supported their conclusion of EtO-induced disease by discussing the time course, the details of the neuropsychological tests, and the patterns of cognitive and peripheral neuropathic changes in this patient mitigating against Dretchen et al.'s claim (Grober et al., 1992) (see Neuropsychological Diagnosis section).

Neurophysiological Diagnosis

Electroencephalography (EEG) and *event-related evoked potentials* (EPs) have been useful in evaluating patients with symptoms due to EtO exposure. A diffusely slow EEG was reported in a 28-year-old man who developed an acute encephalopathy with major motor seizures after he had worked as an EtO sterilizer operator for only 3 weeks. Similarly, increased amounts of theta activity were noted on the EEG recording of a 27-year-old man who developed a sensorimotor neuropathy 2 years after he began working as an EtO sterilization unit operator. Nonspecific scattered theta activity was seen on the EEG of a 17-year-old boy who developed peripheral neuropathy 1.5 years after he began working 20 hours per week as an EtO sterilization unit operator (Gross et al., 1979). Conversely, the EEG was normal in a 23-year-old man who developed peripheral neuropathy following exposure to EtO (Finelli et al., 1983).

Studies of two separate cohorts (Estrin et al., 1987, 1990) did not show differences in the EEG patterns of workers exposed to low levels of EtO, compared with non-exposed controls. However, Estrin et al. (1990) did find significantly ($p = 0.0008$) lower P-300 amplitudes on EP testing in the EtO-exposed workers. Although P-300 latencies were prolonged in the exposed workers from both cohorts, this difference was not found to be statistically significant in either study (Estrin et al., 1987, 1990).

The EEG of a 29-year-old woman exposed to low levels of EtO for 10 years was suggestive of mild temporal lobe dysfunction, greater on the left side, 2 months after cessation of exposure. At a follow-up 6 months later, the EEG was reported as showing mild slowing of the background activity (Crystal et al., 1988). The EEG of this patient was normal at a follow-up examination 5 years after cessation of exposure (Dretchen et al., 1992).

Electromyographic (EMG) recordings and *nerve conduction studies* (NCS) can be used to document the severity, persistence, and reversibility of the neuropathy associated with EtO exposure. Needle electrode (EMG) recordings of leg and foot muscles reveal denervation potentials, while NCS reveal decreased conduction velocities in motor and sensory nerve fibers of the distal peripheral nerves (see Table 19-3). These electrophysiological findings generally parallel the patient's clinical presentation, but may also be used to detect cases of subclinical neuropathy (Gross et al., 1979; Finelli et al., 1983; Zampollo et al., 1984). Kuzuhara et al. (1983) reported the EMG and NCS results of two patients who developed peripheral neuropathy following occupational exposure to EtO at concentrations of 50 to 700 ppm. The first patient was a 33-year-old man who developed a peripheral neuropathy within 6 months after he began working as an EtO sterilizer operator. The EMG of this patient revealed denervation patterns in the distal limb muscles. Nerve conduction studies were not performed in this patient. The second patient was a 21-year-old man who developed a peripheral neuropathy 6 months after he began a new job loading and unloading medical supplies from a sterilizer unit. Needle EMG recordings from the limb muscles of this patient revealed long-duration and high-amplitude units in the triceps, along with reduced motor nerve conduction velocity in the right median and superficial peroneal nerves. In addition, sensory conduction velocity in the distal sural nerve was slowed, but remained normal in the distal median nerve. The left sural nerve was biopsied and confirmed the presence of neuropathy with loss of myelin and axonal changes.

Gross et al. (1979) reported the nerve conduction studies findings from four cases of EtO-induced peripheral neuropathy. The first patient (Case 1) was a 28-year-old man who developed an acute encephalopathy with major motor seizures after he had worked as an EtO sterilizer operator for only 3 weeks (see paragraphs on electroencephalography, above). Nerve conduction studies were not performed at the time of the initial examination, so it is impossible to compare these with the findings found 2 months after removal from exposure, when the patient's neurological exam and NCS were normal. Cases 2 (27-year-old man) and 3 (31-year-old man) presented with symptoms of peripheral neuropathy including numbness and weakness in the extremities. The NCS in Case 2 revealed generalized sensorimotor polyneuropathy, and the EMG revealed fibrillations in the intrinsic muscles of the feet. Nerve conduction studies in Case 3 were also compatible with a sensorimotor neuropathy. EMG studies of this patient revealed decreased numbers and increased amplitude and duration of motor unit potentials in the distal muscles. The fourth patient (30-year-old man) was asymptomatic, but his NCS revealed a subclinical sensorimotor neuropathy. Motor and sensory nerve conduction velocities were normal at a follow-up examination 4 years after cessation of exposure. The decreased amplitudes of muscle action potentials, moderately decreased conduction velocities, and signs of denervation seen in the latter three cases are compatible with a reversible axonal degenerative type of neuropathy.

Neurophysiological findings in the three patients with EtO-induced polyneuropathy demonstrated mild slowing of motor NCVs, with positive sharp waves and fibrillations potentials on EMG during the active disease state, indicating axonal neuropathy (Finelli et al., 1983). In Case 1, the NCS showed no response to stimulation of the left peroneal nerve, slowing of motor conduction velocities over the right peroneal and the right posterior tibial nerves, and absence of both right tibial H-reflex and the right sural nerve sensory action potential. The EMG showed scattered positive sharp waves and fibrillation potentials, with increased polyphasic activity in the intrinsic foot muscles and, to a lesser extent, in the leg muscles. Repeated examination 5 weeks and 7 months later showed the return of normal conduction velocities and a disappearance of denervation potentials, as well as the recording of giant potentials as signs of reinnervation. The left H-reflex remained suppressed. In Case 2, the EMG initially showed positive sharp waves, fibrillation potentials, and small-amplitude motor unit potentials in leg and foot muscles. Follow-up studies showed the disappearance of the denervation potentials and the appearance of giant potentials indicating reinnervation. Case 3 showed absent evoked potentials from the extensor digitorum brevis muscle on stimulation of the right peroneal nerve. The right tibial conduction velocity was slowed, and the tibial H-reflex was absent on the right and delayed on the left. The right sural nerve sensory evoked potential amplitude was normal, but delayed. Leg and foot muscle EMG studies showed denervation potentials. Repeat studies 7 months later showed mild slowing and active denervation on EMG but some polyphasic and giant potentials were also seen.

Neuropsychological Diagnosis

Neuropsychological testing has been used to document the clinical and subclinical CNS effects associated with exposure to EtO (Estrin et al., 1987, 1990; Crystal et al., 1988; Klees et al., 1990; Garry et al., 1979). Workers with chronic exposure to EtO exhibit memory disturbances, attention and executive function deficits, and slowing of psychomotor speed (Estrin et al., 1987, 1990; Crystal et al., 1988; Klees et al., 1990). The CNS effects of chronic low-level (TWA: 4.7 ppm) exposure to EtO were assessed in 22 hospital workers using a neuropsychological test battery (Klees et al., 1990). The workers had a mean EtO exposure duration of 6.13 years (range: 1 to 11 years). Analysis of the neuropsychological testing results revealed a significantly higher frequency of cognitive impairment and/or personality dysfunction among the EtO-exposed workers as compared with 24 nonexposed age- and sex-matched controls, indicating a possible relationship to low levels of EtO exposure.

The two following studies demonstrate that performance is affected in certain neurobehavioral domains and not others; in addition, there is a suggestion of an exposure-dose–response effect. In one study eight female (age: 33 to 66 years) hospital workers were exposed to low levels of EtO for durations of 5 to 20 years, working around gas sterilizers using either 12% EtO and 88% chlorodifluoromethane (Freon) or 100% EtO (Estrin et al., 1987). The exposed workers were compared with eight age and sex-matched controls. Computer-based neurobehavioral tests administered included simple reaction time, digit span, digit symbol, pattern memory, horizontal addition, eye–hand coordination, and continuous performance test. Performance of the exposed workers on the hand–eye coordination test was significantly ($p = 0.03$) impaired. In addition, a significant ($r = 0.67$; $p \leq 0.05$) dose–response relationship was found between decreasing performance on the continuous performance test and years of exposure to EtO. These findings indicate that EtO affects attention and visuomotor functioning. In a second study, a cohort of ten female workers (age: 30 to 60 years) had detected the odor of EtO during routine operation of sterilization equipment (Estrin et al., 1990). These workers had been employed in the sterilization department for 0.5 to 10 years (mean: 5 years) and were exposed to 12% EtO and 88% Freon. Industrial hygiene samples from the past 2 years showed EtO concentrations of 15 to 250 ppm. The subjects were examined using both computer- and hand-administered neuropsychological test batteries. Neuropsychological domains assessed included memory, verbal ability, visuospatial ability, psychomotor speed, and visuomotor performance. The exposed workers were compared with a group of age-matched controls. The hand-administered neuropsychological test battery revealed significant impairment of performance in the exposed workers on the Trails Test A (significant at $p = 0.04$). A highly significant difference in performance on the computer-based finger-tapping test was found between the exposed and nonexposed subjects. Furthermore, the exposed workers performed less well, although not statistically significantly, on the Cancellation Test ($p = 0.06$) and on the visual reproduction subtest of the Wechsler Memory Scale (WMS) ($p = 0.07$). The findings of this study by Estrin et al. show that exposure to EtO impairs performance on tests of visuomotor tracking, psychomotor-speed, memory, and attention. No significant difference in the performance of the exposed workers was revealed by the computer-based tests of verbal and visuospatial abilities.

Diminished intellectual function, impaired memory, and attention as well as perceptual and cognitive slowing were noted on neuropsychological testing in a 29-year-old woman who worked adjacent to an EtO sterilization tank (Crystal et al., 1988). A 35-point discrepancy was noted between her current verbal intelligence quotient (VIQ) of 81 measured by the Wechsler Adult Memory Scale (WAIS) and her predicted VIQ of 116 estimated by the New Adult Reading Test (NART). Visual memory tested by having the subject draw geometric patterns from memory, was impaired; as was spatial memory, tested by having her recall the spatial location of previously presented pictures. Disturbance of attention was noted by visual digit span testing. Perceptual and cognitive slowing for both visual and verbal material was demonstrated by testing. Also, an unusual pattern of forgetting was noted. On a cued recall she was able to retrieve all items on each of four trials, but 1 hour later she was able to retrieve only seven items. This patient showed a pattern of intact learning and profound forgetting strikingly different from the pattern of impaired initial learning and modest forgetting that occurs in most mildly demented subjects and depressed patients. Following cessation of exposure, these symptoms improved over a month, but did not disappear. Evidence in this case that chronic EtO exposure can result in cognitive decline included (a) borderline intelligence in a subject whose premorbid intelligence was estimated to be in the bright normal range, (b) impaired performance on tests of visual and verbal memory and on auditory and visual attention, (c) perceptual and cognitive slowing in the processing of verbal and visual information, (d) symptoms lessening over weekends, only to increase over a workweek, and (e) improvement after EtO exposure had ceased. Nevertheless, in a review of this patient's case by Dretchen et al. (1992), a causal relationship between her clinical manifestations, neuropsychological findings, and exposure to EtO was seriously questioned.

Biochemical Diagnosis

Alveolar air and blood EtO concentrations can be used to monitor worker exposure, since alveolar air and blood EtO concentrations correlate with environmental air sample concentrations (Brugnone et al., 1986). However, the *American Conference of Governmental Industrial Hygienists* (ACGIH) has not determined or recommended biological exposure indices (BEIs) for EtO (ACGIH, 1995) (Table 19-4). Environmental air, alveolar air, and blood samples analyzed during and at the end of the work shift in ten EtO sterilizer workers showed that the blood concentration measured at the fourth and eighth hours of the work shift correlated significantly with ambient air EtO levels. Blood EtO concentrations were on average 3.3 times higher than that of the environmental concentrations and 12 times the alveolar concentrations, reflecting the high solubility of EtO in blood (Brugnone et al., 1986; Florack and Zielhuis, 1990).

Determination of urinary thioethers such as mercapturic acid can be used to qualitatively monitor exposure to EtO. Total urinary thioethers are elevated in EtO-exposed sterilization workers, indicating that these workers had been exposed to EtO (Burgaz et al., 1992). However, urinary thioethers are not considered a sensitive quantitative measure of exposure dose. For example, although total urinary thioethers were elevated in the EtO-exposed workers studied by Burgaz et al. (1992), the difference in excretion of

TABLE 19-4. *Biological exposure indices for ethylene oxide*

	Urine	Blood	Alveolar air
Determinant:	Thioethers	EtO	EtO
Start of shift:	Not established	Not established	Not established
During shift:	Not established	Not established	Not established
Prior to last shift of workweek:	Not established	Not established	Not established

Data from ACGIH, 1995–1996.

total urinary thioethers among the sterilization unit operators was not significantly higher than that of workers involved only in the packing and stocking of sterilized materials.

Measurement of EtO-alkylated amino acids in hemoglobin (hemoglobin adducts) is a more sensitive biomarker technique for detecting EtO exposure. Ethylene oxide is an electrophilic alkylating agent that binds with hemoglobin at the nucleophilic centers of the amino acids cysteine, histidine, and N-terminal valine (Segerbäck, 1990). Hemoglobin adducts can be used to estimate previous exposures for a period equal to the lifetime of a red blood cell, or 120 days (van Sittert et al., 1993). Ethylene from endogenous and exogenous sources is biotransformed to EtO *in vivo*. Low levels of hemoglobin adducts have been reported in nonexposed individuals, suggesting that exogenous ethylene from cigarette smoke, pollution, and possibly dietary factors may contribute to nonoccupational EtO exposure (Törnqvist et al., 1986). Background levels of alkylated cysteines and histidines are higher than are those of N-terminal valines, suggesting that the latter two should show greater affinity for and sensitivity to low-level EtO exposure (Walker et al., 1990). The formation of hemoglobin adducts may also vary interindividually so that this parameter could be less suitable for biological monitoring than DNA adducts in lymphocytes (Föst et al., 1995).

Because EtO is an alkylating agent, it also reacts with DNA, thereby forming *DNA adducts* which can be used as biological markers of exposure. EtO primarily reacts with DNA at guanine to yield 7-hydroxyethyl guanine (7-HEG), which represents approximately 90% of the alkylated DNA sites (Walker et al., 1990). No other DNA adducts have been quantified in tissues following *in vivo* exposure to EtO. Persistent DNA lesions may be due to repair deficiencies. Pero et al. (1982) reported depressed DNA repair capability following *in vivo* EtO exposure.

The cytogenetic changes occurring in peripheral blood lymphocytes as a result of EtO binding to DNA, including an increase in the frequency of sister chromatid exchanges (SCEs), chromosomal aberrations, and micronuclei, have also been used to document EtO exposure (Schulte et al., 1992, 1995; Lerda and Rizzi, 1992). The frequency of SCE is a very sensitive indicator for detecting acute and chronic past exposures to EtO and, thus, can be used for ongoing monitoring of workers exposed to EtO. The frequency of SCE was determined in three workers who developed clinical symptoms following an accidental exposure to EtO at concentrations of more than 700 ppm for 30 minutes during a sterilization process (Laurent, 1988); the frequencies of SCEs were determined at 5 days and at follow-up 2 years later. All three workers initially showed a similar increase in the mean number of SCE per cell after the accident (SCE/cell: exposed = 13.8 vs. control = 8.6). The mean frequencies of SCE among these workers had returned to preaccident levels at 2-year follow-up. SCE frequencies were examined in a group of 14 hospital workers exposed to EtO for an average of only 3.6 minutes per sterilizing task. The workers performed the task between six to 120 times during the 6-month study period. An exposure-related increase was observed in frequency of SCEs both in relation to EtO exposure and in relation to cigarette smoking, since smokers in both the exposed and control groups had cells containing the highest frequencies of SCEs. SCE frequency was studied in exposed hospital sterilization workers with a maximum measured peak EtO exposure of 36 ppm (Garry et al., 1979). These workers were found to have higher frequencies of SCEs when compared with nonexposed controls. The SCE frequencies of the exposed workers remained elevated at 3 weeks and 8 weeks after cessation of exposure. A possible cumulative or persistent effect on SCEs is noted in workers exposed daily to low levels of EtO (Laurent et al., 1984; Galloway et al., 1986; Laurent, 1988). Schulte et al. (1992) reported that the frequency of SCE and hemoglobin adducts increased with cumulative exposure to EtO. Workers exposed daily had a 17-fold increase in SCEs, whereas controls exposed occasionally to EtO had only a three- to fourfold increase in SCEs (Tates, 1991). These findings suggest that the frequency and rate of decline of SCEs depends on the duration and intensity of exposure (Laurent, 1988). Other factors affecting the frequency of SCEs include (a) new lymphocytes which may circulate and lower the SCE average by a dilution effect and (b) accumulation of a large amount of DNA lesions due to a brief exposure to EtO at high concentrations which may induce SCEs.

The peripheral lymphocytes of seven workers were observed to have elevated *chromosomal aberrations* (CAs) for as long as 18 months after a one-time accidental exposure to approximately 1,500 ppm for a period of 2 hours (Ehrenberg et al., 1981). An increased frequency of CAs has been observed in workers with relatively low levels (<1 ppm) of EtO exposure, although a significant effect of EtO on the frequency of micronuclei (MN) per cell was not found at this level of exposure (Högstedt et al., 1983). However, a significant ($p = 0.02$) increase in the frequency of MN was seen in sterilization workers exposed to EtO concentrations above 32 ppm (Schulte et al., 1995).

Neuroimaging

Magnetic resonance imaging (MRI) and *computer-assisted tomography* (CT) scans were both normal at the time of a 4-year follow-up examination of a 39-year-old man who developed persistent symptoms resembling Parkinson's disease after being acutely exposed to a high dose of EtO (Barbosa et al., 1992). The brain CT scan of a 19-year-old man who developed acute encephalopathy and peripheral neuropathy following exposure to EtO for 6 weeks also did not reveal any abnormalities (Endo et al., 1984). MRI revealed slightly enlarged ventricles in a 29-year-old woman who developed symptoms after working for 7 years adjacent to an EtO chemical sterilizer (Crystal et al., 1988; Dretchen et al., 1992).

Neuropathological Diagnosis

Neuropathological changes attributable to EtO exposure have been documented for both the central and peripheral nervous systems (Kuzuhara et al., 1983; Schröder et al., 1985; Ohnishi et al., 1985, 1986; Ohnishi and Murai, 1993; Matsuoka et al., 1990). Neuropathological studies demonstrate that EtO exposure induces a distal axonopathy. Histological studies of the sural nerve biopsies of three patients revealed decreased density of large myelinated fibers, reduction of cross-sectioned area of axons, reduction of axonal circularity, and the presence of myelin ovoids and Büngner bands compatible with a mild degree of axonal degeneration and regeneration (Ohnishi and Murai, 1993). A sural nerve biopsy was done in a 23-year-old man exposed to EtO at concentrations of up to 500 ppm for 5 months and who had experienced distal weakness of the lower extremities (Schröder et al., 1985). Light microscopy of a transverse section showed a moderate decrease in large myelinated nerve fibers, an increase in thin myelinated fibers, and, occasionally, disintegrated myelin fragments and bands of Büngner (i.e., a bundle of Schwann cell processes enclosed in the tube-like remnants of the original Schwann cell basal lamina). The Schwann cells were increased in number within the bands of Büngner. Several atropic axons were also seen. Some endoneurial cells showed vacuoles. No inflammatory infiltrates were seen, and many nerve fibers appeared to be normal. Endoneurial connective tissue was not increased (Fig. 19-3). Electron

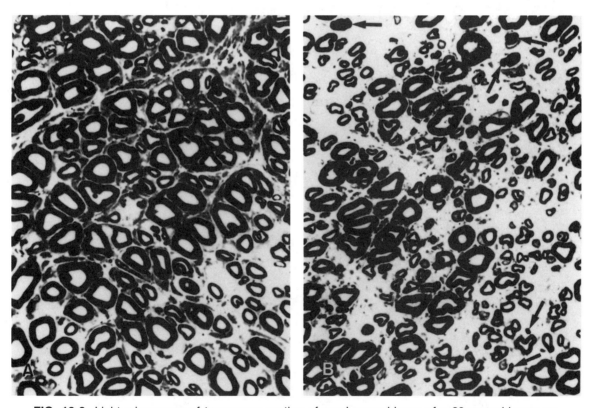

FIG. 19-3. Light microscopy of transverse section of sural nerve biopsy of a 23-year-old man exposed to ethylene oxide. **A:** Control sural nerve biopsy from 26-year-old unexposed man. **B:** Patient's sural nerve biopsy showing a loss of thick myelinated fibers and an increase of thin myelinated fibers. Myelin ovoids (*arrows*) and bands of Büngner are also seen.

microscopy of this patient's sural nerve biopsy revealed unusual cisternae with introverted hemidesmosomes in an endoneural fibroblast (Fig. 19-4A and 19-3B). Bands of Büngner were also visible (Fig. 19-4C). The electron micrograph of a longitudinal section of the nodes of Ranvier revealed small foci of vesicular disintegration in the para-

nodal myelin lamellae; these changes were noted in the proximal and distal paranodes (Fig. 19-5A and 19-5B). The vesicles were at least 20 to 30 nm and had no contract with the axoplasm. Accumulation of mitochondria was seen only on one side of the node of Ranvier (Fig. 19-5C). Most nodes of Ranvier were of normal width. There were no

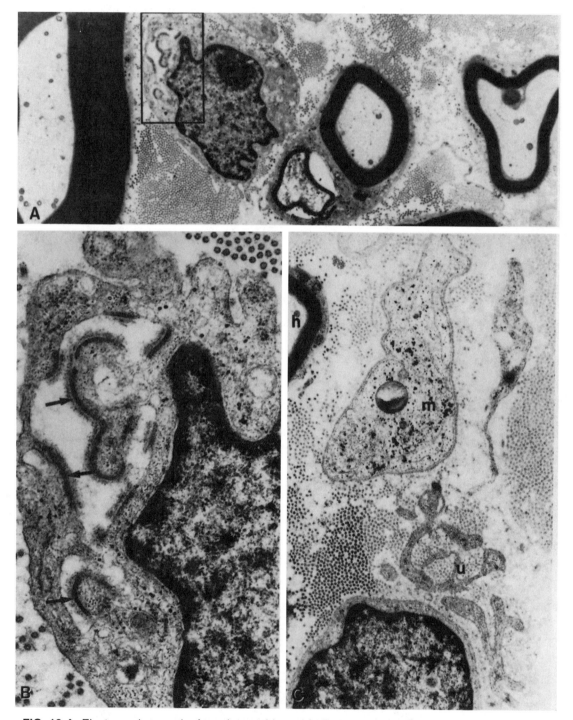

FIG. 19-4. Electron micrograph of sural nerve biopsy. **A:** Endoneurial fibroblasts (original magnification, ×8,700) showing dilated cisternae. **B:** The area in the insert of figure **A** at higher magnification (original magnification, ×40,000) showing inverted hemidesmosomes (*arrows*). **C:** Bands of Büngner (original magnification, ×14,000) from myelinated (*m*) and unmyelinated (*u*) nerve fibers which are seen adjacent to a hypomyelinated axon (*h*). (From Schröder et al., 1985, with permission.)

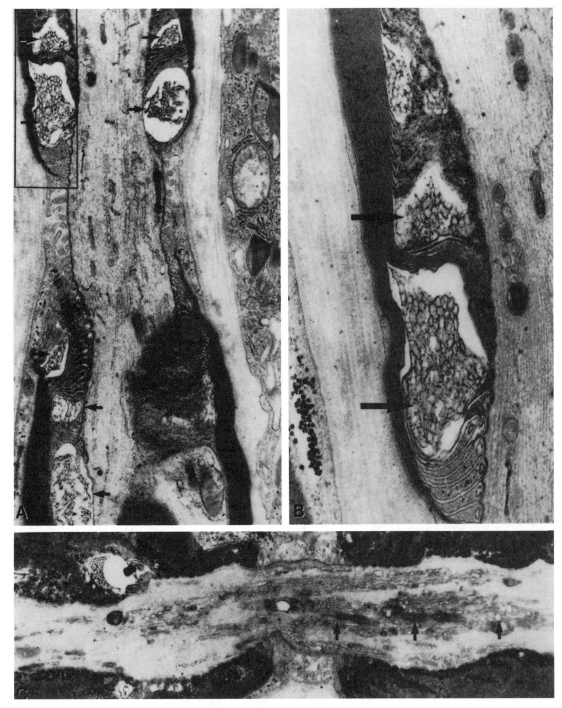

FIG. 19-5. Electron micrograph (original magnification, ×16,000) of longitudinal section of sural nerve biopsy. **A:** The paranodal myelin lamellae show several small foci of vesicular disintegration (*arrows*). **B:** Higher magnification (original magnification, ×27,000) of the area indicated by arrows in **A** demonstrating focal vesicular myelin disintegration at the site of the myelin loops. **C:** Axon at node of Ranvier contains vesicular and tubular membranous profiles with accumulated mitochondria seen only on one side of the node (*arrows*). (From Schröder et al., 1985, with permission.)

paranodal or segmentally demyelinated axons or onion bulb formation, suggesting that these paranodal myelin changes are reversible.

Two employees of a medical supplies factory developed distal symmetrical polyneuropathies after being exposed to EtO for approximately 6 months (Kuzuhara et al., 1983). The nerve biopsies of both patients showed axonal degeneration and regeneration. Light microscopy of a teased sural nerve from patient 2 (21-year-old man) revealed many myelin ovoids and balls along the length of the fiber.

In addition, several nodes of Ranvier appeared widened. Light microscopy of a transverse epon section of the sural nerve biopsy of patient 1 (33-year-old man) revealed a loss of myelinated fibers, several degenerating fibers, and occasional Schwann cell cytoplasms containing myelin fragments. Swollen Schwann cells containing numerous filaments, myelin fragments, debris, and vacuoles with and without granules were seen on the electron micrograph of the sural nerve biopsy of patient 1. Bands of Büngner were also visible indicating regeneration of axons.

Light microscopy of transverse sections of muscle biopsies of both patients showed atrophic fibers, scattered or grouped, with many target fibers. The electron micrograph of longitudinal sections of the muscle biopsies of both patients revealed smearing and distortion of the Z-bands. In addition, occasional myofibers showed electron-dense zones consisting of disrupted myofibrils, tightly packed thick filaments surrounded by normal myofibrils, and absence of mitochondria. Furthermore, the cytoplasm of several myofibers of both patients contained vacuoles, membranous bodies, and myelin fragments. Enzyme histochemistry of muscle from patient 2 revealed atrophy of both type 1 and type 2 fibers on myosin ATPase reaction and revealed dark angulated fibers, target, targetoid, and moth-eaten fibers on NADH-TR reaction, indicating denervation.

Experimental EtO neuropathy was produced in rats exposed to a one-time dose of 6 hours at 500 ppm or five doses over a week of 250 ppm for 6 hours. In both experiments, distal axonal degeneration was found both in peripheral and central myelinated axons of lumbar primary sensory neurons of rats. In hindleg nerves and in the fasciculus gracilis, myelinated fibers showed axonal degeneration sparing the nerve cell body of the lumbar dorsal root ganglion and myelinated fibers of lumbar dorsal and ventral roots. The rats exposed to 250 ppm also showed a retardation of growth and maturation of myelinated fibers in the presence of mild axonal degeneration (Ohnishi et al., 1985, 1986).

The exact mechanism of EtO neurotoxicity is unknown. However, due to its epoxide structure, EtO is a highly reactive alkylating agent (Högstedt et al., 1983; Segerbäck, 1983, 1990; Katoh et al., 1989). Because EtO is electrophilic, it reacts directly with the nucleophilic centers of cellular macromolecules such as the DNA, RNA, proteins, and lipids of biological systems without requiring metabolic activation (Ehrenberg and Osterman-Golkar, 1980; Ehrenberg and Hussain, 1981; Segerbäck, 1983, 1990; Katoh et al., 1989; Walker et al., 1990). Targets of EtO alkylation include nucleophilic amino acids such as guanine and adenine. Quantification of alkylated amino acids (adduct) formation (a marker of EtO exposure) suggests that the alkylation of the amino acids in cellular proteins and DNA occurs to the same extent in all tissues including the brain (Ehrenberg et al., 1974; Walker et al., 1990). Ethylene oxide binds covalently to DNA at the nucleophilic centers of guanine and adenine to form the adducts 7-(2-hydroxy-ethyl) guanine (7-HEG), O^6-(2-hydroxyethyl) guanine (O^6-HEG), and 3-(2-hydroxyethyl) adenine (3-HEAde) (Walker et al., 1990; Segerbäck, 1983, 1990). Reaction of EtO with DNA may be the basis for EtO to induce mutagenic effects and genotoxicity in a number of biological systems by producing point mutations, sister chromatid exchanges, and chromosomal aberrations (Halliwell, 1989; Walker et al., 1990; Schulte et al., 1995). DNA damage can lead to a consequent activation of poly(ADP-ribose) synthetase, a decrease in cellular ATP content, and an increase in intracellular free Ca^{2+} possibly damaging neurons (Halliwell, 1989). In addition, damage to the DNA of cells including neurons can induce cell death via apoptosis (Corcoran et al., 1994).

Impairment of creatine kinase activity, which is partially responsible for maintaining ATP levels in cells including neurons, may also be involved in the genesis of the encephalopathy and distal axonopathy associated with exposure to EtO. Serum creatine kinase activity was lowered by approximately 40%, and serum triglyceride levels were decreased by 20% in rats exposed to EtO at a concentration of 500 ppm 6 hours per day three times a week for 12 weeks (Matsuoka et al., 1990). Creatine kinase activity was decreased by 10% in the brain of these animals after a single 6-hour exposure to EtO at 500 ppm. The in vivo activity of creatine kinase was also decreased in the brain, spinal cord, and muscles after the fourth week of exposure to EtO. Duration of exposure was related to the decrease in creatine kinase activity, which was lowest after 12 weeks of exposure to EtO. Tissue levels of creatine kinase were shown to recover with time after cessation of exposure.

Another possibility is that lipid peroxidation occurs, as evidenced by an increase in the biological marker, malondialdehyde, in the livers of rats after exposure to EtO. A significant increase of malondialdehyde was not found in the brains of these same animals, although EtO crosses the BBB (Applegren et al., 1977; Katoh et al., 1989; Walker et al., 1990).

The aldehyde and acid metabolites of EtO have also been implicated in its neurotoxicity (Parry and Wallach, 1974). Glycoaldehyde and glyoxal inhibit oxidative phosphorylation, cellular respiration, and glucose metabolism. In addition, these aldehydes have been shown to depress serotonin metabolism and alter CNS amine levels (Jofre de Breyer et al., 1970; LaBorit et al., 1971).

PREVENTATIVE AND THERAPEUTIC MEASURES

The OSHA requires training at the time of initial assignment and at least annually thereafter for employees who are at risk for exposure to EtO concentrations at or above the action level. Training must include ways to detect EtO, information on the hazards of exposure, and methods to protect employees from hazardous exposures. An employer in operations using EtO is required to perform an initial monitoring of personal exposure levels to assess typical exposure concentrations per work shift. Periodic monitoring is required if employees are exposed to EtO concentrations which are at or above the action level (TWA = 0.5 ppm). Medical surveillance is required for those individuals exposed to concentrations at or above the action level for 30 days or more per year. This includes medical and work histories as well as a physical examination by a licensed physician, with emphasis on detecting EtO's effects on the nervous, pulmonary, hematological, and reproductive systems. Respirators, impermeable clothing, and face shields must be worn in areas where there is potential exposure to high concentrations of EtO. Splash-proof eye protection is required in areas where pure EtO liquid is stored or used (OSHA, 1995).

Risk of EtO exposure can be reduced by the use of technical and engineering controls and emergency warning systems to alert employees of sudden gas releases. Hazard warning signs are required on all EtO containers. The proper sealing of manufacturing and sterilization systems is imperative. EtO containers and transport pipes should be stored or in nonenclosed areas with adequate ventilation.

Aerating is necessary to remove EtO and its by-products from sterilized materials. The length of time required for aeration depends on the physical properties of the item, the type and temperature of the aeration process, and the intended use of the item. The more porous an item, the more difficult the EtO removal process. Nonporous metal and glass do not absorb EtO during sterilization and require no aeration if sterilized unwrapped. Items that do not come into direct contact with patients require less aeration; a lower level of EtO residue is required for implantable prostheses or surgical instruments than for equipment that does not come into direct contact with patients.

Since the odor of EtO is detectable only at concentrations above the established and recommended exposure limits, an employee noticing its smell is already at risk of exposure to toxic levels. With inhalation exposure, the patient should be immediately removed from the source to a well-ventilated area. Medical management is symptomatic for syncope and seizures. Vomiting should be induced in cases of oral ingestion of EtO (OSHA, 1995). Clothing that becomes wet with EtO should immediately be removed to prevent local injury to the skin as well as dermal absorption. Skin should also be washed immediately.

When symptomatic cases of EtO-induced polyneuropathy or encephalopathy are identified in the workplace, other employees should be assessed clinically as well as neuropsychologically and neurophysiologically for subclinical effects of exposure. Neuropsychological and neurophysiological examinations can be used to identify persons who are more susceptible to the effects of EtO and for whom removal from exposure would be advisable (Finelli et al., 1983). Individuals who have developed peripheral neuropathy or encephalopathy following exposure to EtO should avoid future contact with it and therefore may require vocational retraining.

CLINICAL EXPERIENCES

Group Studies

Clinical Effects and the Exposure Duration

Two groups of sterilizer gas (12% EtO and 88% Freon)-exposed workers that demonstrate the effects of duration of exposure and EtO levels were reported by Estrin et al. (1987, 1990). One group of ten women was exposed to ambient air EtO concentrations that were usually <15 ppm, with breathing zone levels as high as 250 ppm for a mean duration of 5 years. The other group was exposed to ambient air levels of levels <3 ppm, with occasional breathing zone peak exposures in excess of 200 ppm, for a mean duration of 11.6 years.

Each subject in the 5-year mean-exposure-duration group completed a symptoms check list, underwent a complete neurological examination, had an EEG, nerve conduction studies, and a neuropsychological assessment including an event-related potential test of cognitive function (P-300). Exposed workers reported more symptoms and more severe degrees of fatigue, confusion, depression, and anxiety than did nonexposed controls. Neuropsychological findings included poorer performance on neuropsychological tests involving psychomotor speed (e.g., finger-tapping test) and lower P-300 amplitude. In addition, the exposed group had diminished vibratory sensation and bilaterally hypoactive reflexes in the lower extremities. Nerve conduction studies and spectral analysis of EEG revealed no intergroup differences.

The eight hospital workers who had been chronically exposed to EtO while operating gas sterilizers for 5 to 20 years (mean: 11.6 years) were evaluated using a computerized psychometric test battery (CPTB), nerve conduction studies, P-300 event-related potentials, EEG spectral analysis, and a standardized neurological examination. Among these eight EtO-exposed workers there were four pertinent findings: (a) hand–eye coordination was significantly ($p = 0.03$) less accurate; (b) there was a significant ($r = 0.67$, $p \leq 0.05$) relationship between years of exposure and decreasing performance on the CPTB; (c) the exposed group performed more poorly than the control on all eight psychometric subtests; and (d) there was a significant ($r = -0.58$; $p \leq 0.05$) relationship between years of exposure and slowing of sural nerve conduction velocity.

Effects of Continuing Exposure After Ignoring the Odor of EtO

Three young men (ages: 17 to 23 years), who had been employed as EtO sterilization unit operators, developed symptoms including eye irritation, headaches, nausea, nervousness, insomnia, and signs of peripheral neuropathy (Finelli et al., 1983). Two of the men were employed as sterilization operators at the same surgical supply company; one worker had been employed for 1 year and the other had worked part time for 1.5 years before developing symptoms.

Both of these men reported noticing an odor at their workplace, suggesting they had been exposed to relatively high concentrations of EtO. These two workers experienced eye irritation, numbness and weakness in their distal lower extremities, and difficulty with gait. The third man worked 6 days per week at a plastics manufacturing company, where he was required to work in a sterilization tank for about 40 minutes. In addition, he had to unload the sterilized materials into a decontamination area for one half-hour each day. He too was aware of gas fumes but reportedly only wore a safety mask 75% of the time when he worked in the sterilization tank. His symptoms began approximately 3 months after he started working at the shop and included nervousness, insomnia, tingling sensations in both feet, and cramps in his hands and calves. One month later he began to experience difficulty with his gait, including repeated instances of stumbling. Neurological examination of these workers showed decreased vibratory sensation in the lower distal extremities, distal weakness which was more pronounced in the lower extremities, absent ankle jerks, flexor plantar response, dorsiflexor weakness, and bilateral footdrop with steppage gait. EMG and nerve conduction studies revealed abnormalities in all three workers (see Neurophysiological Diagnosis section). Marked clinical improvement was seen in all three men following removal from exposure to EtO.

Individual Studies

Chronic EtO Exposure Associated with Peripheral Neuropathy

A 24-year-old man began employment in a factory producing medical appliances as a sterilization worker after working in a factory producing synthetic rubber (Fukushima et al., 1986). Twenty-two months later, he began to experience numbness and weakness in both feet. He contacted an orthopedist who diagnosed his condition as ischialgia. Seven months later, the numbness had spread to his knees, at which time he consulted a physician who treated him for neuritis. His symptoms continued to progress, and 4 months later he was admitted to the hospital with gait difficulties, disturbed urinary function, and numbness of his fingers. His preliminary diagnosis was a suspected tumor of the spinal cord. Neurological examination revealed diminished sensation to pain, touch, and vibration. In addition, he had a steppage gait and a positive Romberg's sign, and his ankle jerk reflexes were absent. Urination was delayed. Within 2 days after admission to the hospital, his symptoms began to improve and he left the hospital 20 days later with the numbness limited to the soles of his feet and calves.

Subacute EtO Exposure Associated with Delirium, Dysarthria, and Neuropathy

A 19-year-old male sterilization worker began to feel general malaise, loss of appetite, and numbness of the fingers after 2 weeks of exposure to EtO (Endo et al., 1984; Fukushima et al., 1986). Over the course of the next 2 weeks he began to develop weakness of the lower limbs. He consulted a physician who diagnosed him as simply overworked. However, his symptoms continued to progress as he began to experience gait disturbances and dysarthria. On two occasions, he became delirious. He was admitted to a local university hospital 2 days later. Neurological examination was performed upon admission and revealed steppage gait and postural instability. Muscle tone was reduced in both legs. Diminished sensation to pain, touch, and vibration was noted in the lower extremities. He was also dysarthric. Brain CT scan and cerebrospinal fluid were normal (Endo et al., 1984).

Although the patient had been well oriented upon admission, that evening he had a visual hallucination in which the bodies of a man and woman were being sawed into pieces. He also claimed to smell a foul odor of blood and believed that he had to remove the bodies from his hospital room. During the next day he remained anxious about the events of the night before. That night, he had an auditory hallucination that he claimed directed him to wander around naked and then to urinate on his bed. Following this episode, he began packing up to leave, convinced that he should not remain in the hospital in his condition. He was medicated with antipsychotic drugs, and these symptoms faded within 3 days. His mental status continued to be normal thereafter. He was treated with multiple vitamins.

A follow-up neurological examination 3 months later revealed reduced numbness and weakness. However, diminished vibration sensation and hyperactive muscle stretch reflexes were noted in the distal lower extremities. Nerve conduction studies performed at this time were also abnormal.

Clinical Neuropathy and "Normal" Nerve Conduction Studies Following a Single Acute EtO Exposure

A 35-year-old man was referred to a medical clinic because of asthma. He was a nonsmoker and claimed that he did not use alcohol. While working as a repairman in a railway station, he had been exposed to a leak of EtO from a wagon about 18 meters from him, at which time he was not wearing protective equipment. He had been exposed to EtO for 4 hours per day for 4 days when he began to develop a cough, shortness of breath, and wheezing. He reported no clinically obvious symptoms of the central or peripheral nervous system. However, a neurological exam at the time revealed abnormal position sense in the toes and decreased ankle jerks. EMG and nerve conduction studies were normal except H-reflex amplitudes were markedly diminished compared to those elicited by a direct soleus response (Deschamps et al., 1992).

EtO and Reversible Peripheral Neuropathy

Case 1. A 38-year-old woman with no past medical history had been working in a sterilization center of a hospital in Italy for 2 years when she began to notice conjunctival irritation, and developed lower limb weakness, and distal paresthesias in both the upper and lower limbs (Zampollo et al., 1984). Her neurological exam was notable for slight distal vibratory hypesthesia of the lower limbs and decreased ankle jerk. EMG data revealed diffuse neuropathic damage, both sensory and motor, mainly in the lower limbs. A large reduction of mean action potential amplitude (4.2 mV in the left posterior tibial nerve and 3.2 mV in the right common peroneal nerve), a modest reduction of motor conduction velocities (43.8 milliseconds and 44.8 m/sec, respectively), and H-reflexes of 34.2 msec with only a 68% index were noted. These findings along with peripheral signs of denervation, evidenced by fibrillations of the lower limb muscles, pointed to an axonal neuropathy. Follow-up study 6 months later revealed a mean action potential amplitude of 6 and 6.5 mV for the left posterior tibial nerve and the right common peroneal nerve, respectively, with NCV improving to 48.2 and 59.2 m/sec. H-reflex improved to 29.5 with a 98% index.

Case 2. A 32-year-old female worker from the same hospital was also employed in the sterilization center for 2 years (Zampollo et al., 1984). She complained of headache, conjunctival irritation, and persistent distal paresthesias of the upper limbs. The neurological examination was negative. EMG showed signs of sensory impairment in the upper extremities. Sensory nerve conduction velocity (SCV) of the right ulnar nerve was 46.1 m/sec with an amplitude of 5.2 mV. EMG of the lower extremities revealed no abnormalities. Follow-up 6 months later revealed improved SCV of 53.4 m/sec and a sensory amplitude of 7 mV.

Case 3. A 23-year-old man had been exposed two to three times a day for several months to high levels of EtO (up to 500 ppm) while working in a food and medical sterilization factory prior to his admission to a hospital (Schröder et al., 1985) (see Neuropathological Diagnosis section). He complained of increasing weakness in his lower extremities and had decreased pinprick sensation in his legs. In addition, he reported experiencing a period of lethargy which was accompanied by memory impairment and difficulty thinking. This episode occurred after about 2 months of exposure. Neurological examination revealed normal mental status and an unsteady and cautious gait. The patient had slight weakness of the upper right face and symmetrical distal limb weakness. Muscle stretch reflexes were normal except for absent ankle jerks. Pinprick sensation was diminished in the lower extremities. On examination 1 year after cessation of exposure, the patient's condition had markedly improved. Although there was a slight symmetrical hypersensitivity and hypesthesia, the weakness in his lower limbs had disappeared.

Case 4. A 33-year-old man began to experience paresthesias and weakness in the distal-most portions of his upper and lower extremities after operating a sterilizer for approximately 3 months in a factory that produced medical supplies (Kuzuhara et al., 1983). The air EtO levels to which he was exposed were estimated to exceed 700 ppm for several minutes each time the sterilizer door was opened. The

previous operator of the sterilizer had left the job complaining of paresthesias and weakness in his extremities. The patient continued to work despite his early symptoms of polyneuropathy, and soon he also began to have mild difficulty with his gait. He continued to work for another 3 months, because he still could use his upper extremities.

When he could no longer walk well and his hands were numb and weak, the patient sought medical attention. He was admitted to a local hospital, where a neurological examination revealed symmetrical weakness of his distal extremities and loss of cutaneous sensory perception. The patient was removed from his job for several weeks and his symptoms subsided. However, as soon as he felt able, he returned to the same job and within a few weeks his symptoms began to return. He was readmitted to the hospital, where the neurological examination revealed moderate bilateral weakness of the lower extremities but no muscle wasting. Patellar reflexes were decreased and ankle jerks were absent bilaterally. Sensations of touch, pain, temperature, and vibration were decreased in the feet. Laboratory data were normal. Electromyography revealed denervation in the distal lower extremities. Sural nerve biopsy studies confirmed the diagnosis of peripheral neuropathy associated with exposure to EtO. The patient's symptoms cleared 2 months after no further exposure to EtO.

Case 5. A 21-year-old man started to notice symptoms 6 months after he began loading and unloading the sterilizers at the same factory as Case D (Kuzuhara et al., 1983). He continued to work and his symptoms continued to progress. He was admitted to the hospital 1 month after the onset of his symptoms, at which time a neurological examination revealed staggering gait and moderate weakness in the distal extremities. Touch, pain and temperature, and vibration sensations were also reduced in the distal portions of the upper and lower extremities. Position sensation was normal. Deep tendon reflexes were normal and plantar response was flexor. All laboratory data including cerebrospinal fluid were normal. Nerve conduction, EMG, and sural nerve biopsy studies confirmed the diagnosis of peripheral neuropathy associated with exposure to EtO. His symptoms cleared 1 month after his removal from exposure to EtO.

EtO and Parkinsonism

A 39-year-old man was comatose for 3 days following an intense acute exposure to EtO. When he regained consciousness he showed a global parkinsonian syndrome including bradykinesia, resting tremor, and severe motor disability. Symptoms were partially controlled with levodopa. Neurological exam 4 years after the incident disclosed moderate bradykinesia, rigidity, resting tremor, shuffling gait, poor facial mimic, stooped posture, and brisk deep tendon reflexes. MRI scans, CT scans, and cerebrospinal fluid were normal. Alternative etiologies for this patient's condition could not be identified, suggesting that the acute intense EtO exposure resulted in this patient's acute onset of an irreversible parkinsonian syndrome (Barbosa et al., 1992).

REFERENCES

American Conference of Governmental Industrial Hygienists (ACGIH). *Threshold limit values (TLVs) for chemical substances and physical agents and biological exposure indices (BEIs)*. Cincinnati: ACGIH, 1995.

Alomar A, Camarasa JMG, Noguera J, Aspinolea F. Ethylene oxide dermatitis. *Contact dermatitis* 1981;7:205–207.

Amoore JE, Hautala E. Odor as an aid to chemical safety: odor thresholds compared with threshold limit values and volatilities for 214 industrial chemicals in air and water dilution. *J Appl Toxicol* 1983;3:272–290.

Applegren LE, Eneroth G, Grant C. Studies on ethylene oxide, whole body autoradiography and dominant lethal test in mice. *Proc Eur Soc Toxicol* 1977;18:315–317.

Barbosa ER, Comerlatti LR, Haddad MS, Scaff M. Parkinsonism secondary to ethylene oxide exposure: case report. *Arq Neurosiquiatr* 1992;50(4):531–533.

Baumbach N, Herzog V, Schiller F. *In-vitro* study of permeation of ethylene oxide through human skin. *Dermatol Monschr* 1987;173:328–322.

Biro L, Fischer AA, Price E. Ethylene oxide burns. *Arch Dermatol* 1974;110:924–925.

Brown CD, Wong BA, Fennell TR. *In vivo* and *vitro* kinetics of ethylene oxide metabolism in rats and mice. *Toxicol Appl Pharmacol* 1996;136:8–19.

Brugnone F, Perbellini L, Faccini G, Pasini F, Bartolucci GB, DeRosa E. Ethylene oxide exposure: biological monitoring by analysis of alveolar air and blood. *Int Arch Occup Environ Health* 1986;58:105–112.

Bryant HE, Visser ND, Yoshida K. Ethylene oxide sterilizer use and short-term symptoms amongst workers. *J Soc Occup Med* 1989;39:101–106.

Burgaz S, Rezanko R, Kara S, Karakaya AE. Thioethers in urine of sterilization personnel exposed to ethylene oxide. *J Clin Pharmacol Ther* 1992;17:169–172.

Clay KL, Murphy RC. On the metabolic acidosis of ethylene glycol intoxication. *Toxicol Appl Pharmacol* 1977;39:39–49.

Coen G, Weiss B. Oxidation of ethylene glycol to glycoaldehyde by mammalian tissues. *Enz Biol Clin (Basal)* 1966;6:288–296.

Corcoran GB, Fix L, Jones DP, et al. Contemporary issues in toxicology. Apoptosis: molecular control point in toxicity. *Toxicol Appl Pharmacol* 1994;128:169–181.

Crystal HA, Schaumburg HH, Grober E, Fuld PA, Lipton RB. Cognitive impairment and sensory loss associated with chronic low level ethylene oxide exposure. *Neurology* 1988;38:567–569.

Dellarco VL, Generoso WM, Saga GA, Fowle JR, Jacobsen-Kram D. Review of the mutagenicity of ethylene oxide. *Environ Molec Mutat* 1990;16:85–103.

Deschamps D, Rosenberg N, Soler P, et al. Persistent asthma after accidental exposure to ethylene oxide. *Br J Ind Med* 1992;49:523–525.

Dretchen KL, Balter NJ, Schwartz SL, et al. Cognitive dysfunction in a patient with long term exposure to EtO: role of EtO as a causal factor. *J Occup Med* 1992;34:1106–1113.

Dunkelberg H. Carcinogenicity of ethylene oxide and 1,2-propylene oxide upon intragastric administration to rats. *Br J Cancer* 1982;46:924–933.

Ehrenberg L, Hussain S. Genetic toxicity of some important epoxides. *Mutat Res* 1981;86:1–113.

Ehrenberg L, Hiesche KD, Osterman-Golkar S, Wennberg I. Evaluation of genetic risks of alkylating agents: tissue doses in mouse from air contaminated with ethylene oxide. *Mutat Res* 1974;24:83–103.

Ehrenberg L, Osterman-Golkar S, Segerback D, Svensson K, Calleman CJ. Evaluation of genetic risks of alkylating agents. III. Alkylation of haemoglobin after metabolic conversion of ethene to ethene oxide *in vivo*. *Mutat Res* 1977;45:175–184.

Ehrenberg L, Osterman-Golkar S. Alkylation of macromolecules for detecting mutagenic agents. *Teratogen Carcinogen Mutagen* 1980;1:105–127.

Ehrenberg L, Hällström T, Osterman-Golkar S. *Etylenoxid. Kriteriedokument för Gränsvärden*. Stockholm: Arbetarskyddsverket, 1981:1–33.

Endo M, Sato T, Umaki I, Note S. Correspondence: ethylene oxide withdrawal delirium. *Biol Psychiatry* 1984;19:1731–1734.

Estrin WJ, Cavalieri S, Becker C, Wald P, Jones J. Evidence of neurological dysfunction related to long term ethylene oxide exposure. *Arch Neurol* 1987;44:1283–1286.

Estrin WJ, Bowler RM, Lash A, Becker CE. Neurotoxicological evaluation of hospital sterilizer workers exposed to ethylene oxide. *Clin Toxicol* 1990;28:1–20.

Filser JG, Bolt HM. Exhalation of ethylene oxide by rats on exposure to ethylene. *Mutat Res* 1983;120:57–60.

Filser JG, Denk B, Tornquist M, Kessler W, Ehrenberg L. Pharmacokinetics of ethylene in man; body burden with ethylene oxide and hydroxyethylation of hemoglobin due to endogenous and environmental ethylene. *Arch Toxicol* 1992;66:157–163.

Filser JG, Kreuzer PE, Greim H, Bolt HM. New scientific arguments for the regulation of ethylene oxide residues in skin-care products. *Arch Toxicol* 1994;68:401–405.

Finelli PF, Morgan TF, Yaar I, Granger CV. Ethylene oxide induced polyneuropathy: a clinical and electrophysiological study. *Arch Neurol* 1983;40:419–421.

Fiserova-Bergervova, V. Physiological models for pulmonary administration and elimination of inert vapors and gases. In: Fiserova-Bergervova V, ed. *Modeling of inhalation exposure to vapors: uptake, distribution, and elimination*, vol 1. Boca Raton, FL: CRC Press, 1983:73–100.

Fishbein L. Degradation and residues of alkylating agents. *Ann NY Acad Sci* 1969;163:869–894.

Florack JM, Zielhuis GA. Occupational ethylene oxide exposure and reproduction. *Int Arch Occup Environ Health* 1990;62:273–277.

Föst U, Törnqvist M, Leutbecher M, et al. Effects of variation in detoxication rate on dose monitoring through adducts. *Hum Exp Toxicol* 1995;14:201–203.

Fukushima T, Abe K, Nakagawa A, Osaki Y, Yoshida N, Yamane Y. Chronic ethylene oxide poisoning in a factory manufacturing medical appliances. *J Soc Occup Med* 1986;36:118–123.

Galloway SM, Berry PK, Nichols WW, et al. Chromosome aberrations in individuals occupationally exposed to ethylene oxide, and in a large control population. *Mutat Res* 1986;170:55–74.

Gardiner TH, Waechter JM, Stevenson DE. Epoxy compounds. In: Clayton GD, Clayton FE, eds. *Patty's industrial hygiene and toxicology*, 4th ed. New York: John Wiley and Sons, 1994:4207–4218.

Garry VF, Hozier J, Jacobs D, Wade RL, Gray PG. Ethylene oxide: evidence of human chromosomal effects. *Environ Mutagen* 1979;1:375–382.

Gérin M, Tardif R. Urinary *N*-acetyl-2 hydroxyethyl-L-cysteine in rats as biological indicator of ethylene oxide exposure. *Fundam Appl Toxicol* 1986;7:419–423.

Gessner PK, Parke DV, Williams RT. Studies in detoxification: 86. The metabolites of ^{14}C-labeled ethylene glycol. *Biochem J* 1961;79:482–488.

Gregus Z, Klaassen CD. Mechanisms of toxicity. In: Klaassen CD, ed. *Casarett and Doull's toxicology the basic science of poisons*, 5th ed. New York: McGraw-Hill, 1996:35–74.

Grober E, Crystal H, Lipton RB, Schaumburg H. Author's commentary: ethylene oxide is associated with cognitive dysfunction. *J Occup Med* 1992;34:1114–1116.

Gross JA, Haas ML, Swift TR. Ethylene oxide neurotoxicity: report of four cases and review of the literature. *Neurology* 1979;29:978–983.

Hallier E, Langhof T, Leutbecher M, et al. Polymorphism of glutathione conjugation of methyl bromide, ethylene oxide and dichlormethane in human blood: influence on the induction of sister chromatid exchanges in lymphocytes. *Arch Toxicol* 1993;67:173–178.

Halliwell B. Oxidants and the central nervous system: some fundamental questions. Is oxidant damage relevant to Parkinson's disease, Alzheimer's disease, traumatic injury and stroke? *Acta Neurol Scand* 1989;126:23–33.

Harrison VC. Ethylene, an ovulatory hormone [Letter]? *Lancet* 1981; 21:438.

Högstedt B, Gullberg B, Hedner K, et al. Chromosomal aberration and micronuclei in bone marrow cells and peripheral blood lymphocytes in human exposed to ethylene oxide. *Hereditas* 1983;98:105–113.

Hollingsworth RL, Row VK, Oyen F. Toxicity of ethylene oxide determined on experimental animals. *Arch Ind Health* 1956;13:217–227.

Jay WM, Swift TR, Hull DS. Possible relationship of ethylene oxide exposure to cataract formation. *Am J Ophthalmol* 1982;93:727–732.

Jofre de Breyer IJ, Ortiz A, Soehring K. The effects of aldehydes on serotonin metabolism in rat liver slices. *Pharmacology* 1970;3:85–90.

Jones AR, Wells G. The comparative metabolism of 2-bromoethanol and ethylene oxide in the rat. *Xenobiotica* 1981;11:763–770.

Joyner RE. Chronic toxicity of ethylene oxide: A study of human responses to long term low level exposures. *Arch Environ Health* 1964;8:700–710.

Katoh M, Cachiero NLA, Cornett CV, Cain KT, Rutledge JC, Generoso WM. Fetal anomalies produced subsequent to treatment of zygotes with ethylene oxide or ethylene methane sulfonate are not likely due to the usual genetic causes. *Mutat Res* 1989;210:337–344.

Katoh T, Higashi K, Inoue N. Lipid peroxidation and metabolism of glutathione in rat liver and brain following ethylene oxide inhalation. *Toxicology* 1990;58:1–9.

Klees J, Lash A, Bowler RM, Shore M, Becker CE. Neuropsychological impairment in a cohort of hospital workers chronically exposed to ethylene oxide. *Clin Toxicol* 1990;28:21–28.

Krishnan K, Gargas ML, Fennel TR, Andersen ME. A physiologically based description of ethylene oxide dosimetry in the rat. *Toxicol Ind Hlth* 1992;8:121–140.

Kuzuhara S, Kanazawa I, Nakanishi T, Egashira T. Ethylene oxide polyneuropathy. *Neurology* 1983;33:377–380.

LaBorit H, Baron C, London A, Olympie J. Activité nerveuse centrale et pharmacologie générale comparé du glyoxylate, du glycolate et du glycoaldéhyde. *Agressologie* 1971;12(3):187–211.

Landrigan PJ, Meinhardt TJ, Gordon J, et al. Ethylene oxide: an overview of toxicological and epidemiological research. *Am J Ind Med* 1984;6:103–115.

Laurent C, Frederic J, Leonard AY. Sister chromatid exchanges frequency in workers exposed to high levels of ethylene oxide, in a hospital sterilization service. *Int Arch Occup Environ Health* 1984;54:33–43.

Laurent C. SCE increases after an acute accidental exposure to EtO then recovery to normal after two years. *Mutat Res* 1988;204:711–717.

Lerda D, Rizzi R. Cytogenic study of persons occupationally exposed to ethylene oxide. *Mutat Res* 1992;281:31–37.

Lewis RJ. *Hazardous chemicals desk reference.* New York: Van Nostrand Reinhold, 1993:580–581.

Martis L, Kroes R, Darby TD, Woods EF. Disposition kinetics of ethylene oxide, ethylene glycol, and 2-chloroethanol in the dog. *J Toxicol Environ Health* 1982;10:847–856.

Matsuoka M, Igisu H, Inoue N, Hori H, Tanaka I. Inhibition of creatine kinase activity by ethylene oxide. *Br J Ind Med* 1990;47:44–47.

McKelvey JA, Zemantis MA. The effects of ethylene oxide exposure on tissue glutathione levels in rats and mice. *Drug Chem Toxicol* 1986;9:51–66.

Mortimer VD, Kercher SL. *Control technology for ethylene oxide sterilization in hospitals.* NIOSH Publication No. 89-120. Cincinnati: National Institute for Occupational Safety and Health, 1989.

National Institute of Occupational Safety and Health (NIOSH). Current Intelligence Bulletin 35. *Ethylene oxide.* Cincinnati: US Department of Health and Human Services, May 22, 1981.

National Institute of Occupational Safety and Health (NIOSH). *Pocket guide to chemical hazards.* Cincinnati: US Department of Health and Human Services, CDC, June 1994.

Occupational Safety and Health Administration (OSHA). Occupational exposure to ethylene oxide: final standard. *Federal Register* 1984;49:25767.

Occupational Safety and Health Administration (OSHA). *Code of federal regulations,* 29, 1910.1000/.1047. Washington, DC: Office of the Federal Register, National Archives and Records Administration, 1995:411–431.

Ohnishi A, Murai Y. Polyneuropathy due to ethylene oxide, propylene oxide, and butylene oxide. *Environ Res* 1993;60:242–247.

Ohnishi A, Inoue N, Yamamoto T, et al. Ethylene oxide induces central peripheral distal axonal degeneration of the lumbar primary neurones in rats. *Br J Ind Med* 1985;42:373–379.

Ohnishi A, Inoue N, Yamamoto T, et al. Ethylene oxide neuropathy in rats: exposure to 250 ppm. *J Neurol Sci* 1986;74:4215–221.

O'Leary RK, Guess WL. Toxicological studies on certain medical grade plastics sterilized by ethylene oxide. *J Pharm Sci* 1968;57:12–17.

Osterman-Golkar S, Bergmark E. Occupational exposure to ethylene oxide. Relation between *in vivo* dose and exposure dose. *Scand J Environ Health* 1988;58:105–112.

Parkinson A. Biotransformation of xenobiotics. In: Klaassen CD, ed. *Casarett and Doull's toxicology the basic science of poisons,* 5th ed., New York: McGraw-Hill, 1996:113–186.

Parry MF, Wallach R. Ethylene glycol poisoning. *Am J Med* 1974;57:143–150.

Pero RW, Bryngelsson T, Witdegren G, Godstedt B, Welinder H. A reduced capacity for unscheduled DNA synthesis from individuals exposed to propylene oxide and ethylene oxide. *Mutat Res* 1982;104:193–200.

Poothullil J, Shimizu A, Day RP, Dolovich J. Anaphylaxis from products and ethylene oxide gas. *Intern Med* 1975;82:58–63.

Rowe VK, Wolf MA. Glycols. In: Clayton GD, Clayton FE, eds. *Patty's industrial hygiene and toxicology,* vol IIc, 3rd ed. New York: John Wiley and Sons, 1982:3817–3908.

Salinas E, Sasich L, Hall DH, Kennedy RM, Morriss H. Acute ethylene oxide intoxication. *Drug Int Clin Pharm* 1981;15:384–386.

Sax NI. *Dangerous properties of industrial chemicals,* 5th ed. New York: Van Nostrand Reinhold, 1979.

Schmiedel G, Filser JG, Bolt HM. Rat liver microsomal transformation of ethane to oxirane *in vitro. Toxicol Lett* 1983;19:293–297.

Schröder JM, Hoheneck M, Weis J, Deist H. Ethylene oxide polyneuropathy: clinical follow up study with morphometric and electron microscopic findings in a sural nerve biopsy. *J Neurol* 1985;232:83–90.

Schröder JM, Hallier E, Peter H, Bolt HM. Dissociation of a new glutathione *S*-transferase activity in human erythrocytes. *Biochem Pharmacol* 1992;43:1671–1674.

Schulte PA, Boeniger M, Walker JT, et al. Biological markers in hospital workers exposed to low levels of ethylene oxide. *Mutat Res* 1992;278:237–251.

Schulte PA, Walker JT, Boeniger MF, Tsuchiya Y, Halperin WE. Molecular, cytogenetic, and hematological effects of ethylene oxide on female hospital workers. *J Occup Environ Med* 1995;37:313–320.

Segerbäck D. Alkylation of DNA and hemoglobin in the mouse following exposure to ethene and ethene oxide. *Chem Biol Interact* 1983;45: Segerbäck D. Reaction products in hemoglobin and DNA after *in vitro* treatment with ethylene oxide and *N*-(2-hydroxyethyl)-*N*-nitrosourea. *Carcinogenesis* 1990;11:307–312.

Sheikh K. Adverse health effects of ethylene oxide and occupational exposure limits. *Am J Ind Med* 1984;6:117–127.

Tardif R, Goyal R, Brodeur J, Gérin M. Species differences in the urinary disposition of some metabolites of ethylene oxide. *Fundam Appl Toxicol* 1987;9:448–457.

Tates AD, Grummt T, Törnqvist M, et al. Biological and chemical monitoring of occupational exposure to ethylene oxide. *Mutat Res* 1991;250:483–497.

Törnqvist MÅ, Osterman-Golkar S, Kautiainen A, Jensen S, Farmer PB, Ehrenberg L. Tissue doses of ethylene oxide in cigarette smokers determined from adduct levels in hemoglobin. *Carcinogenesis* 1986;7:1519–1521.

Törnqvist MÅ, Almberg JG, Bergmark EN, Nilsson S, Osterman-Golkar SM. Ethylene oxide doses in ethene-exposed fruit store workers. *Scand J Work Environ Health* 1989;15:436–438.

Törnqvist MÅ. Is ambient ethene a cancer risk factor? *Environ Hlth Perspect* 1994;102[Suppl 4]:157–160.

United States Environmental Protection Agency (USEPA): Ethylene oxide: tolerances for residues. US Code Federal Register Title 40, Part 185.2850, 1992:456.

United States Environmental Protection Agency (USEPA). Drinking water regulations and health advisories. EPA 822-R-96-001. Washington, DC: Office of Water, 1996.

United States Food and Drug Administration (USFDA). US Code Federal Register Title 21, Parts 175.105, 176.180, 176. 210, 176.300, 178.1010, 178.3520, 178.3570; 1993:129–144, 196–200, 202–206, 317–325, 355–358.

van Sittert NJ, Beulink GDJ, van Vliet EWN, van der Waal H. Monitoring occupational exposure to ethylene oxide by the determination of hemoglobin adducts. *Environ Health Perspect* 1993;99:217–220.

Walker VE, Fennell TR, Boucheron JA, et al. Macromolecular adducts of ethylene oxide: a literature review and time-course study on the formation of 7-(2-hydroxyethyl) guanine following exposure of rats by inhalation. *Mutat Res* 1990;233:151–164.

Wesley F, Rourke B, Darbishire O. The formation of persistent toxic chlorohydrins in foods fumigated with ethylene oxide and propylene oxide. *J Food Sci* 1965;30:1037–1042.

Windebank AJ, Blexrud MD. Residual ethylene oxide in hollow fiber hemodialysis units is neurotoxic *in vitro. Ann Neurol* 1989;26:63–68.

Wolfs P, Durieux M, Scailteur V, Haxhe J-J, Zumofen M, Lauwerys R. Monitoring of workers exposed to ethylene oxide in a plant distributing sterilizing gases and in units for sterilizing medical equipment. *Arch Mal Prof* 1983;44:321–328.

World Health Organization (WHO). *Ethylene oxide. IARC monographs on the evaluation of carcinogenic risks to humans,* 60. Geneva: WHO, 1994.

Zampollo A, Zacchetti O, Pisati G. On ethylene oxide neurotoxicity: report of two cases of peripheral neuropathy. *Ital J Neurol Sci* 1984;V:59–62.

CHAPTER 20

Carbon Monoxide

Carbon monoxide (CO) is an odorless, colorless, nonirritating, combustible gas (Sax, 1979; Hardy and Thom, 1994), commonly formed as a byproduct of incomplete combustion of organic materials and petroleum fuels (Beard, 1982; Gajdos et al., 1991). CO binds to hemoglobin and interferes with the delivery of oxygen from the lungs to the various tissues of the body (Bernard, 1927). The hypoxemia resulting from the binding of CO to hemoglobin (carboxyhemoglobin) is associated with numerous deaths each year and with nonfatal but severely disabling damage to the nervous system (Winter and Miller, 1976; Dolan, 1985; Cobb and Etzel, 1991; Risser and Schneider, 1995). From 1979 through 1988, there were 56,133 CO exposure-related deaths in the United States (Cobb and Etzel, 1991).

Most occupational exposures occur in industries where CO production is expected, but where improper ventilation of the workplace allows the gas to accumulate. The most tragic reports tell of unsuspecting families who were killed or suffered permanent neurological damage because CO was released from faulty gas heating units or indoor wood- or coke-burning stoves while they slept (MMWR, 1992, 1993).

Acute and chronic nonfatal exposures to CO have been associated with both reversible and persistent neurological effects (Thom and Keim, 1989; White et al., 1992). Neuropathological abnormalities and developmental behavioral deficits have been reported in children born to pregnant mothers exposed to CO (Norman and Halton, 1990). The consequential central nervous system effects of CO-induced hypoxemia are frequently more severe among persons who are more vulnerable to the effects of hypoxia, such as those with preexisting coronary arteriosclerosis or cerebrovascular disease (Aronow and Isbell, 1973; Aronow, 1976; Winter and Miller, 1976). Because many of the symptoms associated with mild acute CO poisoning are transient and nonspecific, the potential of greater harm from continuing and cumulative exposures to CO frequently goes unrecognized. CO exposure should be considered in patients presenting with nonspecific situation-related flulike symptoms, lethargy, confusion, seizures, somnolence, syncope, or

coma (Grace and Platt, 1981; Neufeld et al., 1981; Fisher and Rubin, 1982; Dolan, 1985; Thom and Keim, 1989).

SOURCES OF EXPOSURE

CO is ubiquitous. Natural sources include gaseous emissions from volcanoes, forest fires, and photochemical degradation of organic compounds in the atmosphere (Jaffe, 1970). CO produced by marine brown algae is released into the ocean and subsequently into the atmosphere. It has also been detected in fresh water samples (Swinnerton et al., 1970). Incomplete combustion of coal, wood, tobacco, and petroleum products is the principal source of CO in the environment (Russell et al., 1976; Beard, 1982; Gajdos et al., 1991). Exposure to CO occurs around barbecues that use charcoal briquettes; around stoves and heating appliances that use organic gases; and from fumes that escape from wood stoves and fireplaces, kerosene- and oil-fired portable home heating appliances, and the gasoline-powered small engines used in generators and other small engine–powered equipment (Grace and Platt, 1981; Gajdos et al., 1991; Cobb and Etzel, 1991; Madani et al., 1992; MMWR, 1993; Chung et al., 1994). Unintentional exposures to CO are more common during cold weather when these appliances are used without adequate ventilation (Chung et al., 1994; Risser and Schneider, 1995; Cook et al., 1995). For example, in Korea, where charcoal briquettes (Yeontan) are commonly used to heat homes, improper installation or inadequate ventilation of the Yeontan heating system (Ondol) has been implicated in many cases of unintentional CO poisoning (Chung et al., 1994). Iron foundry workmen who work near the blast furnaces are exposed to high levels of CO (Virtamo and Tossavainen, 1976; Lewis et al., 1992). Professional and volunteer firefighters as well as the victims of fires are exposed to high levels of CO during building fires (Brown et al., 1992; Cook et al., 1995). Of the 981 cases of CO poisoning reported in Colorado from 1986 through 1991, 355 were related to fires (Cook et al., 1995). Intentional nonoccupational exposures to CO occur during successful and failed suicide attempts (Shimosegawa et al., 1992; Zagami et al., 1993).

Exposure to organic gases such as methane, butane, propane, and *natural gas* [i.e., a naturally occurring gas composed of 85% methane, 10% ethane, and small amounts (less than 5%) of propane, butane, and nitrogen] produces tissue hypoxia. Organic gases are asphyxiants and cause hypoxia by directly excluding oxygen from entering the lungs (Sax, 1979). In addition, the incomplete combustion of these organic gases yields CO as a byproduct (Finck, 1966; Sax, 1979; Baron et al., 1989). Hockey players and recreational ice skaters are exposed to CO emitted from fuel-powered ice resurfacing equipment, and warehouse workers are exposed to CO emitted from propane-fueled forklift engines (Fawcett et al., 1992; Lee et al., 1994). The use of propane-powered floor refinishing equipment has been associated with high indoor air concentrations of CO (MMWR, 1993). High indoor ambient air concentrations of CO can also occur during the use of defective or improperly installed cooking stoves that use liquid propane as fuel (see Clinical Experiences section).

CO formed by incomplete combustion of gasoline is released in automobile exhaust fumes. Although the establishment of the Clean Air Act and the subsequent development of more efficient automobile engines has resulted in significant decreases in automobile-related CO exposures (Cobb and Etzel, 1991), automotive repair persons and especially do-it-yourselfers can be exposed to high levels of CO while operating inefficiently running engines in poorly ventilated areas (MMWR, 1992). Professional drivers and ordinary persons are exposed to CO when operating the gas or diesel engines of their automobiles, trucks, buses, or boats. Carbon monoxide levels inside a car or truck frequently exceed those in the ambient air, particularly if the vehicle's exhaust system is faulty (Weisel et al., 1992). In addition, tollbooth workers and police officers on traffic duty are frequently exposed to neurotoxic levels of CO (Gilbert and Glaser, 1959; Burgess et al., 1977; Stern et al., 1988). High levels of CO occur in tunnels and enclosed parking garages (Finck, 1966; Stern et al., 1988; Kamada et al., 1994). Carbon monoxide may invade the indoor residential air from a garage located under the living areas (Kamada et al., 1994).

CO results from breakdown of dihalomethanes (e.g., methylene chloride) (Carlsson and Hultengren, 1975; Kubic and Anders, 1975; Stewart and Hake, 1976); craftspersons and hobbyists who use methylene chloride-based paint removers are thus exposed (Stewart and Hake, 1976). Nonsmoking triacetate fiber–production workers exposed to methylene chloride at levels of up to 90 ppm had blood COHb levels of up to 4.0%; COHb levels in exposed workers who also smoked cigarettes were as high as 6.4% (Soden et al., 1996). Exposure to methylene chloride at an 8-hour time-weighted average (TWA) concentration of 150 ppm is equivalent to an 8-hour TWA exposure of 35 ppm of CO (DiVincenzo and Kaplan, 1981). The *Occupational Safety and Health Administration's* (OSHA) established 8-hour TWA permissible exposure limit (PEL) for methylene chloride is 500 ppm, but the OSHA PEL for CO is 50 ppm,

indicating that significant exposures to CO can occur among persons using methylene chloride (DiVincenzo and Kaplan, 1981; OSHA, 1995) (see Exposure Limits and Safety Regulations section).

EXPOSURE LIMITS AND SAFETY REGULATIONS

CO is toxic at very low concentrations; exposure to 0.1% CO in air results in a carboxyhemoglobin (COHb) level of 50% (Smith, 1996). Therefore, monitoring of ambient air CO levels is necessary to prevent neurotoxicity. Since the odor threshold for CO is 100,000 ppm (Amoore and Hautala, 1983), several thousand times higher than the concentration at which severe neurotoxic effects can occur, the odor of CO cannot be relied on to provide an adequate warning of exposure. OSHA has established an 8-hour TWA PEL of 50 ppm (OSHA, 1995). The *National Institute for Occupational Safety and Health* (NIOSH) recommends a 10-hour TWA exposure limit (REL) of 35 ppm, with a 15-minute short-term exposure ceiling of 200 ppm, which should not be exceeded during any part of the work day. The NIOSH immediately dangerous to life and health concentration for CO is 1,200 ppm (NIOSH, 1997). The *American Conference of Governmental and Industrial Hygienists* (ACGIH) recommends an 8-hour TWA threshold limit value (TLV) of 25 ppm (ACGIH, 1995) (Table 20-1).

TABLE 20-1. *Established and recommended occupational and environmental exposure limits for carbon monoxide in air and water*

	Air (ppm)[a]	Water (mg/L)[a]
Odor threshold*	100,000	2.7
OSHA		
PEL (8-hr TWA)	50	—
PEL ceiling (15-min TWA)	—	—
PEL ceiling (5-min peak)	—	—
NIOSH		
REL (10-hr TWA)	35	—
STEL (15-min TWA)	—	—
STEL ceiling	200	—
IDLH	1,200	
ACGIH		
TLV (8-hr TWA)	25	—
STEL (15-min TWA)	—	—
USEPA		
MCL	—	—
MCLG	—	—

[a]Unit conversion: 1 ppm = 1.16 mg/m³; 1 ppm 1 mg/L.
OSHA, Occupational Safety and Health Administration; PEL, permissible exposure limit; TWA, time-weighted average; NIOSH, National Institute of Occupational Safety and Health; REL, recommended exposure limit; STEL, short-term exposure limit; IDLH, immediately dangerous to life or health; ACGIH, American Conference of Governmental Industrial Hygienists; TLV, threshold limit value; USEPA, U.S. Environmental Protection Agency; MCL, maximum contamination level; MCLG, maximum contamination level goal.
Data from *Amoore and Hautala, 1983; OSHA, 1995; ACGIH, 1995; and NIOSH, 1997.

METABOLISM

Tissue Absorption

CO is a gas at room temperature, and inhalation is the principal route of intake in humans (Sax, 1979). Inhaled CO is absorbed across the pulmonary alveolar membranes into the blood, after which it diffuses across the cell membranes of erythrocytes, where it combines with hemoglobin to yield COHb (Fig. 20-1). The rate of uptake and the total amount of pulmonary absorption is determined by the ambient air concentrations of CO and oxygen, the duration of exposure, the pulmonary ventilatory rate, and the cardiac output (Roughton and Darling, 1944; Forbes, 1970). Thus, an increase in physical activity while in a contaminated area increases a person's total pulmonary absorption of the gas (Roughton and Darling, 1944). As the concentrations in the blood and ambient air approach equilibrium, the rate of pulmonary absorption of CO decreases.

As COHb levels rise, alveolar ventilation rate increases and vasodilation occurs. This compensatory augmentation of blood flow increases the supply of oxygen to the brain and other tissues (Jones and Traystman, 1984; Sinha et al., 1991; Benignus et al., 1992). However, there is considerable individual variation in CO absorption rates and in the extent to which brain blood flow compensation occurs. These differences in absorption rates and physiological compensatory responses to CO influence an individual's susceptibility to the neurotoxic effects of CO exposure (Forbes, 1970; Benignus et al., 1992).

Dermal absorption of CO is influenced by the state of hydration of the skin, as well as the condition of the stratum corneum (Rozman and Klaassen, 1996). Overall, percutaneous absorption of CO does not contribute significantly to total exposure dose (Coburn et al., 1963).

Tissue Distribution

Most of the CO absorbed into the body binds to hemoglobin in erythrocytes and is distributed throughout the body by the systemic circulation. Extravascular distribution is determined by the tissue's blood perfusion and the partial pressure of CO in the various tissues of the body. Because the solubility of CO in water is low and its partial pressure small even when COHb levels are elevated, less than 1% of the absorbed dose is found dissolved in the body fluids. Ten to 15% of an absorbed dose is located in the extravascular tissues chemically bound to other heme proteins such as myoglobin and cytochrome P-450. Hepatic tissue stores of CO are significantly increased by chemicals that induce production of microsomal heme compounds such as cytochrome P-450 (Coburn, 1970). During hypoxemia, 20% to 40% of the intravascular CO is redistributed from hemoglobin to myoglobin and other hemeproteins (Coburn, 1970; Coburn and Mayers, 1971). CO readily crosses the placenta, exposing the fetus to increased levels, which can disrupt cellular respiration (Longo, 1970; Norman and Halton, 1990; Farrow et al., 1990). Furthermore, the fetus is at greater risk of hypoxic tissue damage than the mother during CO exposures because the fetal blood attains higher COHb levels (Longo, 1970; Mactutus, 1989; Farrow et al., 1990).

COHb reduces the oxygen-carrying capacity of blood by 40%, with subsequent tissue hypoxia. The sympathetic nervous system responds to brain hypoxia by increasing regional brain blood flow through dilation of the cerebral vasculature. In addition, the microvasculature of the brain adjusts to accommodate for hypoxia by presenting a larger surface area and reduced diffusion distance for oxygen. For example, increases in blood flow were found in the cerebral cortex (126%) and lower brainstem [pons (45%) and medulla (39%)] of rats (Sinha et al., 1991). The distribution and effects of CO in human brain tissue can be estimated only in retrospect by the residual functional impairments that correlate clinically with neuroimaging and postmortem studies to indicate where damage to brain tissues was most significant (Geschwind et al., 1968; Lapresle and Fardeau, 1967; Shimosegawa et al., 1992) (see Neuroimaging and Neuropathological Diagnosis sections). For example, positron emission tomography (PET) scans performed after acute exposure has ended and the patient's hypoxia has been corrected show a reduction in blood flow to those areas of the brain damaged by COHb-induced hypoxia. In addition, PET studies reveal that the damaged brain regions are unable to maintain normal glucose metabolism (Shimosegawa et al., 1992) (see Neuroimaging section, Table 20-3). Anatomical localization and extent of gray and white matter damage depend on the

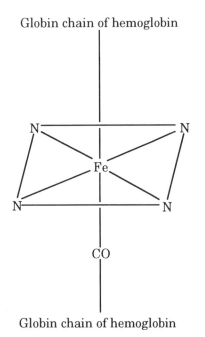

FIG. 20-1. Chemical structure of a single heme moiety in a molecule of carboxyhemoglobin. Carbon monoxide binds at the site usually occupied by oxygen.

concentration of CO in blood, the duration of exposure, and other concomitant factors of the circumstances and the premorbid condition of the exposed person (Lapresle and Fardeau, 1967) (see Neuropathological Diagnosis section, Table 20-4).

Tissue Biochemistry

Because CO is a nucleophilic compound, it reacts with electrophilic compounds. The four ferrous (Fe^{2+}) heme-binding sites of hemoglobin are the most common electrophilic sites in the human body. CO also reacts with the ferrous sites of other heme proteins (Coburn, 1970; Gregus and Klaassen, 1996). The reaction of CO with hemoglobin leads to the formation of COHb. The affinity of CO for the ferrous binding sites of hemoglobin in human blood varies among individuals but typically ranges from 200 to 250 times that of oxygen (Douglas et al., 1912; Roughton and Darling, 1944). As a result, the numbers of available oxygen binding sites are decreased during exposure to CO. In addition, binding of a molecule of CO to the heme of hemoglobin increases the affinity of its other heme moieties for oxygen, thereby shifting the oxygen dissociation curve to the left and resulting in a decrease in the release of oxygen to the various tissues of the body—including the brain (Douglas et al., 1912; Roughton and Darling, 1944). Furthermore, CO binds to the ferrous atoms of cytochrome A3 in mitochondria, thereby interfering with the electron transport chain and cellular respiration (Chance et al., 1970). The tissue hypoxia resulting from this reaction is especially harmful to the cells of the brain, which normally require a high rate of oxidative metabolism and cannot endure substantial periods of anaerobic metabolism (Murray, 1985; Scott and Jankovic, 1996). The globus pallidus, for example, which has a particularly high rate of oxygen consumption, appears to be especially vulnerable to the tissue hypoxia induced by CO exposure (Ginsberg et al., 1974; Sanchez-Ramos, 1993) (see Neuropathological Diagnosis section).

A small amount of CO is released endogenously in humans during the catabolism of heme proteins into bile pigments. The CO formed in this reaction is derived through the catabolic actions of heme oxygenase from the α-methene carbon atom in the protoporphyrin ring of hemoglobin and other heme-containing proteins (Coborn et al., 1963, 1967). There are two forms of heme oxygenase in the human body. Heme oxygenase-1, which is inducible, is found in high concentrations in the liver, where it is responsible for catabolism of the hemoglobin in red blood cells. Heme oxygenase-1 is also synthesized in the brain in response to oxidative stress and other noxious stimuli. Heme oxygenase-1 catalyzed heme breakdown liberates free iron, and CO may contribute to mitochondrial electron transport chain deficiencies (Schipper et al., 1998). The second, heme oxygenase-2, is not inducible, but is distributed throughout the various tissues of the body including the brain (Sun et al., 1990). High concentrations of heme oxygenase-2 are found in the hippocampus (Marks et al.,

1991; Ewing and Maines, 1992; Verma et al., 1993; Zhuo et al., 1993; Hawkins et al., 1994; Nathanson et al., 1995). Inhibitors of heme oxygenase-2 deplete endogenous cyclic guanosine 3′,5′-monophosphate (cGMP) and block induction of long-term potentiation (LTP) in the CA1 neurons of the hippocampus (Verma et al., 1993; Hawkins et al., 1994). CO elevates cGMP and stimulates cytochrome A3-Na, K-ATPase activity in hippocampal neurons *in vitro* (Nathanson et al., 1995). In addition, CO also induces a long-lasting alteration in A3-Na, K-ATPase in the Purkinje neurons of the cerebellum; this alteration is also associated with an increase in cGMP (Nathanson et al., 1995). These findings suggest that in the brain endogenous CO may function as a retrograde messenger in the synaptic alterations of LTP, which has been proposed as the mechanism for memory and learning (Hebb, 1949; Marks et al., 1991; Ewing and Maines, 1992; Verma et al., 1993; Zhuo et al., 1993; Hawkins et al., 1994; Nathanson et al., 1995).

Excretion

CO is bound reversibly to hemoglobin, and therefore it readily leaves the blood following cessation of exposure (Selvakumar et al., 1993). Most of an absorbed dose of CO is exhaled unchanged. A small portion is oxidized to carbon dioxide before excretion (Coburn, 1970). Elimination rate depends on the partial pressures of oxygen and CO in the alveolar capillaries and the pulmonary ventilation rate. The rate of elimination is faster immediately after cessation of exposure than later (Selvakumar et al., 1993). The elimination half-life of CO is 7 hours when the subject is breathing ambient air, approximately 2 hours when 100% oxygen is administered, and is reduced to approximately 50 minutes when hyperbaric oxygen is administered at 2.5 atm (Winter and Miller, 1976). Because of the low solubility of CO in water, excretion of unchanged CO via the urine or sweat is not significant. Fecal excretion of CO has not been demonstrated (Coburn et al., 1963).

CLINICAL MANIFESTATIONS AND DIAGNOSIS

Symptomatic Diagnosis

The severity of the acute effects produced by CO-induced tissue hypoxia is determined by the atmospheric concentration of CO, duration of exposure, individual COHb levels reached during the exposure, and preexposure health status (Stewart et al., 1973; Merideth and Vale, 1988) (Fig. 20-2). Because CO produces hypoxemia, the symptoms of exposure are essentially those of tissue hypoxia and manifest first in those organ systems with the greatest oxygen requirements (e.g., brain and heart) (Winter and Miller, 1976; Scott and Jankovic, 1996). Subjective symptoms are rarely reported at blood COHb levels of less than 5%; however, objective tests of vision demonstrate impairments at and below this level of exposure (Beard and Grandstaff, 1970). Subjective awareness of the effects

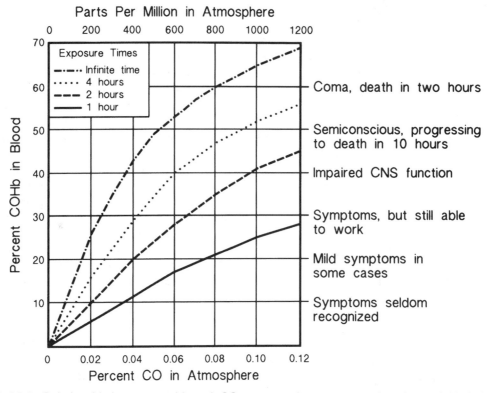

FIG. 20-2. Relationship between ambient air CO concentration, percent carboxyhemoglobin in blood (COHb), and clinical manifestations after 1 hour, 2 hours, 4 hours, and an infinite duration of exposure. Symptoms vary among individuals, with headache being the most common manifestation of exposure. Subjective awareness of symptoms does not usually occur below a blood COHb level of 10%. Neurobehavioral tests show impairments at levels of less than 5%. (Modified from Forbes, 1970, with permission.)

of CO poisoning varies among individuals, but generally occurs at blood COHb levels between 10 and 15%. CO in cigarette smoke leads to elevated baseline blood COHb levels among smokers and those nearby. Symptoms are experienced sooner among smokers than nonsmokers when exposure to additional sources of CO occurs (Stewart and Hake, 1976). A slight increase in physical activity at a COHb level above 40% can rapidly exhaust existing oxygen reserves and result in overt symptoms in the exposed individual (Roughton and Darling, 1944).

The symptoms of CO-induced hypoxia are nonspecific and are often mistaken for flulike viral illnesses (Grace and Platt, 1981; Dolan et al., 1987). Although CO exposure is often difficult to recognize, absence of fever, sore throat, and adenopathy can aid in differentiating CO poisoning from a viral illness. In addition, the skin of patients with elevated COHb levels is bright pink (Jefferson, 1976; Pulst et al., 1983; Hayashi et al., 1993). CO poisoning should be suspected and a source of exposure sought if several persons in a common environment have similar symptoms (Kales, 1993).

Acute Exposure

The early acute symptoms include headache, dizziness, fatigue, weakness, nausea, vomiting, irritability, disorien-

tation, difficulty thinking, increased heart rate, and hyperventilation (Stewart et al., 1973; Jefferson, 1976; MMWR, 1993). The symptoms associated with acute low-level CO exposures are usually ameliorated following cessation of exposure. With continuing exposure the severity of these symptoms increases and others emerge, including headache, memory loss, visual disturbances, chest pain, hypertonia, seizures, somnolence, coma, and death (Richardson et al., 1959; Jefferson, 1976; Stewart and Hake, 1976).

Nonfatal acute exposures to higher levels of CO, which produce severe central nervous system (CNS) effects, often result in permanent CNS damage (Jefferson, 1976; Jaeckle and Nasrallah, 1985; Walton, 1994). These permanent effects appear after a period of apparent but not lasting (pseudo) recovery (Raskin and Mullaney, 1940; Richardson et al., 1959; Jaeckle and Nasrallah, 1985; Hayashi et al., 1993; Choi et al., 1993). Persistent residual symptoms following acute high-level CO intoxication include incontinence, dystonia, and parkinsonism, as well as prominent neurobehavioral features such as emotional lability, disorientation, memory impairment, aphasia, akinetic mutism, agnosia, dementia, cortical blindness, ataxia, and apraxia (Raskin and Mullaney, 1940; Richardson et al., 1959; Ringel and Klawans, 1972; Geschwind et al., 1968; Fisher, 1982; Jaeckle and Nasrallah, 1985; Perry, 1994). In a 3-year follow-up of 63 patients surviving acute exposure to CO, 27 reported deterioration of memory function, 21 deterioration in personality, and 8 clinical improvement. The most commonly reported changes in personality were increased irritability, aggression, and moodiness. Deterioration of memory and personality were significantly correlated ($r = 0.423$; $p < 0.001$). In addition, complaints of memory impairment were significantly correlated ($r = 0.441$; $p < 0.001$) with a low memory quotient on neuropsychological testing (Smith and Brandon, 1973) (see Clinical Experiences section).

A 22-year-old woman remained in a coma for 17 days following a severe acute exposure to CO (Geschwind et al., 1968). When she regained consciousness, her spontaneous speech was confined to a few stereotyped phrases, and although she exhibited echolalic repetition and excellent articulation, she was apparently unable to comprehend language. In addition, she had seizures. Neurological examination revealed normal grip strength and coordination in both arms, but both legs were spastic, with hyperactive deep tendon reflexes, which were slightly greater on the left. Plantar responses were flexor. The patient was also incontinent. Over time, she gradually became more dystonic until she was immobile, in a position of severe paraplegia-in-flexion. She died 10 years after the CO exposure. This patient had also experienced hypoxia-induced cardiac arrest, suggesting that her symptoms may have been partially induced by the cardiac arrest (see Neuropathological Diagnosis section).

Chronic Exposure

Symptoms of chronic CO exposure include headache, emotional lability, fatigue, weakness, nausea, increased sweating, difficulty thinking, memory disturbances, aphasia, anxiety, personality disturbances, anorexia, weight loss, cardiac arrhythmia and angina, episodes of loss of consciousness, seizures, apraxia, ataxia, and parkinsonism (Gilbert and Glaser, 1959; Ringle and Klawans, 1972). Symptoms associated with chronic CO exposure are exacerbated by additional short-duration peak exposures. Diagnosis of the effects of chronic exposure requires careful consideration of all potential proximate sources of CO exposure. Furthermore, a biochemical diagnosis may be difficult to confirm because blood sample COHb levels more closely reflect the most recent exposure than cumulative exposure. Higher blood COHb levels, which are associated with symptoms, may have been reached during brief periods of higher CO exposures. These may go undetected at the time of sampling. However, this does not mean that the exposure did not occur (Gross et al., 1989) (see Biochemical Diagnosis section).

Neurophysiological Diagnosis

Electroencephalographic (EEG) changes following exposure to CO were first described by Berger in 1934, in a patient who had lost consciousness during the exposure. High-voltage slow rhythms of 3.5 to 5 Hz were seen on the initial EEG. The EEG improved when the patient regained

consciousness, but the slow waves remained prominent. Serial EEG recordings were performed in a 24-year-old man after he attempted suicide by inhalation of exhaust fumes (Richardson et al., 1959). The initial EEG recording performed 9 days after the exposure showed complete absence of normal frequencies with diffuse high-voltage slow waves. A second tracing 4 months later revealed improvement, with return of alpha activity, but many slow waves of 3 to 6 Hz were still visible. Follow-up EEG 6 months after the incident showed further normalization. The EEG recording 43 days after a 29-year-old man was acutely exposed to CO emitted by a charcoal briquette heater showed generalized slowing of the background activity as well as theta waves of 4 to 4.5 Hz, which were primarily seen in the frontal areas bilaterally (Kobayashi et al., 1984).

EEG recording of 33 patients acutely exposed to CO revealed that the most severe abnormalities occurred in those 13 patients who were either over 50 years of age or who had remained unconscious for more than 7 hours following removal from CO exposure (Lennox and Petersen, 1958). Five of these 13 died and only 2 recovered fully. In another study of 12 patients with documented COHb blood levels of 15 to 45%, the EEG recordings of 3 showed diffuse slowing on the day of admission to the hospital (Denays et al., 1994). An 18-year-old man developed focal seizures after he was exposed to CO (blood COHb: 62%) and was found comatose in the closed garage where he had been repairing his car; the initial EEG showed repetitive sharp waves, recorded most prominently over the anterior right hemisphere (Neufeld et al., 1981). The sharp wave activity was also seen (less frequently) in the left frontocentral region. The background rhythm consisted of medium-amplitude, 1- to 1.5-Hz, polymorphic waves, with 3- to 5-Hz waves superimposed and more predominant over the right hemisphere. Serial EEGs taken 48 hours and 8 weeks later showed improvement. Although clinical improvement was notable, irregularities persisted in the EEG (Fig. 20-3).

A quantitative EEG of two patients acutely exposed to CO showed elevated absolute power of all EEG frequencies, increased delta activity over the temporal–parietal–occipital cortex bilaterally, increased relative power of alpha activity most pronounced over the prefrontal cortex, and marked decreases in the interhemispheric coherence for most frequency bands (Fitz-Gerald and Patrick, 1991). Although these findings do not parallel those reported by other authors, many of the quantitative features found in these two patients are not easily recognizable with visual interpretation of an EEG. These findings indicate that topographic quantitative EEG recordings may be useful in elucidating the acute and long-term effects of exposure to CO.

Visual evoked potential (VEP) wave patterns were recorded during acute exposure to CO in 12 male volunteers whose blood COHb levels ranged from 20% to 22%. The VEPs of these volunteers were not affected at blood COHb levels of 14% (Hosko, 1970). VEPs have been used as a neurophysiological method for documentation of overt clinical effects following CO poisoning, as shown in the

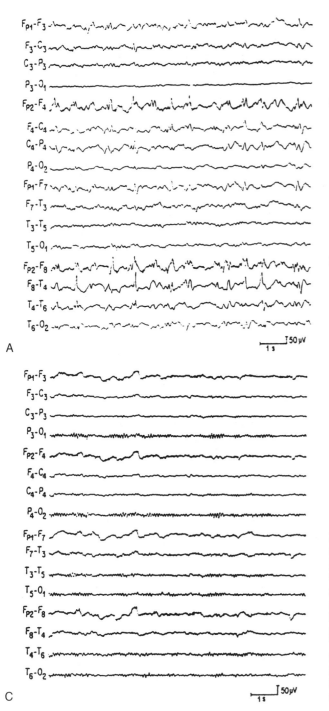

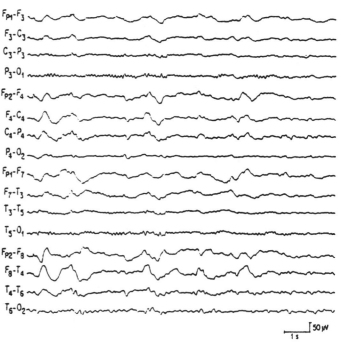

FIG. 20-3. Serial EEG studies in an 18-year-old man who developed seizures after a severe acute exposure to CO. **A:** The initial EEG 8 hours after removal from exposure shows repetitive sharp waves in the left central frontal region and even more pronounced over the anterior right hemisphere. The background activity consisted of medium-amplitude 1- to 1.5-Hz, polymorphic waves, and 3- to 5-Hz waves. **B:** EEG 48 hours after the incident shows intermittent slow-wave abnormalities in the anterior right hemisphere. The sharp waves have disappeared and the background activity in the posterior right and left hemispheres has improved. **C:** The EEG 8 weeks after exposure shows low-voltage theta waves in the right posterior temporal region. (From Neufeld et al., 1981, with permission.)

following case summaries. The first patient, a 19-year-old man, developed parkinsonism following an acute exposure to CO because of defective heating equipment. His blood COHb level on admission to the hospital was 22%. At follow-up examination 4 months after the exposure he was considered clinically recovered, but his VEP latencies were prolonged (right: 128 milliseconds; left: 126 milliseconds). The second was a 30-year-old woman who also developed parkinsonism following exposure to CO emitted by defective heating equipment. Blood COHb levels for this patient

were not reported. At follow-up examination 18 months after the exposure, the patient presented with hypomimia and awkward alternating movements of the left upper extremity. VEP studies at this time showed prolongation of latency (right: 120 milliseconds; left: 122 milliseconds). VEPs documented the effects of CO exposure on visual system functioning in a 20-year-old woman 12 days after she had been found unconscious in a burning building (Zagami et al., 1993). On admission to the hospital, her blood COHb level was 38%. VEP studies performed at this time were abnormal, with no identifiable P100 wave. She had difficulty reading and identifying colors. The patient improved clinically over the course of the next few weeks. Follow-up VEP studies showed the gradual return of P100 wave. The initial EEG of this patient showed diffuse slow activity with no lateralization or proximal features. Follow-up EEG was normal.

Neuropsychological Diagnosis

Neurobehavioral test batteries should be selected on the basis of previously demonstrated sensitivities to the effects of CO exposure (Laties and Merigan, 1979). Neuropsychological testing can reveal cerebral dysfunction associated with CO exposure and can document the severity of poisoning, track recovery, and predict prognosis (Myers and Britten, 1989). Messier and Myers (1991) have recommended a brief neuropsychological test battery for emergency assessment of patients exposed to CO. Suggested tests include (a) verbal assessment of general orientation; (b) Digit Span; (c) Trail Making; (d) Digit Symbol; (e) Aphasia Screening; and (f) Block Design. The accuracy of these tests for detecting CNS impairments following CO exposure was assessed by administering the battery to 66 CO-exposed patients and 66 controls. The exposed patients performed significantly less well than did the control group on all six tests, with the most marked differences (p <0.001) seen on Trail Making, Digit Symbol, Aphasia Screening, and Block Design tests. The mean performance level for the CO-exposed patients on Block Designs and Trails tests was at the dysfunctional level on admission to the hospital. In addition, comparison of the CO-exposed patients' performance on this test battery before and after hyperbaric oxygen therapy (HBO$_2$) revealed a significant improvement in performance after HBO$_2$ therapy.

The subtle neurobehavioral effects associated with acute low-level exposure to carbon monoxide may be overlooked when using low-demand neuropsychological performance tasks (Bender et al., 1971, 1972; Putz, 1979; Mihevic et al., 1983; Myers and Britten, 1989). For example, a blood COHb level of approximately 2.5% was associated with decrements on tests of vigilance (i.e., sustained attention) and time estimation (Beard and Wertheim, 1967); 18 nonsmoking subjects (aged: 20 to 30 years) showed no decrements in vigilance at blood COHb levels of 5% (Roche et al., 1981). However, dual-task performance tests that required subjects to monitor the intensity of a light while performing a visual-tracking task revealed attentional deficits at blood COHb of 5%. Performance deficits were most notable on the more difficult tasks, and analysis of variance showed that the relationship between tracking difficulty and exposure time and level was significant at p < 0.01 (Putz, 1979). Motor performance was not impaired at blood COHb levels up to 5% (Mihevic et al., 1983). However, a 2.5-hour exposure to 100 ppm CO (blood COHb: 7%) resulted in performance deficits on two ver-

sions of the Purdue Pegboard test, one of which included concurrent performance of a verbal task (Bender et al., 1971, 1972). Reaction times (RT) during low-level CO exposure have been measured using driving simulators and suggest that RTs begin to deteriorate at COHb levels as low as 6% (Ray and Rockwell, 1970; Rummo and Sarlanis, 1974). In contrast to these findings, significant performance deficits were not found in volunteers at blood COHb levels of 11% to 13% on hand and foot RT in a driving simulator. In addition, no significant performance deficits were noted at this exposure level in these same volunteers on the Flanagan coordination test; Crawford collar test; pin and screw test; Ortho-rator visual tests of depth perception, visual acuity, and color vision; auditory test of time estimation; and tests of steadiness (Stewart et al., 1970).

The encephalopathy following severe acute CO exposures includes altered mood and deficits in memory and psychomotor function (Beard and Grandstaff, 1970; Mihevic et al., 1983; Deckel, 1994). For example, a 51-year-old man and his 52-year-old sister were acutely exposed to CO while driving home from Maine to Connecticut in an automobile with a faulty exhaust system (Deckel, 1994). The man and his sister briefly lost consciousness shortly after exiting the car when they arrived home. Both patients were admitted to the local hospital. Blood COHb levels were 23.8% in the man and 20.1% in his sister. The man was initially treated with 100% oxygen and HBO$_2$ therapy until his neurological status improved. The woman was treated with 100% oxygen and discharged 8 hours after admission to the hospital. Neuropsychological assessment 2 years after exposure revealed deficits in memory (Wechsler Memory Scale and California Verbal Learning Test) and executive functioning (Wisconsin Card Sorting Task and Digit Symbol Test). By contrast, neuropsychological assessment of four patients who were acutely exposed to CO (blood COHb: 1 to 39.1%) but were asymptomatic 6 months after exposure failed to reveal performance deficits (Weaver et al., 1996). However, two of these four patients, including the one with the highest COHb levels (blood COHb: 39.1%), were hypothermic on admission to the hospital. These findings may reflect the neuroprotective effects of hypothermia (Craig et al., 1959; Carlson et al., 1976; Duhaine and Ross, 1990).

Biochemical Diagnosis

The blood COHb level increases with dose and duration of CO exposure and therefore is the most sensitive biological marker for determining CO levels in the body and confirming exposure. Endogenous production of CO is 0.4 mL/hr, providing a baseline CO level of less than 1% COHb (Coburn et al., 1963); it is increased in patients with hemolytic anemia (Coborn et al., 1966). The ACGIH recommends that end of shift blood COHb levels not exceed 3.5% (ACGIH, 1995). Tobacco smokers have elevated

TABLE 20-2. *Biological exposure indices for carbon monoxide*

	Urine	Blood	Alveolar air
Determinant	CO	COHb	CO
Start of shift	Not established	Not established	Not established
During shift	Not established	Not established	Not established
End of shift at end of workweek	Not established	3.5% of hemoglobin	20 ppm

CO, carbon monoxide; COHb, carboxyhemoglobin.
Data from ACGIH, 1995.

baseline COHb levels, which range from 5% to 13% (Mactutus, 1989). Since blood COHb levels decrease rapidly after cessation of exposure, the reported measurement may not reflect the maximum levels reached during the exposure period. Therefore, prognosis cannot be based on COHb levels alone, particularly if oxygen has been administered or if a sufficient period of time has passed between cessation of exposure and sampling, allowing a decline in the blood COHb levels (Gross et al., 1989). Since tissue COHb levels persist after death, they can be used to document CO exposures posthumously (Farrow et al., 1990).

Measurement of alveolar air CO concentrations can also be used to monitor for CO exposure. The ACGIH biological exposure index for CO in end-exhaled air at the end of the work shift is 20 ppm (ACGIH, 1995) (Table 20-2). Baseline alveolar CO levels are elevated in tobacco smokers (Mactutus, 1989).

Neuroimaging

Magnetic resonance imaging (MRI), *computed tomography* (CT), *single-photon emission topography* (SPECT), PET, and *magnetic resonance spectroscopy* (MRS) can be used to document the neuropathological and metabolic effects of CO noninvasively. The neuropathological findings and thus the neuroimaging findings can vary depending on the amount of time that has passed since an acute CO exposure incident (Vieregge et al., 1989; Gotoh et al., 1993). Neuroimaging studies of the human brain following CO exposure often show lesions in the globus pallidus and periventricular white matter (Gotoh et al., 1993; Kamada et al., 1994). Neuroimaging studies reveal unilateral differences in the severity of the brain tissue lesions (Vieregge et al., 1989) (Fig. 20-4). Serial neuroimaging studies are needed to correlate the clinical picture with the changes seen by neuroimaging (Vieregge et al., 1989; Gotoh et al., 1993; Jones et al., 1994). For example, a 40-year-old man who developed parkinsonism 4 weeks after a severe acute exposure to CO (blood COHb: 30%) had an initial CT scan on the day of admission to the hospital which revealed no abnormalities (Jaeckle and Nasrallah, 1985). Neurological examination at that time was also normal. However, 4 weeks after exposure, the patient exhibited signs of parkinsonism (see Clinical Experiences section), and his follow-up CT scan revealed bilateral necrosis of the globus pallidus and bilateral symmetrical lesions in the white matter

of the posterior limbs of the internal capsules. At follow-up CT scans 12 weeks and 6 months after the incident, the appearances of the lesions in the globus pallidus remained unchanged, whereas the lesions in the internal capsule appeared less marked. Neuroimages of the pallidal lesions immediately after exposure to CO correlate poorly with prognosis. The overall prognosis in cases of CO poisoning is correlated better with neuroimages of white matter lesions than with lesions of the globus pallidus (Vieregge et al., 1989; Bruno et al., 1993; Choi et al., 1993; Gotoh et al., 1993; Jones et al., 1994). However, the prognosis in patients who show a period of pseudo-recovery followed by development of parkinsonian features may correlate better with the neuroimages seen in the globus pallidus (Jaeckle and Nasrallah, 1985).

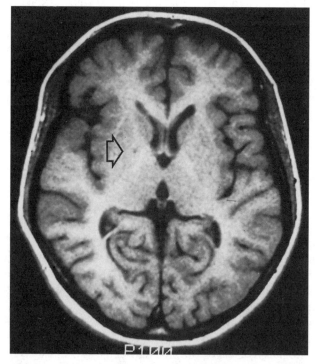

FIG. 20-4. MRI of the brain of a 30-year-old woman who developed parkinsonism and memory deficits following exposure to carbon monoxide. The T_1-weighted image 18 months after exposure shows a small lesion in the left globus pallidus (arrow). This lesion was not visible on a CT scan performed at this time. (From Vierregge et al., 1989, with permission.)

A   B   C   D

T$_1$-weighted images

T$_2$-weighted images

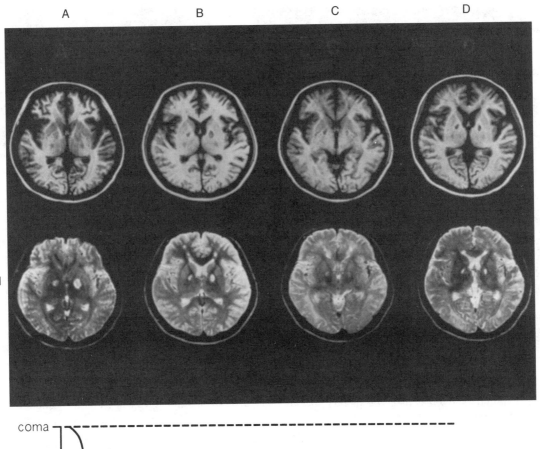

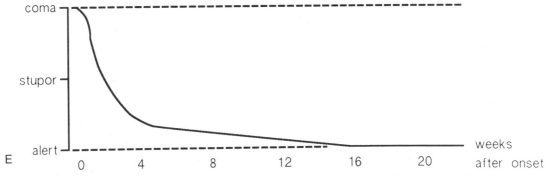

E

FIG. 20-5. Changes in the level of consciousness and the MRI images of a 20-year-old woman acutely exposed to CO. The disappearance of the lesions in the cerebral white matter coincided with amelioration of the patient's clinical neurological condition. The globus pallidus lesions, which became obscure on MRI images at 2 months after exposure, reappeared on the MRI images at 4 months after the incident. **A:** The T$_1$-weighted images 4 days after exposure demonstrating areas of hypointensity in the globus pallidus bilaterally; areas appear hyperintense on the T$_2$-weighted images. **B:** The T$_1$-weighted images at 1 month after exposure still show distinct, but diminished, areas of hypointensity in the globus pallidus bilaterally. In addition, areas of abnormal signal intensity are seen in the subcortical white matter; areas are more clearly seen and appear hyperintense on T$_2$-weighted images. **C:** The T$_1$- and T$_2$-weighted images at 2 months after exposure showing diminution of the lesions in the globus pallidus and the subcortical white matter. **D:** The T$_1$- and T$_2$-weighted images at 4 months after exposure showing distinct lesions in the globus pallidus bilaterally. **E:** Graph showing levels of consciousness at 4,8,12,16, and 20 weeks after onset of exposure. (From Gotoh et al., 1993, with permission.)

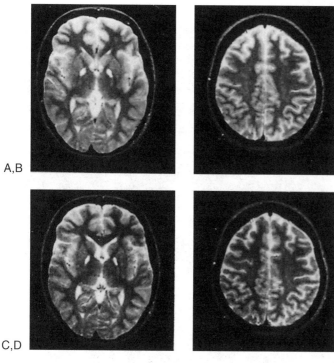

A,B

C,D

FIG. 20-6. Brain MRI images in a 29-year-old woman after intentional exposure to CO. **A and B:** T$_2$-weighted axial images at 6 months show lesions in the globus pallidus bilaterally. There were no visible lesions in the cortical gray matter, subcortical white matter, or hippocampus in this patient. **C and D:** No morphological changes in the pallidal lesions are seen on the T$_2$-weighted axial images at follow-up 1 year after the CO exposure incident. (From Shimosegawa et al., 1992, with permission.)

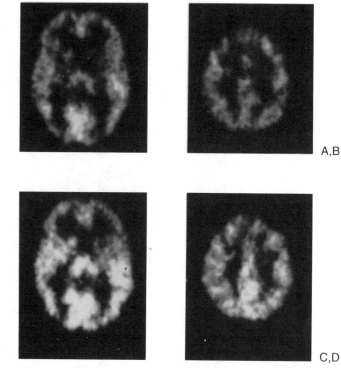

A,B

C,D

FIG. 20-7. Brain PET images of cerebral blood flow in a 29-year-old woman after intentional exposure to CO. **A and B:** The initial PET scan in this patient 6 months after exposure revealed 41% decrease in regional cerebral blood flow (rCBF) in the basal ganglia and a 32% decrease in the frontal cortex. No decrease in rCBF was noted in the centrum semiovale. **C and D:** At the follow-up 1 year after the CO exposure, PET scan showed CBF to the basal ganglia was 10% below normal; in the frontal cortex, CBF was 20% below normal. (From Shimosegawa et al., 1992, with permission.)

Serial MRIs demonstrated sequential changes in the brain of a 20-year-old woman who became comatose following an acute exposure to CO (Gotoh et al., 1993). The woman was treated with 100% oxygen and regained consciousness within 24 hours. However, when she awoke she exhibited akinetic mutism. Initial brain MRI was performed 4 days after the exposure and showed bilateral lesions in the globus pallidus (Fig. 20-5A). The MRI 1 month later revealed bilateral lesions of the globus pallidus and areas of abnormal signal intensity in the periventricular white matter (Fig. 20-5B). The lesions to the globus pallidus appeared diminished 2 months after the exposure (Fig. 20-5C). The follow-up MRI 4 months after the incident still showed bilateral lesions in the globus pallidus, although the areas of abnormal signal intensity in the periventricular white matter had disappeared (Fig. 20-5D). The disappearance of the white matter lesions correlated with the patient's pattern of neurological and neuropsychological recovery.

Serial neuroimaging (MRI and PET) studies were performed in a 29-year-old woman who had been acutely exposed to CO when she attempted suicide by inhaling automobile exhaust fumes (Shimosegawa et al., 1992). Blood COHb

was not determined. On admission to the hospital her responses to stimulation were impaired and she was given hyperbaric oxygen (HBO$_2$) therapy, but her neurological status did not improve. She remained poorly responsive at 6-month and 1-year follow-up. No focal neurological deficits were noted. Brain MRI images 6 months after the incident revealed lesions in the globus pallidus bilaterally. There were no visible lesions in the subcortical white matter in this patient (Fig. 20-6A and B). No changes were noted on the MRI images 1 year after the CO exposure incident (Fig. 20-6C and D). The initial PET scan in this patient 6 months after exposure revealed a 41% decrease in regional cerebral blood flow (rCBF) in the basal ganglia and a 32% decrease in the frontal cortex (Fig. 20-7A and B). At the follow-up 1 year after the CO exposure, PET scan showed that rCBF to the basal ganglia was 10% below normal; in the frontal cortex, rCBF was 20% below normal (Fig. 20-7C and D). PET of regional glucose metabolism (rCMRGlu) 6 months after exposure showed bilateral hypometabolism of glucose in the basal ganglia and frontal cortex (Fig. 20-8A and B). At follow-up 1 year after the incident, hypometabolism of glucose

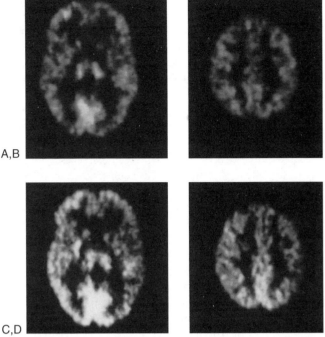

FIG. 20-8. Brain PET images of regional glucose metabolism (rCMGlu) in a 29-year-old woman after intentional exposure to CO. **A and B:** PET of rCMGlu at 6 months after exposure show bilateral hypometabolism of glucose in the basal ganglia and frontal cortex. No decrease in rCMRGlu was noted in the centrum semiovale. **C and D:** At follow-up 1 year after the incident, hypometabolism of glucose was still evident and was 22% below normal in the frontal cortex. (From Shimosegawa et al., 1992, with permission.)

was still evident and was 22% below normal in the frontal cortex (Fig. 20-8C and D). No decrease in rCBF or rCMRGlu was noted in the centrum semiovale of this patient (Table 20-3). These findings indicate that PET is a sensitive tool for detecting subtle changes in neurological functioning that may not be morphologically evident on MRI or CT.

Kamada et al. (1994) used MRI, MRS, and SPECT to assess the neuropathological changes in a 55-year-old woman who developed akinetic mutism, ataxia, incontinence, and bizarre behavior following a severe acute exposure to CO. She was found unconscious in her living room, which contained automobile exhaust fumes from an underground parking garage in the basement of her apartment building. Her blood COHb level was 47.6% on admission to the hospital. Although the MRI revealed no abnormalities 29 days after the exposure, on day 45 the MRI revealed areas of high signal intensity in the periventricular white matter bilaterally. On day 151, the MRI revealed abnormalities in the globus pallidus; the areas of high signal intensity previously noted in the white matter appeared less marked. MRS documented the neurochemical correlates of CO exposure in the brain of this patient by detecting the protons in choline-containing compounds (Cho), creatine and phosphocreatine (Cr), and N-acetylaspartate (NAA). The MRS showed markedly lower levels of NAA relative to Cr and Cho 29 days after the exposure, when the clinical picture was severe. In addition, the ratio of Cho to Cr was slightly increased at this time. These ratios returned to normal with clinical recovery. The increase in Cho may reflect an increase in phosphocholine and glycerophosphocholine, both of which are reported to fluctuate when cell membranes are degraded, as occurs during demyelination (Murata et al., 1995). Although the exact role of the amino acid NAA in the clinical symptomology of CO intoxication remains unknown, NAA is present in neurons and has been shown to enhance the transport of high-energy phosphates; a decrease in NAA has been suggested to reflect a loss of neurons (Nadler and Cooper, 1972; Nakada, 1991; Menon et al., 1990; Murata et al., 1995). These findings demonstrate that MRS can be used to correlate neuronal activity with the clinical severity of the symptoms of CO poisoning and suggest that this technique may be useful in determining neuronal viability and prognosis early in the course of CO poisoning (Murata et al., 1995).

SPECT performed on the 2nd, 11th, 24th, and 42nd days after exposure revealed no abnormalities in this case (Kamada et al., 1994); however, Silverman et al. (1993) reported bilateral posterior occipital lobe hypoperfusion on the SPECT in a 20-year-old patient who developed bilateral congruous central scotomas following exposure to CO, documenting a cortical origin to the patient's visual loss.

TABLE 20-3. *Changes in regional cerebral blood flow and glucose metabolism after exposure to carbon monoxide[a]*

	rCBF			rCMGlu		
	Normal[b]	6 months	12 months	Normal[b]	6 months	12 months
Cortex (mean)	52.2 ± 9.9	40.6	50.4	6.19 ± 0.65	5.68	5.81
Frontal cortex	48.6 ± 8.0	33.1	39.1	6.40 ± 0.70	4.50	5.02
Basal ganglia	59.3 ± 12.9	35.0	53.7	6.20 ± 0.61	5.09	5.46
Centrum semiovale	26.4 ± 5.3	23.4	24.3	3.22 ± 0.28	3.14	2.63

[a]Positron emission tomography findings in a 29-year-old woman at 6 months and 1 year after a severe acute exposure to CO: exposure-associated decreases in regional cerebral blood flow (rCBF) and regional glucose metabolism (rCMGlu).
[b]Normal values including standard deviations.
(Modified from Shimosegawa et al., 1992, with permission.)

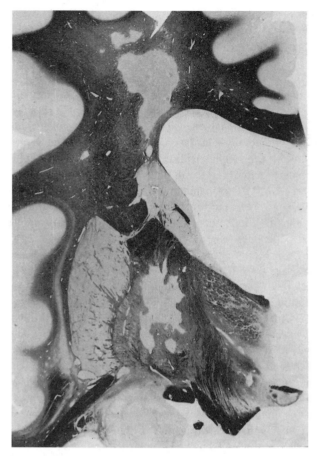

FIG. 20-9. Transverse section through the gray nuclei demonstrating necrosis in the globus pallidus extending to the internal capsule and patchy demyelination in the centrum semiovale. (Original magnification, ×2; Wölke's stain.) (From Lapresle and Fardeau, 1967, with permission.)

Neuropathological Diagnosis

The neuropathological and neurobehavioral correlates of CO-induced hypoxia develop insidiously over the course of days and weeks if the patient survives the acute effects of CO poisoning. Edema and petechial hemorrhages are the earliest neuropathological manifestation of CO exposure (Hill and Semerak, 1918; Richardson et al., 1959; Lapresle and Fardeau, 1967; Somogyi et al., 1981). Necrosis can be seen at autopsy in those areas that are particularly sensitive to the effects of hypoxia, such as Sommer's sector of Ammon's horn of the hippocampus, the globus pallidus and putamen of the basal ganglia, the internal capsule, and the centrum semiovale of the white matter of the cerebral hemispheres (Richardson et al., 1959; Lapresle and Fardeau, 1967; Geschwind et al., 1968; Ginsberg et al., 1974; Okeda et al., 1981; Kobayashi et al., 1984; Jones et al., 1994) (Fig. 20-9). The damage to Ammon's horn may involve the entire structure or may be limited to the pyramidal cell layer of Sommer's sector (Lapresle and Fardeau, 1967). Successive CO exposures produce a consistent pattern of neuronal degeneration in the CA1 pyramidal neurons of the hippocampus of mice (Ishimaru et al., 1991). The neuropathological effects of CO poisoning differ from those associated with other forms of brain tissue hypoxia in that an increase is seen in the frequency of necrosis in the globus pallidus and leukoencephalopathy in the centrum semiovale (Grinker, 1926; Lapresle and Fardeau, 1967; Kobayashi et al., 1984; Poirier et al., 1990). The area of necrosis in the globus pallidus varies with the circumstances of exposure. However, the damage is frequently limited to the anterior portion and rarely affects both pallidi completely. Lesions in the white matter vary from small isolated areas, which give a patchy appearance on microscopic examination, to more extensive damage producing a macroscopically evident softening of the cerebral hemispheres. Lesions are also seen in the corpus callosum and anterior commissure (Lapresle and Fardeau, 1967). Lesions in the cortex are distributed throughout the cortical layers, although damage is primarily found in the third, fifth, and sixth layers of the neocortex, especially in the parietal and occipital lobes. Damage to the cerebellum includes necrosis of the Purkinje cells of the cerebellar cortex and focal demyelination (Grinker, 1926; Lapresle and Fardeau, 1967; Geschwind et al., 1968; Poirier et al., 1990). The subcortical U fibers, hypothalamus, substantia nigra, and brain stem are usually spared (Grinker, 1927; Lapresle and Fardeau, 1967).

Grinker (1927) described the macro- and microscopic neuropathological findings in a 58-year-old woman who survived for 2 months after a severe acute exposure to CO. This patient regained consciousness after a few hours in the hospital, but following a 26-day period of pseudo-recovery, her clinical condition deteriorated. Macroscopic examination of coronal sections of the brain revealed symmetrical yellow-brownish areas of necrosis in the globus pallidus bilaterally. The areas of necrosis extended from the anterior tip of the globus pallidus to its center; its caudal portions appeared normal. Microscopic examination of the brain revealed areas of necrosis and demyelination in the globus pallidus and demyelination of the ansa lenticularis. The globus pallidus was entirely devoid of myelin at the anterior ends, where there was a marked increase in glial cells with numerous free microglia, which were filled with lipoid material and lymphocytic infiltration. There was slight demyelination of the finer fibers of the striatum, but no definite lesions were noted. The subthalamic nucleus and the red nucleus were thinned. The lateral pontine bundle from the pallidus to the substantia nigra was partially degenerated. Microscopic examination of the subcortical white matter revealed areas of demyelination with a flecklike or patchy appearance, which was especially notable in the centrum semiovale. There were also numerous lipid-filled glia cells in this area. The subcortical U fibers, perivascular white matter, internal capsule, and corpus callosum appeared normal.

The neuropathological findings in a 65-year-old woman who developed mutism, ataxia, and incontinence following exposure to CO emitted from a charcoal briquette heater revealed demyelination in the centrum semiovale and bilateral necrosis of the globus pallidus (Fig. 20-10). Demyelination with fibrillary gliosis was noted in the white matter in the frontal lobes (Kobayashi et al., 1984) (Fig. 20-11). Microscopically, the demyelination had a

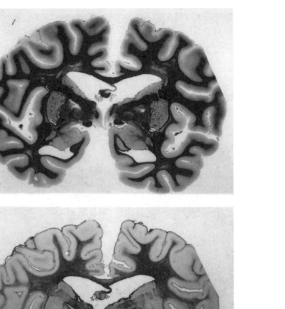

A

B

FIG. 20-10. Coronal sections through the infundibulum following exposure to CO. **A:** Woelcke-stained section reveals demyelination in the centrum semiovale and bilateral necrosis of the globus pallidus. **B:** Holzer-stained section showing diffuse fibrillary gliosis. (From Kobayashi et al., 1984, with permission.)

flecked appearance. The subcortical U fibers were spared. Other microscopic changes noted in this region included destruction of axons, hypertrophic astrocytes, and numerous lipid droplets. The cytoarchitecture of the frontal cortex was unremarkable (Fig. 20-12).

The autopsy of a 32-year-old woman who was exposed to CO and then had a hypoxia-induced cardiac arrest revealed damage to the globus pallidus and the frontal lobes, especially the leg area of the sensory–motor cortex, with relative preservation of the Rolandic cortex (Geschwind et al., 1968). There was extensive damage to the fibers connecting the posterior parietal association cortex to Wernicke's and Broca's areas; the auditory pathways up to and including Heschl's gyrus, Wernicke's and Broca's areas, and the arcuate fasciculus were well preserved. In addition, with the exception of Sommer's sector, the hippocampus was relatively well preserved. This patient developed mixed transcortical aphasia and severe dystonic paraplegia-in-flexion following the exposure incident, indicating that the extensive damage to the fibers connecting the posterior parietal association cortex to Wernicke's and Broca's areas and the damage to the globus pallidus and the frontal lobes, especially the leg area of the sensory–motor cortex, may have been involved in her clinical presentation.

The neuropathological findings following exposure to CO can be categorized according to the site of the lesions and reflect the patient's clinical course (Lapresle and Fardeau, 1967). Patients presenting with coma and surviving for shorter durations (less than 5 days) show more severe damage in all areas of the brain, especially in the white matter and globus pallidus. In addition, damage is frequently seen in Ammon's horn, and the cerebral cortex of these patients. By contrast, the neuropathological find-

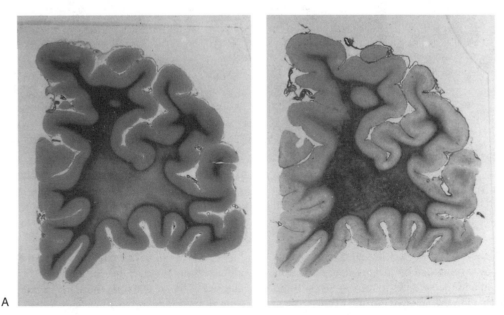

A

B

FIG. 20-11. Coronal sections through the left frontal lobe following exposure to CO. **A:** Demonstrates demyelination of the white matter (Woelcke stain). **B:** Holzer stain reveals marked fibrillary gliosis in astrocytes. (From Kobayashi et al., 1984, with permission.)

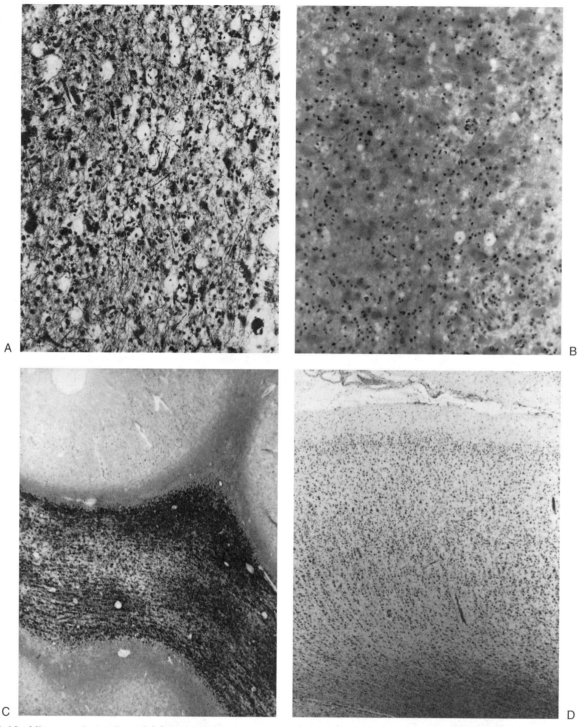

FIG. 20-12. Microscopic studies of CO-induced white matter lesions. **A:** Swollen and destroyed axis cylinders (original magnification, ×200). **B:** Hypertrophic astrocytes (original magnification, ×500). **C:** Lipid droplets. **D:** Preservation of neuronal cytoarchitecture in the cerebral cortex. (From Kobayashi et al., 1984, with permission.)

ings in those patients who present a period of pseudo-recovery followed by a relapse show patchy demyelination of the white matter, and the necrosis to the globus pallidus is frequently confined to the anterior portion (Table 20-4).

The neuropathological changes seen following exposures to CO have primarily been attributed to the com-

bined effects of CO, hypoxemia, and hypotension. CO alone cannot induce the morphological changes seen at autopsy. The severity of the early white matter changes seen in the brains of cats has been correlated with hypoxemia and decreases in cerebral blood pressure (Okeda et al., 1981; Okeda et al., 1982). The shift to anaerobic respi-

TABLE 20-4. *Carbon monoxide poisoning in 22 cases: clinical correlates of neuropathological findings*

Clinical course	Neuropathological findings
Uninterrupted evolution	
Short duration coma (<5 days)	If death occurs within 24 hours after exposure to CO, only cerebral edema is noted, but no significant lesions are seen. At 4 days after exposure, edema, severe necrosis of the globus pallidus extending to the internal capsule, multifocal necrosis in the centrum semiovale and interhemispheric commissures, focal lesions in the gray matter, and numerous hemorrhagic foci are seen. Damage may also be seen in the putamen, thalamus, cerebellum, and Ammon's horn.
Prolonged coma (>7 days)	Edema, necrosis of the globus pallidus, necrosis of the centrum semiovale, discrete lesions in the cerebral cortex, intact Ammon's horn.
Interrupted evolution	Edema, necrosis of the anterior internal globus pallidus, patchy demyelination of white matter particularly notable in the centrum semiovale; the cortex appears normal, the subcortical U fibers are spared, and Ammon's horn is intact.

Data from Lapresle and Fardeau, 1967.

ration and the release of lactate that occurs during hypoxia results in intracellular acidosis in the tissues of the brain (Ginsberg and Meyers, 1974; Wallace and Waugh, 1985; Murata et al., 1995). Exposure to CO also increases the extracellular levels of catecholamines such as dopamine and the production of free radicals, both of which have been associated with cell damage (Halliwell, 1989; Hiramatsu et al., 1994; Nathanson et al., 1995). In addition, reuptake of catecholamines is an adenosine triphosphate (ATP)-dependent process, and hypoxia has been shown to deplete ATP (Hansen, 1985). Therefore, the increased levels of catecholamines may reflect hypoxia-induced depletion of ATP (Hiramatsu et al., 1994). The *N*-methyl-D-aspartate (NMDA) receptor/ion channel complex has also been implicated in the mechanism of neuronal degeneration associated with CO exposure. NMDA stimulates the release of dopamine from dopaminergic nerve terminals (Imperato et al., 1990; Ishimaru et al., 1992; Hiramatsu et al., 1994). The administration of NMDA antagonists decreases the release of dopamine, thereby providing protection against the neurodegenerative effects of CO (Ishimaru et al., 1992; Hiramatsu et al., 1994). Increases in extracellular dopamine are mediated *in vivo* by glutamate, which stimulates NMDA and non-NMDA receptors (Hiramatsu et al., 1994). Although glutamate can induce an increase in intracellular calcium as well as the release of dopamine, Chow and Haddad (1998) have shown that the response of cultured neurons exposed to glutamate is morphologically and biochemically different than that induced by anoxia. Increased release of dopamine has also been associated with increased oxidative stress. Increased oxidative stress has been shown to induce heme oxygenase-1 activity (Schipper et al., 1998). Increased levels of heme- derived free iron resulting from heme oxygenase-1 overactivity may contribute to the pathogenesis of idiopathic Parkinson's disease as well as the parkinsonism seen in persons chronically exposed to low levels of CO (see Clinical Experiences section).

PREVENTION AND THERAPEUTIC MEASURES

OSHA has established PELs for workers at risk of exposure to CO (OSHA, 1995). Nevertheless, occupational exposures resulting in neurological manifestations continue to occur (Fawcett et al., 1992). Work areas such as smelters and automotive repair shops must be properly ventilated. Automobile and truck mechanics should be alerted to the risk of CO exposure from exhaust fumes and instructed on the proper use of exhaust ventilation systems. Small gasoline engine-powered compressors and generators should be located in well-ventilated areas and equipped with external exhaust elimination hoses. Firefighters entering burning buildings should wear self-contained air supply respirators as well as protective clothing. Safety precautions and optimal flue functioning must be used when burning wood in fireplaces or wood stoves. Gas stoves and heaters should be periodically inspected and maintained to ensure proper combustion of the gas and adequate elimination of combustion products. Persons with coronary arteriosclerosis or cerebrovascular disease are more vulnerable to the effects of CO and therefore should be monitored more closely (Aronow and Isbell, 1973; Aronow, 1976; Winter and Miller, 1976).

CO poisoning should be considered in the differential diagnosis of patients presenting with acute or persistent nonspecific flulike symptoms or coma, in association with a history suggesting a possible source of CO exposure (Grace and Platt, 1981; Fisher and Rubin, 1982; Dolan, 1985; Thom and Keim, 1989). Persons rendered unconscious by CO exposure should be immediately removed from the exposure source and placed in a well-ventilated area. Oxygen therapy should begin as soon as possible (Gross et al., 1989). The patient may require endotracheal intubation and mechanical ventilation. HBO_2 therapy increases the amount of oxygen dissolved in the blood and should be administered to those patients not responding to 100% oxygen and to any patient with a COHb level greater than 20% (Gross et al., 1989; Hardy and Thom, 1994). In addition, CO-exposed pregnant women should be administered HBO$_2$ to prevent injury to the fetus (Brown et al., 1992; Hardy and Thom, 1994).

The prognosis in cases of CO poisoning depends on the severity and duration of the exposure. Patients who do not lose consciousness have a better prognosis than those who do. Most patients who develop reversible neurobehavioral manifestations following exposure show full recovery within 1 year; others may retain disabilities permanently (Geschwind, 1968; Min, 1986). Patients who also experience cardiac arrest during the acute stages of CO poisoning have the worst prognosis (Geschwind, 1968; Mathieu et al., 1985; Norkool and Kirkpatrick, 1985).

CLINICAL EXPERIENCES

Group Studies

Paraoccupational Exposure: A Propane-Powered Floor Refinisher and Carbon Monoxide Poisoning

Nine employees (age range: 17 to 42 years) of a Vermont pharmacy were exposed to CO on two separate occasions, 4 days apart (MMWR, 1993). On both days, a subcontractor had cleaned and polished the pharmacy's floors with a propane-powered floor refinishing machine before the employees arrived for work. During the first exposure incident, one employee lost consciousness, but CO poisoning was not suspected at this time, and the patient was diagnosed with vasovagal syncope. On the second occasion, two employees lost consciousness approximately 4 hours after arriving for work. This second incident raised suspicion of CO poisoning. The pharmacy was immediately evacuated and the other employees transported to a local hospital for evaluation. Blood COHb levels were documented in six of the nine employees and ranged from 6.7% to 25.3%. Symptoms reported included headache (nine), lightheadedness (seven), constriction of visual fields (five), nausea and vomiting (four), syncope (two), chest pain (two), difficulty breathing (two), and hearing impairment (one).

Although the floor refinisher did not report experiencing symptoms during use of the machine, investigations by the Vermont Department of Health (VDH) revealed that CO concentrations in the exhaust from the machine's engine ranged from 3,000 ppm at idle to 50,000 ppm at full throttle. CO levels in the pharmacy on the two mornings after the floor refinisher had been used were estimated to have ranged from 507 to 1,127 ppm, or 10 to 22 times the OSHA exposure limit of 50 ppm. The cause of CO poisoning was therefore determined to be failure to maintain the floor refinishing equipment adequately and inadequate ventilation of the work area. Based on these findings, the VDH recommended that the subcontractor replace the propane-powered machines with electric floor refinishers and/or that CO alarms be used whenever the propane-powered machines were used.

Warehouse Workers Exposed to Carbon Monoxide from Propane-Fueled Forklifts

Seventeen warehouse workers developed neurological symptoms following exposure to propane-fueled forklift exhaust fumes (Fawcett et al., 1992). Sixteen of the workers were forklift operators. Investigations showed that the forklifts were not malfunctioning and were producing normal CO emissions from an efficient running forklift engine (range: 1.0% to 1.5%). However, this level of CO in exhaust emissions can rapidly result in a high ambient air concentration of CO in an unventilated area. Not surprisingly, 15 of the 17 cases occurred in the winter months in closed warehouses; the remaining two cases occurred in midsummer in air-conditioned warehouses. The average duration of exposure to exhaust fumes was 4.4 hours. Average blood COHb levels were 19.1% (nonsmokers) and 23.3% (smokers). The one exposed worker who was not a forklift operator was a nonsmoker and had a COHb level of 4.2%.

The most common complaints among all 17 of the exposed workers were headache, lightheadedness, and nausea. In addition, three workers experienced syncope, and one worker reportedly lost consciousness as a result of exposure to CO gas emitted from the forklift. All patients were treated with HBO$_2$ therapy following which their symptoms quickly resolved. No long-term sequelae were detected at follow-up. These results indicated that high levels of CO can be reached in enclosed areas where propane-powered equipment is used and that proper ventilation of these areas and education of equipment operators is necessary for worker safety.

A Family Chronically Exposed to Carbon Monoxide Emitted by a Defective Liquid-Propane Gas Stove

Three adults, a 42-year-old woman, her 44-year-old husband, and their pregnant 20-year-old daughter lived together and spent most of their day working in the kitchen of their home where a new liquid propane gas-fueled stove had recently been installed (R. G. Feldman, personal observation). The man worked as an electrician and his business was run out of this room, with the phone and paperwork done by his wife and daughter. The women worked in the kitchen most of the day, while he came and went from here to his jobs. All three people often suffered from headaches, fatigue, shortness of breath, dizziness, and lightheadedness, all of which were exacerbated while they were in the kitchen. In addition to these symptoms, the wife reported clumsiness and a sense of being "off-balance" much of the time. She also noticed increased emotional irritability, and difficulty concentrating on her work and her hobby of needlework. These symptoms were worse on the days she had sat at the kitchen table and done bookkeeping all day. During the same period her husband began to have noticeable problems with memory and headaches. He had poor concentration, slept poorly, and felt drugged at times, especially when at home during the evening. At these times his speech seemed "all screwed up." He often worked in the kitchen with his wife and noted that he felt better on the days he was out of the house on jobs. The daughter had similar complaints of headache and dizziness; on one occasion she became stuporous and lost consciousness while driving her car. A diagnosis of seizures was made. It was also during this time that her pregnancy came to term. The common symptoms prompted the family physician to suspect CO poisoning.

The only potential source of exposure in the family's kitchen was the liquid propane gas stove, which had been installed just before the family's symptoms began. Investigations revealed that the gas stove had been functioning with half of its burner ports unignited. The TWA CO concentration emitted by the stove during 100 minutes of operation was determined to be 226 ppm. CO concentrations emitted from a properly operating stove of this type would not exceed 10 ppm. The ambient air CO level in the family's kitchen rose from 0 ppm prior to the test to 50 ppm after the 100-minute test. Further inspection and testing of the stove revealed that its regulator, which controls the stove's manifold pressure, was defective and was causing the stove to operate less efficiently, thereby increasing the appliance's output of CO. In addition, this defect caused the burner to discharge high levels of unburned propane. It was concluded that the stove's gas regulator was defective or improperly designed and manufactured.

Neuropsychological testing of the husband 10 months after cessation of exposure revealed problems with short-term memory involving both visuospatial and verbal information. Constructional deficits were observed. Psychomotor control problems, with a tendency to be tremulous, were noted. He also showed problems with cognitive tracking and cognitive flexibility. Despite these difficulties, his basic language and verbal skills were intact. Follow-up neuropsychological assessment showed significant improvement in cognitive flexibility, and visual memory and visuospatial analysis. However, finger-tapping speed decreased. It was concluded that the patient showed good recovery from the effects of CO poisoning, although visual memory deficits and sensitivity to interference on tests of verbal memory remained.

Neuropsychological testing of the wife 10 months after cessation of exposure to CO revealed cognitive inflexibility on tests of inferential reasoning. Occasionally perseveration and loss of set was seen on tests of executive function. Visual attention spans were inferior to verbal attention spans. Deficits were seen on tasks assessing visuospatial analysis and organization. She was sensitive to interference on verbal learning tasks. Mood was anxious, depressed, and irritable. Follow-up neuropsychological assessments showed marked improvement in executive functioning at 1-year follow-up but less marked improvements at 3 years. Marked improvement in performance on tests of verbal and visual

memory was noted at 3-year follow-up. Performance on psychomotor tests (Digit Symbol) also showed improvement at this time. However, her manual dexterity and her ability to inhibit interference on tests of memory remained below expectation.

Neuropsychological assessment of the daughter revealed difficulties on tasks of visuospatial analysis and organization. Performance scores on visual spans were lower than on verbal spans. In addition, she was sensitive to interference on verbal learning tasks.

Neuropsychological assessment of the daughter's son, who was born while the family was being exposed to CO, was performed at the time of the 3-year follow-up; the child was 3 years old at this time. Testing revealed poor speech articulation.

The test results seen in this family with chronic CO exposure suggest that neuropsychological testing can reveal persistent subclinical effects of CO exposure after the clinically overt symptoms have ameliorated.

Individual Studies

Reversible Effects of Acute Carbon Monoxide Exposure

Case 1

A 30-year-old man was found unconscious in a running car in a closed garage (Zink et al., 1994). The patient's blood COHb level was determined by the paramedics immediately after cessation of exposure and was found to be 53%. On arrival at the hospital, the patient was comatose and had extensor posturing. Reflexes were symmetrical, and the patient had a positive Babinski response bilaterally. HBO_2 therapy was administered twice in the first 24 hours but did not improve the patient's neurological status. Brain CT scan revealed no edema or lesions at this time. The patient regained consciousness 17 days after the incident, at which time he had difficulty following commands. After 3 months of rehabilitative therapy, his speech was fluent and he was able to walk with a cane. At follow-up 1 year after the incident, the patient was living independently and was able to play recreational basketball, although his performance on the court was not what it was before his exposure to CO.

Case 2

A 19-year-old woman was found unconscious in a running car in a closed garage (Zink et al., 1994). On arrival at the hospital, she was comatose, with extensor posturing. Her blood COHb level was 55%. Urine toxicology screen was positive for opiates and barbiturates. The patient received HBO_2 therapy three times in the first 24 hours after her removal from exposure to CO, but her neurological status did not improve. The patient regained consciousness after 10 days but did not interact with her environment until day 35 post-exposure, at which time she began to speak and to follow simple commands. After 1 year of rehabilitation therapy, the patient's speech was fluent, and she ambulated without difficulty. Although her cognitive abilities remained mildly impaired, she was able to manage her own financial and legal affairs.

Parkinsonism and Carbon Monoxide Exposure: Effects of L-Dopa Therapy

Case 1

A 40-year-old man developed parkinsonism 4 weeks after a severe acute exposure to CO (Jaeckle and Nasrallah, 1985). The man had been found alone in his home in an obtund state, following which he was admitted to the local hospital. CO poisoning was suspected, and blood COHb level 1 hour after admission was 30%. The patient was treated with oxygen therapy and within 8 hours after admission to the hospital had regained full consciousness. Further investigations revealed that the furnace in the patient's home was emitting 0.02% CO, which accumulated because of improper ventilation. Although the duration and maximum exposure levels could not be determined, it was decided that the CO poisoning was unintentionally caused by the malfunctioning of his furnace. No abnormalities were noted on the neurological examination at this time. Four weeks later, neurological examination revealed bradykinesia, shuffling gait, stooped posture, cogwheel rigidity in all four extremities, resting tremor, masked facies, micrographia, hypophonia, and slow monotonous speech. There was no history of neurological illness prior to his exposure to CO. A diagnosis of delayed-onset parkinsonism secondary to CO intoxication was made. Clinical improvement following L-dopa was reported.

Case 2

A 48-year-old man developed parkinsonian symptoms after chronic exposure to CO (Ringle and Klawans, 1972). The man had been exposed while using a gas-powered concrete saw, which he frequently operated in closed or unventilated rooms. On two occasions he was found comatose as a result of using the saw in an unventilated area. Four years after his last incident of CO-induced unconsciousness, he began to experience difficulty walking, and his speech became slower, monotonous, and lower in volume. During the course of the next few months, his speech gradually became inaudible, his walking grew progressively slower, and sometimes he would freeze while turning or when rising to get out of a chair. He experienced constant profuse sweating and sialorrhea. Eventually the patient was unable to feed or bathe himself. The patient had no history of head trauma or neurological disease. Neurological examination revealed marked rigidity of all extremities and the neck. The patient had a slight coarse resting tremor in both upper extremities, and finger dexterity was poor bilaterally. Deep

tendon reflexes were symmetrical, and the plantar responses were flexor. Extraocular movements were normal. The patient was treated with and responded acutely to L-dopa.

Case 3

A 50-year-old woman who attempted suicide by inhalation of automobile exhaust was found unconscious by a family member (Klawans et al., 1982). Eight hours after her admission to the hospital she awoke, and initially felt well. However, 3 days later, she began to experience tremulousness in her lower extremities and imbalance without syncope or vertigo. A neurological examination 3 months later revealed tremor, simian posture, micrography, bradykinesia, and propulsion. The patient's symptoms were unresponsive to L-dopa.

Recurrent Carbon Monoxide Exposures and Episodes of Impaired Consciousness

A 50-year-old police officer with 18 years of service developed transient episodes of loss of consciousness while he was directing automobile traffic (Gilbert and Glaser, 1959). These episodes appeared once every 2 to 3 months, always began with mild lightheadedness, and progressed to include dizziness and ataxia, after which he would lose consciousness for 15 to 90 minutes. He requested a transfer to the police garage, where he subsequently worked as a mechanic. It was often necessary for him to run the car engines during repairs. When the garage doors were closed, he again experienced episodes of loss of consciousness. During one of these episodes, which typically occurred toward the end of his work shift, he was taken to the hospital. He regained consciousness by the time he reached the hospital. His examination showed poor memory, ataxic gait, and a fine rapid tremor of the fingers. Laboratory studies reported a positive test for albumin in urine; blood COHb level was 20% of the total hemoglobin on the day after admission. A diagnosis of CO poisoning was made, and anticonvulsant medications were discontinued; these had been prescribed 2 years earlier when a diagnosis of psychomotor seizures was made following one of these episodes. The patient was discharged recovered. However, following his discharge, the patient experienced two additional episodes of confusion and staggering gait after he used a gasoline-powered tractor, which was found to have its exhaust pipe located near his breathing space. The patient was advised to avoid further exposure to CO, and he remained asymptomatic thereafter.

REFERENCES

American Conference of Governmental Industrial Hygienists (ACGIH). *Threshold limit values (TLVs) for chemical substances and physical agents and biological exposure indices (BEIs)*. Cincinnati, OH: ACGIH, 1995–1996.

Amoore, JE, Hautala E. Odor as an aid to chemical safety: odor thresholds compared with threshold limit values and volatilities for 214 industrial chemicals in air and water dilution. *J Appl Toxicol* 1983;3:272–290.

Aronow WS. Effect of cigarette smoking and carbon monoxide on coronary heart disease. *Chest* 1976;70:514–518.

Aronow WS, Isbell MW. Carbon monoxide effect on exercise-induced angina pectoris. *Ann Intern Med* 1973;79:392–395.

Baron RC, Backer RC, Sopher IM. Fatal unintended carbon monoxide poisoning in West Virginia from nonvehicular sources. *Am J Public Health* 1989;79:1656–1658.

Beard RR. Inorganic compounds of oxygen, nitrogen, and carbon. In: Clayton GD, Clayton FE, eds. *Patty's industrial hygiene and toxicology,* 3rd ed., vol. IIc. New York: John Wiley & Sons, 1982:4114–4124.

Beard RR, Wertheim GA. Behavioral impairment associated with small doses of carbon monoxide. *Am J Public Health* 1967;57:2012–2022.

Beard RR, Grandstaff N. Carbon monoxide exposure and cerebral function. *Ann NY Acad Sci* 1970;174:385–395.

Bender W, Göthert M, Malorny G, Sebbesse P. Wirkungsbild neidriger Kohlenoxid-Konzentration beim Menschen. *Arch Toxicol* 1971;27:142–158.

Bender W, Göthert M, Malorney G. Effect of low carbon monoxide concentration on psychological functions. *Staub Reinhalt Luft* (English) 1972;32:54–60.

Benignus VA, Petrovisk MK, Newlin-Clapp L, Prah JD. Carboxyhemoglobin and brain blood flow in humans. *Neurotoxicol Teratol* 1992;14:285–290.

Berger H. Uber das elektroephalogram des Menschen IX. *Arch Psychiatr Nervenkr* 1934;102:538.

Bernard C. *An introduction to the study of experimental medicine.* New York: Macmillan, 1927:159–162.

Brown DB, Mueller GL, Golich FC. Hyperbaric oxygen treatment for carbon monoxide poisoning in pregnancy: a case report. *Aviation Space Environ Med* 1992;63:1011–1014.

Bruno A, Wagner W, Orison WW. Clinical outcome and brain MRI four years after carbon monoxide intoxication. *Acta Neurol Scand* 1993;87:205–209.

Burgess WA, Diberardinis L, Speizer FE. Health effects of exposure to automobile exhaust—V. Exposure of toll booth operators to automobile exhaust. *Am Ind Hyg J* 1977;38:184–191.

Carlson C, Hagerdal M, Siesjo BK. Protective effect of hypothermia in cerebral oxygen deficiency caused by arterial hypoxia. *Anesthesiology* 1976;44:27–35.

Carlsson A, Hultengren M. Exposure to methylene chloride. III. Metabolism of ^{14}C-labelled methylene chloride in rat. *Scand J Work Environ Health* 1975;1:104–108.

Chance B, Erecinska M, Wagner M. Mitochondrial responses to carbon monoxide toxicity. *Ann NY Acad Sci* 1970;174:193–204.

Choi IS, Kim SK, Choi YC, Lee SS, Lee MS. Evaluation of outcome after acute carbon monoxide poisoning by brain CT. *J Korean Med Sci* 1993;8:78–83.

Chow E, Haddad GG. Differential effects of anoxia and glutamate on cultured neocortical neurons. *Exp Neurol* 1998;150:52–59.

Chung Y, Park SE, Lee K, Yanagisawa Y, Spengler JD. Determinations of personal carbon monoxide exposure and blood carboxyhemoglobin levels in Korea. *Yonsei Med J* 1994;35:420–428.

Cobb N, Etzel RA. Unintentional carbon monoxide-related deaths in the United States, 1979–1988. *JAMA* 1991;266:659–663.

Coburn RF. The carbon monoxide body stores. *Ann NY Acad Sci* 1970;174:11–22.

Coburn RF, Blakemore WS, Forster RE. Endogenous carbon monoxide production in man. *J Clin Invest* 1963;42:1172–1178.

Coburn RF, Williams WJ, Kahn SB. Endogenous carbon monoxide production in patients with haemolytic anaemia. *J Clin Invest* 1966;45:460–468.

Coburn RF, Mayers LB. Myoglobin O_2 tension determined from measurements of carboxyhemoglobin in skeletal muscle. *Am J Physiol* 1971;220:66–74.

Cook M, Simon PA, Hoffman RE. Unintended carbon monoxide poisoning in Colorado, 1986 through 1991. *Am J Public Health* 1995;85:988–990.

Craig TV, Hunt W, Atkinson R. Hypothermia—its use in severe carbon monoxide poisoning. *N Engl J Med* 1959;261:854–856.

Dawson TM, Snyder SH. Gases as biological messengers: nitric oxide and carbon monoxide in the brain. *J Neurosci* 1994;14:5147–5159.

Deckel AW. Carbon monoxide poisoning and frontal lobe pathology: two case reports and a discussion of the literature. *Brain Injury* 1994;8:345–356.

Denays R, Makhoul E, Dachy B, et al. Electroencephalographic mapping and ^{99m}Tc HMPAO single-photon emission computed tomography in carbon monoxide poisoning. *Ann Emerg Med* 1994;24:947–952.

DiVincenzo GD, Kaplan CJ. Effect of exercise or smoking on the uptake, metabolism, and excretion of methylene chloride vapor. *Toxicol Appl Pharmacol* 1981;59:141–148.

Douglas CG, Haldane JS, Haldane JBS. The laws of combination haemoglobin with carbon monoxide and oxygen. *J Physiol* 1912;44:275–304.

Dolan MC. Carbon monoxide poisoning. *Can Med Assoc J* 1985;133:392–399.

Dolan MC, Haltom TL, Barrows GH, Short CS, Ferriell KM. Carboxyhemoglobin levels in patients with flu-like symptoms. *Ann Emerg Med* 1987;16:782–786.

Duhaine AC, Ross D. Degeneration of hippocampal CA1 neurons following transient ischemia due to raised intracranial pressure: evidence of a temperature-dependent excitotoxic process. *Brain Res* 1990;512:169–174.

Ewing JF, Maines MD. In situ hybridization and immunohistochemical localization of heme oxygenase-2 mRNA and protein in normal rat brain: differential distribution of isozyme 1 and 2. *Mol Cell Neurosci* 1992;3:559–570.

Farrow JR, Davis GJ, Roy TM, McCloud LC, Nichols GR. Case report. Fetal death due to nonlethal maternal carbon monoxide poisoning. *J Forens Sci* 1990;35:1448–1452.

Fawcett TA, Moon RE, Fracica PJ, Mebane GY, Theil DR, Piantadosi CA. Warehouse workers' headache. *J Occup Med* 1992;34:12–15.

Finck PA. Exposure to carbon monoxide: review of the literature and 567 autopsies. *Mil Med* 1966;131:1513–1539.

Fisher J, Rubin KP. Occult carbon monoxide poisoning. *Arch Intern Med* 1982;142:1270–1271.

Fitz-Gerald MJ, Patrick G. Longitudinal quantitative EEG findings after acute carbon monoxide exposure: two case studies. *Clin Electroencephalogr* 1991;22:217–224.

Forbes WH. Carbon monoxide uptake via the lungs. *Ann NY Acad Sci* 1970;174:72–75.

Gajdos P, Conso F, Korach JM, et al. Incidence and causes of carbon monoxide intoxication: results of an epidemiological survey in a French department. *Arch Environ Health* 1991;46:373–376.

Geschwind N, Quadfasel FA, Segarra JM. Isolation of the speech area. *Neuropsychologia* 1968;6:327–340.

Gilbert GJ, Glaser GH. Neurological manifestations of carbon monoxide poisoning. *N Engl J Med* 1959;261:1217–1220.

Ginsberg MD, Myers RE, McDonagh BF. Experimental carbon monoxide encephalopathy in the primate. II. Clinical aspects, neuropathology, and physiologic correlation. *Arch Neurol* 1974;30:209–216.

Gotoh M, Kuyama H, Asari S, Ohmoto T, Akioka T, Lai M-Y. Sequential changes in MR images of the brain in acute carbon monoxide poisoning. *Comput Med Imaging Graph* 1993;17:55–59.

Grace TW, Platt FW. Subacute carbon monoxide poisoning. Another great imitator. *JAMA* 1981;246:1698–1700.

Gregus Z, Klaassen CD. Mechanisms of toxicity. In: Klaassen KD, ed. *Casarett and Doull's toxicology. The basic science of poisons,* 5th ed. New York: McGraw-Hill, 1996:35–74.

Grinker RR. Parkinsonism following carbon monoxide poisoning. *J Nerve Ment Dis* 1926;64:18–28.

Gross PL, Weber-Bornstein N, Castronovo FP, Baker AS. Environmental hazards. In: Wilkins EW, ed. *Emergency medicine. Scientific foundations and current practices,* 3rd ed. Baltimore: Williams & Wilkins, 1989:184–186.

Halliwell B. Oxidants and the central nervous system: some fundamental questions. Is oxidant damage relevant to Parkinson's disease, Alzheimer's disease, traumatic injury and stroke? *Acta Neurol Scand* 1989;126:23–33.

Halperin MH, McFarland RA, Niven JI, Roughton FJW. The time course of the effects of carbon monoxide on visual thresholds. *J Physiol* 1959;146:583–593.

Hansen AJ. Effects of anoxia on ion distribution in the brain. *Physiol Rev* 1985;65:101–148.

Hardy KR, Thom SR. Pathophysiology and treatment of carbon monoxide poisoning. *Clin Toxicol* 1994;32:613–629.

Hawkins RD, Zhuo M, Arancio O. Nitric oxide and carbon monoxide as possible retrograde messengers in hippocampal long-term potentiation. *J Neurobiol* 1994;25:652–665.

Hayashi R, Hayashi K, Inoue K, Yanagisawa N. A serial computerized tomographic study of the interval form of CO poisoning. *Eur Neurol* 1993;33:27–29.

He F, Liu X, Yang S, et al. Evaluation of brain function in acute carbon monoxide poisoning with multimodality evoked potentials. *Environ Res* 1993;60:213–226.

Hebb DO. *The organization of behavior: A neuropsychological theory.* New York: John Wiley & Sons, 1949.

Hill E, Semerak CB. Changes in the brain in gas (carbon monoxide) poisoning. *JAMA* 1918;71:644–648.

Hiramatsu M, Yokayama S, Nebeshima J, Kameyama T. Changes in concentrations of dopamine, serotonin, and their metabolites induced by carbon monoxide (CO) in rat striatum as determined by in vivo microdialysis. *Pharmacol Biochem Behav* 1994;48:9–15.

Hosko MJ. The effect of carbon monoxide on the visual evoked response in man. *Arch Environ Health* 1970;21:174–180.

Imperato A, Honoré T, Jensen LH. Dopamine release in the nucleus caudate and in the nucleus accumbens is under glutamatergic control through non-NMDA receptors: a study in freely moving rats. *Brain Res* 1990;530:223–228.

Ishimaru H, Katoh A, Suzuki H, Fukuta T, Kameyama T, Nebeshima T. Effects of N-methyl-D-aspartate receptor antagonists on carbon monoxide-induced brain damage in mice. *J Pharmacol Exp Ther* 1992;261:349–352.

Ishimaru H, Nebeshima T, Katoh A, Suzuki H, Fukuta T, Kameyama T. Effects of successive carbon monoxide exposures on delayed neuronal death in mice under the maintenance of normal body temperature. *Biochem Biophys Res Commun* 1991;179:836–840.

Jaeckle RS, Nasrallah HA. Single case study. Major depression and carbon monoxide-induced parkinsonism: diagnosis, computerized axial tomography, and response to L-dopa. *J Nerve Ment Dis* 1985;173:503–508.

Jaffe LS. Carbon monoxide in the environment. Sources, characteristics, and fate of atmospheric carbon monoxide. *Ann NY Acad Sci* 1970;174:76–88.

Jefferson JW. Subtle neuropsychiatric sequelae of carbon monoxide intoxication: two case reports. *Am J Psychiatry* 1976;133:961–964.

Jones JS, Lagasse J, Zimmerman G. Computed tomographic findings after acute carbon monoxide poisoning. *Am J Emerg Med* 1994;12:448–451.

Jones MD, Traystman RJ. Cerebral oxygenation of the fetus, newborn, and adult. *Semin Perinatol* 1984;8:205–216.

Kales SN. Carbon monoxide intoxication. *Am Fam Phys* 1993;48:1100–1104.

Kamada K, Houkin K, Aoki T, et al. Cerebral metabolic changes in delayed carbon monoxide sequelae studied by proton MR spectroscopy. *Neuroradiology* 1994;36:104–106.

Klawans HL, Stein RW, Tanner CM, Goetz CG. A pure parkinsonian syndrome following acute carbon monoxide intoxication. *Arch Neurol* 1982;39:302–304.

Kobayashi K, Isaki K, Fukutani Y, et al. CT findings of the interval form of carbon monoxide poisoning compared with neuropathological findings. *Eur Neurol* 1984;23:34–43.

Kubic VL, Anders MW. Metabolism of dihalomethanes to carbon monoxide. II. In vitro studies. *Drug Metab Dispos* 1975;3:104–112.

LaPresle J, Fardeau M. The central nervous system and carbon monoxide poisoning. II. Anatomical study of brain lesions following intoxication with carbon monoxide (22 cases). *Prog Brain Res* 1967;24:31–74.

Laties VG, Merigan WH. Behavioral effects of carbon monoxide on animals and man. *Annu Rev Pharmacol Toxicol* 1979;19:357–392.

Lee K, Yanagisawa Y, Spengler JD, Nakai S. Carbon monoxide and nitrogen dioxide exposures in indoor ice skating rinks. *J Sports Sci* 1994;12:279–283.

Lennox MA, Petersen PB. Electroencephalographic findings in acute carbon monoxide poisoning. *EEG Clin Neurophysiol* 1958;10:63–68.

Lewis S, Mason C, Srna J. Carbon monoxide exposure in blast furnace workers. *Aust J Public Health* 1992;16:262–268.

Longo LD. Carbon monoxide in the pregnant mother and fetus and its exchange across the placenta. *Ann NY Acad Sci* 1970;174:313–341.

Mactutus CF. Developmental neurotoxicity of nicotine, carbon monoxide, and other tobacco smoke constituents. *Ann NY Acad Sci* 1989;562:105–122.

Madani IM, Khalfan S, Khalfan H, Jidah J, Aladin MN. Occupational exposure to carbon monoxide during charcoal meat grilling. *Sci Tot Environ* 1992;114:141–147.

Marks G, Brien J, Nakatsu K, McLaughlin B. Does carbon monoxide have a physiological role? *Trends Pharmacol Sci* 1991;1:185–188.

Mathieu D, Nolf M, Durocher A, et al. Acute carbon monoxide poisoning: risk of late sequelae and treatment by hyperbaric oxygen. *Clin Toxicol* 1985;23:315–324.

Menon DK, Sargentoni J, Peden CJ, et al. Proton MR spectroscopy in herpes simplex encephalitis: assessment of neuronal loss. *J Comput Assist Tomogr* 1990;14:449–452.

Meredith T, Vale A. Carbon monoxide poisoning. *BMJ* 1988;296:77–78.

Messier LD, Myers RAM. A neuropsychological screening battery for emergency assessment of carbon-monoxide-poisoned patients. *J Clin Psychiatry* 1991;47:675–684.

Mihevic PM, Gliner JA, Horvath SM. Carbon monoxide exposure and information processing during perceptual-motor performance. *Int Arch Occup Environ Health* 1983;51:355–363.

Min SK. A brain syndrome associated with delayed neuropsychiatric sequelae following acute carbon monoxide intoxication. *Acta Psychiatr Scand* 1986;73:80–86.

Morbidity and Mortality World Report (MMWR). *Unintentional death from carbon monoxide poisoning—Michigan, 1987–1989.* Washington: US Department of Health and Human Services, CDC, vol. 41, no. 47, 1992.

Morbidity and Mortality World Report (MMWR). *Unintentional carbon monoxide poisoning following a winter storm—Washington, January 1993.* Washington: US Department of Health and Human Services, CDC, vol. 42, no. 6, 1993.

Morbidity and Mortality World Report (MMWR). *Carbon monoxide poisoning associated with a propane-powered floor burnisher—Vermont, 1992.* Washington: US Department of Health and Human Services, CDC, vol. 42, no. 37, 1993.

Murata T, Itoh S, Koshino Y, et al. Serial proton magnetic resonance spectroscopy in a patient with the interval form of carbon monoxide poisoning. *J Neurol Neurosurg Psychiatry* 1995;58:100–103.

Murray JF. Respiration. In: Smith LH, Thier SO, eds. *Pathophysiology. The biological principles of disease,* 2nd ed. Philadelphia: WB Saunders, 1985:753–844.

Myers RAM, Britten JS. Are arterial blood gases of value in treatment decisions for carbon monoxide poisoning? *Crit Care Med* 1989;17:139–142.

Nadler JV, Cooper JR. N-acetyl-L-aspartic acid content of human neural tumours and bovine peripheral nervous tissues. *J Neurochem* 1972;19:313–319.

Nathanson JA, Scavone C, Scanlon C, McKee M. The cellular Na+pump as a site of action for carbon monoxide and glutamate: a mechanism for long-term modulation of cellular activity. *Neuron* 1995;14:781–794.

National Institute of Occupational Safety and Health (NIOSH). *Pocket guide to chemical hazards.* Washington: US Department of Health and Human Services, CDC, June 1997.

Neufeld Y, Swanson JW, Klass DW. Localized EEG abnormalities in acute carbon monoxide poisoning. *Arch Neurol* 1981;38:524–527.

Norkool DM, Kirkpatrick JN. Treatment of acute carbon monoxide poisoning with hyperbaric oxygen: a review of 115 cases. *Ann Emerg Med* 1985;14:1168–1171.

Norman CA, Halton DM. Is carbon monoxide a workplace teratogen? A review and evaluation of the literature. *Ann Occup Hyg* 1990;34:335–347.

Occupational Safety and Health Administration (OSHA). Code of Federal Regulations, 29, 1910.1000/.1047. Washington: Office of the Federal Register, National Archives and Records Administration, 1995:411–431.

Okeda R, Funata N, Song SY, Higashino F, Takano T, Yokohama K. Comparative study on pathogenesis of selective cerebral lesions in carbon monoxide poisoning and nitrogen hypoxia in cats. *Acta Neuropathol* 1982;56:265–272.

Okeda R, Funata N, Takano T, et al. The pathogenesis of carbon monoxide encephalopathy in acute phase—physiological and morphological correlation. *Acta Neuropathol* 1981;54:1–10.

Perry GF. Occupational medicine forum. What are the potential delayed health effects of high-level carbon monoxide exposure? *J Occup Med* 1994;36:595–597.

Pitt BR, Radford EP, Gurtner GH, Tryastman RJ. Interaction of carbon monoxide and cyanide on cerebral circulation and metabolism. *Arch Environ Health* 1976;34:345–349.

Poirier J, Gray F, Escourolle R. *Manual of basic neuropathology,* 3rd ed. Philadelphia: WB Saunders, 1990:164–179.

Pulst S-M, Walshe TM, Romero JA. Carbon monoxide poisoning with features of Gilles de la Tourette's syndrome. *Arch Neurol* 1983;40:443–444.

Putz VR. The effects of carbon monoxide on dual-task performance. *Hum Fact* 1979;21:13–24.

Ray AM, Rockwell TH. An exploratory study of automobile driving performance under the influence of low levels of carboxyhemoglobin. *Ann NY Acad Sci* 1970;174:396–408.

Richardson JC, Chambers RA, Heywood PM. Encephalopathies of anoxia and hypoglycemia. *AMA Arch Neurol* 1959;1:178–190.

Ringel SP, Klawans HL. Carbon monoxide-induced parkinsonism. *J Neurol Sci* 1972;16:245–251.

Risser D, Schneider B. Carbon monoxide-related deaths from 1984 to 1993 in Vienna, Austria. *J Forensic Sci* 1995;40:368–371.

Roughton FJW, Darling RC. The effect of carbon monoxide on the oxyhemoglobin dissociation curve. *Am J Physiol* 1944;141:17–31.

Rozman KK, Klaassen CD. Absorption, distribution and excretion of toxicants. In: Klaassen KD, ed. *Casarett and Doull's toxicology. The basic science of poisons,* 5th ed. New York: McGraw-Hill, 1996:91–112.

Rummo N, Sarlanis K. The effect of carbon monoxide on several measures of vigilance in a simulated driving task. *J Safety Res* 1974;6:126–130.

Russell MA, Feyerabend C, Cole PV. Plasma nicotine levels after cigarette smoking and chewing nicotine gum. *BMJ* 1976;1:1043–1046.

Sanchez-Ramos JR. Toxin-induced parkinsonism. In: Stern MB, Koller WC, eds. *Parkinsonian syndromes.* New York: Marcel Dekker, 1993:155–171.

Sax NI. *Dangerous properties of industrial chemicals,* 5th ed. New York: Van Nostrand Reinhold, 1979.

Schipper HM, Liderman A, Stopa EG. Neural heme oxygenase-1 expression in idiopathic Parkinson's Disease. *Exp Neurol* 1998;150:60–68.

Scott BL, Jankovic J. Delayed-onset progressive movement disorders after static brain lesions. *Neurology* 1996;46:68–74.

Selvakumar S, Sharan M, Singh MP. A mathematical model for the elimination of carbon monoxide in humans. *J Theor Biol* 1993;162:321–336.

Shimosegawa E, Hatazawa J, Nagata K, et al. Cerebral blood flow and glucose metabolism measurements in a patient surviving one year after carbon monoxide intoxication. *J Nucl Med* 1992;33:1696–1698.

Silverman IE, Galetta SL, Gray LG, et al. SPECT in patients with cortical visual loss. *J Nucl Med* 1993;34:1447–1451.

Sinha AK, Klein J, Schultze P, Weiss J, Weiss HR. Cerebral regional capillary perfusion and blood flow after carbon monoxide exposure. *J Appl Physiol* 1991;71:1196–1200.

Smith JS, Brandon S. Morbidity from acute carbon monoxide poisoning at three-year follow-up. *BMJ* 1973;1:318–321.

Smith RP. Toxic responses of the blood. In: Klaassen KD, ed. *Casarett and Doull's toxicology. The basic science of poisons,* 5th ed. New York: McGraw-Hill, 1996:335–354.

Soden KJ, Marras G, Amsel J. Carboxyhemoglobin levels in methylene chloride–exposed employees. *J Occup Environ Med* 1996;38:367–371.

Somogyi E, Balogh I, Rubányi G, Sótonyi P, Szegedi L. New findings concerning the pathogenesis of acute carbon monoxide (CO) poisoning. *Am J Forensic Med Pathol* 1981;2:31–39.

Stern FB, Halperin WE, Hornung RW, et al. Heart disease mortality among bridge and tunnel officers exposed to carbon monoxide. *Am J Epidemiol* 1988;128:1276–1288.

Stewart RD, Hake CL. Paint-remover hazard. *JAMA* 1976;235:398–401.

Stewart RD, Peterson JE, Baretta ED, Bachand RT, Hosko MJ, Herrmann AA. Experimental human exposure to carbon monoxide. *Arch Environ Health* 1970;21:154–164.

Stewart RD, Peterson JE, Fisher TN, et al. Experimental human exposure to high concentrations of carbon monoxide. *Arch Environ Health* 1973;26:1–7.

Sun Y, Rotenberg MO, Maines MD. Developmental expression of heme oxygenase isozymes in rat brain. Two HO-2 mRNAs are detected. *J Biol Chem* 1990;265:8212–8217.

Swinnerton JW, Linnenborn VJ, Lamontagne RA. Distribution of carbon monoxide between the atmosphere and the ocean. *Ann NY Acad Sci* 1970;174:96–101.

Thom SR, Keim LW. Carbon monoxide poisoning: a review of epidemiology, pathophysiology, clinical findings, and treatment options including hyperbaric oxygen therapy. *Clin Toxicol* 1989;27:141–156.

United States Environmental Protection Agency (USEPA). *Drinking water regulations and health advisories.* EPA 822-R-96-001. Washington: Office of Water, 1996.

Verma A, Hirsch DJ, Glatt CE, Ronnett GV, Snyder SH. Carbon monoxide: a putative neural messenger. *Science* 1993;259:381–384.

Vieregge P, Klostermann W, Blumm RG, Borgis KJ. Carbon monoxide poisoning: clinical, neurophysiological, and brain imaging observations in acute disease and follow-up. *J Neurol* 1989;236:478–481.

Virtamo M, Tossavainen A. Carbon monoxide in foundry air. *Scand J Work Environ Health* 1976;2:37–41.

Wallace AG, Waugh RA. The pathophysiology of cardiovascular disease. In: Smith LH, Thier SO, eds. *Pathophysiology. The biological principles of disease,* 2nd ed. Philadelphia: WB Saunders, 1985:855–1003.

Walton JN. *Brain's diseases of the nervous system,* 10th ed. Oxford: Oxford University Press, 1994.

Weaver LK, Hopkins RO, Larson-Lohr V. Neuropsychological and functional recovery from severe carbon monoxide poisoning without hyperbaric oxygen therapy. *Ann Emerg Med* 1996;27:736–740.

Weisel CP, Lawryk NJ, Lioy PJ. Exposure to emissions from gasoline within automobile cabins. *J Exp Anal Environ Epidemiol* 1992;2:79–96.

White RF, Feldman RG, Proctor SP. Neurobehavioral effects of toxic exposures. In: White RF, ed. *Clinical syndromes in adult neuropsychological diagnosis: the practitioner's handbook.* New York: Elsevier Science Publishers, 1992:1–51.

Winter PM, Miller JN. Carbon monoxide poisoning. *JAMA* 1976;236:1502–1504.

Zagami AS, Lethlean AK, Mellick R. Delayed neurological deterioration following carbon monoxide poisoning: MRI findings. *J Neurol* 1993;240:113–116.

Zhuo M, Small SA, Kandel ER, Hawkins RD. Nitric oxide and carbon monoxide produce activity-dependent long-term synaptic enhancement in hippocampus. *Science* 1993;260:1946–1950.

Zink RS, Adkinson CD, Davies SF. Neurological recovery after prolonged coma from carbon monoxide poisoning. *Am J Emerg Med* 1994;12:607–610.

CHAPTER 21

Carbon Disulfide

Carbon disulfide (CS_2; carbon bisulfide) is a clear liquid that evaporates at room temperature and off-gases a faintly sweet, ethereal aroma. Pure CS_2 is highly flammable and will autoignite at 194°F; combustion releases sulfur dioxide, which is also highly toxic (Sax, 1979). Commercial production of CS_2 involves reacting sulfur with methane, ethane, and/or ethylene (Windholz, 1994). Alternatively, CS_2 can be produced by reacting sulfur with charcoal at high temperatures (Seppäläinen and Haltia, 1980). Carbon disulfide is formed in active volcanoes, in marshes, and in the ocean (Lovelock, 1974; Aneja et al., 1980; Rasmussen et al., 1982).

Careful monitoring of workplace exposure levels and replacement of CS_2 with other less toxic substances has not eliminated the risk of hazardous exposures, particularly where there may be improper ventilation of work areas and unhygienic work practices (Peterson, 1892; Gordy and Trumper, 1938; Manu et al., 1970; Aaserud et al., 1990; Chu et al., 1995; Drexler et al., 1995). Occupational exposures have been associated with reports of toxic effects including peripheral neuropathy, encephalopathy, parkinsonism, and microangiopathy (Gordy and Trumper, 1938; Braceland, 1942; Hänninen, 1971; Tolonen, 1975; Sugimoto et al., 1976a; Vasilecu and Florescu, 1980; Seppäläinen and Haltia, 1980; Aaserud et al., 1992; Chu et al., 1995). Differences in susceptibility to the effects of CS_2 contribute to the range of presenting symptoms and affect prognosis of recovery in certain individuals (Hänninen, 1971; Lieben and Williams, 1974; Besarabic, 1978; Drexler et al., 1995).

SOURCES OF EXPOSURE

CS_2 has been used as a solvent for the cold vulcanization of rubber products and for extracting fats and oils (Gordy and Trumper, 1938; ATSDR, 1995). Most occupational exposures occur in the textile industry during the manufacture of viscose rayon. Viscose rayon workers are constantly exposed to low levels of CS_2 in the ambient air; higher levels of exposure occur during the spinning process and during equipment malfunctions and repairs (Vigliani, 1954; Manu et al., 1970; Cirla et al., 1978; Chu et al., 1995; Drexler et al., 1995; Liss and Finkelstein, 1996; Vanhoorne et al., 1995, 1996). It is also used in the manufacture of cellophane packaging materials (Seppäläinen and Haltia, 1980).

Exposure to CS_2 can occur during the synthesis of other chemicals such as carbon tetrachloride and dithioacetic acids and their derivatives (Timmerman, 1978; R. G. Feldman, personal observation). Exposure occurs during the manufacture and application of dithiocarbamate pesticides, which are metabolized to CS_2 (Peters et al., 1988; Brugnone et al., 1993; Valentine et al., 1995). CS_2 is also a component in pesticide mixtures used to fumigate grains (Peters et al., 1988).

Persons taking disulfiram for alcohol dependence may acquire significant levels of its metabolite, CS_2 (Kane, 1970; Ansbacher et al., 1982; Laplane et al., 1992). CS_2 is a byproduct of biological degradation and incineration of sewage (ATSDR, 1995), and it is emitted into the environment during volcanic eruptions (Rasmussen et al., 1982). Low levels have been detected in ocean waters (Lovelock, 1974). It can be taken in by consumption of contaminated grains and produce (Daft, 1988a,b). Individuals living nearby workplaces where CS_2 is used are often exposed to concentrations high enough to result in measurable uptake (Helasova, 1969). Accidental ingestion of liquid CS_2 has also been reported in humans (Lecousse and Dervillée, 1934; Yamada, 1977). It has been detected in the blood and urine of individuals without an identifiable source of CS_2 exposure (Brugnone et al., 1993, 1994).

EXPOSURE LIMITS AND SAFETY REGULATIONS

Recognition of its odor can serve as a warning of the presence of CS_2 for individuals at risk for exposure. The olfactory threshold for detecting the mild sweet, nonirritating odor of CS_2 in air is 0.11 ppm, a level well below the established and recommended exposure limits (Amoore and Hautala, 1983) (Table 21-1). The *Occupational Safety*

TABLE 21-1. *Established and recommended occupational and environmental exposure limits for carbon disulfide in air and water*

	Air (ppm)[a]	Water (mg/L)[a]
Odor threshold*	0.11	0.00039
OSHA		
PEL (8-hr TWA)	20	—
STEL ceiling (15-min TWA)	30 (100)[b]	—
NIOSH		
REL (10-hr TWA)	1[c]	—
STEL (15-min TWA)	10[c]	—
IDLH	500[c]	—
ACGIH		
TLV (8-hr TWA)	10[c]	—
STEL (15-min TWA)	—	—
USEPA		
MCL	—	—
MCLG	—	—

[a]Unit conversion: 1.0 ppm = 3.16 mg/m^3; 1 ppm 1 mg/L.

[b]See text for discussion of OSHA STEL ceiling exposure limit.

[c]SKIN designation assigned by NIOSH and ACGIH: indicates that the potential exists for significant dermal absorption of this solvent.

OSHA, Occupational Safety and Health Administration; PEL, permissible exposure limit; TWA, time-weighted average; NIOSH, National Institute of Occupational Safety and Health; REL, recommended exposure limit; STEL, short-term exposure limit; IDLH, immediately dangerous to life or health; ACGIH, American Conference of Governmental Industrial Hygienists; TLV, threshold limit value; USEPA, U.S. Environmental Protection Agency; MCL, maximum contamination level; MCLG, maximum contamination level goal.

Data from *Amoore and Hautala, 1983; OSHA, 1995; ACGIH, 1995; USEPA, 1996; NIOSH, 1997.

and Health Administration (OSHA) has established an 8-hour time-weighted average (TWA) permissible exposure level (PEL) for CS$_2$ vapor of 20 ppm, with a 15-minute TWA ceiling of 30 ppm. Because individual workers are intermittently exposed to higher peak levels during some job tasks, a maximum 30-minute TWA exposure level of CS$_2$ of 100 ppm is allowable but should not be exceeded. Furthermore, all exposures above the 15-minute TWA ceiling must be compensated for by exposures to lower levels and/or break time away from exposure, so that the TWA exposure level for the entire work shift does not exceed 20 ppm (OSHA, 1995).

The *National Institute for Occupational Safety and Health's* (NIOSH) recommended inhalation exposure limit (REL) for CS$_2$ vapor is a 10-hour TWA of 1 ppm, with a 15-minute TWA short-term exposure limit (STEL) of 10 ppm, which should not be exceeded at anytime during the work shift. NIOSH has determined that dermal absorption of CS$_2$ is significant; therefore, to prevent exposures by this route, it has assigned CS$_2$ a dermal absorption warning designation (SKIN). In accordance with this ruling, NIOSH recommends that protective clothing such as

gloves and coveralls be worn by all employees who work in areas where the potential for dermal contact with CS$_2$ exists (NIOSH, 1997). The NIOSH immediately dangerous to life or health (IDLH) concentration for CS$_2$ is 500 ppm. The *American Conference of Governmental Industrial Hygienists'* (ACGIH) recommended threshold limit value for CS$_2$ is an 8-hour TWA of 10 ppm. The ACGIH has also assigned CS$_2$ a SKIN designation (ACGIH, 1995).

The odor threshold for CS$_2$ in water is 0.00039 mg/L (Amoore and Hautala, 1983). The *United States Environmental Protection Agency* (USEPA) has not established a maximum contamination level (MCL) for CS$_2$ in drinking water (USEPA, 1996). However, the Comprehensive Environmental Response Compensation and Liability Act of 1980 requires companies and or individuals spilling or releasing 100 pounds or more of CS$_2$ into the environment within any given 24-hour period to notify the National Response Center (CFR, 1996).

METABOLISM

Absorption

CS$_2$ vaporizes easily (vapor pressure: 400 mm at 82°F), and inhalation is the main route of intake during exposure (Sax, 1979; Rosier et al., 1987a; Riihimäki et al., 1992). Pulmonary absorption correlates with the ambient air concentration of CS$_2$ (Teisinger and Soucek, 1949; Lam and DiStefano, 1982; Riihimäki et al., 1992). Total pulmonary absorption of CS$_2$ increases with physical activity (Drexler et al., 1995). However, the percentage of the inhaled CS$_2$ dose retained decreases as the blood and body tissues become saturated (Teisinger and Soucek, 1949; Rosier et al., 1987a). For example, Teisinger and Soucek (1949) found that 80% of an inhaled dose was retained in human volunteers exposed to CS$_2$ concentrations of 17 to 51 ppm during the first 15 minutes of an exposure period but that retention dropped to approximately 40% after 45 minutes of exposure. Retention of CS$_2$ is positively correlated with the exposed individual's percentage of body fat (Rosier et al., 1987a).

CS$_2$ is readily absorbed through the gastrointestinal mucosa if swallowed (Lecousse and Dervillée, 1934; Yamada, 1977).

Dermal absorption of CS$_2$ readily occurs on contact with unprotected skin and contributes significantly to an individual's total uptake of the solvent (Dutkiewicz and Baranowska, 1967; Drexler et al., 1995). In addition, prolonged dermal contact with CS$_2$ disrupts the stratum corneum, leading to an increase in dermal absorption (Drexler et al., 1995) (see Exposure Limits and Safety Regulations section).

Tissue Distribution

CS$_2$ is found in both free and bound forms. Approximately 90% of the CS$_2$ in the blood is transported by the red blood cells; the remaining 10% circulates bound to other blood proteins (Lam et al., 1986; Lam and DiStefano, 1986). CS_2, a lipophilic compound, is rapidly distributed by systemic circulation to the various lipid-rich tissues of the body, where it subsequently binds with available amino and sulfhydryl substrates (McKenna and DiStefano, 1977a; Lam and DiStefano, 1982; Lam and DiStefano, 1986). Distribution of the free and bound forms reflects the different concentrations of amino and sulfhydryl groups in the various body tissues. Most of an exposed individual's body burden of bound CS_2 is found associated with proteins and thiols in the brain, liver, kidneys, skeletal muscles, and heart (Bartonicek, 1959; McKenna and DiStefano, 1977a; Snyderwine et al., 1988). Although no reports are available on tissue distribution of CS_2 in humans, McKenna and DiStefano (1977a) reported high concentrations in the brains of rats exposed to CS_2 vapor. In addition, approximately one-third of the absorbed dose was still present in the brains of these animals 16 hours after cessation of exposure, suggesting that CS_2 accumulates in the brain and other tissues with repeated exposures (McKenna and DiStefano, 1977a; Lam and DiStefano 1986). By contrast, tissue concentrations of free (unbound) CS_2 are greatest in the lipid-rich adipose tissue, which has a relatively low concentration of available substrates to which it can bind (McKenna and DiStefano, 1977a). Because this particular tissue is not as well perfused with blood as the parenchymal organs, it is correspondingly not as readily saturated with CS_2 (McKenna and DiStefano, 1977a; Rosier et al., 1987a). However, higher concentrations can be reached during chronic exposures, and redistribution of free CS_2 released from adipose tissue serves as a continuous source of exposure (McKenna and DiStefano, 1977a).

Because free CS_2 is lipophilic, it also readily passes through the lipid bilayer of neuronal cell membranes and subsequently binds to proteins of intracellular macromolecules (Savolainen et al., 1977; Pappolla et al., 1987). For example, in the neurons of the peripheral system, CS_2 metabolites are found covalently bound to the neurofilaments (Jirmanová and Lukas, 1984; Pappolla et al., 1987; DeCaprio et al., 1992; Graham et al., 1995) (see Neuropathological Diagnosis section).

Tissue Biochemistry

CS_2 is a bifunctional electrophilic compound that readily reacts with amines, sulfhydryls, and hydroxyl groups in biological systems (WHO, 1979; Lam and DiStefano, 1986; Graham et al., 1995) (Fig. 21-1). Reaction of CS_2 with amino acids leads to the formation of thiocarbamides, thiocarbamates, and dithiocarbamates (Bartonicek, 1957; Cohen et al., 1959; Pergal et al., 1972a,b). Dithiocarbamates are subsequently cyclized to 2-thio-5-thiazolidinones (Bartonicek, 1957; Cohen et al., 1959). Reaction of CS_2 with sulfhydryl groups of cysteine or glutathione yields trithiocarbonates, which are cyclized to form 2-thio-thiazolidine-

4-carboxylic acid (TTCA) (Van Doorn et al., 1981; Cambell et al., 1985; Rosier et al., 1987b; Meuling et al., 1990; Valentine et al., 1992; Graham et al., 1995). Because of a greater proportion of basic amino groups relative to cysteinyl groups in biological systems, dithiocarbamate formation predominates over formation of trithiocarbamates *in vivo;* less than 5% of an absorbed dose of CS_2 is conjugated with the sulfhydryl groups of glutathione to form TTCA (Rosier et al., 1987b; Riihimäki et al., 1992). Approximately 5% of an absorbed dose of carbon disulfide is metabolized by the cytochrome P-450 mixed function oxidase system to carbonyl sulfide (COS) and then carbon dioxide (CO_2); two reactive sulfur atoms are released during this reaction (de Matteis and Seawright, 1973; Dalvi et al., 1974, 1975; McKenna and DiStefano, 1977a; Snyderwine et al., 1988; Graham et al., 1995).

The reactive sulfur atoms formed during oxidative metabolism of CS_2 primarily exert their toxic effects by immediately binding with and suppressing the activity of the cytochrome P-450 enzymes. Suppression of cytochrome P-450 enzyme activity inhibits oxidative metabolism of additional amounts of CS_2, thereby increasing blood levels of the parent compound (Orzechowska-Juzwenko et al., 1984).

When exposure to CS_2 occurs concurrently with exposure to other chemicals, additive or synergistic effects may occur. For example, oxidative metabolism of CS_2 is enhanced by chronic exposure to chemicals such as ethanol and phenobarbital which have been shown to induce cytochrome P-450 enzymatic activity; thus chronic exposure to these chemicals can potentiate the toxic effects of CS_2 by increasing the formation of reactive sulfur atoms (de Matteis and Seawright, 1973; Dalvi et al., 1974; Savolainen and Vainio, 1976; Orzechowska-Juzwenko et al., 1984; Wronska-Nofer et al., 1986; Snyderwine et al., 1988). Conversely, inhibition of cytochrome P-450 by CS_2 can prevent detoxification of benzene and its derivatives (e.g., toluene), thereby potentiating the effects of these commonly used solvents (Gregus and Klaassen, 1996). CS_2 has been shown to potentiate the effects of amphetamines, which are metabolized by cytochrome P-450 (Caroldi et al., 1987; Parkinson, 1996). By contrast, exposure to CS_2 decreases the toxicity of solvents such as trichloroethylene and carbon tetrachloride, which are metabolically activated to toxic intermediates by cytochrome P-450 (Siegers and Younes, 1984; Gregus and Klaassen, 1996). Carbon disulfide has also been shown to inhibit the activity of the enzyme aldehyde dehydrogenase; thus concurrent exposure to CS_2 and ethanol can increase blood acetaldehyde levels (Freundt et al., 1976).

Excretion

Ten to 30% of an absorbed dose of CS_2 is exhaled unchanged in humans (Teisinger and Soucek, 1949; Soucek and Pavelkova, 1953; Demus, 1964; Petrovic and Djuric,

1966) (Fig. 21-1). Another 5% is metabolized by cytochrome P-450 oxidative enzymes to CO_2 before it is exhaled (de Matteis and Seawright, 1973; Dalvi and Neal, 1978). Respiratory elimination of unchanged free and bound CS_2 has a fast and slow component, reflecting elimination from the blood and well-perfused tissue stores, respectively (Lam and DiStefano, 1982; Cambell et al., 1985; Rosier et al., 1987a). For pulmonary elimination, the half-times of the fast and slow phases of free CS_2 in humans were reported to be 1.1 and 109.7 minutes,

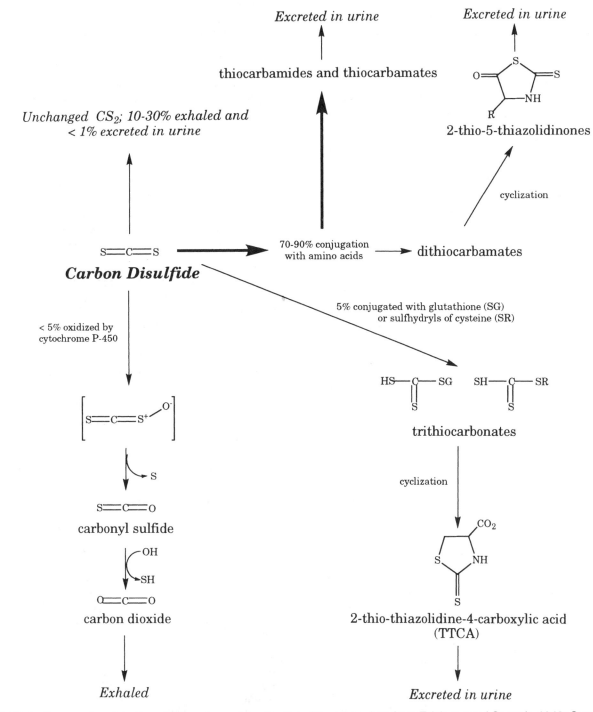

FIG. 21-1. Proposed metabolic pathways for carbon disulfide (Based on data from Teisinger and Soucek, 1949; Soucek and Pavelkova, 1953; Toyama and Kusano, 1953; Soucek, 1957; Cohen et al., 1958; Demus, 1964; Petrovic and Djuric, 1966; Pergal et al., 1972a,b; de Matteis and Seawright, 1973; Dalvi et al., 1974, 1975; Dalvi and Neal, 1975; Van Doorn et al., 1981; Rosier et al., 1982; Cambell et al., 1985; Rosier et al., 1987; Snyderwine et al., 1988; Meuling et al., 1990; Riihimäki et al., 1992; Valentine et al., 1992; Graham et al., 1995; Drexler et al., 1995).

respectively. Half-times for the slow phase of the pulmonary elimination curve for free CS_2 are influenced by differences in individual body fat content and are prolonged for obese individuals (Rosier et al., 1987a).

Less than 1% of an absorbed dose of CS_2 is excreted unchanged in the urine (Teisinger and Soucek, 1949; Toyama and Kusano, 1953). Most CS_2 (70% to 90%) binds with amino acids and is excreted in the urine primarily as thiourea, and to a lesser extent as 2-thio-5-thiazolidinone (Pergal et al., 1972; Riihimäki et al., 1992; Drexler et al., 1995). Less than 5% of an absorbed dose is conjugated with glutathione and is subsequently excreted in the urine as the water-soluble metabolite TTCA (Cambell et al., 1985; Riihimäki et al., 1992) (see Biochemical Diagnosis section). Urinary excretion of TTCA correlates with the cumulative exposure dose and reflects intake by inhalation, dermal absorption, and oral routes (Cambell et al., 1985: Riihimäki et al., 1992; Drexler et al., 1995).

Urinary excretion of CS_2 metabolites also follows a biphasic pattern. The half-time of the fast component is approximately 6 hours and reflects elimination from the well-perfused parenchymal organs (e.g., liver and kidneys); the half-time for the slow phase is 68 hours, reflecting elimination of CS_2 metabolites from the less well-perfused adipose tissues (McKenna and DiStefano, 1977a; Lam and DiStefano, 1982; Riihimäki et al., 1992). Like pulmonary excretion, urinary output is delayed in obese individuals, who retain the solvent for longer periods (McKenna and DiStefano, 1977a; Rosier et al., 1987b). Delayed excretion of CS_2 metabolites has also been reported to contribute to the development of symptoms in susceptible individuals (Besarabic, 1978).

CLINICAL MANIFESTATIONS AND DIAGNOSIS

Symptomatic Diagnosis

Acute Exposure

Exposures to CS_2 vapor for hours or weeks results in nonspecific symptoms, usually beginning with transient irritation of the conjunctiva of the eye, mucous membranes, oral pharynx, and upper airway. Eye irritation is a common nonspecific acute complaint among individuals who work in industries in which the chemical vapors of solvents such as CS_2 are present in the ambient air, especially when the exposed workers do not wear protective goggles. In the viscose rayon industry, CS_2 is often used concurrently with H_2S, which is also a very strong eye irritant; therefore exposed workers may experience an additive lacrimatory effect (Vanhoorne et al., 1995). CS_2 contact with exposed skin produces a burning sensation, followed by anesthesia of the affected area (Gordy and Trumper, 1938). Lieben and Williams (1974) reported clinical findings in a group of 12 workers who were acutely exposed to high levels of CS_2 when the manufacturing machinery at a viscose rayon plant malfunctioned.

These workers developed nonspecific symptoms of exposure including tinnitus, confusion, irritability, emotional instability, and atypical behavior. Similarly, more than half of the 27 persons in a group of workers exposed to CS_2 that had spilled from a railroad tanker car experienced nonspecific acute symptoms including headache, dizziness, and nausea, which persisted for several days after cessation of exposure (Spyker et al., 1982) (Table 21-2).

Recurrent short-term exposure over several months may lead to more evident and persistent pulmonary ventilation abnormalities, nausea, vomiting, headache, lightheadedness, dizziness, emotional irritability, confusion, disorientation, vertigo, tinnitus, auditory hallucinations, nightmares, insomnia, and loss of consciousness (Gordy and Trumper, 1938; Braceland, 1942; Kane, 1970; Manu et al., 1970; Lieben and Williams, 1974; Knave et al., 1974; Feldman et al., 1980; Spyker et al., 1982; Peters et al., 1988; Aaserud et al., 1990; Laplane et al., 1992; Vanhoorne et al., 1995). Braceland (1942) described a 33-year-old man who began experiencing hallucinations, intense emotional irritability, and a slight tremor of the hands after approximately 2 months of daily exposure to undetermined concentrations of CS_2. At 3 months after removal from exposure to CS_2, the patient showed full clinical recovery. Gordy and Trumper (1938), described a 27-year-old woman who had worked in a viscose rayon factory for 6 years without developing any overt neurological or health effects despite her probable recurrent episodes of exposure to low levels of CS_2. She then experienced a severe acute exposure while handling several spools of incompletely dried viscose rayon; she developed a severe headache, felt dizzy, and lost consciousness a few minutes later. When she regained consciousness she was stuporous and remained so for the rest of the day; she soon developed persistent symptoms including numbness and paresthesia in her extremities and experienced auditory hallucinations.

One of our patients, a very bright 29-year-old female chemistry graduate student, experienced mild burning of her eyes, a feeling of inebriation, and difficulties with con-

TABLE 21-2. *Acute symptoms of exposure to carbon disulfide*

	Aaserud et al., 1990	Spyker et al., 1982
Number of subjects	24	27
Exposure level (ppm)	3–16	20
Symptoms (%)		
Headache	63	59
Dizziness/vertigo	63	59
Inebriation	69	
Irritation of conjunctiva/ mucous membranes	50	40
Dyspnea	81	15
Nausea	81	52
Vomiting	69	4

centration and problem solving. These symptoms were associated with certain times when she worked in the laboratory. Her laboratory work involved the synthesis of a dithioacetic acid derivative that required the base-catalyzed reaction of a tagged isotope of CS_2 with picoline methiodides. The fumes from the reaction were released directly into the room air; no ventilation hood was used. During the first 5 months she worked in the laboratory, she assumed that her symptoms were part of her laboratory experience. After another month, her symptoms became progressively worse and persisted after she left the room. By this time, she had nausea, occasional vomiting, dizziness, unsteady gait, and tremulousness in the extremities. In addition, numbness, initially in the toes and feet, spread to involve the hands as well. She was removed from further exposure, but her symptoms of peripheral neuropathy continued to progress over the next 3 months. Neurophysiological studies revealed impaired sensory nerve conduction velocities, and clinical examination showed signs of reduced perception of vibration sensation indicating neuropathy. The neuropathy receded, and her attention and concentration over the next 9 months improved (see Clinical Experiences section).

Chronic Exposures

Exposures to CS_2 for durations of months to years has been associated with the same nonspecific symptoms seen acutely, in addition to more severe and persistent ones including headache, dizziness, impaired short-term memory, emotional lability, depression, fatigue, decreased libido, visual disturbances, nightmares, auditory hallucinations, insomnia, anorexia, perfuse perspiration, hypertension, and angina (Gordy and Trumper, 1938; Braceland, 1942; Manu et al., 1970; Hänninen, 1971; Mancusa and Locke,

1972; Lilis, 1974; Tolonen et al., 1975; Aaserud et al., 1990). Clinically overt symptoms of the extrapyramidal system include tremor, bradykinesia, and cogwheel rigidity (Richter, 1945; Vigliani, 1950, 1954; Laplane et al., 1992; Peters et al., 1988; Chu et al., 1995). Symptoms associated with peripheral nervous system dysfunction include distal muscle weakness, numbness, and painful paresthesias (Vigliani, 1954; Manu et al., 1970; Lilis, 1974; Seppäläinen et al., 1972; Seppäläinen and Haltia, 1980; Corsi et al., 1983; Johnson et al., 1983). Symptoms of peripheral nervous system dysfunction have also been reported in persons taking disulfiram, which is metabolized to CS_2 (Morki et al., 1981). Exposure duration as well as intensity of CS_2 air concentration appears to be related to frequency of symptoms among three selected and comparable groups of chronically exposed workers. Headache was especially prominent among the workers exposed to levels greater than 70 ppm, for durations up to 6 years (Manu et al., 1970). This finding contrasts with the lower frequency of headache among workers exposed to lower levels for longer durations (Table 21-3).

A 32-year-old female viscose rayon worker developed chronic headaches, dizziness, diplopia, memory problems, fatigue, and numbness and paresthesia in her extremities after 7 years on the job (Gordy and Trumper, 1938). She frequently forgot what she was doing and complained that she was unsure of her footing when she walked. As her symptoms progressed, her memory impairment became so severe that she had to write down the simplest things so as not to forget what she was supposed to do. In addition, she became more irritable, anorexic, and lost all sexual interest.

The effects of chronic exposure to CS_2 on ocular microcirculation (and probably the brain's vascular system as well) have been documented by ophthalmoscopy, fluorescein angiography (FAG), and color fundus photography

TABLE 21-3. *Prevalence of symptoms of chronic exposure to carbon disulfide*

	Aaserud et al., 1990	Seppäläinen et al., 1972	Manu et al., 1970
Number of subjects	24	36	84
Exposure level (ppm)	3–16	10–40	> 75
Duration of exposure (years)	10–35	2–27	1–6
Symptoms (%)			
Central nervous system			
Headache	38	54	77
Dizziness/vertigo	50		
Irritability	63		56
Loss of libido/impotence	50		
Sleep disturbances	63	74	
Nightmares			26
Fatigue	63	69	72
Decreased memory	75		35
Peripheral nervous system			
Paresthesia	31	74	80
Muscle weakness			56
Muscle pain	31		88
Gait disturbance	38		40

(CFP). FAG revealed microaneurysms in 55.9% (109 of 195) of CS_2-exposed Japanese workers, compared with 15.4% (26 of 39) of unexposed control subjects (Goto et al., 1971). CFP revealed retinopathy in 30.8% of 289 exposed workers; retinopathy was detected in only 4.1% of a 49-member unexposed control group (Sugimoto et al., 1976b). A trend was reported toward a greater incidence of retinal vasculopathy in workers exposed to higher concentrations of CS_2 compared with those who had lower levels of exposure. Raitta et al. (1974) did not find a significantly greater degree of retinal artery narrowing in 100 CS_2-exposed workers compared with 97 nonexposed control subjects using routine ophthalmologic examination. However, FAG studies of the same two groups revealed disturbed choroidal circulation in 68% of the exposed workers while similar findings were seen in only 39% of the unexposed controls; these changes were not related to aging or raised intraocular pressure.

The results of a 5-year follow-up study of angiopathy in 214 male CS_2 workers showed progression in 23.1% with continued exposure and 11.7% of those removed from further chronic exposure; no progression was found after cessation of short duration (less than 10 years) or remote exposure (Sugimoto et al., 1976a). Improvement or disappearance of retinopathy was seen in 11.3% of workers removed from further exposure, and improvement was seen in only 1.5% of those still exposed to CS_2. Using CFP, Sugimoto et al. (1977, 1978) compared the incidence of retinopathy among 420 Japanese viscose rayon workers (mean age: 41.1 years; mean exposure duration: 17.0 years) with long-term low-level exposure to CS_2 with that of 390 nonexposed age-matched control subjects. Although no correlation was found between duration of exposure to CS_2 and the incidence of retinopathy, a significant ($p < 0.01$) correlation was found between exposure dose and incidence of retinopathy. Exposure to CS_2 has been associated with disturbances of glucose and lipid metabolism (Tolonen, 1975), but no relationship was found between the development of retinopathy and the incidence of diabetes mellitus, elevated serum cholesterol, triglyceride, or β-lipoprotein levels, obesity, hypertension, or heart disease, among this group of CS_2-exposed workers. Nevertheless, these findings suggest that the alterations in retinal vessels are important in early detection of the effects of chronic CS_2 exposure, which may parallel hemodynamic and structural disturbances in brain blood vessels and circulation (Raitta et al., 1974; Vanhoorne et al., 1996). A history of exposure to CS_2 may add to an individual's risk of developing coronary heart disease (Tolonen et al., 1975, 1979).

Chronic exposure to CS_2 is also associated with disturbances of vision including decreased visual acuity, central scotoma, and dyschromatopsia (Grant and Schuman, 1993; Merigan et al., 1988). Disturbances in color vision following exposure may be due to a loss of central retinal ganglion cells or demyelination of nerve fibers (Raitta et al., 1981; Merigan et al., 1988; Eskin et al., 1988) (see Neuropathological and Neuropsychological Diagnosis sections).

Although many of the symptoms are ameliorated after cessation of CS_2 exposure, others may be permanent. For example, 12 of 33 viscose rayon workers with previously diagnosed peripheral neuropathy still had clinically overt symptoms as well as subclinical markers of peripheral neuropathy at a 10-year follow-up (Seppäläinen and Tolonen, 1974; Corsi et al., 1983) (see Neurophysiological Diagnosis section).

Neurophysiological Diagnosis

Neurophysiological techniques have been used to document the effects of CS_2 exposure. The various sensitive electrodiagnostic measures of peripheral nerve and central nervous system (CNS) functioning often provide early detection of subclinical and possibly reversible neurological effects of acute exposure to CS_2 before permanent damage occurs with intense repeated brief exposures or prolonged periods of continuous exposure.

Electroencephalography (EEG) documents the CNS effects of exposure. The variances in the EEG findings reported in the literature may be explained by many factors, including differences in the ambient air concentrations of CS_2, the presence of other chemicals, the length of exposure, the latency between the most recent exposure to CS_2 and the time of the EEG testing, the age of the subjects, and the effects of underlying cerebrovascular disease or previous brain injury. Nevertheless, collectively these published findings suggest that alterations in brain electrical activity are associated with exposure to CS_2. Abnormal brain wave activity in CS_2-exposed workers appears to develop over time with chronic exposure. For example, 23 of 54 EEG recordings were abnormal in a group of 54 workers exposed to CS_2 at ambient air levels of 10 to 60 ppm for durations of 1 to 27 years; for the previous decade, ambient air concentrations had been less than 30 ppm (Seppäläinen and Tolonen, 1974). Findings in the exposed workers included diffuse slow waves (12 of 54), focal slow waves (8 of 54), and paroxysmal activity (3 of 54). By comparison, only 6 of 50 members of a nonexposed control group, with no history of exposure to CS_2, had similar EEG abnormalities (i.e., diffuse and/or focal slowing). Aaserud et al. (1990) reported dysrhythmia of uncertain significance on the EEG recordings in 2 of 16 workers previously exposed to CS_2 while employed in the spinning department of a viscose rayon factory. Although none of these workers had been exposed to CS_2 during a 4-year period between ending their employment (and thus their exposure) and the date of their EEG recording, the two workers with abnormal EEGs had been exposed for at least 12 years, at average daily ambient air concentrations ranging from 3 to 28 ppm, with peaks in air CS_2 concentrations ranging from 189 to 316 ppm. The persistently abnormal EEGs in these two workers clearly relate to the previous prolonged exposure to CS_2.

EEGs were made in 250 CS_2-exposed viscose rayon workers (mean age: 40.8 years; range: 19 to 58 years) with a mean CS_2 exposure duration of 11.2 years (range: 0.5 to 29 years) (Stýblová, 1977). The exposed workers were divided into high (TWA: 44 ppm or less) and low (TWA: 22 ppm or less) exposure groups, based on individual exposure history by work site. Spinners comprised the high-exposure group, and all other workers were assigned to the low-exposure group. The EEG recordings of both groups were compared with those of 61 healthy nonexposed controls (mean age: 35 years; range: 19 to 50 years) and with those of 47 patients with cerebrovascular disease (mean age: 63.2). EEG abnormalities were seen in 38.7% of the high-exposure group and 27.1% of the low-exposure group. These recordings revealed a general slowing of alpha activity (below 10 Hz in 40.0%). By comparison, only 13% of the recordings in unexposed controls showed a similar alpha frequency slowing. EEG abnormalities were seen in only 6.6% of the healthy controls, whereas 63.83% of the patients with cerebrovascular disease had EEG abnormalities, probably due to areas of ischemic change or tissue infarction. The EEG abnormalities seen in the group with cerebrovascular disease could be expected, but the difference in prevalence of EEG abnormalities among CS_2-exposed persons is quite remarkable when compared with nonexposed control subjects (Table 21-4).

Maj and Czeczótko (1995) conducted a longitudinal study in workers exposed to a mixture of CS_2 (0 to 20 ppm) and hydrogen sulfide (0 to 30 ppm). The exposed workers were compared with a group of nonexposed control subjects. The exposed workers received their initial EEGs before beginning employment at the plant and again after 5 years of continuous work-related exposure to CS_2. Initial baseline and 5-year follow-up EEGs were also made in the controls. A 14% increase in the number of abnormal EEG recordings was seen in the exposed workers, compared with only 2% in the control subjects over the same 5-year period. An increase in diffuse slow waves was the most frequently found abnormality in the exposed workers. There was no obvious explanation for the slight increase in EEG abnormalities among the control subjects; the modest (14%) increase in abnormalities among the exposed workers was attributed to CS_2.

EEG abnormalities were also observed in four of six grain storage workers exposed to a pesticide mixture that contained 80% carbon tetrachloride and 20% CS_2 (Peters et al., 1982). Because carbon tetrachloride has a depressant effect on CNS functioning (Torkelson and Rowe, 1981), its contribution to these changes must be taken into account.

Evoked potentials have also been used to document the subclinical CNS effects of chronic exposure to CS_2. Hirata et al. (1992) measured the *brain stem auditory evoked potentials* (BAEP) in 74 viscose rayon manufacturing workers (age range: 40 to 55 years). All workers were currently or previously employed in the spinning department, where ambient air levels of CS_2 ranged from 3.3 to 8.2 ppm. The workers were divided into three groups: (a) currently employed spinners with at least 19 years of exposure ($n = 34$; mean age: 47 years); (b) currently employed spinners with 2 to 8.5 years of exposure ($n = 24$; mean age: 44 years); and (c) former spinners with at least 7 years of exposure ($n = 16$; mean age 49). Workers with diabetes mellitus, renal dysfunction, or neurological disease were excluded from the study. The exposed workers were compared with a group of unexposed nylon filament factory workers ($n = 40$; mean age: 46 years). BAEPs were analyzed for prolongation of latencies in wave components I, III, and V and for interpeak latencies (IPL) of wave components I–III, III–V, and I–V. The latencies of wave component V were significantly ($p < 0.01$) prolonged in the currently exposed workers from group A. In addition, the IPLs of wave components III–V and I–V in group A were significantly ($p < 0.05$) greater. These results showed impaired BAEPs in currently exposed workers whose duration of employment was at least 19 years.

Aaserud et al. (1990) also recorded evoked potentials in 15 workers from the spinning department of a viscose rayon factory, 4 years after they had been removed from further exposure to CS_2. The overall results of this study did not reveal convincing evidence of persistent neurological effects of CS_2 exposure in workers tested several or more years after removal from exposure. In this study, spinning room workers had been exposed to ambient air CS_2 vapor concentrations ranging from 3 to 28 ppm, with frequently reported peak concentrations of 189 to 316 ppm. Individual exposure durations ranged from 10 to 35 years. The BAEPs were abnormal in only one member of the group. *Visual evoked potentials* (VEPs) were bilaterally

TABLE 21-4. *Electroencephalographic abnormalities in workers exposed to carbon disulfide[a]*

EEG findings	Exposed ($n = 250$)	Controls ($n = 61$)	Cerebral arteriosclerosis patients ($n = 47$)
Paroxysmal activity	84 (33.6)	5 (8.2)	7 (14.9)
Diffuse abnormalities	74 (29.6)	4 (6.6)	14 (29.8)
Focal abnormalities	5 (2.0)	1 (1.6)	22 (46.8)

[a]Data are numbers, with percent in parentheses.
Data from Stýblová, 1977.

abnormal in 2 of 15 workers and unilaterally abnormal in 1 of 15. *Sensory evoked potentials* (SEPs) were considered abnormal at the cervical spinal cord level in 1 of 15 workers and at the level of the brachial plexus in another. Actual changes in the peak to peak latencies and waveforms of the evoked potentials were not reported in this study.

Nerve conduction studies (NCS) documented 17 cases of peripheral neuropathy in workers who were currently exposed to CS_2 vapor at relatively high concentrations (150 to 300 ppm), while working in the fiber cutting department of a viscose rayon manufacturing plant (Chu et al., 1995). Nine of the 17 workers had clinically overt neurological signs of peripheral neuropathy including numbness, muscle weakness, and hyporeflexia or areflexia. Motor and sensory NCS in the median and ulnar nerves revealed significantly decreased conduction velocities and amplitudes, as well as significantly increased distal latencies. Sensory NCS in the sural nerves of these workers revealed significantly decreased amplitudes and significantly increased distal latencies, but the sensory nerve conduction velocities were not significantly different from controls. Distal latency and nerve conduction velocity in motor nerves and action potentials amplitudes in sensory nerves are sensitive indicators of CS_2-induced polyneuropathy (see Clinical Experiences section).

To determine whether chronic exposure was associated with electrodiagnostic evidence of peripheral neuropathy, Seppäläinen and Tolonen (1974) performed NCS in 118 viscose rayon workers (mean age: 50 years; age range: 33 to 68 years) who were exposed to CS_2 for a median of 15 years (range: 1 to 27 years) at concentrations ranging from 10 to 60 ppm. Exposure levels during the previous 10 years had averaged less than 30 ppm in all work areas, including the spinning rooms. Of the exposed workers, 53 had been removed from exposure for as little as 3 months to as long as 15 years (median: 7 years). For the 5-year period prior to testing, the exposed workers had been taking a daily dose of 80 to 120 mg of pyridoxine hydrochloride, a vitamin that was believed to prevent the development of polyneuropathy in persons exposed to CS_2. The workers were compared with a control group of 100 paper mill workers (mean age: 48 years) with no history of exposure to CS_2.

Motor NCS were made in the median, ulnar, peroneal, and posterior tibial nerves, and sensory NCS recordings were made only in the median and ulnar nerves. These measurements were made in a routine manner from the skin surface; determinations of conduction velocity of the slower fibers (CVSF) in ulnar and deep peroneal nerves required use of the partial antidromic block technique. The lower extremities were more affected than the upper. The maximal motor conduction velocities (MMCV) were significantly reduced in the posterior tibial ($p < 0.005$) and deep peroneal ($p < 0.0025$) nerves of the CS_2-exposed workers, whereas MMCVs in the ulnar and median nerves of the exposed workers were not significantly reduced be-

low those of the unexposed control subjects. Motor distal latencies were significantly ($p < 0.0005$) longer in the exposed workers, but sensory distal latencies were similar in both groups. No differences in NCS were found in the testing results between workers currently exposed to CS_2 and workers who had been exposed for many years before being removed from exposure, suggesting that the damage to peripheral nerve fibers resulting from exposure to CS_2 is persistent. CVSFs of the ulnar and deep peroneal nerves were also significantly ($p < 0.0005$) reduced. Using cumulative percentage distribution of CVSFs of the ulnar nerve, a CVSF of less than 40 m/sec was recorded for 50% of the exposed subjects and only 14% of the control subjects. These findings indicate that measuring CVSFs is a sensitive parameter for detecting cases of subclinical CS_2-induced polyneuropathy.

Similar electrodiagnostic measures were made in 156 male viscose rayon factory workers exposed to ambient air CS_2 vapor concentrations of 1 to 20 ppm for a mean duration of 12.1 years (Johnson et al., 1983). The workers were divided into three exposure groups: high (more than 7.1 ppm); medium (3 to 7.1 ppm); and low (less than 3 ppm), based on individual job task-related exposure history. Significant reductions were noted in the sural nerve sensory conduction velocities and the peroneal nerve motor conduction velocities. The reductions in peroneal nerve conduction velocities were related to cumulative exposure dose. Measures of distal latency and muscle and nerve action potential amplitudes did not differ significantly between the two groups at this level of exposure, in contrast to what had been shown by Seppäläinen and Tolonen (1974) in the median and ulnar nerves. This difference may be a matter of recording technique.

A group of 33 viscose rayon factory workers were tested 10 years after they had been diagnosed with CS_2-induced peripheral neuropathy (Corsi et al., 1983). CS_2 concentrations in the factory during the time the workers had been exposed ranged from 10 to 70 ppm. All subjects were screened for concomitant factors such as diabetes or nutritional deficiencies, which could also produce peripheral neuropathy. The subjects were divided into high (spinners: $n = 20$) and low (maintenance workers: $n = 13$) exposure groups. Although no specific data on CS_2 exposure levels in the plant were reported in this study, spinners are generally considered to be among the most highly exposed workers in the viscose rayon manufacturing industry (Manu et al., 1970; Cirla et al., 1978; Aaserud et al., 1990, 1992; Chu et al., 1995). The motor and sensory nerve conduction velocities of the ulnar and peroneal nerves were measured. Nineteen (95%) of the workers from the high-exposure group and three (23%) from the low-exposure group had abnormal NCS. These findings are in agreement with those of Seppäläinen and Tolonen (1974) and demonstrate persistent evidence of peripheral neuropathy, even 10 years later, which was most prominent in those workers who had had higher levels of exposure in the past.

Neuropsychological Diagnosis

Acute Exposure

Acute exposure to CS$_2$ vapor is likely to be sufficiently irritating to the eyes and upper respiratory system that an exposed person will leave the contaminated area before experiencing transient symptoms of dizziness, inebriation, or confusion. However, individuals who remain in contaminated areas may have altered consciousness and other acute effects persisting for various length of time (Gordy and Trumper, 1938; Knave et al., 1974; Lieben and Williams, 1974). Furthermore, subtle behavioral changes associated with acute exposures to CS$_2$ may go unrecognized by the exposed individual until they become severe and observable by other people.

Neuropsychological testing is sensitive to the acute and chronic effects of CS$_2$; therefore periodic testing of exposed workers is warranted in an attempt to detect effects that are not yet severe or persistent (Hänninen, 1971; Herbig, 1973). CS$_2$ affects performance on tests of specific neuropsychological domains including measures of intelligence quotient (IQ), motor functioning, attention, memory, verbal skills, visuospatial ability, affect, and personality (Hänninen, 1971; Feldman et al., 1980; Aaserud et al., 1988; Matthews et al., 1990; White et al., 1992). Hänninen (1974) found a correlation between decreased performances on tests of motor speed and dexterity and reduced motor nerve conduction velocities in the arms of exposed workers, indicating that performance on motor skill tests is affected by peripheral nerve functioning. The results of tests of verbal functioning in CS$_2$-exposed persons have been equivocal (Hänninen, 1971; Peters et al., 1982; White et al., 1992).

Although no studies specifically assessing the acute neuropsychological effects of CS$_2$ at the time of exposure in humans have been reported (ATSDR, 1995), performance would be expected to parallel excitatory, depressive, and sedative effects of CS$_2$ on CNS functioning. Few data exist on the effects of acute CS$_2$ exposure on neurobehavioral functioning in humans.

Subchronic Exposure

Subchronic exposures to relatively high concentrations of CS$_2$ produce neurobehavioral effects similar to those seen following chronic exposure to relatively lower concentrations. For example, one of our patients, a 28-year-old man, was exposed to CS$_2$ several times a day several days a week for 3 months, while he worked as a contract electrician repairing equipment and power lines in a rayon manufacturing plant (Feldman et al., 1980). On several occasions, his clothing was doused with CS$_2$, which was leaking from the pipes around which he worked while installing CS$_2$ monitors in the solution room of the plant. His shirts disintegrated where the solvent had soaked the cloth. In addition, he was frequently exposed to the vapors emit-

ted from pools of CS$_2$ that had accumulated in a regeneration pit behind extruder machines, where he sometimes had to work. He frequently would stop working because of severe acute eye irritation, nausea, and difficulty breathing. His family began to notice behavioral symptoms at home, which included irritability, forgetfulness, and depression approximately 2 months after he began working at the plant. He reportedly had trouble remembering the names of familiar people, and it was difficult for him to follow a conversation. He lost interest in his favorite recreational activities. In addition, he developed a tremor that made it difficult for him to hold his tools steady while working. The tremor and memory impairment made it necessary for him to stop working.

A neuropsychological evaluation was performed after cessation of work (and therefore further exposure). His verbal IQ at that time was 96 and his performance IQ 88. His performance on a vigilance test was impaired, suggesting a decreased ability to sustain attention. His scores on the Digit Symbol test were impaired, suggesting deficits in motor skills. Performance deficits in visuospatial functioning were noted on the Block Design and Picture Completion tests. His performance on Trails A and Trails B, which have been shown to be sensitive to the effects of CS$_2$, revealed significant impairments. Tests of short-term memory, including paired associates and logical memory, revealed deficits in acquiring new information. His remote memory was relatively well preserved. The lower performance IQ and the decreased performance on the Digit Symbol test, Trailmaking tests of attention and executive functioning, and short-term memory tests seen in this patient are consistent with the toxic encephalopathy subsequent to CS$_2$ exposure and documents the neurobehavioral elements of his day to day practical and social adjustment problems.

At a follow-up examination 5 years after cessation of exposure the patient was considerably less irritable; he was not able to work because of persistent tremor, impaired ability to sustain attention, and short-term memory problems. Only mild improvements in visuomotor functioning were found on a neuropsychological assessment performed at that time. His performance on attention and executive function tasks and on tests of short-term memory was still impaired.

Chronic Exposure

Hänninen (1971) used a comprehensive neuropsychological test battery to assess cognitive functioning in 50 former viscose rayon workers diagnosed with CS$_2$ poisoning (group I) and compared their test performances with those of 50 viscose rayon workers who were employed at the time of testing but were asymptomatic (group II) and with a group of 50 unexposed controls (group III). Ambient air levels of CS$_2$ in the factory ranged from 10 to 44 ppm. The workers in group I had previously been exposed to CS$_2$ for durations of 0.5 to 20 years (mean: 9 years). Of the group I workers, 20 had been diagnosed within 1 year of testing, 15 had been diagnosed within the previous 1 to 4 years, and 15 had been diagnosed more than 5 years previously. All workers in group II were currently exposed to CS_2 and had been exposed consistently for durations of 5 to 20 years (mean: 11 years). The control workers (group III) were from the same viscose rayon factory but had little or no contact with CS_2. The cognitive domains assessed included general intelligence, vigilance, visual memory, psychomotor functioning, manual dexterity, visuospatial ability, and personality. Group I workers showed significant ($p < 0.001$) performance deficits on tests of vigilance and on the psychomotor skills (Digit Symbol). The Santa Ana Dexterity test was particularly sensitive ($p < 0.001$) to the effects of CS_2 on motor skills and revealed significant deficits among the group I and the group II workers. The Picture Completion test revealed significant ($p < 0.01$) deficits in both groups of exposed workers. CS_2 produced neuropsychological deficits in those exposed workers including decreased vigilance, reduced psychomotor speed, and impaired manual dexterity. Psychomotor functioning was markedly impaired in the group I workers but only moderately impaired in group II. These findings indicate that neuropsychological testing can reveal slight functional disturbances before clinically overt symptoms manifest. The development of clinically overt symptoms among some workers while others remain clinically asymptomatic can be attributed to individual differences in susceptibility to the long-term effects of CS_2.

A well-designed longitudinal study by Cassitto et al. (1993) documented acute and persistent neurobehavioral effects of chronic exposure to CS_2 and confirmed the early findings of Hänninen (1971). These investigators made serial neuropsychological assessments, over a 15-year period from 1974 to 1990, in a group of 493 viscose rayon workers. The average ambient air CS_2 concentrations ranged from 20 to 40 ppm in 1974. Due to improvements in the industrial hygiene protocol, average exposure levels had been reduced to less than 10 ppm by 1990. Behavioral domains assessed included perceptual ability, visuospatial ability, visuomotor skills, attention, and memory. The results of this study revealed a marked improvement in neurobehavioral performance following reductions of ambient air concentrations of CS_2 vapor. However, neurobehavioral functioning in those workers exposed to higher levels of CS_2 before improvements in industrial hygiene was markedly worse than that of workers employed since exposure had been reduced, indicating that neurobehavioral functioning is related to past as well as current CS_2 exposures. Furthermore, assessment of workers who had been employed only since the reductions in ambient air CS_2 concentrations were made showed impaired performance on tests of memory and perceptual ability, indicating that subtle neurobehavioral effects of CS_2 occur at exposure levels below the current OSHA PEL of 20 ppm.

Putz-Anderson et al. (1993) assessed neuropsychological functioning in 131 workers exposed to an ambient air CS_2 concentration of less than 20 ppm, much lower than the highest CS_2 exposures experienced by the workers in the two studies cited above; they did not find as strong an effect of CS_2 exposure. The neuropsychological test battery used by Putz-Anderson et al. (1983) included tests of personality and affect (Profile of Mood States and an abbreviated mania scale from the Minnesota Multiphasic Personality Inventory), psychomotor functioning (simple and choice reaction times and an eye–hand coordination test), and cognitive–perceptual functioning (Neisser Test and Digit Span). In addition, the exposed workers and the controls completed a subjective symptoms questionnaire. Significant differences were not demonstrated between the neuropsychological test performance of the CS_2-exposed workers and the unexposed controls on the tests administered; however, the exposed workers reported more subjective symptoms than the unexposed controls.

Raitta et al. (1981) used the Farnsworth-Munsell 100-Hue test to study color discrimination and visual perception in a group of 62 viscose rayon workers (age range: 30 to 58 years) exposed to CS_2 and H_2S for a mean duration of 16 years (range: 6 to 36 years). The average ambient air concentrations of CS_2 and H_2S were 20 and 10 ppm, respectively. The exposed workers were compared with 40 age matched nonexposed control subjects. The exposed workers had significantly impaired color discrimination and visual perception compared with controls. Similarly, Vanhoorne et al. (1996) assessed color vision in a group of 123 viscose rayon workers (median age: 33.5 years; range: 31 to 60 years) exposed to CS_2 and H_2S at vapor concentrations of less than 35 and less than 7 ppm, respectively. Individual exposure levels were associated with job tasks, many of which required workers to breathe air containing CS_2 vapor concentrations in excess of 10 ppm. A significant association was found between exposure to CS_2 and decreased color discrimination. Furthermore, color vision loss was associated with a prevalence of retinal microaneurysms, suggesting a pathological relationship.

Ruijten et al. (1990) assessed color discrimination in a group of 45 male viscose rayon workers (mean age: 49 years; mean exposure duration: 20 years) exposed to CS_2 levels of less than 10 ppm. The exposed subjects were compared with a group of 37 age- and sex-matched controls. In this study, no significant difference in color discrimination was found between the exposed and the control groups at CS_2 exposure levels of less than 10 ppm. However, color discrimination was assessed using the Lanthony D-15 color vision test, which is considered a less sensitive measure of color discrimination than the Farnsworth-Munsell test. Although the color discrimination studies by these investigators failed to reveal effects of CS_2 on color vision at exposure concentrations of less than 10 ppm, NCS in these same viscose rayon workers did document evidence of peripheral neuropathy, demonstrating the importance of using several sensitive measures of neurological, neurophysiological, and neuropsychological functioning for confirmation of a diagnosis (see Neurophysiological Diagnosis section).

Biochemical Diagnosis

Individual differences in absorption of CS_2 have been detected (Rosier et al., 1987a; Drexler et al., 1995). In addition, individuals may be exposed to other chemicals that are metabolized to CS_2 such as disulfiram and its derivatives. Therefore, simply monitoring ambient air levels of CS_2 is not an adequate method for determining total individual exposure dose, and personal biological marker testing is essential to the health of workers exposed to this solvent.

The concentration of CS_2 in exhaled air reflects the individual's exposure to CS_2 vapor levels at the time immediately preceding the sampling. Because the half-time for CS_2 elimination by exhalation is relatively short and the exhaled CS_2 levels quickly fall after ending exposure, alveolar air levels of CS_2 have not been recommended for monitoring an individual's daily cumulative exposure to CS_2 (Cambell et al., 1985; Rosier et al., 1987b; ACGIH, 1995). CS_2 exposure can be documented more accurately by monitoring blood and urine levels of unchanged CS_2 (Lam and diStefano, 1982; Brugnone et al., 1993, 1994).

The blood concentration of free and bound CS_2 increases linearly with exposure dose. The concentration of protein-bound CS_2 in the blood continues to rise for at least 32 hours after cessation of exposure (Lam and DiStefano, 1982). Elimination of CS_2 from the blood is biphasic, with half-times of 2 hours for the free CS_2 and 43 hours for the bound form. Blood levels of free and total (i.e., bound plus free) CS_2 in 208 unexposed individuals were 438 and 2,407 ng/L, respectively. The mean concentration of unchanged CS_2 in 126 urine samples from unexposed individuals was 459 ng/L. These blood and urine concentrations represent exposure to background levels of CS_2 in the environment (Brugnone et al., 1994).

Determining urinary concentrations of the metabolite TTCA is recommended for monitoring individuals exposed to CS_2 (ACGIH, 1995) (Table 21-5). Although less than 5% of an absorbed dose of CS_2 is excreted in the urine as TTCA, urinary TTCA levels nevertheless correlate well with an individual's cumulative exposure dose (Cambell et al., 1985; Riihimäki et al., 1992; Krstev et al., 1993; Drexler et al., 1995) (Fig. 21-2). For example, the urine TTCA levels in an individual who had worked two consecutive shifts continued to increase despite a 50% reduction in ambient air CS_2 levels (Riihimäki et al., 1992). Urine samples should be obtained at the end of the work shift, and urine TTCA concentrations should not exceed 5 mg/g creatinine (ACGIH, 1995).

Urine TTCA levels ranging from 0.05 to 0.17 mg/g creatinine (geometric mean: 0.09 mg/g creatinine) have been reported in unexposed individuals. However, urine TTCA is not specific to CS_2, and consumption of foods such as cabbage and cauliflower is associated with increased background levels of urinary TTCA (Simmon et al., 1994), indicating that dietary sources of TTCA should be considered as a confounder when monitoring workers suspected of exposure to low levels of CS_2.

Serum thyroxine (T_4), an indicator of thyroid functioning, has been suggested as a surrogate diagnostic marker of CS_2 poisoning (Cavalleri, 1975; Cirla et al., 1978). The mean serum T_4 level in workers exposed to CS_2 (3.0 µg/100 mL) was significantly lower than that in a group of unexposed control subjects (4.5 µg/100 mL). This reduction was correlated with longer durations of exposure to CS_2. Greater CS_2 exposure is associated with decreases in serum levels of the protein-bound fraction of T_4. A dose–response relationship has been reported between serum T_4 levels and CS_2 exposure concentration (Cirla et al., 1978). In those workers with previous exposures to high levels of CS_2, serum T_4 levels were similar to those seen in the low-exposure group. However, the occurrence of clinical hypothyroidism, as documented by the thyroid hormone binding ratio and free thyroxine index, was not seen in these workers. The serum concentration of the free T_4, which is considered to be responsible for the clinical manifestations associated with hyper- and hypothyroidism, is influenced by binding of T_4 to thyroxine-binding globulin (TBG), suggesting that TBG may be affected by CS_2 in a similar way as it is by diphenylhydantoin and salicylates (Cirla et al., 1978). Other alterations in endocrine levels following CS_2 exposure have been noted by Cirla et al. (1978), who studied the relationship between CS_2 exposure and blood levels of luteinizing hormone (LH), follicle-stimulating hormone (FSH), prolactin, and

TABLE 21-5. *Biological exposure indices for carbon disulfide*

	Urine	Blood	Alveolar air
Determinant	TTCA	CS_2	CS_2
Start of shift	Not established	Not established	Not established
During shift	Not established	Not established	Not established
End of work shift	0.05 mg/g creatinine	Not established	Not established

TTCA, 2-thio-thiazolidine-4-carboxylic acid; CS_2, carbon disulfide.
Data from ACGIH, 1995.

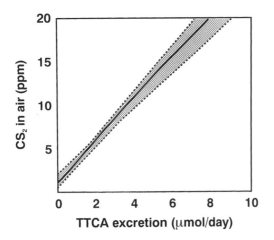

FIG. 21-2. Correlation between 8-hour TWA CS_2 exposure dose, as determined by personal air samples and end of shift TTCA level in 20 viscose rayon workers. Regression line and 95% confidence intervals (shaded area). (Data from Riihimäki et al., 1992.)

testosterone. Levels of the hypophyseal hormones (LH and FSH) but not testosterone were significantly reduced in CS_2-exposed persons.

Identification of cross-linked α- and β-subunits of spectrin (α, β-heterodimers) has been suggested as a novel biomarker of CS_2 neurotoxicity (Graham et al., 1995). In CS_2 toxicity the accumulation of spectrin dimers is proportional to exposure dose and can be detected prior to clinical evidence of neurotoxicity (Valentine et al., 1992). Based on these findings CS_2-promoted modifications of hemoglobin have been proposed as a sensitive and practical biomarker of risk of CS_2 neurotoxicity (Valentine et al., 1998).

Neuroimaging

Neuroimaging studies have been reported in cases of CS_2 exposure, but often the value of such studies is in detecting evidence of primary cerebrovascular disease or other pathologies of non-CS_2 origin for use in the differential diagnosis. *Computed tomography* (CT) scans were abnormal in 12 of 20 CS_2 workers, showing cortical and subcortical atrophy with changes predominantly in the frontal lobes. Workers were selected for imaging because they had shown the greatest morbidity on serial neuropsychological tests and EEG recordings, which were initially made at the time they began employment at the factory and again after 5 years of exposure to air containing 0 to 20 ppm CS_2 and 0 to 30 ppm H_2S (Maj and Czeczótko, 1995) (Table 21-6).

Aaserud et al. (1990) considered exposure to CS_2 to be at least partly responsible for cerebral atrophy found on the CT scans 4 years after cessation of exposure in 13 of 24 Norwegian viscose rayon workers (median age: 58 years; range: 43 to 65 years; mean exposure duration: 17 years; range: 10 to 35 years). The workers had been exposed to ambient air CS_2 vapor concentrations ranging from 3 to 28 ppm but were generally within the exposure limit of 20 ppm and may have been as low as 10 ppm during the 10-year period immediately prior to ending exposure approximately 4 years before the CT scans were done. However, peak concentrations as high as 316 ppm were recorded during certain machine failures. CT scans revealed three cases with moderate cerebral atrophy and nine cases in which the atrophy was considered only slight. Six of these workers had generalized cerebral atrophy, two had focal cerebral changes, and three had focal and generalized atrophy. One worker from the spinning department showed moderate central and severe cortical atrophy (Fig. 21-3). Only one case showed cerebellar atrophy. No areas of infarction due to vascular occlusion were observed, and ultrasound (Doppler) studies did not reveal current evidence of extracranial vessel occlusions. Areas of low density on CT scans in 8 of 14 Japanese workers exposed to CS_2 were attributed to possible vascular ischemic effects (Sugimura et al., 1979). However, such areas of low density were not present on the CT scans of the Norwegian workers (Aaserud et al., 1990).

The CT scans of three patients who were receiving disulfiram (Antibuse), which is metabolized to CS_2, showed lesions in the lentiform nuclei (i.e., globus pallidus and putamen) of the basal ganglia (Laplane et al., 1992). These patients had all developed features of motor and postural control usually associated with basal ganglia disease. In one patient, a 42-year-old alcoholic woman, symptoms developed 5 days after she ingested 75 500-mg disulfiram tablets (total oral dose: 37.5 g). Initial symptoms included nightmares and hallucinations, followed in 3 weeks by development of a resting tremor, dysarthria, dysphagia, and buccofacial apraxia. Her clinical appearance resembled idiopathic Parkinson's disease. However, she also had signs

TABLE 21-6. *Brain computed tomography scans in carbon disulfide workers[a]*

Type of atrophy	Number of workers with atrophy in specific brain regions ($n = 20$)			
	Frontal lobes	Temporal lobes	Parietal lobes	Diencephalon
Cortical	3	3	—	—
Subcortical	7	—	1	1

[a]Twenty workers were exposed to CS_2 vapor at ambient air concentrations of 0–20 ppm for 5 years. Total number of CT scans revealing pathological changes equals 12.
Data from Maj and Czeczótka, 1995.

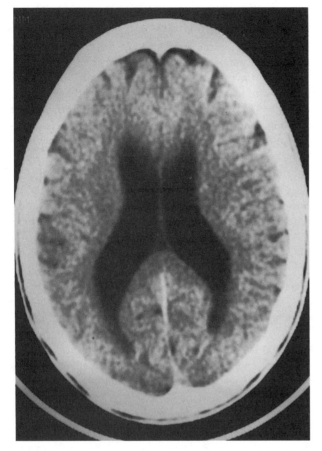

FIG. 21-3. CT scan of a 59-year-old viscose rayon spinning room worker who developed polyneuropathy and encephalopathy after he was exposed to CS$_2$ for 32 years. Demonstrates diffuse prominence of ventricular system, disproportionate to cortical sulci, consistent with white matter atrophy. (Courtesy of Olaf Aaserud)

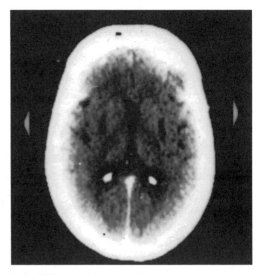

FIG. 21-4. CT scan showing bilateral lesions in the putamen of a 42-year-old woman, 5 days after she ingested 75 500-mg disulfiram tablets (total oral dose: 37.5 g). (From Laplane et al., 1992, with permission.)

of peripheral neuropathy including painful dysesthesias. A sural nerve biopsy documented acute axonopathy. The CT scan of this patient revealed bilateral lesions in the putamen (Fig. 21-4). Lesions of the lentiform nuclei have also been reported in primates experimentally exposed to CS$_2$ (Richter, 1954) (see Neuropathological Diagnosis section).

Single-photon emission computerized tomography (SPECT) was done in the same 24 spinning workers from the viscose rayon plant mentioned above (Aaserud et al., 1992). On the basis of findings from neurological, neuropsychological, CT, and EEG studies, a diagnosis of toxic encephalopathy was related to previous chronic CS$_2$ exposures in 14 of these same 24 workers. All 14 of the 24 workers diagnosed with encephalopathy received SPECT scan studies of regional cerebral blood flow (rCBF). Although seven showed modest reductions in rCBF in the right hemisphere, the differences in mean hemispheric cerebral blood flow, flow asymmetry, and anterior–posterior flow ratio were not significantly different from a reference group. The significance of these findings is uncertain,

as the validity of SPECT scan as an indicator or chronic neurotoxic effect is still unknown.

Neuropathological Diagnosis

The paucity of neuropathological descriptions of the toxic effects of CS$_2$ on the CNS in humans was noted by Seppäläinen and Haltia in 1980, and it still exists. Our current knowledge of histopathology following CS$_2$ exposure is based on old reports and animal studies.

Abe (1933) described diffuse loss of cortical ganglion cells, nonspecific neuronal changes, and mild lesions in the basal ganglia of a patient exposed to CS$_2$. Alpers (1939) also performed postmortem examination on the brain of a patient who was exposed to CS$_2$. In this case there was marked atherosclerosis of the cerebral arteries, marked necrosis in the globus pallidus, putamen, and cortex, and patchy loss of ganglion cells, most noticeable in the frontal lobes. The autopsy of this patient also revealed evidence of peripheral neuropathy. Vigliani (1954) described neuropathological findings in the brain of a 46-year-old man with a history of occupational exposure to CS$_2$. Marked diffuse cerebral atherosclerosis was noted. Areas of necrosis were seen throughout the brain, most marked in the basal ganglia. The morphological changes were attributed to atherosclerosis.

Neuropathological examination of the brains of nonhuman primates that developed parkinsonism following experimental exposure to CS$_2$ revealed marked bilateral symmetrical areas of necrosis and demyelination in the globus pallidus and necrosis of the zona compacta of the substantia nigra (Richter, 1954). Occasionally, the lesions in the globus pallidus extended into the ansa lenticularis and the internal capsule. There was generalized atrophy of the cerebral hemispheres, and the cerebellum appeared morphologically normal.

Vigliani (1954) studied a muscle biopsy in a 52-year-old man who developed symptoms of peripheral neuropathy after 16 years of exposure to CS_2 but nevertheless had continued to work for an additional 10 years before seeking medical attention. The patient complained of subjective symptoms including headache, loss of libido, gastric disturbances, paresthesia, and painful cramps and rigidity in the calf muscles. On neurological examination the patient's calf muscles were contracted and tender, and his Achilles tendon reflexes were absent. Muscle biopsy of the patient's gastrocnemius muscle showed denervation atrophy and degeneration of muscle fibers (Fig. 21-5).

Jirmanová and Lukas (1984) studied the effects of chronic CS_2 exposure on the morphology of the peripheral nerves, neuromuscular junctions, and skeletal muscles of rats experimentally exposed to CS_2 vapor at a concentration of 760 ppm for 6 months. The proximal paranodal and internodal regions of the myelinated neurons were swollen, and numerous giant axons were seen on transverse sections. Axonal enlargements were apparently due to accumulation of tightly packed neurofilaments; other organelles typically seen in the axoplasm such as neurotubules, mitochondria, and profiles of smooth endoplasmic reticu-

lum were markedly reduced. The myelin sheaths were thinned at most of the affected paranodes; at others, complete demyelination was seen. Many neurons had degenerated entirely, and others showed evidence of regeneration marked by the presence of Büngner's bands. Filamentous swelling was also seen in nerve terminals at the neuromuscular junction. However, the postsynaptic part of the neuromuscular junction was spared. Muscle fibers were atrophic and degenerated.

The effects of CS_2 on the visual system have been attributed to the neurological and vascular effects (Raitta et al., 1981; Pappolla et al., 1984; Eskin and Merigan, 1986; Vanhoorne et al., 1996). Eskin and Merigan (1986) performed pathological examinations in primates that had developed marked losses in visual acuity and contrast sensitivity following exposure to CS_2 at a vapor concentration of 256 ppm for 6 hours a day, 5 days a week for 36 to 86 days. Evidence of a vascular pathology was not seen in these animals, suggesting that the damage to the visual system was not dependent on structural changes in the retinal blood vessels. However, the pathological studies in these animals did reveal distal neurofilamentous swelling in the retinogeniculate axons and neuronal loss in the central retinal ganglion cells, especially those cells projecting to the parvocellular lateral geniculate nucleus. The neuropathological findings in these animal studies are consistent with the

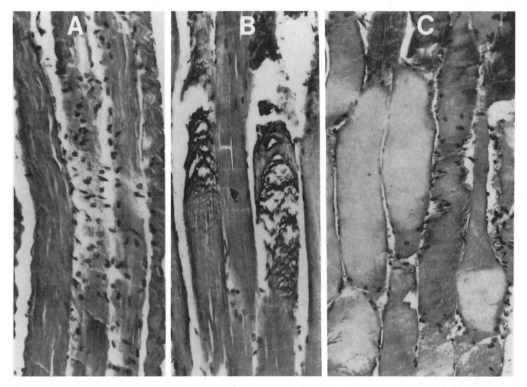

FIG. 21-5. Gastrocnemius muscle biopsy of a 52-year-old man exposed to carbon disulfide for 26 years. Demonstrating denervation atrophy associated with peripheral neuropathy (original magnification, ×200). **A:** Sarcolemma nuclei invading a muscle fiber. **B:** Degeneration of two muscle fibers. **C:** Swelling and waxy degeneration of muscle fibers. (From Vigliani, 1954, with permission.)

color vision losses seen in humans exposed to CS_2, which indicate impaired receptiveness of ganglion cells for polarizing and depolarizing signals generated by the cones (Raitta et al., 1981). Only minimal effects were noted on the other neurons in the retina. Distal neurofilamentous swelling of optic tract axons and degeneration of ganglion cells has also been reported in primates exposed to acrylamide and 2,5-hexanedione (Eskin et al., 1985, Eskin and Merigan, 1986; Lynch et al., 1986). CS_2 and 2,5-hexanedione have both been demonstrated to bind to neurofilaments, thereby inducing neurofilamentous swelling and axonal degeneration in the neurons of the peripheral nervous system (Graham et al., 1995). Neurofilamentous axonopathy has also been found in the optic nerve fibers of rats exposed to CS_2 (Pappolla et al., 1984).

Although the biochemical mechanisms of CS_2 neurotoxicity and the pathogenesis of tissue damage remains unknown, several hypotheses have been raised, including interference with lipid metabolism, chelation of copper, and binding to cellular macromolecules. For example, CS_2 has been shown to alter lipid metabolism and to induce hypercoagulation of blood. Increased levels of serum cholesterol, particularly of the β-fraction, have been associated with exposures to CS_2 (Vigliani, 1954; Harashima et al., 1960; Cavalleri, 1975; Tolonen, 1975). Inhibition of lipid metabolism can significantly increase an exposed worker's risk of developing atherosclerotic disease and vascular encephalopathy (Vigliani, 1954; Tolonen, 1975). The morphological changes seen in the brains of patients exposed to CS_2 have been attributed at least partly to arteriopathic effects (Quensel, 1904; Abe, 1933; Vigliani, 1954). Quensel (1904) noted chromatolysis of the cortical ganglion cells of the human brain following exposure to CS_2. However, CS_2 has been shown to cross the blood–brain barrier readily, and chromatolysis of neurons has also been shown to occur in response to axonal damage; it may therefore reflect interruptions in axonal transport of neurofilaments, a phenomenon that has been associated with peripheral neuropathy following exposure to CS_2 (McKenna and DiStefano, 1977b; Anthony et al., 1996).

CS_2 enters the body as an electrophilic compound and therefore, unlike many other solvents, such as styrene, perchloroethylene, and trichloroethylene, it does not require metabolic activation before it can bind to cellular macromolecules. Experimental evidence suggests that CS_2 reacts with the nucleophilic sulfhydryl and amino groups of cellular macromolecules (Lam and DiStefano, 1986; Graham et al., 1995; Valentine et al., 1995). Binding of CS_2 to amino and sulfhydryl groups leads to the formation of dithiocarbamates and trithiocarbonates, respectively. Dithiocarbamates have been demonstrated to chelate copper (Lam and DiStefano, 1986).

Chelation of copper ions can inactivate metalloenzymes such as dopamine β-hydroxylase, an enzyme important to norepinephrine synthesis (Magos and Jarvis, 1970; McKenna and DiStefano, 1977b). Exposure to CS_2 is asso-

ciated with decreases in norepinephrine in the brains of rats, supporting the contention that CS_2 inhibits the synthesis of norepinephrine (McKenna and DiStefano, 1977b). Female workers chronically exposed to CS_2 had lower blood levels of dopamine, decreased activity of serum dopamine β-hydroxylase, and lower urinary excretion of adrenaline and noradrenaline (Stanosz et al., 1994). Alterations in brain catecholamine and monoamine levels may be involved in the neurobehavioral and physiological effects of exposure to CS_2 (Bus, 1985; Stanosz et al., 1994).

Carbon disulfide is metabolized via microsomal oxidation to two electrophilic sulfur atoms, which, like the parent compound, can covalently bind to cellular macromolecules (Savolainen and Vianio, 1976). Although a clear relationship between the formation of reactive sulfur compounds and the neurotoxicity of CS_2 has not been established, the formation of these reactive sulfur compounds has been associated with the hepatotoxic effects of CS_2 (Bus, 1985; Halliwell, 1989; Corcoran et al., 1994; Graham et al., 1995). Electrophilic compounds such as CS_2 and its reactive metabolites can covalently bind to DNA and lead to cell death (Savolainen and Vianio, 1976; Halliwell, 1989; Corcoran et al., 1994).

Oxidative coupling of two dithiocarbamates yields a bis (thiocarbamoyl) disulfide. Both dithiocarbamates and bis (thiocarbamoyl) disulfides are subsequently metabolized to isothiocyanates, which can covalently bind with and cross-link the nucleophilic centers of cytoskeletal proteins such as axonal neurofilaments (Sayre et al., 1985; Graham et al., 1995; Valentine et al., 1995; Gregus and Klaassen, 1996). The formation of dithiocarbamates may also alter the structural integrity of amino acids and proteins (Lam and DiStefano, 1986).

CS_2 has also been shown to react with pyridoxamine, a biologically active form of B_6, and to deplete the activity of pyridoxamine-requiring enzymes such as transaminases and amine oxidases (Teisinger, 1974). However, the neurotoxic effects of this reaction are uncertain, and although a vitamin B_6 deficiency has been associated with peripheral neuropathy and behavioral effects, decreased levels of vitamin B_6 have not been shown to induce accumulation of neurofilaments within the axon, as occurs in CS_2 neuropathy (Teisinger, 1974; Calabrese, 1980; Graham et al., 1995).

PREVENTATIVE AND THERAPEUTIC MEASURES

Safety training programs that educate workers about the hazards of exposure to CS_2 and the importance of ventilation hoods and fans should be available in all occupational settings. Respirators should be provided for workers at risk of exposure to high concentrations of CS_2. Ambient air concentrations should be measured periodically, and workers should be monitored for individual exposure dose on a regular basis (see Biochemical Diagnosis section).

Individuals suspected of acute exposure to high concentrations of CS_2 should immediately be moved to a well-ventilated area. Hyperventilation with fresh air or an oxygen supply increases displacement and elimination of the CS_2 vapors. If liquid CS_2 has been ingested, controlled stomach gavage should be used to remove the stomach contents. Hemodialysis and blood transfusion for acute renal failure and hepatic dysfunction may be necessary following ingestion.

Irritation of conjunctive membranes of the eyes can be prevented by wearing goggles, and nasopharyngeal irritation can be reduced by wearing a filtered face mask. Dermal exposures to liquid CS_2 should be avoided by wearing protective clothing and washing off accidental skin contamination as soon as possible.

Administration of disulfiram to individuals with potential for exposure to CS_2 has been suggested as a preemployment screening method to evaluate an individual's ability to metabolize sulfur compounds and thus to handle a risk of CS_2 exposure (Djuric et al., 1973; Besarabic, 1978). Workers who excrete more than 150 μg of diethyldithiocarbamate/mg creatinine in their urine following intake of a 0.5-g oral dose of disulfiram can be expected to develop significantly fewer symptoms of CS_2 exposure than those who excrete lower quantities (Besarabic, 1978).

Recovery from acute CS_2 intoxication depends on the intensity and duration of the exposure. Workers who develop persistent symptoms, behavioral manifestations, or peripheral neuropathy following recurrent exposure to CS_2 may require transfer to another department or vocational retraining to prevent further exposures (White et al., 1992). Symptomatic pharmacological treatment for anxiety, sleeplessness, and even acute psychosis may be needed. Use of the B-complex vitamins, including B_6, may have empirical merit.

CLINICAL EXPERIENCES

Group Studies

A Sentinel Case Leading to Discovery of Others Exposed to CS_2 in a Viscose Rayon Factory

A 48-year-old male viscose rayon factory fiber cutter, with 23 years of experience as a fiber cutter, developed peripheral neuropathy and came to the attention of management (Chu et al., 1995). A walk-through survey and ambient air measurements were made at the factory and revealed that exposure levels varied between departments, with the highest air concentrations found in the fiber cutting (range: 150 to 300 ppm) and spinning (range: 15 to 100 ppm) departments. Repairpersons who were repairing equipment in the fiber cutting and spinning departments were also exposed to relatively high concentrations. The factory employed a total of 163 workers. For purposes of the study the workers were divided into three exposure groups: (a) *high*: fiber cutters ($n = 17$); (b) *medium*: spinners and repairpersons ($n = 69$); and (c) *low*: other jobs including cellulose production, viscose II production, and CS_2 production and recycling ($n = 77$).

The investigation revealed nine workers (53%) from the fiber-cutting department with clinically overt muscle weakness, numbness, paresthesia, and hyporeflexia or areflexia, documented by NCS. In addition, NCS documented subclinical peripheral neuropathy in another 19 workers including two additional fiber cutters, seven repairpersons, three viscose II production workers, two spinners, four CS_2 production and recycling workers, and one cellulose production worker. No parkinsonian signs or symptoms were seen in these workers.

This occupational health hazard evaluation attributed the outbreak of CS_2 poisoning to four specific factors: (a) lack of a well-organized and -instituted employee industrial hygiene education program; (b) nonuse of respirators or gloves in workers who developed peripheral neuropathy; (c) recent increases in product production; and (d) recent plant layoffs, which led to longer individual working hours and thus greater cumulative exposure to CS_2.

Peripheral Neuropathy and Subjective Symptoms in CS_2-Exposed Workers

Eighty-four young (mean age: 24.5 years) male workers from a viscose rayon factory developed neurological signs and symptoms following exposure to CS_2 vapor at ambient air concentrations of 70 to 95 ppm (Vasilescu and Florescu, 1972). Brief exposures to higher CS_2 vapor concentrations often occurred during technical accidents and equipment repairs. Nonspecific symptoms included headache (77%), irritability (56%), depression (35%), loss of memory (35%), insomnia (34%), and nightmares (26%). Symptoms of peripheral neuropathy included paresthesias (80%), muscle pain (88%), and diminished muscle strength (56%). The subjective onset of peripheral neuropathy was signaled by fatigue while walking, muscle pain in the calves, and distal paresthesias, particularly in the lower extremities.

As the neuropathy progressed, the workers noted diminution of muscle power in their hands, which made it difficult for them to handle commonly used tools properly. Neurological examination revealed hypoesthesia in 56 of the 84 workers. In 21 cases the hypoesthesia extended to the forearms and calves in a stocking-glove pattern. Tendon reflexes were diminished or absent in the lower extremities of 26 workers. Muscle atrophy was seen in the hands of 9 workers, in the calves of 2, and in the quadriceps of 1. Electromyography (EMG) documented lower motor neuron injury in 72 of 81 workers tested.

Follow-up examinations of 28 of these workers at 3 and 14 months after cessation of exposure revealed clinical improvement in all cases, but in no case was complete recovery documented on EMG studies. These findings demonstrate the importance of early detection of peripheral neuropathy in CS_2-exposed patients, since prognosis in more advanced cases is generally poor.

Individual Case Studies

Reversible Neurological and Thyroid Effects in a Graduate Chemistry Student Exposed to CS_2

A 29-year-old chemistry doctoral student began to notice symptoms of eye and pharyngeal irritation, headache, nausea, vomiting, and sleeplessness. She sought medical attention for anxiety and sleep disturbances, but no connection was made between her work in the laboratory (synthesizing a CS_2-containing chemical) and her symptoms. Notably, the compound she worked with was radiolabeled with the β-emitting S35, and thus the patient was exposed to both CS_2 and β-emitting radiation. Her exposure to CS_2 began in January of 1994 and was daily (8 to 12 hrs/day) or at least biweekly until July of 1994, at which time she had the greatest exposure because of the stage of her work. It was at this time that she began testing the pharmacological properties of the chemical on laboratory mice. Two hours after injection, only 20% of the radioactive sulfur compound was present in the organs, blood, and urine of the injected mice she was studying, indicating that a significant percentage of the CS_2 had been exhaled into the room. By mid-July, her physical symptoms had progressed to include dizziness, tremors, limb weakness, difficulty breathing, slurred speech, and weakness in her legs. Her gait became progressively more unsteady, and she sometimes lost her footing. She continued to work in the laboratory until October, at which time she finished her experimental work. Although she was removed from further exposure, she continued to experience symptoms throughout the month of November. At this time her gait difficulties resulted in a fall from which she suffered a broken ankle. Because of her symptoms, especially the weakness in her legs, she was referred for neurological assessment. The examination was performed after she had recovered from her broken ankle; it showed significant stocking distribution sensory diminution and vibration loss symmetrically in the lower extremities; pinprick and joint position was intact. She had equal and symmetrical reflexes bilaterally. She walked well, with a normal base, and Romberg sign was negative.

NCS showed prolonged latencies in the upper and lower extremities, suggestive of early polyneuropathy. EMG was done in the left lower extremity and selective muscle testing on the right lower extremity, limited by her inability to withstand the discomfort of the needle insertions. Evidence of denervation was not found in the muscles tested. Laboratory tests 6 months after cessation of exposure showed normal electrolytes, blood glucose, complete blood count, and blood urea nitrogen. Free T_4 was normal. Thyroid uptake was normal, but thyroid-stimulating hormone was suppressed at 0.09 μU/mL (normal range: 0.46 to 3.59 μU/mL).

The history and examination of this patient indicated that she had been exposed to CS_2 as a byproduct of her chemical experiments for 10 months (January through October 1994) and that she had developed symptoms consistent with acute polyneuropathy and encephalopathy. The laboratory tests were suggestive of secondary hypothyroidism (see Biochemical Diagnosis section). Additional studies were done at follow-up in November 1995, a year later, and consisted of magnetic resonance imaging (MRI), posturogram for balance, neuroophthalmological examination, EEG, EMG, NCS, and neuropsychological assessment. Posturogram, MRI, and EEG were normal. NCS in the ulnar, peroneal, and posterior tibial nerves were now normal, although NCS in the median nerves were consistent with mild carpal tunnel entrapments. The neuropsychological assessment performed at this time showed no evidence of continued cognitive impairment. Follow-up thyroid function tests revealed that thyroid-stimulating hormone levels had returned to normal (2.03 μU/mL).

It was concluded that the patient had developed acute polyneuropathy and encephalopathy consistent with her exposure to CS_2. The laboratory tests in this patient suggest effects of CS_2 on thyroid functioning consistent with previous reports; her spontaneous recovery following removal from exposure without specific thyroid hormone replacement therapy indicates that CS_2 was responsible for her symptoms. She received her degree and has pursued a career outside the laboratory.

REFERENCES

Aaserud O, Hommeren J, Tvedt B, et al. Carbon disulfide exposure and neurotoxic sequelae among viscose rayon workers. *Am J Ind Med* 1990;18:25–37.

Aaserud O, Russell D, Nyberg-Hansen R, et al. Regional cerebral blood flow after long-term exposure to carbon disulfide. *Acta Neurol Scand* 1992;85:266–271.

Abe M. Beitrag zur pathologischen Anatomie der chronischen Schwefelkohenstoffvergiftung. *Jpn J Med Sci* 1933;3:1.

Agency for Toxic Substances and Disease Registry (ATSDR). *Toxicological profile for carbon disulfide.* Washington: US Department of Health and Human Services, 1995.

Alpers BJ. Changes in the nervous system in carbon disulfide poisoning. *Neurol Psychiatry* 1939;42:1173.

American Conference of Governmental Industrial Hygienists (ACGIH). *Threshold limit values (TLVs) for chemical substances and physical agents and biological exposure indices (BEIs).* Cincinnati, OH: ACGIH, 1995–1996.

Amoore JE, Hautala E. Odor as an aid to chemical safety: odor thresholds compared with threshold limit values and volatilities for 214 industrial chemicals in air and water dilution. *J Appl Toxicol* 1983;3:272–290.

Aneja VP, Overton JH Jr, Cupitt LT, et al. Measurements of emission rates of carbon disulfide form biogenic sources and its possible importance to the stratospheric aerosol layer. *Chem Eng Commun* 1980;4:721–727.

Ansbacher LE, Bosch P, Cancilla PA. Disulfiram neuropathy: neurofilamentous distal neuropathy. *Neurology* 1982;32:424–428.

Anthony DC, Montine TJ, Graham DG. Toxic responses of the nervous system. In: Klaassen CD, ed. *Casarett and Doull's toxicology: the basic science of poisons,* 5th ed. New York: McGraw-Hill, 1996:463–486.

Bartonicek V. [Distribution of free carbon disulfide in the whole blood, the brain, adrenal glands over a given period with parenteral administration to white rats]. *Prac Lek* 1957;9:28–30.

Bartonicek V. Distribution of free carbon disulfide and bound carbon disulfide liberated by acid hydrolysis in the organs of white rats. *Prac Lek* 1959;10:504–510.

Besarabic M. Antabuse test and absenteeism in workers exposed to carbon disulfide. *Arh Hig Rada* 1978;29:323–326.

Braceland FJ. Mental symptoms following carbon disulphide absorption and intoxication. *Ann Intern Med* 1942;16:246–261.

Brugnone F, Maranelli G, Guglielmi G, Ayyad K, Soleo L, Elia G. Blood concentrations of carbon disulfide in dithiocarbamate exposure and in the general population. *Int Arch Occup Environ Health* 1993;64:503–507.

Brugnone F, Perbellini L, Giuliari C, Cerpelloni M, Soave M. Blood and urine concentrations of chemical pollutants in the general population. *Med Lav* 1994;85:370–389.

Bus JS. The relationship of carbon disulfide metabolism to development of toxicity. *Neurotoxicology* 1985;6:73–80.

Calabrese EJ. Does use of oral contraceptives enhance the toxicity of carbon disulfide through interactions with pyridoxine and tryptophan metabolism? *Med Hy* 1980;6:21–33.

Cambell L, Jones AH, Wilson HK. Evaluation of occupational exposure to carbon disulfide by blood, exhaled air, and urine analysis. *Am J Ind Med* 1985;8:143–153.

Caroldi S, Magos L, Jarvis J, et al. The potentiation of the non-behavioral effects of amphetamine by carbon disulfide. *J Appl Toxicol* 1987;7:63–66.

Cassitto MG, Camerino D, Imbriani M, Contrardi T, Masera L, Gilioli R. Carbon disulfide and the central nervous system: A 15-year neurobehavioral surveillance of an exposed population. *Environ Res* 1993;63: 252–263.

Cavalleri A. Serum thyroxine in the early diagnosis of carbon disulfide poisoning. *Arch Environ Health* 1975;30:85–87.

Chu C-C, Huang C-C, Chen R-S, Shih T-S. Polyneuropathy induced by carbon disulfide in viscose rayon workers. *Occup Environ Med* 1995;52:404–407.

Cirla AM, Bertazzi PA, Tomasini M, et al. Study of endocrinological functions and sexual behavior in carbon disulfide workers. *Med Lav* 1978;69:118–129.

Code of Federal Regulations (CFR). Protection of environment. 40: Parts 300 to 399. Washington: Office of Federal Register, National Archives and Records Administration, 1996.

Cohen AE, Scheel LD, Kopp JF, et al. Biochemical mechanisms in chronic carbon disulfide poisoning. *Am Ind Hyg Assoc J* 1959;20: 303–323.

Corcoran GB, Fix L, Jones DP, et al. Contemporary issues in toxicology. Apoptosis: molecular control point in toxicity. *Toxicol Appl Pharmacol* 1994;128:169–181.

Corsi G, Maestrelli P, Picotti G, Manzoni S, Negrin P. Chronic peripheral neuropathy in workers with previous exposure to carbon disulfide. *Br J Ind Health* 1983;40:209–211.

Daft JL. Fumigant contamination during large-scale food sampling for analysis. *Arch Environ Contam Toxicol* 1988a;17:177–182.

Daft JL. Rapid determination of fumigant and industrial chemical residues in food. *J Assoc Off Anal Chem* 1988b;71:748–760.

Dalvi RR, Neal RA. Metabolism in vivo of carbon disulfide to carbonyl sulfide and carbon dioxide in the rat. *Biochem Pharmacol* 1978;27: 1608–1609.

Dalvi RR, Poore RE, Neal A. Studies of the metabolism of carbon disulfide by rat liver microsomes. *Life Sci* 1974;14:1785–1796.

Dalvi RR, Hunter AL, Neal RA. Toxicological implications of the mixed-function oxidase catalyzed metabolism of carbon disulfide. *Chem Biol Interact* 1975;10:347–361.

DeCaprio AP, Spink DC, Chen X, Fowke JH, Zhu M, Bank S. Characterization of isothiocyanates, thioureas, and other lysine adduction products in carbon disulfide-treated peptides and protein. *Chem Res Toxicol* 1992;5:496–504.

de Matteis F, Seawright AA. Oxidative metabolism of carbon disulfide by the rat; effect of treatments which modify the liver toxicity of carbon disulfide. *Chem Biol Interact* 1973;7:375–388.

Demus H. On the reception, chemical transformation and excretion of carbon disulfide by the human body. *Int Arch Gewerbepath Gewerbehyg* 1964;20:507–536.

Djuric D, Postic-Grujin A, Graovac-Leposavid L, Delic V. Disulfiram as an indicator of human susceptibility to carbon disulfide excretion of diethyldithiocarbamate sodium in the urine of workers exposed to CS_2 after oral administration of disulfiram. *Arch Environ Health* 1973;26:287–289.

Drexler H, Gõen T, Angerer J. Carbon disulfide. II. Investigations on the uptake of CS_2 and the excretion of its metabolite 2-thiothiazolidine-4-carboxylic acid after occupational exposure. *Int Arch Occup Environ Health* 1995;67:5–10.

Dutkiewicz T, Baranowska B. The significant of absorption of carbon disulfide through the skin in the evaluation of exposure. In: Brieger H,

Teisinger J, eds. *Toxicology of carbon disulfide.* Amsterdam: Excerpta Medica, 1967:50.

Eskin TA, Lapham LW, Maurissen JPJ, Merigan WH. Acrylamide effects on the macaque visual system: II. Retinogeniculate morphology. *Invest Ophthalmol Vis Sci* 1985;26:317.

Eskin TA, Merigan WH. Selective acrylamide-induced degeneration of color opponent ganglion cells in macaques. *Brain Res* 1986;378:379.

Eskin TA, Merigan WH, Wood RW. Carbon disulfide effects on the visual system. II. Retinogeniculate degeneration. *Invest Ophthalmol Vis Sci* 1988;29:519–527.

Feldman RG, Ricks NL, Baker EL. Neuropsychological effects of industrial toxins: a review. *Am J Ind Med* 1980;1:211–227.

Freundt KJ, Lieberwirth K, Netz H, et al. Blood acetaldehyde in alcoholized rats and humans during inhalation of carbon disulfide vapor. *Int Arch Occup Environ Health* 1976;37:35–46.

Gordy ST, Trumper M. Carbon disulfide poisoning with a report of six cases. *JAMA* 1938;110:1543–1549.

Goto S, Hotta R, Sugimoto K. Studies on chronic carbon disulfide poisoning: pathogenesis of retinal microaneurysm due to carbon disulfide, with special reference to a subclinical defect of carbohydrate metabolism. *Int Arch Arbeitsmed* 1971;28:115–126.

Graham DG, Amarath V, Valentine WM, Pyle SJ, Anthony DC. Pathogenic studies of hexane and carbon disulfide neurotoxicity. *Crit Rev Toxicol* 1995;25:91–112.

Grant WM, Schuman JS. *Toxicology of the eye: effects on the eyes and visual system from chemicals, drugs, metals, minerals, plants, toxins and venoms; also systemic side effects from eye medications.* 4th ed. Charles C Thomas, Springfield, IL. 1993:318–323.

Gregus Z, Klaassen CD. Mechanisms of toxicity. In: Klaassen KD, ed. *Casarett and Doull's toxicology. The basic science of poisons,* 5th ed. New York: McGraw-Hill, 1996:35–74.

Halliwell B. Oxidants and the central nervous system: some fundamental questions. Is oxidant damage relevant to Parkinson's disease, Alzheimer's disease, traumatic injury and stroke? *Acta Neurol Scand* 1989;126:23–33.

Hänninen H. Psychological picture of manifest and latent carbon disulfide poisoning. *Br J Ind Med* 1971;28:374–381.

Hänninen H. Behavioral study of the effects of carbon disulfide. In: Xintaras C, Johnson BL, deGroot I, eds. *Behavioral toxicology: early detection of occupational hazards.* Washington: US Department of Health Education and Welfare, NIOSH, HEW publ. no. 74-126, 1974:73–80.

Harashima S, Toyama T, Sakurai T. Serum cholesterol level of viscose rayon workers. *Keijo J Med* 1960;9:81–90.

Helasova P. Observations on a group of children from an area polluted by carbon disulfide and hydrogen sulfide exhalation compared with a control group of children. *Cs Hyg* 1969;14:260–265.

Herbig C. Psychological investigation into CS_2 effects on female workers. *Med Lav* 1973;64:272–275.

Hirata M, Ogawa Y, Okayama A, Goto S. A cross-sectional study on the brainstem auditory evoked potential among workers exposed to carbon disulfide. *Int Arch Occup Environ Health* 1992;64:321–324.

Jirmanová I, Lukas E. Ultrastructure of carbon disulfide neuropathy. *Acta Europathol* 1984;63:255–263.

Johnson BL, Boyd J, Burg JR, Lee ST, Xintaras C, Albright BE. Effects on the peripheral nervous system of workers' exposure to carbon disulfide. *Neurotoxicology* 1983;4:53–66.

Kane FJ. Carbon disulfide intoxication from overdose of disulfiram. *Am J Psychiatry* 1970;127:690–694.

Knave B, Kolmodin-Hedman B, Persson HE, Goldberg JM. Chronic exposure to carbon disulfide: effects on occupationally exposed workers with special reference to the nervous system. *Work Environ Health* 1974;11:49–58.

Krstev S, Perunicic B, Farkic B. The effects of long-term occupational exposure to carbon disulfide on serum lipids. *Eur J Drug Metab Pharmacokinet* 1992;17:237–240.

Krstev S, Perunicic B, Farkic B, Varagic M. Environmental and biological monitoring in carbon disulfide exposure assessment. *Med Lav* 1993;84: 473–481.

Lam CW, DiStefano V. Behavior and characterization of blood carbon disulfide in rats after inhalation. *Toxicol Appl Pharmacol* 1982;64: 327–334.

Lam CW, DiStefano V. Characterization of carbon disulfide binding in blood and other biological substances. *Toxicol Appl Pharmacol* 1986;86:235–242.

Lam CW, DiStefano V, Morken DA. The role of the red blood cell in the transport of carbon disulfide. *J Appl Toxicol* 1986;6:81–86.

Laplane D, Attal N, Sauron B, de Billy A, Dubois B. Lesions of basal ganglia due to disulfiram neurotoxicity. *J Neurol Neurosurg Psychiatry* 1992;55:925–929.

Lecousse H, Dervillée P. Intoxication aiguë par ingestion accidentelle d'un mélange à base de sulfure de carbone. *J Me Bordeaux* 1934;111:71.

Lieben J, Williams RA. Five years of experience with CS$_2$. In: Xintaras C, Johnson BL, de Groot I, eds. *Behavioral Toxicology: early detection of occupational hazards.* Washington: US Department of Health Education and Welfare, CDC, HEW publ. no. (NIOSH) 74-126, 1974:60–63.

Lilis R. Behavioral effects of occupational carbon disulfide exposure. In: Xintaras C, Johnson BL, deGroot I, eds. *Behavioral toxicology.* Cincinnati, OH: National Institute for Occupational Safety and Health, 1974:51–60.

Liss GM, Finkelstein MM. Mortality among workers exposed to carbon disulfide. *Arch Environ Health* 1996;51:193–200.

Lovelock JE. CS$_2$ and the natural sulphur cycle. *Nature* 1974;248:625–626.

Lynch JJ, Eskin TA, Merigan WH. Visual toxicity of 2,5-hexanedione: are effects different in felines and primates? *Toxicologist* 1986;6:72.

Magos L, Jarvis JAE. Effects of diethyldithiocarbamate and carbon disulfide on brain tyrosine. *J Pharm Pharmacol* 1970;22:936–938.

Maj JC, Czeczótko B. The evaluation of the health state of the workers occupationally exposed to low concentration of carbon disulfide (CS$_2$). Part two: The complex way of the examination of the central nervous system. *Przeg Lek* 1995;52:252–256.

Mancusa TF, Locke BZ. Carbon disulphide as a cause of suicide. Epidemiological study of viscose rayon workers. *J Occup Med* 1972;14:595–606.

Manu P, Lilis R, Lancranjan I, Ionescu S, Vasilescu I. The value of electromyographic changes in the early diagnosis of carbon disulfide peripheral neuropathy. *Med Lav* 1970;61:102–108.

Matthews CG, Chapman LJ, Woodard AR. Differential neuropsychologic profiles in idiopathic versus pesticide-induced parkinsonism. In: Johnson BL, ed. *Advances in neurobehavioral toxicology.* Chelsea, MA: Lewis Press, 1990:323–330.

McKenna MJ, DiStefano V. Carbon disulfide. I. Metabolism of carbon disulfide in the rat. *J Pharmacol Exp Ther* 1977a;202:245–252.

McKenna MJ, DiStefano V. Carbon disulfide. II. A proposed mechanism for the action of carbon disulfide on dopamine β-hydroxylase. *J Pharmacol Exp Ther* 1977b;202:253–266.

Merigan WH, Wood RW, Zehl D, Eskin TA. Carbon disulfide effects on the visual system. I. Visual threshold and ophthalmoscopy. *Invest Ophthalmol Vis Sci* 1988;29:512–518.

Meuling WJA, Bragt PC, Brun CLJ. Biological monitoring of carbon disulfide. *Am J Ind Med* 1990;17:247–254.

Mokri B, Ohnishi A, Dyck PJ. Disulfiram neuropathy. *Neurology* 1981;31:730–735.

National Institute of Occupational Safety and Health (NIOSH). *Pocket guide to chemical hazards.* Washington: US Department of Health and Human Services, CDC, 1997.

Occupational Safety and Health Administration (OSHA). Code of Federal Regulations, 29, 1910. 1000/.1047. Washington: Office of the Federal Register, National Archives and Records Administration, 1995:411–431.

Orzechowska-Juzwenko K, Wronska-Nofer T, Wiela A, et al. Effect of chronic exposure to carbon disulfide on biotransformation of phenazone in rabbits. *Toxicol Lett* 1984;22:171–174.

Pappolla M, Monaco S, Weiss H, et al. Slow axonal transport in carbon disulfide (CS$_2$) axonopathy. *J Neuropathol Exp Neurol* 1984;43:305.

Pappolla M, Penton R, Weiss HS, et al. Carbon disulfide axonopathy. Another experimental model characterized by acceleration of neurofilament transport and distinct changes in axonal size. *Brain Res* 1987;424:272–280.

Parkinson A. Biotransformation of xenobiotics. In: Klaassen KD, ed. *Casarett and Doull's toxicology. The basic science of poisons,* 5th ed. New York: McGraw-Hill, 1996:113–186.

Pergal M, Vukojevic N, Djuric D. Carbon disulfide metabolites excreted in the urine of exposed workers. I. Isolation and identification of 2-mercapto-2-thiazolinone-5. *Arch Environ Health* 1972a;25:38–41.

Pergal M, Vukojevic N, Djuric D. Carbon disulfide metabolites excreted in the urine of exposed workers. II. Isolation and identification of thiocarbamide. *Arch Environ Health* 1972b;25:42–44.

Peters HA, Levine RL, Matthews CG, Chapman LJ. Carbon disulfide-induced neuropsychiatric changes in grain-storage workers. *Am J Ind Med* 1982;3:373–391.

Peters HA, Levine RL, Matthews CG, Sauter S, Chapman LJ. Synergistic neurotoxicity of carbon tetrachloride/carbon disulfide (80/20 fumigants) and other pesticides in grain storage workers. *Acta Pharmacol Toxicol* 1986;59[Suppl 7]:535–546.

Peters HA, Levine RL, Matthews CG, Chapman LJ. Extrapyramidal and other neurological manifestations associated with carbon disulfide fumigant exposure. *Arch Neurol* 1988;45:537–540.

Peterson F. Three cases of acute mania from inhaling carbon disulfide. *Boston Med Surg J* 1892;127:325–326.

Petrovic D, Djuric D. Carbon disulphide in the exhaled air of exposed workers. *Arh Hig Rada Toksikol* 1966;17:159–163.

Putz-Anderson V, Albright BE, Lee ST, et al. A behavioral examination of workers exposed to carbon disulfide. *Neurotoxicology* 1983;4:67–78.

Quensel F. Neue erfahrungen über geistesstörungen nach schwefelkohlenstoffvergiftung. *Monatsschr Psych Neurol* 1904;16:246.

Raitta C, Tolonen M, Nurminen M. Microcirculation of ocular fundus in viscose rayon workers exposed to carbon disulfide. *Albrecht von Graefes Arch Klin Ophthalmol* 1974;191:151–164.

Raitta C, Tier H, Tolonen M, Nurminen M, Helpiö E, Malmström S. Impaired color discrimination among viscose rayon workers exposed to carbon disulfide. *J Occup Med* 1981;23:189–192.

Rasmussen RA, Khalil MAK, Dalluge RW, Carbonyl sulfide and carbon disulfide from eruptions of Mount St. Helens. *Science* 1982;215:665–667.

Richter R. Degeneration of the basal ganglia in monkeys from carbon disulfide poisoning. *J Neuropathol Exp Neurol* 1945;4:324–353.

Riihimäki V, Kivistö H, Peltonen K, Helpiö E, Aitio A. Assessment of exposure to carbon disulfide in the viscose production workers from urinary 2-thiothiazolidine-4-carboxylic acid determinations. *Am J Ind Med* 1992;22:85–97.

Rosier J, Van Doorn R, Grosjean R, Van de Walle A, Billemont G, Van Peteghem C. Preliminary evaluation of urinary 2-thio-thiazolidine-4-carboxylic acid levels as a test for exposure to carbon disulphide. *Int Arch Occup Health* 1982;51:159–167.

Rosier J, Veulemans H, Masschelein R, Vanhoorne M, Van Peteghen C. Experimental human exposure to carbon disulfide. I. Respiratory uptake and elimination of carbon disulfide under rest and physical exercise. *Int Arch Occup Environ Health* 1987a;59:233–242.

Rosier J, Veulemans H, Masschelein R, Vanhoorne M, Van Peteghen C. Experimental human exposure to carbon disulfide. II. Urinary excretion of 2-thiothiazolidine-4-carboxylic acid (TTCA) during and after exposure. *Int Arch Occup Environ Health* 1987b;59:243–250.

Ruijten MWMM, Sallé HJA, Verbeck MM, Muijser H. Special nerve functions and colour discrimination in workers with long term low level exposure to carbon disulphide. *Br J Ind Med* 1990;47:589–595.

Savolainen H, Vainio H. High binding of CS$_2$ sulphur in spinal cord axonal fraction. *Acta Neuropathol* 1976;36:251–257.

Savolainen H, Lehtonen E, Vainio H. CS$_2$ binding to rat spinal neurofilaments. *Acta Neuropathol* 1977;37:219–223.

Sax NI. *Dangerous properties of industrial chemicals,* 5th ed. New York: Van Nostrand Reinhold, 1979.

Sayre LM, Autilio-Gambetti L, Gambetti P. Pathogenesis of giant neurofilamentous axonopathies: a unified hypothesis based on chemical modification of neurofilaments. *Brain Res Rev* 1985;10:69–83.

Seppäläinen AM, Haltia M. Carbon disulfide. In: Spencer PS, Schaumburg HH, eds. *Experimental and clinical neurotoxicology.* Baltimore: Williams & Wilkins, 1980:356–373.

Seppäläinen AM, Tolonen M. Neurotoxicity of long-term exposure to carbon disulfide in the viscose rayon industry. A neurophysiological study. *Work Environ Health* 1974;11:145–153.

Seppäläinen AM, Tolonen M, Karli P, et al. Neurophysiological findings in chronic carbon disulfide poisoning. *Work Environ Health* 1972;9:71–75.

Siegers CP, Younes M. Protection by diethydithiocarbamate, a CS$_2$-liberating agent, against different models of experimentally induced liver injury. *G Ital Med Lav* 1984;6:135–137.

Simon P, Nicot T, Dieudonné M. Dietary habits, a non-negligible source of 2-thiothiazolidine-4-carboxylic acid and possible overestimation of carbon disulfide exposure. *Int Arch Occup Environ Health* 1994;66:85–90.

Snyderwine EG, Kroll R, Rudin RJ. The possible role of the ethanol-inducible isozyme of cytochrome P_{450} in the metabolism and distribution of carbon disulfide. *Toxicol Appl Pharmacol* 1988;93:11–21.

Soucek B, Pavelkova E. Absorption, metabolism and action of carbon disulfide in the organism. IV. Resorption and excretion of carbon disulfide in man in long-term experiments. *Prac Lek* 1953;5:181.

Soucek B. Transformation of carbon disulfide in the organism. *J Hyg Epidemiol Microbiol Immunol* 1957;1:10–22.

Spyker DA, Gallanosa AG, Suratt PM. Health effects of acute carbon disulfide exposure. *J Toxicol Clin Toxicol* 1982;19:87–93.

Stanosz S, Kuligowski D, Pieleszek A, Zuk E, Rzechula D, Chlubek D. Concentration of dopamine in plasma activity of dopamine beta-hydroxylase in serum and urinary excretion of free catecholamines and vanillylmandelic acid in women chronically exposed to carbon disulfide. *Int J Occup Med Environ Health* 1994;7:257–261.

Stýblová V. Die elektroencephalographie in der diagnotik der frühzeitigen hirnschädigung durch schwefelkohlenstoff. *Int Arch Environ Health* 1977;38:263–282.

Sugimoto K, Goto S, Hotta R. Studies on chronic carbon disulfide poisoning. A 5-year follow-up study on retinopathy due to carbon disulfide. *In Arch Occup Environ Health* 1976a;37:233–248.

Sugimoto K, Goto S, Hotta R. An epidemiological studies on retinopathy due to carbon disulfide: CS_2 exposure level and development of retinopathy. *Int Arch Occup Environ Hlth* 1976b;37:1–8.

Sugimoto K, Goto S, Kanda S, et al. Ocular fundus photography of workers exposed to carbon disulfide—a comparative epidemiological study between Japan and Finland. *Int Arch Occup Environ Health* 1977;39: 97–101.

Sugimoto K, Goto S, Kanda S, Taniguchi H, Nakamura K, Baba T. Studies on angiopathy due to carbon disulfide. Retinopathy and index of exposure dosages. *Scand J Work Environ Health* 1978;4:151–158.

Sugimura K, Kabashima K, Tatetsu S, et al. Computerized tomography in chronic carbon disulfide poisoning. *Brain Nerve (Tokyo)* 1979;31:1245–1253.

Teisinger J. New advances in the toxicology of carbon disulfide. *Am Ind Hyg Assoc J* 1974;35:55–61.

Teisinger J, Soucek B. Absorption and elimination of carbon disulfide in man. *J Ind Hyg Toxicol* 1949;31:67–73.

Timmerman RW. Carbon disulfide. In: Grayson M, ed. *Kirk-Othmer encyclopedia of chemical technology,* vol 4, 3rd ed. New York: John Wiley & Sons, 1978:743.

Tolonen M. Vascular effects of carbon disulfide. A review. *Scand J Work Environ Health* 1974;1:63–77.

Tolonen M, Hernberg S, Nurminen M, TiiTola K. A follow-up study of coronary heart disease in viscose rayon workers exposed to carbon disulphide. *Br J Ind Med* 1975;32:1–10.

Tolonen M, Nurminen M, Hernberg S. Ten-year coronary mortality of workers exposed to carbon disulfide. *Scand J Work Environ Health* 1979;5:109–114.

Torkelson TR, Rowe VK. Halogenated aliphatic hydrocarbons. In: Clayton GD, Clayton FE, eds. *Patty's industrial hygiene and toxicology,* 3rd ed., vol IIB. New York: John Wiley & Sons, 1981:3472–3478.

Toyama T, Kusano H. An experimental study on absorption and excretion of carbon disulfide. *Jpn J Hyg* 1953;8:10.

United States Environmental Protection Agency (USEPA). *Drinking water regulations and health advisories.* EPA 822-R-96-001. Washington: Office of Water, 1996.

Valentine WM, Amarnath V, Graham DG, Anthony DC. Covalent cross-linking of proteins by carbon disulfide. *Chem Res Toxicol* 1992;5: 254–262.

Valentine WM, Amarnath V, Amarnath K, Rimmele F, Graham DG. Carbon disulfide mediated cross-linking by N,N-diethyldithiocarbamate. *Chem Res Toxicol* 1995;8:96–102.

Valentine WM, Amarnath V, Amarnath K, et al. Covalent modification of hemoglobin by disulfide: III. A potential biomarker of effect. *Neurotoxicology* 1998;19:99–107.

Van Doorn R, Leijdekkers CM, Henderson P, Vanhoorne M, Vertin PG. Determination of thio compounds in urine of workers exposed to carbon disulfide. *Arch Environ Health* 1981;36:289.

Vanhoorne M, de Douck A, Bacquer D. Epidemiological study of eye irritation by hydrogen sulphide and/or carbon disulphide exposure in viscose rayon workers. *Ann Occup Hyg* 1995;39:307–315.

Vanhoorne M, de Douck A, Bacquer D. Epidemiological study of the systemic ophthalmological effects of carbon disulfide. *Arch Environ Health* 1996;51:181–188.

Vasilescu C. Nerve conduction velocity and electromyogram in carbon disulfide poisoning. *Rev Roum Neurol* 1972;9:63–71.

Vasilescu C, Florescu A. Clinical and electrophysiological studies of carbon disulfide polyneuropathy. *J Neurol* 1980;224:59–70.

Vigliani EC. Clinical observations on carbon disulfide intoxication in Italy. *Ind Med Surg* 1950;19:240–242.

Vigliani EC. Carbon disulphide poisoning in viscose rayon factories. *Br J Ind Med* 1954;11:235–244.

White RF, Feldman RG, Proctor SP. Neurobehavioral effects of toxic exposures. In: White RF, ed. *Clinical syndromes in adult neuropsychology: the practioners handbook.* New York: Elsevier Science Publishers, 1992:1–51.

Windolz M, ed. *The Merck index,* 10th ed. Rahway, NJ: Merck, 1994:251.

World Health Organization (WHO). *Environmental health criteria 10: carbon disulfide.* Geneva: WHO, 1979.

Wronska-Nofer T, Klimczak J, Wisnieweska-Knypl JM, et al. Combined effects of ethanol and carbon disulfide on cytochrome P-450 monooxygenase, lipid peroxidation and ultrastructure of the liver in chronically exposed rats. *J Appl Toxicol* 1986;6:297–302.

Yamada Y. A case of acute carbon disulfide poisoning by accidental ingestion (author's transl). *Ind Health* 1977;19:140–141.

CHAPTER 22

Organophosphorus Compounds

Organophosphorus (OP) compounds consist of a central pentavalent phosphorus atom to which are bonded either an oxygen or a sulfur atom, two organic radicals (R and R′), and an inorganic or organic leaving group (X) (Fig. 22-1). When the phosphorus atom is double-bonded to oxygen, the compound is called an organophosphate. When the oxygen atom is replaced with a sulfur atom, the compound is called a phosphorothioate. The R and R′ positions can be occupied by either alkyl, aryl, or amide groups. The substituents that can occupy the X position include alkyl and aryl groups, cyanide, and the halides. The numerous OP compounds synthesized for commercial use result from the myriad of possible substituents that occupy the R, R′, and X positions of the molecule, making it very difficult for a clinician to be familiar with the uses and toxic potential of all the available OP compounds.

Attempts to give order to the seemingly unlimited number of different OP compounds have resulted in the publication of lists of OP compounds, which separate the various compounds into categories, classes, and subclasses, based upon chemical species and structural differences and/or the demonstrated capacity of the parent compound to inhibit the action of the enzyme acetylcholinesterase (AChE). The fact that bioactivation can result in significant similarities in neurotoxic potential between structurally unrelated parent compounds makes these lists difficult to interpret. For example, the phosphorothioates have significantly less anticholinesterase activity than do the organophosphates. However, microsomal oxidation of the parent phosphorothioate compound enhances its anticholinesterase activity *in vivo*. The capability of a particular OP compound to inhibit acetylcholinesterase activity is dependent first on the affinity of the compound or its metabolites for acetylcholinesterase and then on the total duration of time for which the enzyme's activity is inhibited by the attached OP compound (Lotti et al., 1993).

The ease with which the compound dissociates (i.e., loses its leaving group) after its binding to AChE is directly related to its neurotoxic potential in humans. Four major categories of OP compounds can be defined based on the properties of the compound's leaving group (X): (a) *phosphorylcholines,* within which X contains a quaternary nitrogen, are highly toxic to humans (e.g., phospholine); (b) *fluorophophorus compounds,* within which X is fluorine (e.g., sarin), are the second most highly toxic group of OP compounds; (c) *cyano- and halophosphorus compounds,* within which X is a cyanide group or a halogen other than fluorine (e.g., tabun), are the third most toxic group; (d) *alkyl and arylphosphorus compounds,* within which the X moiety is attached to the molecule by an oxygen or sulfur atom (e.g., dichlorvos) (see Fig. 22-1). The compounds in the fourth category have the lowest AChE activity and can be further divided into seven toxicity subgroups based on the substituents at the R and R′position; these OP compounds are commonly used as insecticides (Holmstedt, 1963).

There are literally thousands of commercial preparations that contain OP compounds either alone or in combination with other OP compounds, other chemicals known to have pesticidal capacity (e.g., carbamates), and various solvent carriers (i.e., inerts) that facilitate dispersion and absorption. Many of these so-called inert ingredients are also toxic to humans. In 1987 the Environmental Protection Agency (EPA) determined that 57 of the chemicals used as inert ingredients (e.g., perchloroethylene, trichloroethylene, *n*-hexane, and methyl *n*-butyl ketone) are highly toxic to humans, and warning labels are required on those OP compounds that contain these chemicals. The EPA also strongly encourages manufacturers to remove these and other potentially toxic inert ingredients (e.g., toluene, xylene, and 1,1,1-trichloroethane) from those OP compounds that contain them (EPA, 1987). (See respective chapters in this volume for the neurotoxic effects associated with exposures to the above-mentioned chemicals.)

There are nearly 2.7 million agriculture workers in the United States, many of whom are either migrant or seasonal farm workers (Midtling et al., 1985). The prevalence of pesticide-induced illness including that resulting from exposure to OPs among farm workers is estimated to range

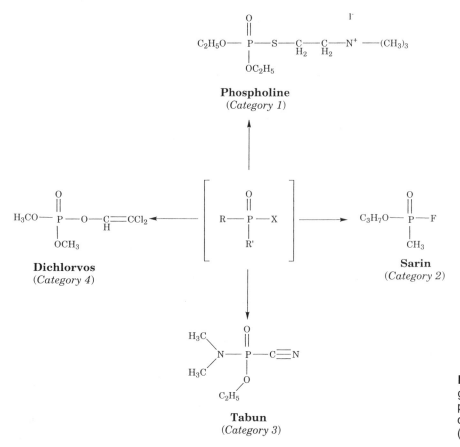

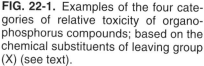

FIG. 22-1. Examples of the four categories of relative toxicity of organophosphorus compounds; based on the chemical substituents of leaving group (X) (see text).

from 150,000 to 300,000 cases annually (Barnes, 1961; Coye, 1985). Of these, less than 2% is estimated to be reported to public health authorities (Coye, 1985). In addition, there are approximately 1.3 million certified pesticide applicators in the United States, many of whom, although trained, are nevertheless at risk for exposure to OPs (DHHS, 1980; EPA, 1988; Ames et al., 1995). Thus, the possibility of exposure to OP compounds is quite widespread.

OP compounds constitute almost 40% of all pesticides used in the United States; and while careful application of these potentially dangerous chemicals is of great medical, public health, and economic value, it is of greater importance that indiscriminate human and wildlife exposure to OP compounds be avoided because of the neurotoxic and other hazardous properties (e.g., carcinogenesis) of these compounds (Brown et al., 1990; Schwarz et al., 1995). The action of inhibiting cholinesterase results in an excess of available acetylcholine at particular central nervous system (CNS) receptors and at neuromuscular junctions. The latter situation leads to paralysis of insect flight muscles. Because certain OP compounds can also disable humans by paralyzing their striated muscles and their diaphragm and by causing symptoms of severe parasympathetic nervous system effects on smooth muscle (e.g., diarrhea, nausea, and vomiting), they have been used as chemical warfare agents (Sidell, 1997). Anticholinesterase properties of OP compounds are also used in certain medical conditions in

which neuromuscular relaxation is desirable. Studies by Kaufer et al. (1998) indicate that cholinesterase inhibitors can induce changes in the expression of proteins mediating brain cholinergic neurotransmission.

Once neurotoxic effects occur, it is essential that they are recognized and differentiated from other disorders of neuromuscular transmission and disruptions of cholinergic synaptic activity (e.g., Eaton–Lambert syndrome, myasthenia gravis, and botulism). The carbamates also inhibit AChE and thus the possibility that the patient has been exposed to one of these compounds must be considered in the differential diagnosis (see Chapter 23). Two other classes of pesticides, the chlorinated hydrocarbons and the synthetic pyrethroids, are in common use, but neither of these chemical groups has been shown to inhibit AChE activity. The results of blood cholinesterase activity assays are used as indicators of OP-induced neurotoxicity.

SOURCES OF EXPOSURE

Employees involved in the manufacture of OP compounds are chronically exposed to low levels and are also at risk for episodes of acute exposure to high peak levels depending on production volume. Farmers, pesticide handlers (mixers, loaders, appliers, flaggers, equipment maintenance workers), and forest, nursery, and greenhouse workers are exposed to OP compounds (Metcalf and Holmes, 1969). Accidents caused by mechanical failure or hose breakage can lead to large-scale spillage, resulting in severe acute exposures among workers and bystanders. Pilots flying planes (crop dusting) involved in the application of OP pesticides are at risk for exposure (Quinby et al., 1958). Likewise, overflying a flagger during aerial spraying may result in acute exposure. Excessive levels of OP compounds resulting from violations of workplace safety precautions and hygienic measures (such as failure to provide or utilize proper mixing/loading devices, personal protective clothing, and/or washing facilities) can result in significant contributions to total worker exposure (Midtling et al., 1985). Unique circumstances may be associated with OP exposure. For example, museum personnel were exposed to OP compounds used to protect specimens from insect damage (Deer et al., 1993).

In addition to the agricultural industry, there are other opportunities for hazardous exposure to these chemicals for humans and animals. Ingestion of OP compounds is a common method of suicide (Yeh et al., 1993; Bentur et al., 1993; Betrosian et al., 1995; Futagami et al., 1995). Accidental ingestion by children as well as adults is also common (Zwiener and Ginsburg, 1988; Muldoon and Hodgson, 1992; Aiuto et al., 1993; Laynes Bretones, et al., 1997). Illegal application of highly toxic OP compounds not licensed for indoor use, such as methyl parathion, has also been reported (Esteban et al., 1996). Thousands of unsuspecting persons were exposed through the intake of cooking oil and ethanol extracted from ginger (i.e., "Jamaica Ginger") that was adulterated with OP compounds and many of them suffered significant and persistent adverse health effects (Senanayake and Jeyaratnam, 1981; Morgan and Penovich, 1978; Woolf, 1995). Airplane passengers have been acutely exposed to OP insecticides used to fumigate planes (Jensen et al., 1965). OP compounds are used as fire retardants in polyurethane foams (Petajan et al., 1975). OP compounds have been detected in foods, including milk and cheese (Mallatou et al., 1997). OP poisoning has been associated with consumption of contaminated produce (Goh et al., 1990). OP compounds are considered environmentally nonpersistent because they readily undergo nonenzymatic hydrolysis (WHO, 1986). Nevertheless, contamination of water supplies through improper disposal of OP compounds has also been reported and contributes to the elevated background tissue levels in some nonoccupationally exposed populations (Virtue and Clayton, 1997; Miliadis and Malatou, 1997; García-Repetto et al., 1997; Serrano et al., 1997).

EXPOSURE LIMITS AND SAFETY REGULATIONS

The *Occupational Safety and Health Administration* (OSHA), the *National Institute for Occupational Safety and Health* (NIOSH) and the *American Conference of Governmental Industrial Hygienists* (ACGIH) have established and recommended occupational exposure limits for many OP compounds. However, due to the great number of

compounds that fall into this chemical category, it is only possible to consider the exposure limits for a few of the more commonly used ones here; for current information on a specific carbamate compound consult the *NIOSH Pocket Guide to Chemical Hazards* (NIOSH, 1997) or access the NIOSH Internet homepage at <http://www.cdc.gov/niosh/homepage.html>.

The OSHA had established an 8-hour time-weighted average (TWA) permissible exposure limit (PEL) of 0.2 mg/m³ for chlorpyrifos, but this limit was vacated in July 1992 (OSHA, 1995). The NIOSH recommended exposure limit (REL) for chlorpyrifos is a 10-hour TWA ambient air concentration of 0.2 mg/m³. The NIOSH has also established a 15-minute TWA short-term exposure limit (STEL) of 0.6 mg/m³ for chlorpyrifos. The NIOSH has not determined an immediately dangerous to life and health (IDLH) concentration for chlorpyrifos (NIOSH, 1997). The ACGIH threshold limit value (TLV) for chlorpyrifos is an 8-hour TWA ambient air concentration of 0.2 mg/m³ (ACGIH, 1995). The NIOSH, and the ACGIH have both assigned chlorpyrifos a "SKIN" designation, indicating that dermal absorption contributes significantly to the exposed individual's total body burden (NIOSH, 1997; ACGIH, 1995) (Table 22-1).

THE OSHA has established a PEL of 1.0 mg/m³ for dichlorvos (OSHA, 1995). The NIOSH REL for dichlorvos is 1.0 mg/m³. The NIOSH has recommended an IDLH concentration for dichlorvos of 100 mg/m³ (NIOSH, 1997). The ACGIH TLV for dichlorvos is 0.9 mg/m³ (ACGIH, 1995). The OSHA, NIOSH, and ACGIH have all assigned dichlorvos a "SKIN" designation (NIOSH, 1997; ACGIH, 1995; OSHA, 1995).

The OSHA has established a PEL of 15 mg/m³ for malathion (OSHA, 1995). The NIOSH REL for malathion is 10 mg/m³. The NIOSH IDLH concentration for malathion is 250 mg/m³ (NIOSH, 1997). The ACGIH TLV for malathion is 10 mg/m³ (ACGIH, 1995). The OSHA, NIOSH, and ACGIH have all assigned malathion a "SKIN" designation (NIOSH, 1997; OSHA, 1995; ACGIH, 1995).

The OSHA PEL for parathion is 0.1 mg/m³ (OSHA, 1995). The NIOSH REL for parathion is 0.05 mg/m³. The NIOSH IDLH concentration for parathion is 10 mg/m³ (NIOSH, 1997). The ACGIH TLV for parathion is 0.1 mg/m³ (ACGIH, 1995). The OSHA, NIOSH, and ACGIH have all assigned malathion a "SKIN" designation (NIOSH, 1997; OSHA, 1995; ACGIH, 1995).

Restricted entry intervals (REIs) have been established that restrict entry into a field that has been treated with an OP compound until a specified duration of time has elapsed. Reentry intervals are set only for the active OP ingredient, and there are no set standards for the inert ingredients of pesticide preparations. Entering a sprayed field without proper personal protective equipment prior to the expiration of the reentry interval exposes the workers to the pesticide that is still active and hazardous. Such exposures can be prevented by proper notification of pesticide application and use of personal protection equipment. Dry

TABLE 22-1. *Established and recommended occupational and environmental exposure limits for selected organophosphorus compounds in air and water*

	Air (mg/m³)[a]	Water (mg/L)[a]
Odor threshold*	—	—
OSHA		
Chlorpyrifos		
PEL (8-hr TWA)	0.2[b]	—
Dichlorvos		
PEL (8-hr TWA)	1	—
Malathion		
PEL (8-hr TWA)	15	—
Parathion		
PEL (8-hr TWA)	0.1	—
NIOSH		
Chlorpyrifos		
REL (10-hr TWA)	0.2	—
STEL (15-min TWA)	0.6	—
Dichlorvos		
REL (10-hr TWA)	1	—
Malathion		
REL (10-hr TWA)	10	—
IDLH	250	—
Parathion		
REL (10-hr TWA)	0.05	—
IDLH	10	—
ACGIH		
Chlorpyrifos		
TLV (8-hr TWA)	0.2	—
Dichlorvos		
TLV (8-hr TWA)	0.9	—
Malathion		
TLV (8-hr TWA)	10	—
Parathion		
TLV (8-hr TWA)	0.1	—
EPA[c]		
MCL	—	—
MCLG	—	—

[a]Unit conversion: Chlorpyrifos, not available; dichlorvos, 1 ppm = 9.19 mg/m3; malathion, 1 ppm = 13.73 mg/m3; parathion, 1 ppm = 12.11 mg/m3; 1 ppm = 1 mg/L.

[b]Vacated PEL (see text).

[c]See text for EPA drinking water health advisory levels.

OSHA, Occupational Safety and Health Organization; PEL, permissible exposure limit; TWA, time-weighted average; NIOSH, National Institute for Occupational Safety and Health; REL, recommended exposure limit; STEL, short-term exposure limit; IDLH, immediately dangerous to life and health; ACGIH, American Conference of Governmental Industrial Hygienists; EPA, Environmental Protection Agency; MCL, maximum contamination level; MCLG, maximum contamination level goal.

Data from *Amoore and Hautala, 1983; OSHA, 1995; ACGIH, 1995; NIOSH, 1997.

weather may reduce non-enzymatic hydrolysis of OP compounds and prolong the decay time of the organophosphate beyond the reentry interval, thereby increasing the risk for exposure. Toxic compounds may persist on the foliage for several weeks, especially in dry climates (EPA, 1992) (see Clinical Experiences section).

REIs are established according to the relative toxicity of the OP compound and are as follows: (a) Category I pesticides: REI = 48 hours; the REI is increased to 72 hours in arid areas; (b) Category II pesticides: REI = 24 hours; (c) Category III and Category IV pesticides: REI = 12 hours. With few exceptions, workers are restricted from entering the pesticide treated area during the REI period. However, a worker wearing proper protective clothing may enter an area before termination of the REI for short-term tasks that do not require contact with the treated surfaces (EPA, 1992).

The *Environmental Protection Agency* (EPA) has not established maximum contamination levels (MCLs) or maximum contamination level goals (MCLGs) for chlorpyrifos, dichlorvos, malathion, or parathion. OP compounds are considered to be nonpersistent in water because they readily undergo nonenzymatic hydrolysis (WHO, 1986). However, the EPA has established drinking water health advisories for chlorpyrifos (lifetime intake: 0.02 mg/L) and malathion (lifetime intake: 0.02 mg/L). These limits represent the drinking water concentrations of chlorpyrifos and malathion not expected to cause any adverse noncarcinogenic health effects over a lifetime of exposure (EPA, 1996).

The environmental exposure limits for the nerve agents tabun, sarin, and VX have all been set at 0.000003 mg/m³, while for occupationally exposed workers the 8-hour TWA limits are 0.0001 mg/m³ for GA and GB, and 0.00001 mg/m³ for VX (MMWR, 1988).

METABOLISM

Tissue Absorption

Most OPs are highly lipid-soluble and thus are readily absorbed after inhalation and oral and dermal exposures. The inhaled dose is easily absorbed across the pulmonary alveoli into the blood as was shown by plasma cholinesterase activity levels which were promptly depressed to 75% to 80% of normal in human volunteers who were acutely exposed to dichlorvos by inhalation at an air concentration of 1 mg/m³ for durations of 7.5 to 8.5 hours, respectively (Hester, 1988). Bronchial irritation and mucous membrane reactions to direct contact with OP compounds result in bronchorrhea, bronchial constriction, and dyspnea following respiratory exposure (Midtling et al., 1985).

Oral intake can result in a prompt and dramatic symptomatic response with diarrhea, vomiting, and abdominal cramps followed by muscle weakness and CNS effects (Senanayake and Johnson, 1982). Acute symptoms of AChE inhibition reported in a 22-year-old woman who ingested 100 mL of parathion included lacrimation and excessive salivation, miosis, bradycardia, and hypotension, followed by coma and then the OP intermediate syndrome and neuropathy (Yeh et al., 1993) (see Symptomatic Diagnosis section).

OP compounds readily penetrate all external surfaces of the body, including the mucous membranes and the epidermis (Gaines, 1969; Shah and Guthrie, 1983). Dermal absorption is enhanced by the vehicle (Sortorelli et al., 1997). Total dermal absorption is influenced by the size, temperature, and level of hydration of the exposed area of skin, and uptake is higher when the skin surface is broken (e.g., abrasions or cuts). Dermal absorption reduces hepatic metabolism; thus, OP compounds which do not require metabolic activation (i.e., toxification via *in vivo* oxidation) are considerably more toxic when absorbed via dermal routes than are those compounds that do require metabolic activation (Gaines et al., 1966; Gaines, 1969; Chang et al., 1994) (see Tissue Biochemistry section). Gershon and Shaw (1961) reported the case of a scientific field officer who was acutely poisoned in the course of checking the potency of OP insecticides. He handled treated branches and leaves without protective gloves on several occasions, after which he experienced symptoms including dizziness, fatigue, nausea, muscle cramps, hallucinations, and concentration and memory deficits.

Tissue Distribution

OP compounds readily cross the blood–brain barrier (BBB). The concentration of OP compounds in lipid-rich tissues such as the brain and adipose tissue reflects the relative lipophilicity of the various OP compounds. Following subcutaneous injection of mice with radio-labeled parathion, the highest level of radioactivity was found in the brown fat and the salivary glands; high levels were found in the ordinary adipose tissues, liver, and kidney; fairly high levels were in the walls of the gastrointestinal

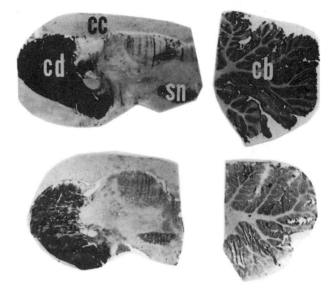

FIG. 22-2. Acetylcholinesterase activity levels in the brain of an unexposed control (**top**) and in the brain of a 36-year-old man who committed suicide by ingesting parathion (**bottom**). Left sagittal sections of exposed individual and control show reduction in staining intensity in the molecular layer of the cerebellum, substantia nigra, and caudate nucleus, along with preservation of staining in the corpus callosum and anterior commissure of the exposed patient. cb, cerebellum; cc, corpus callosum; cd, caudate; sn, substantia nigra. (From Finkelstein et al., 1988b, with permission.)

tract, spleen, lungs, and thyroid; lower levels were detected in the CNS and muscles (Fredriksson and Bigelow, 1961). Postmortem examinations in humans who died after intentional ingestion of fenthion showed higher levels of OP compounds in kidney and fat than in blood and vitreous humor (Tsatsakis et al., 1996).

It is suggested that different forms of AChE predominate in different regions of the brain, leading to different regional sensitivities to different OP compounds (Finkelstein et al., 1988a, 1988b). Distribution of OP compounds within the brain reflects region specific differences in cholinergic activity. Exposure to parathion resulted in a significant decrease in AChE activity in the cerebral cortex (occipital lobe and cingulate gyrus), and in the molecular layer, and dentate nucleus of the cerebellum; reductions were also noted in the basal ganglia and the thalamus. No significant reduction was seen in AChE activity in the white matter (Table 22-2 and Fig. 22-2). The regional variation in AChE inhibition may determine the CNS symptoms following exposure. Significant reduction in the AChE in the frontal cortices may correlate with psychomotor slowing, impaired reading comprehension, and expressive language defects with pauses and perseverations, whereas reductions in the AChE activity in the cerebellum may be associated with the poor coordination, ataxia, and slurred speech caused by parathion intoxication.

TABLE 22-2. *Acetylcholinesterase activity levels in the brain of a 19-year-old woman who committed suicide by ingesting parathion and in an unexposed control*

Brain region	Exposed patient	Unexposed control	Percent reduction
Cerebral gyri:			
Frontal lobe			
Superior frontal	3	10	70
Middle frontal	4	9	56
Inferior frontal	1	7	86
Temporal lobe			
Superior temporal	5	10	50
Middle temporal	6	9	33
Inferior temporal	4	8	50
Insula			
Gyrus longus	6	13	54
Gyri breves	4	10	60
Basal ganglia			
Putamen	38	50	24
Caudate	35	49	39
Claustrum	2	6	67
Centrum semiovale	1	1	0

Data from Finkelstein et al., 1988b.

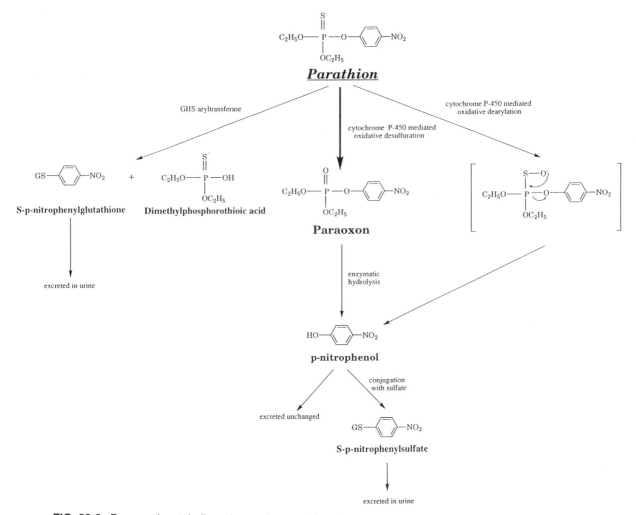

FIG. 22-3. Proposed metabolic pathways for parathion. Parathion was selected as a prototype because this particular compound is metabolized via several pathways and is metabolically activated to a more toxic metabolite (paraoxon).

Knowledge about tissue distribution and storage properties of OP compounds contributes to the understanding of the clinical course following exposure to a particular compound. Compounds that are initially stored in the fat tissues and in certain organs may continue to be released into circulation and to be redistributed to target sites where they continue to cause toxicity directly or through their active metabolites. This has significant therapeutic implications, especially with regards to anticipating a relapse in an apparently treated patient, making it essential that an observation period is sufficiently long to avoid delayed crisis. For example, parathion-poisoned animals relapsed several hours after initial successful treatment with pralidoxime. This rapid relapse was attributed to the formation of an active and toxic metabolite from parathion (Svetlicic and Vandekar, 1960); however, it may also be due to continuing absorption from exposure surfaces and/or from storage tissues of the direct toxicant as well as continuing metabolic activation of an indirect toxicant as in the case of parathion. In humans, it may be difficult to distinguish between the toxicant that continues to be absorbed from the initial contact surface (skin, intestinal tract, respiratory tract, etc.) and the one that is released from the storage tissues after the initial exposure (Hodgson et al., 1986).

Tissue Biochemistry

The majority of an absorbed dose of an OP compound is metabolized in the liver, but metabolism has been demonstrated in brain tissue as well. Phase I of *in vivo* biotranformation precedes via hydrolysis and oxidation and/or through the actions of glutathione transferase. Phase II involves conjugation of the Phase I metabolites with glucuronic acid, glutathione, and/or sulfate. These conjugated forms have increased water solubility and thus are readily excreted in the urine through the kidneys (Fig. 22-3).

Considering that OPs are the esters of phosphoric acid, they are targets for hydrolytic enzymes during Phase I. Hydrolysis cleaves the R groups and inactivates the OP compound (see Fig. 22-3). The hydrolytic enzymes involved in the metabolism of OP compounds include arylesterases, carboxyamidases, carboxylesterases, phosphorylphosphatases, and phosphotriesterases. Other enzymes that can induce hydrolysis of OP compounds include AChE and butyrylcholinesterase, otherwise known as plasma cholinesterase or pseudocholinesterase. Butyrylcholinesterase, which is synthesized primarily in the liver and detected mainly in the plasma, normally scavenges anticholinesterase compounds such as those with OP and thus prevents inhibition of AChE (Taylor and Radic, 1994). The cholinergic manifestations associated with OP exposure emerge when tissue stores of butyrylcholinesterase are depleted.

Oxidative metabolism of OP compounds occurs via the actions of the cytochrome P-450 monooxygenase system. Examples of oxidative biotransformation include oxidative dealkylation and dearylation, desulfuration, and thioether oxidation (Ma and Chambers, 1994; Butler and Murray, 1997). Oxidation can enhance or reduce the toxicity of OP compounds (O'Shaughnessy and Sultatos, 1995). Oxidative dealkylation and dearylation reduce the toxicity of all OP compounds. However, the oxidative desulfuration of sulfur-containing OP compounds (phosphorothioates) such as parathion results in the formation of the corresponding oxygen-containing compound (e.g., paraoxon) and enhanced anticholinesterase activity. Thus, the metabolites of OP desulfuration are more toxic than the parent molecule (O'Shaughnessy and Sultatos, 1995; Butler and Murray, 1997). The active metabolite (e.g., paraoxon) formed via oxidative desulfuration subsequently undergoes hydrolysis (see Fig. 22-3). OP compounds that undergo oxidative activation are called indirect inhibitors, whereas those compounds that need no metabolic conversion for full toxicity are known as direct inhibitors. The clinical effects of direct inhibitors develop faster than indirect inhibitors at the contact sites, such as the lungs, eyes, or the gastrointestinal system. Monooxygenase-induced activation is also seen with certain phosphothioether compounds such as thimet. The oxidation of these compounds proceeds in two steps, each producing a more potent compound than the preceding one (Metcalf et al., 1957; Bowman and Casida, 1958; Bull, 1965; Eto, 1974). Chronic exposures to chemicals which induce cytochrome P-450 activity such as ethanol enhance the metabolism of OP compounds and thus may increase the toxicity of indirect inhibitors such as parathion while decreasing the toxicity of the direct inhibitors (O'Shaughnessy and Sultatos, 1995).

The phosphothioate esters (e.g., dichlovos and parathion) can be dealkylated via the actions of glutathione transferase (GHS-transferase). Glutathione aryltransferases can accept the aryl group from phosphorothioates. Metabolism of parathion via this pathway leads to the formation of *S-p*-nitrophenylglutathione (Hollingworth et al., 1973) (see Fig. 22-3).

Phase II detoxification conjugates the active metabolite with glutathione, glucuronic acid, and/or sulfate. For ex-

ample, parathion is conjugated with glucuronide and sulfate to yield paranitrophenyl glucuronide and paranitrophenyl sulfate, respectively (Oneto et al., 1995) (see Fig. 22-3). Exposure to OP compounds that are conjugated with glutathione depletes tissue stores of this Phase II enzyme and thus may decrease the ability of the exposed individual to detoxify other toxins (Della Morte et al., 1994).

AChE can be synthesized by a variety of cells, including neurons, muscle cells, and erythrocytes. The enzyme is found in the perikaryon, dendrites, and axons of cholinergic neurons, in the cholinergic synapses, and at the surface and infoldings of the postjunctional motor end plates. A separate gene encodes for butyrylcholinesterase, also known as plasma cholinesterase or pseudocholinesterase. Butyrylcholinesterase is detected in the liver, plasma, and glial cells of the nervous system (Lockridge et al., 1987). AChE hydrolyzes acetylcholine (ACh) faster than butyrylcholinesterase, but both enzymes are inhibited by OP compounds. The function of butyrylcholinesterase is not fully understood, but it appears that it acts as a scavenger of AChE inhibitors such as OP compounds and carbamates (Loewenstein-Lichtenstein et al., 1995).

AChE has two subsites that react with acetylcholine: (a) an esteric site and (b) a negatively charged anionic center. The esteratic site of the enzyme covalently binds the carbonyl carbon of the acetate moiety of ACh, while the anionic center attracts the positively charged quaternary nitrogen of the choline moiety in ACh (Schwarz et al., 1995; Cooper et al., 1996). Acetylation of AChE is followed by cleavage of the ester link and the release of choline. The acetylated enzyme then reacts with water, thereby releasing acetic acid and thus restoring or regenerating the active enzyme (Massoulie et al., 1993; Taylor and Radic, 1994). Most OP compounds lack a positively charged acidic group and therefore do not react with the anionic site of AChE. Nevertheless, the chemical similarity between ACh and the OP compounds does allow for bonding at the esteric site and the formation of a phosphate ester bond (OP–AChE complex), resulting in inhibition of AChE activity (Ordentlich et al., 1996). Inhibition of AChE results in accumulation of endogenous ACh at the synaptic cleft resulting in symptoms of cholinergic overstimulation.

The binding of the OP compounds to AChE results in very stable phosphorylated enzyme–substrate complex. The phosphorous atom of an OP compound is attached to AChE's esteratic site, analogous to that seen between carbonyl carbon of acetate of ACh and the same esteratic site of AChE. The acidic group is subsequently cleaved from the OP–AChE complex, a mechanism that is analogous to the separation of choline for ACh. The phosphorylated enzyme then reacts with water to form a hydroxylated complex. However, dephosphorylation and hydroxylation of AChE is a very slow process that can take up to 40 days; the speed of this step depends on the particular OP compound. For example, if the alkyl groups in the phosphorylated enzyme complex are methyl or ethyl, AChE regeneration requires only several hours. Organophosphorus compounds with secondary or tertiary alkyl groups cause the formation of extremely stable phosphorylated enzyme complexes, the hydrolysis of which is insignificant. Consequently AChE inhibition by many OP compounds is essentially irreversible, and thus any restoration of AChE activity is essentially dependent on *de novo* synthesis of the enzyme.

As the duration of OP-induced AChE inhibition lengthens, an exponentially higher proportion of the phosphorylated enzyme becomes entirely resistant to dephosphorylation (reactivation) (Hobbiger, 1955, 1956). This phenomenon is referred to as *aging* (i.e., irreversible binding with, and thus inhibition of, the enzyme). Aging is caused by the hydrolysis of one alkoxy group, leading to the formation of a monoalkoxy phosphate–enzyme complex that is resistant to oximes and other nucleophilic agents (Berends et al., 1959; Harris et al., 1966). The speed of aging is affected by the type of enzyme affected and the OP compound involved. Butyrylcholinesterase ages five to ten times faster than AChE regardless of the OP compound involved. The estimated decreasing order of AChE aging capacity for the various OP compounds is: isopropylphosphoryl-methyl-AChE > dimethylphosphoryl-AChE = diisopropylphosphoryl-AChE > diethylphosphoryl-AChE (Davies and Green, 1956; Witter and Gaines, 1963). In the light of the relationship between the irreversible inhibition of esterases and the occurrence of neuropathy among persons exposed to OP compounds, it is considered necessary to start treatment with oximes as early as possible in order to increase enzyme reactivation, to minimize aging, and to reduce the risk of subsequently developing peripheral neuropathy (see Neuropathological Diagnosis section).

Reactivation of the phosphorylated enzyme can be hastened by nucleophilic agents such as hydroxylamine, hydroxamic acids, and oximes (e.g., pralidoxime and obidoxime chloride), all of which have quaternary nitrogen atoms with a positive charge (Wilson, 1951). The electrophilic reaction between the positively charged quaternary nitrogen and the negatively charged (anionic) active center of the enzyme brings the nucleophilic oxime in close proximity with the phosphorus atom of the OP compound that has phosphorylated the enzyme. This facilitates a nucleophilic substitution reaction with the formation of an oximephosphonate, which then readily separates from AChE and thus regenerates the active AChE enzyme (Wilson, 1959). Although oximes are used in the treatment of OP intoxication, they do not readily cross the BBB and thus are relatively less effective at reversing CNS toxicity (see Preventive and Therapeutic Measures section).

Excretion

OP compounds that have undergone hydrolysis are eliminated in the urine free and/or conjugated with glutathione, glucuronic acid, and sulfate. Paranitrophenyl sulfate, pa-

ranitrophenyl glucuronide, and free paranitrophenol were detected in human urine following acute suicidal parathion ingestion. Studies showed that approximately 81% of the total dose was excreted as paranitrophenyl sulfate conjugates. Total paranitrophenol excreted by this patient was equivalent to 76 mg parathion (lethal dose in humans: 20 to 100 mg) (Oneto et al., 1995). The excretion of chlorpyrifos and its principal metabolite, 3,5,6-trichloro-2-pyridinol (3,5,6-TCP), was investigated in six healthy male volunteers given a single oral dose of 0.5 mg/kg and, 2 or more weeks later, a 0.5 or 5.0 mg/kg dermal dose of chlorpyrifos. No unchanged chlorpyrifos was found in the urine following either route of administration. Mean blood 3,5,6-TCP concentrations peaked at 0.93 μg/mL 6 hours after ingestion of the oral dose and at 0.063 μg/mL 24 hours after the 5.0 mg/kg dermal dose. The 3,5,6-TCP was cleared from the blood and eliminated in the urine with a half-life of 27 hours following both oral and dermal intake. An average of 70% of the oral dose but less than 3% of the dermal dose was excreted in the urine as 3,5,6-TCP, indicating that only a small fraction of the dermally applied chlorpyrifos was absorbed. These findings indicate that chlorpyrifos and its principal metabolite 3,5,6-TCP are rapidly eliminated and therefore have a low potential to accumulate in humans with repeated or chronic exposures. In addition, these findings demonstrate that urine 3,5,6-TCP concentrations can be used to quantify the amount of chlorpyrifos absorbed (Nolan et al., 1984) (see Biochemical Diagnosis section and Fig. 22-3).

CLINICAL MANIFESTATIONS AND DIAGNOSIS

Symptomatic Diagnosis

The neurotoxic effects of exposure to organic phosphorous compounds occur in three successive clinical stages (a) *acute cholinergic crisis;* (b) *intermediate syndrome;* and (c) *delayed peripheral neuropathy,* which is also known as organophosphate-induced delayed neuropathy (OPIDN). The acute cholinergic crisis is frequently followed by a brief symptom-free period lasting 1 to 4 days subsequent to which the intermediate syndrome develops. Although overlapping of the clinical pictures of the acute cholinergic crisis and that of the intermediate syndrome is also seen, recognition of the brief period of recovery that frequently occurs is critical in the management of OP intoxication and should not be misinterpreted as the termination of the toxic offense. Those patients with mild cholinergic crisis may never develop the intermediate syndrome or neuropathy (De Bleecker, 1995). Conversely, when the exposure is sufficient, treatment with anticholinergic medications (e.g., atropine) does not prevent or reverse the emergence of the later two stages (Wadia et al., 1974; Yeh et al., 1993; De Bleecker et al., 1993). The clinical presentation of these three stages reflects the different pathophysiological mechanisms that underlie each stage of OP poisoning.

Depending on the particular OP compound present and the severity of the intoxication, the acute stage may resolve with or without treatment and the later stages may never develop.

Acute Cholinergic Crisis

The *acute cholinergic crisis* develops within hours of exposure to OPs and may last as long as 96 hours. The signs and symptoms are due to the inhibition of neural AChE and reflect excessive nicotinic (excitatory) and muscarinic (inhibitory) receptor stimulation by accumulating ACh (Wadia et al., 1974; Midtling et al., 1985; De Bleecker et al., 1993). Muscle fasciculations and weakness as well as tachycardia are common nicotinic effects of OP exposure, while miosis, lacrimation, and excessive salivation are symptoms of stimulation of muscarinic receptors. Commons effects of excessive OP-exposure-induced cholinergic stimulation in the CNS include altered visual acuity, lethargy, ataxia, seizures, and sometimes coma. Hyperthermia is also a common acute manifestation of OP poisoning in humans (Gordon, 1994). The following two cases are good examples of the acute cholinergic crisis.

An example of an acute cholinergic crisis is that of a 22-year-old woman who ingested 100 mL of parathion. She experienced acute cholinergic effects including lacrimation and excessive salivation, miosis, bradycardia, and hypotension before she became comatose (Yeh et al., 1993). The initial erythrocyte AChE and plasma cholinesterase activity levels in this patient were depressed but within the lab normal range at 26 μmol/L-sec and 20 μmol/L-sec, respectively (lab normals: erythrocyte AChE: 20 to 46 μmol/L-sec; plasma cholinesterase: 20 to 61 μmol/L-sec). She subsequently recovered from coma but went on to develop the intermediate syndrome and neuropathy associated with OP exposure (see below).

CNS symptoms persisted longer than did the acute muscarinic and nicotinic symptoms in a 22-year-old man who was found unconscious after he attempted suicide by ingesting approximately 80 mL of methamidophos; blurred vision was the last acute symptom to disappear in this patient (Senanayake and Johnson, 1982).

The Intermediate Syndrome

The *intermediate syndrome* follows the acute cholinergic crisis, develops within the first 24 to 96 hours after exposure, and persists for up to 6 weeks. The intermediate syndrome is characterized by muscle weakness predominantly affecting the proximal limbs and neck muscles (Wadia et al., 1987; De Bleecker, 1995) (Table 22-3). Muscle weakness involving the neck, shoulder, and hip muscles may become evident by the patient's failure to raise his or her head from the pillow, difficulty sitting up in bed, and/or difficulty abducting the arms. The clinical picture is similar to that of Eaton–Lambert syndrome, hyperkalemic peri-

TABLE 22-3. *Frequency of intermediate syndrome symptoms in 101 patients following exposure to organophosporus compounds*

Symptom	Frequency (%)
Inability to sit up	98
Inability to lift neck	86
Limb weakness (proximal more than distal)	85
Facial weakness	51
Areflexia	51
Slow eye movement	39
Respiratory paralysis	37
Death	33
Ophthalmoparesis	27
Swallowing difficulty	14

Data from Wadia et al., 1987.

odic paralysis, and myasthenia gravis (De Bleecker et al., 1992). Depressed tendon reflexes and flexor plantar responses can be seen. A physical examination restricted to testing the strength of distal muscle groups may fail to demonstrate the paresis involving the proximal muscles. Cranial nerve palsies and weakness of respiratory muscles are also common. Cranial nerve palsies are most apparent in external ocular, facial, and palatal muscles. Palatal and respiratory muscle weakness poses a great risk for aspiration and its complications. Weakness in respiratory muscles including the diaphragm may necessitate intubation and respiratory support. Death may occur in the most severe cases. Recovery is gradual, and complete recovery is expectable. A clinical report written before the concepts of an OP-induced intermediate syndrome and OPIDN were defined shows how the clinical picture of OP neurotoxicity could be diagnosed as Guillain–Barré syndrome (Fisher, 1977) (see Clinical Experiences section). Prolonged ACh stimulation at the neuromuscular junction is the main neurophysiological mechanism responsible for the intermediate syndrome. In more severe cases, the overstimulation of muscle fibers induced by exposures OPs may result in muscle fiber necrosis (Wadia et al., 1974; Dettbarn, 1984; Senanayake and Kalliedde, 1987; Yeh et al., 1993; De Bleecker, 1995). This pathological event may prolong the duration of the syndrome and slow recovery (Namba et al., 1971; Wadia et al., 1974, 1987; Senanayake and Karalliedde, 1987; Yeh et al., 1993; Shailesh et al., 1994) (see Neurophysiological Diagnosis and Neuropathological Diagnosis sections).

Organophosphate-Induced Delayed Neuropathy

As its name implies, *organophosphorus-induced delayed neuropathy* (OPIDN) is characterized by the onset of neuropathy that becomes apparent after a delay of 1 to 5 weeks after an acute exposure to sufficient doses of certain OP compounds. The clinical presentation of OPIDN was first recognized in the United States during prohibition when an estimated 50,000 persons consumed tainted "Jamaica Ginger." The batch of Jamaica Ginger responsible for the outbreak had been diluted with Lindol, a solvent containing the organophosphate compound tri-ortho-cresyl phosphate (TOCP). Shortly after consuming the TOCP-contaminated Jamaica Ginger the victims experienced acute nausea and diarrhea. A few weeks later they developed malaise, tingling sensations, and weakness beginning in the lower extremities and progressing to involve the upper extremities as well. The bilateral footdrop commonly seen was referred to as "Jake leg" palsy (Aring, 1942; Woolf, 1995).

Although this OP compound (i.e., TOCP) lacks anticholinesterase activity, the development of OPIDN following exposure to other OP compounds which do have anticholinesterase activity (e.g., mipafox, leptophos, and trichlorfon) stimulated extensive research to elucidate the biochemical mechanisms and the pathophysiology of this phenomenon. It appears to involve inhibition of neuropathy target esterase (NTE) but may also involve an intermediate metabolite, possibly an electrophilic alkylating agent, capable of disrupting axonal transport mechanisms and inducing a distal dying-back neuropathy (Abou-Donia, 1993; Jokanović et al, 1998) (see Neuropathological Diagnosis section).

The clinical features of OPIDN include flaccid paralysis of distal muscles (which affect the legs more than the arms with preservation of cranial nerves) and respiratory muscles, as well as cutaneous sensation. The distal neuropathy is contrasted with proximal myopathy seen in the intermediate syndrome. Initially the patients experience numbness, tingling, coldness, tenderness in legs, pricking sensation in the soles of the feet, and muscle pain that is worse while walking or exercising. Cramp-like sensations develop in the legs, which are then followed by the emergence of flaccid paralysis of the legs with weak dorsiflexion. In more severe cases, tenderness and weakness of thigh muscles, along with weakness and hypotonia in the upper extremities (forearm and hand), also appear about 1 week after the onset in the legs. Muscle atrophy in the affected hand muscles, along with wristdrop, may develop subsequently. If the intoxication is mild, the arms may never be affected.

Stocking and glove distribution paresthesias may develop; however, pain, temperature, and pressure sensation is usually preserved. Deep tendon reflexes become diminished to absent, whereas plantar reflexes remain flexor. In some patients with greater CNS involvement the decreased reflexes become increased and the plantar reflexes become extensor (see below). Recovery of function proceeds in the reverse order of the development of the above signs and symptoms. Thus, the earliest recovery begins in the hands and then occurs in the arms and thighs. Recovery is slow, requiring at least several months and often requiring several years; recovery may be incomplete, especially in the legs and the feet in the most severe cases

(Bidstrup et al., 1953; Vasilescu et al., 1984) (see Clinical Experiences section).

Signs and symptoms indicative of CNS pathology are also noted in patients with OPIDN (Aring, 1942). Morgan and Penovich (1978) described the neurological findings 47 years after the exposure and onset of OPIDN in four patients. Their flaccid weakness affecting the distal muscles of arms and legs was replaced by hypertonicity, spasticity, hyperreflexia, clonus, and extensor plantar responses, indicating an upper motor neuron syndrome and permanent damage to the spinal cord pathways in patients exposed to TOCP. One of the patients became paralyzed 8 days after ingesting Jamaica Ginger adulterated with TOCP. The paresis gradually improved over the next year to the point that he was able to walk while using two canes. At 47-year follow-up the patient, now 71 years old, was alert and oriented and his cranial nerve function was normal, but he could walk only with support. Walking was initiated from the hips, and footdrop was noted bilaterally. When standing, he hyperextended his knees for added support. Muscle strength was reduced and there was atrophy in the upper and lower extremities. No muscle fasciculations were observed. Spasticity and hyperactive deep tendon reflexes were noted in the lower extremities. Plantar responses were extensor (Babinski sign). No clonus was noted. Sensation to light touch and pinprick was normal, but vibratory and proprioceptive sense was slightly decreased in the toes bilaterally. Together these findings indicate damage to corticospinal tracts, posterior columns, and lower motor neurons, as well (see Neuropathological Diagnosis section).

Neurophysiological Diagnosis

Electroencephalograms (EEGs) can document acute spike waves associated with seizure activity induced by an overabundance of the excitatory neurotransmitter ACh following severe acute exposures to OP compounds (Metcalf and Holmes, 1969; Burchfiel et al., 1976; Hatta et al., 1996). In contrast, there was an increase in theta activity without an increase in spike activity on the EEGs in OP manufacturing workers who developed mild signs and symptoms of AChE inhibition (Metcalf and Holmes, 1969). A 23-year-old farm worker who had been periodically exposed to malathion for 4 years and who was admitted to the hospital following a fugue state also showed excessive slowing on his EEG. The patient appeared apathetic, was sweating excessively, and had blurred vision. His blood cholinesterase activity level was 60% of normal. He recovered clinically and 4 weeks later his EEG returned to normal, but the patient still complained of memory problems and sleep disturbances (Gershon and Shaw, 1961). EEGs in a group of 77 workers 1 year after exposure to sarin revealed persistently decreased alpha activity and increased delta, theta, and beta activity (Duffy et al., 1979). These workers had all experienced acute cholinergic symptoms immediately following exposure to sarin and had AChE activity levels that were depressed to less than 75% of baseline. The changes seen on the EEGs of these workers were not readily detected by visual inspection of the EEG record but required computer-derived spectral analysis to detect the abnormalities. In addition, an increased amount of rapid eye movement (REM) sleep was seen in these workers. These findings reflect persistent electroencephalographic and thus neurologic dysfunction in OP-exposed populations, which may also be related to neurobehavioral effects reported by others (Metcalf and Holmes, 1969; Duffy et al., 1979) (see Neuropsychological Diagnosis section).

Evoked potentials (EPs) can also be used to document central nervous effects of OP exposure (see Clinical Experiences section). Metcalf and Holmes (1969) noted lower amplitudes and longer peak-to-peak latencies in auditory and visual EPs in OP manufacturing workers who developed mild symptoms of AChE inhibition.

Nerve conduction studies (NCS) were normal in the popliteal and ulnar nerves of 66 patients who developed an intermediate syndrome with clinical features of severe weakness, following intentional ingestion of OP compounds (diazinon, malathion, fenthion, and sumithion). However, repetitive discharges were noted on the compound muscle action potential (CMAP) following a single fiber stimulation (Fig. 22-4). In addition, decrementing (i.e., a decrease in the amplitude of the CMAP with a train of stimuli) was noted on the CMAPs in two cases at 3 Hz, four cases at 10 Hz, and 18 cases at 30 Hz (Wadia et al., 1987) (Fig. 22-5). The decrement phenomenon is characteristic of more severe intoxication and correlates with the stage of clinical weakness (Besser et al., 1989). The presence of excess ACh in the synaptic cleft, due to AChE inhibition, is responsible for prolongation of ion channel open time. This condition induces repetitive discharges during initial stimulation, and it leads to the decrement phenome-

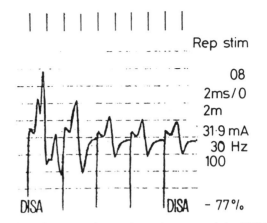

FIG. 22-5. Compound muscle action potentials (CMAPs) measured during organophosphorus intermediate syndrome showing decrementing at 30 Hz. The first two responses show a small repetitive response. (From Wadia et al., 1987, with permission.)

non seen during repetitive stimulation on CMAP studies (Besser and Gutmann, 1994).

In another study by Misra et al. (1988) the subclinical effects of OP exposure were assessed in a group of 24 workers (mean age: 31.7 years; range: 22 to 52) who were chronically and recurrently exposed to fenthion for mean durations of 8.5 years (range: 1 to 19 years) and who at the time of testing had depressed plasma cholinesterase activity levels but no clinical evidence of neuropathy. Nerve conduction studies in these workers showed significantly ($p < 0.01$) reduced motor conduction velocities and prolonged terminal motor latencies in the peroneal nerves. In addition, the F responses and H reflexes (late responses) in 12 of these workers were significantly prolonged compared to unexposed controls. Sensory conduction velocities, and distal latencies in the sural and median nerves were within normal ranges. CMAP studies showed repetitive discharges in 29% (7 of 24) of the exposed workers. A follow-up study was made 3 weeks after the end of the spraying season and showed improvement in motor conduction velocities, along with late responses. Furthermore, the repetitive activity seen on the CMAP studies was no longer present, indicating recovery of neuromuscular synapse function. These findings indicate the presence of subclinical neuropathy in workers chronically exposed to OP compounds, and they also indicate that nerve conduction studies can reveal effects of OP exposure before overt symptoms of neuropathy develop and possibly before irreversible damage to peripheral and CNS functioning occurs. In addition, these findings demonstrate reversible anticholinesterase effects of OP compounds on neuromuscular synapses as documented by the disappearance of repetitive discharges following removal from OP exposure.

Electromyograms (EMGs) can be used to document muscle fiber denervation and reinnervation associated with

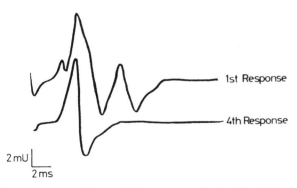

FIG. 22-4. Repetitive activity seen on single stimulation of compound muscle action potentials in organophosphorus poisoning. (From Wadia et al., 1987, with permission.)

OPIDN. However, the EMGs of patients with intermediate syndrome typically do not reveal any abnormalities. (Wadia et al., 1987). OPIDN with severe axonal degeneration leads to denervation and neurogenic muscle atrophy. Electromyographic studies at this stage of OP poisoning are consistent with denervation and show the characteristic findings of fibrillation, reduced amplitude of compound muscle action potentials, and reduced numbers of motor unit potentials on volitional contraction (interference pattern) and with regeneration polyphasic potentials (Senanayake, 1981; Vasilescu et al., 1984).

Neuropsychological Diagnosis

Acute and persistent neurobehavioral effects have been associated with OP intoxication. Agitation, irritability, insomnia, nervousness, forgetfulness, confusion and depression, hallucinations, psychoses, and combativeness are seen during the acute stage of the intoxication. Certain neurobehavioral problems including irritability, mood swings, anxiety, lethargy, difficulty in concentrating, impaired short-term memory function, and depression may persist indefinitely after acute intoxication (see Clinical Experiences section). Epidemiological studies have collectively revealed various neurobehavioral impairments involving attention and executive functioning, psychomotor skills, and memory (Gershon and Shaw, 1961; Metcalf and Holmes, 1969; Savage et al., 1988; Cole et al., 1997; Fiedler et al., 1997). Depression, anxiety, fatigue, and confusion are significantly more common among individuals with toxic exposure to OP compounds. These impairments have been detected up to years after cessation of exposure, suggesting permanent effects (Savage et al., 1988; Steenland et al., 1994).

The above findings are contrasted by those of Fiedler et al. (1997), who used neuropsychological testing to determine the effects of chronic OP exposure in farmers with no history of acute poisoning. The farmers were divided into high- and low-exposure groups based on the total number of acres treated per year and the total number of years of exposure. The workers from the high-exposure group showed significantly slower reaction times when compared to a group of unexposed controls. These findings suggest that chronic exposure to OP compounds without the occurrence of symptoms of acute poisoning produces only subtle changes in neuropsychological performance. It is questioned whether higher mortality rates among farm workers due to motor vehicle accidents, crop dusting aircraft accidents, farm machinery accidents, and workplace accidents is related to acute or chronic neurobehavioral impairments due to the effects of OP exposure (Quinby et al., 1958; OTA, 1990). However, caution must be raised about studies of groups that may consist of subjects that are heterogeneous with regard to age, extent of exposure, prior head injury, or other brain disorders.

Serial testing in well-documented individual cases, such as the following, often provide the most information about acute effects and follow-up status after exposure to OP compounds. While driving in his car with the windows down on a June day, a 44-year-old field inspector for the EPA was sprayed with liquid released from an overflying crop duster airplane (R. G. Feldman, personal observation). The solution was later determined to contain the OP, phosmet and two carbamates, benomyl and polyram. All three pesticides were in a solvent solution of kerosene and petroleum products. His car, clothing, and face were saturated with the pesticide. He had inhaled a large amount of the mist via nostrils and mouth. He immediately experienced a stinging sensation over his entire face and nasalpharynx and soon after became nauseous and drowsy. Nevertheless, he managed to drive himself to a nearby emergency room where he reported feeling nauseous and was sweating and salivating excessively. He also complained of blurred vision and generalized headache. Although he had severe abdominal cramps, he did not have diarrhea. He was interviewed, generally examined, and sent home, with instructions to shower thoroughly. No cholinesterase levels in blood or plasma were done. He went to bed feeling very weak and having photophobia. These symptoms lasted for several days, during which time he also could not sleep. He contacted his family physician who prescribed diazepam because he complained of a "racing feeling," mood changes, and irritability. Although he recovered from his acute symptoms, the patient began to have recurrent symptoms of blurred vision, dizziness, and difficulty concentrating and maintaining his attention on his work. He was examined by a neurologist who found no overt physical abnormalities. EEGs, brain-stem evoked potentials, nerve conduction studies, and results of magnetic resonance imaging were all normal. A brief neuropsychological assessment was performed 6 months after the exposure, at which time a normal performance was found on Digit Spans (attention and short-term memory), Benton Visual Retention (visual memory), Block Designs (visuospatial skills), the Purdue Pegboard (motor speed and coordination), and an executive function task. Despite the reassurance that he was cognitively "normal," the patient continued to experience difficulty with his activities of daily living because of his difficulty with ongoing discomfort.

A more detailed neuropsychological assessment was then performed by another examiner at 24 months after the exposure. At testing the patient's full-scale intelligence quotient (IQ) (Wechsler Adult Intelligence Scale-Revised) was 121; his verbal IQ (126) was significantly greater than his performance IQ (106). Deficits were noted in specific cognitive domains. For example, performance on several tests of attention and executive function including Trails B was impaired. His answers tended to be concrete, and he missed the Gestalt on tests of complex verbal reasoning. Visuomotor speed and incidental learning of associations on the Digit Symbol tests were both below expectation. Memory deficits were noted on delayed recall of both visual and verbal material; immediate recall was within expectation. The patient reported significant affective symptoms of depression, anger, fatigue, and attention problems on the Profile of Mood States (POMS).

A follow-up neuropsychological battery was done 13 months after the second neuropsychological battery (3 years and 4 months after the OP exposure incident). Overall improvement was noted on tests of executive function, visuomotor speed, and retrieval of information on delayed recall. However, he continued to show mild attention deficits and had difficulty with recall of verbal paired associates. His major problem on this testing continued to be difficulty with complex verbal reasoning tasks. The POMS revealed only irritability. It was concluded that the overall improvement in cognitive functioning seen in this patient with some residual impairments is consistent with recovery from acute toxic encephalopathy that could have resulted from OP exposure. Of interest in this case is that the patient went on to complete law school and his only residual complaints reported 10 years after the OP exposure were that he had occasionally experienced unexplained symptoms of nausea, blurred vision, and anxiety. Such an instance occurred when he became ill upon entering a local grocery store for a brief period of time and became nauseous and had blurred vision. He went home and contacted the store manager by telephone and inquired about the possibility that he might have been exposed to a chemical used in the store. The manager informed him that the store had been sprayed with an insecticide earlier that same day. In addition, he has recognized that he feels anxious and has nonspecific discomfort at those times when he can also detect aromatic substances in the air such as perfumes, petroleum products, or auto exhaust. He adjusted to his apparent chemical sensitivities by avoiding such circumstances as best as he could.

Biochemical Diagnosis

Biochemical diagnosis of exposure to OP compounds can be achieved directly by measuring levels of the parent compound and/or metabolites in blood, urine, and/or tissue samples (Lores et al., 1978; ACGIH, 1995). Indirect biochemical diagnosis is made by determining the amount of erythrocyte and plasma cholinesterase activity inhibition, which is a biological marker of OP toxicity. Plasma cholinesterase is a butyrylcholinesterase, whereas erythrocyte cholinesterase is acetylcholinesterase. Plasma cholinesterase is a nonspecific scavenger of anticholinesterases; thus, plasma cholinesterase activity levels are more sensitive to low level OP exposures, but erythrocyte AChE activity is considered to be a better indicator of neuronal AChE inhibition (Durham and Hayes, 1962; Midtling et al., 1985; Schwarz et al., 1995; Loewenstein-Lichtenstein et al., 1995; ACGIH, 1995). No signs or symptoms of neurotoxicity or changes in erythrocyte AChE activity were observed in six healthy male volunteers given a single oral dose of 0.5 mg/kg or a 5.0 mg/kg dermal dose of chlorpyrifos. Plasma cholinesterase activity

levels were depressed to 85% of predose levels by the 0.5 mg/kg oral dose but were essentially unchanged following the 5.0 mg/kg dermal dose (Nolan et al., 1984). The correlation between depression of plasma cholinesterase and erythrocyte cholinesterase activity is low, and the relationship between the degree of plasma cholinesterase inhibition and severity of symptoms is only of clinical value in the initial stages of acute poisoning (Nouira et al., 1994). Furthermore, although symptoms of poisoning typically begin to emerge when plasma cholinesterase activity is depressed to below 70% of normal, susceptible individuals (i.e., those with mutant butyrylcholinesterase) may experience symptoms at lower levels of exposure to OP compounds, indicating that close monitoring of workers' symptoms and erythrocyte AChE activity levels and not simply measurement of ambient air levels is important to worker health (Namba et al., 1971; Midtling et al., 1985; Schwarz et al., 1995; Loewenstein-Lichtenstein et al., 1995).

Cholinesterase activity levels gradually return to baseline following exposure to OP compounds. Thus, until cholinesterases have regenerated to normal levels, additional exposure to OP compounds can produce symptoms at lower concentrations. Erythrocyte AChE activity levels did not plateau until 66 days after exposure in 16 cauliflower workers poisoned with mevinphos and phosphamidon. This indicates that acute peak exposures during chronic low-level exposure can result in significant inhibition of neuronal AChE activity at OP levels that would not produce symptoms following a single acute exposure to OP compounds (Midtling et al., 1985). Although the anticholinesterase effects of carbamate pesticides are short-lived, they can enhance the effects of OP compounds and exacerbate symptoms in patients recovering from the effects of OP exposure (Jokanović et al, 1998).

Baseline plasma and erythrocyte AChE activity levels vary among individuals. Plasma cholinesterase activity levels have been shown to fluctuate with nutritional status, with pregnancy, and with exposure to opiates, cocaine, ether, chloroquine, thiamine, and xanthine compounds (e.g., tea, coffee, and chocolate) while multiple myeloma, leukemia, and quinine may decrease erythrocyte AChE activity (Vandekar et al., 1968; Howard et al., 1978; Ellenhorn and Barceloux, 1988). Therefore, when monitoring workers at risk for exposure, baseline cholinesterase activity levels should be ascertained (Midtling et al., 1985). Measurement of both plasma cholinesterase and erythrocyte AChE activity increases the accuracy and the effectiveness of OP exposure monitoring and the prevention of neurotoxic effects of exposure. The ACGIH has recommended that OP workers be removed from exposure when their erythrocyte AChE activity levels are at or below 70% of their predetermined individual baseline (ACGIH, 1995) (Table 22-4).

Exposure to a particular OP compound can be verified by analyzing the metabolites in the urine samples (Namba et al., 1971; Lores et al., 1978; ACGIH, 1995). Excretion of the OP metabolites occur at a faster rate compared to re-

TABLE 22-4. *Biological exposure indices for organophosphorus compounds*

	Urine	Blood	Alveolar air
Determinant:	Free and conjugated alcohol derivatives[a]	Erythrocyte cholinesterase	Not established
Start of shift:	Not established	70% of individual's baseline	Not established
During shift:	Not established	70% of individual's baseline	Not established
End of work shift:	Not established	70% of individual's baseline	Not established

[a]See text and Figure 22-3.
Data from ACGIH, 1995.

activation of the AChE. Therefore, although analysis of blood or urine samples for the compound or its metabolites are sensitive for detecting very recent exposures and identifying specific OPs, measurement of erythrocyte AChE is more telling about the accumulated physiological outcome of prolonged, repeated exposures during preceding month(s) (Arterberry et al., 1961; Roan et al., 1969; Lores et al., 1978). Nevertheless, the ACGIH has recommended that the end of shift urine concentration of *p*-nitrophenol (free and conjugated) in parathion-exposed workers not exceed 0.5 mg/g creatinine (ACGIH, 1995) (see Fig. 22-3 and Table 22-4).

Neuroimaging

Neuroimaging studies including magnetic resonance imaging (MRI) and computed tomography (CT) scans have been used in the differential diagnosis of OP poisoning. The initial CT scan in a 3-year-old boy who was accidentally exposed to Dursban (chlorpyrifos) did not reveal any abnormalities (Aiuto et al., 1993). This child subsequently developed OPIDN, but a follow-up CT scan was not performed. The brain MRI was normal in a 44-year-old who developed acute encephalopathy after he was sprayed with phosmet by an overflying crop duster airplane (R. G. Feldman; personal observation) (see Neuropsychological Diagnosis section). The brain MRI and CT of a 35-year-old man acutely exposed to sarin were also normal (Hatta et al., 1996). These findings indicate that gross morphological changes do not occur after acute exposures to OPs. They also indicate that neuroimaging studies can be used to differentiate OP poisonings from acute exposure to other neurotoxins that can induce coma and suppression of respiratory function, such as triethyltin, as well as from other etiologies of these symptoms, such as viral encephalopathies and aseptic meningitis (see Chapter 9).

Neuropathological Diagnosis

Muscle fiber necrosis has been reported in humans and laboratory animals exposed to OP compounds (Ariens et al., 1969; Namba et al., 1971; Wecker et al., 1978; Ahlgren et al., 1979; Yeh et al., 1993; De Bleecker et al., 1994; De Bleecker, 1995). Excessive calcium influx due to cholinergic overstimulation of the postsynaptic membrane has been

proposed as a mechanism for the development of necrosis (Antunes-Madeira and Madeira, 1982; Dettbarn, 1984; De Bleecker et al., 1994). Studies in laboratory animals show marked necrosis in the diaphragm, whereas clinical experience with humans indicates that death following OP exposure results in part from weakness of respiratory muscles (Wecker and Dettbarn, 1976).

Most muscle necrosis occurs during the first 48 hours and is clinically accompanied by myalgia and weakness. Since degeneration of muscle fibers precedes the development of neuropathy in OP-poisoned patients it is not neurogenic. Several authors have concluded that myolysis underlies features of the intermediate syndrome of OP exposure (Senanayake and Karalliedde, 1987; De Wilde et al., 1991; Yeh et al., 1993).

Several OP compounds can induce peripheral–central neuropathy after the clinical signs and symptoms of AChE inhibition have subsided. The neuropathological mechanisms of OPIDN have been studied in humans and in experimental animal models. The distal-most segment of the longest and largest myelinated nerve fibers degenerates first, following which the axon dies back to the perikaryon. This process of distal to proximal axonal degeneration has been referred to as a "distal dying-back neuropathy" (Cavanagh, 1954; Prineas, 1969; Bouldin and Cavanagh, 1979a, 1979b). The sural nerve biopsy in a 22-year-old man who ingested approximately 20 g of Dipterex (trichlorfon) showed a decrease in the number of large myelinated fibers and numerous axons with thin myelin sheaths on light microscopy. Teased fibers showed demyelination and evidence of regeneration. Electron microscopy revealed proliferation of Schwann cells (bands of Büngner) (Vasilescu et al., 1984). These findings are consistent with ongoing degeneration and regeneration of myelinated fibers. Light microscopy studies of a gastrocnemius muscle biopsy in this patient showed evidence of neurogenic atrophy (isolated angular fibers). Electron microscopic studies of the muscle biopsy showed areas of myofibril disorganization and myofibril destruction.

The initial pathological feature visible on teased fiber preparations from the left recurrent laryngeal nerve of the cat are intraaxonal and intramyelin vacuoles. As the neuropathy progresses, the affected axons show paranodal swelling with secondary demyelination. The segment of the axon distal to the area of focal swelling subsequently degenerates (Cavanagh, 1954; Prineas, 1969; Bouldin and Cavanagh, 1979a, 1979b). Neuropathological changes are also seen in the CNS of animals experimentally exposed to OP compounds and are analogous to those seen in the peripheral nerves. Neuropathological studies in cats administered a single intraperitoneal injection of diisopropylfluorophosphate (DFP) revealed degeneration in (a) the distal ends of myelinated long fibers of ascending dorsal columns and spinocerebellar tracts and (b) the distal ends of the descending corticospinal and tectospinal tracts in the gray matter (Cavanagh and Patangia, 1965; Bouldin and Cavanagh, 1979a, 1979b).

Experimental studies in animals have revealed within species variation with regards to susceptibility to OPIDN; younger animals are more resistant to OPIDN. Intraspecies variation in susceptibility to OPIDN has also been noted; hens, cows, lambs, water buffalos, and cats are more susceptible to OPIDN than are rats, mice, guinea pigs, hamsters, gerbils, and rabbits (Abou-Donia, 1981).

Several OP compounds have been identified which can induce OPIDN without inhibiting AChE or butyrylcholinesterase activity (Aldridge et al., 1961). Furthermore, clinical and experimental observations indicate that preventing or reactivating AChE inhibition does not protect against OPIDN, and the clinical course of acute OP intoxication resulting from AChE inhibition does not relate to the occurrence or course of OPIDN (Aldridge et al., 1961; Cavanagh, 1964, 1973; Aldridge and Barnes, 1966). These observations have led to the conclusion that a mechanism other than AChE inhibition probably is involved in the pathogenesis of OPIDN (Aldridge et al., 1969; Johnson, 1969). Two such notions are the neuropathy target esterase hypothesis and the phosphorylation of cytoskeletal proteins.

The NTE Hypothesis

A relation between those OP compounds that induce neuropathy and also react with a specific esterase known as "neuropathy target esterase" (NTE) has led to the suggestion that NTE may be involved in the development of delayed onset neuropathy (i.e., OPIDN) (Aldridge and Barnes, 1969; Johnson, 1969; Jokanović et al, 1998). The degree of inhibition (i.e., phosphorylation) of NTE was found to correlate with the severity of the neuropathy; compounds that do not inhibit NTE also do not induce OPIDN (Olajos and Rosenblum, 1979; Janović et al., 1998). It has also been postulated that OP compounds that undergo aging, such as phosphates, phosphonates, and phospramidates, are capable of permanently inhibiting NTE and, thus, inducing OPIDN (Johnson, 1974). In support of this, it was noted that OPIDN was prevented when compounds that do not irreversibly inhibit NTE (e.g., phenyl phenylcarbamate) were given prior to administration of compounds that do (Johnson and Lauwerys, 1969). Although the exact mechanism of how the inhibition of NTE leads to OPIDN is not known, the degree and dura-

tion of NTE inhibition appears to be related to the development of OPIDN (Jokanović et al, 1998). For example, several compounds that irreversibly inhibit NTE do not cause neuropathy, while repeated administration of reversible NTE inhibitors such as phenyl N-methyl N-benzyl carbamate (PMBC) or phenylmethanesulfonyl fluoride (PMSF) causes OPIDN in the hen, when brain NTE is inhibited to 95%. Both tri-2-ethyl-phenyl phosphate and diphenyl 2-isopropyl-phenyl phosphate induce OPIDN only when NTE inhibition approaches 90%. Mipafox and methamidophos caused OPIDN when they irreversibly inhibited NTE by 80% and 90%, respectively. Lesser inhibition does not cause OPIDN, despite the occurrence of aging. In addition, it was shown that exposure to aging inhibitors such as dichlorvos, methamidophos, DFP, and PMBC, in doses not initially sufficient to cause clinically overt signs of OPIDN, could be promoted to induce OPIDN by subsequent administration of PMSF. This was called the "promotion phenomenon" (Lotti et al., 1993). Three conclusions can be drawn from these findings that "aging" is not necessary for OPIDN to occur based on the following data: (a) Certain OP compounds that do undergo aging do not cause OPIDN; (b) compounds that do not undergo aging (e.g., the carbamates) can cause OPIDN if given in certain mode and dosage; and (c) compounds that are known to cause OPIDN will do so only after a certain percentage of NTE is permanently inhibited. Thus, these findings collectively indicate that it is the "degree" to which NTE is inhibited that is the marker of OPIDN neurotoxicity (see Chapter 23).

Phosphorylation of Cytoskeletal Proteins

Impairment of axonal transport due to abnormal phosphorylation of cytoskeletal proteins has been noted in the pathogenesis OPIDN. Experimental studies by Abou-Donia (1993) revealed that TOCP increases the calcium/calmodulin kinase II–dependent phosphorylation of cytoskeletal proteins including α- and β-tubulin, neurofilaments, and microtubule-associated protein-2 (MAP-2). Hyperphosphorylation of the cytoskeletal proteins causes a decrease in their axonal transport rate, resulting in accumulation of the hyperphosphorylated cytoskeletal proteins and axonal swelling with secondary demyelination associated with OP exposure (Abou-Donia, 1993).

PREVENTIVE AND THERAPEUTIC MEASURES

All workers involved in the handling and application of OP products should be instructed about basic safety measures required regarding pesticides. Posters informing about the pesticide safety issues should be posted at locations throughout the work areas. All workers should have access to the materials data sheets as well as the information on the labeling of the product they are exposed to and should be aware of the associated hazards. OP products should only be handled and applied by properly trained personnel. All workers handling and applying OP products must wear the protective equipment indicated on the package label. Only properly equipped workers and bystanders should be in the area where formulations are mixed and where pesticides are being applied. Care must be taken to prevent drifting of the OP pesticide from the site of application to avoid contact with any other persons. To prevent inadvertent exposures, employers are required to inform all workers about the sites where pesticides have been applied. All workers who may come close to a treated area must be notified, either verbally or by posting warning signs in the area, about pesticide application and the duration of the REI. Persons entering an area treated with OP compounds before the completion of the REI must wear the appropriate protective equipment. Workers should wash and change clothing immediately after they have finished handling an OP compound or entered a treated area before the end of the REI. The employer should monitor any worker who is handling or who may be remotely affected by a pesticide carrying a label with a skull and crossbones symbol on it. The name and location of the nearest emergency medical facility should be posted, and the employer should provide the medical personnel treating an exposed worker with information about the pesticide(s) to which the worker has been exposed.

Effective recognition of an exposed patient is extremely important. Removal from exposure and thorough cleansing and emergency medical care must be provided. Decontamination can significantly shorten the course and reduce the severity of the intoxication by preventing undue continued absorption. If the patient has been splashed with an OP compound, his or her clothing should be removed immediately and the skin thoroughly washed with copious amounts of soap and water. The scalp hair should also be washed. Eyes should be rinsed with normal saline solution. If the patient has ingested an OP compound and has not vomited, gastric lavage should be performed to remove the toxicant from the stomach and to reduce the risk of aspiration of vomitus. Cathartics are also affective in removing part of the ingested toxicant. The importance of maintaining an adequate airway can never be overstated; when necessary, the patient should be intubated. Suctioning of excessive oral secretions may also be necessary. Hemodialysis can prevent renal failure.

OP intoxication is a medical emergency with a risk of death due to paralysis of respiratory muscles. The early recognition of OP intoxication, be it accidental or suicidal, is of paramount importance. The management is largely symptomatic and it should be delivered expectantly regarding the possible life-threatening complications. Patients at high risk for life-threatening complications of intoxication should be transferred to intensive care units for therapy and monitoring. Pulmonary aspiration and hypoventilation are prominent causes of morbidity and mortality. The adequacy of upper airways should be secured, and excessive upper airways secretions and/or vomitus should be suc-

tioned. Patients with impaired consciousness require endotracheal intubation and mechanical ventilation to prevent aspiration and provide sufficient ventilation and oxygenation. Conscious patients should be observed closely for gradual or sudden deterioration in condition, which would require aggressive life support measures. Hypoventilation of central and/or peripheral origin may also develop. Therefore, breathing rate, blood gases, maximal inspiratory pressure, and vital capacity should be checked regularly. Patients may require mechanical ventilation from a few days to more than a month. Excess of cholinergic stimulation may lead to bradycardia and other cardiac arrhythmias. Therefore, continuous cardiovascular monitoring or checking electrocardiogram and blood pressure at regular intervals is necessary. Similarly, cerebral dysrhythmias and convulsions may occur.

Atropine sulfate (atropine) is still the medication of choice in the management of excessive cholinergic stimulation resulting from OP and/or carbamate intoxication. Patients with OP poisoning are more tolerant to atropine sulfate than are those exposed to carbamates; therefore larger doses may be required to obtain a therapeutic result. Atropine counteracts the muscarinic effects of excessive cholinergic stimulation, leading to a decrease in bronchial secretions, salivation, lacrimation, and sweating. Gastric secretion and motility is also inhibited by atropine, which further contributes to preventing pulmonary aspiration. Bradycardia may also be alleviated. Bladder and bowel emptying may be delayed. The mechanism of epileptogenesis following OP poisoning is cholinergic; thus, seizures do not respond to anti-epileptic medications such as phenytoin, diazepam, or barbiturates. Atropine in adequate dosages must be used to stop convulsions in OP-intoxicated patients. Scopolamine has been shown to be even more effective than atropine (Capacio and Shih, 1991). While it prevents many of the acute effects of muscarinic overstimulation, atropine does not reactivate cholinesterases and thus is ineffective on nicotinic receptors at the neuromuscular junction; atropine does not reverse the muscle weakness or twitching associated with OP exposure (Ellenhorn and Barceloux, 1988).

Atropine should be administered every 15 minutes in small incremented subcutaneous doses of 0.5 to 1.0 mg until signs of sufficient atropinization including dilation of pupils, flushing of the face, dryness of mucous membranes, and disappearance of sweating are noted. The effects of intravenous atropine become apparent within minutes. Atropine can be given at a dose of up to 2 mg by intravenous injection every hour over a 4- to 5-day period to suppress upper respiratory secretions (Besser and Gutmann, 1994). Intravenous administration at regular intervals has been shown to be more effective than continuous drip (Ye et al., 1990). If the patient has been atropinized for several days, the medication should be tapered down rather than being discontinued abruptly. Increasing the successive dosage intervals and watching for the recurring signs and symptoms such as excessive salivation and lacrimation, miosis, and respiratory impairment may help titrate and/or taper doses of atropine on an individual basis. Patients exposed via inhalation may need only 12 to 24 hours of full atropinization; however, those patients who have ingested OP compounds (e.g., in a suicide attempt) may require several days of full atropinization due to continued absorption of residual OP compounds that can remain in the gastrointestinal tract even after gastric lavage (Futagami et al., 1995).

The administration of oximes is strongly recommended in the treatment of OP poisoning. The primary mechanism of oxine chemotherapy is reactivation of the AChE enzyme by facilitating removal of the OP compound attached to the enzyme. However, the reactivation of AChE by oximes can only occur before the compound loses its leaving group (i.e., aging phenomenon). Therefore, oximes are most effective when given as soon as possible after OP toxic exposure. Administration via continuous infusion rather than by intermittent intravenous bolus may prevent relapse during the first few days following poisoning. An important property of oximes is their ability to reactivate the enzyme at the neuromuscular junction and autonomic ganglia. Therefore, timely administration of oximes helps to alleviate weakness in respiratory muscles. The use of adequate oxime therapy may prevent the occurrence of the intermediate syndrome (Benson and Tolo, 1992). At high doses, oximes can inhibit AChE and thus cholinergic symptoms may develop if they are administered too rapidly and/or at too high a dose (Ellenhorn and Barceloux, 1988; Thiermann et al., 1997).

CLINICAL EXPERIENCES

Group Studies

Ignorance of Restricted Entry Interval (REI) Results in OP Poisoning Among Cauliflower Workers

Twenty-three cauliflower farm workers began tying leaves over the heads of the cauliflower plants 6 hours after the plants had been sprayed with mevinphos and phosphamidon; the state reentry interval for these two compounds was 72 hours (Midtling et al., 1985). Shortly after beginning the task of tying back the leaves, many of the workers began to experience shortness of breath, eye irritation, and blurred vision. Despite these initial symptoms of OP exposure, they continued to work; and over the course of the next 2 hours, all the workers began to experience dizziness, headache, disorientation, abdominal cramps, and nausea and vomiting. Several workers also experienced cramps in their arms and legs. One worker lost consciousness (patient 1) and another collapsed without losing consciousness (patient 2).

The two collapsed workers were transported to a nearby hospital by another worker (patient 3) who was less severely affected by the exposure. On admission the two most affected workers were bradycardic, salivated exces-

sively, and had muscle fasciculations and miosis. Plasma cholinesterase activity levels were significantly depressed in patients 1 and 2, respectively, at 2.4 and 3.04 IU per liter (laboratory normal range: 8 to 18 IU per liter). The driver (patient 3) had a plasma cholinesterase of 6.06 IU per liter. All three individuals were treated with atropine; in addition, patient 1 also received pralidoxime. Fourteen other cauliflower workers subsequently sought medical attention over the next 24 hours. Of these, three were admitted to the hospital, including one who collapsed at his home the next day, while the 11 other patients were given pralidoxime (2 g) and released. The remaining six workers, who did not actively seek medical attention, were examined in response to the outbreak during the following week.

Sixteen of the exposed cauliflower workers ranging in age from 9 to 72 years old were followed with weekly examinations until symptoms had disappeared and erythrocyte AChE activity levels had returned to normal. The acute symptoms reported most frequently in these workers included dizziness, abdominal pain, nausea and vomiting, and ataxia. These aforementioned symptoms disappeared in all workers by 28 days after exposure. However, more persistent symptoms were reported at follow-up 6 months after exposure and included headache, blurred vision, weakness, and anorexia.

The findings reported in this study demonstrate the risks associated with entering an OP-treated area before the reentry interval has expired and indicate that symptoms can persist for at least 6 months following acute exposure to OPs.

Peripheral Neuropathy and Impaired Short-Term Memory in a Family Exposed to Chlorpyrifos

All four members of a family became acutely ill with headaches, nausea, and muscle cramps immediately after an exterminator sprayed their home with chlorpyrifos (Kaplan et al., 1993). The acute symptoms resolved within days, but over the course of the next month all four persons developed paresthesias and numbness in their lower extremities. In addition, they all noted forgetfulness, and the academic performance of the children, ages 14 and 15 years old, declined. They became concerned and hired investigators who found chlorpyrifos levels of 66 ppm in samples taken from the kitchen of the house.

Neurological examinations of all four patients made 6 months after the onset of their symptoms were unremarkable except for mild short-term memory loss noted on clinical mental status tests. Formal neuropsychological testing was not performed, and the MRI in each case was normal. Nerve conduction studies revealed subclinical sensory neuropathy in the lower extremities of all four patients.

Follow-up clinical examinations made 6 months after the end of exposure revealed marked cognitive and neurophysiological improvements in all but one patient who continued to show subclinical evidence of sensory neuropathy on nerve conduction studies made in the lower extremities.

Terrorist Attack on an Urban Population

Yokoyama and colleagues have reported on the acute and persistent clinical and subclinical effects of sarin after the Tokyo subway attack (Murata et al., 1997; Yokoyama et al., 1996; 1998). Initial examination of 213 patients (139 males and 74 females) revealed acute symptoms including coughing, nasal discharge, pupillary constriction, loss of consciousness, and respiratory failure. Pupillary constriction was seen in 89% of patients and was the most common acute cholinergic symptom (Yokoyama et al., 1996).

Neurophysiological studies were made 6 months after the attack in 18 asymptomatic victims (Murata et al., 1997). Tests included event-related and visual evoked potentials (P-300 and VEPs), brain-stem auditory evoked potentials (BAEPs), and electrocardiographic R-R interval variability (CVRR). In addition, the victims were administered a post-traumatic stress disorder (PTSD) check list. The victims were compared with unexposed control subjects matched for age and sex. P-300 and VEP latencies were significantly prolonged in the sarin-exposed group. The CVRR was significantly related to the acute cholinesterase inhibition levels determined immediately after exposure. PTSD scores were elevated but were not significantly related to any neurophysiological data. These finding indicate that sublinical CNS effects of sarin can persist up to 6 months after exposure has ended and may be permanent.

Posturography performed 6 to 8 months after poisoning documented significant postural stability differences between 18 (nine male and nine female) of the exposed patients and a group of unexposed controls (Yokoyama et al., 1998). Postural sway was related to the acute cholinesterase inhibition levels determined in these patients immediately after their exposure to sarin. In addition, the impairment of postural stability was more marked among the female patients. These findings suggest that persistent vestibulocerebellar dysfunction occurs subsequent to acute sarin poisoning and that women may be more sensitive than men to the effects of sarin.

Individual Case Studies

Acute Cholinergic Crisis Followed by OPIDN

A 22-year-old man was found unconscious a few hours after he ingested approximately 80 mL of Tamaron (methamidophos) (Senanayake and Johnson, 1982). Examination on admission to the hospital found the patient unresponsive and sweating profusely, with miosis and muscle fasciculations. He was given atropine (270 mg/24 hours), furosemide, and penicillin. After 24 hours of unconsciousness, with supportive care he rapidly recovered. He was discharged 5 days after admission with no symptoms other than blurred vision which disappeared 3 days later.

Ten days after discharge and approximately 15 days after he ingested the Tamaron, the patient began to experience muscle pain and paresthesias in his lower extremities. These

symptoms of neuropathy progressed over the following month and included weakness, first in the lower extremities and then in the upper extremities. The patient was readmitted to the hospital, where a routine neurological examination revealed bilateral footdrop with marked weakness of the dorsiflexors and evertors of the feet. Muscle strength in the knee and hip flexors was slightly reduced. In addition, the tone of the more proximal lower-extremity muscles was slightly increased and deep tendon reflexes were hyperactive except for the ankle jerks, which were absent. Plantar responses were flexor. Sensory examination was normal. Cerebrospinal fluid opening pressure was within normal range, as were cell, protein, and glucose levels. Results of routine laboratory tests were unremarkable. Electromyography documented denervation of muscle fibers indicating peripheral neuropathy. The patient was treated supportively and symptomatically with physical therapy and was considered well enough to be released 1 month later.

This case report demonstrates the typical clinical course of OPIDN which is preceded by an acute OP-induced cholinergic crisis, followed by a symptom-free period and then the development of peripheral neuropathy. In addition, this patient showed signs of disinhibition of reflexes and increased muscle tone indicative of CNS involvement.

Guillain–Barré Syndrome or OP Poisoning?

A 28-year-old man was mixing cotton defoliant (merphos) when he accidentally became splashed with a moderate amount of the undiluted OP compound (Fisher, 1977). His bare arms and tee shirt were saturated with the solution. He continued to wear the soaked shirt and he did not wash off the liquid from his exposed skin. He carelessly repeated the procedure on the next 2 days and again had significant amounts of dermal exposure. Approximately 4 days after the initial exposure he noted weakness in his upper extremities. However, he did not seek medical attention until 2 days later, at which time he presented with profound weakness in his upper and lower extremities, but without signs of an acute cholinergic crisis. He was alert and well-oriented but was unable to stand unassisted. His pupils reacted normally, his deep tendon reflexes were absent, and his cranial nerves were normal.

Based on the patient's history and symptoms indicating OP exposure, he was administered atropine and pralidoxime. Nevertheless, he developed shallow, rapid breathing. By 14 days after the initial exposure he had complete facial diplegia. A lumbar puncture revealed normal opening pressure, elevated protein (150 mg/dL), 4 lymphocytes/mm^3, and normal glucose. Neurophysiological studies showed denervation potentials, decreased voltage of muscle action potentials, and delayed motor conduction velocities. The patient's motor function gradually improved and he was discharged at 6 weeks after the initial exposure to merphos, at which time he had residual facial weakness but could grasp objects and walk with a walker. At follow-up 14 weeks after discharge he showed complete clinical recovery.

It is reasonable, with the history of exposure provided by this patient, despite the absence of symptoms of a cholinergic crisis, that presumptive anticholinergic therapy along with oxime treatment was given. The absence of acute cholinergic symptoms in this patient also suggests other etiologies of peripheral motor dysfunction, and the differential diagnosis should include Guillain–Barré syndrome, acute inflammatory demyelinating polyneuropathy, or hyperkalemic periodic paralysis. Although this patient did not report previous symptoms of an acute cholinergic crisis, the clinical, laboratory, and neurophysiological findings are consistent with the OP-induced intermediate syndrome followed by development of OPIDN and indicate that exposure to merphos was responsible for his clinical manifestations.

REFERENCES

Abou-Donia MB. Organophosphorus ester-induced delayed neurotoxicity. *Ann Rev Pharmacol Toxicol* 1981;21:511–548.

Abou-Donia M. The cytoskeleton as a target for organophosphorus ester-induced delayed neurotoxicity (OPIDN). *Chem-Biol Interact* 1993;87:383–393.

Ahlgren JD, Manz HJ, Harvey JC. Myopathy of chronic organophosphate poisoning: a clinical entity? *South Med J* 1979;72(5):555–558.

Aiuto LA, Pavlakis SG, Boxer RA. Life-threatening organophosphate-induced delayed polyneuropathy in a child after accidental chlorpyrifos ingestion. *J Pediatr* 1993;122:658–660.

Aldridge WN, Barnes JM. Further observations on the neurotoxicity of some organophosphorus compounds. *Biochem Pharmacol* 1966;15:549.

Aldridge WN, Barnes JM. Studies on delayed neurotoxicity produced by some organophosphorus compounds. *Ann NY Acad Sci* 1969;160:314–322.

Aldridge WN, Barnes JM, Johnson MK. Neurotoxic and biochemical properties of some triaryl phosphates. *Biochem Pharmacol* 1961;6:177.

American Conference of Governmental Industrial Hygienists (ACGIH). Threshold Limit Values (TLVs) for chemical substances and physical agents and Biological Exposure Indices (BEIs). Cincinnati: ACGIH, 1995.

Ames RG, Steenland K, Jenkins B, et al. Chronic neurologic sequelae to cholinesterase inhibition among agricultural pesticide applicators. *Arch Environ Health* 1995;50:440–444.

Antunes-Madeira MC, Madeira VMC. Interaction of insecticides with the calcium-pump activity of sarcoplasmic reticulum. *Pest Biochem* 1982;17:185–190.

Ariens AT, Meeter E, Wolthuis OL, Van Benthem RMJ. Reversible necrosis at the end plate region in striated muscles of the rat poisoned by cholinesterase inhibitors. *Experientia* 1969;25:57–59.

Aring CD. The systemic nervous affinity of triothocresyl phosphate (Jamaica ginger palsy). *Brain* 1942;65:34–47.

Arterberry JD, Durham WF, Elliot JW, Wolfe HR. Exposure to parathion: Measurement by blood cholinesterase level and urinary *p*-nitrophenol excretion. *Arch Environ Health* 1961;13:476–485.

Barnes JM. Letter. *Lancet* 1961;2:102–103.

Benson B, Tolo D. Is the intermediate syndrome in organophosphate poisoning the result of insufficient oxime therapy? *Clin Toxicol* 1992;30:347–349.

Bentur Y, Nutenko I, Tsipiniuk A, et al. Pharmacokinetics of obidoxime in organophosphate poisoning associated with renal failure. *Clin Toxicol* 1993;31:315–322.

Berends F, Posthumus CH, Sluys IVD, Deierkauf FA. The chemical basis of the "aging process of DFP-inhibited pseudocholinesterase. *Biochim Biophys Acta* 1959;34:576–578.

Besser R, Gutmann L, Dillmann U, Weilemann LS, Hopf HC. End-plate dysfunction in acute organophosphate intoxication. *Neurology* 1989;39:561–567.

Besser R, Gutmann L. Intoxication with organophosphorus compounds. In: de Wolff, ed. *Handbook of clinical neurology, intoxications of the nervous system,* vol 20, part 1. Amsterdam: Elsevier, 1994:151–181.

Betrosian A, Balla M, Kafiri G, et al: Multiple systems organ failure from organophosphate poisoning. *Clin Toxicol* 1995;33:257–260.

Bidstrup PL, Bonnell JA, Beckett AG. Paralysis following poisoning by a new organic phosphorus insecticide (Mipafox). *Br Med J* 1953;1:1068.

Bouldin TW, Cavanagh JB. Organophosphorus neuropathy. I. A teased-fiber study of the spatio-temporal spread of axonal degeneration. *Am J Pathol* 1979a;94:241–252.

Bouldin TW, Cavanagh JB. Organophosphorus neuropathy. II. A fine-structural study of the early stages of axonal degeneration. *Am J Pathol* 1979b;94:253–270.

Bowman JS, Casida JE: Further studies on the metabolism of Thimet by plants, insects and mammals. *J Econ Entomol* 1958;51:838.

Brown LM, Blair A, Gibson R, et al. Pesticide exposures and other environmental risk factors for leukemia among men in Iowa and Minnesota. *Cancer Res* 1990;50:6585–6591.

Bull DA. Metabolism of Disyston by insects, isolated cotton leaves and rats. *J Econ Entomol* 1965;58:249.

Burchfiel JL, Duffy FH, Sim VM. Persistent effect of sarin and dieldrin upon the primate electroencephalogram. *Toxicol Appl Pharmacol* 1976;35:365–379.

Butler AM, Murray M. Biotransformation of parathion in human liver: participation of CYP3A4 and its inactivation during microsomal parathion oxidation. *J Pharmacol Exp Ther* 1997;280:966–973.

Capacio BR, Shih TM. Anticonvulsant actions of anticholinergic drugs in soman poisoning. *Epilepsia* 1991;32:604–615.

Cavanagh JB. The toxic effects of tri-ortho-cresyl phosphate on the nervous system. *J Neurol Neurosurg Psychiatry* 1954;17:163–172.

Cavanagh JB. The significance of the "dying-back" process in experimental and human neurological disease. *Int Rev Exp Biol* 1964;3:219–267.

Cavanagh JB. Peripheral neuropathy caused by chemical agents. *CRC Crit Rev Toxicol* 1973;2:365.

Cavanagh JB, Patangia GN. Changes in the central nervous system in the cat as the result of tri-ortho-cresyl phosphate poisoning. *Brain* 1965;88:165.

Chang SK, Williams PL, Dauterman WC, Riviere JE. Percutaneous absorption, dermatopharmacokinetics and related bio-transformation studies of carbaryl, lindane, malathion, parathion in isolated perfused porcine skin. *Toxicology* 1994;91:269–280.

Cole DC, Crapio F, Julian J, et al. Neurobehavioral outcomes among farm and nonfarm rural Ecuadorians. *Neurotoxicol Teratol* 1997;19:277–286.

Cooper JR, Bloom FE, Robert HR. Acetylcholine. In: Cooper JR, ed. *The biochemical basis of neuropharmacology.* London: Oxford University Press, 1996:194–225.

Coye MJ. The health effects of agricultural production. I. The health of agricultural workers. *J Public Health Policy* 1985;6:349–370.

Davies DR, Green AL. The kinetics of reactivation by oximes of cholinesterase inhibited by organophosphorus compounds. *Biochem J* 1956;63:529–535.

De Bleecker J. The intermediate syndrome in organophosphate poisoning: an overview of experimental and clinical observations. *Clin Toxicol* 1995;33:683–686.

De Bleecker J, Willems J, Van Den Neucker K, et al. Prolonged toxicity with intermediate syndrome after combined parathion and methyl parathion poisoning. *Clin Toxicol* 1992;30:333–345.

De Bleecker J, Van Den Neucker K, Colardyn F. Intermediate syndrome in organophosphorus poisoning: A prospective study. *Crit Care Med* 1993;21:1706–1711.

De Bleecker J, Lison D, Van Den Abeele K, et al. Acute and subacute organophosphate poisoning in the rat. *Neurotoxicology* 1994;15:341–348.

De Wilde V, Vogelaers D, Colardyn F, et al. Postsynaptic neuromuscular dysfunction in organophosphate induced intermediate syndrome. *Klin Wochen* 1991;69:177–183.

Deer HM, Beck ED, Roe AH. Respiratory exposure of museum personnel to dichlorvos insecticide. *Vet Hum Toxicol* 1993;35:226–228.

Della Morte R, Villani GR, Di Martino E, et al. Glutathione depletion induced in rat liver fractions by seven pesticides. *Boll Soc Ital Biol Sper* 1994;70:185–192.

Department of Health and Human Services, United States (DHHS). *1978 Migrant health program target population estimates.* Rockville, MD: Health Services Administration, Bureau of Community Health Services, April 1980.

Dettbarn WD. Pesticide induced muscle necrosis: mechanisms and prevention. *Fundam Appl Toxicol* 1984;4:18–26.

Duffy FH, Burchfiel JL, Bartels PH, Gaon M, Sim VM. Long-term effects of an organophosphate upon the human electroencephalogram. *Toxicol Appl Pharmacol* 1979;47:161–176.

Durham WF, Hayes WJ. Organic phosphorus poisoning and its therapy. *Arch Environ Health* 1962;5:21–43.

Ellenhorn MJ, Barceloux DG. *Medical toxicology: diagnosis and treatment of human poisoning.* New York: Elsevier, 1988:1067–1108.

Environmental Protection Agency (EPA). Inert ingredients in pesticide products. *Federal Register* 1987:13305–13309.

Environmental Protection Agency (EPA). Office of Public Affairs, EPA proposes new worker protection standards for agricultural pesticides, press release June 29, 1988.

Environmental Protection Agency (EPA). Worker protection standard, hazard information, hand labor tasks on cut flowers and ferns exception; final rule, and proposed rules. *Federal Register.* Part III: Environmental Protection Agency, 40 CFR, Parts 156 and 170, 1992.

Environmental Protection Agency (EPA). *Drinking water regulations and health advisories.* EPA 822-R-96-001. Washington, DC: Office of Water, 1996.

Esteban E, Rubin C, Hill R, et al. Association between indoor residual contamination with methyl parathion and urinary para-nitrophenol. *J Exp Anal Environ Epidemiol* 1996;6(3):375–387.

Eto M. *Organophosphorus pesticides: organic and biological chemistry.* Boca Raton, FL: CRC Press, 1974.

Fiedler N, Kipen H, Kelly-McNeil K, Fenske R. Long-term use of organophosphates and neuropsychological performance. *Am J Ind Med* 1997;32:487–496.

Finkelstein Y, Taitelman U, Biegon A. CNS involvement in acute organophosphate poisoning: specific pattern of toxicity, clinical correlates and antidotal treatment. *Ital J Neurol Sci* 1988a;9:437–446.

Finkelstein Y, Wolff M, Biegon A. Brain acetylcholinesterase after acute parathion poisoning: a comparative quantitative histochemical analysis post mortem. *Ann Neurol* 1988b;24:252–257.

Fisher JR. Guillain-Barré syndrome following organophosphate poisoning. *JAMA* 1977;238:1950–1951.

Fredriksson T, Bigelow JK. Tissue distribution of P32-labeled parathion. *Arch Environ Health* 1961;2:633–667.

Futagami K, Otsubo K, Nakao Y, et al. Acute organophosphate poisoning after disulfoton ingestion. *Clin Toxicol* 1995;33:151–155.

Gaines TB. Acute toxicity of pesticides. *Toxicol Appl Pharmacol* 1969;14:515–534.

Gaines TB, Hayes WJ, Linder RE. Liver metabolism of anticholinesterase compounds in live rats: relation to toxicity. *Nature* 1966;209:88–89.

García-Repetto R, Martínez D, Repetto M. Biodisposition study of the organophosphorus pesticide, methyl-parathion. *Bull Environ Contam Toxicol* 1997;59:901–908.

Gershon S, Shaw FH. Psychiatric sequelae of chronic exposure to organophosphorus insecticides. *Lancet* 1961;1371–1374.

Goh KT, Yew FS, Ong KH, Tan IK: Acute organophosphorus food poisoning caused by contaminated green leafy vegetables. *Arch Environ Health* 1990;45:180–184.

Gordon CJ. Thermoregulation in laboratory mammals and humans exposed to anticholinesterase agents. *Neurotoxicol Teratol* 1994;16:427–453.

Harris LW, Fleisher JH, Clark J, Cliff WJ. Dealkylation and loss of capacity for reactivation of cholinesterase inhibited by sarin. *Science* 1966;154:404–407.

Hatta K, Yasuko M, Nozomu A, Yuichi H. Amnesia from sarin poisoning. *Lancet* 1996;347:1343.

Hester C. Communication the TLV committee from Tunstall Laboratory, Sittingbourne, Kent, England. Cited in the American Conference of Governmental Industrial Hygienists (ACGIH). *Documentation of the threshold limit values (TLVs) and biological exposure indices,* 5th ed. Cincinnati: ACGIH, 1988.

Hobbiger F. Effect of nicotinhydroxamic acid methoxide on human plasma cholinesterase inhibited by organophosphates containing a dialkylphosphate group. *Br J Pharmacol Chemother* 1955;10:356–362.

Hobbiger F. Chemical reactivation of phosphorylated human and bovine true cholinesterase. *Br J Pharmacol Chemother* 1956;11:295–303.

Hodgson MJ, Block GD, Parkinson DK. Organophosphate poisoning in office workers. *J Occup Med* 1986;28:434–437.

Hollingworth RM, Alstott RL, Litzenberg RD. Glutathione S-aryl transferase in the metabolism of parathion and its analogs. *Life Sci* 1973;13:191.

Holmstedt B. Structure–activity relationship of the organophosphorus anticholinesterase agents. In: Eichler O, Farah A, eds. *Handbuch der Experimentellen Pharmakologie.* Berlin: Springer-Verlag, 1963:428–485.

Howard JK, East NJ, Chaney JL. Plasma cholinesterase activity in early pregnancy. *Arch Environ Health* 1978;33(5):277–279.

Jensen JA, Flury VP, Schoof HF. Dichlorvos vapour disinsection of aircraft. *Bull WHO* 1965;32:175–179.

Johnson MK. A phosphorylation site in brain and the delayed neurotoxic effects of some organophosphorus compounds. *Biochem J* 1969;111:487.

Johnson MK. The primary biochemical lesion leading to the delayed neurotoxic effects of some organophosphorus esters. *J Neurochem* 1974;23:785–789.

Johnson MK. Delayed neurotoxicity—do trichlorphon and/or dichlorvos cause delayed neuropathy in man or in test animals. *Acta Pharmacol Toxicol* 1981;94[suppl 5]:87–98.

Johnson MK, Lauwerys R. Protection by some carbamates against the delayed neurotoxic effects of di-isopropyl phosphorofluoridate. *Nature* 1969;222(198):1066–1067.

Jokanović M, Stepanovic RM, Maksimovic M, et al. Modification of the rate of aging of diisopropylfluorophosphate-inhibited neuropathy target esterase of hen brain. *Toxicol Lett* 1998;95:93–101.

Kaplan JG, Kessler J, Rosenberg N, et al. Sensory neuropathy associated with Dursban (chlorpyrifos) exposure. *Neurology* 1993;43:2193–2196.

Kaufer D, Friedman A, Seidman S, Soreq H. Acute stress facilitates long-lasting changes in cholinergic gene expression. *Nautre* 393:373–376, 1998.

Laynes Bretones F, Martinez Garcia L, Fernandez Tortosa I, et al. Fatal food poisoning by parathion. *Med Clin* 1997;108:224–225.

Lockridge O, Bartels CF, Vaughan TA, et al. Complete aminoacid sequence of human serum cholinesterase. *J Biol Chem* 1987;262:549–557.

Loewenstein-Lichenstein Y, Schwarz M, Glick D, et al. Genetic predisposition to adverse consequences of anti-cholinesterases in 'atypical' BCHE carriers. *Nature Med* 1995;1:1082–1085.

Lores EM, Bradway D, Moseman RF. Organophosphorus pesticide poisonings in humans: determination of residues and metabolites in tissues and urine. *Arch Environ Health* 1978;33:270–276.

Lotti M, Moretto A, Capodicasa E, et al. Interactions between neuropathy target esterase and its inhibitors and the development of polyneuropathy. *Toxicol Appl Pharmacol* 1993;122:165–171.

Ma T, Chambers JE. Kinetic parameters of desulfuration and dearylation of parathion and chlorpyrifos by rat liver microsomes. *Food Chem Toxicol* 1994;32:763–767.

Mallatou H, Pappas CP, Knodyli E, Albanis TA. Pesticide residues in milk and cheese from Greece. *Sci Tot Environ* 1997;196:111–117.

Marshall E. Bracing for a biological nightmare. *Science* 1997;275:745.

Massouli J, Pezzementi L, Bon S, Krejci E, Vallette FM. Molecular and cellular biology of cholinesterases. *Prog Neurobiol* 1993;41:31–91.

Metcalf RL, Fukuto TR, March RB. Plant metabolism of dithiosystox and thimet. *J Econ Entomol* 1957;50:338.

Metcalf DR, Holmes JH. EEG, psychological, and neurological alterations in humans with organophosphorus exposure. *Ann NY Acad Sci* 1969;160:357–365.

Midtling JE, Barnett PG, Coye MJ, et al. Clinical management of field worker organophosphate poisoning. *West J Med* 1985;142:514–518.

Miliadis GE, Maltou PTh. Monitoring of the pesticide levels in natural waters of Greece. *Bull Environ Contam Toxicol* 1997;59:917–923.

Misra UK, Nag D, Khan WA, Ray PK. A study of nerve conduction velocity, late responses and neuromuscular synapse functions in organophosphate workers in India. *Arch Toxicol* 1988;61:496–500.

Morgan JP, Penovich P. Jamaica ginger paralysis. Forty-seven-year follow-up. *Arch Neurol* 1978;35:530–532.

MMWR. Recommendations for protecting human health against potential adverse effects of long-term exposure to low doses of chemical warfare agents. *MMWR* 1988;37:72–79.

Muldoon SR, Hodgson MJ. Risk factors for nonoccupational organophosphate pesticide poisoning. *J Occup Med* 1992;34:38–41.

Murata K, Araki S, Yokoyama K, et al. Asymptomatic sequelae to acute sarin poisoning in the central and autonomic nervous system 6 months after the Tokyo subway attack. *J Neurology* 1997;244:601–606.

Namba T, Nolte CT, Jackrel J, Grob D. Poisoning due to organophosphate insecticides: acute and chronic manifestations. *Am J Med* 1971;50: 475–492.

National Institute for Occupational Safety and Health (NIOSH). *Pocket guide to chemical hazards.* Cincinnati: US Department of Health and Human Services, CDC, June 1997.

NATO: *Handbook on the Medical Aspects of NBC Defensive Operations, Amed P-6, Part 3-Chemical*; 1984.

Nolan RJ, Rick DL, Freshour NL, Saunders JH. Chlorpyrifos: pharmacokinetics in human volunteers. *Toxicol Appl Pharmacol* 1984;73:8–15.

Nouira S, Abizoug F, Elatrous S, et al. Prognostic value of serum cholinesterase in organophosphate poisoning. *Chest* 1994;106:1811–1814.

Occupational Safety and Health Administration (OSHA). *Code of Federal Regulations*, 29, 1910.1000/.1047. Washington, DC: Office of the Federal Register, National Archives and Records Administration, 1995:411–431.

Office of Technology Assessment (OTA), US Congress. Neurotoxicity: Identifying and Controlling Poisons of the Nervous System. OTA-BA-436. Washington, DC: Governmental Printing Office, 1990:281.

Olajos EJ, Rosenblum I. Measurement of neurotoxic esterase activity in various subcellular fractions of hen brain and sciatic nerve homogenates and the effect of diisopropyl fluorophosphate (DFP) administration. *Ecotoxicol Environ Safety* 1979;3:18–28.

Oneto ML, Basack SB, Kesten EM. Total and conjugated urinary paranitrophenol after an acute parathion ingestion. *Sci J* 1995;35:207–211.

Ordentlich A, Barak D, Kronman C. The architecture of human acetylcholine esterase active center probed by interactions with selected organophosphate inhibitors. *J Bio Chem* 1996;271:11953–11962.

O'Shaughnessy JA, Sultatos LG. Interaction of ethanol and the organophosphorus insecticide parathion. *Biochem Pharmacol* 1995;50:1925–1932.

Petajan JH, Voorhees KJ, Packham SC, et al. Extreme toxicity from combustion products of a fire-retarded polyurethane foam. *Science* 1975;187:742–744.

Prineas J. The pathogenesis of dying-back polyneuropathies. I. An ultrastructural study of experimental tri-ortho-cresyl phosphate intoxication in the cat. *J Neuropathol Exp Neurol* 1969;28:571–597.

Quinby GE, Walker KC, Durham WF. Public health hazard involved in the use of organic phosphorus insecticides in cotton culture in the delta area of Mississippi. *J Econ Entomol* 1958;51:831.

Roan CC, Morgan DP, Cook N, Paschal EH. Blood cholinesterases, serum parathion concentrations and urine p-nitrophenol concentrations in exposed individuals. *Bull Environ Contam Toxicol* 1969;4:362–369.

Savage EP, Keefe TJ, Mounce LM, et al. Chronic neurological sequelae of acute organophosphate pesticide poisoning. *Arch Environ Health* 1988;43:38–45.

Schwarz M, Glick D, Loewenstein Y, Soreq H. Engineering of human cholinesterases explains and predicts diverse consequences of administration of various drugs and poisons. *Pharmacol Ther* 1995;67:283–322.

Senanayake N. Tri-cresyl phosphate neuropathy in Sri Lanka: a clinical and neurophysiological study with a three year follow up. *J Neurol Neurosurg Psychiatry* 1981;44:775–780.

Senanayake N, Jeyaratnam J. Toxic polyneuropathy due to gingili oil contaminated with tri-cresyl phosphate affecting adolescent girls in Sri Lanka. *Lancet* 1981;1:88–89.

Senanayake N, Johnson MK. Acute polyneuropathy after poisoning by a new organophosphate insecticide. *N Engl J Med* 1982;306(3):155–157.

Senanayake N, Karalliedde L. Neurotoxic effects of organophosphorus insecticides, an intermediate syndrome. *N Engl J Med* 1987;316:761–763.

Serrano R, López FJ, Hernández J, Pena JB. Bioconcentration of chlopyrifos, chlorfenvinphos, and methidathion in mytilus galloprovincialis. *Bull Environ Contam Toxicol* 1997;59:968–975.

Shah PV, Guthrie FE. Percutaneous penetration of three insecticides in rats: a comparison of two methods for *in vivo* determination. *J Invest Dermatol* 1983;80:291–293.

Shailesh KK, Pais P, Vengamma B, Muthane U. Clinical and electrophysiological study of intermediate syndrome in patients with organophosphorus poisoning. *JAPI* 1994;42:451–453.

Sidell FR, Hurst CG. Long-term health effects of nerve agents and mustard. In: Sidel FR, Takafuji ET, Franz DR, eds. *Textbook of military medicine: medical aspects of chemical and biological warfare.* Washington, DC: Borden Institute, Walter Reed Medical Center, 1997:229–246.

Sortorelli P, Aprea C, Bussani R, et al. *In vitro* percutaneous penetration of methyl-parathion from a commercial formulation through the human skin. *Occup Environ Med* 1997;54:524–525.

Spear RC, Popendorf WJ, Spencer WF, et al. Worker poisoning due to paraxon residues. *J Occup Med* 1987;19:411–414.

Steenland K, Jenkins B, Ames RG, et al. Chronic neurological sequelae to organophosphate pesticide poisoning. *Am J Public Health* 1994;84:731–736.

Svetlicic B, Vandekar M. Therapeutic effect of pyridine-2-aldoxime methiodid in parathion poisoned animals. *J Comp Pathol Ther* 1960;70:257–271.

Taylor P, Radic Z. The cholinesterases: from genes to proteins. *Annu Rev Pharmacol Toxicol* 1994;34:281–320.

Thiermann H, Mast U, Klimmeck R, et al. Cholinesterase status, pharmacokinetics and laboratory findings during obidoxime therapy in organophosphate poisoned patients. *Hum Exp Toxicol* 1997;16:473–480.

Tsatsakis AM, Aguridakis P, Mickalodimitrakos MN, et al. Experiences with acute organophosphate poisoning in Crete. *Vet Hum Toxicol* 1996;38:101–107.

United Nations. *Use of chemical weapons by Iraqi regime: report of the specialists appointed by the Secretary General to investigate allegations by Islamic Republic of Iran concerning the use of chemical weapons.* New York: United Nations, 1984.

Vandekar M, Hedayat S, Plestina R, Ahmandy G. A study of the safety of O-isopropoxyphenylmethylcarbamate in an operational field-trial in Iran. *Bull WHO* 1968;38:609–623.

Vasilescu C, Alexiann M, Dan A. Delayed neuropathy after organophosphorus insecticide (Dipterex) poisoning: a clinical, electrophysiological and nerve biopsy study. *J Neurol Neurosurg Psychiatry* 1984;47:543–548.

Virtue WA, Clayton JW. Sheep dip chemicals and water pollution. *Sci Tot Environ* 1997;194–195:207–217.

Wadia RS, Sadagtopan C, Amin RB, Sardesai HV. Neurological manifestations of organophosphorus insecticide poisoning. *J Neurol Neurosurg and Psychiatry* 1974;37:841–847.

Wadia RS, Chitra S, Amin RB, Kiwalkar RS, Sardesai HV. Electrophysiological studies in acute organophosphate poisoning. *J Neurol Neurosurg Psychiatry* 1987;50:1442–1448.

Wecker L, Dettbarn WD. Paraoxon-induced myopathy: muscle specificity and acetylcholine involvement. *Exp Neurol* 1976;51:281.

Wecker L, Laskowski B, Dettbarn WD. Neuromuscular dysfunction induced by acetylcholinesterase inhibition. *Fed Proc* 1978;37:2818–2822.

Widess E. *Neurotoxic pesticides and the farmworker.* Washington, DC: Office of Technology Assessment, 1988.

Wilson IB. Acetylcholinesterase. XI. Reversibility of tetraethylpyrophosphate inhibition. *J Biol Chem* 1951;190:111–117.

Wilson IB. Molecular complementarity and antidotes for alkyl phosphate poisoning. *Fed Proc* 1959;18:752–758.

Witter RF, Gaines TB. Rate of formation in vivo of the unreactivable form of brain cholinesterase in chickens given DDVP or malathion. *Biochem Pharmacol* 1963;12:1421–1427.

Woolf AD. Ginger Jake and the blues: a tragic song of poisoning. *Vet Hum Toxicol* 1995;37:252–254.

World Health Organization (WHO). *Organophosphorus insecticides: a general introduction.* Environmental Health Criteria 63. Geneva: World Health Organization, 1986.

Yang RSH. Enzymatic conjugation and insecticide metabolism. In: Wilkinson CF, ed. *Insecticide biochemistry and physiology.* New York: Plenum Press, 1976:177.

Ye CY, He XH, Chen JS. Prognosis of severe organic phosphorus pesticide intoxication and the effect of atropine treatment: analysis of 506 cases. *Chung-Hua Nei Ko Tsa Chih Chinese J Intern Med* 1990;29:76–78, 125.

Yeh T-S, Wang C-R, Wen C-L, et al. Organophosphate poisoning complicated by rhabdomyolysis [Letter]. *J Toxicol Clin Toxicol* 1993;31:497–498.

Yokoyama K, Yamada A, Nobuhide M. Clinical profiles of patients with sarin poisoning after the Tokyo subway attack. *Am J Med* 1996;100:586.

Yokoyama K, Araki S, Murata K, et al. A preliminary study on delayed vestibulo-cerebellar effects of Tokyo subway sarin poisoning in relation to gender difference: frequency analysis of postural sway. *J Occup Environ Med* 1998;40:17–21.

Zwiener RJ, Ginsburg CM. Organophosphate and carbamate poisoning in infants and children. *Pediatrics* 1988;81:121–126.

CHAPTER 23

Carbamates

Carbamate esters (carbamates) are derivatives of carbamic acid. A naturally occurring carbamate, physostigmine (eserine; calabrine), is extracted from the calabar bean (Taylor, 1990). There are also many synthetic carbamates available for commercial use, including alkyl carbamates, aliphatic oxime carbamates, procarbamates, and mono- and dithiocarbamates. Consideration of the chemical structures of the various synthetic carbamates facilitates an understanding of their individual neurotoxic potential.

Chemical substitutions are typically made at the nitrogen atom and at the ester oxygen atom. In addition, the carbonyl and ester oxygens can be replaced with sulfur atoms. Most carbamate products are methylcarbamates (e.g., carbaryl). The structure of the carbamate precursor molecule, carbamic acid, includes a nitrogen atom with two hydrogen atoms. The methyl carbamate ester derivatives retain the nitrogen atom, but one hydrogen atom has been replaced with a methyl group. The second hydrogen atom, which occupies the R9 position, can also be replaced by other substituents. For example, position R9 might be occupied by another methyl group yielding a dimethyl carbamate (e.g., dimetilan). Various alkyl and aryl substituents (R) can also bind to the ester oxygen. In addition to the differences in the chemical constituents, the length and branching of the alkyl chain of the R groups contribute further to the large number of available carbamate compounds and alter their biological effects and toxicities (Zavon, 1974; Loewenstein et al., 1993) (Fig. 23-1 and Table 23-1).

The solubility of the various carbamates also depends on the properties of the R and R′ groups. For example, 2-isopropoxyphenyl-N-methylcarbamate (common name: propoxur) is relatively lipid-soluble (solubility in water: 0.2% at 20°C) while S-methyl-N-[(methylcarbamoyl)oxy]-thioacetimidate (common name: methomyl) is considerably more polar and as a result is relatively more soluble in water (solubility in water: 5.8% at 25°C) (Kobayashi et al., 1988; Baron, 1991). The difference in the water-solubility of the various carbamates determine the characteristics of

formulations of these compounds (i.e., granules, wettable powder, or liquid spray). For example, methomyl is usually available as water-soluble powders and aqueous solutions, whereas propoxur is frequently found as granules, a wettable powder, or as an oil fog concentrate (Baron, 1991; Moses et al., 1993) (see Sources of Exposure section).

As previously mentioned, the toxicity of the various carbamates depends upon the chemical constituents of the R (e.g., naphthyl as in carbaryl) and R′(e.g., methyl as in primicarb) groups of the molecule (Reiner, 1971; Ryan, 1971; Ferraz et al., 1988; Loewenstein et al., 1993). For example, the aliphatic oxime carbamates have a second nitrogen at the R position to which an alkyl chain is bound by a double bond (see Fig. 23-1). These compounds are among the most toxic of the synthetic carbamates and include 2-methyl-2-(methylthio)-propionaldehyde-O-(methylcarbamoyl)-oxime (common name: aldicarb; trade name: Temik). Procarbamates are derivatives of methylcarbamates and are formed when the hydrogen atom associated with the nitrogen atom in a monomethylcarbamate compound is replaced with a sulfur or an oxygen atom. Examples of procarbamates include carbosulfan and thiodicarb, which are the derivatives of the parent carbamates carbofuran and methomyl, respectively (see Fig. 23-1). Many procarbamates have the same insecticidal potential as the parent carbamate ester; however, the procarbamates are less neurotoxic to humans and other mammals because the metabolism of these compounds favors the formation of nontoxic products (Baron, 1991).

Another commonly used group of carbamates are the dithiocarbamate compounds, which are formed when the two oxygen molecules of a carbamate ester are replaced with sulfur atoms (e.g., tetraethylthiuram disulfide; common name: disulfiram; trade name: Antabuse). The dithiocarbamates are further divided into subgroups (i.e., dimethyldithiocarbamates and ethylenebisdithiocarbamates) based on the specific chemical structure of the dithiocarbamate compound. The dithiocarbamates have relatively low anticholinesterase activity (Baron, 1991). Dithiocarbamates containing a metal atom (e.g., iron, manganese, so-

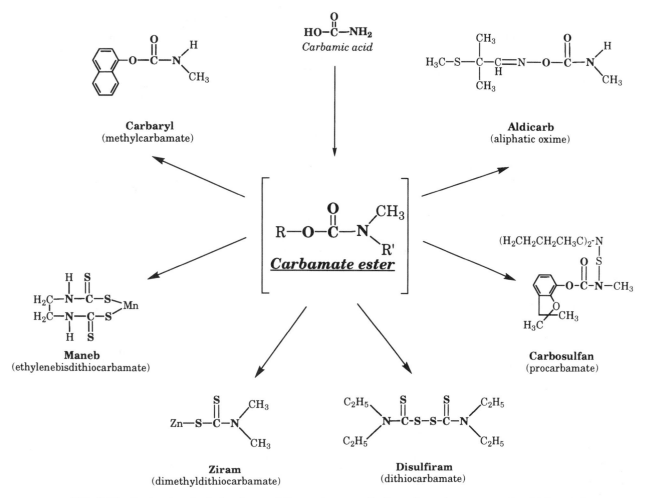

FIG. 23-1. Basic chemical structures of the various synthetic carbamate compounds which are derived from carbamic acid and thus share a common nuclear structure (see text).

dium, or zinc) as an R group are used as herbicides and fungicides (e.g., ziram) (Ferraz et al., 1988). Maneb is an example of an ethylenebisdithiocarbamate used as a fungicide (Edwards et al., 1991) (see Fig. 23-1).

Carbamates, like organophosphorus (OP) compounds, exert their effects by inhibiting cholinesterase enzymes (see Chapter 22). Inhibition of cholinesterase activity results in increased activation of nicotinic, muscarinic, and central nervous system cholinergic synapses (Ecobichon, 1982; Cranmer, 1986; Baron, 1991; Loewenstein et al., 1993). Enzyme inhibition produced by carbamates is of shorter duration than that produced by the OP compounds. Furthermore, in contrast to the poisoning caused by OP compounds, the anticholinesterase effects of the carbamates typically resolve within several hours, and thus there is a rapid disappearance of symptoms following the cessation of exposure. The faster recovery time is a major feature differentiating carbamates from OP compounds and is the primary reason that the former is considered safer and is the preferred pesticide where human exposure is a possibility.

Although the principal *in vivo* effect of all carbamates is the inhibition of the cholinesterase enzymes, there are nevertheless subtle differences in the toxic potential of the various carbamate compounds. The toxicity of carbamates in mammals can be predicted *in vitro,* by the degree to which they inhibit acetylcholinesterase (AChE) activity, and *in vivo,* by the severity of the clinical manifestations (Vandekar et al., 1971; Hudson et al., 1986; Umehara et al., 1991; Loewenstein et al., 1993; Burgess et al., 1994; Grendon et al., 1994; Miller and Mitzel, 1995). Exposure to high concentrations of carbamates for short durations results in dramatic acute clinical manifestations of AChE inhibition; repeated low-level exposure over longer periods of time may cause nonspecific symptoms in susceptible individuals (Miller and Mitzel, 1995; Schwarz et al., 1995a, 1995b).

The broad range of efficacy of these compounds as pesticides along with their lower acute toxicity in mammals and rapid environmental biodegradability has led to widespread use of the various carbamates. The increased use of carbamates, instead of the more toxic OP compounds and

TABLE 23-1. *Common commercial carbamate compounds*

Chemical group	Common name	Trade name[a]
Methylcarbamates	Carbaryl	Sevin
	Carbofuran	Furadan
	Primicarb	Rapid
	Propoxur	Baygon
Aliphatic oximes	Aldicarb	Temik
	Methomyl	Lannate
Procarbamates	Carbosulfan	Advantage
	Mecarbam	Pestan
	Thiodicarb	Larvin
Dithiocarbamates	Disulfiram	Antabuse
	Thiram	Thiosan
	Ziram	Zimate
Ethylenebisdithiocarbamates	Maneb	Dithane M-22
	Zineb	Dithane Z-78

[a]These carbamate compounds may have more than one trade name.

chlorinated hydrocarbons, was originally intended to eliminate adverse health effects. However, a growing body of evidence suggests that carbamates themselves carry significant risks of neurotoxic effects in agricultural and nonagricultural populations and affect humans involved in occupational and nonoccupational endeavors.

SOURCES OF EXPOSURE

Exposure to carbamates occurs among workers involved in the manufacture and formulation, as well as the transportation, handling, and application of these compounds (Best and Murray, 1962; Vandekar et al., 1968; Sidhu and Collisi, 1989; OTA, 1990). While some exposures occur after accidents, others result from ignorance (of the employees and/or their employers) as to the hazards of exposure to the materials being used, inattention to regulations governing use, and/or failure to follow protective measures during handling and application of carbamates (Liddle et al., 1979; Coleman et al., 1990; Hussain et al., 1990; Lima et al., 1995). Agricultural settings are the most likely place for carbamate exposures to occur because of the many tasks that require handling such as during mixing, loading, applying, and equipment cleaning tasks.

It has been estimated that only 1% to 2% of pesticide-related illness is reported and that the actual worldwide incidence of pesticide poisoning is considerably higher (OTA, 1990). Besides the risk to agricultural field workers, those working in a more controlled setting such as greenhouses, tree and shrub nurseries, and home gardens are also in contact with a variety of carbamate pesticides. Carbaryl is rapidly degraded by plants, bacteria, sunlight, and water when it is used outdoors, but indoors it can be stable for long periods of time so that accumulation can be anticipated (Branch and Jacqz, 1986). Nurserymen, foresters, lawn care laborers, highway workers, exterminators, and grain elevator workers are often exposed for short durations to high concentrations of carbamates as well as to other pesticides including OP compounds in the course of

seasonal spraying (Lavy et al., 1993). Bystander exposures affect individuals who happen to be within the vicinity of pesticide applications but who are not directly involved in the application process or even working in the particular field, and they include those living near the target site or who happen to be in the area of drift when crop dusting or tree spraying is being done from overflying aircraft (Vandekar et al., 1968; Grendon et al., 1994; Miller and Mitzel, 1995) (see Clinical Experiences section). Veterinarians and others involved in the use of flea and tick control preparations are also at risk of exposure to carbamates (Sidhu and Collisi, 1989). Polyurethanes (polycarbamates) are a common polymer constituent in many fibers (e.g., spandex), foams, paints, and adhesives (Harris and Sarvadi, 1994).

Small amounts of carbamates are ingested with foods, either as transmitted pesticide residues in food preparations or as a natural ingredient in some foods. Ethyl carbamate (urethane) has been detected in foods such as breads, yogurts, and other acidified milk products, as well as in fermented beverages such as fruit brandy, wine, and beer (Dennis et al., 1989; Battaglia et al., 1990; Vahl, 1993). Chemigation, or the adding of pesticides to irrigation water, is increasingly being used and thus contributes to the content of pesticides on and in produce (Moses et al., 1993). Outbreaks of carbamate poisoning have been reported following consumption of foods containing high concentrations of carbamates. For example, outbreaks have been reported following ingestion of cucumbers (Goes et al., 1980) and melons contaminated with aldicarb (Goldman et al., 1990). Intentional suicidal ingestion of carbamates has also been reported (Dickoff et al., 1987; Umehara et al., 1991; Lima et al., 1995). Carbamate exposures among children are frequently the result of accidental ingestion of carelessly stored or indiscriminately used pesticides in households. Children and domestic animals can put contaminated things into their mouth during their play on floors or carpets that have recently been sprayed with carbamate pesticides (Ramasamy, 1976; Branch and Jacqz, 1986; Zwiener and Ginsburg, 1988; Lima et al., 1995). A sick pet often can be the sentinel case in a household, indicating the presence of the toxic hazard for others (Branch and Jacqz, 1986).

Contamination of ground water with carbamates occurs following accidental spills as well as controlled applications of pesticides (Zaki et al., 1982; Lorber et al., 1990). An enormous problem inherent to the current technology of pesticide application is the problem of "drift" (i.e., dispersal of the pesticide away from the target of application) (Moses et al., 1993). Although early studies had suggested that aldicarb properly applied could not contaminate ground-water supplies, the pesticide was nevertheless found in water samples from 1,121 of 8,404 (13.3%) wells sampled in Suffolk County, New York in 1979 and exceeded the state recommended maximum level of 7 ppb. Aldicarb levels in 52% of the 1,121 contaminated wells ranged from 8 to 30 ppb, 32% had levels between 31 and 75 ppb, and 16% had aldicarb levels greater than 75 ppb. The proximity of the farming activities to the plume feeding the well was determined to be related to the concentration of aldicarb in the water; 94.4% of the wells with detectable levels of aldicarb were within 1,000 feet of a farm (Zaki et al., 1982). Aldicarb was also the most commonly reported man-made ground-water contaminant in Wisconsin (Mirkin et al., 1990).

The reversibility of the AChE inhibition produced by the carbamates has led to medicinal uses of these compounds. For example, urethane is used as an anesthetic agent (Sax, 1979). Disulfiram, a dithiocarbamate compound, with little anticholinesterase activity, is commonly used in the management of patients with a history of alcohol abuse (Christensen et al., 1991). The effectiveness of carbamates (e.g., physostigmine), as compared to tetrahydroaminoacridine (tacrine: common name) or donepezil hydrochloride (Aricept), has also been explored in the symptomatic management of Alzheimer's disease–related dementia, which has been associated with degradation of forebrain cholinergic neurons and, therefore, acetylcholine deficiency (Perry et al., 1978; Collerton, 1986; Iijima et al., 1993; Smith et al., 1997). Pyridostigmine, a quaternary carbamate, is primarily used in the treatment of patients with myasthenia gravis; it has also been administered prophylactically as a pretreatment against irreversible AChE inhibitors such as the OP compounds, which are often used as chemical warfare agents as well as insecticides (Hudson et al., 1986; Friedman et al., 1996; Haley and Kurt, 1997). The risks associated with prophylactic and medicinal uses of carbamates have been noted by Loewenstein-Lichtenstein et al. (1995), who found polymorphisms in butyrylcholinesterase (which in its normal form serves as a scavenger of anticholinesterases) that may contribute to individual differences in susceptibility to the effects of carbamates.

EXPOSURE LIMITS AND SAFETY REGULATIONS

The *Occupational Safety and Health Administration* (OSHA), the *National Institute for Occupational Safety and Health* (NIOSH), and the *American Conference of Governmental Industrial Hygienists* (ACGIH) have determined exposure limits for several of the commonly used carbamates. However, due to the great number of compounds that fall into this chemical category, it is only possible to list exposure limits for a few of the more commonly used ones here; for current information on a specific carbamate compound, consult the *NIOSH Pocket Guide to Chemical Hazards* (NIOSH, 1997) or access the NIOSH Internet homepage at <http://www.cdc.gov/niosh/homepage.html>.

Regulations and/or recommendations for the prevention of toxic effects resulting from occupational exposures to 2-methyl-2(methylthio)-propionaldehyde-*O*-(methylcarbamoyl)-oxime (common name: aldicarb; trade name: Temik) have not been published by the OSHA, NIOSH, or ACGIH (NIOSH, 1997; OSHA, 1995; ACGIH, 1995) (Table 23-2).

The OSHA permissible exposure limit (PEL) for 1-naphthyl-*N*-methylcarbamate (common name: carbaryl; trade name: Sevin) is 5 mg/m^3 (OSHA, 1995). The NIOSH recommended exposure limit (REL) for carbaryl is a 10-hour TWA concentration of 5 mg/m^3. The NIOSH has also recommended an immediately dangerous to life and health (IDLH) exposure limit for carbaryl of 100 mg/m^3 (NIOSH, 1997). The ACGIH recommended threshold limit value (TLV) for carbaryl is an 8-hour TWA exposure of 5 mg/m^3 (ACGIH, 1995).

The OSHA PEL for 2,3-dihydro-2,2-dimethyl-7-benzofuranyl *N*-methylcarbamate (common name: carbofuran; trade name: Furadan) was 0.1 mg/m^3 in 1989, but this value was vacated in 1993 (see AFL-CIO v. OSHA, 965 F.2d 962) (NIOSH, 1997; OSHA, 1995). The NIOSH REL for carbofuran is a 10-hour TWA concentration of 0.1 mg/m^3. The NIOSH has not determined an IDLH exposure limit for carbofuran (NIOSH, 1997). The ACGIH TLV for carbofuran is an 8-hour TWA of 0.1 mg/m^3 (ACGIH, 1995).

The OSHA PEL for *S*-methyl-*N*-[(methylcarbamate)oxy]-thioacetimidate (common name: methomyl; trade name: Lannate) was 2.5 mg/m^3 in 1989, but this value was vacated in 1993 (see AFL-CIO v. OSHA, 965 F.2d 962) (NIOSH, 1997; OSHA, 1995). The NIOSH REL for methomyl is a 10-hour TWA concentration of 2.5 mg/m^3. The NIOSH has not determined an IDLH exposure limit for methomyl (NIOSH, 1997). The ACGIH TLV for methomyl is an 8-hour TWA of 2.5 mg/m^3 (ACGIH, 1995).

The OSHA PEL for 2-isopropoxyphenyl-*N*-methylcarbamate (common name: propoxur; trade name: Baygon) was 0.5 mg/m^3 in 1989, but this value was vacated in 1993 (see AFL-CIO v. OSHA, 965 F.2d 962) (NIOSH, 1997; OSHA, 1995). The NIOSH REL for propoxur is a 10-hour TWA concentration of 0.5 mg/m^3. The NIOSH has not determined an IDLH exposure limit for propoxur (NIOSH, 1997). The ACGIH TLV for propoxur is an 8-hour TWA of 0.5 mg/m^3 (ACGIH, 1995).

The *Environmental Protection Agency* (EPA) has established water contamination levels guidelines for many car-

TABLE 23-2. *Established and recommended occupational and environmental exposure limits for selected carbamates in air and water*

	Air (mg/m^3)	Water (mg/L)
Odor threshold	—	—
OSHA		
PEL (8-hr TWA)		
Aldicarb	—	—
Carbaryl	5[a]	—
Carbofuran	0.1[a]	—
Methomyl	2.5[a]	—
Propoxur	0.5[a]	—
NIOSH		
REL (8-hr TWA)		
Aldicarb	—	—
Carbaryl	5	—
Carbofuran	0.1	—
Methomyl	2.5	—
Propoxur	0.5	—
IDLH		
Aldicarb	—	—
Carbaryl	100	—
Carbofuran	—	—
Methomyl	—	—
Propoxur	—	—
ACGIH		
TLV (8-hr TWA)		
Aldicarb	—	—
Carbaryl	5	—
Carbofuran	0.1	—
Methomyl	2.5	—
Propoxur	0.5	—
EPA		
MCL		
Aldicarb	—	—
Carbaryl	—	0.04
Carbofuran	—	—
Methomyl	—	—
Propoxur	—	—

[a] Vacated OSHA exposure limit; see text.
Unit conversion: 1 mg/m^3 = 0.001 mg/L.
OSHA, Occupational Safety and Health Administration; PEL, permissible exposure limit; TWA, time-weighted average; NIOSH, National Institute for Occupational Safety and Health; IDLH, immediately dangerous to life and health; ACGIH, American Conference of Governmental Industrial Hygienists; TLV, threshold limit value; EPA, Environmental Protection Agency; MCL, maximum contamination limit.
Data from OSHA, 1995; ACGIH, 1995; EPA, 1996; NIOSH, 1997.

TABLE 23-3. *Acceptable adult daily intake for carbamate compounds*

Compound	Daily intake (mg/kg)	Reference
Carbaryl	0.0–0.001	FAO/WHO, 1974
Aldicarb	0.0–0.005	FAO/WHO, 1983
Carbofuran	0.0–0.01	FAO/WHO, 1981
Methomyl	0.0–0.01	FAO/WHO, 1986
Propoxur	00.0–0.02	FAO/WHO, 1974

METABOLISM

Tissue Absorption

Pulmonary absorption of carbamates is a major route of intake in humans; the more readily a carbamate compound crosses the pulmonary alveoli and enters into the circulation, the greater is its toxicity (Best et al., 1962; Hussain et al., 1990). Best et al. (1962) reported that employees involved in the packaging of carbaryl were exposed to higher local air concentrations of the pesticide and had higher urine levels of 1-naphthol, a carbaryl metabolite. In addition, these workers occasionally showed a mild depression of whole blood cholinesterase activity despite following what were considered proper industrial hygienic practices. Pulmonary intake of carbaryl in rats resulted in greater total absorption and severity of toxic effect than did exposure of rats to this carbamate via oral or dermal routes (Ladics et al., 1994).

Gastrointestinal absorption after oral ingestion of carbamate compounds has been demonstrated in humans and laboratory animals (Andrawes et al., 1967; Wills et al., 1968; Sen Gupta and Knowles, 1970; van Hoof and Heyndrickx, 1975; Declume and Benard, 1977; Challis and Adcock, 1981; Ahdaya et al., 1981; Osman et al., 1983; May et al., 1992). In addition to the solubility of the particular carbamate compound, its gastrointestinal absorption is influenced by the vehicle (i.e., carrier solvents) in which the carbamate is mixed or is in solution with. An oil vehicle enhances absorption and increases oral toxicity in mammals (Vandekar et al., 1971).

Incidents of accidental and intentional swallowing of carbamates have resulted in a wide range in severity of neurotoxicity depending on the rate of intake, the total amount ingested, absorption kinetics, and the chemical structure of the particular carbamate compound ingested (Zwiener and Ginsburg, 1988; Lima et al., 1995). Oral intake of carbaryl and propoxur by human volunteers resulted in significant suppression of AChE activity, indicating that these two carbamate compounds are readily absorbed across the gastrointestinal mucosa and have a relatively high affinity for AChE (May et al., 1992). A single oral dose of 1.5 mg/kg of propoxur administered to a 42-year-old male volunteer produced mild symptoms that lasted approximately 2 hours and then completely resolved. During the subject's symptomatic period, there had

bamates. Health advisory warning levels have been established for carbaryl, carbofuran, methomyl, and propoxur. In addition, the EPA has established maximum drinking water contamination levels (MCLs) of 0.04 mg/L (40 ppb) for carbofuran and 0.007 mg/L (7 ppb) for aldicarb (EPA, 1996) (see Table 23-2).

The World Health Organization has recommended acceptable daily intake levels for carbamates (Table 23-3).

been an initial prompt fall in erythrocyte AChE activity without depression of plasma cholinesterase activity. Within minutes after ingestion the subject's erythrocyte AChE activity level was depressed to 27% of normal, following which the erythrocyte AChE activity level began to rise so that at 30 and 45 minutes after ingestion of the propoxur the erythrocyte AChE activity was recorded at 50.4% and 55.5% of its normal level, respectively. A less dramatic effect on blood cholinesterase activity levels was observed when a higher dose was ingested over a prolonged period of time, indicating that absorption and the development of neurotoxic effects are determined by the rate of ingestion and the total amount of carbamate taken in (Vandekar et al., 1971) (see Symptomatic Diagnosis and Clinical Experiences sections).

Dermal absorption of carbamates also occurs and contributes significantly to an exposed individual's total body burden (Vandekar et al., 1968; Gaines, 1969; Feldmann and Maibach, 1974; Shah et al., 1981; Ecobichon, 1982; Hussain et al., 1990; Ladics et al., 1994). Total dermal absorption of carbamates is influenced in part by the physical state of the compound (i.e., dry wettable powder or aqueous solution), the lipid-solubility of the carbamate compound, and the presence of solvents (i.e., the vehicle). For example, approximately 70% of an applied dose of carbaryl, using acetone as vehicle, was absorbed through the intact skin of humans; using the same vehicle, only 19.6% of an applied dose of propoxur was absorbed (Feldmann and Maibach, 1974). Other factors affecting dermal absorption include the size, temperature, and level of hydration of the exposed area of skin (Feldmann and Maibach, 1974; Baron, 1991). Eighty-seven percent of the total body burden absorbed through the skin in grain farmers exposed to carbofuran was taken in through the skin of the hands and wrists, while only 12.8% was absorbed through those areas of skin that were protected by work clothing, indicating that wearing protective clothing and gloves can signifi-

cantly reduce total exposures to carbamates and thus reduce the risk of neurotoxic effects (Hussain et al., 1990).

Under controlled conditions it is possible to make reasonable estimates of the contribution of dermal absorption to an exposed individual's total body burden of carbamates; however, it is difficult to do this following an uncontrolled occupational or accidental exposure. In such cases, circumstantial evidence is relied upon to ascertain the occurrence and significance of dermal absorption. Vandekar et al. (1968) reported fewer symptoms among those workers using propoxur who washed their hands and face more frequently than among those who did not. Similar observations were made in two bystanders who were soaked through their clothing to their skin when sprayed with carbaryl during an aerial pesticide application. One victim examined did not have the opportunity to remove his clothing until 3 hours later, and the second wore his wet clothes for almost 12 hours. The duration of persistent nausea, vomiting, and frequent bowel movements was longer in the second victim than it was in the first person. It would seem reasonable to conclude that more dermal absorption had occurred in the second man than had in the first, thereby contributing to the greater severity of his symptoms (R. G. Feldman, personal observation). Ecobichon (1982) reported a similar case of a 55-year-old man who developed severe and persistent neurological manifestations after he was soaked with carbaryl while spraying a vegetable garden (see Symptomatic Diagnosis and Clinical Experiences sections).

Tissue Distribution

Carbamates readily cross the blood–brain barrier (BBB) and the placenta (Declume and Benard, 1977). Carbamates are distributed to all tissues, with highest concentrations found in the liver, kidneys, and spleen. Lower concentrations are detected in the lungs, heart, skeletal muscles, and fat (Table 23-4). Studies of excretion in workers chroni-

TABLE 23-4. *Time–distribution relationship of radioactivity levels in a dam and her fetus following exposure to radio-labeled carbaryl*

Tissue		\multicolumn{7}{c}{Hours after exposure}						
		1	5	8	24	48	72	96
Brain	Dam	0	0 to TR	0 to TR	TR	TR	0 to TR	0 to TR
	Fetus	0 to TR	TR	TR	+	+	+	+
Blood	Dam	TR	+	TR	TR	TR	0 to TR	0 to TR
	Fetus	TR	TR	+	+	NA	TR	TR
Skeletal muscle	Dam	TR	TR	TR	TR	TR	TR	TR
	Fetus	TR	TR	+	+	+	+	TR
Cardiac muscle	Dam	TR	TR	TR	TR	+	+	+
	Fetus	TR	TR	+	+	+	TR	TR
Adipose	Dam	TR	+	+	++	+	+	+
	Fetus	TR	TR	TR	+	+	+	+
Liver	Dam	+	++	+++	+++	++	+	+
	Fetus	TR	TR	+	+	+	+	+

Radioactivity scale: NA, not available; 0, none; TR, trace; +, low; ++, medium; +++, high.
Data from Declume and Benard, 1977.

cally exposed to carbamates suggest that accumulation in tissues does not occur with repeated exposures (Best and Murray, 1962; Lavy et al., 1993). The permeability of the BBB is increased by stress and distribution of carbamates to the brain (Friedman et al., 1996).

The distribution of carbamates in the brain can be inferred from the observed effects. A single injection of propoxur caused a decrease in brain acetylcholine and AChE in mice (Kobayashi et al., 1988). Furthermore, chronic exposure to propoxur caused a decrease in high-affinity choline uptake in the brains of these animals. Loss of cholinergic neurons and a possible disruption of acetylcholine synthesis have been associated with a decrease in erythrocyte AChE activity (Chipperfield et al., 1981). These findings suggest that accumulation of acetylcholine at the synaptic cleft is not the sole mechanism of carbamate neurotoxicity (see Neuropathological Diagnosis section).

Tissue Biochemistry

The metabolism of a carbamate ester involves two pathways (Fig. 23-2). The first pathway (**A**), oxidation, occurs via cytochrome P-450 microsomal monooxygenases at the R or R' groups, resulting in aromatic hydroxylation, aliphatic hydroxylation, N-dealkylation, O- and S-dealkylation, and sulfoxidation (Ryan, 1971; Chin et al., 1979;

Kulkarni and Hodgson, 1980). The metabolites of these oxidative processes are subsequently conjugated with glutathione, glucuronic acid, and/or sulfate and are excreted in the urine (Ryan, 1971; Chin et al., 1979; Chen and Dorough, 1979). In most cases, microsomal oxidation results in detoxification of carbamates. However, in some cases (e.g., propoxur and aldicarb), oxidation results in the formation of metabolites that are more toxic than the parent compounds (Oonithan and Casida, 1968; Ryan, 1971; Marshall et al., 1987). For example, oxidation of aldicarb yields sulfoxide and sulfone, which are both significantly more effective at inhibiting cholinesterase activity than the parent compound, whereas the oxidation of carbaryl leads to the formation of an epoxide intermediate which can react with cellular macromolecules (Metcalf et al., 1967; Ryan, 1971).

The second pathway (**B**) utilizes hydrolysis of carbamates by esterases, to yield a hydroxylated R group and N-methylcarbamic acid (Sakai and Matsumura, 1971). Hydrolysis of carbaryl liberates 1-naphthol and N-methylcarbamic acid (Hassan et al., 1966). Similarly, hydrolysis of propoxur (2-isopropoxyphenyl-N-methylcarbamate) yields 2-isopropoxyphenol and N-methylcarbamic acid (Dawson et al., 1964). The majority of the hydroxylated R group is conjugated with glutathione, glucuronic acid, and/or sulfate and excreted in the urine. These conjugated metabo-

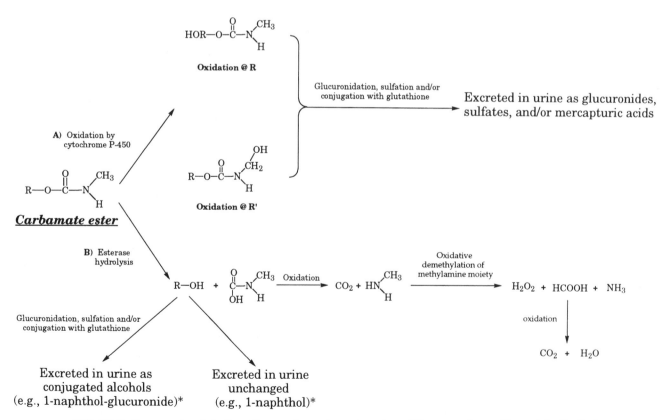

FIG. 23-2. Proposed metabolic pathways for carbamate esters. *Compound-specific metabolite that can be used as a biological marker of exposure.

lites are relatively specific to the particular carbamate compound and thus can be used in the biochemical diagnosis of exposures (see Biochemical Diagnosis section). In addition, the oxidation of *N*-methylcarbamic acid yields methylamine and carbon dioxide. The methylamine moiety is subsequently demethylated via oxidation to yield formate, hydrogen peroxide, and ammonia. The oxidation of formate yields carbon dioxide and water (Hassan et al., 1966) (see Fig. 23-2).

The presence of structural similarities between many carbamates and acetylcholine renders both as substrates for AChE. Thus, carbamates can be hydrolyzed by AChE. The reaction between carbamates and AChE proceeds in three steps: (a) reversible formation of an AChE–carbamate complex; (b) irreversible carbamylation of an AChE–carbamate complex in which AChE loses a hydrogen and the carbamate compound loses its leaving group (e.g., alcohol, phenol, or oxime); and (c) decarbamylation, in which hydrolysis of AChE results in release of the carbamate moiety; the carbamate moiety is unstable and rapidly degrades to carbon dioxide and a methylated amine (Reiner, 1971). The rate at which decarbamylation occurs has a significant impact on neurotoxicity. Reiner (1971) noted that carbamates with longer substituents (e.g., isopropyl versus methyl) in the R′ position on the nitrogen atom form more stable AChE–carbamate complexes with significantly longer reactivation half-lives and thus have the potential to cause neurotoxic effects which last for longer durations. Organophosphate esters also act as substrates for AChE. However, while decarbamylation of most carbamates proceeds rapidly *in vivo,* resulting in acute symptoms that typically resolve within hours after removal from exposure, *in vivo* dephosphorylation is so slow that AChE inhibition by organophosphate esters is practically irreversible, resulting in persistent neurotoxic effects (Reiner and Aldridge, 1967; Reiner, 1971) (see Chapter 22).

Carbamates have also been shown to inhibit the activity of butyrylcholinesterase, an enzyme closely related to AChE. Butyrylcholinesterase appears to function as a scavenger of toxins, thereby protecting acetylcholine-binding proteins such as AChE. Butyrylcholinesterase polymorphisms have been used to explain individual differences in susceptibility to the effects of carbamates and other anticholinesterases (Schwarz et al., 1995b; Loewenstein-Lichtenstein et al., 1995) (see Neuropathological Diagnosis section).

Acute and chronic exposure to other chemicals will alter the metabolism of carbamates. Acute consumption of ethanol has been shown to inhibit the metabolism of ethyl carbamate (i.e., urethane) (Kurata et al., 1991). Simultaneous acute exposure to ethanol and disulfiram and/or its dithiocarbamate analogs inhibits the activity of aldehyde dehydrogenase and increases blood levels of acetylaldehyde, thereby producing characteristic face flushing, headache, nausea, and vomiting (Christensen et al., 1991; Johnsen et al., 1992). Chronic exposure to carbamates and

other chemicals such as ethanol and phenobarbital, which induce cytochrome P-450 enzymatic activity, enhance the metabolism of carbamates (Neskovic et al., 1978; Kurata et al., 1991). For example, mice exposed to phenobarbital showed increased resistance to the anticholinesterase effects of carbaryl, demonstrating that enhanced metabolism reduces the anticholinesterase action of this carbamate (Neskovic et al., 1978). Chronic exposure to benomyl, a carbamate fungicide, has been shown to deplete glutathione stores and to induce lipid peroxidation in rats; this may enhance the neurotoxicity of other chemicals (such as styrene and acrylamide) that are detoxified by conjugation with glutathione (Dixit et al., 1981, 1982; Banks and Soliman, 1997).

The carbonyl carbon of the carbamate compound binds at the esteric site of the various cholinesterases, thereby inhibiting the activity of these enzymes. Inhibition of AChE depends on the length and structure of the alkyl substituents on the amide group. Branched-chain alkyl groups are not accommodated due to steric interference (Loewenstein et al., 1993). The nitrogen atom of the aliphatic oxime carbamate compounds can react with the anionic site of AChE, a mechanism that may account for the increased toxicity of this group of carbamate compounds (Ecobichon, 1982; Cranmer, 1986; Baron, 1991). The lower neurotoxicity of the procarbamates is due to the rapid metabolism of these compounds to "relatively" nontoxic products. The dithiocarbamates are considerably more toxic than thiocarbamates. These compounds are metabolized to carbon disulfide, and it is likely that the neurotoxic effects of these compounds result in part from the actions of carbon disulfide (Edwards et al., 1991; Johnson et al., 1996) (see Chapter 21).

Excretion

A small amount of the parent carbamate is excreted in the urine unchanged. Metabolites of carbamates that have undergone microsomal oxidation or esterase-mediated hydrolysis are eliminated in the urine either as free metabolites or conjugated with glutathione, glucuronic acid, and/or sulfates as mercapturic acids, glucuronides, and sulfates, respectively (Hassan et al., 1966; Ryan, 1971; Lavy et al., 1993) (see Fig. 23-2). Carbamate-derived mercapturic acids are also excreted in the bile and feces (Knaak, 1971; Ryan, 1971; Chen and Dorough, 1979). The carbon dioxide derived from hydrolysis of carbamates is exhaled almost immediately following exposure, as shown by radio-labeled studies of carbaryl exposure in rats (Hassan et al., 1966).

Metabolism of the various carbamate compounds yields a myriad of specific and nonspecific urinary metabolites. Specific metabolites of methylcarbamates reflect hydrolytic cleavage of the molecule at the ester oxygen. For example, free and conjugated 1-naphthol can be detected in the urine of workers exposed to carbaryl (1-naphthyl-*N*-

methylcarbamate), whereas 2-isopropoxyphenol is the principal free and conjugated urinary metabolite of propoxur (2-isopropoxyphenyl-*N*-methylcarbamate) (Best and Murray, 1962; Dawson et al., 1964). The compound 2-isopropoxyphenol can be detected by a colorimetric method in human urine at a dose of about 70 mg (1 mg/kg) when the urine sample is taken within 8 hours of absorption of propoxur (Dawson et al., 1964). Urinary metabolites specific to the dithiocarbamates include carbon disulfide and thiourea (Toyama and Kusano, 1953; Pergal et al., 1972; Riihimäki et al., 1992; Drexler et al., 1995) (see Biochemical Diagnosis section).

CLINICAL MANIFESTATION AND DIAGNOSIS

Symptomatic Diagnosis

Much of the early knowledge about the clinical effects of carbamates on the human nervous system was learned from Africans, who used the naturally occurring carbamate physostigmine as a poison to induce central, peripheral, and autonomic nervous system dysfunction (Holmstedt, 1972). Reversible initial symptoms of burning eyes, mouth, and throat result from direct contact with the carbamate compound and its carrier solvent, whereas the subsequent neurological features arise after sufficient absorption has led to inhibition of AChE and the accumulation of excess amounts of acetylcholine at muscarinic and nicotinic sites including neuromuscular junctions. An acronym "MUDDLES" (i.e., miosis, urination, diarrhea, diaphoresis, lacrimation, excitation of CNS, and salivation) has been proposed to characterize the principal effects of AChE inhibition whether caused by carbamates or OPCs (O'Malley, 1997). The occurrence of persistent peripheral and central nervous system symptoms in some patients does not appear to be caused by the direct anticholinesterase effects of carbamates, thereby suggesting the involvement of other and unexplained secondary mechanisms (see Neuropathological Diagnosis section).

Acute Exposure

The symptoms associated with acute carbamate exposure include lacrimation, excessive salivation and sweating, headache, blurred vision, abdominal cramps, nausea, vomiting, diarrhea, respiratory problems, fecal and urinary urgency and/or incontinence, cardiac irregularities, hypotension, pyrexia, myoclonic spasms, generalized muscle weakness, ataxia, paralysis, loss of consciousness, respiratory apnea, seizures, and death (Wills et al., 1968; Liddle et al., 1979; Zwiener and Ginsburg, 1988; Sofer et al., 1989; Burgess et al., 1994; Grendon et al., 1994; Gordon, 1994; Lima et al., 1995; Lifshitz et al., 1997). Death usually results from respiratory failure due to paralysis of respiratory muscles (Liddle et al., 1979). In nonfatal cases, acute symptoms of cholinesterase inhibition typically resolve

within hours to days (Vandekar et al., 1968, 1971). Mild symptoms including abdominal cramps and insomnia were reported by male volunteers exposed to carbaryl daily for 6 weeks at a dose of 0.06 mg/kg (Wills et al., 1968).

The acute antiacetylcholinesterase activity of carbamates and the associated symptoms are documentable by determining erythrocyte AChE activity. However, the observed duration of depression of erythrocyte AChE activity, its recovery, and the appearance of symptoms are not coincident. This is illustrated by the study by Vandekar et al. (1971), who exposed a male volunteer to 1.5 mg/kg of propoxur. Symptoms were not noted by the subject within 15 minutes after dosing, when erythrocyte AChE activity levels were lowest (27% of normal). Twenty minutes after dosing, when the erythrocyte AChE activity levels were recovering (30% of normal), the subject began to experience symptoms including blurred vision, nausea, and excessive sweating. In addition, his face was pale and his pulse rate had increased from 76 to 140/min. After another 10 minutes, at which time the erythrocyte AChE activity level was at approximately 40% of normal, the subject began to vomit. These symptoms persisted for an additional 15 minutes, during which time the subject's erythrocyte AChE activity level increased to 55.5% of its normal value. One hour after exposure, at which time the erythrocyte AChE activity level was greater than 60% of its normal value, the subject had stopped vomiting but was still nauseous and sweating profusely. The subject was symptom-free within 2 hours after exposure, at which time his erythrocyte AChE activity level had risen to 90% of its normal value. These findings demonstrate that erythrocyte AChE activity levels are depressed before there are subjective or observable clinical manifestations of carbamate effect and that these levels had actually begun to return toward normal values as symptoms evolved, indicating that symptoms can be present when biological markers of exposure have begun to return to normal. In addition, these findings indicate that the severity of an acute exposure can be underestimated when only erythrocyte AChE activity is considered, which may have improved considerably by the time a blood sample is taken, and that the clinician's recognition of the acute effects of cholinergic inhibition may be the only evidence upon which the diagnosis of carbamate exposure can be made (see Biochemical Diagnosis section).

The central nervous system (CNS) effects are more severe in children than in adults exposed to carbamates (Lima et al., 1995; Lifshitz et al., 1997). Lifshitz et al. (1997) reviewed the clinical course in 36 children (age: 1 to 8 years) and 24 adults (age: 17 to 41 years) who had been acutely exposed to either aldicarb or methomyl and who had similar depression of plasma cholinesterase as a marker of dose. The predominant symptoms included miosis and muscle fasciculations in the adults, while the children were more likely to experience CNS effects of stupor and/or coma in addition to diarrhea and hypotonia (Table 23-5). This difference in susceptibility may reflect differ-

TABLE 23-5. *Acute symptoms of carbamate poisoning in adults and children exposed to aldicarb and methomyl*

Symptom	Percent of patients presenting with symptoms	
	Adults ($n = 24$)	Children ($n = 36$)
Stupor/coma[a]	0.0	100.0
Hypotonia[a]	0.0	100.0
Miosis	91.7	55.0
Fasciculations[a]	83.3	5.5
Bradycardia	33.3	16.0
Diarrhea[a]	0.0	33.0
Salivation	8.3	0.0
Seizures	0.0	8.0
Bronchorrhea[a]	16.6	0.0

[a]Significant ($p < 0.05$ by χ^2) difference between groups in frequency of these symptoms; children have more central nervous system effects than adults.

Data from Lifshitz et al., 1997.

ences in the permeability of the BBB of children and adults.

Identifying the anticholinesterase chemicals that are responsible for the various symptoms in a complex clinical picture may be difficult when the pesticide formulations contain a mixture of organophosphorus compounds as well as carbamates and the organic carrier solvents. For example, a veterinary technician was exposed to a commercial formulation intended for use as pesticide to control fleas and ticks, which contained carbamates and OPCs (Sidhu and Collisi, 1989). It contained isopropyl (2E-4E)11-methoxy-3,7,11-trimethyl-2,4-dodecadienoate (methoprene), 2-isopropoxyphenyl-*N*-methylcarbamate (propoxur), and 0.0-dimethyl-0,2,2-dichlorovinyl phosphate (dichlorovos), and dichlormethane (methylene chloride), 1,1-difluoroethane (ethylene fluoride), and 1,1,1-trichloroethane (methyl chloroform) as carrier solvents. This mixture was contained in a pressurized can which exploded in the face of the technician when he opened it. The contents of the container were released into the air, and the solution splashed on the technician's face, arms, hands, and neck. The exposed technician's clothing, including his socks and shoes, was also soaked with the pesticide solvent mixture. Although immediate emergency measures including flushing out the eyes and a shower were undertaken, only a partial change of clothing was possible until 6 hours later when a second shower was taken and a complete change in clothes was made. Acute symptoms of headache, nausea, vomiting, diarrhea, and difficulty breathing began soon after the exposure and persisted for over 4 days before subsiding. The clinical course was complicated by chemical pneumonia which resulted from the inhaled mist and pesticide–solvent droplets. The chemical pneumonia was attributed to the inhalation of the organic solvents which were used as vehicles. The patient's plasma cholinesterase activity was assayed on the seventh day after the exposure (by which time his symptoms had subsided) and was found to

be "normal." From this rapid recovery and the lack of persistently depressed plasma cholinesterase activity, it might be concluded that the main neurotoxicant was the carbamate rather than the OPC.

Persistent symptoms have also been reported following severe acute exposures to carbamates and include photophobia, memory deficits, respiratory problems, lethargy, paresthesia, muscle weakness, and sensory loss in the extremities. Ecobichon (1982) reported the case of a 55-year-old man who was soaked with carbaryl, as a water-wettable powder, while spraying his vegetable garden. Three days after the exposure the patient was admitted to a local hospital where he was given a diagnosis of meningitis and treated with antibiotics. He was considered well enough to be discharged several days later. Approximately 3 weeks later, however, the patient was still experiencing symptoms including headaches, irritability, fatigue, blurred vision, photophobia, memory problems, and weakness, numbness, and paresthesias in his extremities. He consulted his physician, who diagnosed carbaryl poisoning after connecting the patient's complaints with his gardening activities. At follow-up 1 year after exposure the patient continued to experience photophobia, memory impairment, fatigue, and paresthesia and muscle weakness in his extremities despite his avoidance of any additional contact with pesticides. Similar persistent symptoms were also reported among a group of men who had been acutely exposed to aldicarb (Grendon et al., 1994). Three years after exposure, five of six men were still experiencing symptoms and two of them developed persistent respiratory problems that were exacerbated by exposure to other chemicals such as perfumes and hairsprays. Two additional examples of chronic symptoms following acute carbamate exposure are the cases of two men who were directly sprayed by an airplane flying overhead applying carbaryl. Both men had symptoms that persisted for more than 6 years after the exposure incident. One, a 35-year-old man, had developed and continued to have hoarseness, bronchorrhea, dizziness, and peripheral neuropathy; the second, a 53-year-old man, had recurrent bouts of abdominal cramps and diarrhea, accompanied by anxiety attacks with associated flashback memories of the spraying incident (see Clinical Experiences section).

Peripheral neuropathy (i.e., sensory impairment, muscle weakness, and reduced or absent tendon reflexes) affecting the lower extremities more than the upper extremities is seen after carbamate exposure in some persons. For example, a 53-year-old man who was sprayed with carbaryl by a pesticide-applying airplane developed fatigue and numbness in his feet. This gradually affected his fingers. By 3 months after exposure, his gait was clumsy and his lower extremities had reduced sensation to mid-calf. These symptoms of peripheral neuropathy were not confirmed by neurophysiological studies at that time, but residual slowing was found at follow-up 5 years later (see Neurophysiological Diagnosis section). Other clinical examples of peripheral neuropathy after acute exposure to methylcarbamates have been reported in the literature. This includes the case of a 55-year-old housewife, with no previous medical history but troubled by family problems, who attempted suicide by ingesting 200 mL of *m*-tolyl methyl carbamate (common name: metolcarb) (Umehara et al., 1991). The patient was found in a state of stupor a few hours later and was immediately taken to the emergency room. She lost consciousness shortly after her arrival at the hospital. The patient was subsequently treated with atropine sulfate and gastric lavage. Nevertheless, she remained comatose for an additional 72 hours and then began to recover. When she was fully alert, about 6 to 10 days after exposure, she noted numbness in the distal portions of her legs. Examination revealed muscle weakness and sensory loss in the distal lower and upper extremities with slight involvement of facial and neck muscles. Deep tendon reflexes were absent in the upper and lower extremities, and the Babinski sign was absent bilaterally. Cerebral and cerebellar functions were normal. Routine laboratory studies and cerebrospinal fluid were also normal. The neuropathy was confirmed by electrophysiological studies and a sural nerve biopsy that revealed a decrease in the density of large and small myelinated fibers. At 3 and 6 months after exposure, the patient showed marked improvement in muscle strength and sensory perception, although deep tendon reflexes remained absent (see Neurophysiological Diagnosis and Neuropathological Diagnosis sections).

In a third case, a 23-year-old man ingested a small amount of rat poison containing an anticoagulant (dicumarol), without disastrous effect (Dickoff et al., 1987). The next day he consumed an unreported quantity of boric acid and 100 mL of Sevin (27% carbaryl and 73% water). He was found unconscious 3 hours later and was immediately taken to the emergency room. On admission, the patient was unresponsive to auditory or tactile stimulation and his pupils did not react to light. He presented with spontaneous eye movements and rhythmic eyelid twitches, but there were no spontaneous limb movements. Corneal reflexes were present. Tendon reflexes were normal and there was ankle clonus, but extensor plantar responses were absent bilaterally. The patient's muscarinic signs resolved within 12 hours, and by 24 hours after exposure he was able to respond to verbal commands. He had abdominal cramps, persistent diarrhea, and excreted dark brown heme-negative urine for the 24 hours. On the third day, he began to complain of painful paresthesias in his feet which progressed to involve the hands by the fourth day. His whole-blood cholinesterase level at this time was within normal range at 4 U/mL (lab normal: 3 to 8 U/mL). On day 5, the patient could not move his legs, but there was occasional rapid involuntary flexion of the knee and hip. Motor signs were seen in the upper extremities the next day. By the third week after exposure, finger strength was severely impaired and the patient could not stand. Position sense was absent in the toes, and pain and vibration sensations were markedly reduced below the knee. Plantar responses were

flexor. Electrophysiological studies performed at this time confirmed the diagnosis of peripheral neuropathy. At follow-up, 9 months after exposure, muscle strength was still reduced in the ankles and toes. Pain and touch sensations were reduced in the mid-calf bilaterally, and loss of proprioception and diminished vibration sensation were noted bilaterally in the toes.

That prolonged exposure to carbamates has the potential to induce peripheral neuropathy has been suggested by experimental studies (Smalley et al., 1968; Johnson and Lauwerys, 1969). The clinical and electrophysiological findings in the patients presented above also suggest that peripheral neuropathy can also follow severe acute exposure to carbamates. While not all persons exposed to carbamates develop peripheral neuropathy, the growing number of cases reported in the literature indicate that it is associated with severe acute exposures. Attributing these findings to the "vehicle" is not reasonable, at least in the third case because the vehicle was reported to be "water." Furthermore, the other chemicals ingested by this patient are not known to produce neuropathy. That either of the patients who attempted suicide might have consumed other unreported neurotoxicants is certainly plausible, but again the routine toxicological studies of urine and blood in the third case were normal. In addition, the first patient presented was not exposed to any other chemicals, further supporting the hypothesis that peripheral neuropathy can follow severe acute exposures to carbamates.

Chronic Exposure

Chronic exposure to low levels of carbamates is not associated with the dramatic cholinergic symptoms as are seen after high level exposure. For example, workers chronically exposed to carbaryl (at ambient air concentrations of 0.03 to 40 mg/m³) did not report symptoms of exposure (Best and Murray, 1962). Acute cholinergic symptoms may appear and/or recur when a chronically exposed individual experiences a peak acute exposure. At such times, the subclinical depression of cholinesterase activity associated with ongoing exposure is augmented by the additional acute dose allowing symptoms to emerge. The same exposure concentration may not be sufficient to illicit an effect in an unexposed individual whose basal cholinesterase activity levels are higher. The following case illustrates the effects of chronic exposure with fluctuating degrees of intensity of dosing with carbaryl.

A 75-year-old man developed acute symptoms of toxicity, including headache, malaise, epigastric discomfort, and muscle spasms, immediately after treatment of his basement with carbaryl (Branch and Jacqz, 1986). The pesticide control company he had hired to fumigate his basement had used a 10% carbaryl dusting preparation rather than the 2% carbaryl formulation recommended for indoor use. The carbaryl dust was subsequently picked up by the central air-conditioning system (which was located in the basement) and dispersed throughout the house. The patient noted acute symptoms within 3 days of the pesticide application. The patient's basement was dusted with carbaryl (10%) six additional times over the next 6 months. After each dusting the patient's symptoms, which had not completely cleared since the first spraying, were exacerbated. In addition, the patient began to lose weight and he developed symptoms of peripheral neuropathy including muscle weakness. Carbamate poisoning was not suspected as the cause of his illness until after there had been 8 months of ongoing exposure. At that time the patient's plasma cholinesterase activity levels were found to be depressed. Removal of the patient from exposure resulted in an overall improvement in his acute symptoms of cholinesterase inhibition, but signs and symptoms of peripheral neuropathy and encephalopathy persisted (see Neuroimaging and Clinical Experiences sections).

Although pyridostigmine has been used successfully to treat myasthenia gravis, its administration as a prophylactic against the potential effects of nerve-gas on troops in the Persian Gulf has been implicated in Persian Gulf War Illness (Loewenstein-Lichtenstein et al., 1995; Friedman et al., 1996; Chaney et al., 1997; Haley and Kurt, 1997). Sharabi and colleagues (1991) noted a greater incidence of CNS symptoms among Gulf War veterans as compared with individuals who had been exposed to pyridostigmine under nonstressful conditions. Although the increase in symptom frequency may have been due to anxiety, Friedman et al. (1996) have suggested that stress-associated alterations in the permeability of the BBB may have been responsible for this finding. The amount of pyridostigmine required to inhibit brain AChE activity by 50% was reduced to less than 0.01% of the usual dose in mice simultaneously subjected to a forced swim, indicating that stress can augment the CNS effects of pyridostigmine (Friedman et al., 1996). Simultaneous exposure to pyridostigmine and selected adrenergic agents or caffeine also potentiates the effects of pyridostigmine in mice (Chaney et al., 1997). Rats chronically exposed to pyridostigmine developed symptoms and neuropathological changes similar to those seen after acute exposure to organophosphates (Meshul et al., 1985). These findings in humans and animals indicate that exposure to carbamates such as pyridostigmine induces neurological and neuropathological effects, especially in genetically susceptible individuals and possibly under concomitant stress situations (Branch and Jacqz, 1986; Sharabi et al., 1991; Loewenstein-Lichtenstein et al., 1995; Friedman et al., 1996; Kaufer et al., 1998) (see Neuropathological Diagnosis section).

Neurophysiological Diagnosis

Electroencephalographic (EEG) studies in male volunteers exposed to carbaryl at dosages of 0.06 to 0.12 mg/kg per day for 6 weeks did not reveal any changes (Wills et al., 1968). An EEG 36 days following exposure was nor-

mal in a 55-year-old woman after recovery from coma which lasted for 72 hours after she ingested 200 mL of *m*-tolyl methyl carbamate (metolcarb) (Umehara et al., 1991). Her blood cholinesterase activity was normal at that time. In contrast, an EEG in a 23-year-old man taken 1 week after he ingested 100 mL of carbaryl showed symmetrical diffuse theta activity (4 to 6 Hz) (Dickoff et al., 1987). Follow-up EEG made approximately 3 weeks later showed a better organized background but showed persistent abnormality of intermittent episodes of slowing not explained by drowsiness. After 6 months the EEG was normal. Similar reductions in the fast-frequency (beta) activity and increases in amounts of slow waves were recorded in EEGs made in nonhuman primates exposed to carbaryl at doses of 0.01 to 1.0 mg/kg per day for 18 months (Santolucito and Morrison, 1971).

Nerve conduction studies (NCS) were performed in a 55-year-old housewife with no previous medical history who attempted suicide by ingesting 200 mL of *m*-tolyl methyl carbamate (Umehara et al., 1991). She was found in a state of stupor a few hours later and was immediately taken to the emergency room, where she progressed to unconsciousness shortly after her arrival. She was treated with atropine sulfate and gastric lavage. She remained comatose for an additional 72 hours and then began to recover. By the sixth day after exposure she had shown overall improvement, but then she noted numbness in the distal portions of her legs. She had marked muscle weakness, sensory loss in her extremities, and slight facial and neck muscles weakness. Tendon reflexes were absent in the upper and lower extremities; Babinski signs were absent. Cerebral and cerebellar functions were normal. Routine laboratory studies and cerebrospinal fluid were normal. Peripheral neuropathy was confirmed by motor nerve conduction velocity in the tibial nerve (24.6 m/sec) and by sensory conduction in the sural nerve (35.5 m/sec). The amplitudes of the electrically evoked nerve responses of the tibial (3.6 mV) and sural nerve (1.9 mV) were reduced. In the upper extremity her median nerve motor conduction velocity (50.9 m/sec) and amplitude of the motor evoked potentials (14.8 mV) were normal. Sensory conduction velocity of the median nerve was normal (52.3 m/sec), as was the amplitude of the sensory evoked potentials (8.9 mV). A sural nerve biopsy revealed a decrease in the density of large and small myelinated fibers (see Neuropathological Diagnosis section).

Peripheral neuropathy was also documented by neurophysiological studies in a 53-year-old man who was sprayed with carbaryl by a pesticide-applying airplane (R. G. Feldman, personal observation). He experienced acute cholinergic muscarinic symptoms. Peripheral nerve conduction studies were performed in this patient 4.5 years after he first complained of persistent numbness in his extremities and 5 years after his exposure to carbaryl. The motor nerve conduction velocity of the right peroneal nerve was slowed to 38.6 m/sec; the left peroneal nerve showed marked slowing across the fibular head (20.8 m/sec), indicating a local compression, as well as a slowed nerve conduction velocity (41.6 m/sec). The maximal evoked muscle action potential amplitude was at the lower limit of normal (4 to 6 mV). Sural sensory conduction velocities were bilaterally slowed (35.7 m/sec). Prolonged peroneal F-waves bilaterally, along with prolonged H-reflex latencies (34 milliseconds on the right and 33 milliseconds on the left), were recorded.

Electromyographic (EMG) studies were also made in the 53-year-old man described above. Recordings from the right lower extremity showed reduced motor units and large-amplitude potentials. These indicated evidence of peripheral neuropathy with chronic denervation and reinnervation in the distal muscle of the right lower extremity. A sural nerve biopsy confirmed the presence of neuropathy in this patient. EMG studies in the 55-year-old woman who developed clinically overt neuropathy after she ingested 200 mL of metolcarb, also described above, revealed fibrillation potentials and sharp waves at rest. A volitional recruitment pattern revealed reduced numbers of motor units with giant motor unit action potentials (Umehara et al., 1991). These findings were consistent with denervation and reinnervation of motor units associated with the peripheral neuropathy and the muscle atrophy seen clinically. The neuropathy in this patient was also documented by nerve biopsy (see Neuropathological Diagnosis section).

Neuropsychological Diagnosis

Detailed reports of neuropsychological testing following carbamate exposure in humans have not been found in the literature. Carbamates have been suggested by some authors as a means to improve memory function in patients with Alzheimer's disease (Iijima et al., 1993; Smith et al., 1997), whereas other authors have reported persistent memory deficits following human exposure to carbamates (Ecobichon, 1982). Experimental studies in laboratory animals indicate that carbamates have both memory-enhancing and memory-impairing effects. Rats exposed to carbamates initially took less time to complete a maze than did unexposed control animals. However, with continued exposure the carbamate-exposed animals took longer, suggesting that memory deficits may result from chronic or higher-level acute exposures to carbamate compounds (Dési et al., 1974; Ecobichon, 1982). The therapeutic value of anticholinesterases in the treatment of Alzheimer's disease appears to be limited by low oral bioavailability, a short duration of action, and the anticholinesterase (cholinergic) effects that occur at higher doses (Weinstock, 1995).

Neuropsychological testing can reveal acute and/or persistent effects of carbamate compounds on cognitive functioning in humans. Whenever possible, a complete neuropsychological test battery, such as the Wechsler Adult Intelligence Scale (WAIS), should be administered to assess overall cognitive functioning. Selected tests sensitive to the functioning of those cognitive domains typically impaired or spared following toxic exposures should also be administered. Tests of verbal functioning can be used to estimate premorbid ability. Digit Spans and the California Verbal Learning Test can be used to detect and document verbal memory deficits associated with carbamate exposure. Trails A and B are sensitive to deficits in attention and executive functioning, whereas Block Designs and the Digit Symbol Test can be used to assess visuospatial and psychomotor functioning, respectively. Neuropsychological testing can be performed both during and following removal from exposure to assess for and differentiate the acute and chronic CNS effects of the particular carbamate compound (White et al., 1992).

Neuropsychological tests were done in a 35-year-old man 6 years after he had been sprayed with carbaryl by a pesticide-applying airplane (R. G. Feldman, personal observation). At the time of his exposure, the acute symptoms included confusion, cognitive disturbances, and memory problems. Over time he showed clinical improvement in these functions; however, he persisted in having recurrent anxiety attacks and mood changes, which were diagnosed as being related to posttraumatic stress, since he would recall being sprayed with pesticide from an airplane and would also experience abdominal discomfort and nausea on those occasions. The neuropsychological assessment included the Wechsler Adult Intelligence Scale–Revised (WAIS-R), which revealed a discrepancy between verbal and performance intelligence quotients (VIQ = 114; PIQ = 86). Performance on tests of verbal reasoning and verbal fluency tasks were within expectation, but performance on a confrontation naming task (Boston Naming Test) was impaired. Performance on the Continuous Performance Test, a vigilance task, was not impaired. Digit Spans were within expectation (8 forward; 7 backward) and mental control was superior. Memory quotient (Wechsler Memory Scale) was 92 and below expectation for verbal IQ. Performance on memory testing showed a greater loss of verbal and visual information on delayed recall relative to immediate recall. Psychomotor slowing was noted on the Digit Symbol Test. Performance on visual spatial tasks was poor, and deficits were noted on tasks of visual spatial organization and reasoning. Profile of Mood States (POMS) and the Minnesota Multiphasic Personality Inventory (MMPI) revealed depression and anxiety. These results were considered consistent with an unresolved chronic posttraumatic stress syndrome. The severity of the symptoms of depression and anxiety clearly contributed to deficits in performance seen in neuropsychological testing of this patient. Nevertheless, the psychomotor slowing, memory deficits on delayed recall, and visuospatial deficits seen in this patient are consistent with those seen in other patients exposed to carbamates.

A second person, a 53-year-old man who was similarly sprayed by a pesticide-applying airplane, also had confusion and memory impairment within hours of exposure that improved over months; however, he continued to have problems of concentration and fatigue as well as bronchial difficulties for many years afterward (R. G. Feldman, personal observation). Neuropsychological testing done 5 years after exposure revealed normal IQ, with similar verbal and performance IQ scores. Reading comprehension and performance on tests of verbal fluency were normal, but his performance on tests of verbal reasoning was mildly impaired. A handwriting sample was tremulous. Mild difficulties were seen on tests of mental control. The Digit–Symbol test revealed slowing in psychomotor speed, as did his performance on the Santa Ana formboard task. Performance on visual sequencing of pictures was uneven; the sequences did not always match. Visual organization skills were low average, and performance on Block Designs was slow and rotational errors were seen. Memory quotient (Wechsler Memory Scale) was "bright normal," although there was a slight loss of visual and verbal material on delayed recall. POMS showed fatigue with some anxiety, but no evidence of depression. The most striking findings on these neuropsychological tests were psychomotor slowing with mild difficulties on tasks of visual organization and cognitive tracking. The neuropsychological tests were repeated 1 year later and continued to demonstrate marked psychomotor slowing and mild difficulties on tasks of visual organization and cognitive tracking, along with a very mild decline in visual memory function. It was concluded that there was no evidence of a progressive dementia, such as might be due to an Alzheimer-type degenerative process, and that the persistent findings in this patient were due to carbaryl exposure.

Biochemical Diagnosis

Biological monitoring of workers at risk for carbamate poisoning and the documentation of acute carbamate poisoning can be accomplished by measuring erythrocyte AChE activity (Wills et al., 1968; Vandekar et al., 1968, 1971; Umehara et al., 1991; Burgess et al., 1994) (Table 23-6). The time course of acute antiacetylcholinesterase (cholinergic) symptoms and recovery is reflected best by changes in erythrocyte AChE activity. Although plasma cholinesterase activity can also be measured, plasma cholinesterase is a nonspecific butyryl-type cholinesterase,

and thus erythrocyte AChE activity is much more sensitive for documenting the effects of carbamate exposure than is plasma cholinesterase activity (Adams, 1949; Adams and Whitaker, 1949). In addition, plasma cholinesterase activity levels have been shown to fluctuate in response to hepatic dysfunction, malnutrition, pregnancy, and exposure to opiates (Vandekar et al., 1968; Ellenhorn and Barceloux, 1988). Symptoms of exposure usually occur when erythrocyte AChE activity is depressed below 60% of normal. However, the development of acute symptoms does not correlate directly with erythrocyte AChE activity. For example, the erythrocyte AChE activity levels in a 42-year-old male volunteer who ingested propoxur (1.5 mg per kilogram body weight) were lowest 15 minutes after exposure, at which time the subject's only symptom was "pressure in the head" (Vandekar et al., 1971). The most severe symptoms and signs of toxicity were seen in this subject when his erythrocyte AChE activity levels were between 50.4% and 55.5% of normal. These findings indicate that symptoms of acute poisoning do not develop until the carbamate compound has been distributed from the blood to the various tissues of the body, where it can produce effects, and that erythrocyte AChE activity levels may not necessarily reflect contemporaneous toxicity (see Symptomatic Diagnosis section). Furthermore, both erythrocyte AChE and plasma cholinesterase activity levels rapidly return to normal after cessation of exposure to carbamates. For example, whole blood cholinesterase (erythrocyte AChE plus plasma cholinesterase) activity levels were not depressed several hours after exposure in a woman who developed acute symptoms of cholinesterase inhibition after she ate a cucumber that was tainted with aldicarb (Goes et al., 1980) (see Clinical Experiences section).

Because erythrocyte AChE activity levels rapidly return to normal following cessation of exposure to carbamates and because cholinesterase inhibition is not specific to a particular carbamate or OP compound, adjunctive measures including blood and urine analyses should be used to confirm exposure and to identify the anticholinesterase chemical. Blood levels of the parent carbamate and/or its metabolites can be used to confirm exposures to a particular carbamate compound. For example, the measurement of blood levels of the parent carbamate and its metabolites documented exposure in a 43-year-old man who developed severe symptoms including profuse sweating, miosis,

TABLE 23-6. *Biological exposure indices for carbamates*

	Urine	Blood	Alveolar air
Determinant:	Free and conjugated alcohol derivatives[a]	Erythrocyte cholinesterase	Not established
Start of shift:	Not established	Not established	Not established
During shift:	Not established	Not established	Not established
End of work shift:	Not established	Not established	Not established

[a]See Fig. 23-2 and text.
Data from ACGIH, 1995.

weakness, incontinence, and muscle fasciculations approximately 20 minutes after he ingested food contaminated with aldicarb (Burgess et al., 1994). Blood aldicarb concentration was 0.1 μg/mL, while the blood aldicarb sulfoxide and aldicarb sulfone levels in this patient were 1.7 and 3.4 μg/mL, respectively (see Clinical Experiences section).

Urinary concentrations of the metabolites of carbamate hydrolysis can also be used to monitor for and document specific carbamate exposures and may be of special value for documenting exposures when whole-blood cholinesterase levels are no longer markedly depressed (Dawson et al., 1964; Knaak, 1971; Chen and Dorough, 1979). For example, whole-blood cholinesterase activity was slightly depressed in those carbaryl-exposed workers who also had the highest urinary concentrations of 1-naphthol (ambient air concentrations in this study ranged from 0.23 to 31 mg/m³), but the workers with normal blood cholinesterase activity also excreted this metabolite, confirming that exposure to carbaryl had occurred in these workers as well. The average total (free and conjugated) urinary excretion of 1-naphthol among these workers was 18.5 ppm. Assuming that these workers had an average daily air intake of 10 m³, the average pulmonary exposure dose could be estimated from these results to be 3.9 mg/m³ (Best and Murray, 1962). Dawson et al. (1964) monitored the exposure of volunteers to propoxur by determining the urinary concentration of 2-isopropoxyphenol. These investigators initially determined the 2-isopropoxyphenol in ten unexposed subjects and estimated that the urine concentration of 2-isopropoxyphenol in the general population would not exceed 35 μg/mL. By comparison, the urine concentration of 2-isopropoxyphenol in a subject who ingested 100 mL of propoxur was 102 μg/mL approximately 8 hours after dosing and 11 μg/mL by 12 hours after exposure, indicating that urine levels decline rapidly following cessation of exposure and that the biological monitoring of carbamate-exposed workers by this method should be performed at the end of the work shift.

Neuroimaging

Magnetic resonance imaging (MRI) and computed tomography (CT) scans can be used in the differential diagnosis of carbamate poisoning and other conditions resulting in symptoms of brain-stem dysfunction (see Clinical Experiences section). The CT scan of a 43-year-old man who was exposed to aldicarb (blood aldicarb level: 0.1 μg/mL; aldicarb sulfoxide: 1.7 μg/mL; aldicarb sulfone: 3.4 μg/mL) did not reveal any abnormalities (Burgess et al., 1994). A normal CT scan was obtained within 24 hours after a 23-year-old man intentionally ingested 100 mL of Sevin (27% carbaryl and 73% water) (Dickoff et al., 1987). A CT scan 5 years after exposure in a 53-year-old man acutely exposed to carbaryl was normal. In contrast, the head CT scan in a patient who developed peripheral neuropathy and encephalopathy during chronic exposure to carbaryl revealed cerebral atrophy 5 months after the onset

of his exposure, along with a sufficiently enlarged ventricle, to justify a radionuclide cysternogram which was normal. These findings were contrasted with a normal head CT scan done several months before the onset of exposure because of a minor automobile accident. This remarkable change in cerebral mass cannot be attributed to the previous automobile accident; it must rather be considered as probably related to this man's prolonged exposure to carbaryl and his apparent increased susceptibility that the authors related to his concurrent intake of cimetidine (Branch and Jacqz, 1986).

Neuropathological Diagnosis

CNS pathology associated with carbamate poisoning in humans has not been reported. Results of neuropathological studies in the brains of swine who developed weakness and ataxia following chronic exposure to carbaryl at doses of 150 to 300 mg/kg per day showed edema and disruption of the integrity of myelin sheaths in the brain stem, cerebral peduncles, and upper spinal cord (Smalley et al., 1968).

A sural nerve biopsy revealed evidence of demyelination and remyelination in a 53-year-old man who was sprayed with carbaryl by a pesticide-applying airplane (R. G. Feldman, personal observation). The teased fiber preparation showed short internodal segments with thin myelin coverings among 6% of the fibers counted. In a similar case, of a 55-year-old woman who attempted suicide by ingesting 200 ml of m-tolyl methyl carbamate (metolcarb), transverse sections and a histogram of the sural nerve biopsy showed a marked decrease in the density of large and small myelinated fibers; the unmyelinated fiber density was moderately decreased (Fig. 23-3A). Teased fibers showed linear rows of myelin ovoids and evidence of remyelination. Electron microscopy revealed degenerating axons of myelinated fibers, Schwann cell clusters, and collagen pockets (Umehara et al., 1991). Although these findings suggest that carbamates can induce peripheral neuropathy, the contribution of the carrier solvent to the pathology seen in these patients cannot be ruled out entirely.

The neuromuscular junction of the diaphragm in rats that were either acutely or subacutely exposed to pyridostigmine, a quaternary carbamate compound, showed dose-dependent presynaptic morphological changes including (a) changes in organelle ultrastructure, (b) alterations in the relationship of the presynaptic nerve terminal to the postsynaptic folds, and (c) invasion of Schwann cell fingers into the synaptic cleft (Hudson et al., 1986). These ultrastructural observations suggest that pyridostigmine, a compound also administered prophylactically to Persian Gulf War troops to protect against the effects of irreversible AChE inhibitors such as the organophosphates, can produce irreversible changes at the neuromuscular junction in the rat diaphragm.

Kaufer et al. (1998) have suggested that cholinesterase inhibitors can induce changes in the gene coding c-FOS

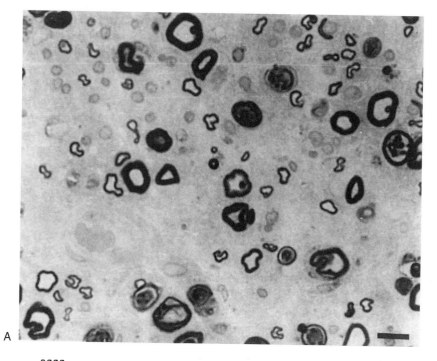

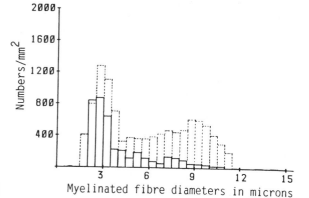

FIG. 23-3. Sural nerve biopsy in a 55-year-old woman exposed to metolcarb. **A:** Transverse section of sural nerve demonstrating decreased density of myelinated fibers and evidence of degeneration (toluidine blue; scale bar represents 10 μm). **B:** Histogram of fiber size distribution. *Solid lines* represent exposed subject; *broken lines* represent control subject. (From Umehara et al., 1991, with permission.)

and that elevated levels of c-FOS might activate regulatory pathways leading to long-term changes in the expression of proteins mediating brain cholinergic neurotransmission.

The mechanism of carbamate neuropathy is not known. One possibility involves the actions of a nonspecific esterase, neuropathy target esterase (NTE), which has been implicated in the development of delayed neuropathy associated with exposure to OP compounds and may be involved in the induction of the delayed neuropathy associated with exposure to carbamate compounds as well (Johnson and Lauwerys, 1969; Dickoff et al., 1987; Umehara et al., 1991). Carbaryl is metabolized to an epoxide, but the relationship of this electrophilic intermediate to the neurotoxicity of carbaryl has not been elucidated (Ryan, 1971). Exposure to disulfiram, a dithiocarbamate that does not appreciably inhibit cholinesterase activity has, however, been associated with the development of peripheral neuropathy and CNS pathology in humans (Laplane et al., 1992). The neurotoxicity of the dithiocarbamates has been attributed in part to carbon disulfide, which is a common metabolite of all dithiocarbamates (Edwards et al., 1991; Johnson et al., 1996) (see Chapter 21). The neuropathological changes associated with carbamates that are not dithiocarbamates or effective inhibitors of acetylcholinesterase may be attributable to the action of free radicals. Rats exposed to methyl-1-(butylcarbamoyl)-2-benzimidazole-carbamate (benomyl), a carbamate compound with relatively low anticholinesterase activity, had an increase in serum hydroperoxides and a significant decline in hepatic reduced glutathione levels. These findings indicate that the *in vivo* toxicity of this carbamate compound is due, at least in part, to free radical metabolites and oxidative stress.

PREVENTIVE AND THERAPEUTIC MEASURES

Warning signs indicating the risk for neurotoxic effects associated with exposure to carbamates should be posted in the work area and on all premises that have been treated with carbamates. Workers at risk for exposure to carbamates should avoid dermal contact and should shower and change their clothing before leaving the work area. Monitoring of ambient air concentrations and biological exposure indices can prevent increased body burdens and the acute effects of higher levels of exposure (Best and Murray, 1962). Pesticides should be applied only under conditions with proper ventilation. Workers at risk for exposure to high concentrations of carbamates should be supplied with respirators. Persons at risk should have periodic monitoring of erythrocyte AChE activity levels. Workers experiencing early acute symptoms of cholinesterase inhibition such as lacrimation, excessive salivation and sweating, blurred vision, respiratory problems, fecal and urinary urgency and/or incontinence, cardiac irregularities, myoclonic spasms, generalized muscle weakness, and ataxia should notify the company physician, who should immediately determine the patient's erythrocyte AChE activity levels. When evidence of depression of erythrocyte AChE activity occurs, it should signal the necessity for taking preventive measures and removing those at risk from further exposure. Erythrocyte AChE activity levels should be determined immediately in all patients presenting symptoms of cholinesterase inhibition and suspected of having been exposed to carbamates (Table 23-7).

The same basic precautions and proactions recommended above should be followed by anyone using carbamates in a nonoccupational setting. The clinician treating at-risk persons should be aware of the clinical signs of toxicity. Patients who use carbamates for pest control in their homes and/or gardens should be informed of the risks and symptoms associated with carbamate exposures. Carbamate insecticides should only be stored in labeled containers and should always be kept out of the reach of children.

Individuals accidentally sprayed with carbamates during pesticide applications should remove their clothing and then shower immediately with highly effective surfactants to prevent dermal absorption. Eye flush and oral pharynx lavage should be done to remove any residual amounts of pesticide and solvent carrier. Gastric lavage, rather than induced vomiting, should be performed in those patients who have accidentally or intentionally ingested carbamates, so as to avoid aspiration of the pesticide and its vehicle. Identification of the pesticide as well as the vehicle (i.e., carrier solvent) should be made whenever possible to determine appropriate treatment because the vehicle may also be a neurotoxicant. Measures including ventilation and vasomotor support may be necessary in severe acute poisonings.

Therapeutic intervention using atropine sulfate (atropine) which competitively blocks acetylcholine from binding to muscarinic receptors should be used to treat acute carbamate poisoning. Atropine should be administered every 15 minutes in small subcutaneous doses of 0.5 to 1.0 mg until signs of sufficient atropinization including dilation of pupils, flushing of the face, and disappearance of sweating are noted. Atropine prevents many of the acute effects of carbamates; however, it is ineffective against nicotinic overstimulation presenting as muscle weakness and twitching because it does not reactivate cholinesterases (Ellenhorn and Barceloux, 1988). Because the carbamate–AChE complex dissociates spontaneously within a few hours after removal from exposure, atropinization of the carbamate poisoned patient must be performed with caution to avoid overatropinization, since excess cholinergic effects induce fever, muscle fibrillations, and delirium. Still, due to the possible continued release of tissue stores of the carbamate, the patient's symptoms may reappear after discontinuation of atropine. Thus, to prevent unattended remissions the clinician should ensure that the patient has been free of signs and symptoms for at least 24 hours after discontinuation of atropine before he or she is discharged (Ellenhorn and Barceloux, 1988; Sidhu and Collisi, 1989).

The use of oximes in the management of patients who have been exposed only to carbamates remains controversial. Natoff and Reiff (1973) reported that oximes enhanced the therapeutic efficiency of atropine. Intravenous pralidoxime appeared to be effective in the management of a patient who was exposed to aldicarb (Burgess et al., 1994). Obidoxime chloride therapy did not appear to contribute to recovery of children exposed to aldicarb or methomyl, but these children also showed no adverse effects (Lifshitz et al., 1994). In contrast, several published reports have indicated that oximes may enhance the toxicity of some carbamates (e.g., carbaryl) (Faragó, 1969; Natoff and Reiff, 1973; Harris et al., 1989; Lifshitz et al., 1994). Together these reports support the empirical use of

TABLE 23-7. *Percent erythrocyte acetylcholinesterase inhibition and industrial hygienic actions for the prevention of poisoning in carbamate exposed workers*

Percent inhibition	Action
20–30	Check and correct hygienic conditions to prevent further exposure.
30–50	Workers are at risk for carbamate poisoning. Remove all workers from exposure and correct hygienic conditions.
> 50	Carbamate poisoning has occurred. Remove all workers from exposure and correct hygienic deficiencies.

Data from WHO, 1986.

these compounds in the management of patients exposed to aldicarb and/or other aliphatic oxime carbamates such as methomyl and who have not responded to atropine therapy alone. However, these findings do not support the use of oximes in the management of patients exposed to carbaryl and/or other carbamates which are not aliphatic oximes. Oxime therapy is also not recommended in the treatment of carbamate-exposed individuals with renal insufficiency (Ellenhorn and Barceloux, 1988).

The effect of exposure to a combination of OP compounds and carbamates is different than that of exposure to carbamates alone. Administration of cholinesterase reactivators (oximes) is indicated in the treatment of patients with a known history of combined exposures to OP and carbamate compounds because of their ability to reverse otherwise practically irreversible anticholinesterase effects of the OP compounds. Oximes such as pralidoxime and obidoxime chloride react with cholinesterase by binding at the esteric site, thereby facilitating release of the inhibitor and, thus, reactivation of the enzyme. The usual adult dosage of pralidoxime is 25 mg/kg and should be administered intravenously over 5 minutes (350 mg/min) (Ellenhorn and Barceloux, 1988). At higher doses (e.g., >500 mg/min), oximes can inhibit cholinesterase activity (Taylor, 1990).

CLINICAL EXPERIENCES

Group Studies

The Family Pet Serves as a Sentinel for Carbaryl in the Home

A 75-year-old man contacted a local exterminator to rid his basement of fleas left behind after his dog died of apparently natural causes (Branch and Jacqz, 1986). The company inadvertently dusted the basement with a 10% carbaryl dust preparation intended for outdoor use; a 2% preparation is recommended for indoor use. The dust was subsequently picked up by the central air-conditioning system (which was located in the basement) and dispersed throughout the house via the duct work. Three days after the house was dusted with carbaryl the man, his wife, and his son began to develop flu-like symptoms including headache, nausea, diarrhea, rhinorrhea, malaise, and muscle spasms. The man also noted loss of balance when rising from the floor after doing his morning exercises. The wife and son recovered within several days, but the man's symptoms continued to progress. One month later the exterminator company applied the second of the six treatments deemed necessary to rid the house of the fleas. The husband's symptoms worsened over the following week, at which time he experienced headache, rhinorrhea, tinnitus, vertigo, muscle fasciculations, distal weakness, and mild ataxia of gait. He contacted his physician, who diagnosed a gastric ulcer and prescribed cimetidine; unsuspecting and unquestioning, he was apparently unaware that the patient's basement was being dusted with carbaryl. Applica-

tions of the 10% carbaryl preparation continued once a month for the next 5 months. During this time the man's symptoms persisted, worsening within days of each treatment, but his wife and son remained asymptomatic. After several carbaryl applications the family cat, who lived in the basement, also became extremely ill and was euthanized.

Approximately 8 months after the first application of carbaryl the man's wife noted that there was a heavy deposit of white dust in the basement. State health officials determined that the dust contained carbaryl and recommended a thorough cleaning of the basement while using protective clothing and masks. In the process of reviewing an EPA booklet on carbaryl the patient noted that measurement of cholinesterase activity levels could be used to document exposures to carbaryl. He brought this entire matter to the attention of his family physician, who ordered the tests that documented depression of erythrocyte AChE and plasma cholinesterase activity levels and thus confirmed that the illnesses in this man and his family were due to exposure to carbaryl. After this discovery the basement was thoroughly cleaned.

Nevertheless, the patient continued to have symptoms, and blood tests continued to show depression of cholinesterase activity levels. At this time the patient developed a bilateral inguinal hernia and was admitted to the hospital for surgery. While in the hospital the patient's symptoms of rhinorrhea, bowel discomfort, vertigo, weakness, and mild ataxia began to disappear. After discharge from the hospital and suspecting that carbaryl dust was still elsewhere in the house, the patient hired a cleaning crew to clean his entire home. During this time the patient and his family stayed in a nearby hotel but would go home to supervise the cleaning process, at which time the patient would experience nasal congestion and lacrimation. The other members of the family were not affected as he was.

After the house had been entirely cleaned, the patient moved back in. However, 1 month later he was readmitted to the hospital with mild weakness and sinus bradycardia. Cholinesterase activity levels were again depressed. The patient had continued to be treated with cimetidine.

These findings indicate the occurrence of neuropathy following chronic exposure to carbaryl and emphasize the importance of individual differences in susceptibility between the patient and the other family members. In addition, the interference with the metabolism of carbaryl by cimetidine probably increased the patient's body burden of carbaryl and contributed to the severity of his clinical manifestations.

In frustration the patient and his family moved to a new house, after which his acute symptoms of cholinesterase inhibition remitted. At follow-up his symptoms of cholinesterase inhibition had disappeared, but signs and symptoms of peripheral neuropathy persisted.

Aldicarb and Local Grown Cucumbers

An outbreak of illness occurred among nine residents (six female and three male) of a small Nebraska town, ranging in age from 7 to 80 years, all of whom had eaten hydroponically grown cucumbers (Goes et al., 1980). All nine persons experienced an acute illness that included abdominal pain, diarrhea, nausea, vomiting, excessive perspiration, blurred vision, dyspnea, muscle fasciculations, paralysis, and convulsions within 15 minutes to 2 hours after eating the cucumbers and which persisted for up to 12 hours. The initial diagnoses included influenza and hypersensitivity to cucumbers. Cholinesterase levels were not determined.

Because of the similarity of the symptoms seen among these nine individuals, a toxic substance was suspected and the Nebraska State Health Department was notified. The search for the etiologic agent began with analyses of the cucumbers for arsenic, mercury, lead, and selenium, which were negative. This prompted a closer consideration of the symptoms, which suggested that a cholinesterase inhibitor might be the responsible agent. However, analysis of the cucumbers for organophosphates also came back negative. The investigators had considered the case closed when it was realized that a carbamate compound could also inhibit cholinesterase activity; unfortunately, however, it was too late to test this hypothesis because the cucumbers had been depleted by the previous laboratory tests.

A little over 1 year later, a second outbreak of acute illness occurred in an adjacent Nebraska city. This time five persons (three males and two females) ranging in age from 6 to 49 years were affected and developed acute symptoms including abdominal pain, diarrhea, nausea, vomiting, excessive perspiration, blurred vision, dyspnea, and muscle fasciculations within 1 hour after ingesting hydroponically grown cucumbers. The symptoms in this incident were relatively milder than those seen in the first outbreak. Nevertheless, four of the five exposed persons did seek medical attention for their symptoms at least once. A young man who sought medical attention for his symptoms was told that he had influenza and was sent home. The following day he shared another cucumber with his 6-year-old son, and both of them subsequently became ill. This time the illness lasted approximately 4 hours; but because he had been told the previous day that the symptoms he experienced were due to influenza, he did not seek medical attention this time for either himself or his son. A woman and her husband, with whom she had shared a cucumber, developed symptoms severe enough to warrant seeking medical attention. The woman, who had eaten the greater portion of the cucumber, was the more severely affected of the two. She had her whole-blood cholinesterase level measured several hours after her admission to the hospital, but it was not depressed at that time.

In both instances, the cucumbers had been grown hydroponically in a nearby greenhouse. The greenhouse owner denied using aldicarb. Analysis of the cucumbers obtained from the greenhouse identified aldicarb as the agent responsible for the second outbreak. Aldicarb was also detected in the water-nutrient solution used to nourish the

plants and in gravel from the greenhouse floor. The well supplying the greenhouse was subsequently tested for aldicarb, but none was found, thereby indicating that the well was not the source.

Aldicarb Poisoning Among Sheep and Sheep Herders: A Possible Case of Multiple Chemical Sensitivity

The acute and chronic effects of carbamates were studied in six men exposed to aldicarb in Washington State (Grendon et al., 1994). Shortly after a sheep herder inadvertently moved a flock of 318 sheep into a buckwheat field that was contaminated with aldicarb, many of the animals began to exhibit signs of respiratory distress followed by diarrhea, hypersalivation, miosis, seizures, and death. Two hundred eighty-eight sheep died immediately from the acute effects of aldicarb poisoning. The remaining 30 sheep were administered atropine. Although some clinical improvement was seen in these animals, they all continued to have poor appetites with associated weight loss and within 3 weeks of the exposure all 30 had either died or had to be euthanized.

Laboratory analysis revealed depressed erythrocyte AChE in the five animals tested. In addition, aldicarb was detected at concentrations of 0.19 to 334 ppm in the rumens of 13 of the exposed sheep. Other carbamates, organophosphates, and/or organochlorines were not detected in the rumen contents or in the tissue samples taken from these animals. Soil samples also contained detectable levels of aldicarb, confirming the diagnosis and source of aldicarb poisoning.

The sheep herder who was initially the only person attending the dying sheep experienced difficulty breathing and a burning sensation in his throat, and as a result he left the field shortly after help arrived. Five men including the owner of the sheep herd, a veterinarian, a state wildlife employee, and two hunters subsequently attended to the dead and dying sheep. Except for the veterinarian, who wore gloves when collecting specimens, none of the men wore any protective clothing. All five men reported acute symptoms, which included headache, dizziness, shortness of breath, chest tightness, sore throat, nausea, fatigue, and muscle aches. Several days later, four of the men developed productive coughs. Three months later these same men still had coughs, plus they reported experiencing an abnormal level of fatigue following periods of exertion. Two of the men also noted difficulty breathing when exposed to perfumes or hairsprays, a condition that neither man had prior to his exposure to aldicarb. Three years after the incident, five of the six men were still experiencing symptoms. One man was described by his physician as having difficulty with activities of daily living, while another reportedly suffers from chronic fatigue and experiences chest tightness and difficulty breathing whenever he is exposed to perfume or hairspray. These symptoms are minimized by his avoidance of such fragrances. Subsequently, a physician described his complaints as "multiple chemical sensitivity" (see Chapter 3). Similar symptoms have been reported by Persian Gulf War veterans and may reflect a form of post-traumatic stress disorder (Weiss, 1998).

Individual Case Studies

Long-Term Follow-Up After Carbaryl Exposure: Post-traumatic Stress Syndrome

A 35-year-old man on a hunting trip was perched in a tree while waiting for a bear to appear (R. G. Feldman, personal observation). Suddenly, from overhead a "rainfall" of liquid was sprayed over the area from four airplanes, each of which made three passes while dropping its load. He was partially protected by the leaves of the trees, but still he was soaked with the spray. Within 15 to 20 minutes he experienced blurred vision, sensitivity to light, lightheadedness, chills, abdominal cramping, and the urge to move his bowels. He left the site without washing or changing his clothing and he drove 2 hours to an emergency room (ER). Throughout the drive he had recurrent cramps, burning and tearing eyes, and blurred vision. When examined in the ER, the doctors noted his discomfort and the symptoms of nausea, blurred vision, photophobia, inflamed conjunctivae, and erythematous throat. His body temperature was not recorded in the ER. His past medical history was negative except for the fact that he had been admitted to the hospital only for knee surgery and the removal of some polyps on his throat up to the time of this event.

It was learned by a phone call to the ER from the State of Maine authorities that spraying of a pesticide (carbaryl: Seven-4-oil) for spruce budworms was going on in the area where the hunter had been. However, the ER doctors were told that the concentrations being applied were less than toxic. Therefore, other than being advised to discard his clothing and to bathe thoroughly, no specific therapy was given to him and he was sent home.

The patient continued to have four or five loose stools over the next 24 hours, when he saw his family physician, to whom the patient complained of sore throat, a cough, and fatigue. The symptoms persisted for another 3 days before subsiding, and clearing completely after 6 days. Over the next month he had recurrent episodes of feeling unwell, as if he had a "flu-like" illness. He had difficulties with sleep and had recurrent headaches. On occasions he had acute anxiety attacks associated with a feeling of nausea. Similar episodes occurred randomly over the next 2 years. His symptoms of anxiety were evaluated by a psychiatrist who ascribed them to post-traumatic stress as a consequence of his pesticide dousing.

A detailed neurological examination was performed 6 years after the exposure. No lateralizing or focal signs were seen. An electroencephalogram performed was normal. Neuropsychological testing at that same time showed visuospatial deficits, psychomotor slowing, mild dysnomia, and impaired memory. Depression and anxiety were also noted. The motor slowing, impaired memory, and visuospatial deficits were considered consistent with those seen in patients with similar exposures, while the finding on tests of affect and mood were considered consistent with post-traumatic stress disorder. The patient was treated with psychotherapy and antianxiety drugs (see Neuropsychological Diagnosis section).

Follow-up 18 years after the exposure episode revealed that the patient had continued to have periods of depression and recurrent episodes of anxiety whenever he heard a small airplane engine overhead. The patient continued to experience vivid recollections of the event with nightmares and dreams, sleep disturbances, marked diminished interest in previous activities, feelings of inadequacy in sexual drive, and poor concentration and memory deficits, indicating that he was still suffering post-traumatic stress disorder.

Acute Carbaryl Exposure and Peripheral Neuropathy

One evening in June a 53-year-old man was fishing from a canoe in the middle of a pond in Maine when an airplane flew over and sprayed the area with a liquid (R. G. Feldman, personal observation). It was learned later that the liquid contained carbaryl in kerosene as a solvent carrier (Seven-4-oil). The airplane made a total of six passes, usually turning off the spraying as it flew over the water, but on one pass it did not stop the discharging of the pesticide and thus the pond surface and the fisherman were directly and heavily soaked by the spray from the airplane. The man canoed back to shore and to his campsite, which was also wet from the spray. Because the lake water had a film of oil and pesticide from the spray, he decided not to bathe in it and remained in his wet clothing for the rest of the night. After less than an hour after being sprayed, the fisherman developed nausea, headache, and abdominal discomfort. He had several bowel movements with painful cramping. He was exhausted from the diarrhea and went to sleep, only to awaken throughout the night with cramps and chills. In the morning he had mental confusion and felt flushed and made his way home. He could not recall his daughter's phone number when he tried to call her. Although he showered with ordinary soap and changed his clothes, he did not seek medical attention for 3 days. During this time he continued to have anorexia, nausea, general fatigue, and weakness. He exhibited confusion and memory loss in his interactions with his family.

A family physician found no obvious physical abnormalities on examination, and he sent blood to the laboratory. The red blood cell cholinesterase level was 0.8 (lab normal: 0.4 to 1.1) on the fourth day after exposure to the carbaryl-in-oil spray. He was given an anticholinergic medication to relieve his cramps, with only slight improvement. Over the next 3 weeks the patient continued to have three to four loose stools per day, intermittently every 2 to 3 days. His headaches disappeared, but his fatigue persisted. A barium enema, sigmoidoscope, and stool cultures, which were normal, were performed to rule out other causes for the recurrent bowel symptoms. A past medical history reported malaria 35 years earlier; he was exposed to chlorine gas in a paper mill 26 years ago; and he was allergic to penicillin, but otherwise he enjoyed good health prior to the incident in question as was documented by annual physical exams.

He returned to his job as a maintenance supervisor in the local water department when he felt able. Although he had occasional recurrent abdominal cramps, felt tired all of the time, and had trouble doing his usual duties because of fatigue, he continued to work throughout the following 6 weeks. Also, during this time he began to notice numbness in his feet, which gradually also affected his fingers. By 3 months after the exposure the patient noticed clumsiness in his gait, and his lower-extremity sensation loss moved proximally to about mid-calf. His physician noted that forgetfulness and occasional dizzy spells were affecting the man's work. The condition worsened more as he began to have a hoarseness in his voice and increased secretions in his throat. Within 2 years after the exposure he had a mild tremor in his handwriting. These findings persisted and were confirmed by a neurologist 4.5 years after the exposure incident.

The patient was examined by this author (R. G. Feldman, personal observation) several weeks after the neurological consultation by the initial neurologist and approximately 5 years after the acute illness. A repeat red blood cell cholinesterase activity was done to compare with the one done 4 days after exposure and showed a level of 17.2 U/mL (lab normal: 7 to 19 U/mL). The patient complained of feeling tired all of the time. His voice was slightly hoarse. His arm swing was good bilaterally, but an involuntary tremor of the right thumb, tremulous handwriting with the right hand, and a mild intention tremor of the outstretched right hand were observed. Slight rigidity was present in the right arm, and it was brought out with reinforcement in the left arm. A glabellar reflex was present. These symptoms suggestive of parkinsonism emerged within 2 years after the patient's exposure to carbaryl. He was given a trial of anticholinergic medication (Cogentin), but he could not tolerate its side effects of excessive dryness and mental confusion; levodopa was not instituted.

Neuropsychological tests were done and revealed psychomotor slowing, visuospatial, and memory deficits. Test of affect and mood revealed fatigue with some anxiety, but no evidence of depression. The neuropsychological tests were repeated 1 year later and continued to demonstrate visuospatial, memory, and psychomotor deficits. It was concluded that there was no evidence of a progressive dementia and that the encephalopathy resulted from a severe acute exposure to carbaryl (see Neuropsychological Diagnosis section).

Vestibular tests were performed because of the unsteady gait. The vestibular–ocular response (VOR) showed asymmetry, with slow phase velocities being greater on the right than on the left. An otoneurologist attributed some of the patient's ataxia and dizziness to possible previous noise damage to the auditory/vestibular nerve, but he noted that the unsteadiness seemed to appear after the exposure to carbaryl. A CT scan of his head was done to visualize the cerebellar-pontine angle and the middle ear cavities and was normal.

The patient left his job 6 months later because of poor stamina and inability to perform his tasks. At a follow-up of this man 18 years after his exposure to carbaryl, he reported that he has remained about the same except for developing prostate cancer during this past year. He claims that his memory and concentration are "no worse, a bit better," but that his main difficulty is tripping and falling. He says he especially has difficulty with his right leg not lifting as high as it should when he is out on his walks and that he must pay attention or he will fall down. In addition, he describes his handwriting as awkward and affected by a tremor. A therapeutic trial of antiparkinsonism medications had not been done at this time. It is interesting to associate this patient's parkinson-like symptoms to his carbaryl exposure in light of the evidence suggesting an association between exposure to insecticides and an increased risk of Parkinson's disease; however, such a conclusion cannot be made because of a lack of knowledge about agent-specific chemical risks and individual susceptibility (Butterfield et al., 1993).

A Question of Combined Organophosphate or Carbamate Exposure Effects

A 43-year-old man developed nausea, vomiting, and diarrhea approximately 20 minutes after eating his dinner (Burgess et al., 1994). The paramedics were called and upon arrival found the patient to be mildly confused, with slurred speech, lacrimation, excessive sweating and salivation, and complaining of weakness. The patient was also bradycardic (pulse rate 50 beats per minute). Carbamate poisoning was suspected but OP exposure could not be excluded and he was administered both atropine and pralidoxime en route to the hospital.

On arrival at the hospital the patient was slightly disoriented, his skin was pale, he had miosis, and fasciculations in the facial muscles and tongue. His blood pressure was 130/100 mmHg and his pulse rate 90 beats per minute. The patient's plasma cholinesterase level was not determined until 6 hours after the onset of his symptoms, at which time it was 469 U/L (lab normal: 4,499 to 13,320 U/L). A blood sample drawn 15 hours after the onset of symptoms confirmed aldicarb poisoning (blood aldicarb level: 0.1 µg/mL; aldicarb sulfoxide: 1.7 µg/mL; aldicarb sulfone: 3.4 µg/mL). Urine screening for organophosphates was negative.

Neurological examination revealed muscle weakness and clonus which was more marked on the right than left. He was able to lift his left arm against gravity but was only able to move his finger on the right side. Sensation and deep tendon reflexes were intact. CT scans and lumbar puncture were unremarkable. His symptoms became worse over the next few hours, at which time he was administered a second 1-g dose of pralidoxime. Shortly after receiving this second bolus the patient had a 3-minute tonic–clonic seizure. The patient's condition continued to worsen, to the point that he required intubation. He was administered two additional 1-g intravenous doses of pralidoxime and a bolus of 2 mg atropine, following which he was infused with pralidoxime and atropine drips at dosages of 0.5 g/hr and 0.5 mg/hr, respectively. Less than 1 hour later, approximately 16 hours after the onset of his symptoms, he began to show clinical improvement. He progressed from only being able to move his fingers to having full use of his right arm. The atropine drip was stopped after 20 hours when the patient became severely agitated. The patient's symptoms continued to improve and he was extubated on the fifth day of hospitalization. The remainder of this patient's recovery was uneventful, and follow-up examinations reportedly revealed no residual effects of his exposure to aldicarb.

REFERENCES

Adams DH. The specificity of human blood erythrocyte cholinesterase. *Biochim Biophys Acta* 1949;3:1–14.

Adams DH, Whitaker VP. Cholinesterase of human blood. I: The specificity of the plasma cholinesterase and its relationship to the erythrocyte cholinesterase. *Biochim Biophys Acta* 1949;3:358–366.

Ahdaya SM, Monroe RJ, Guthrie FE. Absorption and distribution of intubated insecticides in fasted mice. *Pestic Biochem Physiol* 1981;16:38–46.

American Conference of Governmental Industrial Hygienists (ACGIH). *Threshold limit values (TLVs) for chemical substances and physical agents and biological exposure indices (BEIs).* Cincinnati: ACGIH, 1995.

Andrawes NR, Dorough HW, Lindquist DA. Degradation and elimination of TEMIK in rats. *J Econ Entomol* 1967;60:979–987.

Banks D, Soliman MRI. Protective effects of antioxidants against benomyl-induced lipid peroxidation and glutathione depletion in rats. *Toxicology* 1997;116:177–181.

Baron RL. Carbamate insecticides. In: Hayes WJ, Laws ER, eds. *Handbook of pesticide toxicology,* vol 3: *Classes of pesticides.* New York: Academic Press, 1991:1125–1189.

Battaglia R, Conacher HB, Page BD. Ethyl carbamate (urethane) in alcoholic beverages and foods: a review. *Food Addit Contam* 1990;7:477–496.

Best EM Jr, Murray BL. Observations on workers exposed to Sevin insecticide: a preliminary report. *J Occup Med* 1962;4:507–517.

Branch RA, Jacqz E. Subacute neurotoxicity following long-term exposure to carbaryl. *Am J Med* 1986;80:741–745.

Burgess JL, Bernstein JN, Hurlbut K. Aldicarb poisoning: a case report with prolonged cholinesterase inhibition and improvement after pralidoxime therapy. *Arch Intern Med* 1994;154:221–224.

Butterfield PG, Valanis BG, Spencer PS, et al. Environmental antecedents of young-onset Parkinson's disease. *Neurol* 1993;43:1150–1158.

Challis IR, Adcock JW. The metabolism of the carbamate insecticide bendiocarb in the rat and in man. *Pestic Sci* 1981;12:638–644.

Chaney LA, Rockhold RW, Mozingo JR, et al. Potentiation of pyridostigmine bromide toxicity in mice by selected adrenergic agents and caffeine. *Vet Hum Toxicol* 1997;39:214–219.

Chen KC, Dorough HW. Glutathione and mercapturic acid conjugations in the metabolism of naphthlene and 1-naphthyl-*N*-ethylcarbamate (carbaryl). *Drug Chem Toxicol* 1979;2:331–354.

Chin BH, Sullivan LJ, Eldridge JM, Tallant MJ. Metabolism of carbaryl by kidney, liver, and lung from human postembryonic fetal autopsy tissue. *Clin Toxicol* 1979;14:489–498.

Chipperfield B, Newman PM, Moyes ICA. Decreased erythrocyte cholinesterase activity in dementia. *Lancet* 1981;2:199.

Christensen JK, Möller IW, Ronsted P, Angelo HR, Johansson B. Dose–effect relationship of disulfiram in human volunteers. I: clinical studies. *Pharmacol Toxicol* 1991;68:163–165.

Coleman AM, Smith A, Watson L. Occupational carbamate pesticide intoxication in three farm workers. Implication and significance for occupational health in Jamaica. *West Ind Med J* 1990;39:109–113.

Collerton D. Cholinergic function and intellectual decline in Alzheimer's disease [Review]. *Neuroscience* 1986;19:1–28.

Cranmer MF. Carbaryl: a toxicological review and risk analysis. *Neurotoxicology* 1986;7:247–328.

Dawson JA, Heath DF, Rose JA, Thain EM, Ward JB. The excretion by humans of the phenol derived *in vivo* from 2-isopropoxyphenyl-*N*-methylcarbamate. *Bull WHO* 1964;30:127–134.

Declume C, and Benard P. Étude autoradiographique de la distribution d'un aganet anticholinéeterasique, le 1-naphtyl-*N*-methyl[¹⁴C]carbamate, chez la ratte gestante. *Toxicol Appl Pharmacol* 1977;39:451–460.

Dennis MJ, Howarth N, Key PE, Pointer M, Massey RC. Investigation of ethyl carbamate levels in some fermented foods and alcoholic beverages. *Food Add Contam* 1989;6:383–389.

Dési I, Gonczi L, Simon G, et al. Neurotoxicologic studies of two carbamate pesticides in subacute animal experiments. *Toxicol Appl Pharmacol* 1974;27:465–476.

Dési I. Neurotoxicological investigation of pesticides in animal experiments. *Neurobehav Toxicol Teratol* 1983;5:503–515.

Dickoff DJ, Gerber O, Turovsky Z. Delayed neurotoxicity after ingestion of carbamate pesticide. *Neurology* 1987;37:1229–1231.

Dixit R, Mukhtar H, Seth PK, Murti CRK. Conjugation of acrylamide with glutathione catalyzed by glutathione-*S*-transferases in rat liver and brain. *Biochem Pharmacol* 1981;30:1739–1744.

Dixit R, Das M, Mushtaq M, Srivastava P, Seth PK. Depletion of glutathione content and inhibition of glutathione-*S*-transferase and aryl hydrocarbon hydroxylase activity of rat brain following exposure to styrene. *Neurotoxicology* 1982;3:142–145.

Drexler H, Gõen T, Angerer J. Carbon disulfide. II. Investigations on the uptake of CS2 and the excretion of its metabolite 2-thiothiazolidine-4-carboxylic acid after occupational exposure. *Int Arch Occup Environ Health* 1995;67:5–10.

Ecobichon DJ. Carbamic acid ester pesticides. In: Ecobichon DJ, Joy RM, eds. *Pesticides and neurological disease.* Boca Raton, FL: CRC Press, 1982:205–233.

Edwards IR, Ferry DG, Temple WA. Fungicides and related compounds. In: Hayes WJ, Laws ER, eds. *Handbook of pesticide toxicology,* vol 3: *Classes of pesticides.* New York: Academic Press, 1991:1436–1451.

Ellenhorn MJ, Barceloux DG. *Medical toxicology: diagnosis and treatment of human poisoning.* New York: Elsevier, 1988:1067–1108.

Environmental Protection Agency (EPA). *Drinking water regulations and health advisories.* EPA 822-R-96-001. Washington, DC: Office of Water, 1996.

Faragó A. Suicidal, fatal Sevin®(1-naphthyl-*N*-methylcarbamate) poisoning. *Arch Toxikol* 1969;24:309–315.

Feldmann RJ, Maibach HI. Percutaneous penetration of some pesticides and herbicides in man. *Toxicol Appl Pharmacol* 1974;28:126–132.

Ferraz HB, Bertolucci PHF, Pereira JS, Lima JGC, Andrade LAF. Chronic exposure to the fungicide maneb may produce symptoms and signs of CNS manganese intoxication. *Neurology* 1988;38:550–553.

Food and Agricultural Organization/World Health Organization (FAO/WHO). *1973 Evaluations of some pesticides residues in food.* The monographs. WHO pesticide residue Ser. no. 3. Geneva: World Health Organization, 1974.

Food and Agricultural Organization/World Health Organization (FAO/WHO). *Pesticides residues in food: 1980 evaluations.* The monographs. FAO Plant Production and Protection Paper no. 26 (Suppl). Rome: Food and Agriculture Organization U.N., 1981.

Food and Agricultural Organization/World Health Organization (FAO/WHO). *Pesticides residues in food: 1982 evaluations.* The monographs. FAO Plant Production and Protection Paper no. 49. Rome: Food and Agriculture Organization U.N., 1983.

Food and Agricultural Organization/World Health Organization (FAO/WHO). *Pesticides residues in food: 1986 report.* FAO Plant Production and Protection Paper no. 77. Rome: Food and Agriculture Organization U.N., 1986.

Friedman A, Kaufer D, Shemer J, Hendler I, Soreq H, Tur-Kaspa I. Pyridostigmine brain penetration under stress enhances neuronal excitability and induces early immediate transcriptional response. *Nat Med* 1996;2:1382–1385.

Gaines TB. Acute toxicity of pesticides. *Toxicol Appl Pharmacol* 1969;14:515–534.

Goes EA, Savage EP, Gibbons G, Aaronson M, Ford SA, Wheeler HW. Suspected foodborne carbamate pesticide intoxications associated with ingestion of hydroponic cucumbers. *Am J Epidemiol* 1980;111:254–260.

Goldman LR, Smith DF, Neutra RR, et al. Pesticide food poisoning from contaminated watermelons in California, 1985. *Arch Environ Health* 1990;45:229–236.

Gordon CJ. Review. Thermoregulation in laboratory mammals and humans exposed to anticholinesterase agents. *Neurotoxicol Teratol* 1994;16:427–453.

Grendon J, Frost F, Baum L. Chronic health effects among sheep and humans surviving an aldicarb poisoning incident. *Vet Hum Toxicol* 1994; 36:218–223.

Haley RW, Kurt TL. Self-reported neurotoxic chemical combinations in the Gulf War: a cross-sectional epidemiological study. *JAMA* 1997; 277:231–237.

Harris LW, Talbot BG, Lennox WJ, Anderson DR. The relationship between oxime-induced reactivation of carbamylated acetylcholinesterase and antidotal efficacy against carbamate intoxication. *Toxicol Appl Pharmacol* 1989;98:128–133.

Harris LR, Sarvadi DG. Synthetic polymers. In: Clayton GD, Clayton FE, eds. *Patty's industrial hygiene and toxicology,* vol II, Part E, 4th ed. New York: John Wiley and Sons, 1994:3918–3924, 3756–3758.

Hassan A, Zayed SMAD, Abdel-Hamid FM. Metabolism of carbamate drugs-I. Metabolism of 1-naphthyl-*N*-methylcarbamate (Sevin) in the rat. *Biochem Pharmacol* 1966;15:2045–2055.

Hayes WJ. Toxicology of pesticides. *General principles: metabolism.* Baltimore: Williams & Wilkins, 1975:107–181.

Holmstedt B. The ordeal bean of old Calabar: the pageant of physostigmine venenosum in medicine. In: Swain T, ed. *Plants in the development of modern medicine.* Cambridge, MA: Harvard University Press, 1972.

Hudson CS, Foster RE, Kahng MW. Ultrastructural effects of pyridostigmine on neuromuscular junctions in rat diaphragm. *Neurotoxicology* 1986;7:167–186.

Hussain M, Yoshida K, Atiemo M, Johnston D. Occupational exposure of grain farmers to carbofuran. *Arch Environ Contam Toxicol* 1990;19: 197–204.

Iijima S, Greig NH, Garofalo P, et al. Phenserine: a physostigmine derivative that is a long-acting inhibitor of cholinesterase and demonstrates a wide dose range for attenuating a scopolamine-induced learning impairment of rats in a 14-unit T-maze. *Psychopharmacology* 1993;112: 415–420.

Johnsen J, Stowell A, Morland J. Clinical responses in relation to blood acetyladehyde levels. *Pharmacol Toxicol* 1992;70:41–45.

Johnson MK, Lauwerys R. Protection by some carbamates against the delayed neurotoxic effect of di-iso-prophylphosphofluoride. *Nature* 1969;222:1066–1067.

Johnson DJ, Graham DG, Amarnath V, Amarnath K, Valentine WM. The measurement of 2-thiothiazolidine-4-carboxylic acid as an index of *in vivo* release of CS2 by dithiocarbamates. *Chem Res Toxicol* 1996;9:910–916.

Kaufer D, Friedman A, Seidman S, Soreq H. Acute stress facilitates long-lasting changes in cholinergic gene expression. *Nature* 1998;393:373–376.

Knaak JB. Biological and nonbiological modifications of carbamates. *Bull WHO* 1971;44:121–131.

Kobayashi H, Yuyama A, Ohkawa T, Kajita T. Effect of single or chronic injection with a carbamate, propoxur, on the brain cholinergic system and behavior of mice. *Jpn J Pharmacol* 1988;47:21–27.

Kulkarni AP, Hodgson E. Metabolism of insecticides by mixed function oxidase systems. *Pharmacol Exp Ther* 1980;8:379–475.

Kurata N, Hurst HE, Kemper RA, Waddell WJ. Studies on induction of metabolism of ethyl carbamate in mice by ethanol. *Drug Metab Dispos Biol Fate Chem* 1991;19:239–240.

Ladics GS, Smith C, Heaps K, Loveless SE. Evaluation of the humoral immune response of CD rats following a 2-week exposure to the pesticide carbaryl by the oral, dermal, or inhalation routes. *J Toxicol Environ Health* 1994;42:143–156.

Laplane D, Attal N, Sauron B, de Billy A, Dubois B. Lesions of basal ganglia due to disulfiram neurotoxicity. *J Neurol Neurosurg Psychiatry* 1992;55:925–929.

Lavy TL, Mattice JD, Massey JH, Skulman BW. Measurements of year-long exposure to tree nursery workers using multiple pesticides. *Arch Environ Contam Toxicol* 1993;24:123–144.

Liddle JA, Kimbrough RD, Needham LL, et al. A fatal episode of accidental methomyl poisoning. *Clin Toxicol* 1979;15:159–167.

Lifshitz M, Rotenberg M, Sofer S, et al. Carbamate poisoning and oxime treatment in early children: a clinical and laboratory study. *Pediatrics* 1994;93(4):652–655.

Lifshitz M, Shahak E, Bolotin A, Sofer S. Carbamate poisoning in early childhood and in adults. *Clin Toxicol* 1997;53(1):25–27.

Lima JS, Alberto C, Reis G. Poisoning due to illegal use of carbamates as a rodenticide in Rio de Janeiro. *Clin Toxicol* 1995;33(6):687–690.

Litvan I, Gomez C, Atack JR, Gillespie M, et al. Physostigmine treatment of progressive supranuclear palsy. *Ann Neurol* 1989;26:404–407.

Loewenstein Y, Danarie M, Zakut H, Soreq H. Molecular dissection of cholinesterase domains responsible for carbamate toxicity. *Chem-Biol Interact* 1993;87:209–216.

Loewenstein-Lichtenstein Y, Schwarz M, Glick D, et al. Genetic predisposition to adverse consequences of anti-cholinesterase in 'atypical' BCHE carriers. *Nature Med* 1995;1(10):1082–1085.

Lorber MN, Cohen S, DeBuchananne G. A national evaluation of the leaching potential of aldicarb. Part 2. An evaluation of ground water monitoring data. *Ground Water Monit Rev* 1990;10(1):127–141.

Marade SJ, Weaver DJ. Monitoring for aldicarb residues in ground water of the central valley of California. *Bull Environ Contam Toxicol* 1994; 52:19–24.

Marshall TC, Dorough HW, Swim HE. Screening of pesticides for mutagenic potential using Salmonella typhimurium mutants. *J Agric Food Chem* 1976;24:560–563.

May DG, Naukam RJ, Kambam JR, Branch RA. Cimetidine-carbaryl interaction in humans: evidence for an active metabolite of carbaryl. *J Pharmacol Exp Ther* 1992;262(3):1057–1061.

Meshul CK, Boyne AF, Deshpande SS, Albuquerque EX. Comparison of the ultrastructural myopathy induced by anticholinesterase agents at the end plates of rat soleus and extensor muscles. *Exp Neurol* 1985;89: 96–114.

Metcalf RL. Mode of action of carbamate synergists. *Annu Rev Entomol* 1967;12:229–256.

Miller CS, Mitzel HC. Chemical sensitivity attributed to pesticide exposure versus remodeling. *Arch Environ Health* 1995;50(2):119–129.

Mirkin IR, Anderson HA, Hanrahan L, et al. Changes in T-lymphocyte distribution associated with ingestion of aldicarb-containing drinking water: a follow-up study. *Environ Res* 1990;51(1):35–50.

Moses M, Johnson ES, Anger WK, et al. Environmental equity and pesticide exposure. *Toxicol Ind Health* 1993;9(5):913–959.

National Institute for Occupational Safety and Health (NIOSH). *Pocket guide to chemical hazards.* Cincinnati: US Department of Health and Human Services, CDC, 1997.

Natoff IL, Reiff B. Effect of oximes on the acute toxicity of anticholinesterase carbamates. *Toxicol Appl Pharmacol* 1973;25:569–575.

Neskovic NK, Terzic M, Vitorovic S. Acute toxicity of carbaryl and propoxur in mice previously treated with phenobarbital and SKF525-A. *Arh Hig Rada Toksikol* 1978;29:251–256.

Occupational Safety and Health Administration (OSHA). *Code of federal regulations,* 29, 1910.1000/.1047. Washington, DC: Office of the Federal Register, National Archives and Records Administration, 1995:411–431.

Office of Technology Assessment (OTA), U.S. Congress. *Neurotoxicity: identifying and controlling poisons of the nervous system.* OTA-BA-436, p 281. Washington, DC: Governmental Printing Office, 1990:360.

O'Malley M. Clinical evaluation of pesticide exposure and poisonings. *Lancet* 1997;349:1161–1166.

Oonithan ES, Casida JE. Oxidation of methyl- and dimethylcarbamate insecticide chemicals by microsomal enzymes and anticholinesterase activity of the metabolites. *J Agric Food Chem* 1968;26:28–44.

Osman AZ, Hazzaa NI, Awad TM. Fate and metabolism of the insecticide ^{14}C-Lannate in farm animals. *Isot Radiat Res* 1983;15:111–120.

Pergal M, Vukojevic N, Djuric D. Carbon disulfide metabolites excreted in the urine of exposed workers. II. Isolation and identification of thiocarbamide. *Arch Environ Health* 1972;25:42–44.

Perry EK, Tomlinson BE, Blessed G, et al. Correlation of cholinergic abnormalities with senile plaques and mental test scores in senile dementia. *Br Med J* 1978;2:1457–1459.

Ramasamy P. Carbamate insecticide poisoning. *Med J Malaysia* 1976;31:150–152.

Reiner E. Spontaneous reactivation of phosphorylated and carbamylated cholinesterases. *Bull WHO* 1971;44:109–112.

Reiner E, Aldridge WN. Effect of pH on inhibition and spontaneous reactivation of acetylcholinesterase treated with phosphorus acids and carbamic acids. *Biochem J* 1967;105:171–179.

Riihimäki V, Kivistö H, Peltonen K, Helpiö E, Aitio A. Assessment of exposure to carbon disulfide in the viscose production workers from urinary 2-thiothiazolidine-4-carboxylic acid determinations. *Am J Ind Med* 1992;22:85–97.

Ryan AJ. The metabolism of pesticidal carbamates. *CRC Crit Rev Toxicol* 1971;1:33–54.

Sakai K, Matsumura F. Degradation of certain organophosphate and carbamate insecticides by human brain esterases. *Toxicol Appl Pharmacol* 1971;19:660–666.

Santolucito JA, Morrison G. EEG of rhesus monkeys following prolonged low-level feeding of pesticides. *Toxicol Appl Pharmacol* 1971;19:147–154.

Sax NI. *Dangerous properties of industrial chemicals,* 5th ed. New York: Van Nostrand Reinhold, 1979.

Schwarz M, Glick D, Loewenstein Y, Soreq H. Engineering of human cholinesterases explains and predicts diverse consequences of administration of various drugs and poisons. *Pharmacol and Ther* 1995a;67(2):283–322.

Schwarz M, Glick D, Loewenstein Y, Soreq H. Genetic predisposition to adverse consequences of anti-cholinesterases in 'atypical' BCHE carriers. *Nat Med* 1995b;1(10):1082–1085.

Sen Gupta AK, Knowles CO. Fate of formetanate-^{14}C acaricide in the rat. *J Econ Entomol* 1970;63:10–14.

Shah PV, Monroe RJ, Guthrie FE. Comparative rates of dermal penetration of insecticides in mice. *Toxicol Appl Pharmacol* 1981;59:414–423.

Shah PV, Guthrie FE. Percutaneous penetration of three insecticides in rats: a comparison of two methods for *in vivo* determination. *J Invest Dermatol* 1983;80:291–293.

Sharabi Y, Danon YL, Berkenstadt H, et al. Survey of symptoms following intake of pyridostigmine during Persian Gulf war. *Isreal J Med Sci* 1991;27:656–658.

Sidhu KS, Collisi MB. A case of accidental exposure to a veterinary insecticide product formulation. *Vet Hum Toxicol* 1989;31:63–64.

Smalley HE, O'Hara PJ, Bridges CH, Radeleff RD. Neuromuscular effects of carbaryl insecticide in swine. *Toxicol Appl Pharmacol* 1968;12:323–324.

Smith CP, Bores GM, Petko W, et al. Pharmacological activity and safety profile of P10358, a novel, orally active acetylcholinesterase inhibitor for Alzheimer's disease. *J Pharmacol Exp Ther* 1997;280(2):710–720.

Sofer S, Tal A, Shahak E. Carbamate and organophosphate poisoning in early childhood. *Pediatr Emerg Care* 1989;5:222–225.

Takahashi RN, Poli A, Morato GS, Lima TCM, Zanin M. Effects of age on behavioral and physiological responses to carbaryl in rats. *Neurotoxicol Teratol* 1991;13:21–26.

Taylor P. Anticholinesterase agents. In: Goodman Gilman A, Rall TW, Nies AS, Taylor P, eds. *Goodman and Gilman's the pharmacological basis of therapeutics,* Eighth ed. Elmsford, NY: Pergamon Press, 1990:131–149.

Teisinger J. New advances in the toxicology of carbon disulfide. *Am Ind Hyg Assoc J* 1974;35:55–61.

Toyama T, Kusano H. An experimental study on absorption and excretion of carbon disulfide. *Jpn J Hyg* 1953;8:10.

Umehara F, Izumo S, Arimura K, Osame M. Polyneuropathy induced by *m*-tolyl methyl carbamate intoxication. *J Neurol* 1991;238:47–48.

Vahl M. A survey of ethylcarbamate in beverages, bread and acidified milks sold in Denmark. *Food Addit Contam* 1993;10:585–592.

Vandekar M, Hedayat S, Plestina R, Ahmandy G. A study of the safety of *O*-isopropoxyphenylmethylcarbamate in an operational field-trial in Iran. *Bull WHO* 1968;38:609–623.

Vandekar M, Plestina R, Wilhelm K. Toxicity of carbamates for mammals. *Bull WHO* 1971;44:241–249.

van Hoof F, Heyndrickx A. Excretion in urine of four insecticidal carbamates and their phenolic metabolites after oral administration to rats. *Arch Toxicol* 1975;34:81–88.

Weinstock M. The pharmacotherapy of Alzheimer's disease based on the cholinergic hypothesis: an update. *Neurodegeneration* 1995;4:349–356.

Weiss B. Neurobehavioral properties of chemical sensitivity syndromes. *Neurotoxicol* 1998;19:259–268.

White RF, Feldman RG, Proctor SP. Neurobehavioral effects of toxic exposure. In: White RF, ed. *Clinical syndromes in adult neuropsychology: the practitioners handbook.* Amsterdam: Elsevier, 1992:1–51.

Wills JH, Jameson E, Coulston F. Effects of oral doses of carbaryl on man. *Clin Toxicol* 1968;1:265–271.

World Health Organization (WHO). *Organophosphorus insecticides: a general introduction. Environmental health criteria,* no. 63. Geneva: World Health Organization, 1986:181.

Zaki MH, Moran D, Harris D. Pesticides in groundwater: the aldicarb story in Suffolk County, NY. *Am J Public Health* 1982;72(12):1391–1395.

Zavon MR. Poisoning from pesticides: diagnosis and treatment. *Pediatrics* 1974;54(3):332–336.

Zwiener RJ, Ginsburg CM. Organophosphate and carbamate poisoning in infants and children. *Pediatrics* 1988;81(1):121–126.

Appendix

Boston Occupational and Environmental Neurology Questionnaire

Please take as much time as needed to complete the questionnaire in its entirety. Please answer all questions. All answers are confidential. If you don't know the answer to a question, indicate this by writing "don't know". If additional space is needed, use the back of a page. Thank you for taking the time to answer these questions.

A. BACKGROUND INFORMATION

1. Name (Last, First, MI): _____
2. Address: _____
    Street
    _____
    Town or City   State   Zip Code
3. Today's date: _____   4. Telephone _____ ( ) _____ - _____
5. Social security number: _____ - _____ - _____
6. Date of birth: _____ / _____ / _____
7. Age: _____   Height: _____   Weight: _____
8. Sex: M _____   F _____
9. Race: _____ White   _____ Black   _____ Native American
             _____ Asian   _____ Hispanic   Other _____
                                                          Please Specify
10. Marital Status: _____ Single   _____ Married   _____ Divorced
                       _____ Separated _____ Widowed

B. INSURANCE INFORMATION

Name and Address of Person Responsible for Payment:

1. Name (Last, First, MI): _____
2. Address: _____
    _____
    Town or City   State   Zip Code
3. Today's date: _____   4. Telephone _____

C. THIRD PARTY PAYOR (IF APPLICABLE)

1. _____
2. Primary-care physician responsible for approving referral:

    _____   _____
    Name   Physician Number

D. REFERRAL INFORMATION

Reason for Referral

(List medical complaints, especially current symptoms. Please use additional pages if necessary and attach medical records, laboratory data and material safety data sheets):

_____

_____

_____

Referring Physician / Agency / Attorney:

_____
Name

Address:

_____

_____
Number   Street

_____
City   State   Zip

Tel: ( ) _____ - _____   **Fax:** ( ) _____

E. EDUCATIONAL INFORMATION

1. Education (highest level completed):
   - _____ Grade 8 or less   _____ Some college or tech school
   - _____ Grade 9–11   _____ College graduate
   - _____ High school   _____ Postgraduate
2. What was your average grade in school? (A+, A, A-, B+, B, B-, etc.): _____
3. How many years of school did your father complete?: _____
4. How many years of school did your mother complete?: _____
5. What was your father's occupation most of his life?: _____
6. What was your mother's occupation most of her life?: _____

F. OCCUPATION

1. Are you currently working?   _____ Yes   _____ No
2. Month, year job began: _____ / _____
3. Month, year job ended (if not currently working): _____ / _____
4. If not currently working, please indicate reason:
   - _____ Laid off   _____ Retired
   - _____ Quit   _____ Unable to work due to medical problems*
   - *Please explain: _____
   - _____

5. Receiving workman's compensation?   _____ Yes   _____ No

Please answer the following questions about your current job or about the job in which you last worked:
6. Occupation: _____
7. Describe this job: _____
   _____

8. Job title: _____
9. Place of employment: _____
   _____
   Describe work activities:
10. Hours per week/shift: _____
11. Specific job tasks (please describe in detail your job tasks): _____
   _____
   _____

12. Please describe in detail any suspected hazardous exposures or conditions on the job (please be as specific as possible. This could be exposures to chemical substances, heat, noise, dust, other):

_____

_____

13. Please list all your previous jobs, starting with the most recent one:

Date (month, year) From - To	Industry	Job title	Job duties	Suspected exposures	Any health problems	Residence at time of this job

14. Have you ever used or worked around any hazardous chemicals either at work or outside of work?

_____ Yes   _____ No   (If no, skip to 29)

Substance	Ever Used		Dates	Description of Use
15. Mercury (scientific instruments, chlorine plants, dental offices)	Yes	No	_____	_____
16. Arsenic (insecticides, wood preservatives)	Yes	No	_____	_____
17. Acrylamide (construction grouting)	Yes	No	_____	_____
18. Hexane (solvents, rubber cements, inks)	Yes	No	_____	_____
19. Trichloroethylene (triclor, "tri"— degreasing)	Yes	No	_____	_____
20. Perchloroethylene (perchlor, "perc"—dry cleaning)	Yes	No	_____	_____
21. Organophosphates (pesticides)	Yes	No	_____	_____
22. Methyl butyl ketone (MBK, ink)	Yes	No	_____	_____
23. Carbon disulfide (rayon manufacturing, rubber industry, labs)	Yes	No	_____	_____
24. Lead (jewelry making, foundries, battery industry, paint removers)	Yes	No	_____	_____
25. Toluene (solvents, lacquers, inks)	Yes	No	_____	_____
26. Methylene chloride (solvents, paint removers)	Yes	No	_____	_____
27. Carbon monoxide (byproducts of combustion)	Yes	No	_____	_____
28. Other Please specify:	Yes	No	_____	_____

29. Does your spouse/housemate work? _____ Yes _____ No
30. Occupation: _____
31. Place of employment: _____
32. Is she/he exposed to any solvents, metals, or chemicals at work? _____ Yes _____ No
33. If yes, please describe: _____
34. Have you ever had a medical problem possibly related to your work? _____ Yes _____ No
35. If yes, please describe: _____
36. Have any of your fellow employees had a medical problem possibly related to work?
    _____ Yes _____ No
37. Do you wear any of the following personal protective equipment in your work?

	Occasionally	$\frac{1}{2}$ Time	All Time	Reason	N/A
Ear plugs, muffs					
Goggles or face mask					
Dust mask					
Respirator (please specify type)					
Gloves					
Apron, gown					

38. If you wear a dust mask, how often do you change masks?
    _____ More than once a shift
    _____ Once a shift
    _____ 1–3 times per week
    _____ Once a week
39. If you wear a respirator, how often do you change the cartridges?
    _____ More than once a shift
    _____ Once a shift
    _____ 1–3 times per week
    _____ Once a week
40. Have you received instructions regarding proper usage and care of the respirator?
    _____ Yes _____ No
41. Do you ever eat or drink at the work site?
    _____ Always _____ Occasionally _____ Never
42. Do you wash before eating or drinking?
    _____ Always _____ Occasionally _____ Never
43. Are there shower and locker facilities at the workplace? _____ Yes _____ No
44. Do you shower before going home from work?
    _____ Always _____ Occasionally _____ Never
45. Do you change your clothes before going home from work?
    _____ Always _____ Occasionally _____ Never
46. Do you use hand-made pottery for eating food or drinking beverages? _____ Yes _____ No

G. HOBBIES AND HOME REPAIR

1. Do you have any hobbies, or do anything outside of work that might expose you to glues, solvents, or other chemicals?
   _____ Yes _____ No (if no, go to H)

Hobby			Dates	Description (substance used)
2. Painting	Yes	No		
3. Furniture refinishing	Yes	No		
4. Lead glass making	Yes	No		
5. Model building	Yes	No		
6. Auto body work	Yes	No		
7. Jewelry making	Yes	No		
8. Pottery making	Yes	No		
9. Use of pesticides in farming, gardening	Yes	No		
10. Other	Yes	No		

H. ALCOHOL INTAKE AND RECREATIONAL DRUG USE

1. Do you regularly drink alcoholic beverages (more than one a month)?

    _____Yes   _____No   (if yes, go to 3)

2. Have you ever regularly drunk alcoholic beverages?

    _____Yes   _____No   (if no, go to 12)

3. How often do/did you drink?

    _____2–3 times per day

    _____1 time per day

    _____4–6 times per week

    _____1–3 times per week

    _____Less than once a week, but more than once a month

    _____Less than once a month

    _____A few times a year

    _____Never

4. When you drink, how many drinks do/did you usually have? (1 drink = 1 beer, 1 glass of wine, or one shot of liquor; 1 quart of beer = 3 drinks; one pint of liquor = 10 drinks; $\frac{1}{2}$ pint of liquor = 5 drinks)

    _____0 drinks   _____9–12 drinks

    _____1–2 drinks   _____12–15 drinks

    _____3–5 drinks   _____more than 20

    _____6–8 drinks

5. How often do/did you drink more than 5 drinks?

    _____More than 4 times per week

    _____1–3 times per week

    _____Less than once a week, but at least once a month

    _____Less than once a month

    _____Never

6. How many years have you been drinking or did you drink alcoholic beverages?

    _____Less than 5 years

    _____5–9 years

    _____10–14 years

    _____15–20 years

    _____More than 20 years

7. Have you ever had a medical problem related to alcohol?   _____Yes   _____No

8. If yes, please specify: _____

9. Has your drinking pattern changed recently?   _____Yes   _____No

10. If yes, please explain: _____

11. Have you had home-made liquor (moonshine) in the past year?   _____Yes   _____No

12. Have you ever tried   _____cocaine   _____heroin   _____other hallucinogen

    If yes, when? _____

13. Have you ever taken any other nonprescribed, psychotrophic drugs (e.g., LSD, Angel dust, amphetamines, etc.)?

    _____Yes   _____No

14. Have you taken any of these in the past year?   _____Yes   _____No

I. SMOKING

1. Do you now smoke?   _____Yes   _____No

2. If you quite, when did you quit? _____

3. If yes, what do you smoke? _____

    _____Cigarettes   _____Pipe   _____Cigar

4. If you smoke cigarettes, how many per day?

    _____Less than $\frac{1}{2}$ pack per day

    _____$\frac{1}{2}$ to 1 pack per day

    _____1–2 packs per day

    _____2–3 packs per day

    _____More than 3 packs per day

5. If you smoke a pipe, how much tobacco do you smoke? _____

6. If you smoke cigars, how many per day? _____
7. How many cups of coffee do you average per day? _____
8. Have you ever smoked marijuana?
   _____ Never   _____ Fewer than 3 times   _____ More than 3 times
9. Do you smoke marijuana?   _____ Yes   _____ No
10. If yes, how often have you smoked marijuana during the past year?
    _____ Daily   _____ Several times per month
    _____ Several times per week   _____ Several times per year

J. MEDICATIONS

1. Have you ever taken any medications for a prolonged period of time (more than one month), other than antibiotics?
   _____ Yes   _____ No
2. Medications for: (make a check mark if *ever* taken)

	Dates Taken	Name of Medication
_____ Seizures	_____	_____
_____ Diabetes	_____	_____
_____ Thyroid	_____	_____
_____ High blood pressure	_____	_____
_____ Heart problems	_____	_____
_____ Depression	_____	_____
_____ Anxiety	_____	_____
_____ Arthritis	_____	_____
_____ Vitamin deficiencies	_____	_____
_____ Problems sleeping	_____	_____
_____ Allergies	_____	_____
_____ Other	_____	_____

K. REPRODUCTIVE HISTORY

Please answer the following questions if you are female (If you are male, go to 17).

Females

1. Have you ever taken birth control pills?   _____ Yes   _____ No
2. If yes, for how long? _____ Years
3. Have you ever had a miscarriage: _____ Yes   _____ No
4. If yes, when? _____
5. Have you ever had a still birth?   _____ Yes   _____ No
6. If yes, when? _____
7. Have you ever had problems getting pregnant?   _____ Yes   _____ No
8. If yes, please describe: _____
9. Have you had other problems with pregnancies or menstrual cycles?   _____ Yes   _____ No
10. If yes, please describe: _____
11. Have you experienced a change in sex drive over the past 6 months?   _____ Yes   _____ No
12. If yes, please describe: _____
13. Do you have any children?   _____ Yes   _____ No
14. If yes, how many? _____
15. Have you ever had a child born with a birth defect?   _____ Yes   _____ No
16. If yes, please describe: _____

Please answer the following questions if you are male (if you are female, go to L).

Males

17. Have you had any problems with erection?   _____ Yes   _____ No
18. If yes, please describe: _____
19. Has your spouse ever had any problems with any of the following:

Please Describe

Miscarriage	Yes	No	
Stillbirth	Yes	No	
Child born with defect	Yes	No	
Inability to get pregnant	Yes	No	

20. Do you have any children? _____ Yes _____ No
21. If yes, how many? _____
22. Have you ever been tested for sperm count; motility? _____ Yes _____ No

L. MEDICAL HISTORY

1. Have you ever had any medical problems? _____ Yes _____ No (if no, go to M)

2. Diabetes	Yes	No
3. Cancer	Yes	No
4. Seizures	Yes	No
5. Headaches	Yes	No
6. Thyroid trouble	Yes	No
7. Stroke	Yes	No
8. Brain tumor	Yes	No
9. Kidney disease	Yes	No
10. Asthma	Yes	No
11. Allergies	Yes	No
12. Chronic bronchitis	Yes	No
13. Stomach problems	Yes	No
14. Arthritis	Yes	No
15. Anemia	Yes	No
16. Gout	Yes	No
17. Back problems/slipped disc	Yes	No
18. Heart problem	Yes	No
19. High blood pressure	Yes	No
20. Vitamin B_{12} deficiency	Yes	No
21. Lead poisoning	Yes	No

22. Other: _____
23. Have you ever been hospitalized? _____ Yes _____ No
24. What was the reason or reasons for hospitalization? _____
25. Have you ever had surgery? _____ Yes _____ No
26. If yes, when was the surgery performed? _____
27. What was the reason for the surgery? _____
28. Have your hands or arms ever been injured by fracture, frostbite, or other event?
_____ Yes _____ No
29. If yes, please describe: _____
30. Have your legs or feet ever been injured by fracture, frostbite, or other event?
_____ Yes _____ No
31. If yes, please describe: _____

M. FAMILY MEDICAL HISTORY

Has anyone in your family ever had any of the following?

Please describe and state relationship

1. Heart problem	Yes	No
2. Diabetes	Yes	No
3. Cancer	Yes	No
4. Seizures	Yes	No
5. Headaches	Yes	No
6. Thyroid trouble	Yes	No
7. Stroke	Yes	No
8. Brain tumor	Yes	No

9. Senility	Yes	No	
10. Kidney trouble	Yes	No	
11. Asthma	Yes	No	
12. Allergies	Yes	No	
13. Chronic bronchitis	Yes	No	
14. Stomach problems	Yes	No	
15. Arthritis	Yes	No	
16. Anemia	Yes	No	
17. Gout	Yes	No	
18. Back problems	Yes	No	
19. High blood pressure	Yes	No	
20. Multiple Sclerosis	Yes	No	
21. Parkinson's disease	Yes	No	
22. Cerebral Palsy	Yes	No	
23. Muscular dystrophy	Yes	No	
24. Tremors	Yes	No	
25. Huntington's disease	Yes	No	
26. Other	Yes	No	

N. YOUR SYMPTOMS

Please answer the following questions concerning your health in the past 6 months. If the answer is yes to any of these items, please give details on back of sheet.

In the past 6 months, have you experienced any of the following:

			Please Describe
1. Mood changes	Yes	No	
2. Difficulty concentrating	Yes	No	
3. Confusion	Yes	No	
4. Trouble remembering	Yes	No	
5. Depression	Yes	No	
6. Irritability	Yes	No	
7. Fatigue	Yes	No	
8. Trouble sleeping	Yes	No	
9. Loss of sexual interest	Yes	No	
10. Headaches	Yes	No	
11. Dizziness	Yes	No	
12. Loss of balance	Yes	No	
13. Change in the way you walk	Yes	No	
14. Numbness and tingling in arms and hands	Yes	No	
15. Numbness and tingling in legs and feet	Yes	No	
16. Muscle weakness in legs and feet	Yes	No	
17. Unusually cold fingers and toes	Yes	No	
18. Nausea and vomiting	Yes	No	
19. Abdominal cramps	Yes	No	
20. Diarrhea	Yes	No	
21. Constipation	Yes	No	
22. Unintentional weight loss (more than 10 pounds)	Yes	No	
23. Joint pains	Yes	No	
24. Lower back pains	Yes	No	
25. Shortness of breath	Yes	No	
26. Chest pain	Yes	No	
27. Visual problems (double vision, irritated eyes, blurred vision	Yes	No	
28. Changes in voice	Yes	No	
29. Tremors	Yes	No	
30. Changes in handwriting	Yes	No	
31. Difficulty turning over in bed	Yes	No	
32. Other	Yes	No	

O. FOOD HABITS

1. How many times a week do you eat red meat?

    _____Never

    _____1–3 times a week

    _____4–6 times a week

    _____7 or more times a week

2. How many times a week do you each chicken, turkey, or fish?

    _____Never

    _____1–3 times a week

    _____4–6 times a week

    _____7 or more times a week

3. How many times a week do you eat eggs?

    _____Never

    _____1–3 times a week

    _____4–6 times a week

    _____7 or more times a week

4. If yes to the previous question, how many at one meal? _____

P. ENVIRONMENTAL EXPOSURE

1. What is your source of drinking water at your residence?

    _____Private well

    _____Surface   _____Deep

    When was it dug? _____

    _____Public municipal town well

    What town? _____

2. How long have you lived at your current residence? _____

3. Where have you lived in the past? (list complete addresses and dates)

    _____

    _____

    _____

    _____

Residential water use

4. How many showers/baths do you take at home?   _____a day   _____a week

    How long does the water run? _____

5. How much tap water do you drink a day? _____

6. Do you have a swimming pool? _____

7. Do you have a dishwashing machine? _____

Surroundings

8. How would you describe the area where you live?

    _____Residential/suburban

    _____Rural

    _____Industrial/commercial

9. Are there any of the following natural or man-made landmarks nearby? (please check and indicate distance from home)

    _____River, lake, stream   _____

    _____Mountain   _____

    _____Railroad tracks   _____

    _____Electrical power lines   _____

    _____Waste site, landfill, dump _____

    _____Sewage treatment plant   _____

    _____Nuclear power plant   _____

*If you wish to include any additional information, you may write on reverse page.

Subject Index

Page numbers followed by "f" indicate figures. Page numbers followed
by "t" indicate tables.